Mastering NEET Series

Second Edition

Volume-1
(Non-Clinical Subjects)

- Anatomy
- Pathology
- Pharmacology
- Physiology
- Microbiology
- Forensic Medicine
- Biochemistry
- Parasitology
- Preventive and Social Medicine

Mastering NEET Series

Second Edition

Volume-1
(Non-Clinical Subjects)

Kamal KV MBBS MS (Orthopaedics)
Ex-Senior Resident: Safdarjung, ESI-Okhla, Fortis-Noida
Ponseti and Ilizarov Techniques Fellow (Akola)
Madhya Pradesh – Indian Orthopaedic Association
Hand Surgery Fellow – Pune, Maharashtra, India

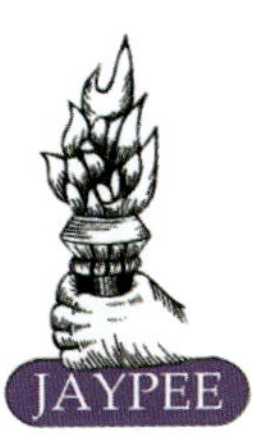

The Health Sciences Publisher
New Delhi | London | Panama

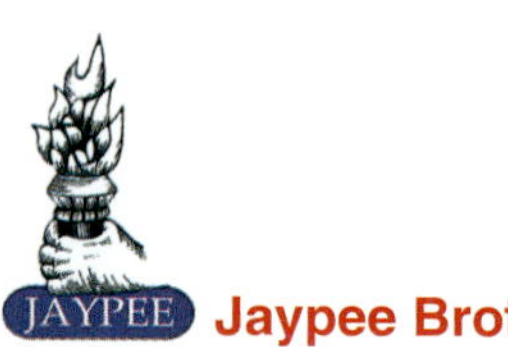

Jaypee Brothers Medical Publishers (P) Ltd

Headquarters

Jaypee Brothers Medical Publishers (P) Ltd
4838/24, Ansari Road, Daryaganj
New Delhi 110 002, India
Phone: +91-11-43574357
Fax: +91-11-43574314
Email: jaypee@jaypeebrothers.com

Overseas Offices

J.P. Medical Ltd
83 Victoria Street, London
SW1H 0HW (UK)
Phone: +44 20 3170 8910
Fax: +44 (0)20 3008 6180
Email: info@jpmedpub.com

Jaypee-Highlights Medical Publishers Inc
City of Knowledge, Bld. 235, 2nd Floor, Clayton
Panama City, Panama
Phone: +1 507-301-0496
Fax: +1 507-301-0499
Email: cservice@jphmedical.com

Jaypee Brothers Medical Publishers (P) Ltd
17/1-B Babar Road, Block-B, Shaymali
Mohammadpur, Dhaka-1207
Bangladesh
Mobile: +08801912003485
Email: jaypeedhaka@gmail.com

Jaypee Brothers Medical Publishers (P) Ltd
Bhotahity, Kathmandu, Nepal
Phone +977-9741283608
Email: kathmandu@jaypeebrothers.com

Website: www.jaypeebrothers.com
Website: www.jaypeedigital.com

Mastering NEET Series (Volume-1)

First Edition: 2017
Second Edition: **2018**

ISBN: 978-93-5270-436-1

Printed at Ajanta Offset & Packagings Ltd., Faridabad, Haryana

Dedication

Before you go through the main content of this book, it is my humble request to devote (at least) few minutes to this particular page and read the name of those brave soldiers who sacrificed their lives to make our lives secure and safe.

Being a son of Honorary Captain/Army Education Corps, I would like to dedicate this title to our brave soldiers who were martyred in Uri (Jammu & Kashmir) terror attack.

Located barely a few kilometres from the Line of Control (LoC) and some 70 km from Srinagar, the base was subjected to the brazen attack by four terrorists at around 5.30 AM, causing heavy casualties in the Dogra Regiment, which lost 17 of its men. About 20 more army personnel were injured, some critically, and were airlifted to the Army Base Hospital in Srinagar.

Here is the full list of jawans who died in the Uri terror attack:

1. Subedar Karnail Singh, r/o Vill Shibu Chak, Teh Bishnah, Dist Jammu, Jammu & Kashmir.
2. Havildar Ravi Paul, r/o Samba, Dist Jammu, Jammu & Kashmir.
3. Sepoy Rakesh Singh, r/o Vill Baddja, Dist Kaimur, Bihar.
4. Sepoy Javra Munda, r/o Vill Meral, Dist Khuti, Jharkhand.
5. Sepoy Naiman Kujur, r/o Vill Chainpur, Dist Gumla, Jharkhand.
6. Sepoy Uike Janrao, r/o Vill Nandgaon (Kh), Dist Amravati, Maharashtra.
7. Havildar NS Rawat, r/o Vill Rajawa, Dist Rajasmand, Rajasthan.
8. Sepoy Ganesh Shankar, r/o Vill Ghoorapalli, Dist Sant Kabir Nagar, Uttar Pradesh.
9. Naik SK Vidarthi, r/o Vill Boknari, Dist Gaya, Bihar.
10. Sepoy Biswajit Ghorai, r/o Vill Ganga Sagar, Dist South 24 Parganas, West Bengal.
11. Lance Naik G Shankar, r/o Vill Jashi, Dist Satara, Maharashtra.
12. Sepoy G Dalai, r/o Vill Jamuna Balia, Dist Howrah, West Bengal.
13. Lance Naik RK Yadav, r/o Vill Balia, Uttar Pradesh.
14. Sepoy Harinder Yadav, r/o Vill Ghazipur, Dist Ghazipur, Uttar Pradesh.
15. Sepoy TS Somnath, r/o Vill Khadangali, Dist Nashik, Maharashtra.
16. Havildar Ashok Kumar Singh, r/o Vill Raktu Tola, Dist Bhojpur, Bihar.
17. Sepoy Rajesh Kumar Singh, r/o Vill Jaunpur, Uttar Pradesh.

Preface to the Second Edition

As I always say, there is nothing more pleasant for an author to release a new edition of his book. This is an indirect indication that this title has been open heartedly accepted by the students. But at the same time it brings a challenge to come up to the expectations of readers in subsequent editions.

In the first edition, I have incorporated many images in the explanations. There were many books in the market, all of which were focussing mainly on explanations and less on illustrations. So I thought of presenting a title which did the reverse, I mean which focus more on illustrations and less on theoretical explanations. This concept was readily accepted by the students because it gave them an opportunity to correlate the theory with illustrations as this helps in understanding the facts clearly. But since the first edition was in single colour, so many images were not that impressive. Moreover at some places, where there were legends for colours (green, red or others), it was very difficult to understand which depiction is in which colour. So this time, we are presenting this title in full colour mode so that each and every image stands out clearly and adds to understanding of the concept.

Hope this title (like my other titles) would serve the purpose.

"To err is human" and being a human, I am bound to commit errors. If you find any such unintentional errors in the book, please do communicate with me on the below given modes of contact.

Since students are the best judge, please do shower me with your necessary feedbacks regarding improvement in the content and presentation of the text.

Good Luck

Kamal KV
drkamalkv's Classes, 116/3,
Near Sribalaji Restaurant, Sudarshan Road,
Gautam Nagar, New Delhi - 49, India
Web: www.drkamalkvgroup.co.in
Mail: drkamalkvgroup@gmail.com
Facebook: Drkamalkvgroup
Twitter handle: drkamalkvgroup
Whatsapp & Cell: 8470004333

Preface to the First Edition

There are many good titles available for PG-standard NBE exams, but the problem is that these are so bulky that the students are in a state of confusion when it comes to revision. They enjoy reading them during the initial few days of studies, but during the last few days, when the exams are near, the students find them very difficult to revise.

Keeping this fact in mind, I have compiled this title, which is comparatively easy to revise during the last few days.

Also earlier the students were always concerned about image-based questions. So, in the explanation part, I have liberally used plenty of images to help the students in this regard.

Related tables had been placed wherever necessity was felt.

MCQs have been categorized into different sections. The sections are the same as those in 'Self Assessment & Review of FMGE', so that the students can read both the titles together sectionwise.

An overall attempt has been made to accommodate much information in minimum space.

Hope this title (like my other titles) would serve the purpose.

"To err is human" and being a human, I am bound to commit errors. If you find any such unintentional errors in the book, please do communicate with me through the below given modes of contact.

Since the students are the best judge, please do shower me with your necessary feedback regarding the improvement in the content and presentation of the text.

Good luck

Kamal KV
116/3, Near A-1 Xerox Shop
Sudershan Road
Gautam Nagar
New Delhi – 110049
India
Web : www.drkamalkvgroup.co.in
Mail : drkamalkvgroup@gmail.com
Facebook : Drkamalkvgroup
Twitter handle : drkamalkvgroup

How to Read this Title

This title should be revised thrice before the exams. The ideal way of reading this title is like this:

- First reading: 3 months
- Second reading: 2 months
- Third reading: 1 month

Content to be studied in different cycles:

- First reading: Read all MCQs with explanations with attached images/tables. Mark some images or tables which seem important and should be revised again.
- Second reading: Read MCQs with explanations only (no attached images or tables) plus marked images or tables.
- Third reading: MCQs and answers only (no explanations) plus marked images or tables.
- Rest of the content needs to be read in all cycles (keynotes, practice MCQs, image-based MCQs and MCQ points).

How to Solve Paper in Examination Hall

Divide the total duration of examination into 2 rounds: 1/3rd and 2/3rd of the time allotted.

1. First round is **'READ ALL QUESTIONS & MARK FEW'**. One should be able to mark the answer by just going through the MCQ statement. Do not try to search for the answers from the options. Read the MCQ statement, think of the answer and if you find any such option, mark it and go ahead. Obviously, ALL EXCEPT/FALSE statement kind of questions should not be attempted, as these questions demand some time to solve them. First reading of all the MCQs should be done within first round (1/3rd duration).
2. Second round is **'SOLVE USING ASSOCIATION/EXCLUSION PRINCIPLE'**. Here MCQs are not straightforward (ALL EXCEPT/FALSE statement kind of questions) and you have to apply your knowledge to choose the best answer. This stage demands a lot of concentration and ability to catch the hints given in the MCQ statement (2/3rd duration).

To minimize the errors, please discard the tendency of changing the answers frequently. Majority of the time, the students will replace a right answer with a wrong one. So, whatever you have marked once, let it be final. No second thoughts please.

Acknowledgments

Most the things (books, classes) I do by my own, singly. So I find it very difficult to write the acknowledgment section as there is no contribution from anyone.

Therefore, I try to pen down few persons/ incidences related to the title or any person who helped me (as a human) in one or other way.

Related to this particular title, I remember one incident.

One day me, Chairman JP Vij sir and Chetna madam were discussing on our FMGE title. In between, Chairman asked me "Kamal, I wish to publish a NBE pattern MCQs bank title. Can you suggest me any good author for the same". I smiled on this particular question. Chairman sir was little surprised as to why I am smiling on this serious question. I said "Sir, one of the best authors is sitting in front of you, and you are telling him to search somebody else". To this Chairman sir replied "I was expecting only this kind of reply from you. Definitely you and only you would be the best person to pen down this title". And that is how; this title was finalized all of a sudden.

So I would like to thank Chairman JP Vij sir for showering me with his blessing and giving me this wonderful opportunity to compile this title.

Chetna madam needs special mention as she never interfered in my work and accepted all my works without any objection. All my suggestions were duly considered and incorporated wherever necessary. Payal madam worked tirelessly to make sure that this title is finished well within the time limit.

I would also like to thank all my FMG (Foreign Medical Graduate) students, who constantly pressurized me to write a DNB/ NEET based title. With their blessings and unconditional support, my FMGE title was already a big hit and therefore they always wanted me to write a PG standard title as well. I would also love to thank them for supporting and promoting the first edition.

Special thanks to all the people who worked tirelessly in publishing the book. There are many, with whom I never met, but they all played a valuable role in putting this book to its final shape. I big thank to the entire unit.

For all my achievements till now, I will always bow my head in the feet of almighty.

Heartfelt thanks to Punit ji & Deepak ji (Arora Book Stall) for their timely help during my struggling days as an author, when they provided me necessary books for references. Words simply cannot pay back the help done by them during the need of hour.

Jain uncle (Jain stationery), Sanjay bhai & Chandarpal (A1 photocopy), and Sonu also need mention for all their timely help.

Special Thanks

I would extend my heartfelt thanks to:

- All the students of "**drkamalkv's classes**". Their faith helped me, survive in this competitive world of the coaching classes.
- My family members: Parents Hon. Capt./AEC ML Verma and Rati Devi, Brothers Ram Kishore and Anil, Sister Deepti, Wife Manju and my lovely daughters Kaakul and Kaavya.

Contents

CHAPTER

1

ANATOMY

KEY POINTS

Sutures and Conditions Associated with Their Closure

- Dolichcocephaly/Scaphocephaly [Closure of sagittal suture (anteroposetrior widening)]
- Brachycephaly [Closure of coronal suture (transverse suture)]
- Oxycephaly/Acrocephaly/Turricephaly [All sutures are closed]

Structures Derived from Neural Crest

- Pia mater
- Dental papillae
- Adrenal medulla
- Schwann
- Melanoblasts
- Dorsal root ganglia
- Autonomic ganglia
- Cells belonging to APUD series
- Bones and connective tissues of craniofacial structures
- Cells of truncoconal; cushions of heart

Structures Derived from Pharyngeal Pouches

- 1st: Middle ear, Eustachian tube.
- 2nd: Tonsil
- 3rd: Upper-Inferior parathyroid; Lower-Thymus
- 4th: Upper-Superior parathyroid; Lower-Ultimobranchial body

Structures Derived from Pharyngeal Clefts

- 1st: External auditory canal
- 2nd, 3rd, 4th: Cervical sinus

Fetal Structures and Adult Remnants

- The extra hepatic portion of umbilical vein: The round ligament of the liver (ligamentum teres hepatic), which lies in the free edge of the falciform ligament
- The intrahepatic portion (ductus venosus): Ligamentum venosum
- Closure of ductus arteriosus: Ligamentum arteriosum
- Closure of distal part of Umbilical arteries: Medial umbilical ligament

Must Know Facts

- Just prior to ovulation, the primary oocyte enters and completes 1st meiotic division.
- During first 24 weeks, there is only fetal hemoglobin; after which adult type Hb appears, at term, 75-80 percent Hb is of fetal type, it is completely replaced by 4 months of age.
- Order of development of paranasal sinuses: Maxillary—Ethmoid—Frontal-Sphenoid.
- Occurrence of acute sinusitis and carcinoma in paranasal sinuses: Maxillary—Ethmoid—Frontal-Sphenoid.

Important Cells

- Gitter cells: Microglia
- Dieter cells: Outer hair cells of organ of Corti
- Hofbauer's cells: Ellipsoidal cells in chorionic villi of placenta
- Juxtaglomerular cells: Smooth muscle cells of afferent arteriole
- Ito cells: Stellate cells in liver
- Langerhans cells: Antigen presenting epithelial dendritic cells
- Glomus cells: Present in carotid bodies

Epithelium

- Simple squamous: Alveoli of lungs, mesothelium of pleura, peritoneum and pericardium, endothelium of heart and blood vessels
- Simple cuboidal: Lining of thyroid follicles, germinal epithelium of ovary
- Simple columnar: Lining of stomach, intestines, gall bladder
- Simple columnar ciliated: Fallopian tubes, uterus, osseous part of Eustachian tube

- Keratinized stratified squamous: Epidermis of skin, external ear, external nose
- Non keratinized stratified: Esophagus, tongue, true vocal cords, cornea, tonsil
- Transitional: Calyces, ureter, urinary bladder, male urethra

Spaces Related to Upper Limb

i. Upper triangular space

- Medial boundary: Teres minor
- Lateral boundary: Long head of triceps
- Inferior boundary: Teres major
- Contents: Circumflex scapular artery

ii. Lower triangular space

- Medial boundary: Long head of triceps
- Lateral boundary: Medial border of humerus
- Superior boundary: Teres major
- Contents: Radial nerve and profunda brachii vessels

iii. Anatomical snuff box/radial fossa

- Anterior boundary: Abductor pollicis longus and extensor pollicis Brevis
- Posterior boundary: Extensor pollicis longus.
- Floor: Scaphoid, trapezium, radial artery
- Roof: Origin of cephalic vein, dorsal cutaneous branch of radial nerve
- Significance: Tenderness is suggestive of Scaphoid fracture

De Quervain's Stenosing Tenosynovitis

- Localized pain over radial styloid process
- Finkelstein's test is positive

Axial Arteries of Limbs

- Axial artery of upper limb: C7 intersegmental artery
- Axial artery of lower limb: L5 intersegmental artery

Infection of Hands and Their Spread to Spaces

- Thumb and index finger infection spreads to Thenar space
- Middle and ring fingers infection spread to Mid-palmar space
- Little finger infection spreads to borearm space of parona

Fascial Compartment of Thigh and Their Nerve-Artery

- Anterior: Femoral artery and Femoral nerve
- Medial: Profunda femoris artery and Obturator nerve
- Posterior: Branches of profunda femoris artery and Sciatic nerve

Fascial Compartment of Leg and Their Nerve-Artery

- Anterior: Anterior tibial artery and Deep peroneal nerve
- Lateral: Branches of peroneal artery and Superficial peroneal nerve
- Posterior: Posterior tibial artery and Tibial nerve

Contents of the Adductor Canal

- Terminal part of femoral artery
- Femoral vein
- Saphenous nerve
- Nerve to vastus medialis
- Terminal part of obturator nerve
- Deep lymph vessels

Must Know Facts

- Nutrient artery to the tibia is the largest nutrient artery in the body
- Housemaid's knee: Prepatellar bursitis
- Clergyman's knee: Infrapatellar bursitis

Bronchopulmonary Segments

- It is an anatomic, functional and surgical unit of the lung.
- As it is separated from rest of the lungs by a connective tissue septum, it can be separated surgically without affecting other segments
- It has a segmental bronchus, a segmental artery, lymph vessels and autonomic nerves.
- There are 10 segments on each side

Esophagus

- It is 10 inches/25 cm long
- Constrictions of esophagus: 15 cm (Cricopharynx); 25 cm (Aortic arch); 27 cm (Left bronchus); 40 cm (Diaphragmatic entry)
- Cricopharynx is the narrowest region of gastrointestinal tract.
- Esophagus shown three indentation on radiographic study; from above downwards they are: Aortic arch; Left bronchus; Left atrium
- Blood supply of esophagus: Upper third-Inferior thyroid artery; Middle third-Branches from descending thoracic aorta; Lower third-Left gastric artery

Diaphragmatic Hiatus

- Esophageal hiatus transmits: Esophagus, anterior and posterior vagal trunks
- Aortic hiatus transmits: Aorta, thoracic duct, Azygos vein

Arterial Supply of Heart

- Right Coronary artery (Main branches are Posterior Descending and Marginal artery) supplies:
  - Right atrium and ventricle
  - Posterior 1/3rd of interventricular septum
  - SA node and AV node
- Left Coronary artery (Main branches are Left Anterior Descending and Circumflex artery) supplies:
  - Anterior 2/3rd of interventricular septum
  - SA node (in 40% cases)
  - Anterior part of right and left ventricle
  - Lateral wall of left ventricle

Venous Drainage

- 10% drains into heart chambers through venae cordis minimis
- 90% drains through Coronary Sinus into right atrium via Great, Small and Middle cardiac veins (GSM)

Length of

- Duodenum: 1 foot
- Jejunum: 8 feet
- Ileum: 12 feet

Liver

- Liver is divided into right and left lobes by the attachment of the peritoneum of the falciform ligament.
- The right lobe is further divided into a quadrate lobe and caudate lobe, by gallbladder, fissure for the ligamentum teres, the inferior vena cava and the fissure for ligamentum vevosum.

Tributaries of Left Renal Vein

- Left gonadal vein
- Left suprarenal vein
- Left inferior phrenic vein

Coverings of Kidney from Inside our

- Fibrous capsule
- Perirenal fat
- Renal fascia (fascia of Gerota)
- Pararenal fat (fascia of Zuckerkandl is the posterior layer of ranal fascia)

The Renal Hilum Transmits Following Structures from Front to Backwards

- Renal vein
- Two branches of the renal artery
- Ureter
- Third branch of the renal artery

Ureter

- 10 inches/25 cm long
- Has three constrictions in its course: Where the renal pelvis joins the ureter; Where it crosses the pelvic brim; Where it enters the bladder wall

Renal Transplantation

- Iliac fossa is the preferred site for transplanted kidney

Prostate

- Prostatic urethra is the widest and the most dilatable part of urethra.
- Lobes of prostate: Anterior lobe; Median/middle lobe (enlarged in BPH); Posterior lobe (most common site of malignancy); Right and left lateral lobes

Superficial Fascia is Divided into

- Camper's fascia: Superficial fatty layer
- Scarpa's fascia: Deep membranous layer

Constituents of Spermatic Cord

- Ductus deferens
- Testicular and cremasteric arteries and artery of the ducts deferens
- Pampiniform plexus of veins
- Lymph vessels from testis
- Plexus of sympathetic nerves around the artery to the ductus deferens
- Remains of processus vaginalis

Coverings of the Spermatic Cord

- External spermatic fascia: Derived from external oblique aponeurosis
- Cremasteric fascia: Derived from internal oblique aponeurosis
- Internal spermatic fascia: Derived from fascia transversalis

Blood Supply of the Stomach

- Right gastric artery (Hepatic artery) supplies: Lower right part of the stomach
- Short gastric artery (Splenic artery) supplies: Fundus
- Left gastric artery (Celiac artery) supplies: Lower third of esophagus, upper right part of the stomach
- Left gastroepiploic artery (Splenic artery) supplies: Upper part of greater curvature

- Right gastroepiploic artery (Gastroduodenal artery) supplies: Lower part of greater curvature

Layers of SCALP

- S: Skin
- C: Connective tissue
- A: Aponeurosis
- L: Loose areolar tissue
- P: Pericranium

Cranial Nerve and Functions

- Olfactory (Sensory): Perceives smell
- Optic (Sensory): Vision
- Oculomotor (Motor): Supplies levator palpebrae superioris, superior rectus, medial rectus, inferior rectus, inferior oblique, supplies sphincter pupillae and ciliary muscle with parasympathetic fibres
- Trochlear (Motor): Supplies superior oblique
- Trigeminal (Mixed): Supplies sensory fibres to the skin of the scalp, face, mouth, teeth, nasal cavity and paranasal sinuses; supplies motor fibres to the muscles of mastication, tensor veli palatini and tensor tympani
- Abducent (Motor): Supplies lateral rectus
- Facial (Mixed): Supplies motor fibres to the muscles of face, scalp with auricle, buccinator, platysma, stapedius, stylohyoid and posterior belly of digastric; gives sensory supply to anterior 2/3rd of tongue, floor of mouth and the palate; gives parasympathetic secretomotor fibres to the submandibular and sublingual salivary glands, lacrimal glands and the glands of the nose and palate.
- Vestibulocochlear (Sensory): Position and movement of head; hearing
- Glossopharyngeal (Mixed): Supplies stylopharyngeus muscle; supplies parasympathetic secretomotor fibres to the parotid gland, sensory and taste fibres to the posterior third of tongue and pharynx.
- Vagus (Mixed): Supplies constrictor muscles of pharynx and intrinsic muscles of larynx involuntary muscles of trachea and bronchi, heart, alimentary tract from pharynx to splenic flexure of colon, liver and pancreas; Afferent fibres from the abdominal structures, taste from epiglottis and velleculae
- Spinal accessory (Motor): Supplies sternocleidomastoid and trapezius
- Hypoglossal (Motor): Supplies muscles of tongue, except palatoglossus.

Cranial Foramen with the Structures Passing Through Them

- Carotid canal: Internal carotid artery
- Foramen rotundum: Maxillary nerve
- Foramen lacerum: Internal carotid artery, nerve of pterygoid canal
- Jugular foramen: Inferior petrosal sinus, 9th, 10th, 11th cranial nerves, internal jugular vein
- Stylomastoid foramen: Facial nerve
- Foramen magnum: Medulla, tonsils of cerebellum, meninges.
  - Through subarachnoid space-Spinal accessory nerve, vertebral artery, posterior spinal artery, anterior spinal artery.
  - Anterior part-Ligament of dens, membrana tectoria.
- Optic canal: Optic nerve
- Superior orbital fissure: Superior ophthalmic vein, lacrimal, frontal, Trochlear, oculomotor, nasociliary, abducent nerves
- Hypoglossal canal: Hypoglossal nerve
- Internal acoustic meatus: Vestibulocochlear and facial nerve
- Foramen spinosum: Middle meningeal artery, nervus spinosus, posterior trunk of middle meningeal artery.
- Foramen ovale: Mandibular nerve, Accessory meningeal artery,Lesser petrosal nerve, vein connecting cavernous sinus with the pterygoid plexus of veins.

Branches of External Carotid Artery

- Anterior: Superior thyroid, Lingual, Facial
- Posterior: Occipital, Posterior auricular
- Medial: Ascending pharyngeal
- Terminal: Maxillary, Superficial temporal.

Sensory Innervation of Tongue [General Sensation (GS); Taste Sensation (TS)]

- Anterior 2/3rd (including circumvallate papillae for taste sensation): Lingual nerve (GS); Chorda tympani branch of facial nerve (TS)
- Posterior 1/3rd (except circumvallate papillae for taste sensation): Glossopharyngeal nerve for GS and TS

Carotid Sheath Contains

- Carotid arteries (within the sheath common carotid divides into external and internal carotids)
- Internal jugular vein
- Vagus nerve

Ocular Muscles (Nerve Supply and Function)

- Superior rectus: Oculomotor nerve; Moves eyeball upward and medially
- Inferior rectus: Oculomotor nerve; Moves eyeball downwards and medially

- Medial rectus: Oculomotor nerve; moves eyeball medially
- Lateral rectus: Abducent; Moves eyeball laterally
- Superior oblique: Trochlear; Moves eyeball downwards and laterally
- Inferior oblique: Oculomotor nerve; Moves eyeball upwards and laterally
- Orbicularis oculi: Facial nerve; Closes eyeball and dilates lacrimal sac
- Levator palpebrae superioris: Oculomotor nerve; Raises upper lid and sympathetic supply
- Sphincter Pupillae: Parasympathetic supply; Constricts pupil by oculomotor nerve
- Dilator pupillae: Sympathetic supply; Dilates pupil
- Ciliary mucle: Parasympathetic supply by oculomotor nerve; controls shape of eye, helps in accommodation

Must Know Facts

- Only cranial nerve to arise from the dorsal aspect of the brain stem is Trochlear nerve
- Facial vein communicates with the cavernous sinus through the superior and inferior ophthalmic veins
- Stenson's duct—Parotid gland
- Wharton's duct—Submandibular gland

Lesion of Visual Pathway

- Optic nerve: Blindness in that eye
- Crossing fibres of optic chiasma: Bitemporal hemianopia
- Lateral parts of chiasma: Binasal hemianopia
- Optic tract/lateral geniculate body: Contralateral homonymous hemianopia
- Meyer's loop of optic radiation: Contralateral superior quadrantic anopia
- Vascular lesion of occipital lobe: Contralateral homonymous hemianopia with macula sparing

Blood-Brain Barrier is Absent at

- Pituitary
- Area postrema
- Organum vasculosum of lamina terminalis
- Subfornical organ
- Ventral part of median eminence of hypothalamus
- Anterior pituitary
- Pineal gland

Sesamoid Bones (in the Tendons of)

- Quadriceps femoris (Patella-largest sesamoid bone)
- Peroneus longus
- Tibialis anterior
- Tibialis posterior
- Lateral head of gastrocnemius

Peculiarities of Sesamoid Bones

- Ossify at birth
- Devoid of periosteum
- Absence of haversian system

Spinal Nerves

- Cervical: 8
- Thoracic:12
- Lumbar: 5
- Sacral: 5
- Coccygeal:1
- Total: 31

Vertebral Levels and Bony Landmarks

- C7: Most prominent spinous process at the base of neck
- T3: Level of the spine of scapula
- T7: Level of lower angle of scapula
- T12: Floating rib
- L4: Level of iliac crests
- S2: Level of posterosuperior iliac supine

Structure and Their Levels in Body

- Xiphoid process: T9
- Celiac trunk: T12 L1
- Spleen: 10th rib
- Superior mesenteric artery: L1
- Stomach pylorus: L1
- Spinal cord ends (adults): L1, L2
- Spinal cord ends (children): L3
- Pancreas: L1, L2
- Inferior mesenteric artery: L3
- Umbilicus: L3, L4
- Highest point of iliac crest: L4
- Transtubercular plane: L5
- ASIS: Sacral promontory

MCQs WITH SHORT EXPLANATIONS

EMBRYOLOGY

1. **Establishment of fetal circulation is by:**
   a. 16th day
   b. 14th day
   c. 21st day
   d. 28th day

Events following fertilization

- Fertilization: 0 hours
- 16 celled stage/ morula enters cavity: 4th day
- Blastocyst formation: 5th day
- Interstitial implantation: 7th day
- Placenta fully established; fetal circulation established & heart formed: 21st day
- Internal gonads formed: 8th weeks
- Swallowing starts: 10–12th weeks
- Fetal breathing movements starts: 11 weeks
- External genital formed; urine formation occurs: 12 weeks

Timetable of some events

Age	Developmental events
3rd week	Blood and vessels forming cells (angioblastic islands) appear. The cardiogenic area, heart tubes and pericardium have formed.
4th week	Heart and pericardium lie ventral to foregut. Subdivisions of heart tube are visible. Heart begins to beat (becomes functional). Heart septa begin to form. Aortic arches begin to establish in cranial to caudal sequence. Most of the first aortic arch disappears at the end of 4th week. Veins start forming.
5th week	The spiral septum is formed. Formation of aortic arches is complete. Lymphatic sacs form. The cardinal, umbilical and vitelline veins are formed. Conduction system of heart forms.
6th week	Coronary circulation is becoming established. Atrio-ventricular valves and papillary muscles are forming.
7th week	Heart septa are completely formed.

Contd...

Contd...

2. **Which of the following is derived from 5th pharyngeal pouch?**
   a. Superior parathyroid
   b. Inferior parathyroid
   c. Thymus
   d. Thyroid (parafollicular cells)

Derivatives of pharyngeal pouches

- **Pharyngeal Pouch 1:** Develops into the auditory tube and middle ear cavity
- **Pharyngeal Pouch 2:** Forms numerous infoldings that become the crypts of the palatine tonsil; later, lymphocytes (from the thymus and bone marrow) infiltrate the underlying lamina propria to establish the definitive palatine tonsil.
- **Pharyngeal Pouch 3:** Divides into a superior (or dorsal) and inferior (or ventral) portion:
  - **Dorsal portion of pouch 3:** Forms the inferior parathyroid glands–the chief (or principal) and oxyphil cells are derived from the endodermal lining of the pouch
  - **Ventral portion of pouch 3:** Forms the thymus – the epithelial reticular cells (including those that comprise the thymic or Hassall's corpuscles) are derived from the endodermal lining of the pouch. T-cell progenitors from the bone marrow infiltrate the cortex to establish the definitive thymus.
- **Pharyngeal Pouch 4:** Also divides into a superior (or dorsal) and inferior (or ventral) portion:
  - **Dorsal portion of pouch 4:** Forms the superior parathyroid glands –the chief (or principal) and oxyphil cells are derived from the endodermal lining of the pouch
  - **Ventral portion of pouch 4:** Forms a diverticulum called the ultimobranchial body, which releases signaling factors to induce the migration and differentiation of nearby neural crest cells into parafollicular (C) cells of the thyroid gland.
- **Pharyngeal pouch 5/Ultimobranchial pouch:** It is generally believed to be incorporated in to the fourth pouch and the two together forming the caudal pharyngeal complex. The superior parathyroid gland arises from this complex. The complex probably also gives origin to the parafollicular cells of the thyroid gland

Ans. 1. **c.** 21st day 2. **d.** Thyroid (parafollicular cells) > a. i.e. Superior parathyroid

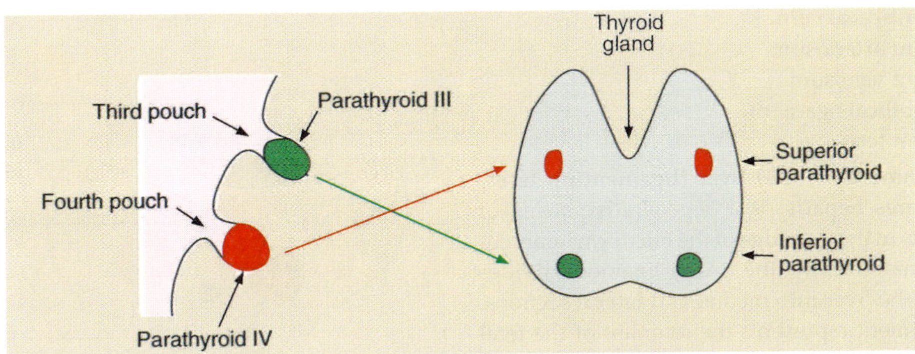

Derivation of superior and inferior parathyroid glands. Note that the relative position of parathyroid III and IV is reversed during development.

3. How many oogonia are present at birth?

a. 1-2 thousands b. 1-2 lakhs
c. 1-2 crores d. 1-2 millions

Number of germ cells/follicles

- Up to the 22nd week of pregnancy, the primordial germ cells multiply along with the resulting oogonia by mitosis.
- The maximum number of germ cells (7 million), found in an ovary, is reached already in the 20th week due to the concomitant massive degeneration of germ cells that begins in the 14th week.

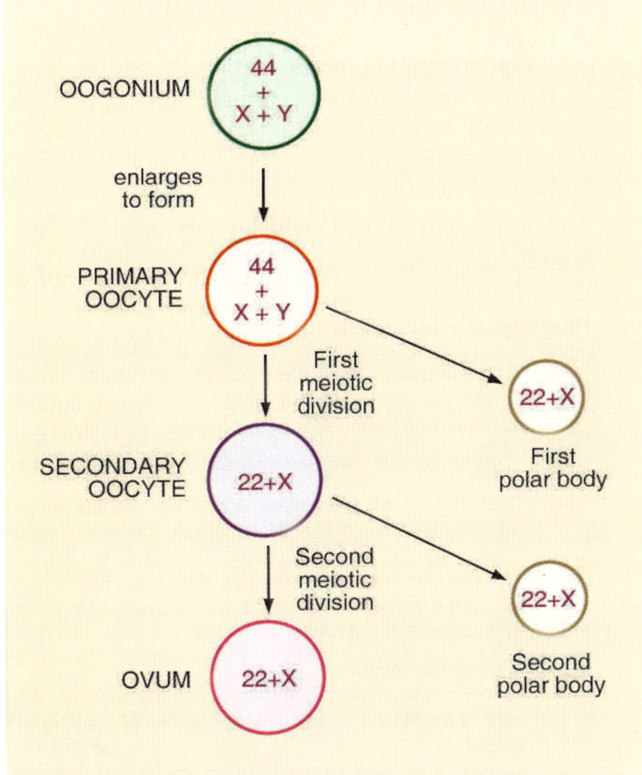

Stages in oogenesis.

- At the time of birth only about 2 million germ cells are still present in the ovary.
- The very first primary oocytes enter the prophase in the 12th week.
- The passage through the various stages, up to the arresting of further development, takes approximately 4 weeks and is accompanied by a restructuring of the epithelial covering (coelomic epithelium → follicular epithelium), so that the first primordial follicle with the primary oocyte, arrested in the dictyotene stage, appears roughly 4 weeks later in the 16th week.
- It is assumed that the generation of the primordial follicles is complete by the time of birth.

4. Which of the following does NOT divide:

a. Spermatogonia b. Primary spermatocyte
c. Secondary spermatocyte d. Spermatid

Spermatids differentiates (NO division) into sperms

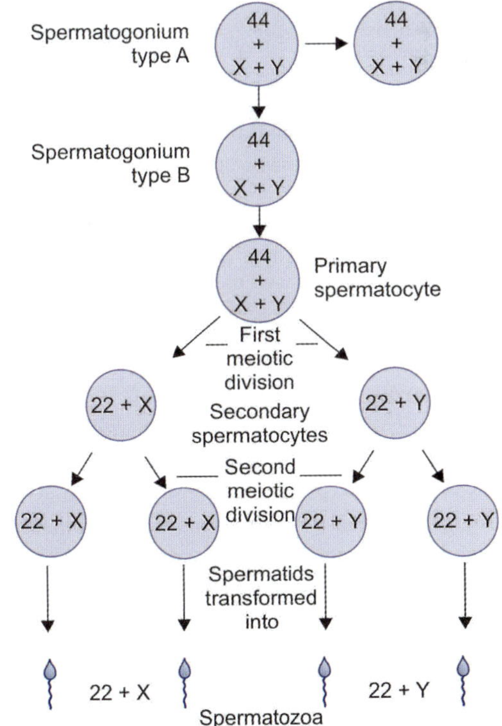

Stages in spermatogenesis. Note the number of chromosomes at each stage.

Ans. 3. **d.** 1-2 millions 4. **d.** Spermatid

5. Remnant of umbilical vein:
 a. Ligamentum arteriosum
 b. Ligamentum venosum
 c. Medial umbilical ligament
 d. Ligamentum teres

The **round ligament of (the) liver (ligamentum teres/ ligamentum teres hepatis)** is a degenerative string of tissue that exists in the free edge of the falciform ligament of the liver. Anatomically, the round ligament divides the left part of the liver into medial and lateral sections. The round ligament represents the remnant of the fetal umbilical vein.

6. Notochord persists as:
 a. Spinous process b. Vertebral foramen
 c. Annulus fibrosus d. Nucleus pulposus

The **notochord** is a flexible rod-shaped body found in embryos of all chordates. It is composed of cells derived from the mesoderm and defines the primitive axis of the embryo. In some chordates, it persists throughout life as the main axial support of the body, while in most vertebrates it becomes the nucleus pulposus of the intervertebral disk. The notochord is found ventral to the neural tube.

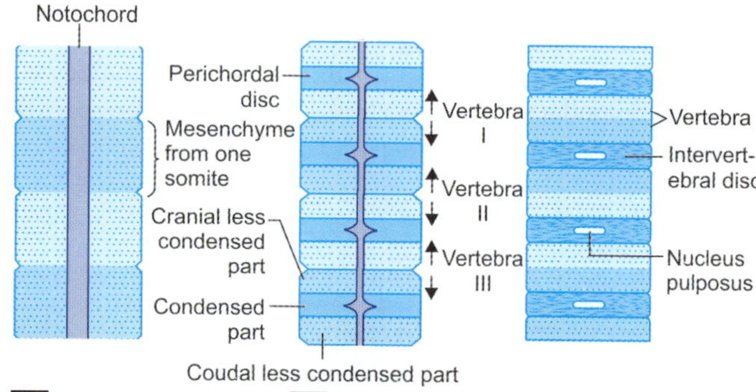

(A) Mesenchyme derived from somites is seen in the form of segments. (B) Each segment has a central condensed part, and cranial and caudal less condensed parts. (C) A vertebra is formed by fusion of adjoining uncondensed parts of two somites. Hence it is an intersegmental structure. Each intervertebral disc is derived from the condensed part of one somite. Hence, it is segmental in position.

7. True regarding umbilical cord:
 a. Two veins b. Two arteries
 c. Covered by amnion and chorion
 d. Umbilical cord pulsation rate equals maternal heart beat

During prenatal development, the umbilical cord is physiologically and genetically part of the fetus and (in humans), normally contains two arteries (the umbilical arteries) and one vein (the umbilical vein), buried within Wharton's jelly. The umbilical vein supplies the fetus with oxygenated, nutrient-rich blood from the placenta. Conversely, the fetal heart pumps deoxygenated, nutrient-depleted blood through the umbilical arteries back to the placenta.

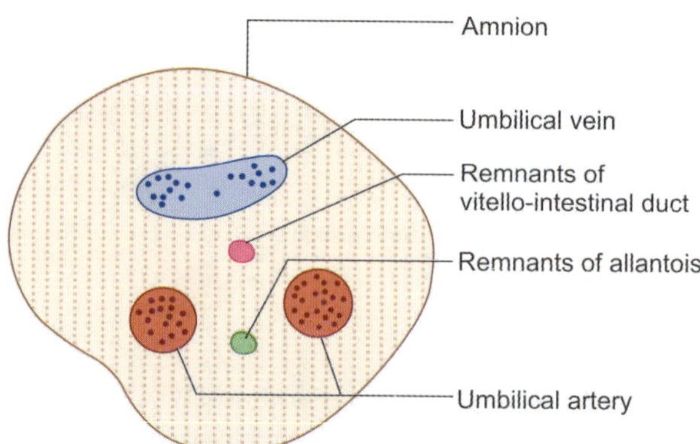

Section through umbilical cord.

8. NOT a derivative of mesonephric duct:
 a. Ureter b. Vas deferens
 c. Prostatic utricle
 d. Trigone of urinary bladder

The prostatic utricle is important primarily because it is the male homologue of the female uterus and vagina, usually described as derived from the Müllerian ducts (paramesonephric duct).

9. Stapes is derived from which pharyngeal arch:
 a. 1st b. 2nd
 c. 3rd d. 4th

Skeletal derivatives of 2nd pharyngeal arch
- Stapes
- Temporal styloid process
- Hyoid (lesser/smaller cornua and upper part of body)
- Stylohyoid ligament
- Reichert's cartilage.

10. Tonsils are derived from which pharyngeal pouch:
 a. 1st b. 2nd
 c. 3rd d. 4th

Pharyngeal pouch derivatives

1st	The endoderm lines the future auditory tube (Pharyngotympanic Eustachian tube), middle ear, mastoid antrum, and inner layer of the tympanic membrane.
2nd	Contributes the middle ear, palatine tonsils
3rd	The third pouch possesses Dorsal and Ventral wings. Derivatives of the dorsal wings include the inferior parathyroid glands, while the ventral wings fuse to form the cytoreticular cells of the thymus. The main nerve supply to the derivatives of this pouch is Cranial Nerve IX, glossopharyngeal nerve.
4th	Derivatives include: Superior parathyroid glands and ultimobranchial body which forms the parafollicular C-cells of the thyroid gland. Musculature and cartilage of larynx (along with the sixth pharyngeal pouch).
5th	Rudimentary structure, becomes part of the fourth pouch contributing to thyroid C-cells

Ans. 5. **d.** Ligamentum teres 6. **d.** Nucleus pulposus 7. **b.** Two arteries 8. **c.** Prostatic utricle
9. **b.** 2nd 10. **b.** 2nd

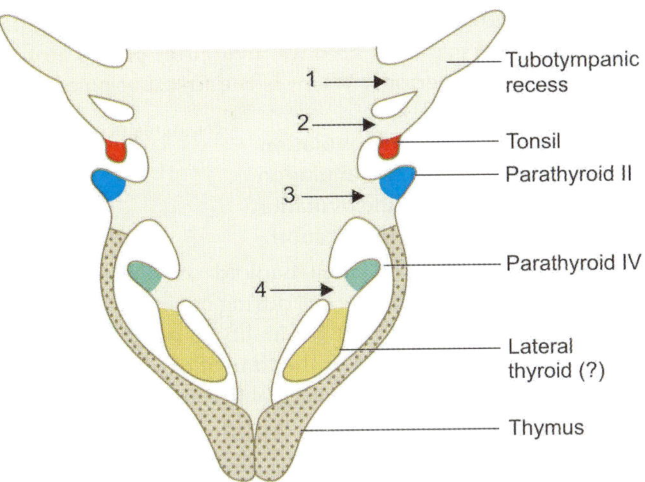

Scheme to show the fate of the pharyngeal pouches (numbered 1 to 4).

11. Muscles of mastication are derived from mesoderm of which pharyngeal arch:

a. 1st b. 2nd
c. 3rd d. 4th

Muscles of mastication, anterior belly of digastrics, mylohyoid, tensor tympani and tensor veli palatini are derived from first pharyngeal arch.

12. The following ocular structure is NOT derived from surface ectoderm:

a. Crystalline lens b. Sclera
c. Corneal epithelium
d. Epithelium of lacrimal glands

Derivatives of head mesenchyme (neural crest and/or mesoderm)

- Blood vessels
- Corneal stroma and endothelium
- Stroma of choroid, ciliary body, and iris
- Ciliary muscle
- Sclera
- Optic nerve sheath (meninges)
- Extraocular muscles and fasciae
- Remainder of the eyelids (orbicularis oculi muscle, tarsus, orbital septum, etc.)
- Vitreous (part).

Summary of derivation of various part of the eyeball.

Part	Derived from
Lens	Surface ectoderm
Retina	Neuroectoderm (optic cup)
Vitreous	Mesoderm
Choroid	Mesoderm (infiltrated by neural crest cells?)
Ciliary body	Mesoderm
Ciliary muscles	Mesenchymal cells covering the developing ciliary body (neural crest?).
Iris	Mesoderm
Muscles of Iris	Neuroectoderm (from optic cup)
Sclera	Mesoderm (infiltrated by neural crest cells?)

Contd...

Contd...

Part	Derived from
Cornea	Surface epithelium by ectoderm, substantia propria and inner epithelium by neural crest
Conjunctiva	Surface ectoderm
Blood vessels	Mesoderm
Optic nerve	Neuroectoderm. Its coverings (pia, arachnoid and dura) are derived from mesoderm

13. All are of mesodermal origin EXCEPT:

a. Sphincter pupillae b. Ciliary muscle
c. Iris d. Ovarian tissue

Within the stroma of the iris, the sphincter pupillae and dilator pupillae muscles develop from optic cup neuroectoderm. In contrast, the ciliary muscle, which is responsible for changing the shape of the lens, is derived from overlying mesenchyme (mesoderm).

14. In hydatidiform mole, blood cell does not develop because of defect in:

a. Primary ectoderm b. Mesoderm
c. Endoderm d. Trophoblast

Blood vessels do not develop in hydatidiform mole due to lack of mesoderm. Blood vessels are mesodermal in origin.

15. True regarding content of umbilical vessels:

a. 2 arteries, 2 veins b. 2 arteries, 1 vein
c. 1 artery, 2 veins d. 1 artery, 1 vein

The umbilical cord contains Wharton's jelly, a gelatinous substance made largely from muco-polysaccharides which protects the blood vessels inside. It contains one vein, which carries oxygenated, nutrient-rich blood to the fetus, and two arteries that carry deoxygenated, nutrient-depleted blood away.

16. Double aortic arch is due to:

a. Persistence of right 4th aortic arch
b. Persistence of left 6th aortic arch
c. Persistence of right 6th aortic arch
d. Persistence of left 4th aortic arch

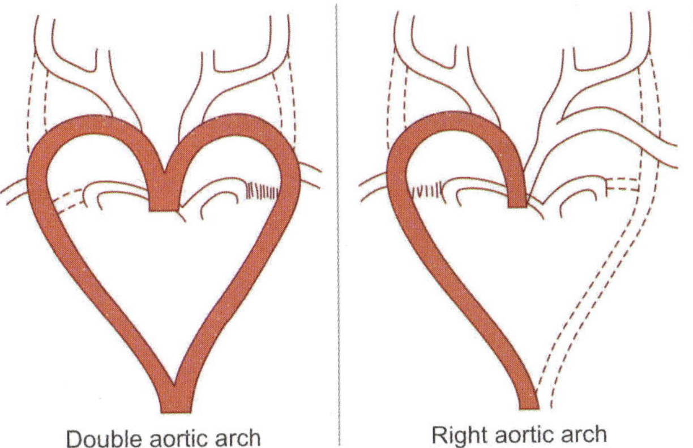

Contd...

MCQs with Short Explanations

Ans. **11. a.** 1st **12. b.** Sclera **13. a.** Sphincter pupillae **14. b.** Mesoderm **15. b.** 2 arteries, 1 vein **16. a.** Persistence of right...

Contd...

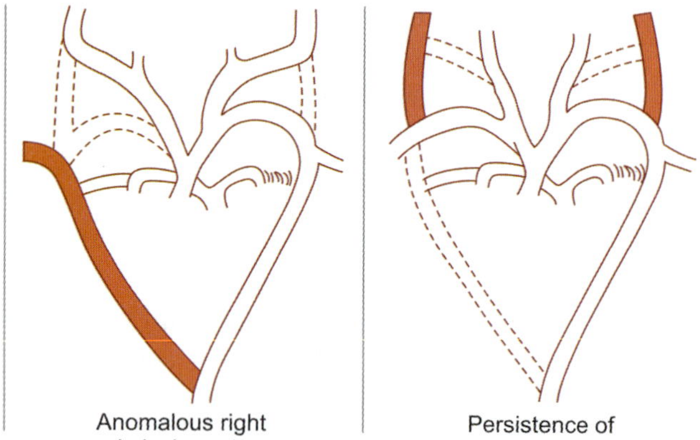

Anomalies associated with the development of aortic arches. The abnormal vessels are shown in red.

The *fourth right arch* forms the right subclavian as far as the origin of its internal mammary branch; while the fourth left arch constitutes the arch of the aorta between the origin of the left carotid artery and the termination of the ductus arteriosus. A double aortic arch; occurs with the development of an abnormal right aortic arch in addition to the left aortic arch, forming a vascular ring around the trachea and esophagus, which usually causes difficult breathing and swallowing.

17. Ectopia cordis is related to:

a. Lungs b. Liver
c. Heart d. Lens

Ectopia cordis (Greek: *'away/out of place' + Latin: 'heart'*) is a congenital malformation in which the heart is abnormally located either partially or totally outside of the thorax.

18. Meckel's diverticulum arises from:

a. Foregut b. Ileum
c. Cecum d. Colon

Meckel's diverticulum is located in the distal ileum, usually within 60–100 cm (2 feet) of the ileocecal valve. This *blind segment* or small pouch is about 3–6 cm long and may have a greater lumen diameter than that of the ileum. It runs anti-mesenterically and has its own blood supply. It is a remnant of the connection from the yolk sac to the small intestine present during embryonic development. It is a *true diverticulum*, consisting of all 3 layers of the bowel wall which are mucosa, submucosa and muscularis propria.

19. Ovary is derived from:

a. Müllerian duct
b. Wolffian duct
c. Genital ridge
d. Genital tubercle

The gonadal ridge (or genital ridge) is the precursor to the gonads.

20. In a young female of reproductive age with regular menstrual cycles of 28 days, ovulation occurs around 14th day of periods. When is the first day polar body extruded:

a. 24 hours prior to ovulation
b. Accompanied by ovulation
c. 48 hours after the ovulation
d. At the time of fertilization

A **polar body** is a small haploid cell that is formed concomitantly as an egg cell during oogenesis, but which generally does not have the ability to be fertilized. First polar body is released at the time of ovulation whereas second polar body is released at the time of fertilization.

21. Primary structural defect is known as:

a. Mutation b. Deformation
c. Anomaly d. Malformation

A **malformation** is associated with a disorder of tissue development. Malformations often occur in the first trimester.

22. Closure of neural tube starts from:

a. Lumbar b. Cephalic
c. Cervical d. Podalic

For a short time, the neural tube is open both cranially and caudally. These openings, called neuropores, close during the fourth week in the human. The closure of the neural tube begins in the cervical area (in the middle of the embryo) and extends from there in both the cranial and caudal directions. Improper closure of the neuropores can result in neural tube defects such as anencephaly or spina bifida.

23. Trigone-urinary bladder develops from:

a. Ectoderm b. Endoderm
c. Mesoderm d. None of the above

Embryologically, the trigone of the bladder is derived from the caudal end of mesonephric ducts, which is of mesodermal origin (the rest of the bladder is endodermal). In the female the mesonephric ducts regresses, causing the trigone to be less prominent, but still present.

24. Auerbach plexus and Meissner plexus are derived from:

a. Epithelial lining of gut b. Mesoderm
c. Endoderm d. Neural crest

The majority of the enteric nervous system is derived from vagal neural crest cells (NCC), which migrate to the developing gut, proliferate, form plexuses and differentiate into neurons and glia.

25. Ureter develops from:

a. Mesonephric duct
b. Paramesonephric duct
c. Urogenital sinus
d. Mesonephric tubules

Ans. 17. **c.** Heart 18. **b.** Ileum 19. **c.** Genital ridge 20. **b.** Accompanied...
21. **d.** Malformation 22. **c.** Cervical 23. **c.** Mesoderm 24. **d.** Neural crest
25. **a.** Mesonephric duct

The **ureteric bud,** also known as the **metanephrogenic diverticulum,** is a protrusion from the mesonephric duct during the development of the urinary and reproductive organs. It later develops into a conduit for urine drainage from the kidneys, which, in contrast, originate from the metanephric blastema.

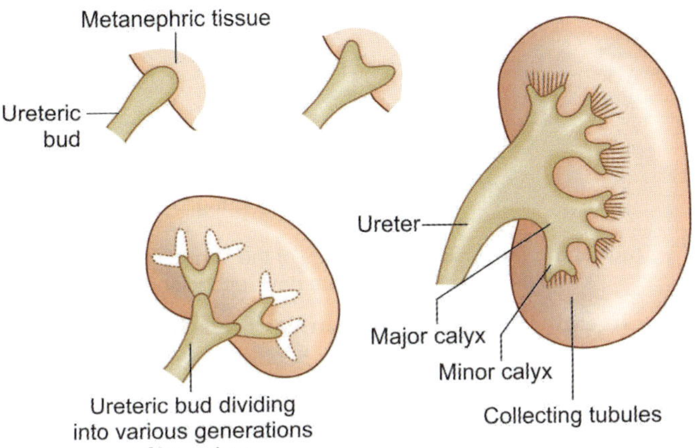

Formation of the collecting system of the kidney, from ramifications of the ureteric bud.

26. Gartner duct is a remnant of:

a. Epoophoron b. Cloacal duct
c. Wolffian duct d. Müllerian duct

The derivatives of the mesonephric duct/Wolffian duct can be remembered using the mnemonic, **'Gardener's SEED'** for **Gartner's** duct, **S**eminal vesicles, **E**pididymis, **E**jaculatory duct and **D**uctus deferens.

Summary of Male and Female Homologues derived from Undifferentiated Genital System.

Structure	*Male Derivative*	*Female Derivative*
Gonad	Testis	Ovary
Sex cords	Sertoli cells (seminiferous tubules)	Granulose cells
Primordial germ cells	Spermatozoa	Ova
Paramesonephric duct	Appendix of testis Utricle of prostate	Uterine tube, uterus Upper vagina
Mesonephric duct	Appendix of epididymis, Epididymis, Ductus deferens, Ejaculatory duct Seminal vesicle	Appendix of ovary Gartner's duct
Mesonephric tubules	Vasa efferentia Paradidymis	Epoophoron Paroophoron
Genital tubercle	Penis	Clitoris
Genital swellings	Scrotum	Labia majora
Urethral folds	Floor of penile urethra	Labia minora

27. NOT a derivative of midgut:

a. Jejunum b. Appendix
c. Ascending colon d. Descending colon

The **hindgut** (or **epigaster**) is the posterior (caudal) part of the alimentary canal. In mammals, it includes the distal third of the transverse colon and the splenic flexure, the descending colon, sigmoid colon and rectum.

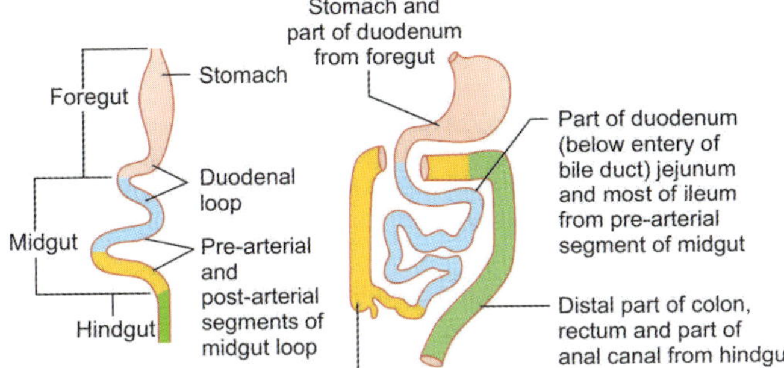

Derivation of various parts of the gut.

28. Clitoris develops from:

a. Genital ridge b. Genital tubercle
c. Wolffian duct d. Müllerian duct

A **genital tubercle** or **phallic tubercle** is a body of tissue present in the development of the reproductive system. It forms in the ventral, caudal region of mammalian embryos of both sexes, and eventually develops into a phallus. In the human fetus, the genital tubercle develops around week 4 of gestation, and by week 9 becomes recognizably either a clitoris or penis.

29. Parathyroid gland develops from:

a. Branchial arch b. Branchial pouch
c. Both d. None

Inferior parathyroid develops from 3rd pharyngeal pouch whereas superior parathyroid gland develops from 4th pharyngeal pouch.

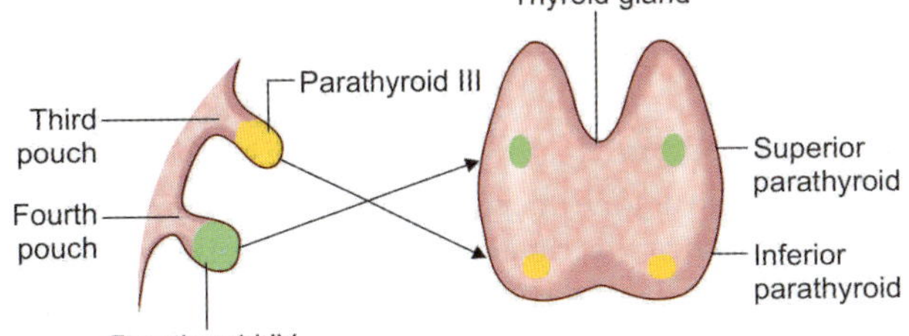

Derivation of superior and inferior parathyroid glands. Note that the relative position of parathyroid III and IV is reversed during development.

30. Appendix of testes is a remnant of:

a. Germ cell b. Urogenital fold
c. Mesonephric duct d. Paramesonephric duct

The **appendix testis** (or **hydatid of Morgagni**) is a vestigial remnant of the Müllerian duct/ paramesonephric duct, present on the upper pole of the testis and attached to the tunica vaginalis. It is present about 90% of the time.

Ans. **26. c.** Wolffian duct **27. d.** Descending colon **28. b.** Genital tubercle **29. b.** Branchial pouch **30. d.** Paramesonephric duct

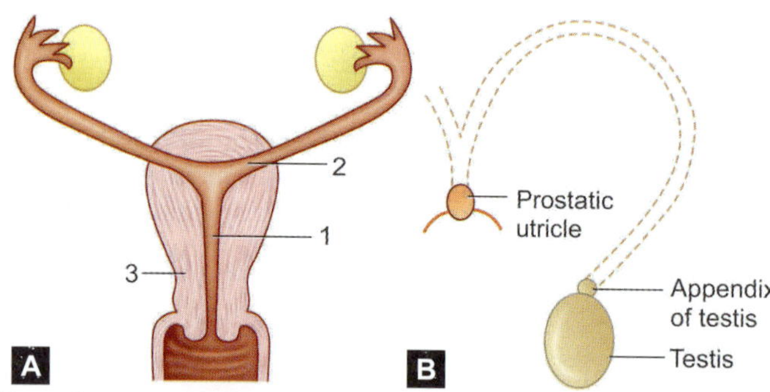

Fate of paramesonephric ducts. (A) In the female they form the uterine tubes, the uterus, and part of the vagina. 1 is epithelium of uterus, 2 is fundus of uterus and 3 is myometrium. (B) In the male most of the duct disappears. Remnants are seen as the appendix of the testis and the prostatic utricle.

31. Lower 1/4th of vagina develops from:

a. Mesonephric duct
b. Paramesonephric duct
c. Genital tubercle
d. Urogenital sinus

Upper 3/4th of vagina develops from Müllerian duct/ paramesonephric duct whereas lower 1/4th develops from urogenital sinus.

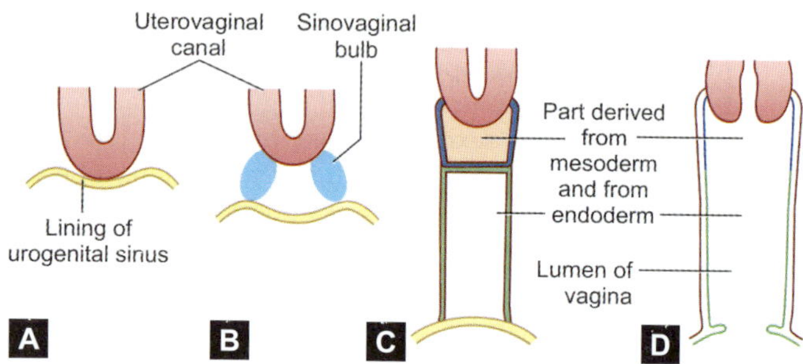

(A) Uterovaginal canal (mesoderm) in contact with lining of UGS (endoderm). (B) Sinovaginal bulbs are formed by proliferation of endodermal lining. (C) Solid vaginal plate derived partly from mesoderm of uterovaginal canal and partly from endoderm of sinovaginal bulbs. (D) Vagina formed by canalisation of vaginal plate.

32. Lens is derived from:

a. Endoderm b. Surface ectoderm
c. Mesoderm d. None of the above

Ocular structures derived from surface ectoderm are lens, cornea, lacrimal gland, tarsal glands and the conjunctiva of the eye.

33. Sympathetic ganglia arise from:

a. Endoderm
b. Neural crest
c. Mesoderm
d. All of the above

Neural crest cells are a transient, multipotent, migratory cell population unique to vertebrates that gives rise to a diverse cell lineage including melanocytes, craniofacial cartilage and bone, smooth muscle, peripheral and enteric neurons and glia.

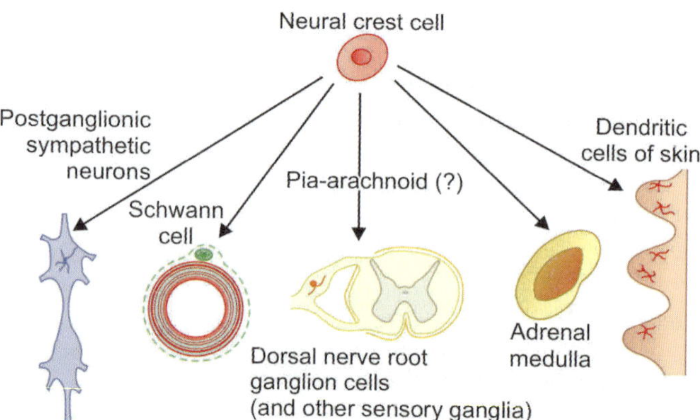

Traditionally recognised derivatives of the neural crest. Some additional derivatives are now recognised.

34. In embryonic life, blood formation is first observed in:

a. Liver b. Bone marrow
c. Yolk sac d. Spleen

In the developing embryos, blood formation occurs in aggregates of blood cells in the yolk sac, called blood islands. As development progresses, blood formation occurs in the spleen and liver. When bone marrow develops (third month), it eventually assumes the task of forming most of the blood cells for the entire organism.

35. CNS cells of mesodermal origin:

a. Microglia b. Sympathetic ganglia
c. Schwann cells d. Neurons

Mesoderm derivatives include the muscle (smooth, cardiac and skeletal), the muscles of the tongue (occipital somites), the pharyngeal arches muscles (muscles of mastication, muscles of facial expressions), connective tissue, dermis and subcutaneous layer of the skin, bone and cartilage, dura mater, endothelium of blood vessels, red blood cells, white blood cells, microglia and Kupffer cells, the kidneys and the adrenal cortex.

Various types of cells are derived from neuroepithelium.

Derivation of nerve cells (neurons) and neuroglial cells		
From neural tube	*From neural crest*	*From mesenchymal cells*
Neurons Fibrous astrocytes Protoplasmic astrocytes Oligodendroglia (?) Ependymal cells	Schwann cells Dorsal n. root ganglion cells Cells of other sensory ganglia Neurons in sympathetic ganglia	Microglia Oligodendroglia (?)

36. Umbilical cord contains:

a. 2 veins, 2 arteries b. 1 vein, 2 arteries
c. 2 veins, 1 artery d. 1 vein, 1 artery

Initially, there are 2 arteries and 2 veins in umbilical cord, but then right umbilical vein disappears and left umbilical vein is left.

Ans. 31. **d.** Urogenital sinus 32. **b.** Surface ectoderm 33. **b.** Neural crest 34. **c.** Yolk sac 35. **a.** Microglia 36. **b.** 1 vein, 2 arteries

37. Salivary glands are derived from:

a. Endoderm
b. Ectoderm
c. Both of the above
d. None of the above

Parotid gland primordia (anlage) arises in weeks 5–6 from ectoderm, followed by submandibular gland primordia in week 6 from endoderm, then sublingual gland primordia in weeks 7–8 from endoderm.

38. Fetal circulation is firstly observed at:

a. 11 days
b. 21 days
c. 31 days
d. 41 days

Uteroplacental circulation is established by 2 weeks and fetoplacental circulation by 3 weeks.

39. After how many days of ovulation implantation of embryo occurs:

a. 3–5 days
b. 6–9 days
c. 10–14 days
d. 15–19 days

In humans, implantation of a fertilized ovum (blastocyst) is most likely to occur about 9 days after ovulation, ranging between 6 and 12 days.

40. Superior parathyroid gland develops from:

a. 1st pharyngeal pouch
b. 2nd pharyngeal pouch
c. 3rd pharyngeal pouch
d. 4th pharyngeal pouch

Inferior parathyroid develops from 3rd pharyngeal pouch whereas superior parathyroid gland develops from 4th pharyngeal pouch.

41. Kidney arises from:

a. Metanephros
b. Ureteric bud
c. Metanephros and ureteric bud
d. None of the above

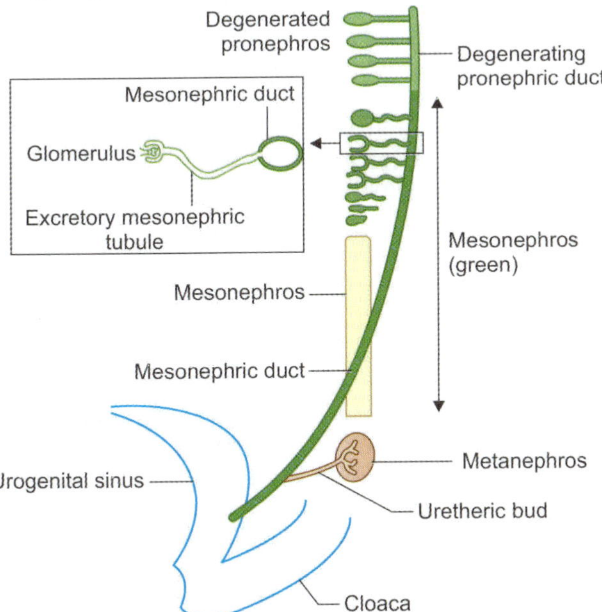

Some details of developing pronephros, mesonephros and metanephros. The pronephros and pronephric duct degenerate soon after formation. The proximal part of the mesonephros shows segmentation (in cranio-caudal sequence). The segments contain functional excretory tubules that drain into the mesonephric duct. Most of these tubules disappear by the time the metanephros forms the definitive kidney.

The development of the kidney proceeds through a series of successive phases, each marked by the development of a more advanced kidney: the pronephros, mesonephros, and metanephros. The pronephros is the most immature form of kidney, while The metanephros is most developed. The metanephros persists as the definitive adult kidney. The elongated stalk of the ureteric bud, called the metanephric duct, later forms the ureter. As the cranial end of the bud extends into the intermediate mesoderm, it undergoes a series of branchings to form the collecting duct system of the kidney. It also forms the major and minor calyces and the renal pelvis.

42. Thymus gland develops from:

a. Brachial arch
b. Brachial cleft
c. Brachial pouch
d. Brachial cyst

Thymus develops from third pharyngeal pouch.

43. Primordial germ cells are derived from:

a. Neural crest
b. Genital ridge
c. Somatopleuritic mesoderm
d. Yolk sac

The primordial germ-cells of Sphenodon originate in the yolk-sac endoderm of the area opaca all round the embryo, but chiefly in a crescentic area in front of it.

44. Second polar body is released:

a. At the time of menstruation
b. At the time of ovulation
c. At the time of fertilization
d. At the time of menopause

First polar body is released at the time of ovulation. Second polar body is released at the time of fertilization.

HISTOLOGY

45. FALSE statement regarding histology of anal canal:

a. Upper 3 cm is lined by mucous membrane
b. Below the pectinate line, whole part is lined by non-keratinized stratified squamous
c. Mucous membrane of upper 15 mm is columnar
d. Sweat & sebaceous glands are present in lower 10 mm

Anal canal

- It represents a transition from features of the lower tract to those of skin.
- The surface changes from a simple columnar epithelium with goblet cells, through a short zone of non-keratinized stratified squamous epithelium, to the typical keratinized stratified squamous epithelium of epidermis.
- Lamina propria and muscularis mucoase disappear distally, and the connective tissue of submucosa changes to the dense fibrous tissue of dermis.
- This connective tissue contains both ordinary eccrine sweat glands and much larger apocrine sweat glands.
- Smooth muscle of the colon changes to striated muscle of the voluntary anal sphincter.

Ans. **37. c.** Both of the above **38. b.** 21 days **39. b.** 6–9 days **40. d.** 4th pharyngeal pouch **41. c.** Metanephros... **42. c.** Brachial pouch **43. d.** Yolk sac **44. c.** At the time of... **45. b.** Below the...

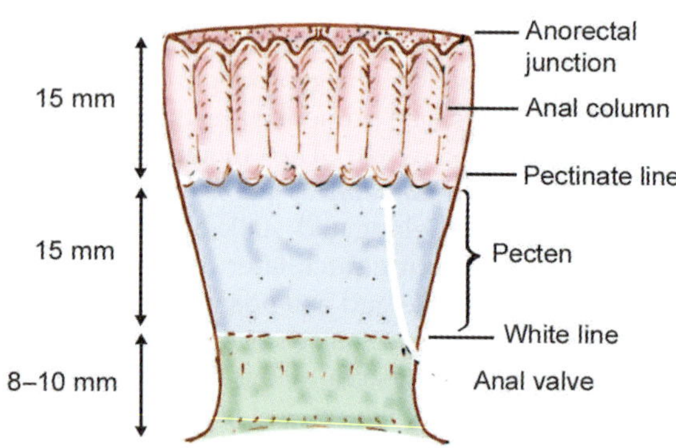

Some features in the interior of the anal canal (Schematic representation)

46. Which of the following is present in kidney cortex?

a. Renal pyramids b. Renal papillae
c. Minor calyces d. Lobules

Structure of a kidney

- The substance, or parenchyma, of the kidney is divided into two major structures: superficial is the renal cortex and deep is the renal medulla.
- Grossly, these structures take the shape of 8 to 18 cone-shaped renal lobes, each containing renal cortex surrounding a portion of medulla called a renal pyramid (of Malpighi).
- Between the renal pyramids are projections of cortex called renal columns (of Bertin). Nephrons, the urine-producing functional structures of the kidney, span the cortex and medulla.
- The initial filtering portion of a nephron is the renal corpuscle, located in the cortex, which is followed by a renal tubule that passes from the cortex deep into the medullary pyramids.
- Part of the renal cortex, a medullary ray is a collection of renal tubules that drain into a single collecting duct.

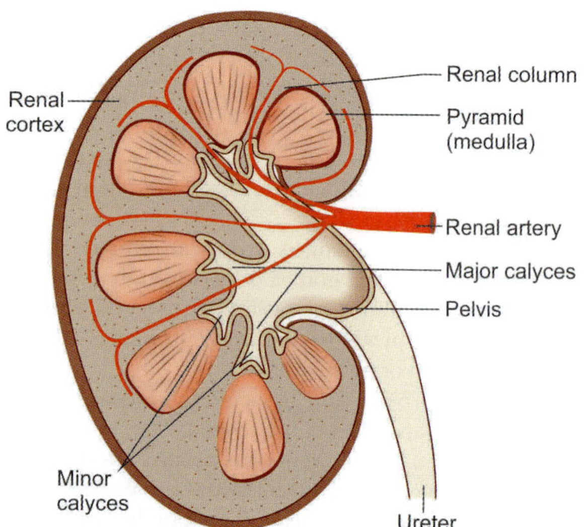

Some features to be seen in a coronal section through the kidney (Schematic representation)

- The tip, or papilla, of each pyramid empties urine into a minor calyx; minor calyces empty into major calyces, and major calyces empty into the renal pelvis, which becomes the ureter.
- At the hilum, the ureter and renal vein exit the kidney while the renal artery enters. Surrounding these structures is hilar fat and lymphatic tissue with lymph nodes.
- The hilar fat is contiguous with a fat-filled cavity called the renal sinus. The renal sinus collectively contains the renal pelvis and calyces and separates these structures from the renal medullary tissue

47. Tip of coracoid is a:

a. Traction epiphysis
b. Atavistic epiphysis
c. Pressure epiphysis
d. Aberrant epiphysis

Atavistic epiphysis: These types of fused bones are called atavistic, *e.g.* the coracoid process of the scapula, which has been fused in humans, but is separate in four-legged animals.

48. All are true for intervertebral disc EXCEPT:

a. Nucleus pulposus is the remnant of notochord
b. Rich vascular supply
c. Prolapse is common in lumbosacral region
d. None of the above

The discs are unique structures in the human body. They have no blood supply of their own. In fact, they are the largest structures in the body without their own blood vessel system. They are able to absorb the nutrients they need from circulating blood by means of osmosis.

49. Following examples are correctly matched *except:*

a. Pressure epiphysis—Head of femur
b. Traction epiphysis—Tubercles of humerus
c. Atavistic epiphysis—Coracoid process of scapula
d. Aberrant epiphysis—Trochanter of femur

Aberrant epiphysis: These epiphyses are deviations from the norm and are not always present. For example, the epiphysis at the head of the first metacarpal bone.

50. Collagen is NOT found in:

a. Tendon b. Aponeurosis
c. Fibroblasts d. Ligament

A **fibroblast** is a type of cell that synthesizes the extracellular matrix and collagen, the structural framework (stroma) for animal tissues, and plays a critical role in wound healing. Fibroblasts are the most common cells of connective tissue in animals.

51. Which of the following is lined by simple cuboidal epithelium:

a. Thyroid b. Trachea
c. Thymus d. Skin

Simple cuboidal epithelia are found on the surface of ovaries, the lining of nephrons, the walls of the renal tubules, and parts of the eye and thyroid.

Ans. **46. d.** Lobules **47. b.** Atavistic... **48. b.** Rich vascular... **49. d.** Aberrant epi... **50. c.** Fibroblasts **51. a.** Thyroid

52. **Cell type NOT found in stomach:**
a. Goblet cells b. Argentaffin cells
c. Parietal cells d. Chief cells

Goblet cells are found scattered among the epithelial lining of organs, such as the intestinal and respiratory tracts. They are found inside the trachea, bronchi, and larger bronchioles in the respiratory tract, small intestines, the large intestine, and conjunctiva in the upper eyelid. Goblet cells are a source of mucus in tears and secrete different types of mucins onto the ocular surface, especially in the conjunctiva. In the lacrimal glands, mucus is synthesized by acinar cells instead.

53. **Urothelium lines all EXCEPT:**
a. Ureters b. Minor calyx
c. Urinary bladder d. Membranous urethra

The epithelium of the urethra starts off as transitional cells as it exits the bladder. Further along the urethra, there are pseudostratified columnar and stratified columnar epithelia, then stratified squamous cells near the external urethral orifice.

54. **Which group has similar kind of epithelium:**
a. Alveoli–Olfactory epithelium
b. Olfactory epithelium–Skin
c. Esophagus–Urinary bladder
d. Lung alveoli–Bowman's capsule

Simple squamous epithelia are found in capillaries, alveoli, glomeruli, and other tissues where rapid diffusion is required.

55. **Mucus-secreting glands are ABSENT in:**
a. Cervix b. Vagina
c. Duodenum d. Esophagus

Vaginal secretions are primarily from the uterus, cervix, and transudation of the vaginal epithelium in addition to miniscule vaginal lubrication from the Bartholin's glands upon sexual arousal.

56. **FALSE about heart muscles:**
a. Acts as syncytium b. Has multiple nuclei
c. Has gap junctions d. Has branching

Cardiac muscle
- In comparison to skeletal myocytes, cardiac myocytes are short in length
- Cardiac myocytes are not tightly packed, there are lots of gaps in between the cells
- Cardiac myocytes have one nucleus per cell unlike skeletal myocytes which are multinucleated
- Cardiac muscle tissue has interclated disks connecting the myocytes together
- Cardiac muscle is involuntary, we do not consciously control it
- Cardiac muscle is striated in appearance.

57. **NOT a feature of skeletal muscle:**
a. Spindle-shaped b. Syncytium
c. Striations d. Hypolemmal nucleus

Smooth muscle
- Called smooth muscle because it lacks striations, just one solid color
- Short cells (fusiform) that have just one nucleus
- This type of muscle is arranged in sheets
- Smooth muscle is involuntary, we do not consciously control it.
- Smooth muscle is mainly found within hollow organs and is used to control the diameter of these organs
- It is found within blood vessels, the GI tract, iris of the eye, the uterus, our airways (bronchioles) and is used to control the openings of sphincters within the body.

58. **Epithelial lining of vagina:**
a. Cuboidal b. Columnar
c. Stratified squamous nonkeratinized
d. Stratified squamous keratinized

Nonkeratinized surfaces must be kept moist by bodily secretions to prevent them from drying out. Examples of nonkeratinized stratified squamous epithelium include cornea (also see corneal epithelium), lining mucosa of oral cavity, esophagus, anal canal, vagina, and the internal portion of the lips.

59. **Brunner's gland is located in:**
a. Duodenum b. Jejunum
c. Ileum d. All of the above

Brunner's glands (or **duodenal glands**) are compound tubular submucosal glands found in that portion of the duodenum which is above the hepatopancreatic sphincter (Sphincter of Oddi). The main function of these glands is to produce a mucus-rich alkaline secretion (containing bicarbonate).

60. **Cartilage in epiglottis:**
a. Hyaline b. Fibrocartilage
c. Elastic d. None

Elastic cartilage or yellow cartilage is a type of cartilage present in the outer ear, Eustachian tube **and** epiglottis. It contains elastic fiber networks and collagen fibers. The principal protein is elastin.

61. **Type of cartilage in auricle (ear):**
a. Elastic b. Hyaline
c. Fibrocartilage d. No cartilage at all

Elastic cartilage or **yellow cartilage** is a type of cartilage present in the outer ear, Eustachian tube and epiglottis. It contains elastic fiber networks and collagen fibers. The principal protein is elastin.

62. **NOT a cell of cerebral cortex:**
a. Granule cells b. Golgi cells
c. Purkinje cells d. Bipolar cells

As a part of the retina, the **bipolar cell** exists between photoreceptors (rod cells and cone cells) and ganglion cells. They act, directly or indirectly, to transmit signals from the photoreceptors to the ganglion cells.

Ans.
52. **a.** Goblet cells 53. **d.** Membranous... 54. **d.** Lung alveoli... 55. **b.** Vagina
56. **b.** Has multiple... 57. **a.** Spindle-shaped 58. **c.** Stratified squamous... 59. **a.** Duodenum
60. **c.** Elastic 61. **a.** Elastic 62. **d.** Bipolar cells

63. Shape of tracheal cartilage is:

a. O-shaped b. C-shaped
c. D-shaped d. V-shaped

There are from fifteen to twenty incomplete C-shaped tracheal rings of cartilage that reinforce the front and sides of the trachea to protect and maintain the airway. This leaves a membranous wall (*pars membranacea*) at the back, without cartilage. The trachealis muscle connects the ends of the incomplete rings and contracts during coughing, reducing the size of the lumen of the trachea to increase the rate of air flow.

64. Example of atavistic epiphysis:

a. Tubercle of humerus
b. Trochanter of femur
c. Coracoid process of scapula
d. Condyles of femur

Atavistic epiphysis: These types of fused bones are called atavistic, *e.g.* the coracoid process of the scapula, which has been fused in humans, but is separate in four-legged animals.

65. Hassall's corpuscles are a histological feature of:

a. Bone marrow b. Lymph node
c. Spleen d. Thymus

In the medullary portion of thymus, the network of reticular cells is coarser than in the cortex, the lymphoid cells are relatively fewer in number, and there are concentric, nest-like bodies called Hassall's corpuscles.

66. NOT lined by urothelium:

a. Urinary bladder b. Minor calyx
c. Ureters d. Collecting duct

Collecting ducts are lined by simple cuboidal epithelium which appears less specialized than that of the proximal or distal tubules.

67. von Brunn nest is related to:

a. Adenocarcinoma
b. Squamous cell carcinoma
c. Transitional cell carcinoma
d. Normal urothelium

Cystitis glandularis arises from and merges with von Brunn's nests, which are groups of urothelial cells (cells of urinary tract) within the lamina propria and submucosa, formed from budding from the surface mucosa. They are considered normal.

68. Fibromuscular stroma is observed in:

a. Urinary bladder b. Liver
c. Testes d. Prostate

The secretory epithelium of prostate is mainly pseudostratified, comprising tall columnar cells and basal cells, which are supported by a fibroelastic stroma containing randomly oriented smooth muscle bundles continuous with the bladder. The epithelium is highly variable and areas of low cuboidal or squamous epithelium are also present, with transitional epithelium in the distal regions of the longer ducts.

69. Peyer's patch is a histological feature of:

a. Stomach
b. Duodenum
c. Jejunum
d. Ileum

Peyer's patches are aggregations of lymphoid tissue that are usually found in the lowest portion of the small intestine, the ileum, in humans; as such, they differentiate the ileum from the duodenum and jejunum. The duodenum can be identified by Brunner's glands. The jejunum has neither Brunner's glands nor Peyer's patches.

70. True for prostate:

a. Muscular structure
b. Fibrous structure
c. Fibroglandular structure
d. None of the above

Histology of prostate

- Glandular cells
- Myoepithelial cells
- Subepithelial interstitial cells

71. PALS (periarteriolar lymphoid sheath) is a histological feature of:

a. Heart b. Brain
c. Liver d. Spleen

Periarteriolar lymphoid sheaths (or **periarterial lymphatic sheaths**, or **PALs**) are a portion of the white pulp of the spleen. They are populated largely by T-cells and surround central arteries within the spleen; the PALs T-cells are presented with blood-borne antigens via myeloid dendritic cells.

72. White fibrocartilage is NOT seen in:

a. Pinna
b. Pubic symphysis
c. Intervertebral disk
d. Temporomandibular joint

Fibrocartilage is found in the pubic symphysis, the anulus fibrosus of intervertebral discs, menisci and the TMJ. It is also present at the tendon bone interface.

73. Does NOT have nonkeratinized stratified squamous epithelium:

a. Cornea
b. Vagina
c. Esophagus
d. Uterus

Simple ciliated columnar epithelia line the uterus.

74. Thyroid follicle is lined by:

a. Squamous epithelium
b. Cuboidal epithelium
c. Columnar epithelium
d. Transitional epithelium

Simple cuboidal epithelia are found on the surface of ovaries, the lining of nephrons, the walls of the renal tubules, and parts of the eye and thyroid.

Ans.				
	63. **b.** C-shaped	64. **c.** Coracoid...	65. **d.** Thymus	66. **d.** Collecting duct
	67. **d.** Normal...	68. **d.** Prostate	69. **d.** Ileum	70. **c.** Fibroglandular structure
	71. **d.** Spleen	72. **a.** Pinna	73. **d.** Uterus	74. **b.** Cuboidal...

75. Coverings of a nerve (from inside to outside):

a. Endoneurium, perineurium, epineurium
b. Perineurium, endoneurium, epineurium
c. Epineurium, perineurium, endoneurium
d. Epineurium, endoneurium, perineurium

Each nerve is a cord-like structure that contains many axons, also called nerve fibers. Within a nerve, each axon is surrounded by a layer of connective tissue called the endoneurium. The axons are bundled together into groups called fascicles, and each fascicle is wrapped in a layer of connective tissue called the perineurium. Finally, the entire nerve is wrapped in a layer of connective tissue called the epineurium.

76. Trachea is lined by:

a. Cuboidal epithelium
b. Stratified squamous keratinized epithelium
c. Stratified squamous nonkeratinized epithelium
d. Pseudostratified ciliated columnar epithelium

Ciliated pseudostratified columnar epithelia are found in the linings of the trachea as well as the upper respiratory tract.

77. Demilunes/crescents are a histological feature of:

a. Lacrimal gland b. Nasal gland
c. Submandibular/sublingual salivary gland
d. Thyroid gland

Serous demilunes are the serous cells at the distal end of mucous tubuloalveolar secretory unit of certain salivary glands. These demilune cells secrete the proteins that contain the enzyme lysozyme, which degrades the cell walls of bacteria.

78. All possess elastic cartilage EXCEPT:

a. Epiglottis b. Thyroid cartilage
c. Lateral part of external acoustic meatus
d. Pinna

Hyaline cartilage exists on the ventral ends of ribs; in the larynx (thyroid, cricoids and arytenoids cartilage), trachea, and bronchi; and on the articular surface of bones.

79. Transitional epithelium is seen in:

a. Gallbladder b. Urinary bladder
c. Thyroid d. Tongue

Transitional epithelium tissue structure type is found in urothelium, including that of the urinary bladder, the ureters, and the superior urethra and gland ducts of the prostate.

80. Stratified squamous epithelium is seen at all the following sites EXCEPT:

a. Skin b. Vagina
c. Esophagus d. Gallbladder

The gallbladder wall's innermost surface is lined by a single layer of columnar cells with an apical brush border of microvilli, very similar to intestinal absorptive cells.

81. Trochanter of femur is:

a. Aberrant epiphysis b. Atavistic epiphysis
c. Pressure epiphysis d. Traction epiphysis

Traction epiphysis: The regions of the long bone which are nonarticular, i.e. not involved in joint formation. Unlike pressure epiphyses, these regions do not assist in weight transmission. However, their proximity to the pressure epiphysis region means that the supporting ligaments and tendons attach to these areas of the bone. Traction epiphyses ossify later than pressure epiphyses. Examples of traction epiphyses are tubercles of the humerus (greater tubercle and lesser tubercle), and trochanters of the femur (greater and lesser).

SUPERIOR EXTREMITY AND BACK

82. Which of the following is NOT a sign of ulnar nerve injury?

a. Weakness of grip
b. Clawing of medial 2 fingers
c. Abductor pollicis brevis palsy
d. Wasting of hypothenar muscles

Abductor pollicis brevis is supplied by median nerve

Ulnar injury at the elbow

- *Common mechanisms of injury:* Cubital tunnel syndrome, fracture of the medial epicondyle (causing cubitus valgus with tardy ulnar nerve palsy)
- *Motor deficit:*
  - Weakness in flexion of the hand at the wrist, loss of flexion of ulnar half of digits, or the 4th and 5th digits, loss of ability to cross the digits of the hand. (Note: Motor deficit is absent or very minor in cubital tunnel syndrome as the ulnar nerve is compressed in the cubital tunnel, rather than transected.)
  - Presence of a claw hand deformity when the hand is at rest, due to hyperextension of the 4th and 5th digits at the metacarpophalangeal joints, and flexion at the interphalangeal joints.
- *Sensory deficit:* Loss of sensation in ulnar half of the palm and dorsum of hand, and the medial 1½ digits on both palmar and dorsal aspects of the hand

Ulnar injury at the wrist

- Common mechanism: Stab wound, Guyon canal cyst
- Motor deficit:
  - Loss of flexion of ulnar half of digits, or the 4th and 5th digits, loss of ability to cross the digits of the hand.
  - Presence of a claw hand deformity when the hand is at rest, due to hyperextension of the 4th and 5th digits at the metacarpophalangeal joints, and flexion at the interphalangeal joints.
  - The claw hand deformity is more prominent with injury at the wrist as opposed to a lesion higher up in the arm, for instance, at the elbow, as the ulnar half of the flexor digitorum profundus is not affected. This pulls the distal interphalangeal joints of the 4th and 5th digit into a more flexed position, producing a more deformed 'claw'. This is known as the ulnar paradox.

Ans. 75. **a.** Endoneurium... 76. **d.** Pseudo... 77. **c.** Subman... 78. **b.** Thyroid... 79. **b.** Urinary bladder 80. **d.** Gallbladder 81. **d.** Traction epiphysis 82. **c.** Abductor pollicis...

- *Sensory deficit:* Loss of sensation in ulnar half of the palm, and the medial 1½ digits on the palmar aspect of the hand, with dorsal sparing. The dorsal aspect of the hand is unaffected as the posterior cutaneous branch of the ulnar nerve is given off higher up in the forearm and does not reach the wrist.

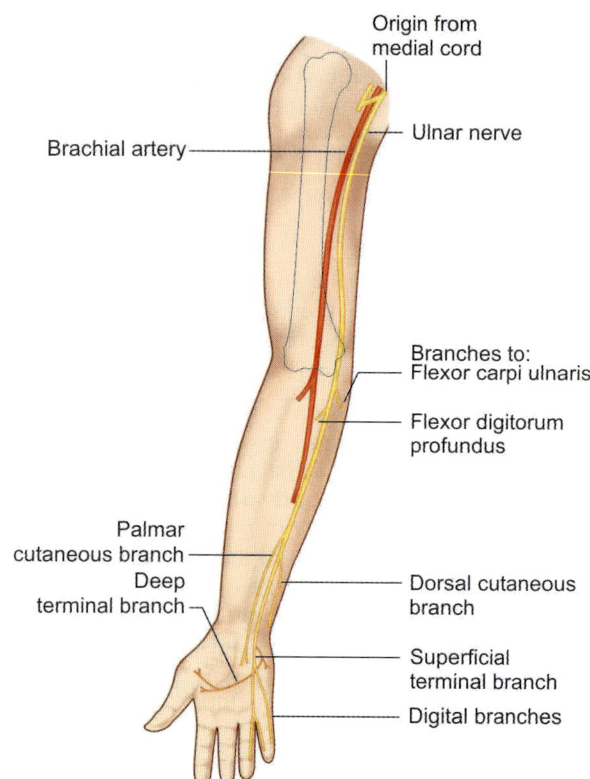

Scheme showing the course and branches of the ulnar nerve

83. Which of the following muscle is NOT supplied by median nerve?

a. Opponens pollicis b. Adductor pollicis
c. 1st lumbricals d. 2nd lumbricals

Adductor pollicis is supplied by ulnar nerve

Median nerve in hand

The median nerve enters the hand through the carpal tunnel, deep to the flexor retinaculum along with the tendons of flexor digitorum superficialis, flexor digitorum profundus (lateral half), and flexor pollicis longus. From there it sends off several branches:

- Recurrent branch to muscles of the thenar compartment (the recurrent branch is also called "the million dollar nerve"). Here it provides motor innervation to opponens pollicis, abductor pollicis brevis and flexor pollicis brevis.
- Digital cutaneous branches to common palmar digital branch and proper palmar digital branch of the median nerve which supply the:
  - Lateral (radial) three and a half digits on the palmar side
  - Index, middle and ring finger on dorsum of the ha
- The median nerve supplies motor innervation to the first and second lumbrical of the hand.

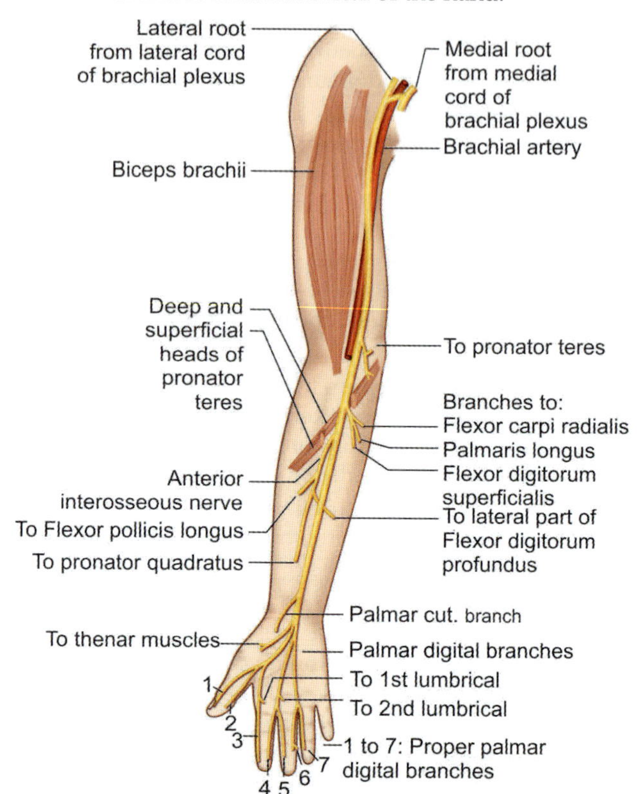

Scheme to show the course and branches of median nerve

84. Which of the following muscle is NOT attached to greater tuberosity of humerus?

a. Supraspinatus b. Infraspinatus
c. Teres minor d. Pectoralis major

The pectoralis major is inserted into the lateral lip of intertubercular sulcus. The insertion is bilaminar

Muscles attached to humerus

- The deltoid originates on the lateral third of the clavicle, acromion and the crest of the spine of the scapula. It is inserted on the deltoid tuberosity of the humerus and has several actions including abduction, extension, and circumduction of the shoulder.
- The supraspinatus also originates on the spine of the scapula. It inserts on the greater tubercle of the humerus, and assists in abduction of the shoulder.
- The pectoralis major, teres major, and latissimus dorsi insert at the intertubercular groove of the humerus. They work to adduct and medially, or internally, rotate the humerus.
- The infrapsinatus and teres minor insert on the greater tubercle, and work to laterally, or externally, rotate the humerus. In contrast, the subscapularis muscle inserts onto the lesser tubercle and works to medially, or internally, rotate the humerus.
- The biceps brachii, branchialis, and brachioradialis (which attaches distally) act to flex the elbow. (The biceps do not attach to the humerus.) The triceps

Ans. 83. **b.** Adductor pollicis 84. **d.** Pectoralis major

brachii and anconeus extend the elbow, and attach to the posterior side of the humerus.

- The four muscles of supraspinatus, infraspinatus, teres minor and subscapularis form a musculo-ligamentous girdle called the rotator cuff. This cuff stabilizes the very mobile but inherently unstable glenohumerial joint. The other muscles are used as counterbalances for the actions of lifting/pulling and pressing/pushing.

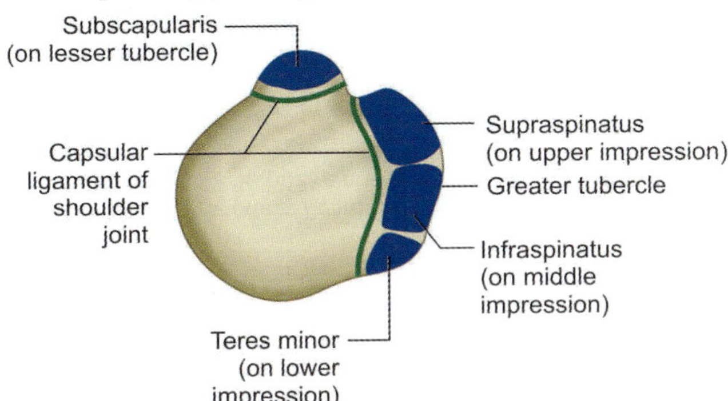

Upper end of right humerus showing attachments seen from above

85. NOT innervated by branches from brachial plexus:

a. Trapezius b. Rhomboid major
c. Serratus anterior d. Subclavius

Trapezius

Origin	External occipital protuberance, nuchal ligament, medial superior nuchal line, spinous processes of vertebrae C7-T12
Insertion	Posterior border of the lateral third of the clavicle, acromion process, and spine of scapula
Artery	Superficial branch of transverse cervical artery or superficial cervical artery
Nerve	Accessory (motor) cervical spinal nerves C3 and C4 (motor and sensation)
Actions	Rotation, retraction, elevation, and depression of scapula
Antagonist	Serratus anterior muscle, Latissimus dorsi

86. NOT a common site of metastasis from carcinoma breast in upper and outer quadrants:

a. Central axillary b. Lateral axillary
c. Parasternal d. Anterior axillary

Lymphatic drainage of the breast assumes great importance to the surgeon because carcinoma of the breast spreads mostly along lymphatics to the regional lymph nodes. About 75% of the lymph from breast drains into the axillary nodes, 20% into the internal mammary/parasternal nodes and 5% into the posterior intercostal nodes.

87. Does NOT pierce clavipectoral fascia:

a. Basilic vein b. Lateral pectoral nerve
c. Thoracoacromial artery d. Cephalic vein

The **clavipectoral fascia** (**costocoracoid membrane; coracoclavicular fascia**) is a strong fascia situated under cover of the clavicular portion of the pectoralis major. The coracoclavicular fascia is pierced by the cephalic vein, thoracoacromial artery and vein, lymphatics and lateral pectoral nerve.

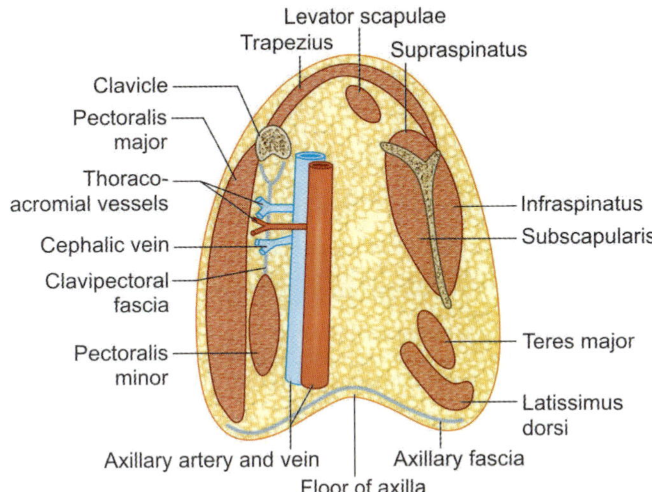

Schematic sagittal section through the axilla to show its anterior and posterior walls and the clavipectoral fascia.

88. Erb's point:

a. C4, C5 b. C5, C6
c. C6, C7 d. C7, C8

Erb's point is formed by the union of the C5 and C6 nerve roots, which later converge. At the nerve trunk, branches of suprascapular nerves and the nerve to the subclavius also merge. The merged nerve divides into the anterior and posterior divisions of C5 and C6.

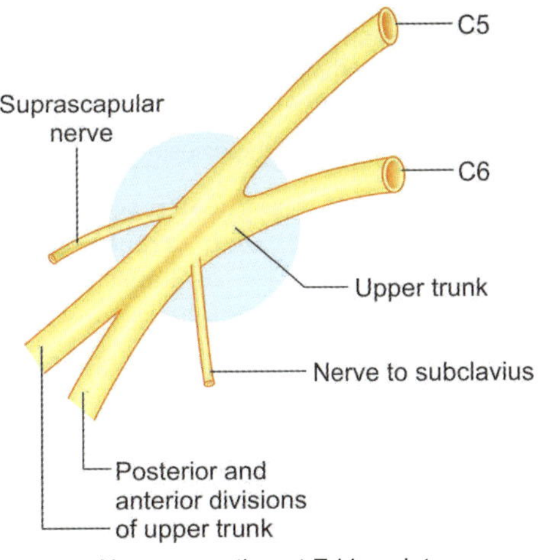

Nerves meeting at Erb's point.

89. Winging of scapula results due to injury to:

a. Ulnar nerve
b. Radial nerve
c. Nerve to serratus anterior
d. Subscapular nerve

Ans. 85. **a.** Trapezius 86. **c.** Parasternal 87. **a.** Basilic vein 88. **b.** C5, C6
89. **c.** Nerve to serratus...

A lesion of the nerve paralyses the serratus anterior to produce winged scapula, which is most prominent when the arm is lifted forward or when the patient pushes the outstretched arm against a wall. However, even winging may not be evident until the trapezius stretches enough to reveal an injury several weeks later.

90. Paralysis of opponens pollicis leads to loss of:

a. Flexion of thumb
b. Abduction of thumb
c. Extension of thumb
d. Pinching action of thumb

Opponens pollicis

Origin	Trapezium and transverse carpal ligament
Insertion	Metacarpal bone of the thumb on its radial side
Artery	Superficial palmar arch
Nerve	Recurrent branch of the median nerve
Actions	Flexion of the thumb's metacarpal at the first carpometacarpal joint, which aids in **opposition** of the thumb

91. Does NOT lead to elevation of scapula:

a. Rhomboid major
b. Latissimus dorsi
c. Levator scapulae
d. Trapezius

Latissimus dorsi

Origin	Spinous processes of vertebrae T7-L5, thoracolumbar fascia, iliac crest, inferior 3 or 4 ribs and inferior angle of scapula
Insertion	Floor of intertubercular groove of the humerus
Artery	Thoracodorsal branch of the subscapular artery
Nerve	Thoracodorsal nerve (C6, 7, 8)
Actions	Adducts, extends and internally rotates the arm when the insertion is moved towards the origin. When observing the muscle action of the origin towards the insertion, the lats are a very powerful rotator of the trunk.
Antagonist	Deltoid and trapezius muscle

92. NOT a boundary of triangle of auscultation:

a. Scapula
b. Trapezius
c. Serratus anterior
d. Latissimus dorsi

Boundaries of triangle of auscultation

- Superiorly and medially, by the inferior portion of the Trapezius
- Inferiorly, by the Latissimus Dorsi
- Laterally, by the medial border of the scapula.

93. Fascia around brachial plexus nerve bundle is derived from:

a. Pectoral fascia
b. Deep cervical fascia
c. Clavipectoral fascia
d. Prevertebral fascia

The prevertebral fascia is prolonged downward and laterally behind the carotid vessels and in front of the scaleni, and forms a sheath for the brachial nerves and subclavian vessels in the posterior triangle of the neck; it is continued under the clavicle as the axillary sheath and is attached to the deep surface of the coracoclavicular fascia.

94. Does NOT retract scapula:

a. Levator scapulae
b. Rhomboideus major
c. Rhomboideus minor
d. Trapezius

Levator scapulae

Origin	Posterior tubercles of transverse processes of C1-C4 vertebrae
Insertion	Superior part of medial border of scapula
Artery	Dorsal scapular artery
Nerve	Cervical nerve (C3, C4) and dorsal scapular nerve (C5)
Actions	Elevates scapula and tilts its glenoid cavity inferiorly by rotating scapula

95. Hypothenar muscles are supplied by:

a. Median nerve
b. Radial nerve
c. Ulnar nerve
d. Posterior interosseus nerve

Four hypothenar muscles are palmaris brevis, abductor digiti minimi, flexor digiti minimi and opponens digiti minimi. Palmaris brevis is supplied by superficial branch of ulnar nerve whereas rest all by deep branch of ulnar nerve.

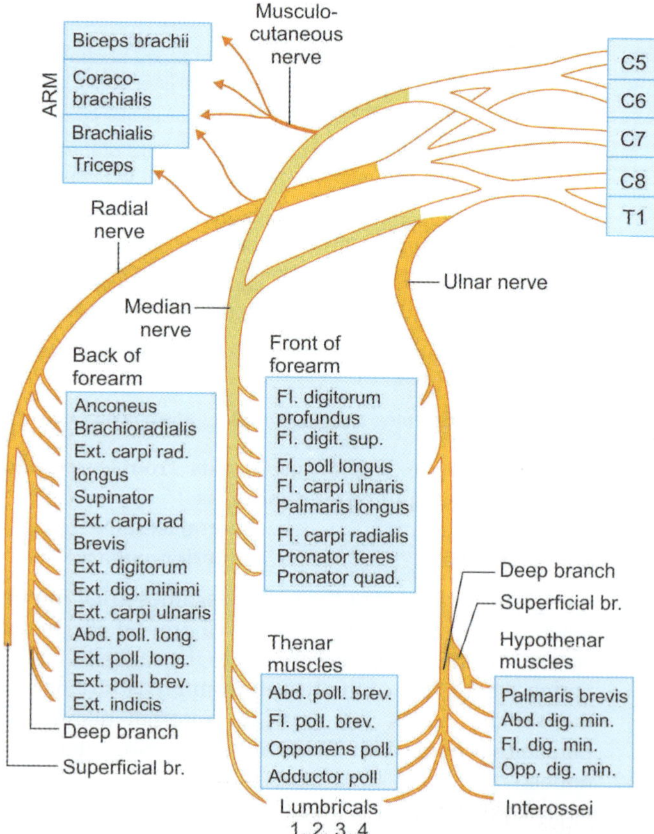

Scheme to show the nerve supply of various muscles of the arm, forearm and hand.

Ans. 90. d. Pinching... 91. b. Latissimus dorsi 92. c. Serratus... 93. d. Prevertebral... 94. a. Levator scapulae 95. c. Ulnar nerve

96. NOT supplied by median nerve:

a. Abductor pollicis brevis b. Opponnens pollicis
c. Flexor pollicis brevis d. Adductor pollicis

Adductor pollicis

Origin	**Transverse head:** Anterior body of the third metacarpal Oblique head: Bases of the second and the third metacarpals and the adjacent trapezoid and capitate bones
Insertion	Medial side of the base of the proximal phalanx of the thumb and the ulnar sesamoid
Artery	Deep palmar arch
Nerve	Deep branch of the ulnar nerve (T1)
Actions	Adducts the thumb at the carpometacarpal joint
Antagonist	Abductor pollicis longus muscle, abductor pollicis brevis muscle

97. NOT involved in median nerve injury above the elbow:

a. Opponens pollicis
b. Flexion at 4th and 5th distal interphalangeal joint
c. Flexion at 2nd and 3rd proximal interphalangeal joint
d. Flexion at 2nd and 3rd metacarpophalangeal joint

Flexor digitorum profundus causes flexion of the distal phalanges after the flexor digitorum superficialis has flexed the middle phalanges. Medial half is supplied by ulnar nerve (hence spared in injury to median nerve) whereas lateral half is supplied by anterior interosseous nerve.

98. NOT supplied by musculocutaneous nerve:

a. Coracobrachialis b. Biceps
c. Brachioradialis d. Brachialis

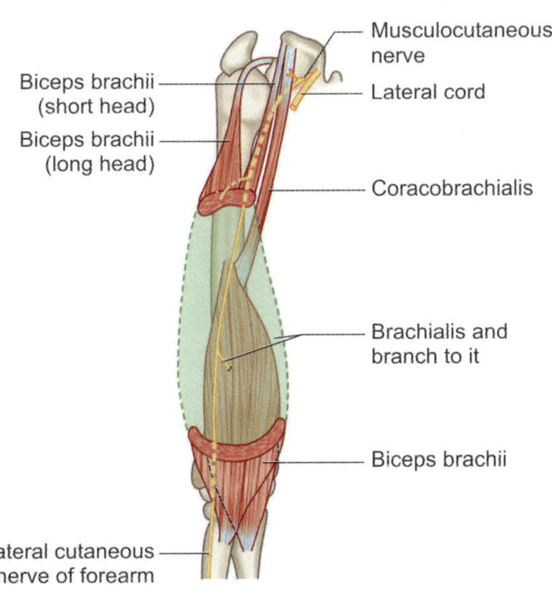

Scheme to show the course and distribution of the musculocutaneous nerve.

Brachioradialis

Origin	Lateral supracondylar ridge of the humerus
Insertion	Distal radius (radial styloid process)
Artery	Radial recurrent artery
Nerve	Radial nerve
Actions	Flexion of elbow and supination

99. NOT a part of posterior wall of axilla:

a. Latissimus dorsi b. Supraspinatus
c. Subscapularis d. Teres major

Axilla is formed posteriorly by the subscapularis above, and teres major and latissimus dorsi below.

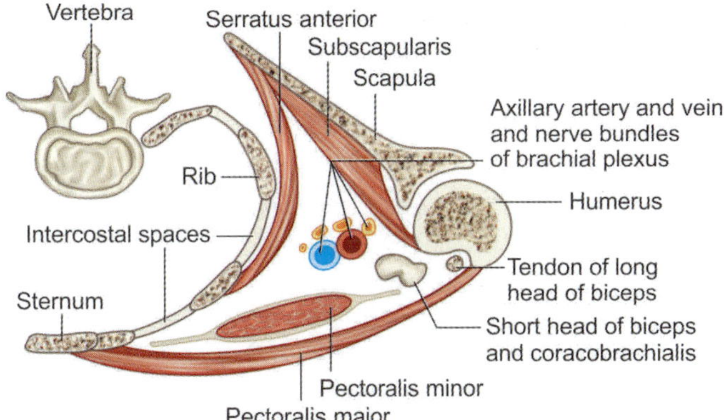

Transverse section through the axilla to show its walls.

100. External level of superficial palmar arch:

a. Distal crease of palm
b. Distal border of extended thumb
c. Proximal border of extended thumb
d. At the level of metacarpophalangeal joint

If one were to fully extend the thumb, the superficial palmar arch would lie approximately at the level of a line drawn from the distal border of the thumb across the palm. The superficial palmar arch extends more distally than the deep palmar arch.

101. Clavipectoral fascia is NOT pierced by:

a. Cephalic vein b. Thora-acromial artery
c. Lateral pectoral nerve d. Middle pectoral nerve

The coracoclavicular fascia is pierced by the cephalic vein, thoracoacromial artery and vein, lymphatics and lateral pectoral nerve.

102. Froment test is positive in lesion of:

a. Radial nerve b. Ulnar nerve
c. Axillary nerve d. Median nerve

Froment's sign is a special test of the wrist. It tests for palsy of the ulnar nerve, specifically the action of adductor pollicis.

103. Winging of scapula is due to:

a. Medial pectoral nerve palsy
b. Lateral pectoral nerve palsy
c. Nerve to serratus anterior palsy
d. Nerve to latissimus dorsi palsy

Ans. 96. **d.** Adductor pollicis 97. **b.** Flexion at 4th... 98. **c.** Brachioradialis 99. **b.** Supraspinatus
100. **b.** Distal border... 101. **d.** Middle pectoral... 102. **b.** Ulnar nerve 103. **c.** Nerve to serratus...

The most common cause of scapular winging is serratus anterior paralysis. This is typically caused by damage (i.e. lesions) to the long thoracic nerve.

104. Nerve related to medial wall of axilla:

a. Long thoracic nerve b. Subscapular nerve
c. Thoracodorsal nerve d. Nerve to latissimus dorsi

Long thoracic nerve descends behind (posterior to) the brachial plexus and the axillary artery and vein, resting on the outer surface of the serratus anterior. It extends along the side of the thorax to the lower border of that muscle, supplying filaments to each of its digitations (finger-like projections).

105. First lumbrical is supplied by:

a. Median nerve b. Ulnar nerve
c. Radial nerve
d. Posterior interosseous nerve

Lumbricals

Origin	Flexor digitorum profundus
Insertion	Extensor expansion
Artery	Superficial palmar arch, common palmar digital arteries, deep palmar arch, dorsal digital artery
Nerve	3rd and 4th deep branches of ulnar nerve, 1st and 2nd median nerve
Actions	Flex metacarpophalangeal joints, extend inter-phalangeal joints

106. Third and fourth lumbricals are supplied by:

a. Radial nerve b. Median nerve
c. Ulnar nerve
d. Posterior interosseous nerve

The first and second lumbricals (the most radial two) are innervated by the median nerve. The third and fourth lumbricals (the most ulnar two) are innervated by the deep branch of the ulnar nerve.

107. Bursa, which may communicate with the shoulder joint cavity:

a. Subacromial bursa b. Subscapularis bursa
c. Bursa related to coracoid process
d. Infraspinatus bursa

The shoulder joint cavity communicates with the subscapular bursa, with the synovial sheath for the tendon of the long head of the biceps brachii, and often the infraspinatus bursa.

108. Abductor of arm:

a. Pectoralis major b. Deltoid
c. Teres major d. Infraspinatus

Deltoid

Origin	The anterior border and upper surface of the lateral third of the clavicle, acromion, spine of the scapula
Insertion	Deltoid tuberosity of humerus
Artery	Thoracoacromial artery, anterior and posterior humeral circumflex artery
Nerve	Axillary nerve
Actions	Shoulder abduction (up to 90 degrees), flexion and extension
Antagonist	Latissimus dorsi

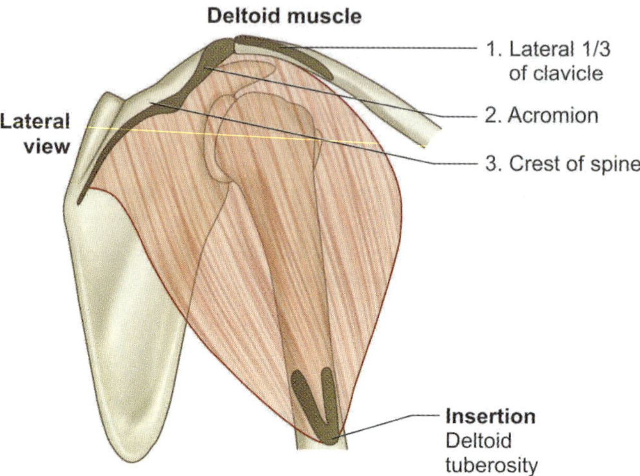

Attachments of deltoid muscle.

109. Injury to upper trunk of brachial plexus results in:

a. Erb's palsy b. Klumpke's palsy
c. Winging of scapula d. Claw hand

Erb's palsy or **Erb-Duchenne palsy** is a paralysis of the arm caused by injury to the upper group of the arm's main nerves, specifically the severing of the upper trunk C5–C6 nerves.

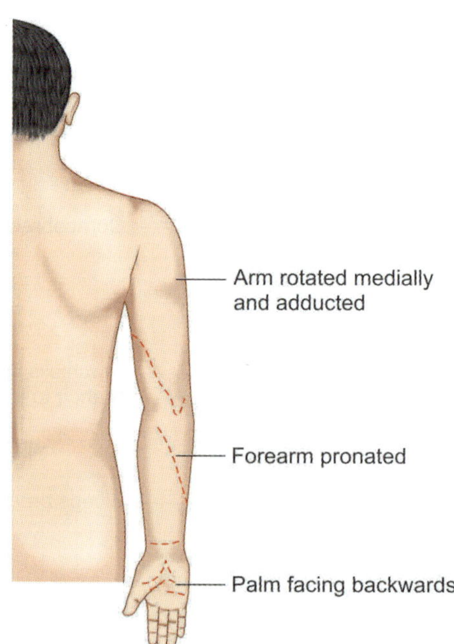

Waiter's tip position of upper limb in Erb's paralysis.

Ans. 104. **a.** Long thoracic... 105. **a.** Median nerve 106. **c.** Ulnar nerve 107. **d.** Infraspinatus bursa 108. **b.** Deltoid 109. **a.** Erb's palsy

110. All the following muscles contribute in rotator cuff EXCEPT:
a. Supraspinatus
b. Infraspinatus
c. Subscapularis
d. Teres major

Teres minor (NOT teres major) is a constituent of rotator cuff.

111. True regarding beginning of superficial palmar arch:
a. At the level of proximal transverse crease of wrist
b. Below distal transverse crease of wrist
c. At the level of proximal palmar crease
d. At the distal border of thumb on palmar surface

The distal point of the arch lies at the same level as the distal border of the thenar eminence when the thumb is fully extended.

112. Nerve involved most commonly in fractures of shaft of humerus is:
a. Ulnar nerve
b. Musculocutaneous nerve
c. Median nerve
d. Radial nerve

The radial sulcus (also known as the musculospiral groove, radial groove, or spiral groove) is a broad but shallow oblique depression for the radial nerve and deep brachial artery. It is located on the center of the lateral border of the humerus bone.

THORAX

113. Which of the following is NOT supplied by right coronary artery:
a. SA node
b. Right atrium
c. Posterior 1/3rd of interventricular septum
d. Anterior interventricular septum

Anterior part of interventricular septum is supplied by left coronary artery

Right coronary artery (RCA)

- It originates above the right cusp of the aortic valve.
- It travels down the right atrioventricular groove, towards the crux of the heart.
- It branches into the posterior descending artery and the right marginal artery.
- At the origin of the RCA is the conus artery.
- In addition to supplying blood to the right ventricle (RV), the RCA supplies 25% to 35% of the left ventricle (LV).
- In 85% of patients (Right Dominant), the RCA gives off the posterior descending artery (PDA). In the other 15% of cases (Left Dominant), the PDA is given off by the left circumflex artery.
- The PDA supplies the inferior wall, ventricular septum, and the posteromedial papillary muscle.
- The RCA also supplies the SA nodal artery in 60% of patients.
- The other 40% of the time, the SA nodal artery is supplied by the left circumflex artery.

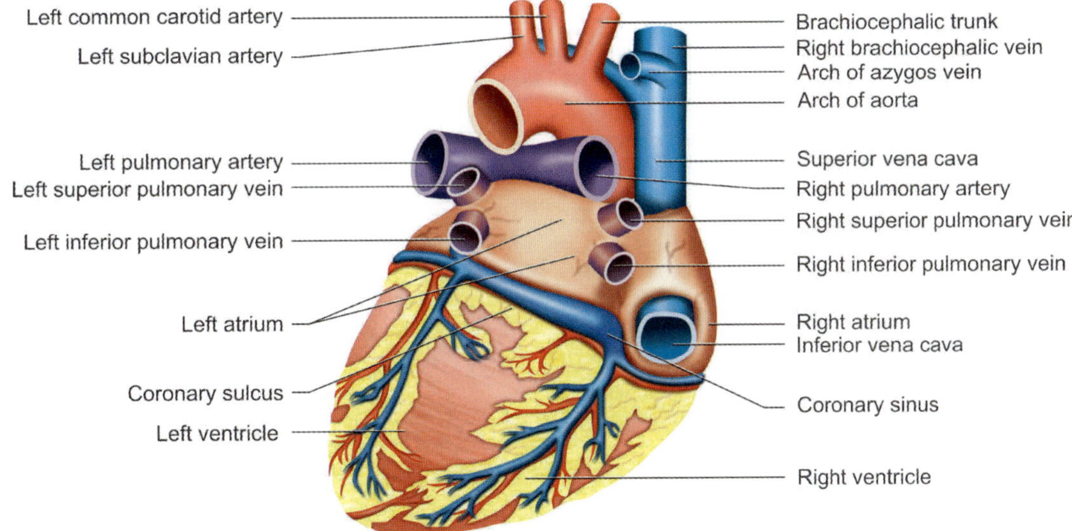

Inferior and basal aspects of heart to show major vessels

114. All of the following are present at C6 vertebral level EXCEPT:
a. Beginning of esophagus
b. End of pharynx
c. End of larynx
d. Bifurcation of trachea

Trachea bifurcates at the level of T4

The transverse thoracic plane

- Plane through T4 & T5 vertebral junction and sterna angle of Louis.
- Marks the:
  - Attachment of rib 2 at the sternal angle;
  - Arch of aorta (beginning and end)

Ans. 110. d. Teres major 111. d. At the distal border... 112. d. Radial nerve 113. d. Anterior inter... 114. d. Bifurcation...

- Upper margin of superior vena cava
- Thoracic duct crossing
- Tracheal bifurcation
- Pulmonary trunk bifurcation

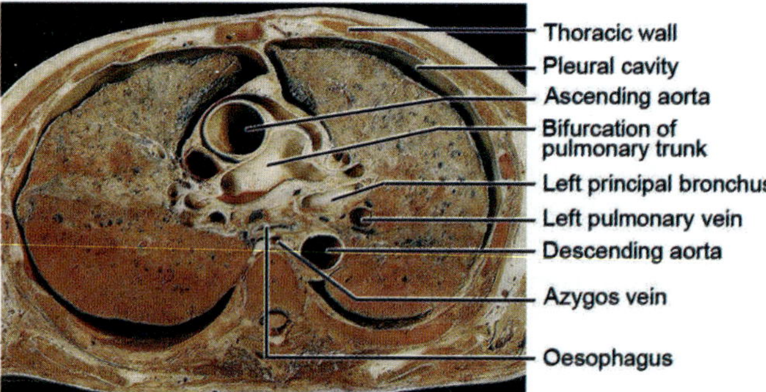

Transverse section of thorax at the level of upper part of T5 vertebra-inferior view

115. Origin of right common carotid artery:

a. Left subclavian artery
b. Arch of aorta
c. Right axillary artery
d. Brachiocephalic artery

The right common carotid originates in the neck from the brachiocephalic trunk; the left arises from the aortic arch in the thoracic region.

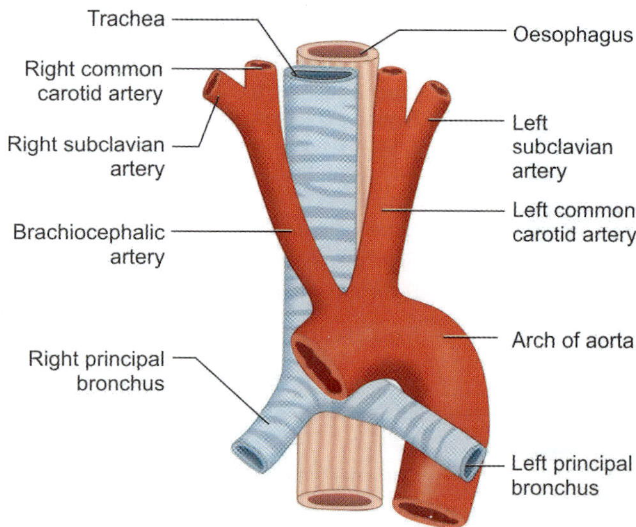

Diagram to show the branches of the arch of the aorta.

116. Sternal angle corresponds to:

a. 1st rib
b. 2nd rib
c. 3rd rib
d. 4th rib

The sternal angle, which varies around 162 degrees in males, marks the approximate level of the 2nd pair of costal cartilages, which attach to the second ribs, and the level of the intervertebral disc between T4 and T5.

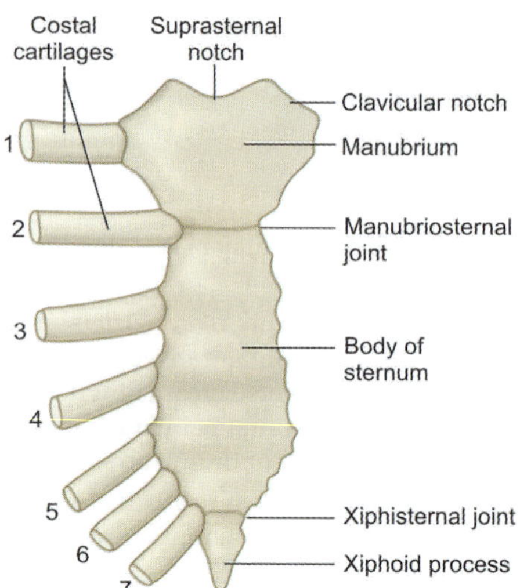

Sternum and costal cartilages seen from front.

117. Muscle of expiration:

a. Diaphragm
b. Rectus abdominis
c. External intercostal
d. All of the above

Rectus abdominis

Origin	Crest of pubis
Insertion	Costal cartilage of ribs 5-7, xiphoid process of sternum
Artery	Inferior epigastric artery
Nerve	Segmentally by thoracoabdominal nerves (T7 to T11)
Actions	Flexion of the lumbar spine
Antagonist	Erector spinae

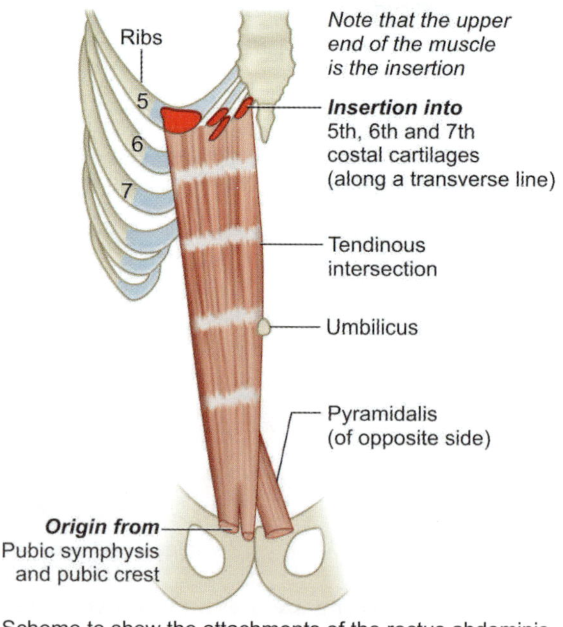

Scheme to show the attachments of the rectus abdominis.

118. Sympathetic supply to heart:

a. T3-T5
b. T1-T3
c. T5-T7
d. T7-T9

The nerves from the sympathetic trunk emerge through the T1-T4 thoracic ganglia and travel to both the sinoatrial

Ans. 115. **d.** Brachiocephalic... 116. **b.** 2nd rib
117. **b.** Rectus... 118. **a.** T3-T5

Volume I Non-Clinical Subjects

and atrioventricular nodes, as well as to the atria and ventricles. The ventricles are more richly innervated by sympathetic fibers than parasympathetic fibers.

119. Base of heart is chiefly formed by:

a. Right atrium b. Right ventricle
c. Left ventricle d. Left atrium

The part of the heart formed mainly by the left atrium and to a lesser extent by the posterior part of the right atrium, directed backward and to the right, and separated from the vertebral column by the esophagus and aorta, is known as base of heart.

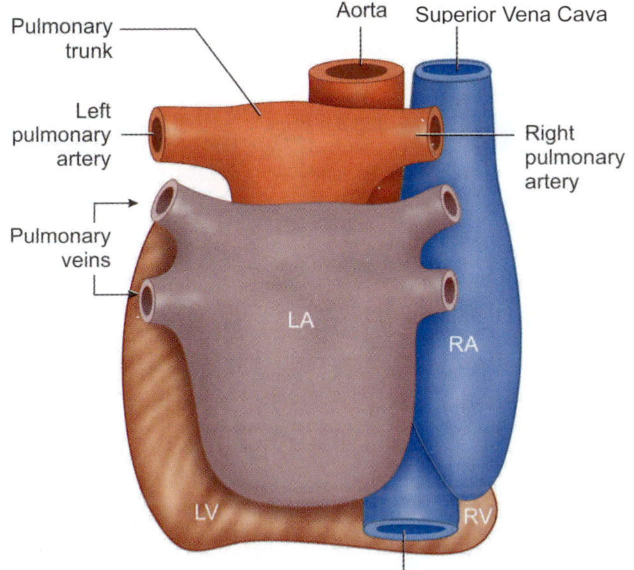

Heart seen from behind to show its base.

120. Left coronary artery supplies all EXCEPT:

a. SA node b. Posterior 1/3rd of septum
c. Left ventricle d. Apex of heart

Posterior one-third of interventricular septum is supplied by right coronary artery. SA node may be supplied by left coronary artery in 40% of cases (usually supplied by right coronary artery).

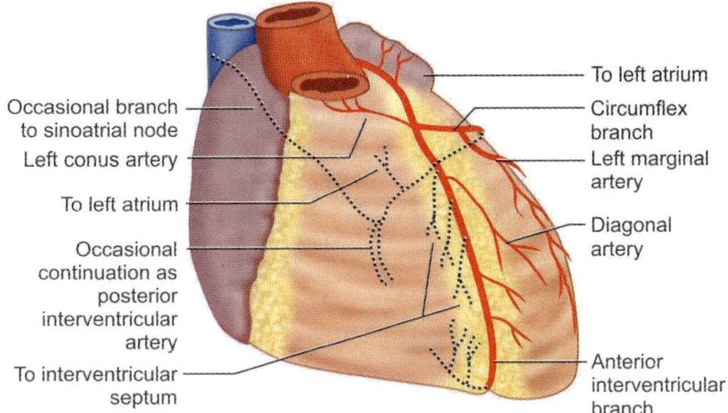

Scheme to show the distribution of the left coronary artery–some small branches given by the anterior interventricular branch to the right atrium are not drawn for sake of clarity.

121. Does NOT pass through aortic hiatus:

a. Azygos vein b. Hemiazygos vein
c. Aorta d. Thoracic duct

Hemiazygos vein usually begins in the left ascending lumbar vein or renal vein, and passes upward through the left crus of the diaphragm to enter the thorax. It continues ascending on the left side of the vertebral column, and around the level of the ninth thoracic vertebra, it passes rightward across the column, behind the aorta, esophagus, and thoracic duct, to end in the azygos vein.

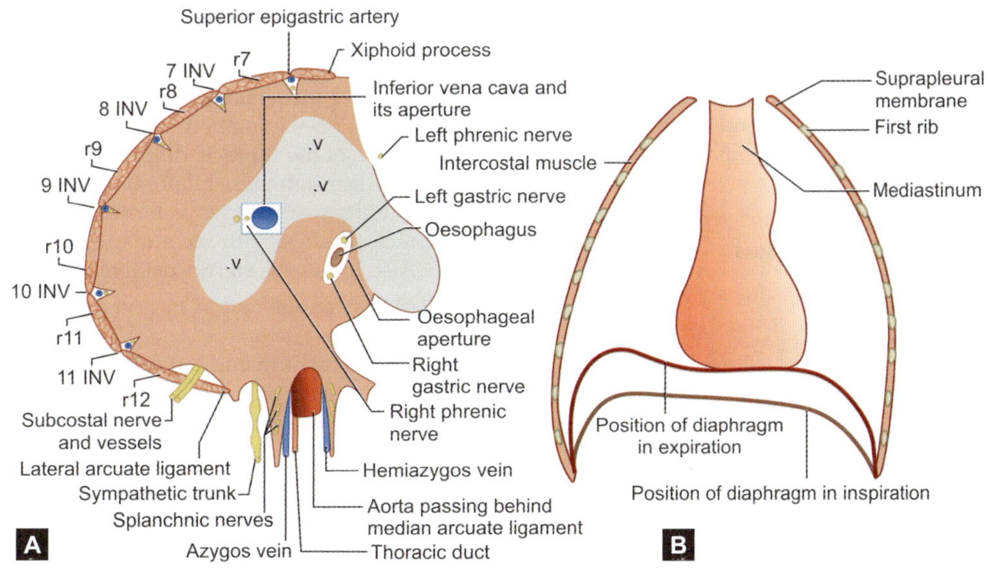

(A) Schematic diagram to show apertures in the diaphragm. INV: Intercostal nerve and vessels; 7th to 12th ribs. (B) Diagram to show change in level of the diaphragm during inspiration and expiration.

Ans. 119. **d.** Left atrium 120. **b.** Posterior 1/3rd...
121. **b.** Hemiazygos vein

122. Structure related to arch of aorta:
a. Bifurcation of pulmonary trunk
b. Tracheal bifurcation
c. Both
d. None

Arch of aorta begins at the level of the upper border of the second sternocostal articulation of the right side, and runs at first upward, backward, and to the left in front of the bifurcation of trachea and above bifurcation of pulmonary trunk; it is then directed backward on the left side of the trachea and finally passes downward on the left side of the body of the fourth thoracic vertebra, at the lower border of which it becomes continuous with the descending aorta.

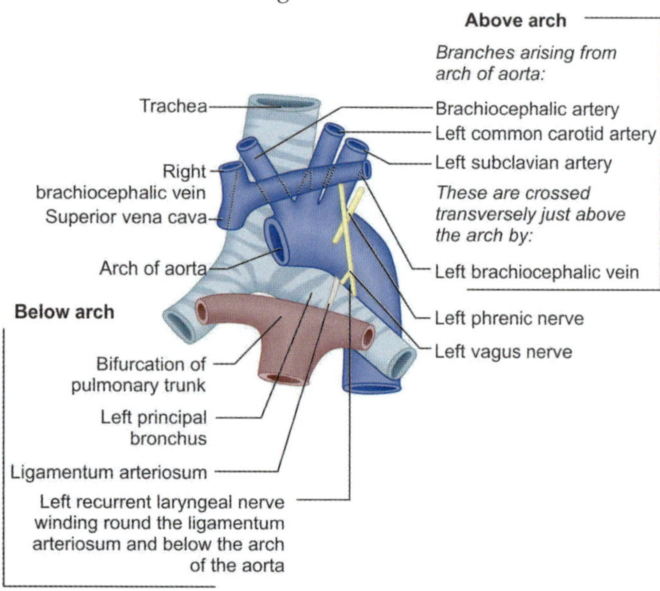

Diagram to show the structures above and below the arch of aorta.

123. Most common site of lodgment of foreign body:
a. Lower lobe right lung b. Lower lobe left lung
c. Apex of right lung d. Apex of left lung

Right bronchus is shorter, wider and more in continuity with trachea; so foreign body tends to pass on to the right side, posterobasal part.

124. NOT a site of esophageal constriction:
a. At the beginning of esophagus
b. Crossing by aortic arch
c. Crossing by thoracic duct
d. Piercing diaphragm

Constrictions of esophagus

- At the start of the esophagus (6 inches from incisor), where the pharynx joins the esophagus, behind the cricoid cartilage
- Where it is crossed on the front by the aortic arch (9 inches from incisor) and the left main bronchus (11 inches from incisor)
- Where it passes through the diaphragm (15 inches from incisor).

125. Termination of thoracic duct into the left brachiocephalic vein is at the junction of:
a. Internal jugular vein and brachiocephalic vein
b. Left internal jugular vein and left subclavian vein
c. External jugular vein and subclavian vein
d. External jugular vein and brachiocephalic vein

Thoracic duct extends vertically in the chest and curves posteriorly to the left carotid artery and left internal jugular vein at the T5 vertebral level to empty into the junction of the left subclavian vein and left internal jugular vein, below the clavicle, near the shoulders.

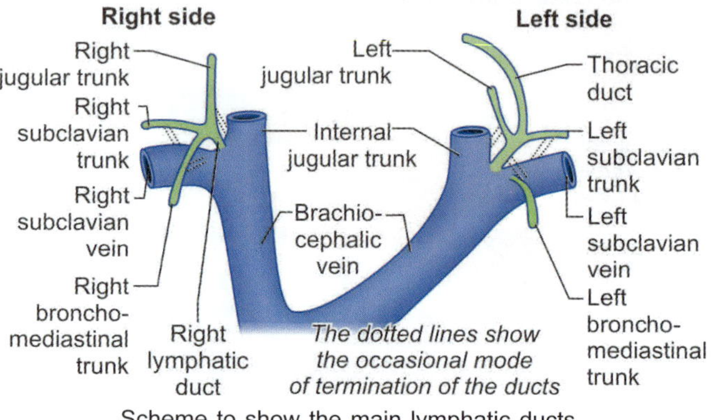

Scheme to show the main lymphatic ducts.

126. Right phrenic nerve passes through which hiatus:
a. Esophageal b. Aortic
c. Vena caval
d. Directly pierces diaphragm

The **right phrenic nerve** passes over the brachiocephalic artery, posterior to the subclavian vein, and then crosses the root of the right lung anteriorly and then leaves the thorax by passing through the vena cava hiatus opening in the diaphragm at the level of T8. The right phrenic nerve passes over the right atrium.

127. Foramen of Morgagni is located in:
a. Lesser omentum b. Greater omentum
c. Diaphragm d. Skull

The **sternocostal triangle** or **foramina of Morgagni** are small zones lying between the costal and sternal attachments of the thoracic diaphragm. Important vessels that pass through these bilateral foramina include the superior epigastric arteries as terminations of the internal thoracic arteries, with accompanying veins and lymphatics. Also known as sternocostal hiatus or (Larrey's) triangle.

128. Membranous part of interventricular septum is located between:
a. Left atrium and left ventricle
b. Left ventricle and right atrium
c. Right ventricle and left atrium
d. Right atrium and right ventricle

Upper and posterior parts of interventricular septum, which separate the aortic vestibule from the lower part of the right atrium and upper part of the right ventricle, thin and fibrous, and are termed the **membranous ventricular septum** (**septum membranaceum**).

Ans. 122. c. Both 123. a. Lower lobe... 124. c. Crossing by... 125. b. Left internal...
126. c. Vena caval 127. c. Diaphragm 128. b. Left ventricle and right atrium

Volume I Non-Clinical Subjects

129. Anterior cardiac vein drains into:

a. Marginal vein b. Coronary sinus
c. Right atrium d. Great cardiac vein

The **anterior cardiac veins** (or **anterior veins of right ventricle)**, comprising three or four small vessels which collect blood from the front of the right ventricle and open into the right atrium.

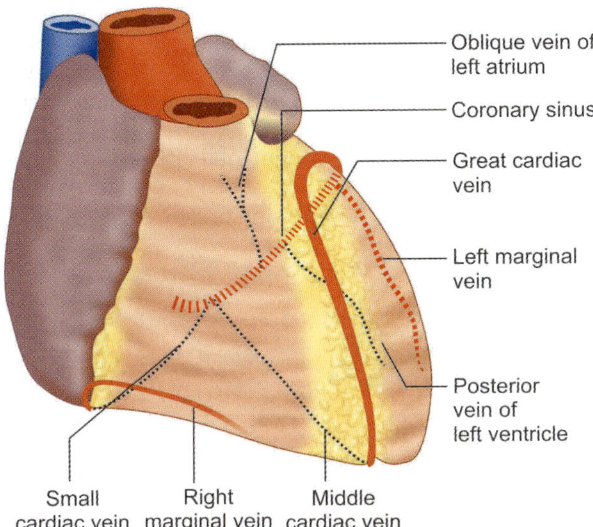

Scheme to show veins of the heart as seen from the front Veins not normally seen from the front are drawn (in dotted lines) as if the walls of the chambers of the heart were transparent.

130. Surface marking of pleura, in mid-axillary line, on left side:

a. 5th intercostal space b. 6th intercostal space
c. 8th intercostal space d. 10th intercostal space

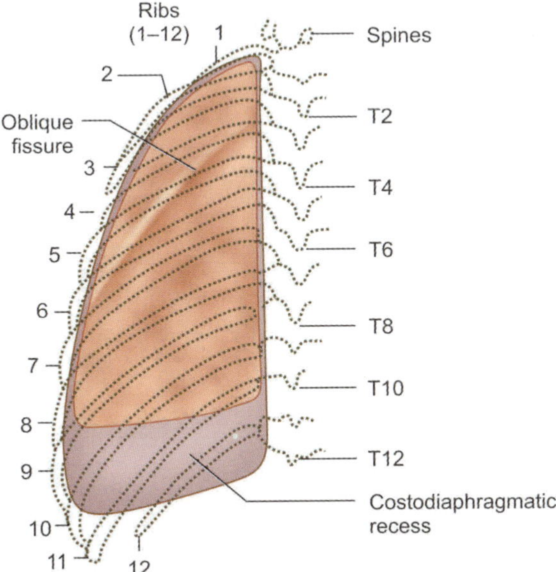

Projection of the pleura (red line) and lung (blue line) on the back of the thorax.

Remember: 2, 4, 6, 8, 10 Lungs

- Each lung extends 3 cm above the clavicle (apex)
- Anterior borders of lungs are closest at the sternal angle – 2nd costal cartilage (cc)
- Both reach to 4th cc
- Left:
  - Moves away from the midline at the 4th cc
- Right:
  - Moves away from the midline at the 6th cc
  - Both cross the midclavicular line at the 8th cc
  - Both cross the midaxillary line at the 10th cc

131. Diaphragm moves to lowermost position during:

a. Sitting b. Standing
c. Supine d. Prone

The height of the diaphragm in the thorax varies considerably with the position of the body. It stands highest when the body is horizontal and the patient on his back, and in this position, it performs the largest respiratory excursions with normal breathing. When the body is erect, the dome of the diaphragm falls, and its respiratory movements become smaller. The dome falls still lower when the sitting posture is assumed, and in this position, its respiratory excursions are smallest. These facts may, perhaps, explain why it is that patients suffering from severe dyspnea are most comfortable and least short of breath when they sit up.

132. Sequestration of lung is seen in:

a. Posterior part of left lung b. Lateral basal
c. Right lower lobe d. Right upper lobe

Lung sequestration consists of a nonfunctioning mass of normal lung tissue that lacks normal communication with the tracheobronchial tree, and that receives its arterial blood supply from the systemic circulation. Two-thirds of the time, the sequestration is located in the paravertebral gutter in the posterior segment of the left lower lobe.

133. Esophagus crosses diaphragm at:

a. T8 level b. T10 level
c. T12 level d. L2 level

Vena caval opening is at the level of T8, esophageal opening at T10 and aortic hiatus at the level of T12.

134. The structures passing posterior to diaphragm are all EXCEPT:

a. Aorta b. Azygos vein
c. Thoracic duct d. Greater splanchnic nerve

Splanchnic nerves

Name	Ganglia	Description
Greater	T5-T9 or T5-T10	The nerve travels through the diaphragm and enters the abdominal cavity, where its fibers synapse at the celiac ganglia. The nerve contributes to the celiac plexus, a network of nerves located in the vicinity of where the celiac trunk branches from the abdominal aorta. The fibers in this nerve modulate the activity of the enteric nervous system of the foregut. They also provide the sympathetic innervation to the adrenal medulla, stimulating catecholamine release.

Contd...

Ans. 129. **c.** Right atrium 130. **d.** 10th intercostal space 131. **a.** Sitting 132. **a.** Posterior part of left lung 133. **b.** T10 level 134. **d.** Greater splanchnic...

Contd...

Name	Ganglia	Description
Lesser	T9-T12, T9-T10, T10-T12, or T10-T11	The nerve travels inferiorly, lateral to the greater splanchnic nerve. Its fibers synapse with their postganglionic counterparts in the superior mesenteric ganglia, or in the aorticorenal ganglion. The nerve modulates the activity of the enteric nervous system of the midgut.
Least or lowest	T12-L2, or T11-T12	The nerve travels into the abdomen, where its fibers synapse in the renal ganglia.

135. An inhaled foreign body is likely to lodge in the right lung due to all of the following features EXCEPT:

a. Right lung is shorter and wider than left lung
b. Right principal bronchus is more vertical than left bronchus
c. Tracheal bifurcation directs the foreign body to the right lung
d. Right inferior lobar bronchus is in continuation with the principal bronchus

An inhaled foreign body lodges in right lung because right bronchus is shorter, wider and more in continuity with trachea.

136. All of the following are characteristic of a bronchopulmonary segment *except:*

a. It is surgically resectable
b. It is named according to the segmental bronchus supplying it
c. It is drained by intrasegmental branch of pulmonary vein
d. It is the largest subdivision of a lobe

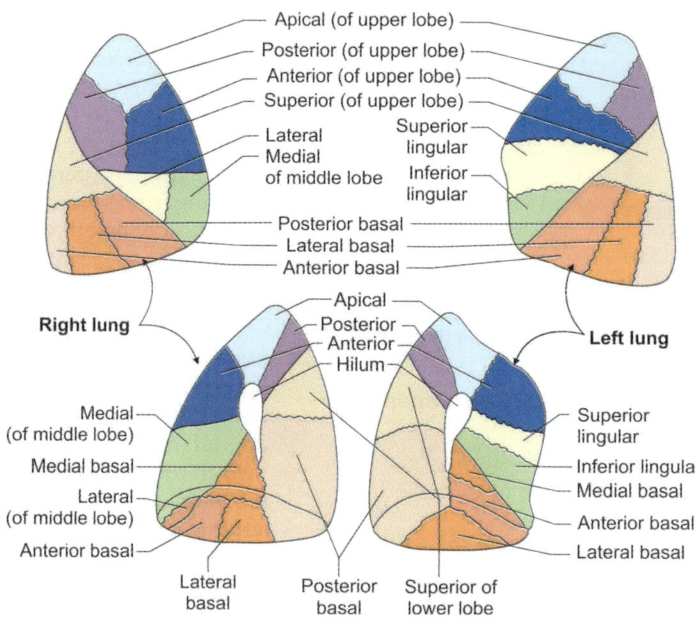

Bronchopulmonary segments of the right and left lungs.

Each of the tertiary bronchi serves a specific **bronchopulmonary segment.** These segments each have their own artery. Thus, each bronchopulmonary segment is supplied by a segmental bronchus, and two arteries, a pulmonary artery and a bronchial artery, which run together through the center of the segment. Veins and lymphatics drain along the edges.

137. The right coronary artery supplies all of the following parts of the conducting system EXCEPT:

a. SA node
b. AV node
c. Right branch of AV bundle
d. Right bundle branch

The right bundle branch receives most of its blood supply from septal branches of the left anterior descending coronary artery, particularly in its initial course. In most patients, it also receives some collateral supply from either the right or circumflex coronary systems depending upon the dominance of the coronary system.

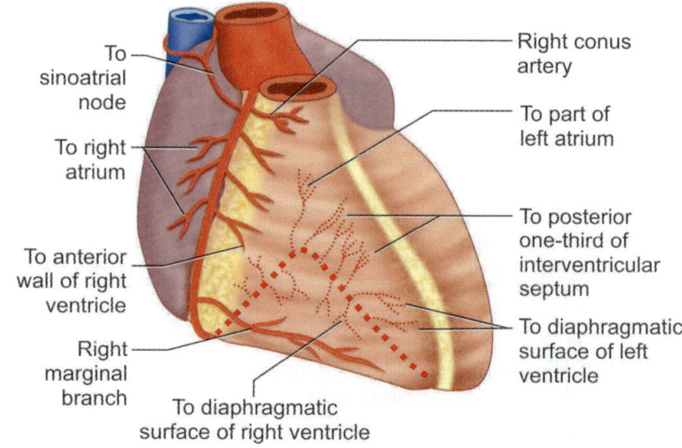

Scheme to show the distribution of the right coronary artery.

Ans. 135. **a.** Right lung is... 136. **c.** It is drained
137. **d.** Right bundle branch

138. Going above downwards, order of neurovascular bundle in intercostal space:

a. Vein, Nerve, Artery
b. Nerve, Artery, Vein
c. Artery, Nerve, Vein
d. Vein, Artery, Nerve

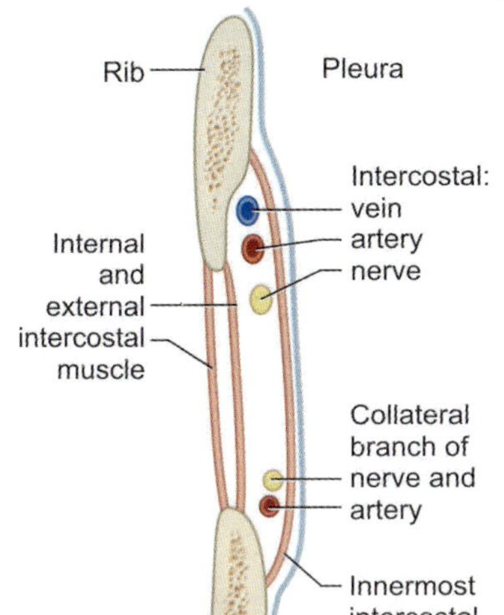

Vertical section through an intercostal space showing the position of nerves and vessels.

Comprehensive insight in the anatomy of the intercostal spaces is mandatory for everyone who practises medicine. One particular concept is that the neurovascular bundle has a strict order: V-A-N, or vein-artery-nerve, from top to bottom. This neurovascular bundle runs high in the intercostal space, and the collateral neurovascular bundle runs just superior to the inferior rib of the space (in the order N-A-V from superior to inferior). Invasive procedures such as thoracentesis are thus performed with oblique entry of the instrument, directly above the upper margin of the relevant rib.

139. Lower angle of scapula corresponds to:

a. D5
b. D6
c. D7
d. D8

The **inferior angle** is covered by latissimus dorsi. It moves forwards round the chest when the arm is abducted. It lies at the level of thoracic vertebra 7.

140. Lingula is related to:

a. Right middle lobe
b. Right upper lobe
c. Left upper lobe
d. Left lower lobe

The left lung, unlike the right, does not have a middle lobe, though it does have a homologous feature, a projection of the upper lobe, termed as the 'lingula'. Its name means 'little tongue'.

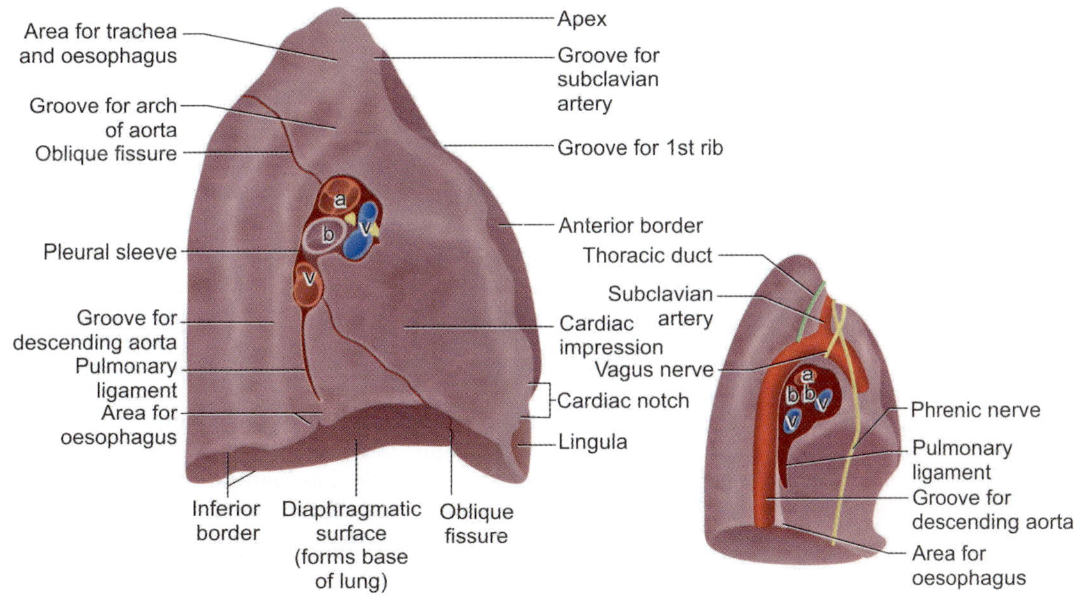

Left lung viewed from the medial side showing areas related to different structures Key: a. Artery b. Bronchus v. Vein.

141. Distance between upper incisors and gastroesophageal junction is:

a. 15 cm
b. 25 cm
c. 40 cm
d. 60 cm

Esophagus

- Length of esophagus is about 25 cm
- Clinically important distance is from incisors to GEJ, which is ~ 40 cm (15 inches)

142. NOT a branch of left coronary artery:

a. Posterior interventricular branch
b. Anterior interventricular branch
c. Left atrial artery
d. Right atrial artery

The **posterior interventricular artery** (**PIV**) or **posterior descending artery** (**PDA**) is an artery running in the posterior interventricular sulcus to the apex of the heart where it meets with the anterior interventricular artery. It supplies the posterior 1/3rd of the interventricular septum. The remaining anterior 2/3rds is supplied by the anterior interventricular artery which is a septal branch

Ans. **138. d.** Vein, Artery, Nerve **139. c.** D7 **140. c.** Left upper lobe **141. c.** 40 cm **142. a.** Posterior interventricular branch of the left anterior descending artery, which is a branch of left coronary artery. It is typically a branch of the right coronary artery (70%, known as right dominance).

143. Lower border of lung in midclavicular plane lies at the level of:

a. 4th rib b. 6th rib
c. 8th rib d. 10th rib

Inferior margins of the lung

- 6th rib at midclavicular plane
- 8th rib at midaxillary plane
- 10th rib posteriorly

144. Structure passing through aortic hiatus:

a. Left vagus and thoracic duct
b. Azygos vein and thoracic duct
c. Thoracic duct and hemiazygos vein
d. Left gastric vein and thoracic duct

Through aortic hiatus passes the aorta, the azygos vein, and the thoracic duct; occasionally the azygos vein and hemiazygos vein pass through the right crus.

145. SA node is usually supplied by:

a. Left coronary artery b. Right coronary artery
c. Left anterior descending artery
d. Posterior interventricular artery

The SA node receives blood supply from the SA node artery (ramus nodi sinuatrialis). Anatomical dissection studies have shown that this supply may be branch of the right coronary artery in the majority (about 60–70%) of hearts, and a branch of the left coronary artery (usually the left circumflex artery) in about 20–30% of hearts.

146. NOT a branch of arch of aorta:

a. Left subclavian b. Right common carotid
c. Left common carotid d. Brachiocephalic

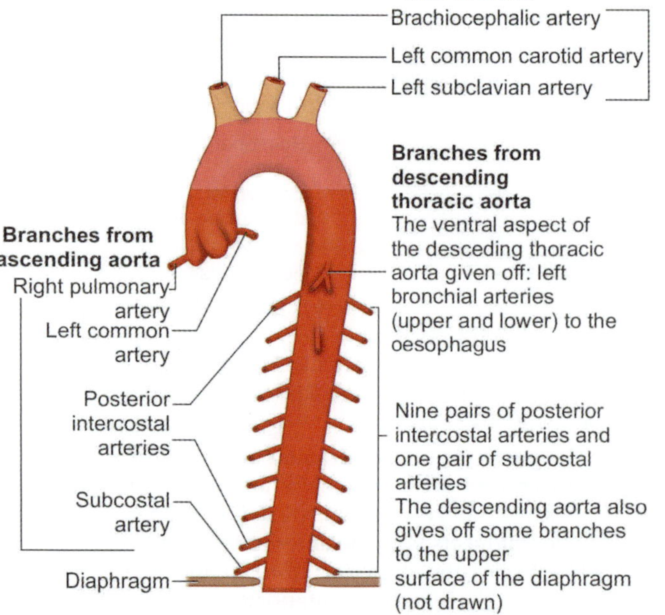

Scheme to show branches arising from the aorta in the thorax.

Common carotid

Precursor	Aortic arch 3
Source	Aortic arch (left), brachiocephalic artery (right)
Branches	Internal carotid artery, external carotid artery
Vein	Internal jugular vein
Supplies	Head and neck

147. Arch of aorta begins at:

a. T1 b. T2
c. T3 d. T4

Arch of aorta begins at the level of the upper border of the second sternocostal articulation of the right side, and runs at first upward, backward, and to the left in front of the trachea; it is then directed backward on the left side of the trachea and finally passes downward on the left side of the body of the fourth thoracic vertebra, at the lower border of which it becomes continuous with the descending aorta.

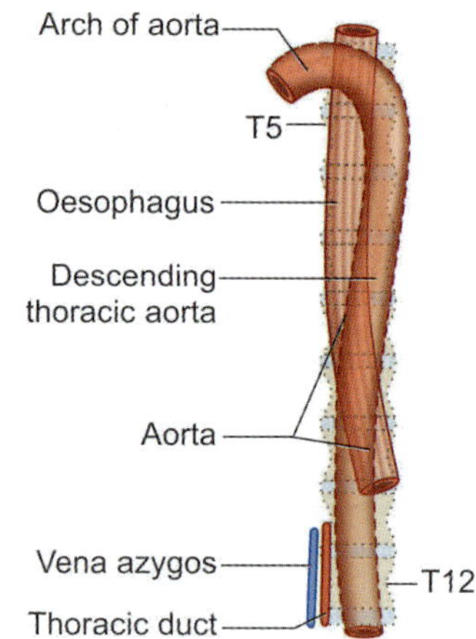

Diagram to show relationship of the aorta to the vertebral column and to the oesophagus.

148. Bronchopulmonary segments in left lung:

a. 6 b. 8
c. 10 d. 12

There are 10 bronchopulmonary segments in the right lung (3 in superior lobe, 2 in middle lobe, 5 in inferior lobe) and 10 segments on the left lung. Some of the segments may fuse in the left lung to form usually 8-9 segments (4-5 in upper lobe, 4-5 in lower lobe).

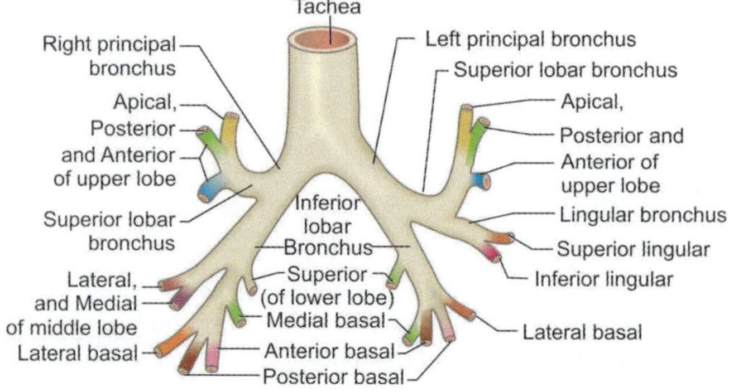

Scheme to show the bronchial tree as seen from the front.

Ans. 143. **b.** 6th rib 144. **b.** Azygos vein and... 145. **b.** Right coronary... 146. **b.** Right common carotid
147. **d.** T4 148. **b.** 8

149. Which of the following is a branch of left coronary artery:

a. Posterior interventricular artery
b. Right atrial artery
c. Infundibular artery
d. Anterior interventricular artery

The left anterior descending artery (also LAD, anterior interventricular branch of the left coronary artery, or anterior descending branch), also known as the 'widow maker', is an artery of the heart.

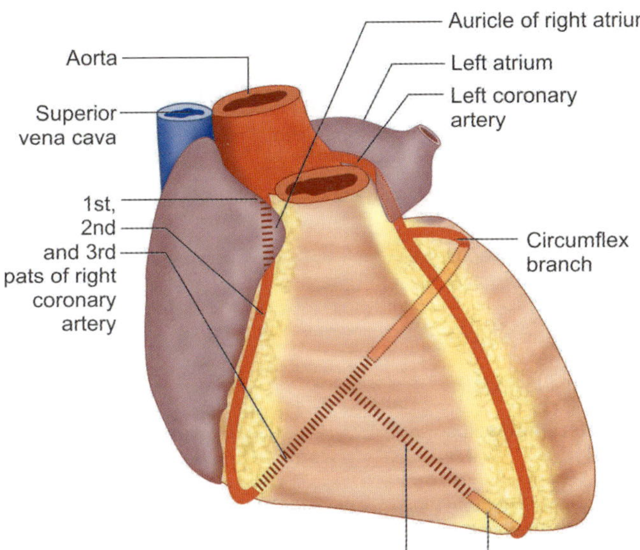

Schematic diagram shows the coronary arteries and their interventricular branches.

150. Posterior-most chamber of heart:

a. Right atrium
b. Left atrium
c. Right ventricle
d. Left ventricle

Posterior-most chamber is left atrium (hence esophagus can be involved, if there is left atria hypertrophy). Most anterior is right ventricle.

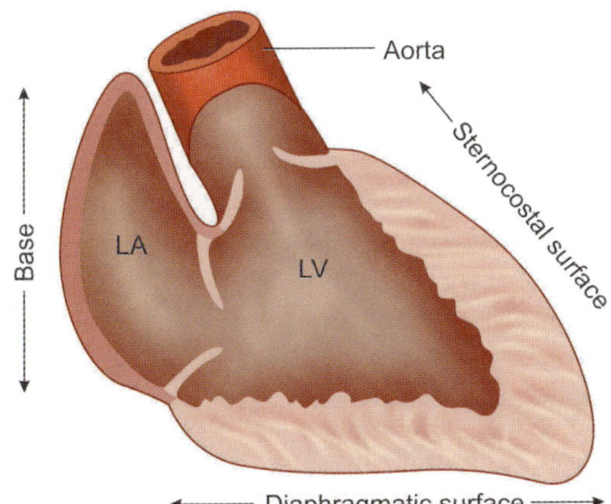

Schematic vertical section, in an oblique plane, passing through the left half of the heart. Note the relationship of the sternocostal and diaphragmatic surfaces to each other.

151. Root value of phrenic nerve:

a. C1, C2, C3
b. C2, C3, C3
c. C3, C4, C5
d. C4, C5, C6

Phrenic nerve

From	C3-C5 of cervical plexus
Innervates	Diaphragm

152. 27 cms from incisors, narrowing in esophagus is due to:

a. Crossing by aortic arch
b. Crossing by left bronchus
c. Piercing through diaphragm
d. Crossing by right bronchus

Esophageal constrictions

- At the start of the esophagus, where the pharynx joins the esophagus, behind the cricoid cartilage
- Where it is crossed on the front by the aortic arch and the left main bronchus
- Where it passes through the diaphragm.

INFERIOR EXTREMITY

153. Which of the following is NOT a branch of femoral artery:

a. Superficial external pudendal artery
b. Inferior epigastric artery
c. Deep external pudendal artery
d. Profunda femoris artery

Inferior epigastric artery arises from the external iliac artery

Branches of femoral artery:

- The superficial circumflex iliac artery is a small branch that runs up to the region of the anterior superior iliac spine.
- The superficial epigastric artery is a small branch that crosses the inguinal ligament and runs to the region of the umbilicus.
- The superficial external pudendal artery is a small branch that runs medially to supply the skin of the scrotum (or labium majus).
- The deep external pudendal artery runs medially and supplies the skin of the scrotum (or labium majus).
- The profunda femoris artery is a large and important branch that arises from the lateral side of the femoral artery about 1.5 in. (4 cm) below the inguinal ligament. It passes medially behind the femoral vessels and enters the medial fascial compartment of the thigh. It ends by becoming the fourth perforating artery. At its origin, it gives off the medial and lateral femoral circumflex arteries, and during its course it gives off three perforating arteries.
- The descending genicular artery is a small branch that arises from the femoral artery near its termination within the adductor canal. It assists in supplying the knee joint.

Ans. 149. **d.** Anterior... 150. **b.** Left atrium 151. **c.** C3, C4, C5 152. **b.** Crossing by... 153. **b.** Inferior...

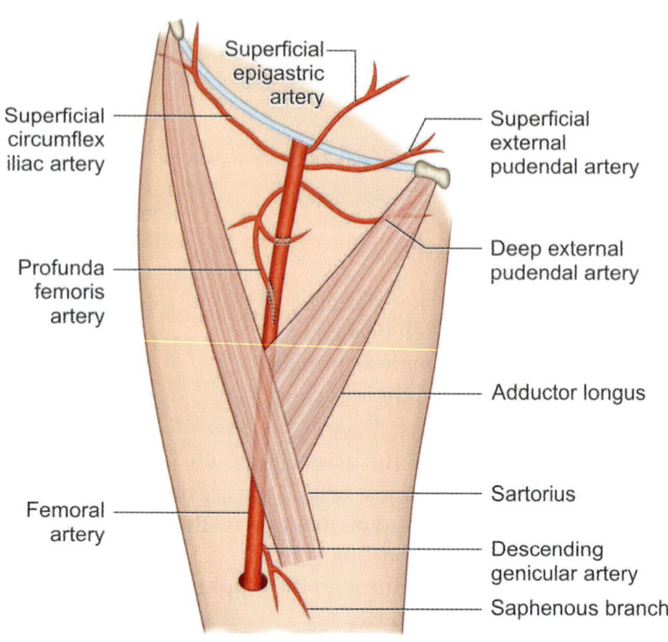

Branches of femoral artery

154. Which of the following is an abductor of lower limb:

a. Gluteus maximus
b. Gluteus medius
c. Adductor magnus
d. Biceps femoris

Gluteus medius

Origin	Gluteal surface of ilium, under gluteus maximus
Insertion	Greater trochanter of the femur
Artery	Superior gluteal artery
Nerve	Superior gluteal nerve (L4, L5, S1 nerve roots)
Actions	Abduction of the hip; preventing adduction of the hip. Medial rotation of the thigh.

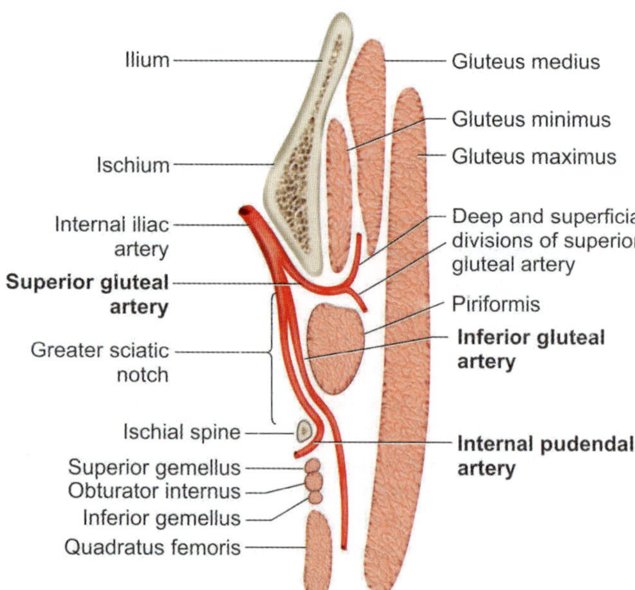

Schematic vertical section of the gluteal region to show the course of some arteries

155. Femoral nerve does NOT supply:

a. Sartorius
b. Rectus femoris
c. Tensor fascia lata
d. Articularis genu

Tensor fascia lata

Origin	Iliac crest
Insertion	Iliotibial tract
Artery	Primarily lateral circumflex femoral artery, superior gluteal artery
Nerve	Superior gluteal nerve (L4, L5, S1)
Actions	Thigh—flexion, medial rotation, abduction Leg—lateral rotation Torso—stabilization

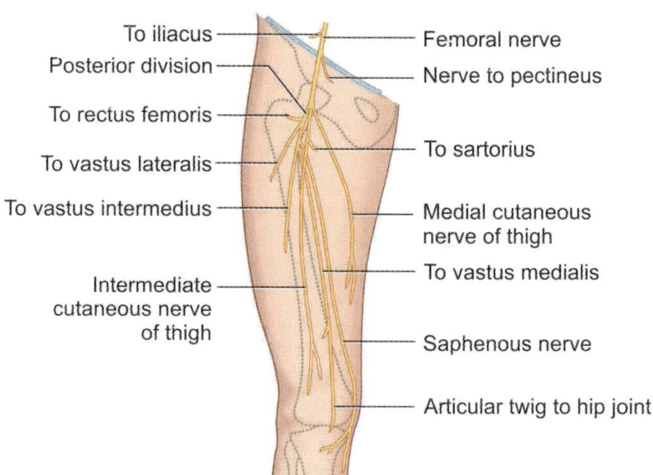

Scheme to show the distribution of the femoral nerve in the thigh.

156. Lateral rotators of hip are all EXCEPT:

a. Piriformis
b. Quadratus femoris
c. Obturator internus
d. Psoas major

Psoas major

Origin	Transverse processes of T12-L5 and the lateral aspects of the disks between them
Insertion	In the lesser trochanter of the femur
Artery	Lumbar branch of iliolumbar artery
Nerve	Lumbar plexus via anterior branches of L1-L3 nerves
Actions	Flexion in the hip joint
Antagonist	Gluteus maximus

157. True about gluteus maximus are all EXCEPT:

a. Supplied by superior gluteal nerve
b. Arises from coccyx, ischium
c. Insertion into iliotibial tract
d. Strong extensor

Ans. 154. b. Gluteus medius **155. c.** Tensor fascia... **156. d.** Psoas major **157. a.** Supplied by superior...

Origin	Gluteal surface of ilium, lumbar fascia, sacrum, sacrotuberous ligament
Insertion	Gluteal tuberosity of the femur and iliotibial tract
Artery	Superior and inferior gluteal arteries
Nerve	Inferior gluteal nerve (L5, S1 and S2 nerve roots)
Actions	External rotation and extension of the hip joint, supports the extended knee through the iliotibial tract, chief antigravity muscle in sitting and abduction of the hip
Antagonist	Iliacus, psoas major and psoas minor

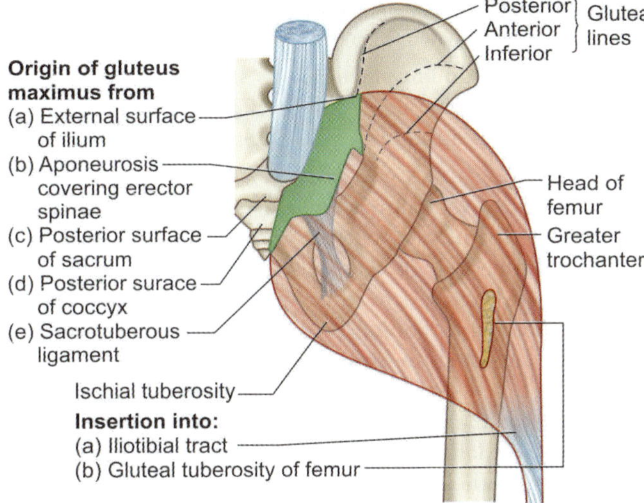

Scheme to show the attachments of the gluteus maximus.

158. Muscle present in first layer of sole:

a. Flexor hallucis longus b. Flexor digitorum brevis
c. Flexor digiti minimi brevis
d. Adductor hallucis

In the first layer, flexor digitorum brevis is the large central muscle located immediately below the plantar aponeurosis. It flexes the second to fifth toes and is flanked by abductor hallucis and abductor digiti minimi.

Contents of the various layers of the sole.

	Muscles	Tendons
First Layer	❑ Flexor digitorum brevis ❑ Abductor hallucis ❑ Abductor digiti minimi	
Second Layer	❑ Flexor digitorum accessorius (Quadratus plantae) ❑ Lumbrical muscles	❑ Flexor hallucis longus ❑ Flexor digitorum longus
Third Layer	❑ Flexor hallucis brevis ❑ Flexor digiti minimi brevis ❑ Adductor hallucis	
Fourth Layer	❑ Plantar interossei ❑ Dorsal interossei	❑ Tibialis posterior ❑ Peroneus longus

159. Structure which passes deep to flexor retinaculum at ankle:

a. Peroneus longus
b. Peroneus brevis
c. Tibialis anterior
d. Tibialis posterior

Enumerated from the medial side of leg, the four canals which it forms transmit the tendons of the tibialis posterior and flexor digitorum longus muscles; the posterior tibial vessels and tibial nerve, which run through a broad space beneath the ligament; and lastly, in a canal formed partly by the talus, the tendon of the flexor hallucis longus.

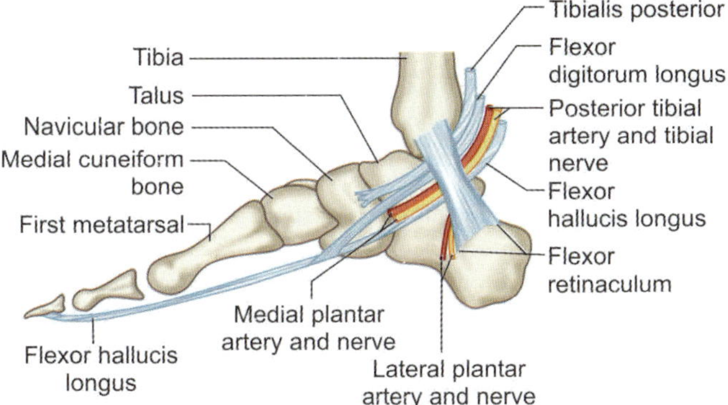

Flexor Retinaculum and structures passing deep to it.

160. NOT an abductor of thigh:

a. Gluteus medius
b. Gluteus maximus
c. Gluteus minimus
d. Sartorius

Gluteus maximus

Origin	Gluteal surface of ilium, lumbar fascia, sacrum, sacrotuberous ligament
Insertion	Gluteal tuberosity of the femur and iliotibial tract
Artery	Superior and inferior gluteal arteries
Nerve	Inferior gluteal nerve (L5, S1 and S2 nerve roots)
Actions	External rotation and extension of the hip joint, supports the extended knee through the iliotibial tract, chief antigravity muscle in sitting and abduction of the hip

161. Which muscle is very important in walking and running:

a. Iliopsoas
b. Tibialis anterior
c. Anterior tibialis
d. Gastrocnemius

Plantar flexion, produced by the gastrocnemius and the soleus, is very important in walking and running. The soleus is more powerful than the gastrocnemius, but the latter is faster acting.

Ans. **158. b.** Flexor... **159. d.** Tibialis posterior **160. b.** Gluteus maximus **161. d.** Gastrocnemius

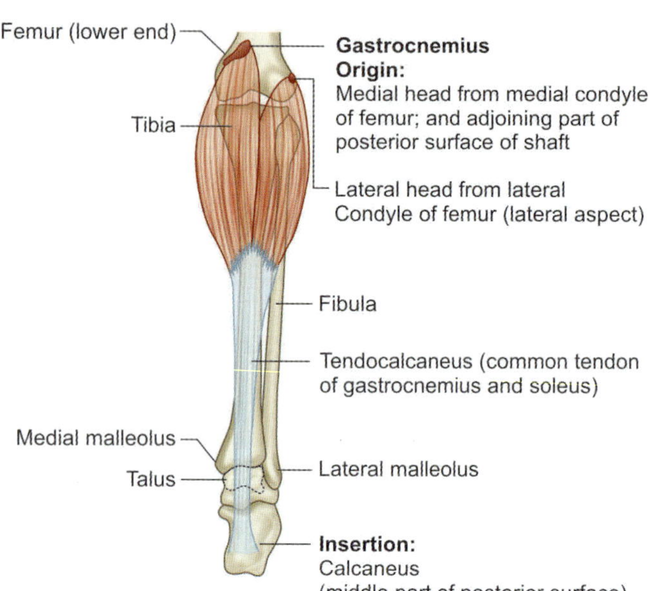

Attachments of the gastrocnemius.

162. Action of superior gemelli:

a. Internal rotation of thigh b. External rotation of thigh
c. Flexion of thigh d. Extension of thigh

Superior Gemelli

Origin	Spine of the ischium
Insertion	Obturator internus tendon
Artery	Inferior gluteal artery
Nerve	Nerve to obturator internus (L5, S1, S2)
Actions	Rotates laterally thigh

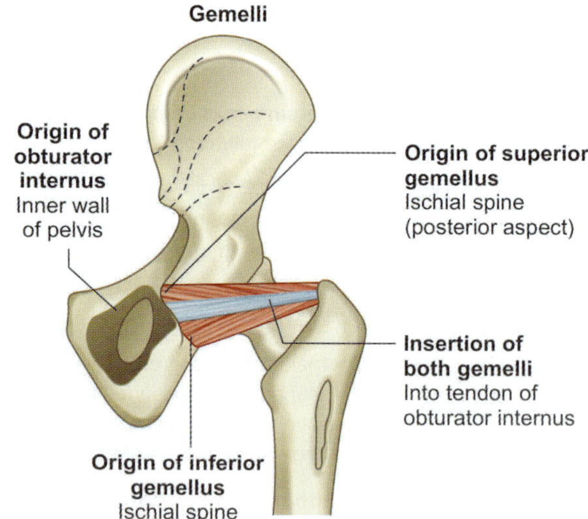

Scheme to show attachments of gemelli.

163. Inversion and eversion occur at:

a. Tibiofibular joint b. Ankle joint
c. Subtalar joint d. Calcaneocuboid joint

The subtalar joint allows inversion and eversion of the foot, but plays no role in dorsiflexion or plantarflexion of the foot.

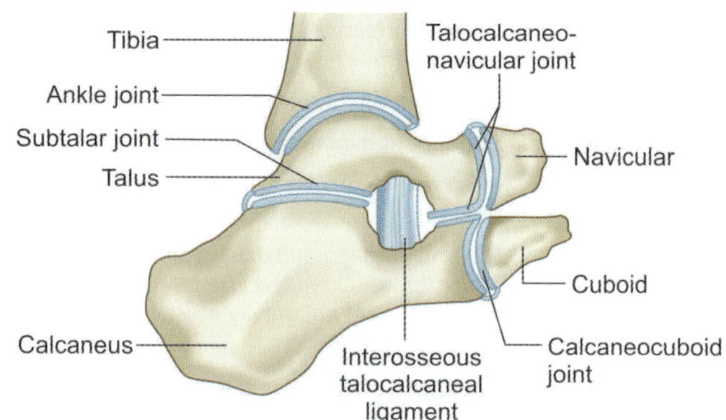

Schematic vertical section along the long axis of the talus to show the various joints formed by it.

164. NOT an abductor of thigh:

a. Gluteus medius b. Gluteus maximus
c. Gluteus minimus d. Sartorius

Action of gluteus maximus

Taking its fixed point from below, it acts upon the pelvis, supporting it and the trunk upon the head of the femur; this is especially obvious in standing on one leg. Its most powerful action is to cause the body to regain the erect position after stooping, by drawing the pelvis backward, being assisted in this action by the biceps femoris (long head), semitendinosus, semimembranosus, and adductor magnus. The gluteus maximus is a tensor of the fascia lata, and by its connection with the iliotibial band steadies the femur on the articular surfaces of the tibia during standing, when the extensor muscles are relaxed. The lower part of the muscle also acts as an adductor and external rotator of the limb. The upper fibers act as abductors of the hip joints.

165. Short saphenous vein is a tributary of:

a. Dorsal venous arch b. Popliteal vein
c. Lateral marginal vein d. Medial marginal vein

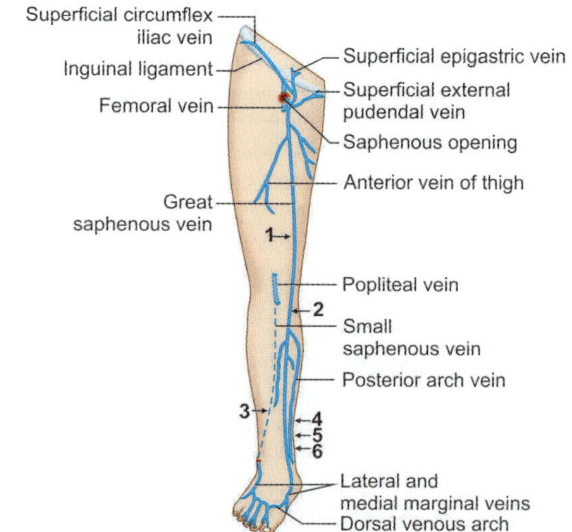

Superficial veins of lower limb. Numbered arrows (from 1 to 6) indicate the position of perforating veins.

Ans. 162. b. External... 163. c. Subtalar joint 164. b. Gluteus maximus 165. b. Popliteal vein

The origin of the small saphenous vein (SSV) is where the dorsal vein from the fifth digit (smallest toe) merges with the dorsal venous arch of the foot, which attaches to the great saphenous vein (GSV). Usually, it drains into the popliteal vein, at or above the level of the knee joint.

166. Muscle NOT arising from ischial tuberosity:

a. Adductor magnus b. Semitendinosus
c. Semimembranosus d. Adductor longus

Adductor longus

Origin	Pubic body just below the pubic crest
Insertion	Middle third of linea aspera
Artery	Deep femoral artery
Nerve	Anterior branch of obturator nerve
Actions	Adduction of hip, flexion of hip joint

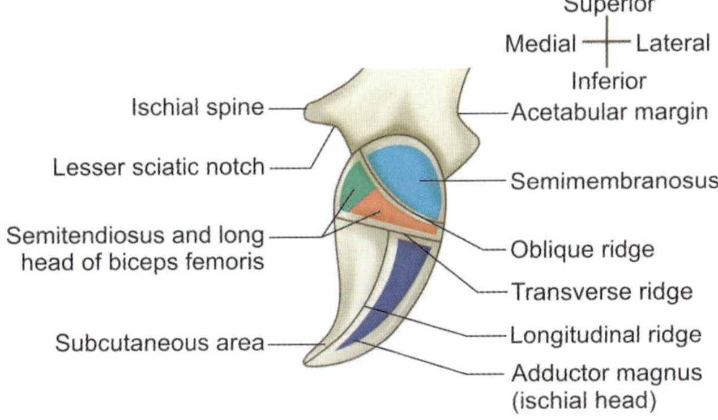

Attachments of ischial tuberosity.

167. NOT a site of attachment of deltoid ligament:

a. Sustentaculum tali b. Medial cuneiform
c. Spring ligament d. Medial malleolus

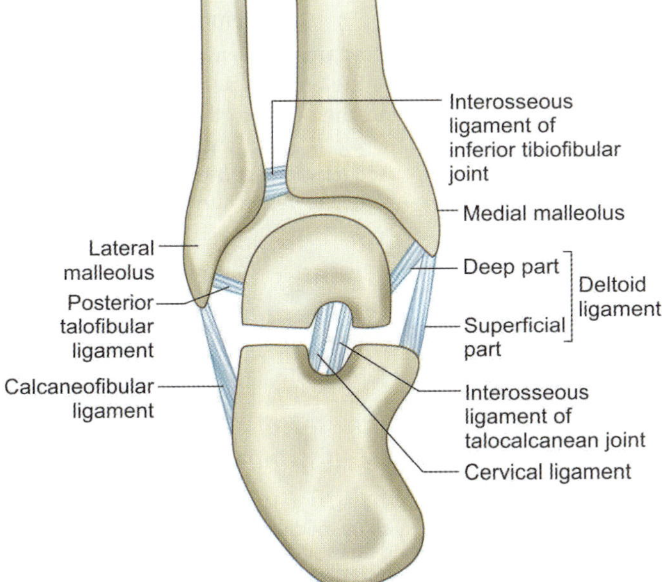

Important ligaments of ankle joint.

The deltoid ligament is composed of the anterior tibiotalar ligament, tibiocalcaneal ligament, posterior tibiotalar ligament and the tibionavicular ligament. It consists of two sets of fibers, superficial and deep.

168. Positive Trendelenburg test indicates injury to:

a. Pudendal nerve b. Obturator nerve
c. Superior gluteal nerve d. Inferior gluteal nerve

In normal gait, the small gluteal muscles on the stance side can stabilize the pelvis in the coronal plane. Weakness or paralysis of these muscles caused by a damaged superior gluteal nerve can result in a weak abduction in the affected hip joint. This gait disturbance is known as Trendelenburg gait. In a positive Trendelenburg's sign, the pelvis sags toward the normal unsupported side (the swing leg).

169. Femoral hernias lie .... to pubic tubercle:

a. Below and medial b. Below and lateral
c. Above and lateral d. Above and medial

The femoral canal is located below the inguinal ligament on the lateral aspect of the pubic tubercle. **Femoral hernias** occur just below the inguinal ligament, when abdominal contents pass through a naturally occurring weakness called the femoral canal.

170. Deep peroneal nerve supplies:

a. 5th webspace of foot
b. 1st webspace of foot
c. Lateral aspect of leg
d. Anterolateral dorsum of foot

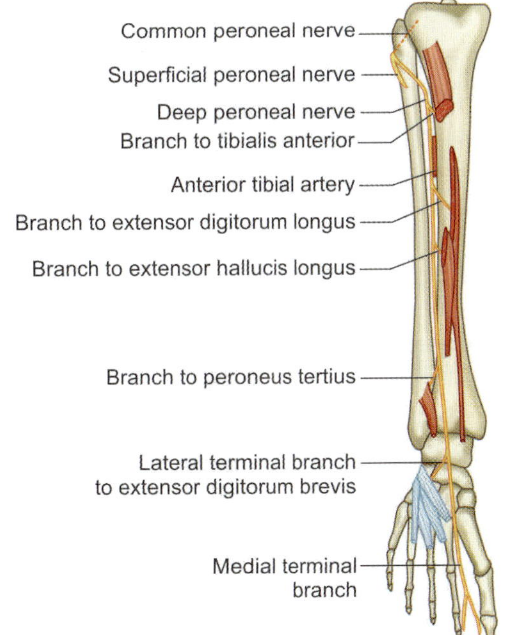

Distribution of deep peroneal nerve.

The **medial terminal branch** (internal branch) of deep peroneal nerve accompanies the dorsalis pedis

Ans. 166. **d.** Adductor... 167. **b.** Medial cuneiform 168. **c.** Superior gluteal... 169. **b.** Below and lateral 170. **b.** 1st webspace...

artery along the dorsum of the foot, and, at the first interosseous space, divides into two dorsal digital nerves (nn. digitales dorsales hallucis lateralis et digiti secundi medialis) which supply the adjacent sides of the great and second toes, communicating with the medial dorsal cutaneous branch of the superficial peroneal nerve.

171. NOT involved in injury to the head of fibula:

a. Common peroneal nerve
b. Superficial peroneal nerve
c. Tibial nerve
d. Anterior tibial nerve

The **tibial nerve** is a branch of the sciatic nerve. The tibial nerve passes through the popliteal fossa to pass below the arch of soleus. Anterior tibial nerve is another term for deep peroneal nerve.

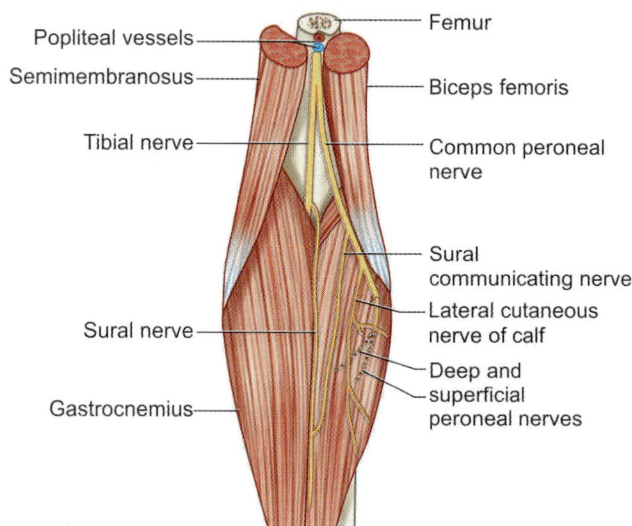

Distribution of the common peroneal nerve.

172. Medial most in the femoral sheath:

a. Vein
b. Artery
c. Nerve
d. Lymphatics

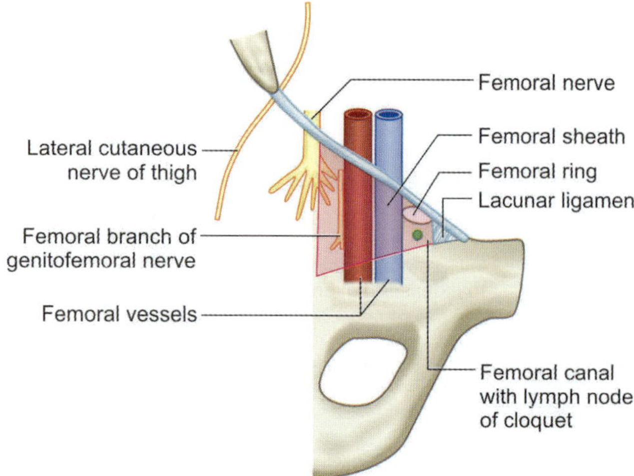

Femoral sheath showing its compartments with their contents (Note that femoral nerve is outside the femoral sheath).

Structures in femoral triangle (from lateral to medial):

- Femoral nerve and its (terminal) branches.
- Femoral sheath and its contents.
- Femoral artery and several of its branches.
- Femoral vein and its proximal tributaries (e.g. the great saphenous and deep femoral veins).
- Deep inguinal lymph nodes and associated lymphatic vessels.

173. Unlocker of knee:

a. Sartorius
b. Popliteus
c. Biceps femoris
d. Adductor magnus

When the knee is in full extension, the femur slightly medially rotates on the tibia to lock the knee joint in place. Popliteus is often referred to as the 'key' to unlocking the knee since it begins knee flexion by laterally rotating the femur on the tibia.

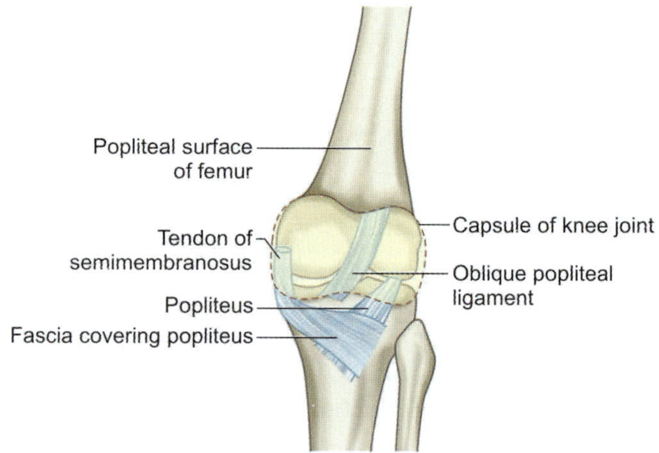

Structures forming the floor of popliteal fossa.

174. NOT a content of adductor canal:

a. Saphenous nerve
b. Nerve to vastus medialis
c. Popliteal artery
d. Femoral artery

The adductor canal contains the femoral artery, femoral vein, and branches of the femoral nerve (specifically, the saphenous nerve, and the nerve to the vastus medialis).

Posterior wall by:
Adductor longus (above)
Adductor magnus (below)

Femoral artery
Femoral vein
Nerve to vastus medialis
Saphenous nerve
Sartorius on antero-medial side
Subsartorial fascia forming roof
Vastus medialis forming anterolateral wall

Femoral vessel in adductor canal; Bounderies of the canal are shown.

Ans. 171. **c.** Tibial nerve 172. **d.** Lymphatics 173. **b.** Popliteus 174. **c.** Popliteal artery

175. Strongest ligament in the body is:

a. Pubofemoral ligament b. Ischiofemoral ligament
c. Ligamentum teres d. Iliofemoral ligament

With a tensile strength exceeding 350 kg (772 lbs), the iliofemoral ligament is not only stronger than the two other ligaments of the hip joint, the ischiofemoral and the pubofemoral, but also the strongest ligament in the human body and, as such, is an important constraint to the hip joint.

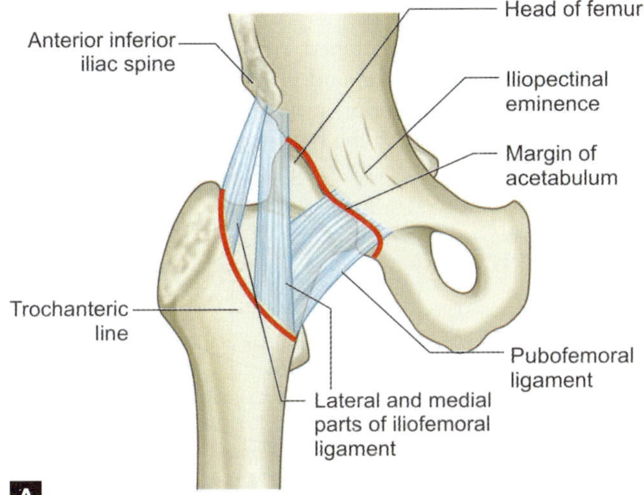

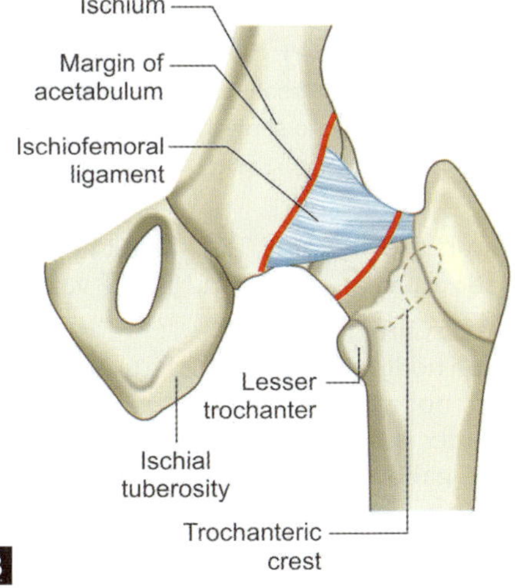

Hip joint (A) Anterior aspect (B) Posterior aspect; The capsular attachments (blue) and epiphyseal lines (magenta) are shown

176. Sacrotuberous ligament is supposed to be a degenerated tendon of:

a. Iliopsoas
b. Coccygeus
c. Short head of biceps femoris
d. Long head of biceps femoris

The lower border of the sacrotuberous ligament was found to be directly continuous with the tendon of origin of the long head of the Biceps femoris in approximately 50% of subjects. Biceps femoris could, therefore, act to stabilize the sacroiliac joint via the sacrotuberous ligament.

177. Tendon occupying groove on the lower surface of sustentaculum tali:

a. Flexor digitorum longus
b. Flexor hallucis longus
c. Tibialis posterior
d. Flexor digitorum accessories

The tendon of FHL lies in a groove which crosses the posterior surface of the lower end of the tibia, the posterior surface of the talus, and the undersurface of the sustentaculum tali of the calcaneus; in the sole of the foot, it runs forward between the two heads of the flexor hallucis brevis, and is inserted into the base of the last phalanx of the great toe.

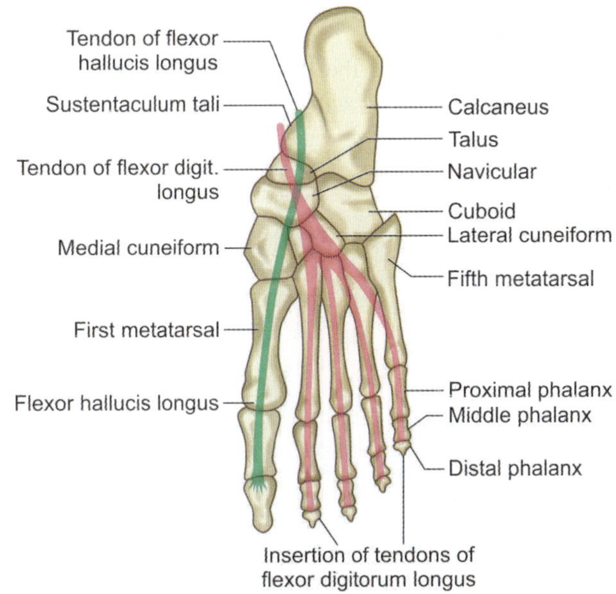

Course and attachments of tendons of flexor hallucis longus and flexor digitorum longus in the sole.

178. Which muscle contributes to medial longitudinal arch of foot:

a. Tibialis anterior b. Tibialis posterior
c. Peroneus longus d. Flexor digitorum brevis

The medial arch is higher than the lateral longitudinal arch. It is made up by the calcaneus, the talus, the navicular, the three cuneiforms, and the first, second, and third metatarsals. Its weakest part (i.e. the part most liable to yield from overpressure), is the joint between the talus and navicular, but this portion is braced by the plantar calcaneonavicular ligament/spring ligament, which is elastic and is thus able to quickly restore the arch to its pristine condition when the disturbing force is removed. The ligament is strengthened medially by blending with the deltoid ligament of the anklejoint,

Ans. 175. **d.** Iliofemoral... 176. **d.** Long head of biceps... 177. **b.** Flexor hallucis 178. **b.** Tibialis posterior

and is supported inferiorly by the tendon of the tibialis posterior, which is spread out in a fan-shaped insertion and prevents undue tension of the ligament or such an amount of stretching as would permanently elongate it.

179. Intersegmental tie of medial longitudinal plantar arch:

a. Deltoid ligament b. Spring ligament
c. Long plantar ligament d. Short plantar ligament

Intersegmental ties

Arch	Tie
Medial longitudinal	Spring ligament
Lateral longitudinal	Long and short plantar ligaments

180. Great saphenous vein is formed by the union of:

a. Medial end of the dorsal venous arch with the medial marginal vein
b. Lateral end of the dorsal venous arch with the lateral marginal vein
c. Medial end of the dorsal venous arch with the lateral marginal vein
d. Lateral end of the dorsal venous arch with the medial marginal vein

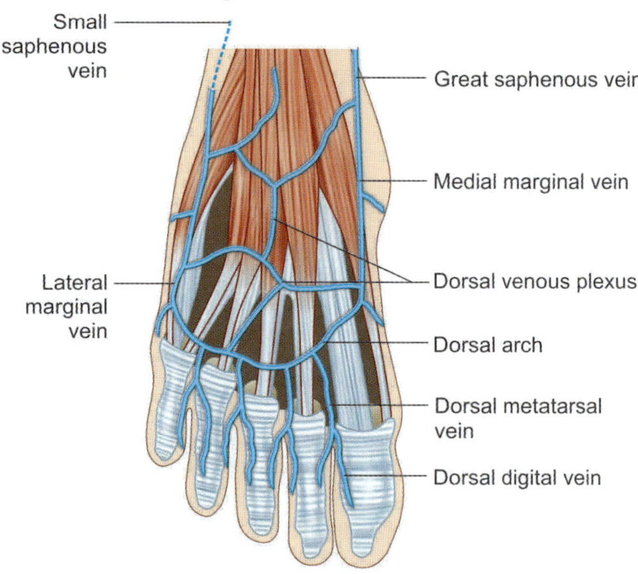

Veins on the dorsum of foot.

The GSV originates from where the dorsal vein of the first digit (the large toe) merges with the dorsal venous arch of the foot. After passing anterior to the medial malleolus (where it often can be visualized and palpated), it runs up the medial side of the leg).

ABDOMEN AND PELVIS

181. Visceral relation of spleen are all EXCEPT:

a. Tail of pancreas b. Left kidney
c. Fundus of stomach d. Duodenum

Spleen visceral surface

- It is divided by a ridge into two regions: an anterior or gastric and a posterior or renal.
- The gastric surface (facies gastrica) is directed forward, upward, and toward the middle, is broad and concave, and is in contact with the posterior wall of the stomach.
- Below this it is in contact with the tail of the pancreas.
- Near to its mid-border is a long fissure, termed the hilum.
- This is pierced by several irregular openings, for the entrance and exit of vessels and nerves. The renal surface (facies renalis) is directed medialward and downward.
- It is somewhat flattened, considerably narrower than the gastric surface, and is in relation with the upper part of the anterior surface of the left kidney and occasionally with the left suprarenal gland.

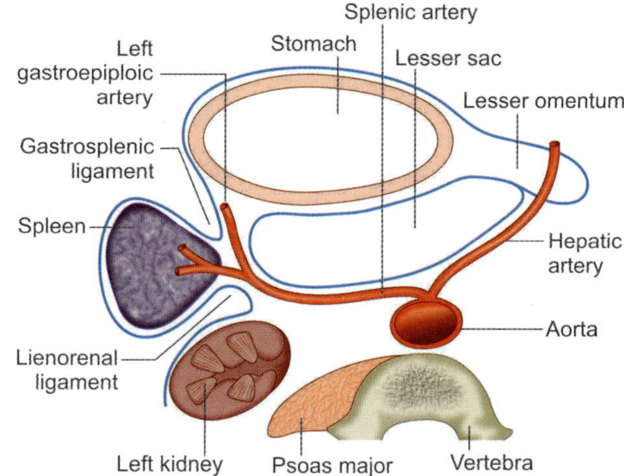

Schematic transverse section to show the course of the splenic artery

182. Which of the following structure is present in Calot's triangle:

a. Lymph node of Lund b. Right hepatic artery
c. Cystic artery d. Portal vein

Content of Calot's triangle

- Lymph node located within the triangle is Mascagni's lymph node or Lund's node.
- The latter is frequently enlarged due to inflammation of the gallbladder (e.g. cholecystitis) or the biliary tract (e.g. cholangitis) and may be removed along with the gallbladder during surgical treatment (cholecystectomy).
- Calot's triangle, containing the cystic artery, may also contain an aberrant / accessory Right Hepatic Artery or anomalous sectoral bile ducts.
- As a result dissection in the triangle of Calot is ill-advised until the lateral-most structures have been cleared and identification of the cystic duct is definitive.
- According to SESAP 12 (produced and distributed by the American College of Surgeons) dissection in the triangle of Calot is the #1 cause of common bile duct injuries.

Ans. **179. b.** Spring ligament **180. a.** Medial end of... **181. d.** Duodenum **182. a.** Lymph node of Lund

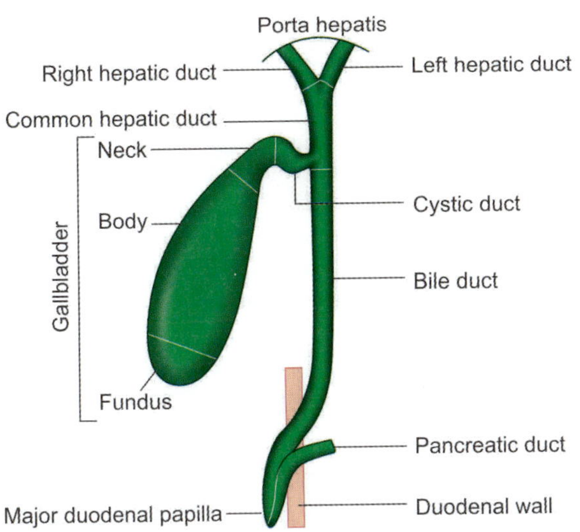

Scheme to show the parts of the extrahepatic biliary apparatus

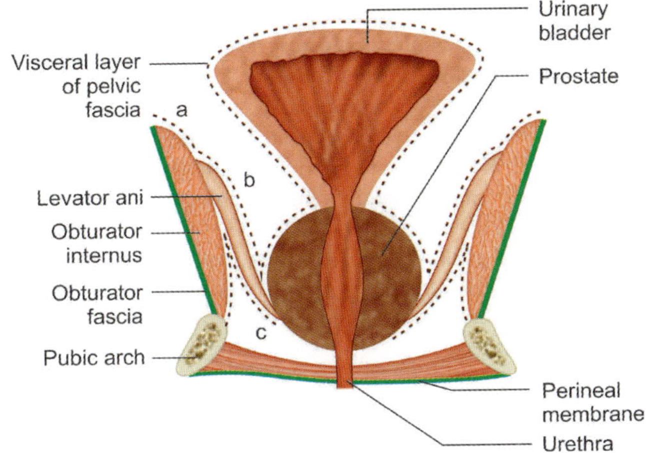

Coronal section through the anterior part of the pelvic diaphragm in the male

Key: a. Greater pelvis **b.** Lesser pelvis **c.** Ischioanal fossa

183. All of the following are true for pelvic floor EXCEPT:
a. Perineal surface of levator ani forms lateral boundary of ischiorectal fossa
b. Consists of levator ani & coccygeus
c. Supports pelvic viscera
d. Helps in maintaining anal continence

Perineal/ inferior surface of levator aniis covered by anal fascia & forms the medial boundary of ischiorectal fossa

Pelvic floor

- The right and left levator ani lie almost horizontally in the floor of the pelvis, separated by a narrow gap that transmits the urethra, vagina, and anal canal.
- The levator ani is usually considered in three parts: pubococcygeus, puborectalis, and iliococcygeus.
- The pubococcygeus, the main part of the levator, runs backward from the body of the pubis toward the coccyx and may be damaged during parturition.
- Some fibers are inserted into the prostate, urethra, and vagina. The right and left puborectalis unite behind the anorectal junction to form a muscular sling.
- Some regard them as a part of the sphincter ani externus.
- The iliococcygeus, the most posterior part of the levator ani, is often poorly developed.
- The coccygeus, situated behind the levator ani and frequently tendinous as much as muscular, extends from the ischial spine to the lateral margin of the sacrum and coccyx.
- The pelvic cavity of the true pelvis has the pelvic floor as its inferior border (and the pelvic brim as its superior border). The perineum has the pelvic floor as its superior border.
- Posteriorly, the pelvic floor extends into the anal triangle.
- The pelvic floor has two hiatuses (gaps): Anteriorly urogenital sinus through which urethra and vagina pass through and posteriorly rectal hiatus through which anal canal passes

184. A content of superficial perineal pouch is:
a. Membranous urethra
b. Sphincter urethrae
c. Bulbospongiosus
d. Bulbourethral glands in male

Superficial perineal pouch

The superficial perineal pouch is a fully enclosed compartment:

- Its inferior border is the fascia of perineum (Gallaudet fascia or deep perineal fascia) is the fasci which covers the muscles of the superficial perineal pouch.
- Its superior border is the perineal membrane

Content

- Muscles
  - Ischiocavernosus muscle
  - Bulbospongiosus muscle
  - Superficial transverse perineal muscle
- Other
  - Crura of penis (males) / crura of clitoris (females)
  - Bulb of penis (males) / vestibular bulbs (females)
  - Greater vestibular glands (female)

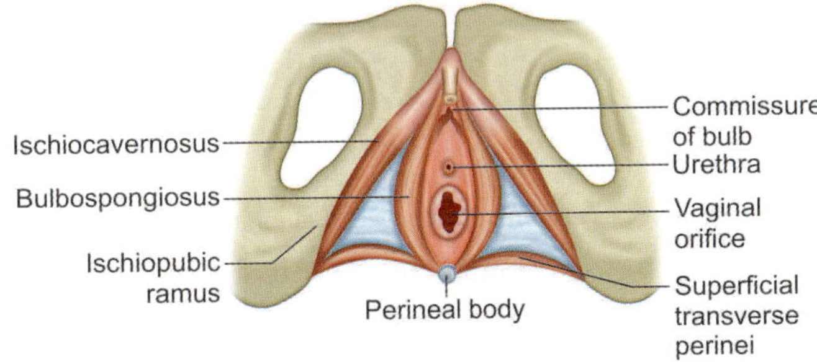

Muscles present in the superficial perineal space in the female

185. Which of the following roots provide parasympathetic supply to urinary bladder?
a. L3-4
b. S2-4
c. L1-L2
d. T11-L2

Ans. 183. a. Perineal surface... **184. c.** Bulbospongiosus **185. b.** S2-4

Parasympathetic system/ PSN

- The pelvic splanchnic nerves, S2-4, work in tandem to innervate the pelvic viscera. Unlike in the cranium, where one PSN was in charge of one particular tissue or region, for the most part the pelvic splanchnics each contribute fibers to pelvic viscera by first traveling to one or more plexuses before being dispersed to the target tissue.
- These plexuses are composed of mixed autonomic nerve fibers (PSN and SN) and include the vesical, prostatic, rectal, uterovaginal, and inferior hypogastric plexus.
- The preganglionic neurons in the neurons do not synapse in named ganglion as in the cranium but rather in the walls of the tissues or organs that they innervate.
- The fiber paths are variable and each individual's autonomic nervous system in the pelvis is unique.
- The visceral tissues in the pelvis that the PSN control include: urinary bladder, ureters, urinary sphincter, anal sphincter, uterus, prostate, glands, vagina and penis.
- Unconsciously, the PSN will cause peristaltic movements of the ureters helping to move urine from the kidneys into the bladder and move feces down the intestinal tract and upon necessity, the PSN will assist excreting urine from the bladder or defecation.
- Stimulation of the PSN will cause the detrusor muscle (urinary bladder wall) to contract and simultaneously relax the internal sphincter urethrae muscle to relax allowing void of urine.

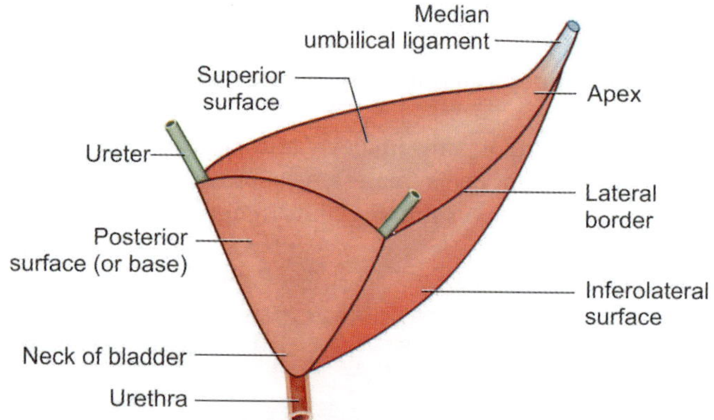

Scheme to show the surfaces of the urinary bladder

186. All of the following are true about rectal canal EXCEPT:

a. Situated in lesser pelvis
b. Taenia coli present
c. 12 cm long
d. Lower one third devoid of peritoneal covering

The three cardinal features of the large intestine (sacculations, appendices epiploicae and taeniae) are ABSENT in rectum

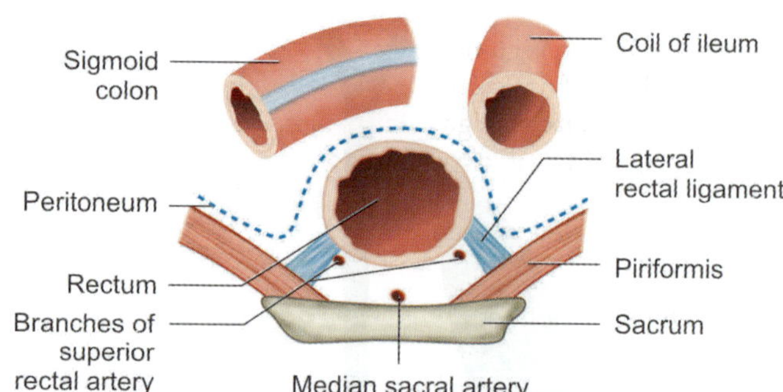

Transverse section through upper one-third of rectum to show some relations

Rectum

- The rectum is a continuation of the sigmoid colon, and connects to the anus. The rectum follows the shape of the sacrum, and ends in an expanded section called the rectal ampulla. Unlike other portions of the colon, the rectum does not have taeniae coli.
- The rectum connects with the sigmoid colon at the level of S3, and connects with the anal canal as it passes through the pelvic floor muscles.

187. All are contents of broad ligament EXCEPT:

a. Paroophoron
b. Ovarian artery
c. Hypogastric nerve
d. Ovarian ligament

Contents of the broad ligament

- Reproductive
  - Uterine tubes (or Fallopian tube)
  - Ovary (some sources consider the ovary to be on the broad ligament, but not in it.)
- Vessels
  - Ovarian artery (in the suspensory ligament)
  - Uterine artery

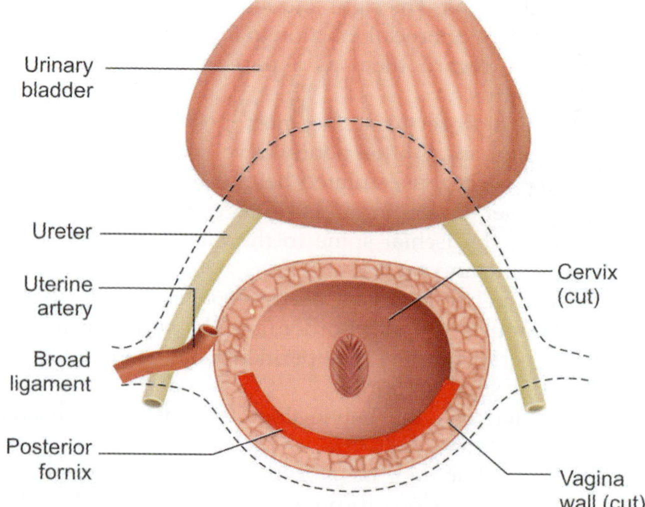

Scheme to show the relationship of the ureters to the cervix of the uterus.

Ans. 186. b. Taenia coli... 187. c. Hypogastric nerve

- Ligaments
  - Ovarian ligament
  - Round ligament of uterus
  - Suspensory ligament of the ovary (Some sources consider it a part of the broad ligament while other sources just consider it a 'termination' of the ligament).

188. NOT a part of posterior wall of inguinal canal:

a. Internal oblique b. External oblique
c. Interfoveolar ligament d. Fascia transversalis

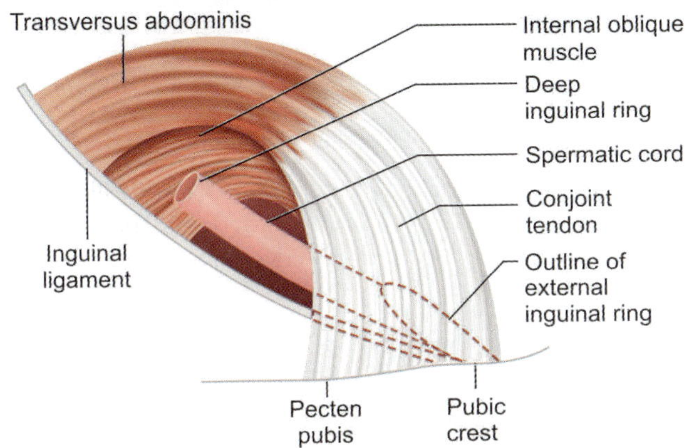

Inguinal canal seen from behind.

Boundaries of inguinal canal

Superior wall (roof): Medial crus of aponeurosis of external oblique Musculoaponeurotic arches of internal oblique and trans-verse abdominal Transversalis fascia		
Anterior wall: Aponeurosis of external oblique Fleshy part of inter-nal oblique (lateral third of canal only) Superficial inguinal ring (medial third of canal only)	(Inguinal canal)	**Posterior wall:** Transversalis fascia conjoint Tendon (Inguinal falx, reflected part of inguinal ligament, medial third of canal only) Deep inguinal ring (lateral third of canal only)
	Inferior wall (floor): Inguinal ligament Lacunar ligament (medial third of canal only) Iliopubic tract (lateral third of canal only)	

189. Does NOT pass through deep inguinal ring:

a. Round ligament
b. Spermatic cord
c. Internal spermatic fascia
d. Ilioinguinal nerve

The ilioinguinal nerve passes through the superficial ring to descend into the scrotum, but does not formally run through the canal.

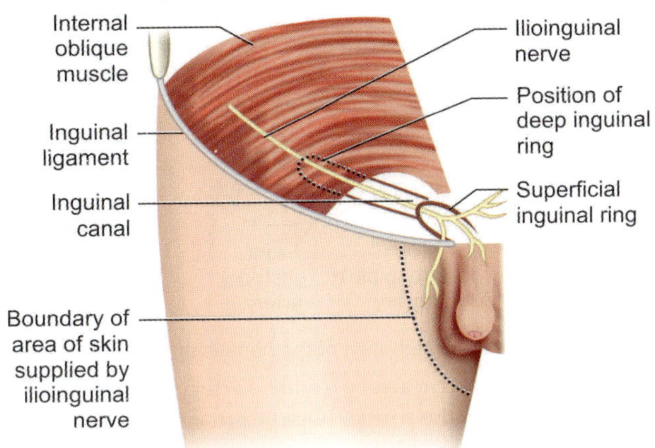

Scheme to show the course of the anterior part of the ilioinguinal nerve.

190. Which pair forms portal vein:

a. Superior mesenteric vein and splenic vein
b. Superior mesenteric vein and inferior mesenteric vein
c. Inferior mesenteric vein and splenic vein
d. Inferior mesenteric vein and hepatic vein

The hepatic portal vein is usually formed by the confluence of the superior mesenteric and splenic veins and also receives blood from the inferior mesenteric, gastric, and cystic veins.

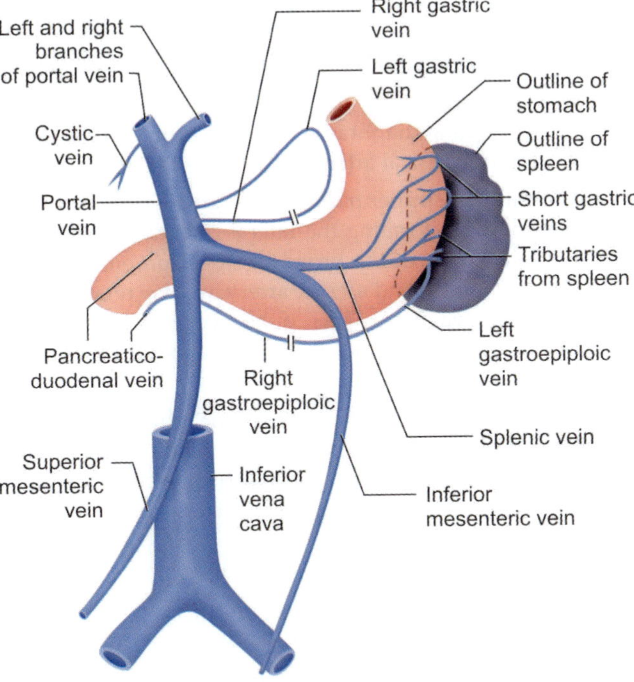

Scheme to show the tributaries of the portal vein.

Ans. 188. **b.** External oblique 189. **d.** Ilioinguinal nerve 190. **a.** Superior mesenteric vein and splenic vein

191. NOT a branch of celiac trunk:

a. Hepatic artery
b. Splenic artery
c. Right gastric artery
d. Left gastric artery

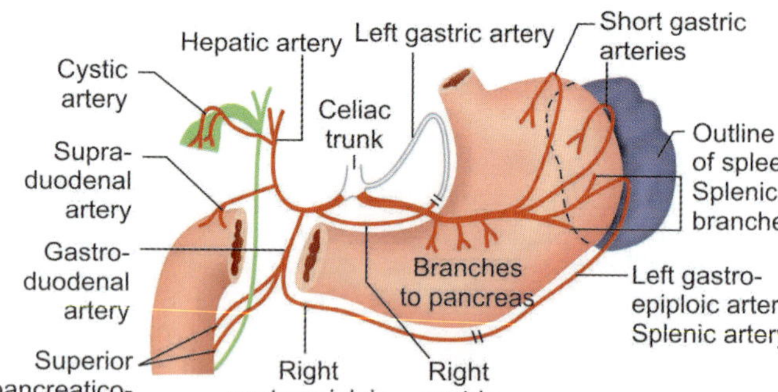

Scheme to show the distribution of the hepatic and splenic arteries.

The **right gastric artery** (pyloric artery) arises above the pylorus from the proper hepatic artery or less frequently from the common hepatic artery, descends to the pyloric end of the stomach, and passes from right to left along its lesser curvature, supplying it with branches, and anastomosing with the left gastric artery.

192. Arterial supply of uterus:

a. Uterine artery
b. Ovarian artery
c. Both of the above
d. None of the above

Uterus

Precursor	Müllerian duct
Artery	Ovarian artery, uterine artery
Vein	Uterine veins
Lymph	Body and cervix to internal iliac lymph nodes, fundus to para-aortic lymph nodes, lumbar and superficial inguinal lymph nodes

193. Structure related to lateral wall of vagina:

a. Urogenital diaphragm
b. Middle rectal artery
c. Inferior vesical artery
d. All of the above

Laterally, the upper part of the vagina is attached to the parametrium forming the lateral cervical ligament and the two layers of the broad ligament on either side of this. The ureter and uterine artery are also related to this part of the vagina. The pubococcygeal portions of the levator ani embrace the vagina about 3 cm above its opening and act as a sphincter.

Below the pelvic diaphragm, the vagina is related laterally to the greater vestibular gland, the bulb of the vestibule, and the bulbospongiosus muscle.

194. Cremasteric reflex is mediated by:

a. Ilioinguinal nerve
b. Genitofemoral nerve
c. Hypogastric nerve
d. None of the above

The genitofemoral nerve is responsible for both the sensory (femoral branch) and motor portions (genital branch) of the cremasteric reflex, which describes contraction of the cremasteric muscle when the skin of the superior medial part of the thigh is touched.

195. Branches of internal iliac artery include all EXCEPT:

a. Uterine artery
b. Middle rectal artery
c. Obturator artery
d. Inferior epigastric artery

Inferior epigastric artery

Source	**External iliac artery**
Branches	Superior epigastric artery, cremasteric branch of inferior epigastric artery, pubic branch of inferior epigastric artery

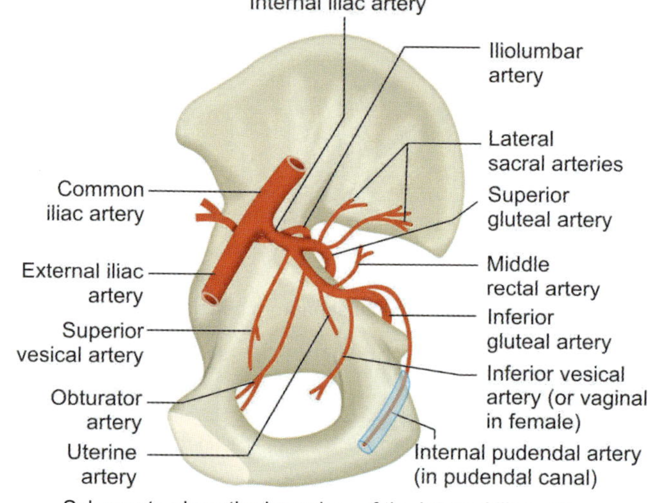

Scheme to show the branches of the internal iliac artery.

196. FALSE about prostate:

a. Surrounds neck of bladder
b. Anterior lobe hypertrophies in old age
c. Median lobe lies between urethra and ejaculatory duct
d. Posterior lobe is prone to carcinomatous changes

Median lobe hypertrophies in old age

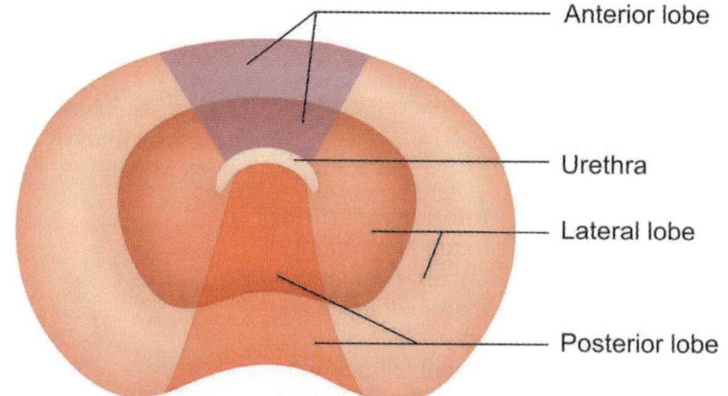

Transverse section through the prostate to show its lobes.

Ans. 191. c. Right gastric... 192. c. Both of... 193. a. Urogenital... 194. b. Genitofemoral... 195. d. Inferior epigast... 196. b. Anterior lobe...

197. Boundaries of Hesselbach's triangle are all EXCEPT:

a. Lateral border of rectus abdominis
b. Inguinal ligament
c. Inferior epigastric artery
d. Medial border of pyramidalis

Boundaries of Hesselbach's triangle (RIP)

- Medial border: Lateral margin of the **R**ectus sheath, also called linea semilunaris
- Superolateral border: **I**nferior epigastric vessels
- Inferior border: Inguinal ligament, sometimes referred to as **P**oupart's ligament.

198. Inferior mesenteric artery supplies all EXCEPT:

a. Ascending colon
b. Transverse colon
c. Descending colon
d. Sigmoid colon

Ascending colon

Precursor	Midgut
Artery	Right colic artery (superior mesenteric artery)
Vein	Right colic vein
Nerve	Celiac ganglia, vagus

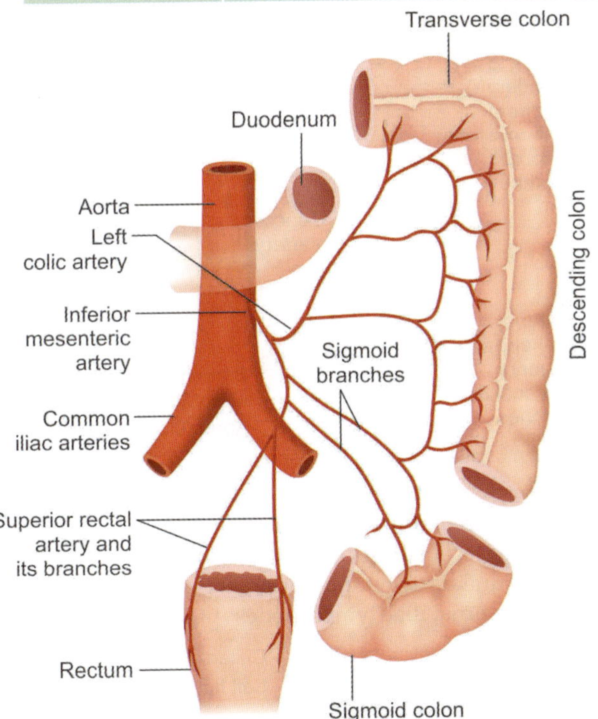

Distribution of inferior mesenteric artery.

199. NOT a tributary of inferior vena cava:

a. Left renal vein
b. Hepatic vein
c. Right suprarenal vein
d. Left gonadal vein

The left gonadal vein drains into the left renal vein, whereas the right drains directly into the inferior vena cava.

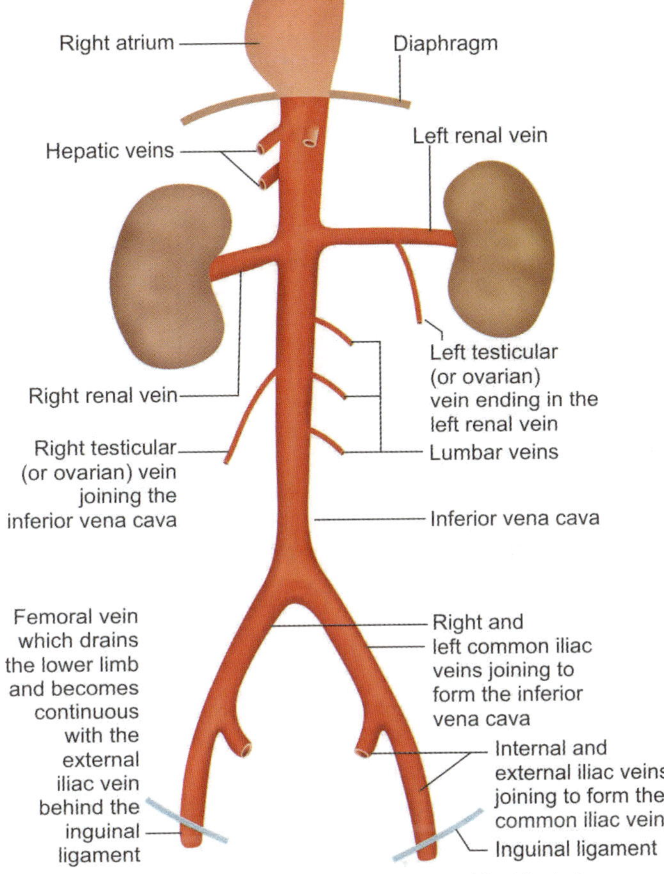

Scheme to show the inferior vena cava and its tributaries.

200. Structure situated in the prostatic part of urethra and unrelated to urethral crest:

a. Colliculus seminalis
b. Bulbourethral gland
c. Prostatic utricle
d. Ejaculatory duct

Bulbourethral glands are located posterior and lateral to the membranous portion of the urethra at the base of the penis, between the two layers of the fascia of the urogenital diaphragm, in the deep perineal pouch. They are enclosed by transverse fibers of the sphincter urethrae membranacea muscle.

201. Does NOT pass through lesser sciatic foramen:

a. Inferior gluteal artery
b. Internal pudendal vessels
c. Nerve to obturator internus
d. Pudendal nerve

The **inferior gluteal artery** (**sciatic artery**), the smaller of the two terminal branches of the anterior trunk of the internal iliac artery, is distributed chiefly to the buttock and back of the thigh. It passes down on the sacral plexus of nerves and the piriformis muscle, behind the internal pudendal artery, to the lower part of the greater sciatic foramen, through which it escapes from the pelvis between the piriformis and coccygeus.

Ans. **197. d.** Medial... **198. a.** Ascending colon **199. d.** Left gonadal vein **200. b.** Bulbourethral gland **201. a.** Inferior...

202. Thickest nerve amongst the following:

a. Axillary b. Median
c. Sciatic d. Radial

Sciatic nerve is the largest and **thickest nerve** of the human body that is the principal continuation of all the roots of the sacral plexus.

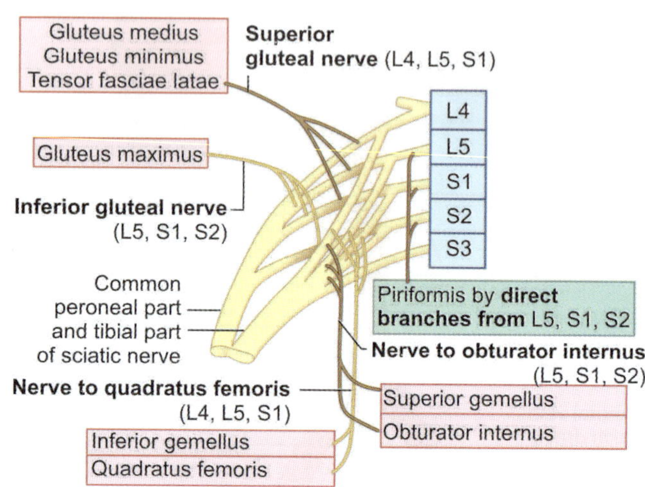

Scheme to show derivation of nerves supplying muscles in the gluteal region.

203. Narrowest part of ureter:

a. At ischial spine b. At pelvic brim
c. Entrance into urinary bladder
d. Pelviureteric junction

On entering the back of the bladder, the ureter is embedded for about 2 cm in the wall of that organ. There the ureteric lumen is narrowest, and the muscular coats of the ureter and bladder are continuous.

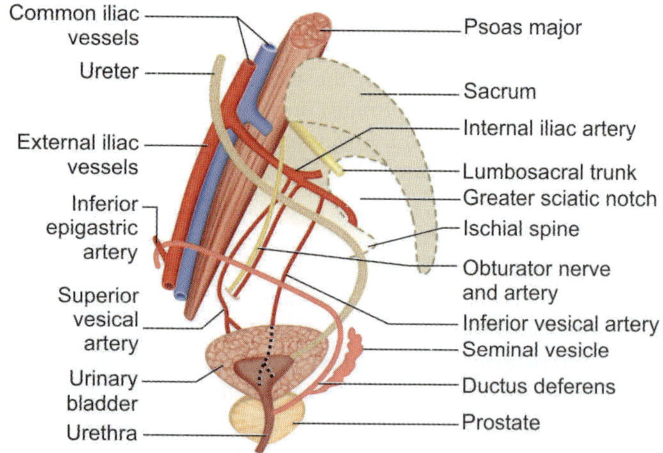

Scheme to show the course and relations of the pelvic part of the ureter in the male.

204. Structure lying posterior to epiploic foramen:

a. Common bile duct b. Hepatic artery
c. Portal vein d. Inferior vena cava

The posterior relations of epiploic foramen include inferior vena cava, the right suprarenal gland and vertebra T12.

205. Does NOT pass through deep inguinal ring:

a. Ilioinguinal nerve b. Round ligament
c. Internal spermatic fascia d. Spermatic cord

The ilioinguinal nerve does not pass through the deep inguinal ring, and, therefore, it only travels through part of the inguinal canal.

206. Which of the following is supplied by superior mesenteric artery:

a. Anus b. Rectum
c. Descending colon d. Ascending colon

The **superior mesenteric artery** (SMA) arises from the anterior surface of the abdominal aorta, just inferior to the origin of the celiac trunk, and supplies the intestine from the lower part of the duodenum through two-thirds of the transverse colon as well as the pancreas.

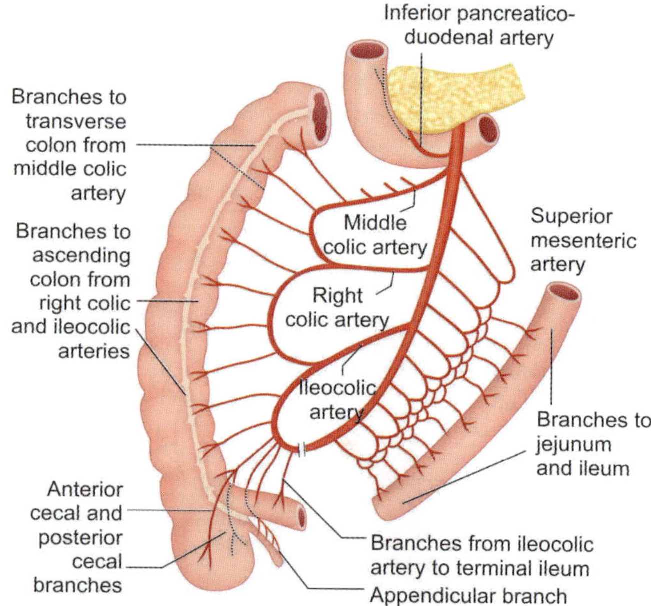

Distribution of superior mesenteric artery.

207. Lymph drainage from testes is to:

a. Deep inguinal lymph nodes
b. Superficial inguinal lymph nodes
c. Para-aortic lymph nodes
d. Internal iliac lymph nodes

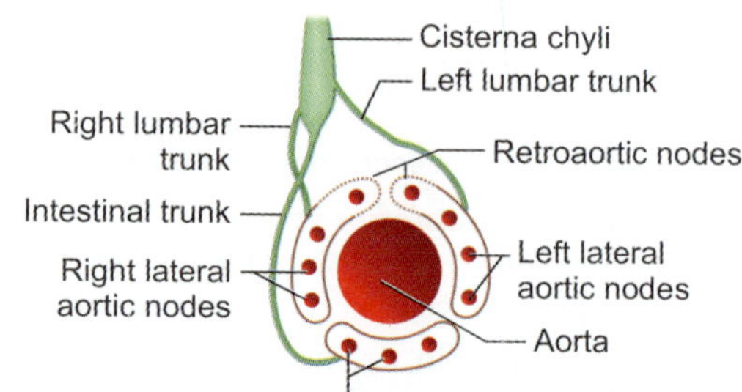

Scheme to show the terminal lymph nodes of the abdomen.

Ans. 202. **c.** Sciatic 203. **c.** Entrance into... 204. **d.** Inferior vena cava 205. **a.** Ilioinguinal... 206. **d.** Ascending... 207. **c.** Para-aortic lymph nodes

Lymphatic drainage of the testes follows the testicular arteries back to the preaortic and para-aortic lymph nodes, while lymph from the scrotum drains to the inguinal lymph nodes.

208. Location of foramen of Winslow:
- a. Pouch of Douglas
- b. Uterine transverse cervical ligament
- c. Hilum of liver
- d. Between lesser and greater sac

The **omental foramen (epiploic foramen, foramen of Winslow** after the anatomist Jacob B Winslow, or uncommonly **aditus** is the passage of communication, or foramen, between the greater sac (general cavity of the abdomen), and the lesser sac.

209. Length of epiploic foramen:
- a. 4–6 cm
- b. 9–12 cm
- c. 10–14 cm
- d. 13–16 cm

The **epiploic foramen** is a potential opening, approximately 4 to 6 cm in **length.**

210. Left testicular vein drains into which of the following:
- a. Superior vena cava
- b. Inferior vena cava
- c. Left renal vein
- d. Portal vein

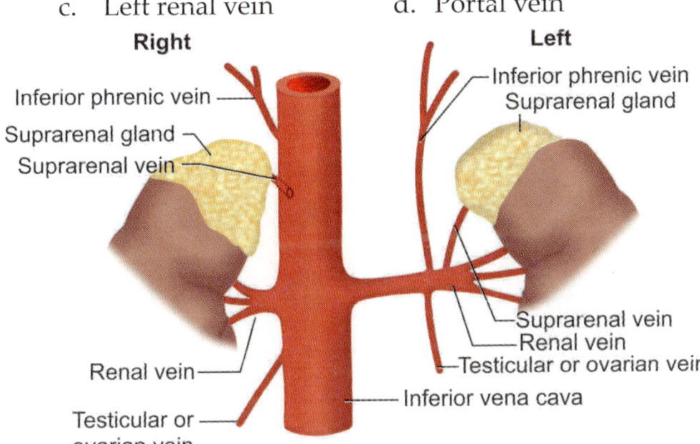

Scheme to show some veins that open on the right side into the inferior vena cava and on the left side into the left renal vein.

The left testicular vein, unlike the right one, joins the left renal vein instead of the inferior vena cava.

211. All are true about inguinal canal EXCEPT:
- a. Conjoint tendon forms part of the posterior wall
- b. Superficial ring is a defect in external oblique aponeurosis
- c. Deep inguinal ring is an opening in transversalis abdominis
- d. Internal oblique forms both anterior and posterior walls

Deep inguinal ring is a defect in fascia transversalis (NOT in the muscle transverses abdominis)

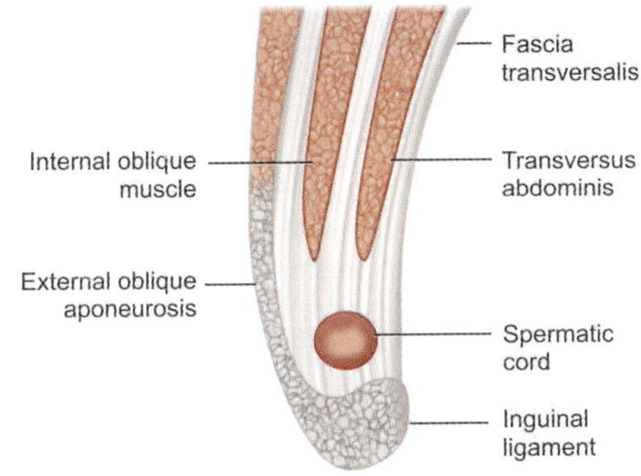

Sagittal section through inguinal canal.

212. Liver is divided into 2 halves by all EXCEPT:
- a. Right hepatic vein
- b. Portal vein
- c. Hepatic artery
- d. Common bile duct

The central area where the common bile duct, hepatic portal vein, and the hepatic artery proper enter is the hilum known as the porta hepatis (gateway to the liver) or the transverse fissure of the liver. The duct, vein, and artery divide into left and right branches, and the areas of the liver supplied by these branches constitute the functional left and right lobes.

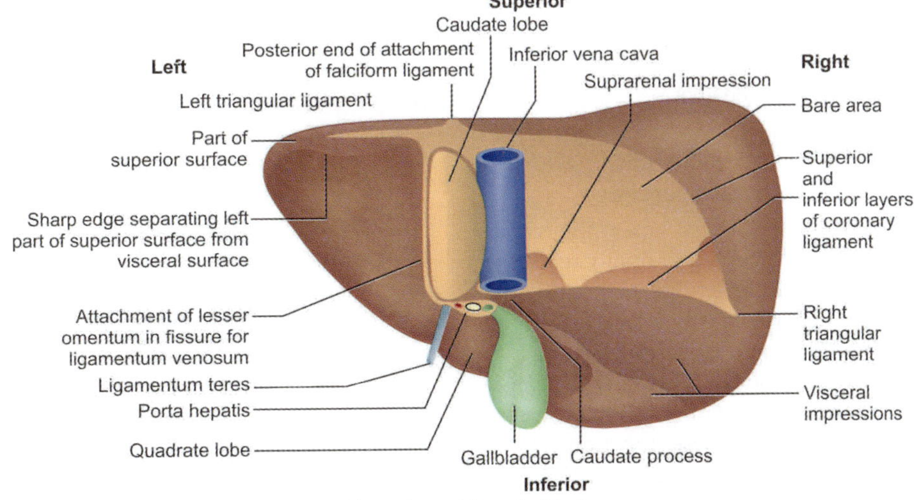

Liver viewed from behind.

Ans.
- 208. **d.** Between transverse cervical ligament
- 209. **a.** 4–6 cm
- 210. **c.** Left renal vein
- 211. **c.** Deep inguinal ring is an opening in transversalis...
- 212. **a.** Right hepatic vein

213. Does NOT drain into portal vein:

a. Superior mesenteric vein b. Splenic vein
c. Renal vein d. Left gastric vein

The **renal veins** are veins that drain the kidney. They connect the kidney to the inferior vena cava.

214. NOT supplied by superior mesenteric artery:

a. Descending colon b. Ascending colon
c. Appendix d. Jejunum

Descending colon

Precursor	Hindgut
Artery	Left colic artery (The **left colic artery** is a branch of the inferior mesenteric artery)

215. Spleen projects into:

a. Intracolic compartment b. Left subhepatic space
c. Greater sac d. Paracolic gutter

Spleen develops in the dorsal mesentery and projects into the greater sac of peritoneal cavity.

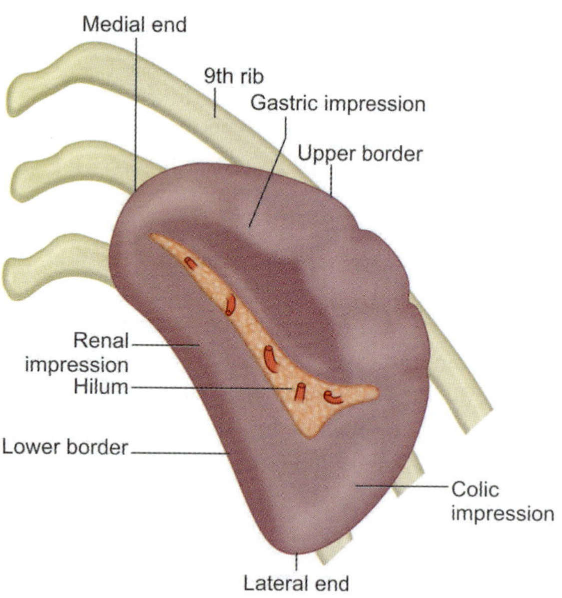

Spleen as seen from the front.

216. Sperm, after formation, is stored in:

a. Sertoli cell b. Epididymis
c. Rete testes d. Seminal vesicle

Spermatozoa formed in the testis enter the caput epididymis, progress to the corpus, and finally reach the cauda region, where they are stored. Sperm entering the caput epididymis are incomplete—they lack the ability to swim forward (motility) and to fertilize an egg. It stores the sperms for 2–3 months. During their transit in the epididymis, sperm undergo maturation processes necessary for them to acquire these functions. Final maturation is completed in the female reproductive tract (*capacitation*).

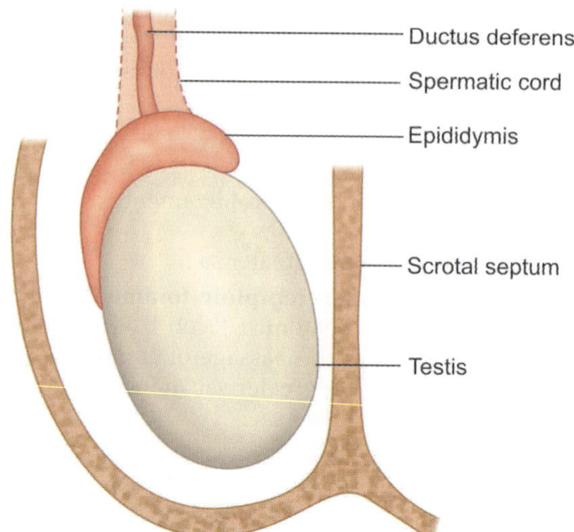

Right testis seen from the front.

217. Lymphatic drainage of ovary:

a. Internal iliac lymph nodes
b. Preaortic and para-aortic lymph nodes
c. Superficial inguinal lymph nodes
d. Deep inguinal lymph nodes

Ovary

Artery	Ovarian artery, uterine artery
Vein	Ovarian vein
Nerve	Ovarian plexus
Lymph	Para-aortic and preaortic lymph node

218. Arterial supply to testes is from:

a. Testicular artery
b. Internal pudendal artery
c. Superficial external pudendal artery
d. Deep external pudendal artery

The **testicular artery** (the male gonadal artery, also called the **internal spermatic arteries** in older texts) is a branch of the abdominal aorta that supplies blood to the testis. It is a paired artery.

219. NOT felt during per-rectal examination:

a. Bulb of penis
b. Prostate
c. Ureter
d. Anorectal ring

During PR examination, areas which can be palpated are: prostate, bulb of penis, urogenital diaphragm, anorectal ring, etc. However, structures like the ureter and urethra cannot be palpated.

220. FALSE regarding prostatic urethra:

a. Contains urethral crest
b. Opening of prostatic ducts
c. Trapezoid in cross-section
d. Presence of verumontanum

Ans. 213. **c.** Renal vein 214. **a.** Descending colon 215. **c.** Greater sac 216. **b.** Epididymis
217. **b.** Preaortic and... 218. **a.** Testicular artery 219. **c.** Ureter 220. **c.** Trapezoid in cross-section

Prostate resembles an inverted cone, measuring about 4 cm transversely at the base (width), 3 cm vertically (length), and 2 cm anteroposteriorly (thickness).

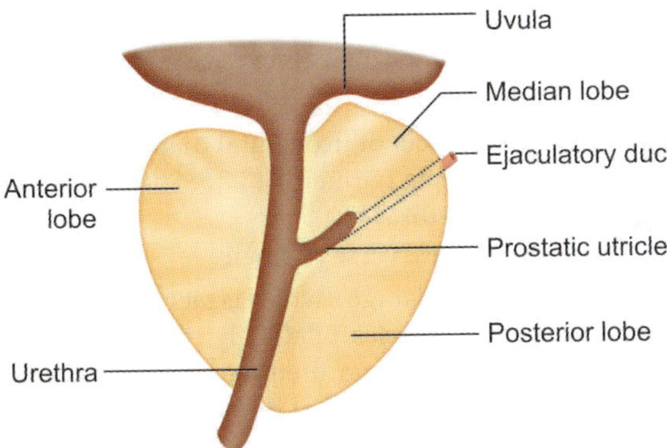

Sagittal section through the prostate to show its lobes.

221. Number of sphincters in sphincter of Oddi:

a. 2
b. 3
c. 4
d. 5

The **sphincter of Oddi** (or **hepatopancreatic sphincter**) is a muscular valve that controls the flow of digestive juices (bile and pancreatic juice) through the ampulla of Vater into the second part of the duodenum. It is named after Ruggero Oddi. The sphincter of Oddi is relaxed by the hormone cholecystokinin (CCK) via vasoactive intestinal peptide (VIP).

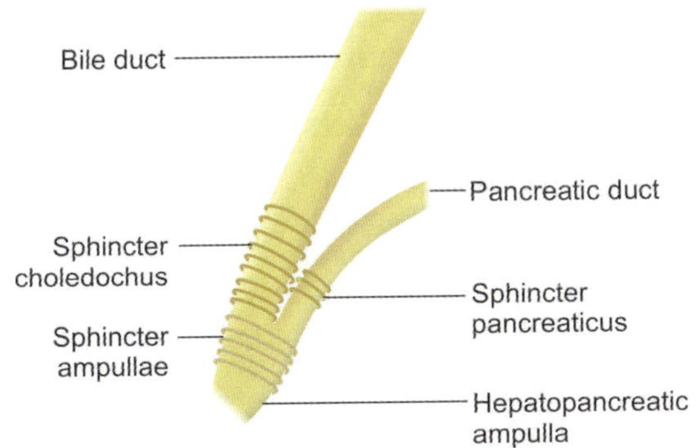

Sphincters around the terminal parts of the bile and pancreatic ducts.

222. Terminal group of lymph nodes for colon:

a. Ileocolic
b. Epicolic
c. Preaortic
d. Paracolic

The **preaortic lymph nodes** lie in front of the aorta, and may be divided into celiac lymph nodes, superior mesenteric lymph nodes, and inferior mesenteric lymph nodes groups, arranged around the origins of the corresponding arteries. Colon is drained by inferior mesenteric lymph nodes.

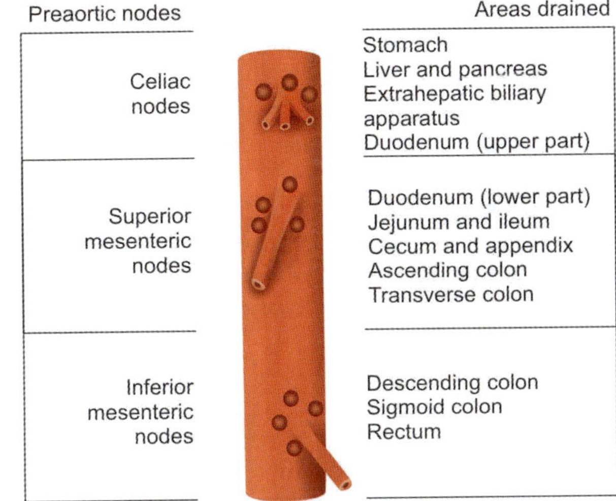

Subgroups of the preaortic lymph nodes, and areas drained by them.

223. NOT a content of vaginal sphincter:

a. Pubovaginalis
b. Bulbospongiosus
c. Internal urethral sphincter
d. External urethral sphincter

Females do not have internal urethral sphincter.

224. Does NOT come into relation of left ureter:

a. External iliac artery
b. Left gonadal vessels
c. Psoas major
d. Quadratus lumborum

Anterior to the quadratus lumborum are the colon, the kidney, the psoas major and (if present) psoas minor, and the diaphragm; between the fascia and the muscle are the twelfth thoracic, ilioinguinal, and iliohypogastric nerves.

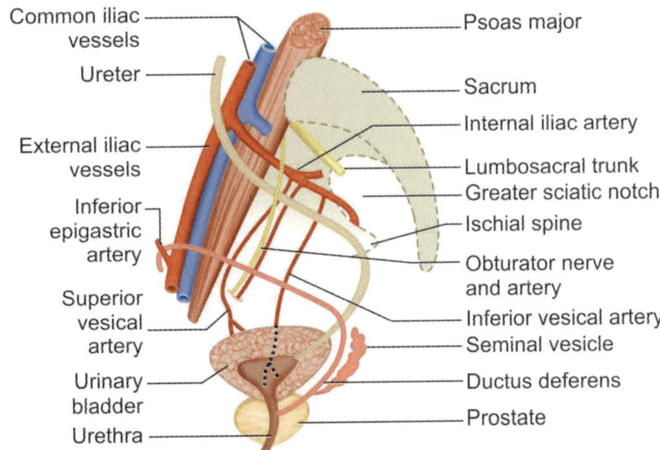

Scheme to show the course and relations of pelvic part of the female ureter.

225. Flexor of abdomen:

a. Pectoralis major
b. Piriformis
c. Gluteus maximus
d. Rectus abdominis

Ans. 221. **b.** 3 222. **c.** Preaortic 223. **c.** Internal urethral... 224. **d.** Quadratus lumborum 225. **d.** Rectus abdominis

Flexion of the trunk/lumbar spine is brought about mainly by the rectus abdominis.

226. Uvula of bladder is:

a. Posterior lobe of prostate
b. Anterior lobe of prostate
c. Lateral lobe of prostate
d. Median lobe of prostate

The mucous membrane immediately behind the internal urethral orifice presents a slight elevation, the uvula of urinary bladder, caused by the middle lobe of the prostate.

227. Azygos vein drains into:

a. Superior vena cava
b. Inferior vena cava
c. Left brachiocephalic vein
d. Right brachiocephalic vein

Superior vena cava

Precursor	Common cardinal veins
Source	Brachiocephalic vein, azygos vein

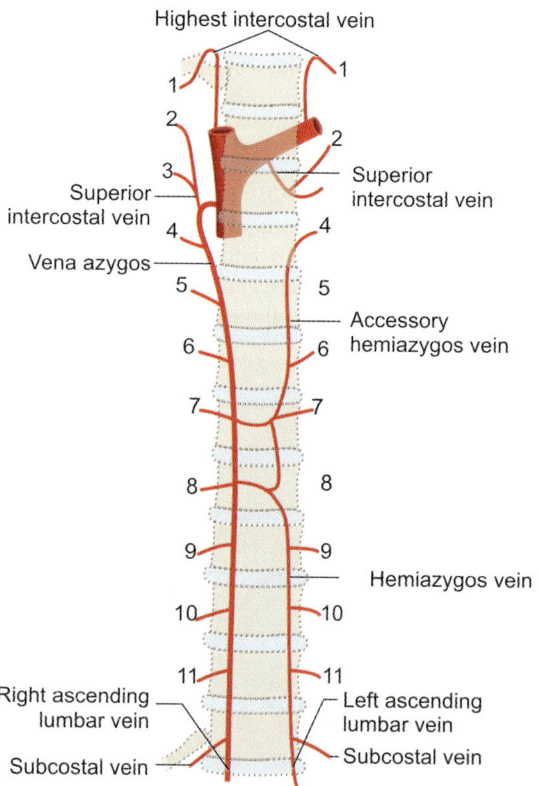

Scheme to show formation of azygos vein 1 to 11— intercostal veins.

228. Medial border of Hesselbach's triangle is formed by:

a. Conjoint tendon
b. Rectus sheath
c. Inferior epigastric artery
d. Linea alba

Hesselbach's traingle

- Medial border: Lateral margin of the rectus sheath, also called linea semilunaris
- Superolateral border: Inferior epigastric vessels
- Inferior border: Inguinal ligament, sometimes referred to as Poupart's ligament.

229. NOT a component of urogenital diaphragm:

a. Superficial fascia of urogenital diaphragm
b. Deep transverse perineii
c. Sphincter urethrae
d. Superficial transverse perineii

The urogenital diaphragm, which is pierced by the urethra, consists of two muscles bilaterally: the deep transverse perineal and the sphincter urethrae. It lies between the inferior fascia of the urogenital diaphragm (perineal membrane) and superior fascia of the urogenital diaphragm.

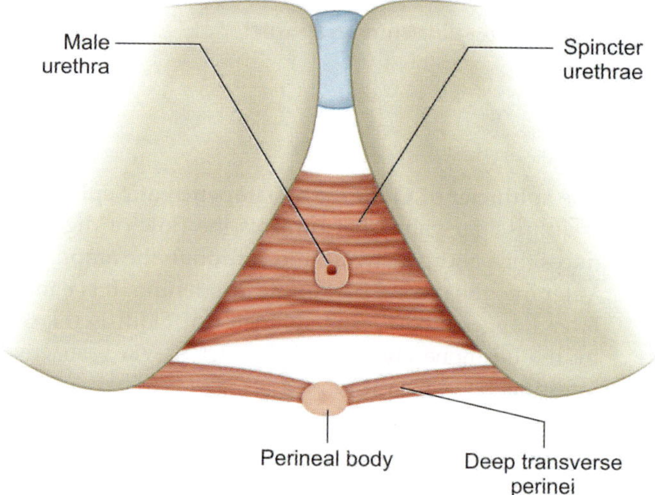

Muscles present in deep perineal space (as seen in the males)

230. Internal spermatic fascia is derived from:

a. External oblique aponeurosis
b. Internal oblique fascia
c. Fascia transversalis
d. All of the above

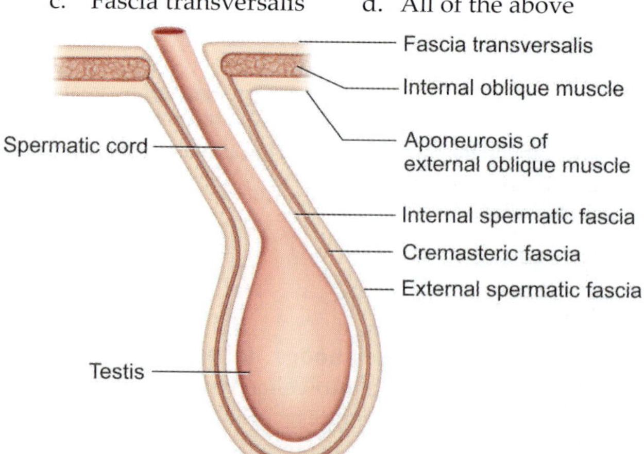

Schematic diagram to show coverings of the spermatic cord and of the testis.

Ans. 226. d. Median lobe... 227. a. Superior vena cava 228. b. Rectus sheath 229. d. Superficial transverse... 230. c. Fascia transversalis

The **internal spermatic fascia (infundibuliform fascia) (Le deuxieme fascia de Webster)** is a thin layer, which loosely invests the cord; it is a continuation downward of the transversalis fascia.

231. NOT a constituent of spermatic cord:

a. Ductus deferens b. Testicular artery
c. Ilioinguinal nerve d. None

Ilioinguinal nerve pierces the internal oblique muscle, distributing filaments to it, and then accompanies (NOT a component) the spermatic cord through the superficial inguinal ring.

232. Does NOT form the stomach bed:

a. Left kidney b. Spleen
c. Transverse mesocolon d. Left lobe of liver

Structures forming stomach bed include the pancreas, spleen (sometimes), left kidney, left suprarenal gland, transverse colon (splenic flexure) and its mesocolon, splenic artery and the diaphragm.

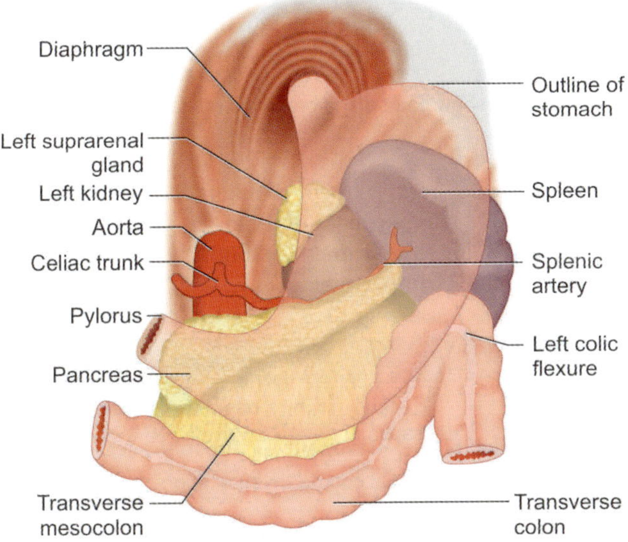

Scheme to show the structures forming the stomach bed. Note that the spleen is separated from the stomach by the gastrosplenic ligament, and is really related to the 'anterior' surface. The remaining structures are separated from the posterior surface of the stomach by the lesser sac.

233. Structure passing through lesser sciatic notch:

a. Tendon of obturator internus
b. Superior gluteal vessels
c. Superior gluteal nerve
d. Inferior gluteal nerve

Lesser sciatic notch is converted into a foramen, the lesser sciatic foramen, by the sacrotuberous and sacrospinous ligaments, and transmits the tendon of the Obturator internus, the nerve which supplies that muscle, and the internal pudendal vessels and pudendal nerve.

234. Lateral wall of ischiorectal fossa is formed by all EXCEPT:

a. Levator ani b. Obturator internus
c. Ischial tuberosity d. Obturator fascia

Levator ani forms the medial wall & superior boundary of ischiorectal fossa.

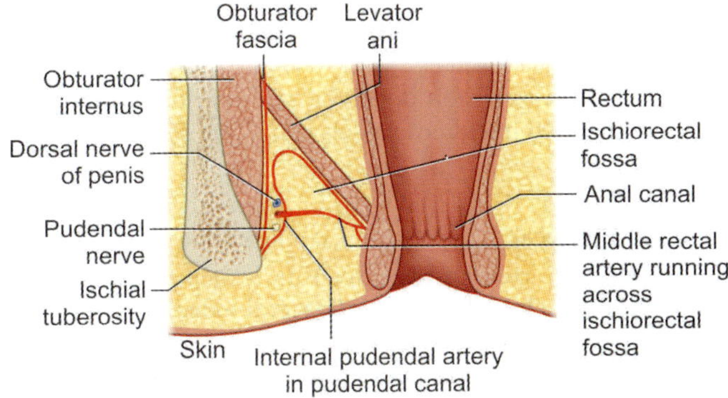

Section through the ischiorectal fossa and the pudendal canal.

235. Transpyloric plane passes through all EXCEPT:

a. 2nd part of duodenum
b. Hilum of both kidneys
c. Spleen
d. Fundus of the stomach

Stomach parts and vertebral levels

- The cardia of the stomach is at the level of the 10th rib
- The fundus of the stomach is in the 5th intercostal space, slightly below the apex of the heart
- Pylorus is usually at the L1 (the transpyloric plane).

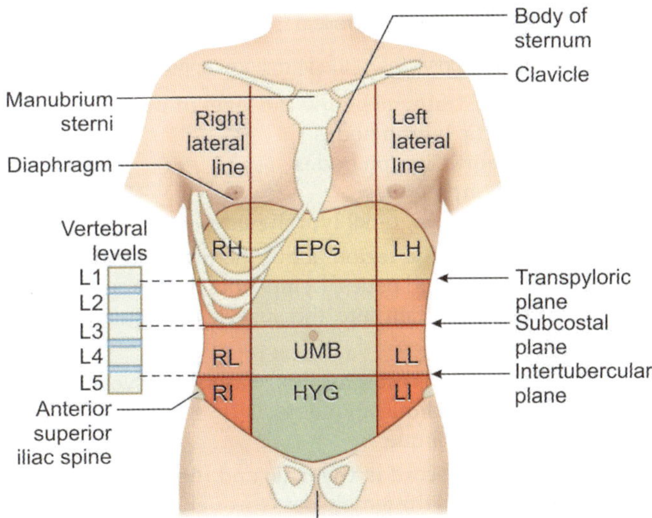

Regions of the abdomen and the lines demarcating them.

236. Organ WITHOUT hilum:

a. Ovary b. Spleen
c. Liver d. Lung

The **hilum** (formerly called **hilus**) is a depression or fissure where structures such as blood vessels and nerves enter an organ. Examples include:

Ans. 231. **c.** Ilioinguinal... 232. **d.** Left lobe of liver 233. **a.** Tendon of obturator 234. **a.** Levator ani
235. **d.** Fundus of... 236. **c.** Liver

- Hilum of kidney, admits the renal artery, vein, ureter, and nerves
- Splenic hilum, on the surface of the spleen, admits the splenic artery, vein, lymph vessels, and nerves
- Hilum of lung, a triangular depression where the structures which form the root of the lung enter and leave the viscus
- Hilum of lymph node, the portion of a lymph node where the efferent vessels exit.

237. MC position of appendix:

a. Pelvic b. Retrocecal
c. Subcecal d. Promontoric

While the base of the appendix is at a fairly constant location—2 cm below the ileocecal valve, the tip of the appendix can be variably located—in the pelvis, outside the peritoneum or behind the cecum/retrocecal (74%).

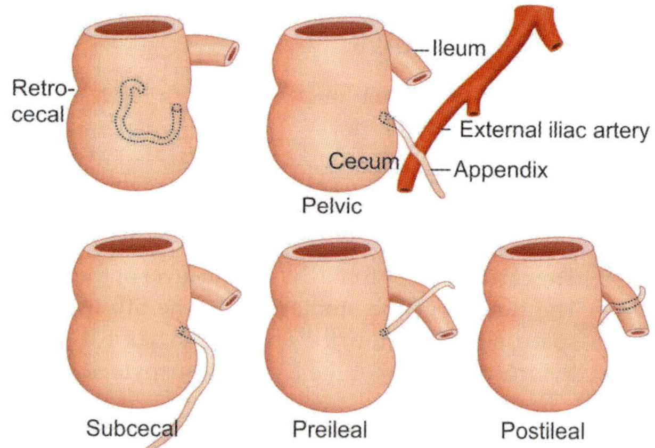

Various positions of the vermiform appendix.

238. Lymphatic drainage below the level of umbilicus:

a. Preaortic lymph nodes
b. Para-aortic lymph nodes
c. Iliac lymph nodes
d. Superficial inguinal lymph nodes

Lymphatics in the region above the umbilicus drain into the axillary lymph nodes. Lymphatics in the region below the umbilicus drain into the superficial inguinal nodes.

239. Deep inguinal ring is a defect in:

a. Transversalis muscle b. Fascia transversalis
c. External oblique aponeurosis
d. Internal oblique

The spermatic cord in the male and the round ligament of the uterus in the female pass through the transversalis fascia at a spot called the deep inguinal ring. This opening is not visible externally, since the transversalis fascia is prolonged on these structures as the internal spermatic fascia.

240. Uterine artery is a branch of:

a. Posterior division of Internal Iliac artery
b. Anterior division of Internal Iliac artery
c. External Iliac artery
d. Abdominal aorta

Uterine artery

Source	Anterior division of Internal iliac artery (i.e. hypogastric artery)
Vein	Uterine veins
Supplies	Round ligament of the uterus, ovary, uterus, vagina, uterine tube

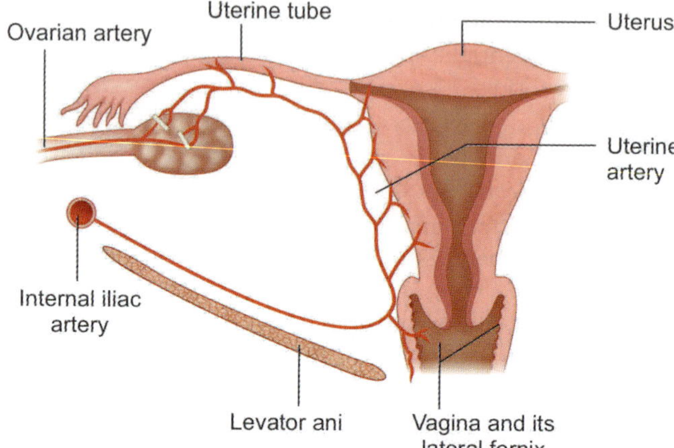

Scheme to show course and branches of the uterine artery.

241. Obturator nerve is the main nerve of:

a. Anterior compartment of thigh
b. Medial compartment of thigh
c. Posterior compartment of thigh
d. All the 3 compartments

Obturator nerve

From	*Lumbar plexus L2-L4*
To	Posterior branch of obturator nerve, anterior branch of obturator nerve
Innervates	Medial compartment of thigh

242. Inferior mesenteric artery supplies:

a. Right 2/3rd of transverse colon
b. Left 1/3rd of transverse colon
c. Jejunum d. Ileum

The **inferior mesenteric artery/IMA**, is the third main branch of the abdominal aorta and arises at the level of L3, supplying the large intestine from the left colic (or splenic) flexure to the upper part of the rectum, which includes the descending colon, the sigmoid colon, and part of the rectum. Proximally, its territory of distribution overlaps (forms a watershed) with the middle colic artery, and therefore the superior mesenteric artery. The SMA and IMA anastomose via the marginal artery of the colon (artery of Drummond) and via Riolan's arcade (also called the 'meandering artery', an arterial connection between the left colic artery and the medial colic artery). The territory of distribution of the IMA is more or less equivalent to the embryonic hindgut.

Ans. 237. **b.** Retrocecal 238. **d.** Superficial... 239. **b.** Fascia... 240. **b.** Anterior...
241. **b.** Medial comp... 242. **b.** Left 1/3rd...

243. Colle's fascia is:

a. Superficial fascia of urogenital region
b. Deep fascia of urogenital region
c. Superficial fascia of kidney
d. Deep fascia of kidney

The **fascia of Colle** is the deeper membranous layer of the superficial perineal fascia. Colle's fascia emerges from the perineal membrane, which divides the base of the penis from t he prostate.

244. Paraduodenal recess is associated with which vessel:

a. Superior mesenteric artery
b. Inferior mesenteric artery
c. Superior mesenteric vein
d. Inferior mesenteric vein

The peritoneum is a serous sac which lines the abdominal cavity and is reflected over the viscera to invest them partially or completely. Duodenum has four parts. The fourth part of the duodenum is related to a number of recesses in the peritoneum known as the peritoneal recesses. They are the superior recess, inferior recess, retro and paraduodenal recesses namely. Paraduodenal recess is a blind sac on the left side and its opening is directed towards the right. Anteriorly, the opening is bounded by the paraduodenal fold which contains the inferior mesenteric vein.

245. Right gastroepiploic artery is a branch of:

a. Splenic artery b. Celiac trunk
c. Abdominal aorta d. Gastroduodenal artery

The **right gastroepiploic artery** (or **right gastro-omental artery**) is one of the two terminal branches of the gastroduodenal artery. It runs from right to left along the greater curvature of the stomach, between the layers of the greater omentum, anastomosing with the left gastroepiploic artery, a branch of the splenic artery.

246. NOT a boundary of foramen of Winslow:

a. Caudate lobe of liver
b. Inferior vena cava
c. 4th part of duodenum
d. Free border of lesser omentum

Borders of foramen of Winslow

- *Anterior*: The free border of the lesser omentum, known as the hepatoduodenal ligament. This has two layers and within these layers are the common bile duct, hepatic artery, and hepatic portal vein. A useful mnemonic to remember these is DAVE: Duct, Artery, Vein, Epiploic foramen.
- *Posterior*: The peritoneum covering the inferior vena cava.
- *Superior*: The peritoneum covering the caudate lobe of the liver.
- *Inferior*: The peritoneum covering the commencement of the duodenum and the hepatic artery, the latter passing forward below the foramen before ascending between the two layers of the lesser omentum.
- *Left lateral*: Gastrosplenic ligament and splenorenal ligament.

247. All of the following forms visceral relations of the spleen EXCEPT:

a. Fundus of stomach b. Duodenum
c. Left kidney d. Splenic flexure of colon

The visceral surface of spleen is related to the fundus of the stomach, the anterior surface of the left kidney, the splenic flexure of the colon and the tail of the pancreas.

HEAD, NECK AND CRANIAL NERVES

248. All of the following structure passes through superior orbital fissure EXCEPT:

a. Nasociliary nerve b. Lacrimal nerve
c. Trigeminal nerve d. Inferior ophthalmic vein

Trigeminal nerve has a large sensory root and a smaller motor root. The roots cross the apex of the petrous temporal bone beneath the superior petrosal sinus to enter middle cranial fossa

Structure passing through superior orbital fissure

- A number of important anatomical structures pass through the fissure, and these can be damaged in orbital trauma, particularly blowout fractures through the floor of the orbit into the maxillary sinus. These structures are:
  - Superior and inferior divisions of oculomotor nerve (III)
  - Trochlear nerve (IV)
  - Lacrimal, frontal and nasociliary branches of ophthalmic (V_1).
  - Abducens nerve (VI)
  - Superior and inferior divisions of ophthalmic vein. Inferior division also passes through the inferior orbital fissure.
  - Sympathetic fibers from cavernous plexus

The nerves passing through the fissure can be remembered with the mnemonic, "**L**ive **F**rankly **T**o **S**ee **A**bsolutely **N**o **I**nsult" - for **L**acrimal, **F**rontal, **T**rochlear, **S**uperior Division of Oculomotor, **A**bducens, **N**asociliary and **I**nferior Division of Oculomotor nerve.

It is divided into 3 parts from lateral to medial:

- *Lateral part transmits:* Lacrimal nerve, frontal nerve, trochlear nerve, meningeal branch of lacrimal artery, anastomotic branch of middle meningeal artery which anastomoses with recurrent branch of the lacrimal artery
- *Middle part transmits:* Upper and lower divisions of the oculomotor nerve, nasociliary nerve between the two divisions of oculomotor nerve and abducent nerve.
- *Medial part transmits:* Superior ophthalmic vein and sympathetic nerves from the plexus around internal carotid artery.

Ans. 243. **a.** Superficial... 244. **d.** Inferior... 245. **d.** Gastroduodenal... 246. **c.** 4th part of...
247. **b.** Duodenum 248. **c.** Trigeminal nerve

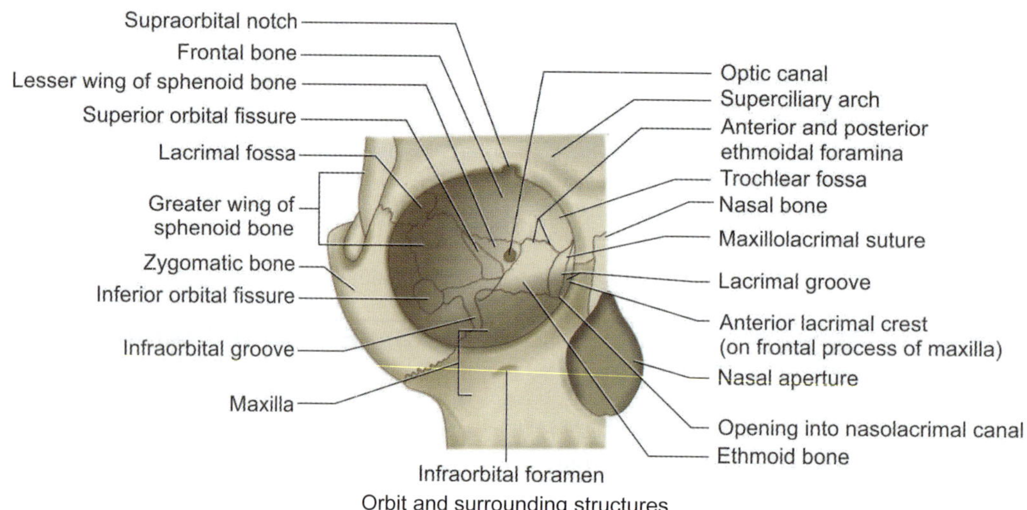

Orbit and surrounding structures

249. Which of the following is the common site of facial nerve injury?

a. Brainstem
b. Parotid gland
c. Temporal bone
d. Neck of mandible

Facial nerve

- The motor part of the facial nerve arises from the facial nerve nucleus in the pons while the sensory and parasympathetic parts of the facial nerve arise from the nervus intermedius.
- Upon reaching the temporal bone, the nerve's path can be divided into the internal auditory canal, labyrinthine segment, intratympanic segment, and descending or vertical segment.
- The labyrinthine segment is the narrowest portion of this pathway and is described to be approximately 0.7 mm in diameter.
- The descending segment is the area where the branches of the chorda tympani and nerve to the stapedius branch from the facial nerve.
- The facial nerve eventually exits via the stylomastoid foramen to enter into the parotid where it branches into its peripheral segments.

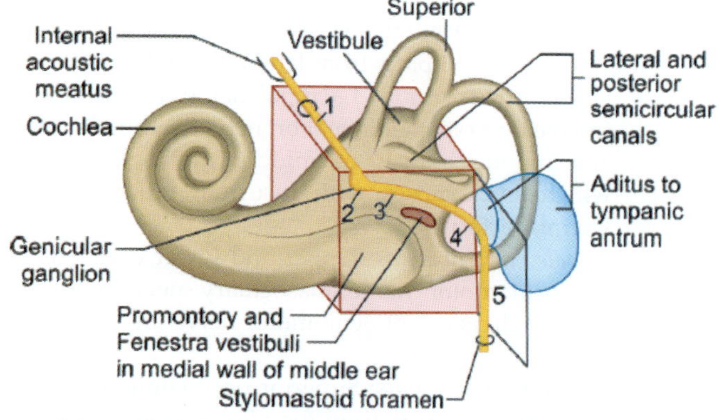

Scheme to show the course of facial nerve within the petrous temporal bone

250. Largest cranial nerve is:

a. Cranial nerve III
b. Cranial nerve IV
c. Cranial nerve V
d. Cranial nerve X

The largest of the cranial nerves, its name ('trigeminal' = *tri-*, or three and *-geminus*, or twin; thrice-twinned) derives from the fact that each trigeminal nerve (one on each side of the pons) has three major branches: the ophthalmic nerve (V_1), the maxillary nerve (V_2), and the mandibular nerve (V_3). The ophthalmic and maxillary nerves are purely sensory, and the mandibular nerve has sensory (or 'cutaneous') and motor functions.

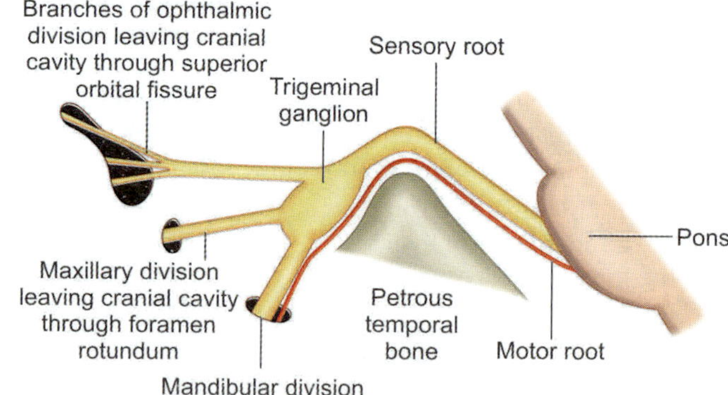

Roots and divisions of trigeminal nerve.

251. Does NOT pass through optic foramen:

a. Ophthalmic nerve
b. Optic nerve
c. Ophthalmic artery
d. Dura mater

Ophthalmic nerve is the smallest of the three divisions of the trigeminal, and arises from the upper part of the trigeminal ganglion as a short, flattened band, about 2.5 cm long, which passes forward along the lateral wall of the cavernous sinus, below the oculomotor and trochlear nerves; just before entering the orbit, through the superior orbital fissure, it divides into three branches, lacrimal, frontal, and nasociliary.

Ans. **249. c.** Temporal bone **250. c.** Cranial nerve... **251. a.** Ophthalmic...

252. Structure passing through foramen spinosum:

a. Meningeal branch of Mandibular nerve
b. Middle meningeal artery
c. Emissary veins
d. All of the above

The middle meningeal artery, middle meningeal vein, and the meningeal branch of the mandibular nerve pass through the foramen spinosum.

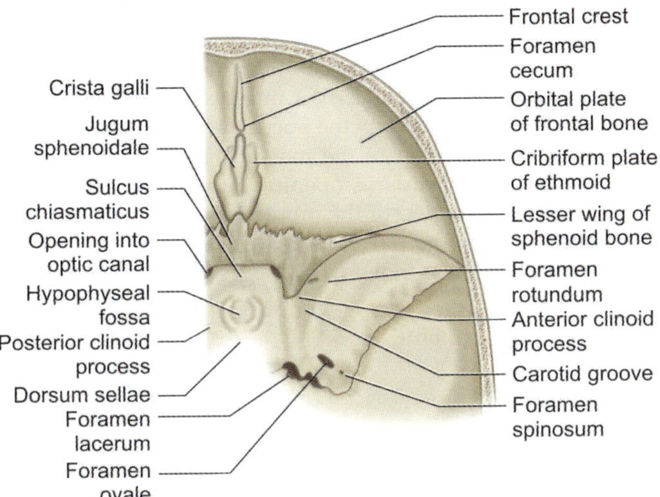

Parts of the anterior and middle cranial fossae.

253. NOT supplied by hypoglossal nerve:

a. Hyoglossus
b. Styloglossus
c. Genioglossus
d. Palatoglossus

Palatoglossus is the only muscle of the tongue that is *not* innervated by the hypoglossal nerve (CN XII). It is innervated by the cranial part of the accessory nerve through the pharyngeal plexus.

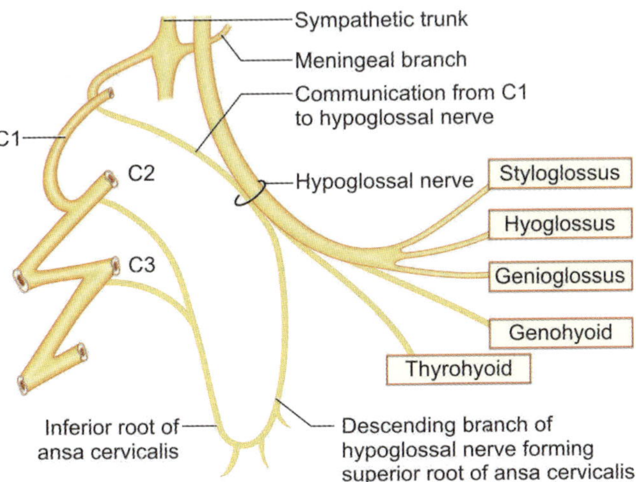

Scheme to show the distribution of the hypoglossal nerve.

254. Nerve carrying taste sensations from posterior 1/3rd of tongue:

a. Vagus
b. Lingual
c. Chorda tympani
d. Glossopharyngeal

Functions of the glossopharyngeal nerve

- It receives general sensory fibers (ventral trigemino-thalamic tract) from the tonsils, the pharynx, the middle ear and the posterior 1/3 of the tongue.
- It receives special sensory fibers (taste) from the posterior one-third of the tongue.
- It receives visceral sensory fibers from the carotid bodies, carotid sinus.
- It supplies parasympathetic fibers to the parotid gland via the otic ganglion.
- It supplies motor fibers to stylopharyngeus muscle, the only motor component of this cranial nerve.
- It contributes to the pharyngeal plexus.

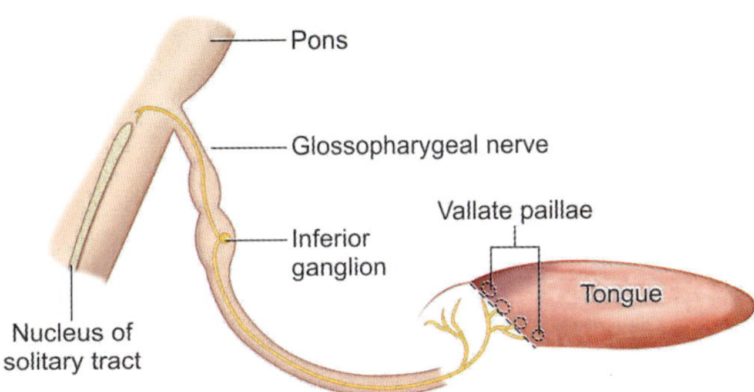

Pathway for taste from the posterior one-third of tongue.

255. Does NOT arise from external carotid artery:

a. Superior thyroid artery
b. Inferior thyroid artery
c. Facial artery
d. Maxillary artery

Inferior thyroid artery arises from the thyrocervical trunk and passes upward, in front of the vertebral artery and longus colli muscle.

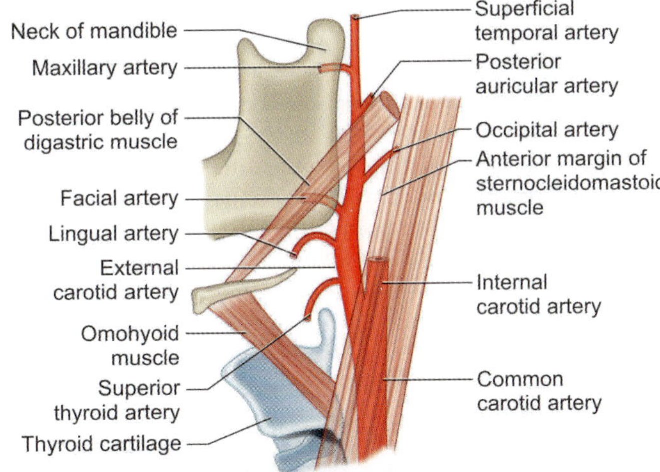

Scheme to show the landmarks to which the external carotid artery and its branches are related—the boundaries of the carotid triangle are shown.

256. Facial nerve supplies:

a. 1st pharyngeal arch
b. 2nd pharyngeal arch
c. 3rd pharyngeal arch
d. 4th pharyngeal arch

Ans. 252. **d.** All of the... 253. **d.** Palatoglossus 254. **d.** Glossopharyngeal 255. **b.** Inferior thyroid artery 256. **b.** 2nd pharyngeal arch

Pharyngeal arches and nerve supply

1st	Trigeminal nerve (part of V_2 and V_3)
2nd	Facial nerve
3rd	Glossopharyngeal nerve
4th	Vagus, superior laryngeal nerve
6th	Vagus, recurrent laryngeal nerve

257. NOT supplied by cranial part of accessory nerve:

a. Tensor veli palati b. Tensor veli tympani
c. Palatopharyngeus d. Palatoglossus

Tensor palati

Origin	Medial pterygoid plate of the sphenoid bone (scaphoid fossa)
Insertion	Palatine aponeurosis
Nerve	Medial pterygoid of mandibular nerve (V_3)
Actions	Tension of the soft palate

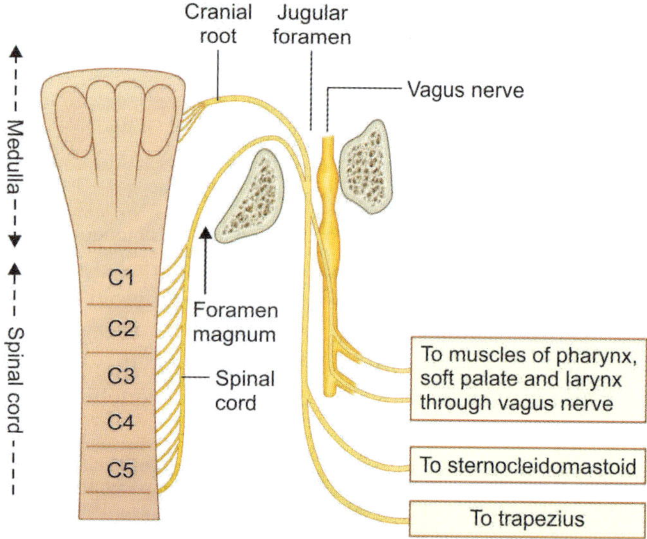

Scheme to show the formation and distribution of accessory nerve.

258. All are tributaries of cavernous sinus EXCEPT:

a. Superficial middle cerebral veins
b. Superior petrosal sinus
c. Inferior ophthalmic vein
d. Sphenoparietal sinus

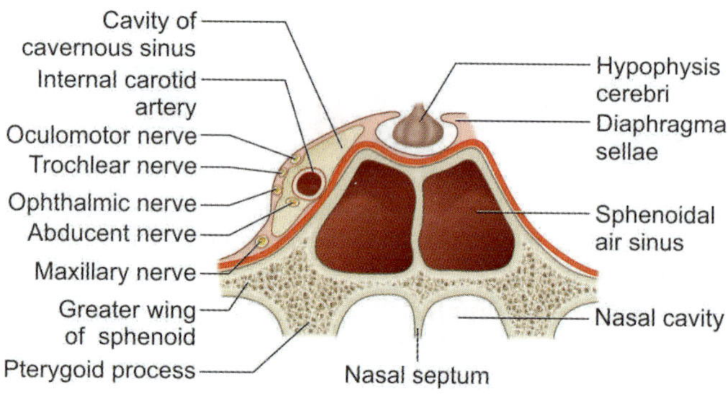

Coronal section through cavernous sinus to show its relations.

The **superior petrosal sinus** is a venous structure located beneath the brain. It receives blood from the cavernous sinus and passes backward and laterally to drain into the transverse sinus.

259. Parotid duct does NOT pass through:

a. Masseterb.Buccal pad of fat
c. Buccinator
d. Buccopharyngeal fascia

The parotid duct is formed when several interlobular ducts—the largest ducts inside the parotid gland—join. It emerges from the gland and runs forward along the lateral side of the masseter muscle. In this course, the duct is surrounded by the buccal fat pad. It takes a steep turn at the border of the masseter and passes through the buccinator muscle, opening into the vestibule of the mouth, the region of the mouth between the cheek and the gums, at the parotid papilla, which lays across the second superior molar tooth.

260. All of the following cranial nerves pass through jugular foramen EXCEPT:

a. 9th b. 10th
c. 11th d. 12th

The hypoglossal nerve arises from the hypoglossal nucleus of the caudal brain stem emerging from the ventromedial medulla oblongata from a number of smaller rootlets in the preolivary sulcus separating the *olive* and the *pyramid*. After passing through the subarachnoid space the nerve then exits the skull-base of the posterior fossa through the hypoglossal canal.

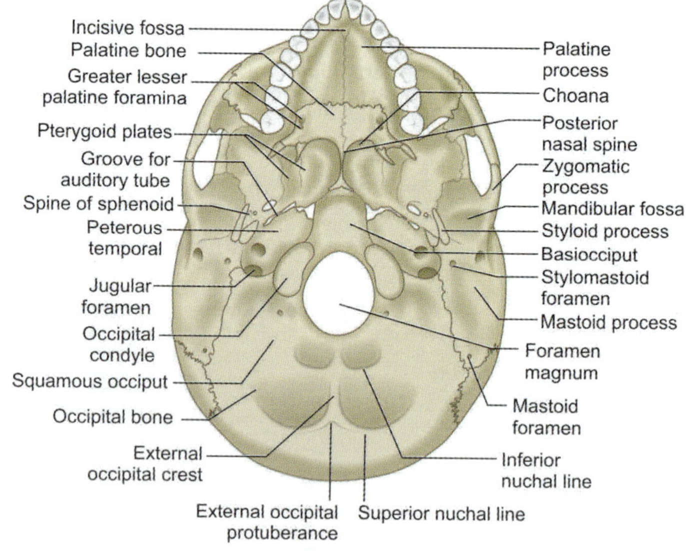

Primary features of base of skull.

261. Structure passing through foramen magnum include all EXCEPT:

a. Spinal accessory nerve b. Spinal cord
c. Vertebral artery d. Vertebral venous plexus

Apart from the transmission of the medulla oblongata (which continue as spinal cord) and its membranes,

Ans. 257. a. Tensor veli... 258. b. Superior petrosal... 259. a. Masseter 260. d. 12th
261. b. Spinal cord

the foramen magnum transmits the vertebral arteries, the anterior and posterior spinal arteries, the tectorial membranes and alar ligaments. It also transmits the spinal component of the accessory nerve into the skull.

262. Sensory supply of the palate is through all of the following EXCEPT:
a. Facial nerve
b. Hypoglossal nerve
c. Glossopharyngeal nerve
d. Maxillary division of trigeminal nerve

The hypoglossal nerve carries axons of general somatic efferent (GSE) type, providing motor control of the extrinsic muscles of the tongue; genioglossus, hyoglossus, styloglossus, and the intrinsic muscles of the tongue.

263. Waldeyer's ring is formed by all EXCEPT:
a. Palatine tonsils
b. Pharyngeal tonsils
c. Tubal tonsils
d. Postauricular nodes

Waldeyer's ring (from superior to inferior)

- 1 (or two) pharyngeal tonsils (or nasopharyngeal tonsil(s), due to the location; also known as 'adenoid(s)' when inflamed/swollen). They are located on the roof of the nasopharynx, under the sphenoid bone.
- 2 tubal tonsils (bilaterally, where each Eustachian tube opens into the nasopharynx) (Usually develops from an accumulation of lymphoid tissue in the pharyngeal tonsil).
- 2 palatine tonsils (commonly called 'the tonsils' in the vernacular, less commonly termed 'faucial tonsils'; located in the oropharynx; also see tonsillitis and tonsillectomy).
- 1 (or many) lingual tonsils (on the posterior tongue).

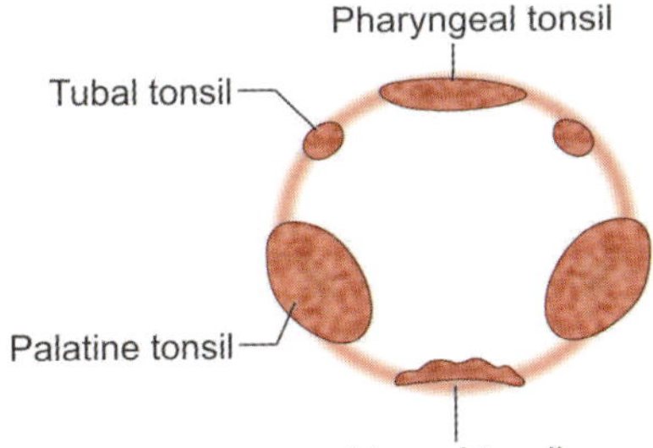

Waldeyer's ring of lymphoid tissue.

264. Does NOT lie within the substance of parotid gland:
a. Facial nerve
b. Facial artery
c. Retromandibular vein
d. External carotid artery

The facial artery arises in the carotid triangle from the external carotid artery a little above the lingual artery and sheltered by the ramus of the mandible, passes obliquely up beneath the digastric and stylohyoid muscles, over which it arches to enter a groove on the posterior surface of the submandibular gland. It then curves upward over the body of the mandible at the anteroinferior angle of the masseter; passes forward and upward across the cheek to the angle of the mouth, then ascends along the side of the nose, and ends at the medial commissure of the eye, under the name of the angular artery.

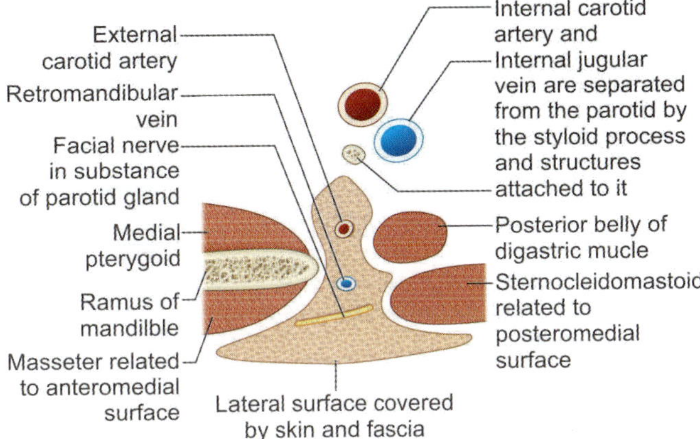

Schematic transverse section through parotid gland to show its relations.

265. Does NOT pierce buccinator muscle:
a. Buccal branch of mandibular nerve
b. Parotid duct
c. Mucus gland of buccopharyngeal fascia
d. Buccal branch of facial nerve

Structures piercing buccinator

Parotid duct (Stenson's duct)
Molar glands of cheeks
Buccal branch of mandibular nerve.

266. Delphi node is another name for:
a. Posterior triangle nodes
b. Supraclavicular nodes
c. Pretracheal nodes
d. Paratracheal nodes

The **Delphian node** (prelaryngeal) along with paratracheal nodes, pretracheal nodes, perithyroidal nodes make up level VI.

267. Involvement of cranial nerve VIII will affect:
a. Smell
b. Touch
c. Taste
d. Equilibrium

The vestibulocochlear nerve carries axons of type SSA, special somatic afferent, which carry the modalities of hearing and equilibrium.

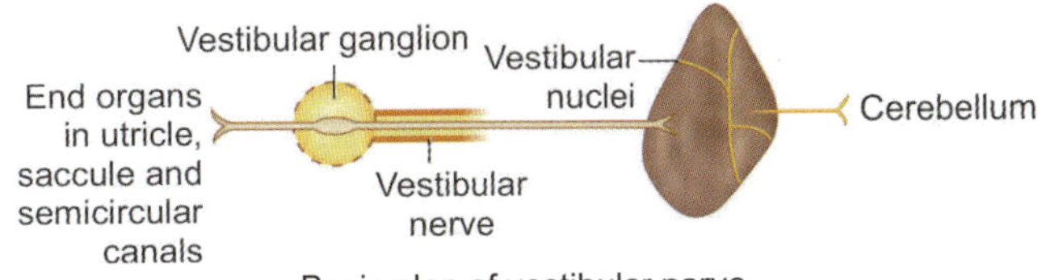

Basic plan of vestibular nerve.

Ans. 262. **b.** Hypoglossal... 263. **d.** Postauricular nodes 264. **b.** Facial artery 265. **d.** Buccal branch of facial... 266. **c.** Pretracheal... 267. **d.** Equilibrium

268. NOT supplied by facial nerve:

a. Parotid gland
b. Posterior belly of digastric
c. Platysma
d. Submandibular gland

Parotid gland

Artery	Transverse facial artery (External carotid artery)
Vein	External jugular vein
Nerve	Glossopharyngeal nerve (IX) otic ganglion
Lymph	Preauricular deep parotid lymph nodes

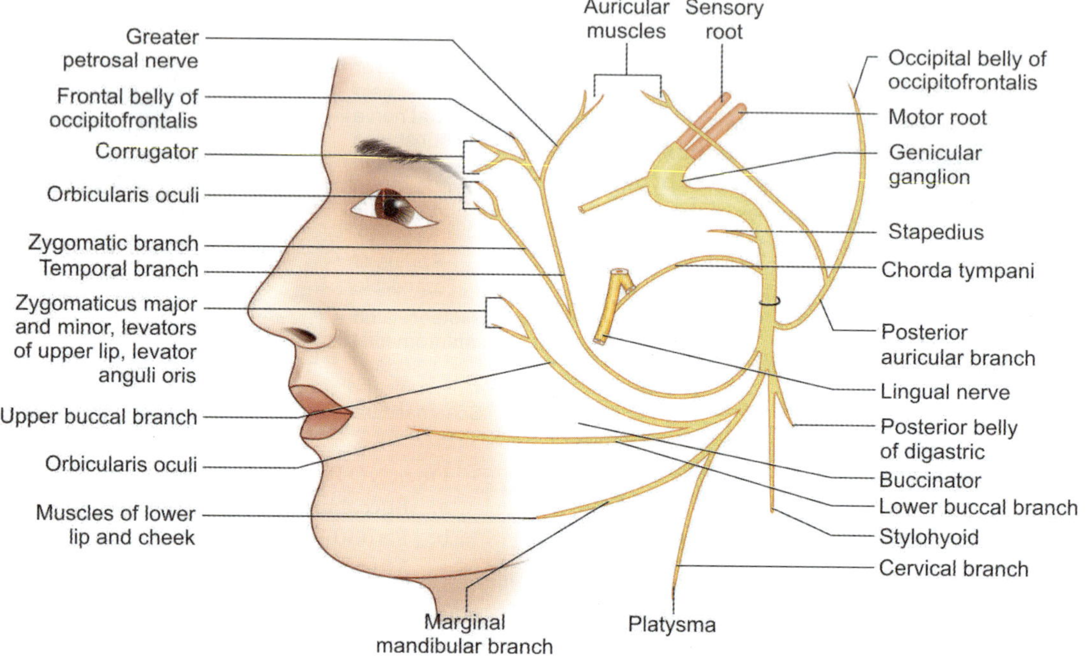

Scheme to show the branches of the facial nerve.

269. NOT a terminal branch of facial nerve:

a. Cervical b. Marginal
c. Mandibular d. Temporal

The **mandibular nerve** (V_3) is the largest of the three branches or divisions of the trigeminal nerve, the fifth (V) cranial nerve.

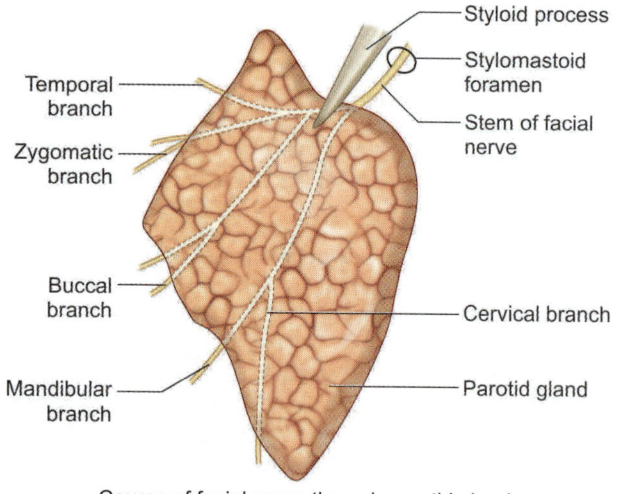

Course of facial nerve through parotid gland.

270. Which bone contributes maximum information of roof of mouth:

a. Palatine
b. Sphenoid
c. Zygomatic
d. Maxillary

Maxilla assists in forming the boundaries of:

- The roof of the mouth
- The floor and lateral wall of the nasal antrum
- The wall of the orbit.

271. NOT supplied by hypoglossal nerve:

a. Palatoglossus
b. Styloglossus
c. Hyoglossus
d. Genioglossus

Palatoglossus

Origin	*Palatine aponeurosis*
Insertion	Tongue
Nerve	Cranial accessory nerve (via pharyngeal branch to pharyngeal plexus)
Actions	Raising the back part of the tongue

Ans. **268. a.** Parotid gland **269. c.** Mandibular **270. d.** Maxillary **271. a.** Palatoglossus

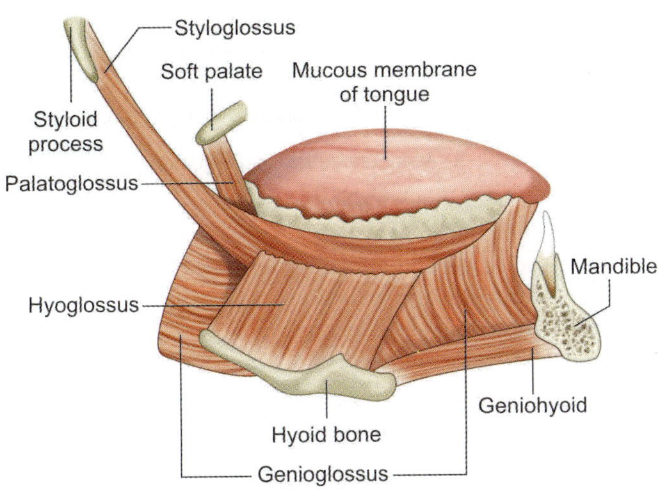

Extrinsic muscles of tongue.

272. In a patient presenting with epistaxis, external carotid artery was ligated but still the patient was bleeding. Source of epistaxis in such a case:

a. Greater palatine artery
b. Facial artery
c. Sphenopalatine artery
d. Anterior ethmoidal artery

Anterior ethmoidal artery arises from ophthalmic artery, a branch of internal carotid artery.

273. Level of mid-tracheostomy:

a. Tracheal rings 1 and 2
b. Tracheal rings 2 and 3
c. Tracheal rings 3 and 4
d. Tracheal rings 4 and 5

A mid-tracheostomy is the preferred one and is done through the II or III rings and would entail division of the thyroid isthmus or its retraction upwards or downwards to expose this part of trachea.

274. Nerve supply to mandible is through:

a. C2, C3 b. C5, C6
c. C7, C8 d. T1, T2

The mandibular nerve (V_3) carries sensory information from the lower lip, the lower teeth and gums, the chin and jaw (except the angle of the jaw, which is supplied by C2, C3), parts of the external ear and parts of the meninges.

275. Intrinsic laryngeal muscles are supplied by:

a. External laryngeal nerve
b. Internal laryngeal nerve
c. Recurrent laryngeal nerve
d. Inferior laryngeal nerve

The **recurrent laryngeal nerve** (RLN) is a branch of the vagus nerve (cranial nerve X) that supplies all the intrinsic muscles of the larynx, with the exception of the cricothyroid muscles (supplied by external laryngeal nerve).

276. Muscle which helps in opening of the mouth:

a. Lateral pterygoid b. Medial pterygoid
c. Temporalis d. Masseter

Lateral pterygoid

Origin	Great wing of sphenoid and pterygoid plate
Insertion	Condyloid process of the mandible
Artery	Pterygoid branches of maxillary artery
Nerve	Lateral pterygoid nerve from the mandibular nerve
Actions	Depresses mandible (opening of mouth), protrude mandible, side-to-side movement of mandible

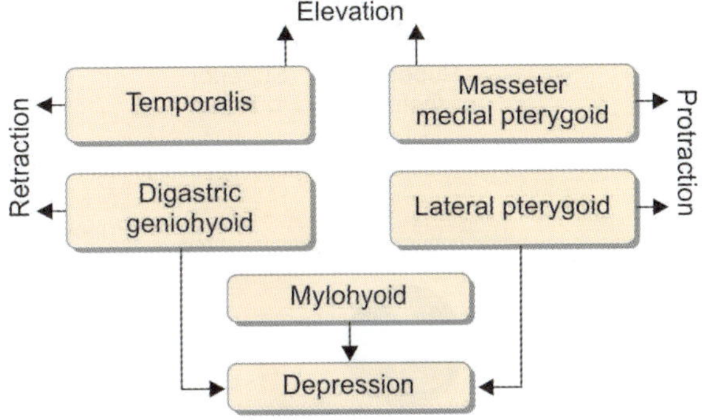

Scheme to show the muscles responsible for movements at the temporomandibular joint.

277. Abductor of vocal cord:

a. Oblique arytenoid b. Transverse arytenoid
c. Lateral thyroarytenoid d. Posterior cricoarytenoid

The cricoarytenoid muscles are the only muscles to open the vocal cords. By rotating the arytenoid cartilages laterally, these muscles abduct the vocal cords and thereby open the rima glottidis.

278. Muscle supplied by glossopharyngeal nerve:

a. Platysma b. Stylopharyngeus
c. Styloglossus d. Genioglossus

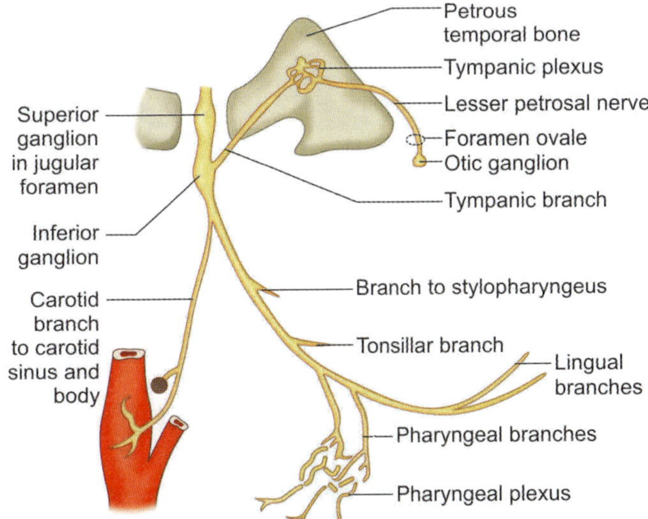

Branches of glossopharyngeal nerve.

Ans. 272. **d.** Anterior... 273. **b.** Tracheal rings 2 and 3 274. **a.** C2, C3 275. **c.** Recurrent...
276. **a.** Lateral pterygoid 277. **d.** Posterior crico... 278. **b.** Stylopharyngeus

Stylopharyngeus

Precursor	3rd branchial arch
Origin	Styloid process (temporal)
Insertion	Thyroid cartilage (larynx)
Nerve	Glossopharyngeal nerve (CN IX)
Actions	Elevate the larynx, elevate the pharynx, swallowing

279. Lateral rectus is supplied by:

a. III cranial nerve b. IV cranial nerve
c. V cranial nerve d. VI cranial nerve

Nerve supply of extraocular muscles: SO_4, LR_6, rest by 3

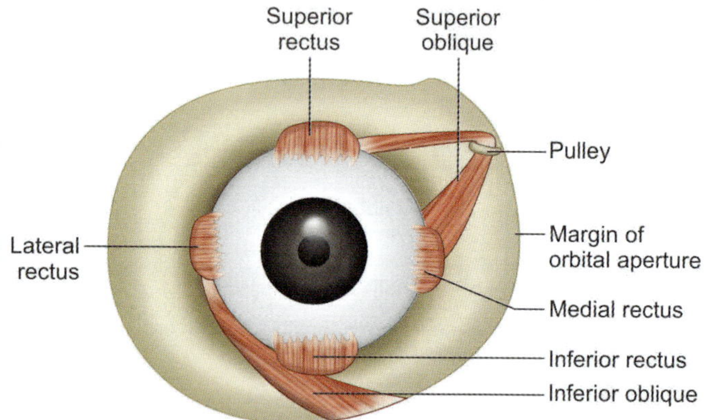

Schematic anterior view of the orbit to show the attachments of extraocular muscles to the eyeball. Particularly note the arrangement of the superior and inferior oblique muscles.

280. Muscle which dilates the palpebral aperture:

a. Orbicularis oculi
b. Orbicularis oris
c. Levator palpebrae superioris
d. Levator labii superioris

Levator palpebrae superioris

Origin	Sphenoid bone
Insertion	Tarsal plate, upper eyelid
Artery	Ophthalmic artery, superior ophthalmic vein
Nerve	Oculomotor nerve
Actions	Retracts/elevates eyelid
Antagonist	Orbicularis oculi muscle

281. Action of ciliary muscle:

a. Constriction of pupil b. Dilatation of pupil
c. Change in shape of lens d. All of the above

Ciliary muscle

Origin	1. Longitudinal fibers → scleral spur; 2) circular fibers → encircle root of iris
Insertion	1. Longitudinal fibers → ciliary process 2. Circular fibers → encircle root of iris
Artery	Long posterior ciliary arteries
Vein	Vorticose vein
Nerve	Short ciliary From oculomotor nerve Through ciliary ganglion
Actions	1) Accommodation, 2) Regulation of trabecular meshwork pore size

282. Action of superior rectus:

a. Abduction and intortion
b. Adduction and extortion
c. Adduction and intortion
d. Abduction and extortion

Superior rectus

Origin	Annulus of Zinn at the orbital apex
Insertion	7.5 mm superior to the limbus
Nerve	Oculomotor nerve
Actions	Elevates, intorsion, and rotates medially the eye

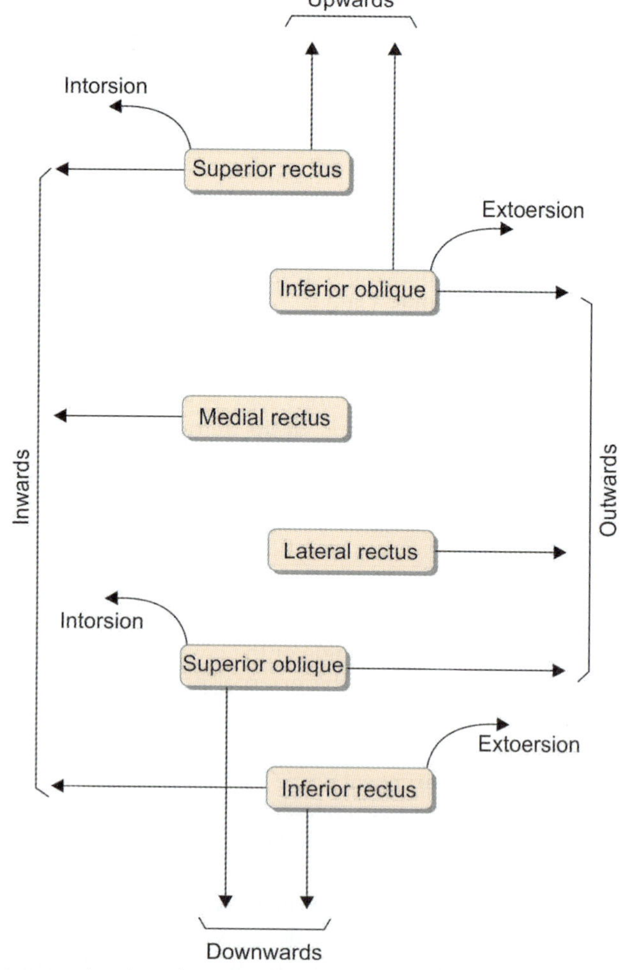

Scheme showing the movements of the eyeball produced by individual extraocular muscles, and the muscles responsible for each movement.

Ans. 279. d. VI cranial nerve 280. c. Levator palpebrae... 281. c. Change in shape... 282. c. Adduction and intortion

283. Suboccipital nerve is derived from:

a. C1 b. C2
c. C3 d. C1, 2, 3, 4

The **suboccipital nerve** is the dorsal primary ramus of the first cervical nerve (C1). It exits the spinal cord between the skull and the first cervical vertebra, the atlas.

284. Only nerve, which emerge from dorsal side:

a. III cranial nerve b. IV cranial nerve
c. V cranial nerve d. VI cranial nerve

The trochlear nerve emerges from the dorsal aspect of the brainstem at the level of the caudal mesencephalon, just below the inferior colliculus.

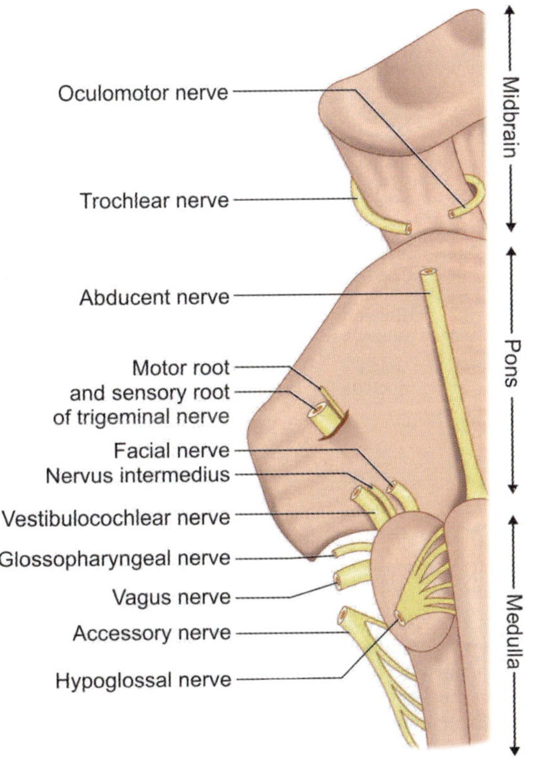

Attachment of cranial nerves to the surface of brainstem.

285. Divisions of trigeminal nerve are all EXCEPT:

a. Ophthalmic b. Maxillary
c. Orbital d. Mandibular

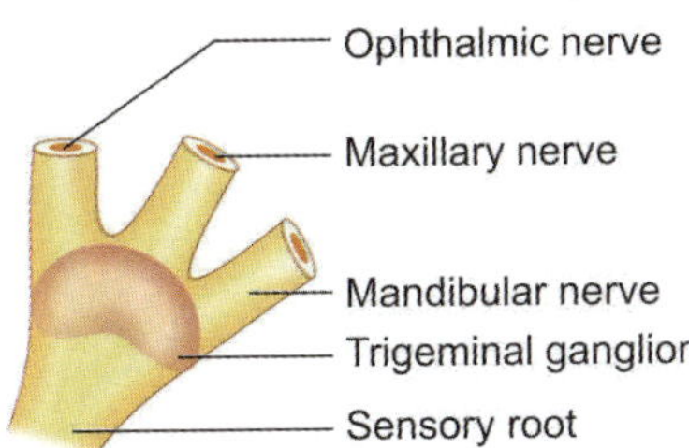

Trigeminal ganglion seen from above.

286. Parotid duct opens:

a. Floor of the mouth
b. Opposite lower second molar tooth
c. Opposite upper second molar tooth
d. At epiglottis border

The parotid duct is formed when several interlobular ducts—the largest ducts inside the parotid gland—join. It emerges from the gland and runs forward along the lateral side of the masseter muscle. In this course, the duct is surrounded by the buccal fat pad. It takes a steep turn at the border of the masseter and passes through the buccinator muscle, opening into the vestibule of the mouth, the region of the mouth between the cheek and the gums, at the parotid papilla, which lays across the second superior molar tooth.

287. True regarding opening of auditory tube in nasopharynx is:

a. Posterior to inferior nasal concha
b. Posterior to middle nasal concha
c. Superior to inferior nasal concha
d. Inferior to inferior nasal concha

The Eustachian tube extends from the anterior wall of the middle ear to the lateral wall of the nasopharynx, approximately at the level of the inferior nasal concha. It consists of a bony part and a cartilaginous part.

A portion of the tube (1/3) proximal to the middle ear is made of bone; this bony part is about 12 mm in length.

288. All of the following are related to facial nerve EXCEPT:

a. Maxillary processes
b. Posterior belly of digastric muscle
c. Stylomastoid foramen
d. Parotid gland

The maxillary process forms the lateral wall and floor of the orbit, and in it is ossified the zygomatic bone and the greater part of the maxilla; it meets with the lateral nasal process, from which, however, it is separated for a time by a groove, the naso-optic furrow, that extends from the furrow encircling the eyeball to the olfactory pit.

289. Trochlear and abducent nerves pass through:

a. Optic canal
b. Superior orbital fissure
c. Inferior orbital fissure
d. Infraorbital foramen

Structures passing through SOF.

- Superior and inferior divisions of oculomotor nerve (III)
- Trochlear nerve (IV)
- Lacrimal, frontal and nasociliary branches of ophthalmic (V_1)
- Abducens nerve (VI)
- Superior and inferior divisions of ophthalmic vein. Inferior division also passes through the inferior orbital fissure.
- Sympathetic fibers from cavernous plexus.

Ans. 283. **a.** C1 284. **b.** IV cranial nerve 285. **c.** Orbital 286. **c.** Opposite upper second...
287. **a.** Posterior to... 288. **a.** Maxillary processes 289. **b.** Superior orbital fissure

290. Which of the following is associated with special somatic afferent nuclei:

a. Cranial nerve V b. Cranial nerve VI
c. Cranial nerve VII d. Cranial nerve VII

Special somatic afferent (**SSA**) refers to afferent nerves that carry information from the special senses of vision, hearing and balance. The cranial nerves containing SSA fibers are the optic nerve (II) and the vestibulocochlear nerve (VIII).

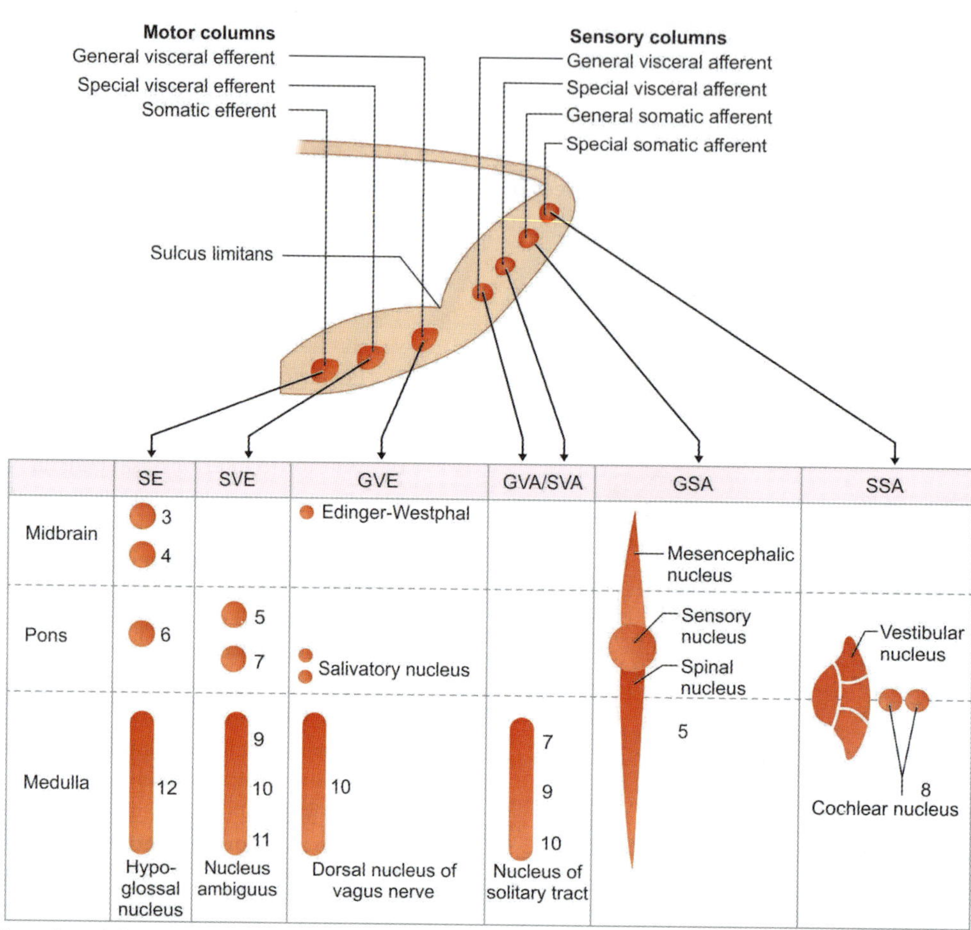

Functional classification of cranial nerve nuclei. The upper figure shows the arrangement of nuclear columns in the brainstem of the embryo. The lower figure shows the nuclei derived from each column. Numbers indicate the cranial nerves connected to the nuclei.
Note that basal lamina consists of motor cell columns: Somatic efferent (SE), special visceral efferent (SVE), general visceral efferent (GVE), and alar lamina consists of sensory columns: General visceral afferent (GVA), special visceral afferent (SVA), general somatic afferent (GSA) and special somatic afferent (SSA).

291. Safety muscle of larynx:

a. Lateral cricoarytenoid
b. Transverse arytenoid
c. Posterior cricoarytenoid
d. Cricothyroids

The posterior arytenoids are called safety muscle because paralysis of the posterior cricoarytenoid muscles may lead to asphyxiation as they are the only laryngeal muscles to open the true vocal folds, allowing inspiration and expiration.

292. NOT a site of attachment of quadrilateral cartilage of nasal septum:

a. Maxilla b. Vomer
c. Sphenoid d. Ethmoid

Main bones taking part in the formation of nasal septum.

Ans. **290. d.** Cranial nerve... **291. c.** Posterior ... **292. c.** Sphenoid

Nasal septum is composed of:

- Perpendicular plate of ethmoid bone
- Vomer bone
- Cartilage of the septum
- Crest of the maxillary bone
- Crest of the palatine bone

293. Cranial nerve supplying secretomotor fibers to submandibular gland:

a. Cranial nerve V
b. Cranial nerve VII
c. Cranial nerve IX
d. Cranial nerve X

Parasympathetic innervation to the submandibular glands is provided by the superior salivatory nucleus via the chorda tympani, a branch of the facial nerve, that becomes part of the trigeminal nerve's lingual nerve prior to synapsing on the submandibular ganglion.

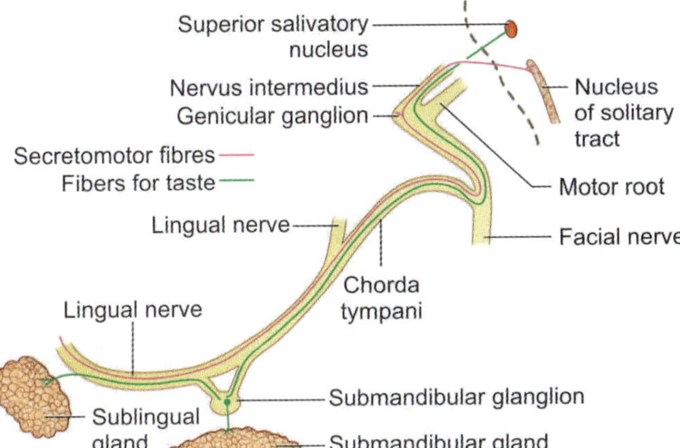

Scheme to show the secretomotor pathway for the submandibular and sublingual glands and the pathway for taste from the anterior two-third of the tongue.

294. NOT at risk in anterior cranial fossa fracture:

a. Root of nose
b. Sphenoid sinus
c. Olfactory bulb
d. Ethmoid sinus

The **anterior cranial fossa** is a depression in the floor of the cranial base which houses the projecting frontal lobes of the brain. It is formed by the orbital plates of the frontal, the cribriform plate of the ethmoid, and the small wings and front part of the body of the sphenoid; it is limited behind by the posterior borders of the small wings of the sphenoid and by the anterior margin of the chiasmatic groove.

295. Chorda tympani is a branch of:

a. Cranial nerve V
b. Cranial nerve VI
c. Cranial nerve VII
d. Cranial nerve VIII

The **chorda tympani** is a branch of the facial nerve that originates from the taste buds in the front of the tongue, runs through the middle ear, and carries taste messages to the brain. It joins the facial nerve (cranial nerve VII) inside the facial canal, at the level where the facial nerve exits the skull via the petrotympanic fissure.

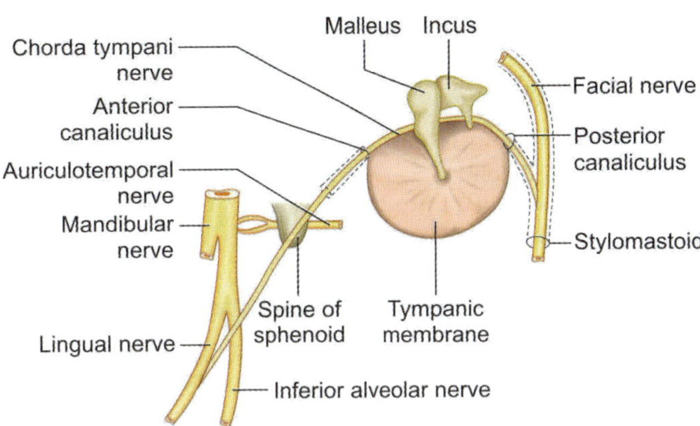

Course of chorda tympani as seen from the medial aspect.

296. Platysma is supplied by:

a. Mandibular nerve
b. Hypoglossal nerve
c. Facial nerve
d. Ansa cervicalis

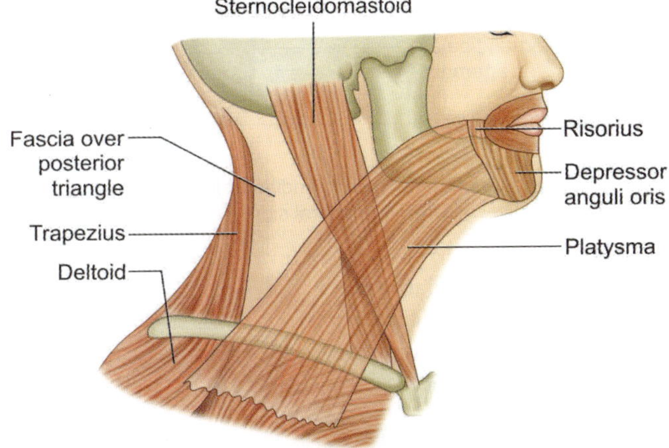

Platysma muscle.

Platysma

Origin	Subcutaneous tissue of infraclavicular and supraclavicular regions
Insertion	Base of mandible; skin of cheek and lower lip; angle of mouth; orbicularis oris
Artery	Branches of the submental artery and suprascapular artery

Contd...

Ans. **293. b.** Cranial nerve... **294. b.** Sphenoid sinus **295. c.** Cranial nerve VII **296. c.** Facial nerve

Contd...

Nerve	Cervical branch of the facial nerve (CN VII)
Actions	Draws the corners of the mouth inferiorly and widens it (as in expressions of sadness and fright). Also draws the skin of the neck superiorly when teeth are clenched
Antagonist	Masseter, temporalis

297. Temporomandibular joint is an example of:

a. Saddle joint
b. Pivot joint
c. Condylar joint
d. Plane joint

TMJ is a synovial joint of the condylar variety.

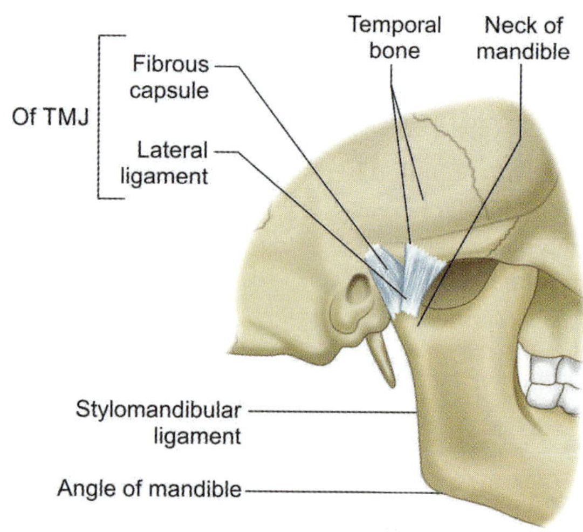

Ligaments of the temporomandibular joint as seen from the lateral side.

298. Nerve supply to skin over the angle of mandible:

a. Great auricular nerve
b. Posterior auricular nerve
c. Auriculotemporal nerve
d. Maxillary nerve

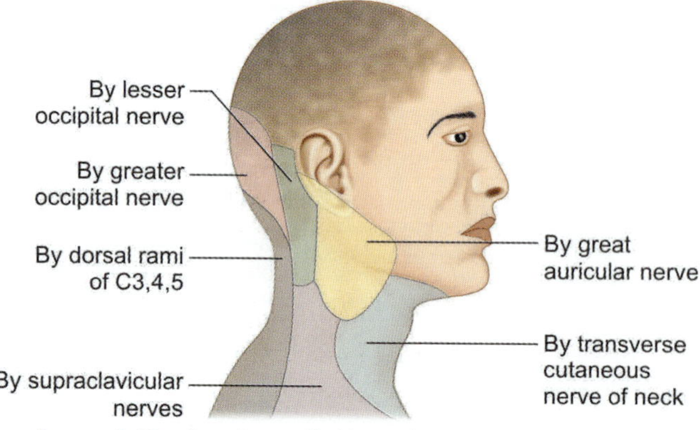

Areas of skin of neck supplied by various cutaneous nerves.

The **great auricular nerve** originates from the cervical plexus, composed of branches of spinal nerves C2 and C3. It provides sensory innervation for the skin over parotid gland and mastoid process, and both surfaces of the outer ear.

299. Origin of superior thyroid artery:

a. Maxillary artery
b. Internal carotid artery
c. External carotid artery
d. Vertebral artery

The **superior thyroid artery** arises from the external carotid artery just below the level of the greater cornu of the hyoid bone and ends in the thyroid gland.

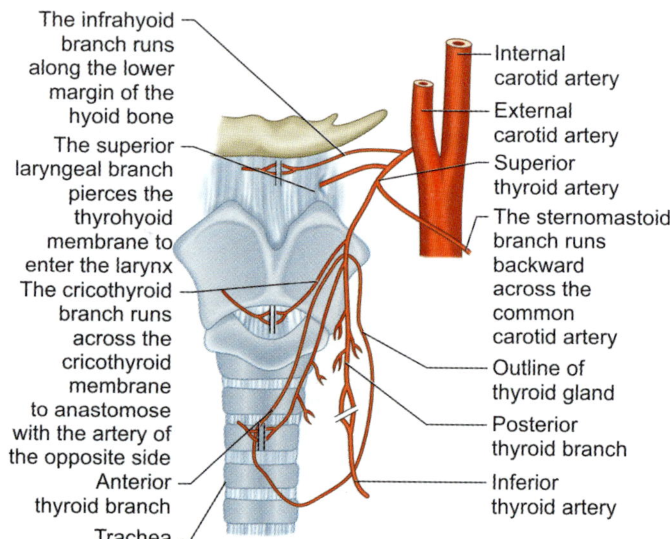

Scheme to show the distribution of the superior thyroid artery.

BRAIN AND SPINAL CORD

300. Lower motor neuron structures are all EXCEPT:

a. Anterior horn cell
b. Anterior nerve root
c. Peripheral ganglia
d. Peripheral nerve

Lower motor neurons (LMNs)

- They are motor neurons located in either the ventral horn of the spinal cord and anterior nerve roots (spinal lower motor neurons) or the cranial nerve nuclei of the brainstem and cranial nerves with motor function (cranial nerve lower motor neurons).
- All voluntary movement relies on spinal lower motor neurons, which innervate skeletal muscle fibers and act as a link between upper motor neurons and muscles.
- Cranial nerve lower motor neurons control movements of the eyes and tongue, and contribute to chewing, swallowing and vocalization.

Ans. **297. c.** Condylar joint **298. a.** Great auricular nerve **299. c.** External carotid... **300. c.** Peripheral ganglia

- Damaged to the lower motor neuron lead to flaccid paralysis.

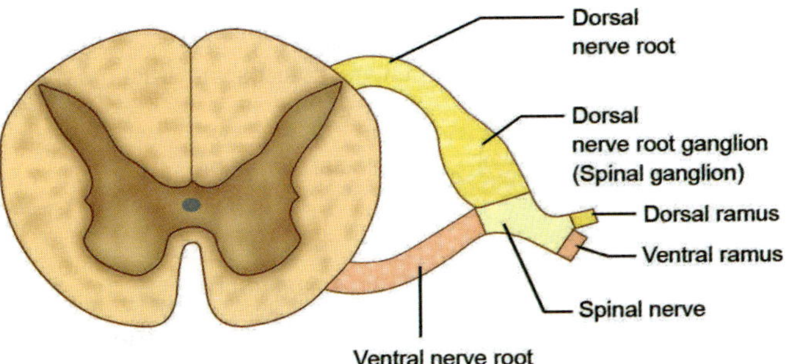

Relationship of a spinal nerve to the spinal cord

301. Taste fibers are relayed in:
a. Red nucleus
b. Nucleus ambiguus
c. Tractus solitarius
d. Nuclei of trigeminal nerve

The solitary tract conveys afferent information from stretch receptors and chemoreceptors in the walls of the cardiovascular, respiratory, and intestinal tracts. Afferent fibers from cranial nerves 7, 9 and 10 convey taste (SVA) in its rostral portion, and general visceral sense (GVA) in its caudal part. Taste buds in the mucosa of the tongue can also generate impulses in the rostral regions of the solitary tract. The efferent fibers are distributed to the solitary tract nucleus.

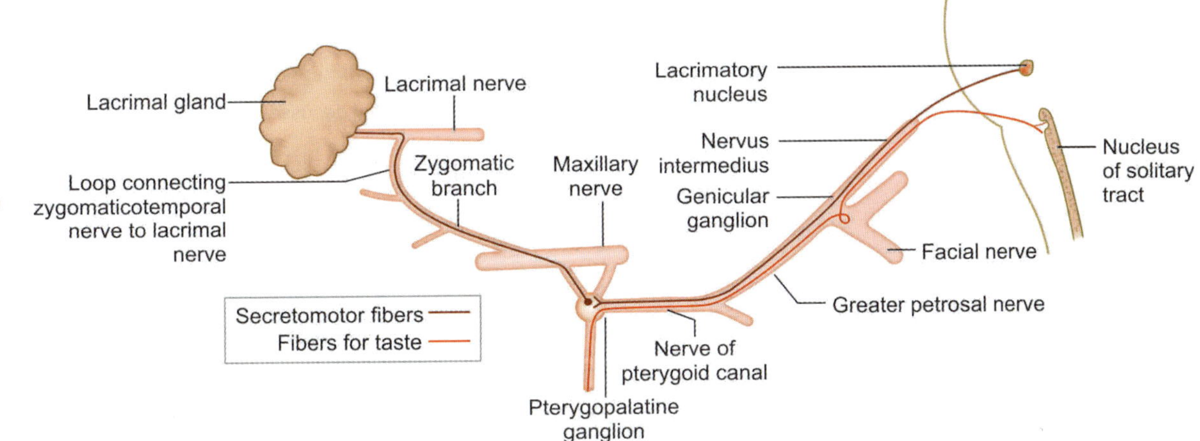

Scheme to show the secretomotor pathway for the lacrimal gland and the pathway for fibres of taste from the soft palate.

302. Rate of formation of CSF:
a. 1400–1500 ml/day
b. 6000–7000 ml/day
c. 8000–9000 ml/day
d. 10000–12000 ml/day

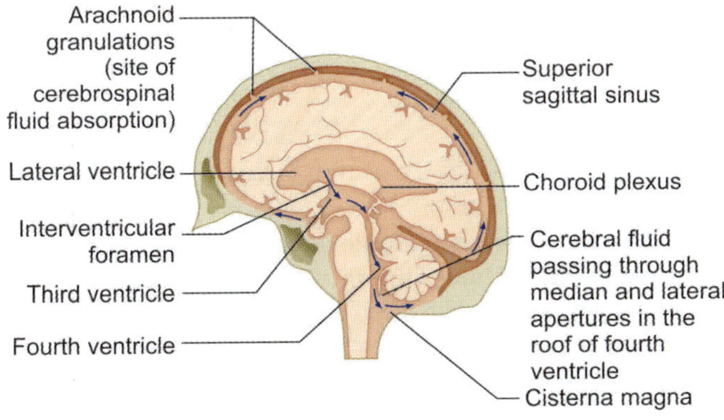

Scheme to show circulation of cerebrospinal fluid.

The brain produces roughly 1500 mL of cerebrospinal fluid per day. This fluid is constantly reabsorbed, so that only 100–160 mL is present at any one time. Ependymal cells of the choroid plexus produce more than two-thirds of CSF.

303. A transection made at the lower end of medulla through the pyramids would cause all EXCEPT:
a. Extensor plantar
b. Involuntary movements
c. Spasticity
d. Increased tendon reflexes

The ventral portion of the medulla oblongata contains the medullary pyramids. The two pyramids contain the motor fibers that pass from the brain to the medulla oblongata and spinal cord. These are the corticobulbar and corticospinal fibers that make up the pyramidal tracts. Extrapyramidal tracts are those motor tracts that do not traverse the medullary pyramids (lesions manifest as involuntary movements).

Ans. 301. c. Tractus solitarius **302. a.** 1400–1500 ml/day **303. b.** Involuntary movements

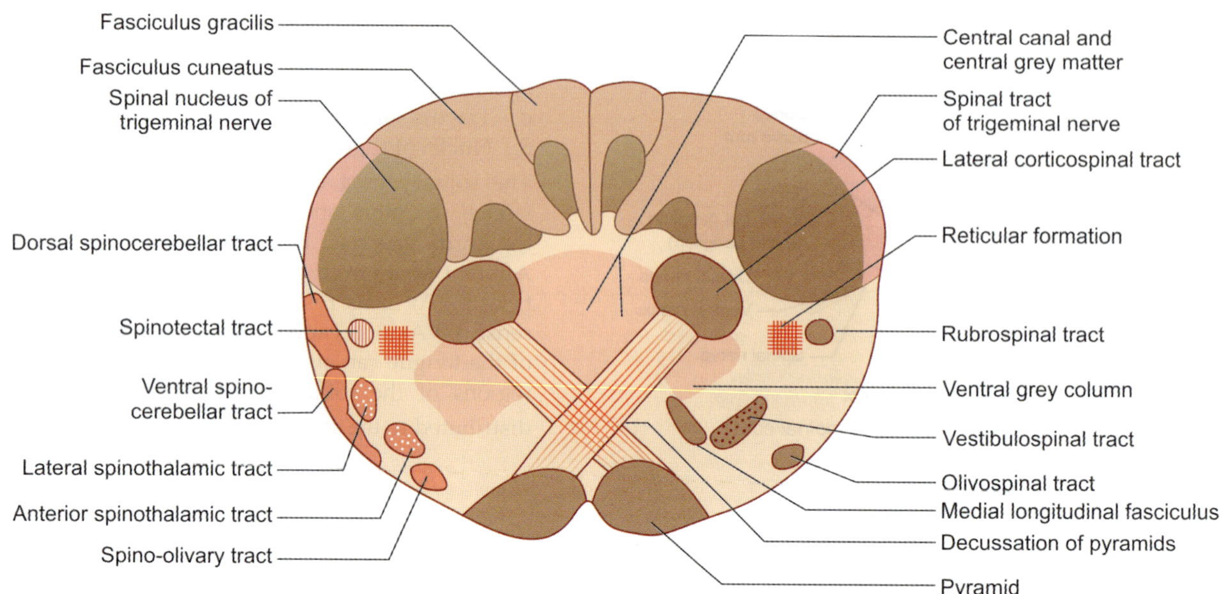

Transverse section through the medulla at the level of the pyramidal decussation.

304. Drainage of CSF from lateral ventricle to third ventricle is through which of the following:

a. Aqueduct of sylvius
b. Foramen of Luschka
c. Foramen of Magendie
d. Foramen of Monro

The **interventricular foramina** (or **foramina of Monro**) are channels that connect the paired lateral ventricles with the third ventricle at the midline of the brain. As channels, they allow cerebrospinal fluid (CSF) produced in the lateral ventricles to reach the third ventricle and then the rest of the brain's ventricular system.

305. Vital point is a feature of:

a. Thalamus
b. Hypothalamus
c. Medulla
d. Cerebellum

Vital point is a point in the medulla oblongata, at the respiratory center, puncture of which causes immediate death.

306. Genu of internal capsule contains:

a. Motor fibers from trunk
b. Motor fibers from upper limb
c. Motor fibers from lower limb
d. Sensory fibers from thalamus to brain

The *genu* is the flexure of the internal capsule. It is formed by fibers from the corticonuclear tracts. The fibers in this region are named the geniculate fibers; they originate in the motor part of the cerebral cortex and, after passing downward through the base of the cerebral peduncle with the cerebrospinal fibers, undergo decussation and end in the motor nuclei of the cranial nerves of the opposite side.

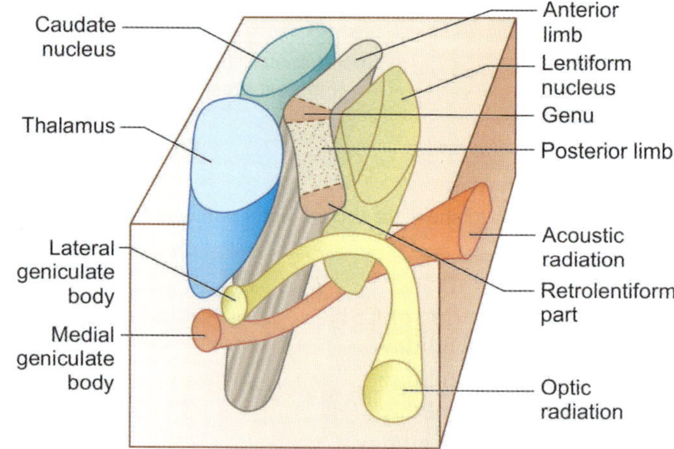

Scheme to show the subdivisions of internal capsule.

307. Basal ganglia consist of all EXCEPT:

a. Caudate nucleus
b. Putamen
c. Thalamus
d. Globus pallidus

The thalamus has multiple functions. It may be thought of as a kind of hub of information. It is generally believed to act as a relay between different subcortical areas and the cerebral cortex. In particular, every sensory system (with the exception of the olfactory system) includes a thalamic nucleus that receives sensory signals and sends them to the associated primary cortical area.

Ans. **304. d.** Foramen of... **305. c.** Medulla **306. d.** Sensory fibers... **307. c.** Thalamus

The thalamus is believed to both process sensory information as well as relay it—each of the primary sensory relay areas receives strong feedback connections from the cerebral cortex.

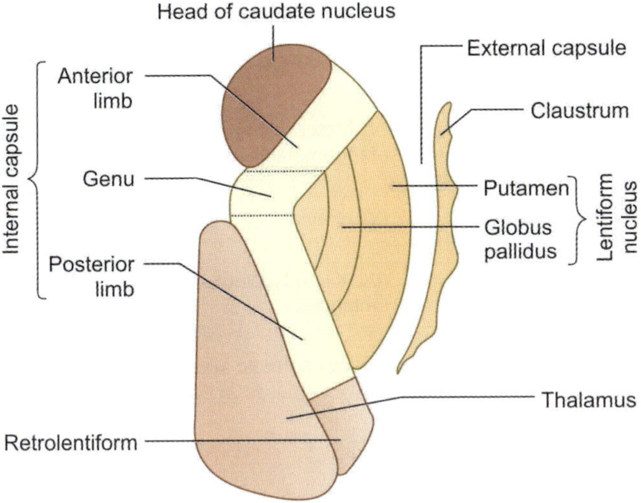

Horizontal section of the cerebral hemisphere showing corpus striatum, thalamus, claustrum and internal capsule.

308. Main factor controlling CSF pressure:

a. Blood pressure
b. Rate of CSF production
c. Rate of CSF absorption
d. Rate of cerebral blood flow

CSF pressure, as measured by lumbar puncture (LP), is 10–18 cm H_2O (8–15 mm Hg or 1.1–2 kPa) with the patient lying on the side and 20–30 cm H_2O (16–24 mm Hg or 2.1–3.2 kPa) with the patient sitting up. In newborns, CSF pressure ranges from 8 to 10 cm H_2O (4.4–7.3 mm Hg or 0.78–0.98 kPa). Rate of absorption is major determinant.

309. Nuclei belonging to general visceral efferent column:

a. Nucleus ambiguus
b. Facial nerve nucleus
c. Trigeminal nerve nucleus
d. Dorsal nucleus of vagus

The cranial nerves containing GVE fibers include the oculomotor nerve (CN III), the facial nerve (CN VII), the glossopharyngeal nerve (CN IX) and the vagus nerve (CN X).

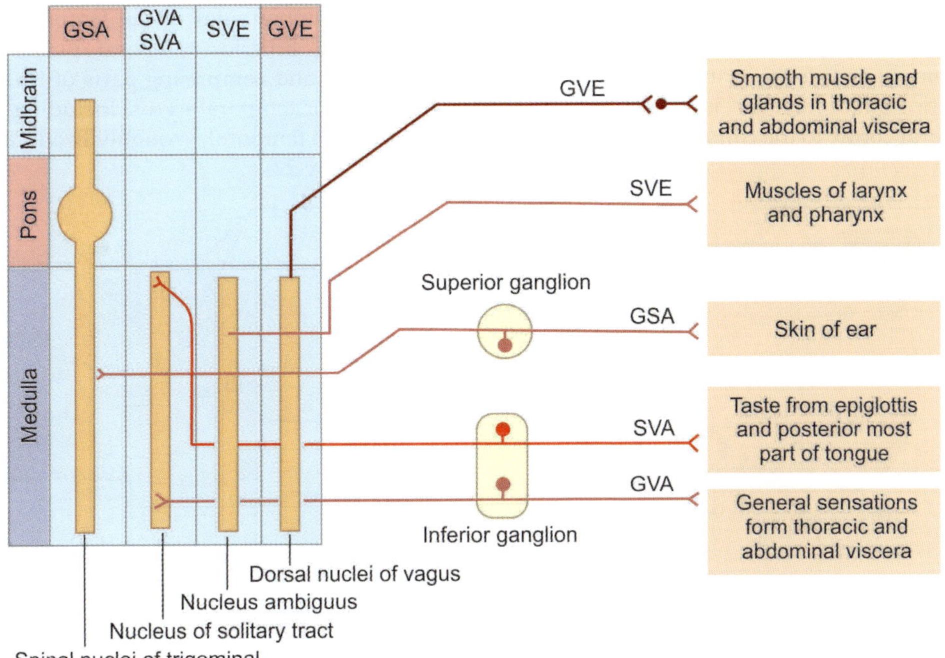

Scheme to show the functional components of vagus nerve.

310. Nuclei in brain common to cranial nerves IX, X and XI:

a. Red nucleus
b. Dentate nucleus
c. Nucleus ambiguus
d. Nucleus solitarius

This nucleus ambiguus gives rise to the branchial efferent motor fibers of the vagus nerve (CN X) and cranial part of accessory nerve terminating in the laryngeal, pharyngeal muscles, and musculus uvulae; as well as to the efferent motor fibers of the glossopharyngeal nerve (CN IX) terminating in the stylopharyngeus muscle.

Ans. **308. c.** Rate of CSF... **309. d.** Dorsal nucleus of... **310. c.** Nucleus ambiguus

The functional nuclear columns and cranial nerve nuclei of brainstem.

	Sensory (Afferent)			*Motor (Efferent)*		
	GVA/SVA	*GSA*	*SSA*	*GSE*	*SVE*	*GVE*
Midbrain		(V) Mesencephalic nucleus of trigeminal nerve		(III) Oculomotor		(III) Edinger-Westphal nucleus
				(IV) Trochlear		
Pons		(V) Sensory nucleus of trigeminal nerve			(V) Motor nucleus of trigeminal nerve	
			(VIII) Vestibulocochlear nuclei	(VI) Abducent	(VII) Facial	Salivatory nuclei (VII, IX)
Medulla	(VII, IX, X) Nucleus of the solitary tract	(V) Nucleus of the spinal tract of the trigeminal nerve	(VIII) Vestibulocochlear nucleus	(XII) Hypoglossal nucleus	(IX, X, XI) Nucleus ambiguus	(X) Dorsal nucleus of vagus

GVA: General visceral afferent; SVA: Special visceral afferent; GSA: General somatic afferent; SSA: Special somatic afferent; GSE: General somatic efferent; SVE: Special visceral efferent; GVE: General visceral efferent.

311. NOT a content of inferior cerebellar peduncle:

a. Pontocerebellar tracts
b. Spinocerebellar tracts
c. Olivocerebellar tracts
d. Vestibulocerebellar tracts

The **pontocerebellar fibers** are the second-order neuron fibers of the corticopontocerebellar tracts that cross to the other side of the pons and run within the middle cerebellar peduncles, from the pons to the contralateral cerebellum. The term 'corticopontocerebellar' is the entire pathway from the cerebral cortex to the contralateral cerebellum.

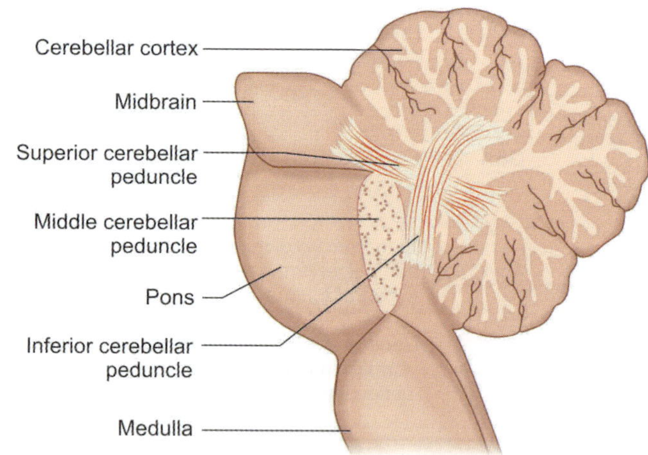

Illustration showing cerebellar peduncles.

312. NOT a pain-sensitive structure in brain:

a. Choroid plexus
b. Falx cerebri
c. Dural sinuses
d. Middle meningeal artery

The cranium, brain parenchyma, ependymal lining of the ventricles, and choroid plexus are all pain-insensitive.

313. Primary auditory area is located in:

a. Frontal cortex
b. Superior temporal cortex
c. Inferior frontal gyrus
d. Occipital cortex

Primary auditory cortex is located bilaterally, roughly at the upper sides of the temporal lobes— in humans on the superior temporal plane, within the lateral fissure and comprising parts of Heschl's gyrus and the superior temporal gyrus, including planum polare and planum temporale (roughly Brodmann areas 41, 42, and partially 22).

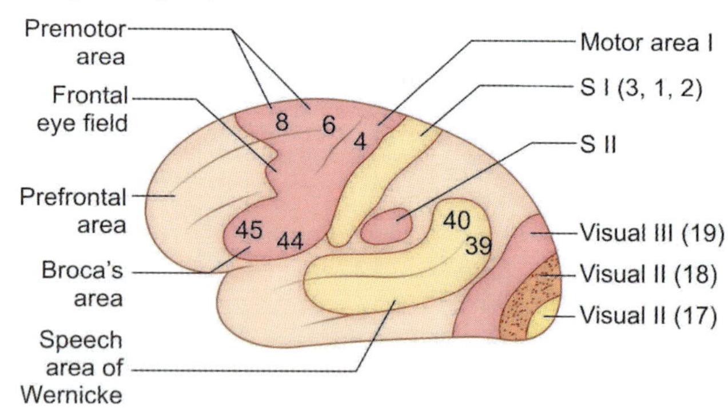

Functional areas on the superolateral aspect of the cerebral hemisphere.

314. Right homonymous hemianopia may be observed in lesions of:

a. Left optic nerve
b. Left optic chiasma (central)
c. Left optic chiasma (peripheral)
d. Left optic radiation

A homonymous hemianopia is the loss of half of the visual field on the same side in both eyes. The visual images that we see to the right side travel from both eyes to the left side of the brain, while the visual images

Ans. **311. a.** Pontocere... **312. a.** Choroid plexus **313. b.** Superior... **314. d.** Left optic radiation

we see to the left side in each eye travel to the right side of the brain. Therefore, damage to the right side of the posterior portion of the brain or right optic tract can cause a loss of the left field of view in both eyes. Likewise, damage to the left posterior brain or left optic radiation can cause a loss of the right field of vision.

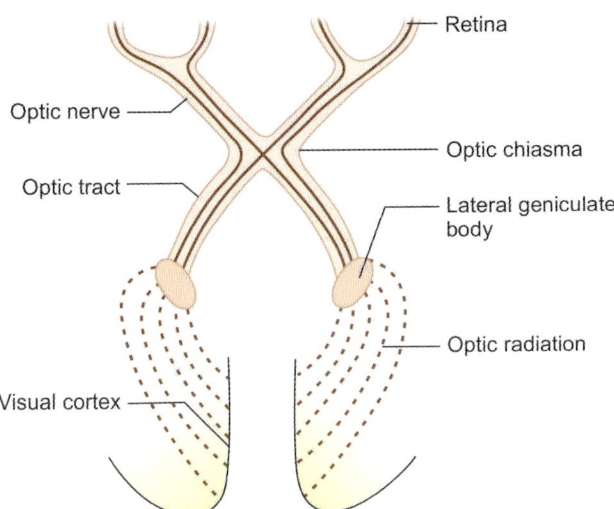

The optic pathway. Note that the fibres from the medial (or nasal) half of each retina cross over to the optic tract of the opposite side.

315. Charcot's artery of cerebral hemorrhage is a branch of:

a. Anterior cerebral artery
b. Posterior cerebral artery
c. Middle cerebral artery
d. Posterior inferior cerebellar artery

One of the lenticulostriate branches is most frequently ruptured (cerebral hemorrhage); it is known as Charcot's artery of cerebral hemorrhage. This lesion also produces hemiplegia with deep coma, and is ultimately fatal.

316. Striae medullares represent fibers passing from ..... to the opposite half of cerebellum:

a. Septal nucleus b. Arcuate nucleus
c. Red nucleus d. Dentate nucleus

Winding around the inferior cerebellar peduncle in the lower part of the fourth ventricle, and crossing the area acustica and the medial eminence are a number of white strands, the **medullary striae**, which form a portion of the cochlear division of the vestibulocochlear nerve and disappear into the median sulcus.

317. Tapetum is a part of:

a. Cerebrum b. Corpus callosum
c. Internal capsule d. Thalamus

On either side of the corpus callosum, the fibers radiate in the white matter and pass to the various parts of the cerebral cortex; those curving forward from the genu into the frontal lobe constitute the *forceps anterior*, and those curving backward into the occipital lobe, the *forceps posterior*. Between these two parts is the main body of the fibers which constitute the **tapetum** and extend laterally on either side into the temporal lobe, and cover in the central part of the lateral ventricle.

318. Spinal cord in children ends at the lower border of:

a. L1 b. L2
c. L3 d. L4

Spinal cord in children ends at the lower border of L3 vertebrae that is why spinal anesthesia is given at the level of L4-5.

JOINTS AND OSTEOLOGY

319. Which of the following ligament is NOT present in temporomandibular joint?

a. Stylomandibular b. Sphenomandibular
c. Temporomandibular d. Malleomandibular

Malleomandibular ligament connects middle ear (malleus) with TM joint

Ligaments of temporomandibular joint

- The major ligament, the temporomandibular ligament, is actually the thickened lateral portion of the capsule, and it has two parts: an outer oblique portion (OOP) and an inner horizontal portion (IHP).
  - The base of this triangular ligament is attached to the zygomatic process of the temporal bone and the articular tubercle; its apex is fixed to the lateral side of the neck of the mandible.
  - This ligament prevents the excessive retraction or moving backward of the mandible, a situation that might lead to problems with the TMJ.
- The two minor ligaments, the stylomandibular and sphenomandibular ligaments are accessory and are not directly attached to any part of the joint.
  - The stylomandibular separates the infratemporal region (anterior) from the parotid region (posterior), and runs from the styloid process to the angle of the mandible; it separates the parotid and submandibular salivary glands. It also becomes taut when the mandible is protruded.
  - The sphenomandibular ligament runs from the spine of the sphenoid to the lingual of the mandible. The inferior alveolar nerve descends between the sphenomandibular ligament and the ramus of the mandible to gain access to the mandibular foramen. The sphenomandibular ligament, because of its attachment to the lingula, overlaps the opening of the foramen. It is a vestige of the embryonic lower jaw, Meckel cartilage. The ligament becomes accentuated and taut when the mandible is protruded.

➤ Other ligaments, called "oto-mandibular ligaments", connect middle ear (malleus) with temporomandibular joint:

- Discomallear (or disco-malleolar) ligament,
- Malleomandibular (or malleolar-mandibular) ligament.

Ans. **315. c.** Middle cerebral artery **316. b.** Arcuate nucleus
317. b. Corpus callosum **318. c.** L3
319. d. Malleomandibular

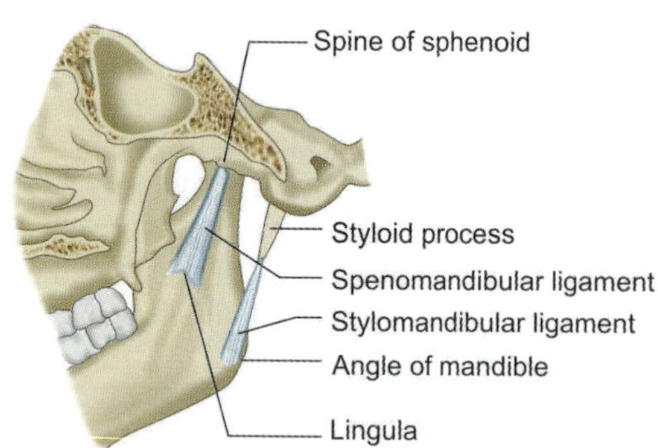

Ligaments of temporomandibular joint as seen from the medial side

320. All of the following are nonpneumatic bones EXCEPT:

a. Clavicle b. Maxilla
c. Humerus d. Femur

Paranasal sinuses are a group of four paired air-filled spaces that surround the nasal cavity. The maxillary sinuses are located under the eyes; the frontal sinuses are above the eyes; the ethmoidal sinuses are between the eyes and the sphenoidal sinuses are behind the eyes.

321. Which of the following is a multipennate muscle:

a. Rectus femoris b. Deltoid
c. Flexor pollicis longus d. Temporalis

If the central tendon branches within a pennate muscle, the muscle is called multipennate, as seen in the deltoid muscle in the shoulder.

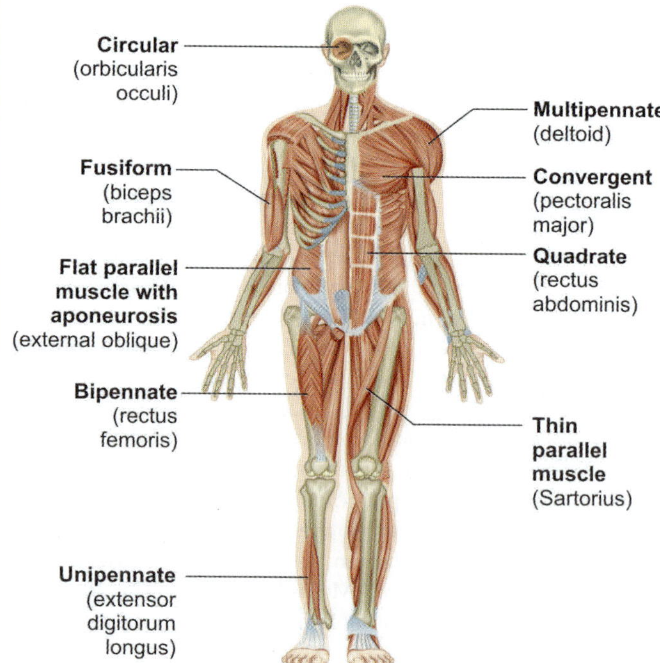

Muscle-shape and architecture.

322. First bone to ossify in body:

a. Upper end of tibia b. Upper end of humerus
c. Lower end of tibia d. Clavicle

It is the first bone to start ossification at around 5th–6th weeks of gestation but finishes around 21–25 years of age. The lateral end has intramembranous ossification.

323. Superior radioulnar joint is an example of:

a. Synchondrosis b. Pivot joint
c. Hinge joint d. Fibrous joint

Examples of a pivot joint

- Proximal radioulnar joint
- Distal radioulnar joint
- Median atlantoaxial joint.

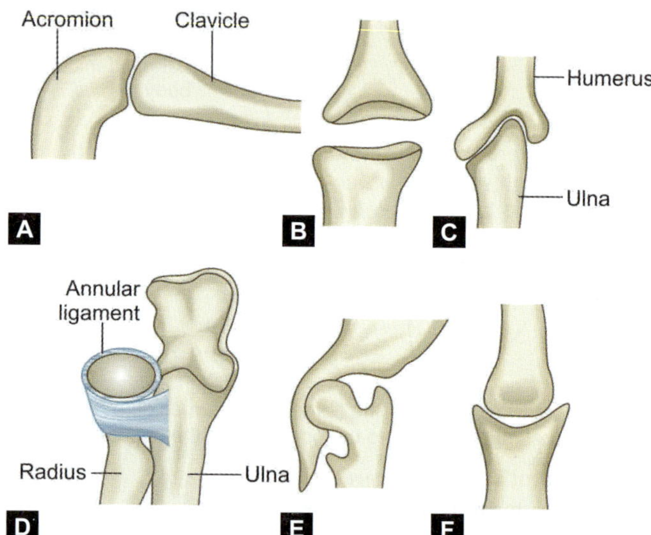

Different types of synovial joints (schematic representation) (A) Plane joint (B) Saddle joint (C) Hinge joint (D) Pivot joint (E) Ball and socket joint (F) Condyloid joint.

324. Movement of inversion and eversion occurs at which of the following joint:

a. Ankle b. Talocalcaneal
c. Inferior tibiofibular d. Tarsometatarsal

Subtalar joint allows inversion and eversion of the foot, but plays no role in dorsiflexion orplantarflexion of the foot.

325. Which movement is NOT possible at lumbar region:

a. Flexion b. Extension
c. Lateral flexion d. Rotation

Flexion and extension occur freely in the cervical and lumbar region, but not in thoracic region. Rotation is free in the thoracic region, and restricted in the lumbar and cervical region.

326. All of the following are pneumatic bones EXCEPT:

a. Maxilla
b. Parietal
c. Ethmoid
d. Mastoid

Pneumatic bone includes maxilla, ethmoid, mastoid, sphenoid and frontal.

Ans. 320. **b.** Maxilla 321. **b.** Deltoid 322. **d.** Clavicle 323. **b.** Pivot joint
324. **b.** Talocalcaneal 325. **d.** Rotation 326. **b.** Parietal

327. NOT a composite muscle:

a. Pectineus
b. Biceps femoris
c. Flexor carpi ulnaris
d. Flexor digitorum profundus

Examples of composite muscles

- Adductor magnus: Adductor part by posterior division of obturator nerve; while the hamstring part is supplied by the tibial part of the sciatic nerve.
- Biceps femoris: Its long head is supplied by the tibial part of sciatic nerve, whereas the short head is supplied by the common peroneal nerve. This reflects the composite derivation from the flexor and extensor musculature.
- Pectineus: Its anterior set of fibers are supplied by the femoral nerve, whereas posterior set of fibers are supplied by the obturator nerve.
- Flexor digitorum profundus: Its radial half of is supplied by the median nerve and the ulnar half is supplied by the ulnar nerve.
- Iliopsoas: It is a composite muscle performing flexion at the hip.
- The tongue is a composite muscle made up of various components like longitudinal, tranverse, horizontal muscles with different parts innervated having different nerve supply.

328. Bone lacking a medullary cavity:

a. Ulna b. Fibula
c. Clavicle d. Radius

Even though it is classified as a long bone, the clavicle has no medullary (bone marrow) cavity like other long bones, though this is not always true. It is made up of spongy (trabecular) bone with a shell of compact bone.

329. Which of the bones ossifies at the earliest:

a. Tibia b. Fibula
c. Talus d. Clavicle

The **clavicle** is the first bone to begin the process of ossification (laying down of minerals onto a preformed matrix) during development of the embryo, during the fifth and sixth weeks of gestation.

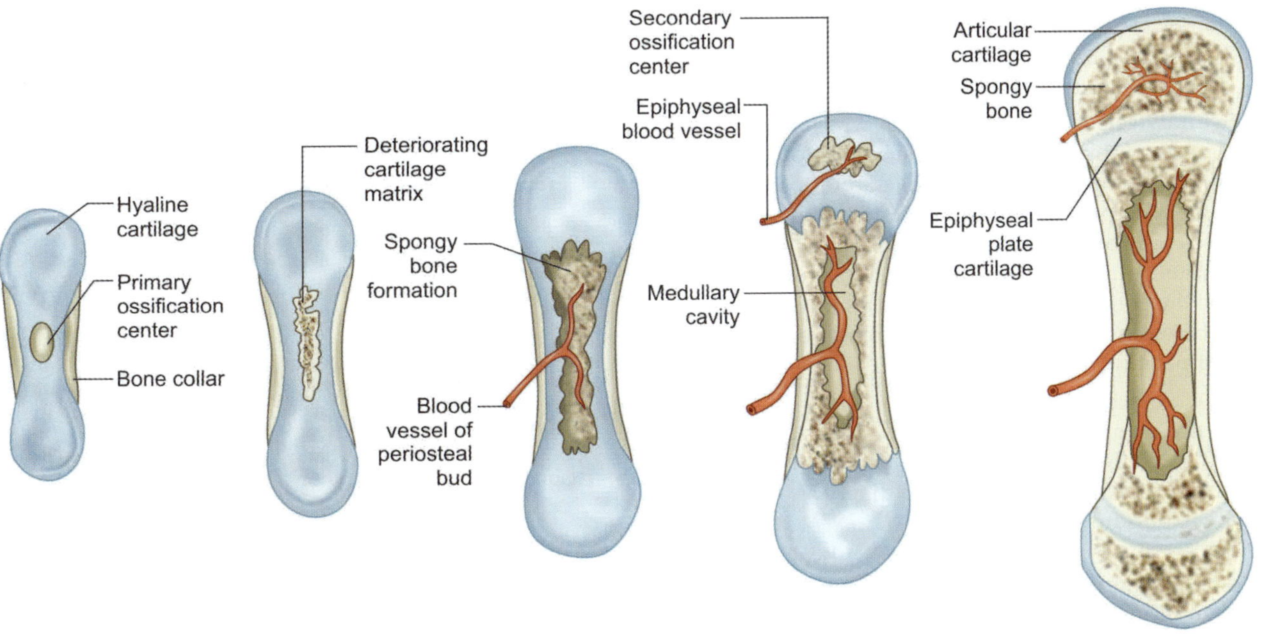

Stages of ossification.

330. NOT a pneumatic bone:

a. Mandible b. Maxilla
c. Mastoid d. Frontal

Pneumatic bone is a **bone** that is hollow or contains many air cells, such as the mastoid process of the **temporal bone**. Also called **hollow bone**. Paranasal air sinuses are also an example of pneumatic bones.

331. FALSE regarding sesamoid bone:

a. Ossify after birth b. Minimize friction
c. Covered by thick periosteum
d. May be seen embedded in joint capsules

Sesamoid bones (Arab. sesame seed) are seed-like bony nodules which develop in certain muscle tendons. They lack haversian system. The sesamoid bones are not classified as true bones as they are not covered by periosteum.

332. Fusion of xiphoid process with body of sternum occurs at:

a. 25 years b. 30 years
c. 35 years d. 40 years

Xiphoid unites with body around **40 years**.

Ans. **327. c.** Flexor carpi... **328. c.** Clavicle **329. d.** Clavicle **330. a.** Mandible
331. c. Covered by... **332. d.** 40 years

333. Bone of axial skeleton:

a. Humerus
b. Sternum
c. Radius
d. Tibia

Axial skeleton consists of 80 bones and is composed of eight parts: the skull bones, the ossicles of the middle ear, the hyoid bone, the rib cage, sternum and the vertebral column.

334. Bone with NO muscular attachment:

a. Calcaneum
b. Intermediate cuneiform
c. Navicular
d. Talus

The second largest of the tarsal bones, it is also one of the bones in the human body with the highest percentage of its surface area covered by articular cartilage. Additionally, it is also unusual in that it has a retrograde blood supply, i.e. arterial blood enters the bone at the distal end.

In humans, no muscles attach to the talus, unlike most bones, and its position, therefore, depends on the position of the neighboring bones.

335. Vomer-sphenoid joint is:

a. Syndesmosis
b. Synchondrosis
c. Schindylesis
d. Synostosis

Schindylesis is an articulation in which two bones are joined by fitting the ridge of one bone into the groove of another. Also known as a 'wedge-and-groove' joint, the name is derived from the Greek 'skhindulesis', meaning 'to cleave', as in cutting with a stump with an axe. This fibrous suture joint can be found between the vomer and the perpendicular plate of the ethmoid bone as well as between the vomer and the gap between the maxilla and palatine.

336. NOT an example of fibrous joint:

a. Inferior tibiofibular joint
b. Tooth in socket
c. Joint between epiphysis and diaphysis
d. Skull suture

Where the connecting medium is hyaline cartilage, a cartilaginous joint is termed a **synchondrosis**. An example of a synchondrosis joint is the first sternocostal joint (where the first rib meets the manubrium). In Such joints are found between the epiphyses and diaphyses of long bones, between the occipital and the sphenoid, and for some years after birth, between the petrous portion of the temporal and the jugular process of the occipital bone.

337. Bigelow's ligament is associated with which joint:

a. Shoulder
b. Hip
c. Elbow
d. Knee

The iliofemoral ligament is a ligament of the hip joint which extends from the ilium to the femur in front of the joint. It is also referred to as the Y-ligament or the ligament of Bigelow.

338. Maximum range of movement is in which joint:

a. Pivot
b. Hinge
c. Ball and socket
d. Saddle

The ball and socket joint (or spheroidal joint) is a type of synovial joint in which the ball-shaped surface of one rounded bone fits into the cup-like depression of another bone. The distal bone is capable of motion around an indefinite number of axes, which have one common center. It enables the bone to move in many planes (almost all directions).

339. Peroneal tubercle lies in:

a. Calcaneum
b. Talus
c. Fibula
d. Tibia

The **trochlear process** (**peroneal trochlea**, or **peroneal tubercle**, or **fibular trochlea of calcaneus**) is an elevated ridge, or tubercle, or projection from the lateral side of the calcaneus (heel bone). It is located between the tendons of the peroneus longus and brevis.

MISCELLANEOUS

340. Which of the following cartilage is present in earlobe:

a. Hyaline
b. Elastic
c. Fibrocartilage
d. All of the above

Elastic cartilage is found in the lobe of the ear, wall of the medial part of the auditory tube, the epiglottis and in some parts of the larynx.

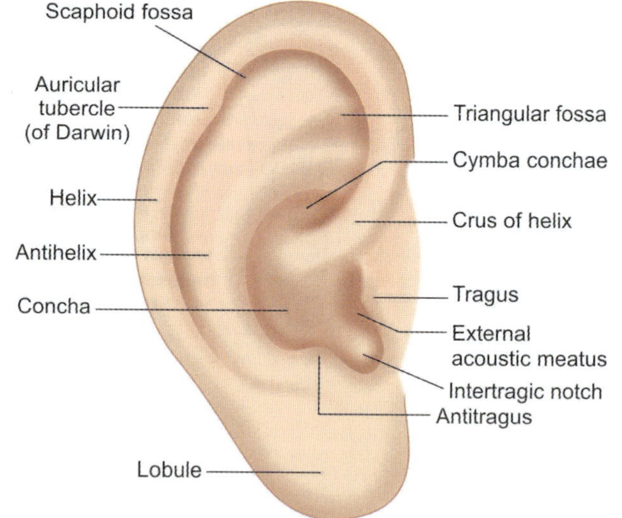

Scheme to show elevations on the external surface corresponding to depressions on the cranial surface of the auricle and vice versa

341. NOT involved in entrapment syndrome:

a. Median
b. Radial
c. Ulnar
d. Femoral

Injury to femoral nerve (rare) by wounds in the groin causes paralysis of the quadriceps femoris and a sensory deficit on the anterior and medial side of thigh. Compression neuropathy is not described for femoral nerve.

Ans. 333. **b.** Sternum; 334. **d.** Talus; 335. **c.** Schindylesis; 336. **c.** Joint between...; 337. **b.** Hip; 338. **c.** Ball and socket; 339. **a.** Calcaneum; 340. **b.** Elastic; 341. **d.** Femoral

ANSWERS WITH REFERENCES

EMBRYOLOGY

1. **Ans. (c)** **21**
Ref: IB Singh's Embryology, 10/e p281

2. **Ans. (d)** **Thyroid (parafollicular cells) > (a) Superior parathyroid**
Ref: IB Singh's Embryology, 10/e p136

3. **Ans. (d)** **1-2 million**
Ref: IB Singh's Embryology, 10/e p24

4. **Ans. (d)** **Spermatid**
Ref: IB Singh's Embryology 10/e p21

5. **Ans. (d)** **Ligamentum teres**
Ref: IB Singh's Embryology 10/e p280

6. **Ans. (d)** **Nucleus pulposus**
Ref: IB Singh's Embryology 10/e p143

7. **Ans. (b)** **Two arteries**
Ref: IB Singh's Embryology 10/e p67

8. **Ans. (c)** **Prostatic utricle**
Ref: IB Singh's Embryology 7/e p284

9. **Ans. (b)** **2nd**
Ref: IB Singh's Embryology 7/e p114

10. **Ans. (b)** **2nd**
Ref: IB Singh's Embryology 10/e p134

11. **Ans. (a)** **1st**
Ref: IB Singh's Embryology 7/e p115

12. **Ans. (b)** **Sclera**
Ref: IB Singh's Embryology 10/e p362

13. **Ans. (a)** **Sphincter pupillae**
Ref: IB Singh's Embryology 7/e p346

14. **Ans. (b)** **Mesoderm**
Ref: Internet resources

15. **Ans. (b)** **2 arteries, 1 vein**
Ref: IB Singh's Embryology 7/e p54

16. **Ans. (a)** **Persistence of right 4th aortic arch**
Ref: IB Singh's Embryology 10/e p258

17. **Ans. (c)** **Heart**
Ref: IB Singh's Embryology 7/e p233

18. **Ans. (b)** **Ileum**
Ref: IB Singh's Embryology 7/e p181

19. **Ans. (c)** **Genital ridge**
Ref: IB Singh's Embryology 7/e p296

20. **Ans. (b)** **Accompanied by ovulation**
Ref: Internet resources

21. **Ans. (d)** **Malformation**
Ref: Internet resources

22. **Ans. (c)** **Cervical**
Ref: IB Singh's Embryology 7/e p304

23. **Ans. (c)** **Mesoderm**
Ref: IB Singh's Embryology 7/e p276

24. **Ans. (d)** **Neural crest**
Ref: Internet resources

25. **Ans. (a)** **Mesonephric duct**
Ref: IB Singh's Embryology 10/e p286

26. **Ans. (c)** **Wolffian duct**
Ref: IB Singh's Embryology 10/e p316

27. **Ans. (d)** **Descending colon**
Ref: IB Singh's Embryology 10/e p189

28. **Ans. (b)** **Genital tubercle**
Ref: IB Singh's Embryology 7/e p285

29. **Ans. (b)** **Branchial pouch**
Ref: IB Singh's Embryology 10/e p136

30. **Ans. (d)** **Paramesonephric duct**
Ref: IB Singh's Embryology 10/e p298

31. **Ans. (d)** **Urogenital sinus**
Ref: IB Singh's Embryology 10/e p299

32. **Ans. (b)** **Surface ectoderm**
Ref: IB Singh's Embryology 7/e p345

33. **Ans. (b)** **Neural crest**
Ref: IB Singh's Embryology 10/e p324

34. **Ans. (c)** **Yolk sac**
Ref: IB Singh's Embryology 7/e p102

35. **Ans. (a)** **Microglia**
Ref: IB Singh's Embryology 10/e p116

36. **Ans. (b)** **1 vein, 2 arteries**
Ref: IB Singh's Embryology 7/e p54

37. **Ans. (c)** **Both of the above**
Ref: IB Singh's Embryology 7/e p163

38. **Ans. (b)** **21 days**
Ref: Internet resources

39. **Ans. (b)** **6–9 days**
Ref: IB Singh's Embryology 7/e p61

40. **Ans. (d)** 4th pharyngeal pouch
Ref: IB Singh's Embryology 7/e p118

41. **Ans. (c)** Metanephros and ureteric bud
Ref: IB Singh's Embryology 10/e p286

42. **Ans. (c)** Branchial pouch
Ref: IB Singh's Embryology 7/e p118

43. **Ans. (d)** Yolk sac
Ref: IB Singh's Histology 5/e p292

44. **Ans. (c)** At the time of fertilization
Ref: IB Singh's Embryology 7/e p34

HISTOLOGY

45. **Ans. (b)** Below the pectinate line, whole part is lined by non-keratinized stratified squamous
Ref: IB Singh's Histology, 7/e p284

46. **Ans. (d)** Lobules
Ref: IB Singh's Histology, 7/e p304

47. **Ans. (b)** Atavistic epiphysis
Ref: IB Singh's Anatomy 6(I)/e p40

48. **Ans. (b)** Rich vascular supply
Ref: GP Pal's General Anatomy 1/e p48

49. **Ans. (d)** Aberrant epiphysis—Trochanter of femur
Ref: IB Singh's Embryology 10/e p40

50. **Ans. (c)** Fibroblasts
Ref: IB Singh's Histology 5/e p65

51. **Ans. (a)** Thyroid
Ref: IB Singh's Histology 5/e p313

52. **Ans. (a)** Goblet cells
Ref: IB Singh's Histology 5/e p246

53. **Ans. (d)** Membranous urethra
Ref: IB Singh's Histology 5/e p278

54. **Ans. (d)** Lung alveoli–Bowman's capsule
Ref: IB Singh's Embryology 5/e p46, 268

55. **Ans. (b)** Vagina
Ref: IB Singh's Histology 5/e p302

56. **Ans. (b)** Has multiple nuclei
Ref: IB Singh's Histology 5/e p133

57. **Ans. (a)** Spindle-shaped
Ref: IB Singh's Histology 5/e p134

58. **Ans. (c)** Stratified squamous non-keratinized
Ref: IB Singh's Histology 5/e p302

59. **Ans. (a)** Duodenum
Ref: IB Singh's Histology 5/e p244

60. **Ans. (c)** Elastic
Ref: IB Singh's Histology 5/e p96

61. **Ans. (a)** Elastic
Ref: IB Singh's Histology 5/e p96

62. **Ans. (d)** Bipolar cells
Ref: IB Singh's Histology 5/e p329

63. **Ans. (b)** C-shaped
Ref: BDC 3(III)/e p160

64. **Ans. (c)** Coracoid process of scapula
Ref: Internet resources

65. **Ans. (d)** Thymus
Ref: IB Singh's Histology 5/e p194

66. **Ans. (d)** Collecting duct
Ref: IB Singh's Histology 5/e p268

67. **Ans. (d)** Normal urothelium
Ref: Internet resources

68. **Ans. (d)** Prostate
Ref: IB Singh's Histology 5/e p289

69. **Ans. (d)** Ileum
Ref: IB Singh's Histology 5/e p197

70. **Ans. (c)** Fibroglandular structure
Ref: IB Singh's Histology 5/e p289

71. **Ans. (d)** Spleen
Ref: IB Singh's Histology 5/e p191

72. **Ans. (a)** Pinna
Ref: IB Singh's Histology 5/e p96

73. **Ans. (d)** Uterus
Ref: IB Singh's Histology 5/e p300

74. **Ans. (b)** Cuboidal epithelium
Ref: IB Singh's Histology 5/e p313

75. **Ans. (a)** Endoneurium, perineurium, epineurium
Ref: IB Singh's Histology 5/e p152f

76. **Ans. (d)** Pseudostratified ciliated columnar epithelium
Ref: IB Singh's Histology 5/e p49

77. **Ans. (c)** Submandibular/sublingual salivary gland
Ref: IB Singh's Histology 5/e p233

78. **Ans. (b)** Thyroid cartilage
Ref: IB Singh's Histology 5/e p95

79. **Ans. (b)** Urinary bladder
Ref: IB Singh's Histology 5/e p50

80. **Ans. (d)** Gallbladder
Ref: IB Singh's Histology 5/e p47

81. **Ans. (d) Traction epiphysis**
Ref: Internet resources

SUPERIOR EXTREMITY AND BACK

82. **Ans. (c) Abductor pollicis brevis palsy**
Ref: IB Singh's Anatomy, 6/e Vol: I, p-208

83. **Ans. (b) Adductor pollicis**
Ref: IB Singh's Anatomy, 6/e Vol: I, p-205

84. **Ans. (d) Pectoralis major**
Ref: IB Singh's Anatomy, 6/e Vol: I, p-103

85. **Ans. (a) Trapezius**
Ref: BDC 3(I)/e p54t

86. **Ans. (c) Parasternal**
Ref: BDC 3(I)/e p35

87. **Ans. (a) Basilic vein**
Ref: IB Singh's Anatomy 6(I)/e p120

88. **Ans. (b) C5, C6**
Ref: IB Singh's Anatomy 6(I)/e p142

89. **Ans. (c) Nerve to serratus anterior**
Ref: BDC 3(I)/e p10

90. **Ans. (d) Pinching action of thumb**
Ref: BDC 3(I)/e p114

91. **Ans. (b) Latissimus dorsi**
Ref: BDC 3(I)/e p54t

92. **Ans. (c) Serratus anterior**
Ref: BDC 3(I)/e p56

93. **Ans. (d) Prevertebral fascia**
Ref: BDC 3(III)/e p53

94. **Ans. (a) Levator scapulae**
Ref: BDC 3(I)/e p54t

95. **Ans. (c) Ulnar nerve**
Ref: IB Singh's Anatomy 6(I)/e p200

96. **Ans. (d) Adductor pollicis**
Ref: BDC 3(I)/e p111

97. **Ans. (b) Flexion at 4th and 5th distal interphalangeal joint**
Ref: BDC 3(I)/e p106

98. **Ans. (c) Brachioradialis**
Ref: IB Singh's Anatomy 6(I)/e p165

99. **Ans. (b) Supraspinatus**
Ref: IB Singh's Anatomy 6(I)/e p133

100. **Ans. (b) Distal border of extended thumb**
Ref: BDC 3(I)/e p148

101. **Ans. (d) Middle pectoral nerve**
Ref: BDC 3(I)/e p39

102. **Ans. (b) Ulnar nerve**
Ref: BDC 3(I)/e p118

103. **Ans. (c) Nerve to serratus anterior palsy**
Ref: BDC 3(I)/e p10

104. **Ans. (a) Long thoracic nerve**
Ref: BDC 3(I)/e p42

105. **Ans. (a) Median nerve**
Ref: BDC 3(I)/e p118

106. **Ans. (c) Ulnar nerve**
Ref: BDC 3(I)/e p117

107. **Ans. (d) Infraspinatus bursa**
Ref: BDC 3(I)/e p134

108. **Ans. (b) Deltoid**
Ref: IB Singh's Anatomy 6(I)/e p151

109. **Ans. (a) Erb's palsy**
Ref: IB Singh's Anatomy 6(I)/e p142

110. **Ans. (d) Teres major**
Ref: BDC 3(I)/e p134f

111. **Ans. (d) At the distal border of thumb on palmar surface**
Ref: BDC 3(I)/e p148

112. **Ans. (d) Radial nerve**
Ref: BDC 3(I)/e p14

THORAX

113. **Ans. (d) Anterior inter-ventricular septum**
Ref: IB Singh's Anatomy, 6/e Vol: II, p-93

114. **Ans. (d) Bifurcation of trachea**
Ref: IB Singh's Anatomy, 6/e Vol: II, p-133

115. **Ans. (d) Brachiocephalic artery**
Ref: IB Singh's Anatomy 6(II)/e p109

116. **Ans. (b) 2nd rib**
Ref: IB Singh's Anatomy 6(II)/e p16

117. **Ans. (b) Rectus abdominis**
Ref: IB Singh's Anatomy 6(II)/e p167

118. **Ans. (a) T3-T5**
Ref: BDC 3(I)/e p229

119. **Ans. (d) Left atrium**
Ref: IB Singh's Anatomy 6 (II)/e p81

120. **Ans. (b) Posterior 1/3rd of septum**
Ref: IB Singh's Anatomy 6(II)/e p107

121. **Ans. (b)** Hemiazygos vein
Ref: IB Singh's Anatomy 6(II)/e p37

122. **Ans. (c)** Both
Ref: IB Singh's Anatomy 6(II)/e p103

123. **Ans. (a)** Lower lobe right lung
Ref: BDC 3(I)/e p204

124. **Ans. (c)** Crossing by thoracic duct
Ref: BDC 3(I)/e p239

125. **Ans. (b)** Left internal jugular vein and left subclavian vein
Ref: IB Singh's Anatomy 6(II)/e p116

126. **Ans. (c)** Vena caval
Ref: BDC 3(I)/e p161

127. **Ans. (c)** Diaphragm
Ref: BDC 3(I)/e p162

128. **Ans. (b)** Left ventricle and right atrium
Ref: BDC 3(I)/e p221

129. **Ans. (c)** Right atrium
Ref: IB Singh's Anatomy 6(II)/e p111

130. **Ans. (d)** 10th intercostal space
Ref: IB Singh's Anatomy 6(II)/e p57

131. **Ans. (a)** Sitting
Ref: BDC 3(I)/e p181

132. **Ans. (a)** Posterior part of left lung
Ref: Internet resources

133. **Ans. (b)** T10 level
Ref: BDC 3(I)/e p239

134. **Ans. (d)** Greater splanchnic nerve
Ref: BDC 3(I)/e p193

135. **Ans. (a)** Right lung is shorter and wider than left lung
Ref: BDC 3(I)/e p204

136. **Ans. (c)** It is drained by intrasegmental branch of pulmonary vein
Ref: IB Singh's Anatomy 6(II)/e p69

137. **Ans. (d)** Right bundle branch
Ref: IB Singh's Anatomy 6(II)/e p106

138. **Ans. (d)** Vein, Artery, Nerve
Ref: IB Singh's Anatomy 6(II)/e p43

139. **Ans. (c)** D7
Ref: Internet resources

140. **Ans. (c)** Left upper lobe
Ref: IB Singh's Anatomy 6(II)/e p66

141. **Ans. (c)** 40 cm
Ref: BDC 3(I)/e p239

142. **Ans. (a)** Posterior interventricular branch
Ref: BDC 3(I)/e p226

143. **Ans. (b)** 6th rib
Ref: BDC 3(I)/e p203

144. **Ans. (b)** Azygos vein and thoracic duct
Ref: BDC 3(I)/e p161

145. **Ans. (b)** Right coronary artery
Ref: BDC 3(I)/e p226

146. **Ans. (b)** Right common carotid
Ref: IB Singh's Anatomy 6(II)/e p105

147. **Ans. (d)** T4
Ref: IB Singh's Anatomy 6(II)/e p104

148. **Ans. (b)** 8
Ref: IB Singh's Anatomy 6(II)/e p69

149. **Ans. (d)** Anterior interventricular artery
Ref: IB Singh's Anatomy 6(II)/e p106

150. **Ans. (b)** Left atrium
Ref: IB Singh's Anatomy 6(II)/e p81

151. **Ans. (c)** C3, C4, C5
Ref: BDC 3(II)/e p269

152. **Ans. (b)** Crossing by left bronchus
Ref: BDC 3(I)/e p239

INFERIOR EXTREMITY

153. **Ans. (b)** Inferior epigastric artery
Ref: IB Singh's Anatomy, 6/e Vol: I, p-321

154. **Ans. (b)** Gluteus medius
Ref: IB Singh's Anatomy, 6/e Vol: I, p-336

155. **Ans. (c)** Tensor fascia lata
Ref: IB Singh's Anatomy 6(I)/e p326

156. **Ans. (d)** Psoas major
Ref: BDC 3(II)/e p277t

157. **Ans. (a)** Supplied by superior gluteal nerve
Ref: IB Singh's Anatomy 6(I)/e p331

158. **Ans. (b)** Flexor digitorum brevis
Ref: IB Singh's Anatomy 6(I)/e p379

159. **Ans. (d)** Tibialis posterior
Ref: IB Singh's Anatomy 6(I)/e p367

160. **Ans. (b)** Gluteus maximus
Ref: BDC 3(II)/e p60

161. **Ans. (d)** Gastrocnemius
Ref: IB Singh's Anatomy 6(I)/e p370

162. **Ans. (b)** **External rotation of thigh**
Ref: IB Singh's Anatomy 6(I)/e p332

163. **Ans. (c)** **Subtalar joint**
Ref: IB Singh's Anatomy 6(I)/e p415

164. **Ans. (b)** **Gluteus maximus**
Ref: BDC 3(II)/e p60

165. **Ans. (b)** **Popliteal vein**
Ref: IB Singh's Anatomy 6(I)/e p266

166. **Ans. (d)** **Adductor longus**
Ref: IB Singh's Anatomy 6(I)/e p275

167. **Ans. (b)** **Medial cuneiform**
Ref: IB Singh's Anatomy 6(I)/e p412

168. **Ans. (c)** **Superior gluteal nerve**
Ref: BDC 3(II)/e p64

169. **Ans. (b)** **Below and lateral**
Ref: BDC 3(II)/e p41

170. **Ans. (b)** **1st webspace of foot**
Ref: IB Singh's Anatomy 6(I)/e p430

171. **Ans. (c) Tibial nerve**
Ref: IB Singh's Anatomy 6(I)/e p430

172. **Ans. (d)** **Lymphatics**
Ref: IB Singh's Anatomy 6(I)/e p309

173. **Ans. (b)** **Popliteus**
Ref: IB Singh's Anatomy 6(I)/e p346

174. **Ans. (c)** **Popliteal artery**
Ref: IB Singh's Anatomy 6(I)/e p320

175. **Ans. (d)** **Iliofemoral ligament**
Ref: IB Singh's Anatomy 6(I)/e p395

176. **Ans. (d)** **Long head of biceps femoris**
Ref: Internet resources

177. **Ans. (b)** **Flexor hallucis longus**
Ref: IB Singh's Anatomy 6(I)/e p373

178. **Ans. (b)** **Tibialis posterior**
Ref: BDC 3(II)/e p141

179. **Ans. (b)** **Spring ligament**
Ref: BDC 3(II)/e p141

180. **Ans. (a)** **Medial end of the dorsal venous arch with the medial marginal vein**
Ref: IB Singh's Anatomy 6(I)/e p265

ABDOMEN AND PELVIS

181. **Ans. (d)** **Duodenum**
Ref: IB Singh's Anatomy, 6/e Vol: II, p-252

182. **Ans. (a)** **Lymph node of Lund**
Ref: IB Singh's Anatomy, 6/e Vol: II, p-241

183. **Ans. (a)** **Perineal surface of levator ani forms lateral boundary of ischiorectal fossa**
Ref: IB Singh's Anatomy, 6/e Vol: II, p-288

184. **Ans. (c)** **Bulbospongiosus**
Ref: IB Singh's Anatomy, 6/e Vol: II, p-187

185. **Ans. (b)** **S2-4**
Ref: IB Singh's Anatomy, 6/e Vol: II, p-306

186. **Ans. (b)** **Taenia coli present**
Ref: IB Singh's Anatomy, 6/e Vol: II, p-297

187. **Ans. (c)** **Hypogastric nerve**
Ref: IB Singh's Anatomy 6(II)/e p326

188. **Ans. (b)** **External oblique**
Ref: IB Singh's Anatomy 6(II)/e p166

189. **Ans. (d)** **Ilioinguinal nerve**
Ref: IB Singh's Anatomy 6(II)/e p170

190. **Ans. (a)** **Superior mesenteric vein and splenic vein**
Ref: IB Singh's Anatomy 6(II)/e p255

191. **Ans. (c)** **Right gastric artery**
Ref: IB Singh's Anatomy 6(II)/e p251

192. **Ans. (c)** **Both of the above**
Ref: BDC 3(II)/e p319

193. **Ans. (a)** **Urogenital diaphragm**
Ref: BDC 3(II)/e p324

194. **Ans. (b)** **Genitofemoral nerve**
Ref: BDC 3(II)/e p278

195. **Ans. (d)** **Inferior epigastric artery**
Ref: IB Singh's Anatomy 6(II)/e p291

196. **Ans. (b)** **Anterior lobe hypertrophies in old age**
Ref: IB Singh's Anatomy 6(II)/e p317

197. **Ans. (d)** **Medial border of pyramidalis**
Ref: BDC 3(II)/e p180

198. **Ans. (a)** **Ascending colon**
Ref: IB Singh's Anatomy 6(II)/e p254

199. **Ans. (d)** **Left gonadal vein**
Ref: IB Singh's Anatomy 6(II)/e p279

200. **Ans. (b)** **Bulbourethral gland**
Ref: BDC 3(II)/e p308

201. **Ans. (a)** **Inferior gluteal artery**
Ref: BDC 3(II)/e p67

202. **Ans. (c)** **Sciatic**
Ref: IB Singh's Anatomy 6(II)/e p338

203. **Ans. (c)** Entrance into urinary bladder
Ref: IB Singh's Anatomy 6(II)/e p305

204. **Ans. (d)** Inferior vena cava
Ref: BDC 3(II)/e p200

205. **Ans. (a)** Ilioinguinal nerve
Ref: BDC 3(II)/e p179

206. **Ans. (d)** Ascending colon
Ref: IB Singh's Anatomy 6(II)/e p253

207. **Ans. (c)** Para-aortic lymph nodes
Ref: IB Singh's Anatomy 6(II)/e p332

208. **Ans. (d)** Between lesser and greater sac
Ref: BDC 3(II)/e p200

209. **Ans. (a)** 4–6 cm
Ref: Internet resources

210. **Ans. (c)** Left renal vein
Ref: IB Singh's Anatomy 6(II)/e p281

211. **Ans. (c)** Deep inguinal ring is an opening in transversalis abdominis
Ref: IB Singh's Anatomy 6(II)/e p166

212. **Ans. (a)** Right hepatic vein
Ref: IB Singh's Anatomy 6(II)/e p234

213. **Ans. (c)** Renal vein
Ref: BDC 3(II)/e p234

214. **Ans. (a)** Descending colon
Ref: BDC 3(II)/e p232

215. **Ans. (c)** Greater sac
Ref: IB Singh's Anatomy 6(II)/e p247

216. **Ans. (b)** Epididymis
Ref: IB Singh's Anatomy 6(II)/e p181

217. **Ans. (b)** Preaortic and para-aortic lymph nodes
Ref: BDC 3(II)/e p313

218. **Ans. (a)** Testicular artery
Ref: BDC 3(II)/e p186

219. **Ans. (c)** Ureter
Ref: BDC 3(II)/e p334

220. **Ans. (c)** Trapezoid in cross-section
Ref: IB Singh's Anatomy 6(II)/e p317

221. **Ans. (b)** 3
Ref: IB Singh's Anatomy 6(II)/e p243

222. **Ans. (c)** Preaortic
Ref: IB Singh's Anatomy 6(II)/e p333

223. **Ans. (c)** Internal urethral sphincter
Ref: Internet resources

224. **Ans. (d)** Quadratus lumborum
Ref: IB Singh's Anatomy 6(II)/e p305

225. **Ans. (d)** Rectus abdominis
Ref: BDC 3(II)/e p171

226. **Ans. (d)** Median lobe of prostate
Ref: BDC 3(II)/e p306

227. **Ans. (a)** Superior vena cava
Ref: IB Singh's Anatomy 6(II)/e p42

228. **Ans. (b)** Rectus sheath
Ref: BDC 3(II)/e p180

229. **Ans. (d)** Superficial transverse perineii
Ref: IB Singh's Anatomy 6(II)/e p188

230. **Ans. (c)** Fascia transversalis
Ref: IB Singh's Anatomy 6(II)/e p167

231. **Ans. (c)** Ilioinguinal nerve
Ref: BDC 3(II)/e p179

232. **Ans. (d)** Left lobe of liver
Ref: IB Singh's Anatomy 6(II)/e p213

233. **Ans. (a)** Tendon of obturator internus
Ref: BDC 3(II)/e p67

234. **Ans. (a)** Levator ani
Ref: IB Singh's Anatomy 6(II)/e p191

235. **Ans. (d)** Fundus of the stomach
Ref: IB Singh's Anatomy 6(II)/e p159

236. **Ans. (c)** Liver
Ref: BDC 3(II)/e p251

237. **Ans. (b)** Retrocecal
Ref: IB Singh's Anatomy 6(II)/e p224

238. **Ans. (d)** Superficial inguinal lymph nodes
Ref: BDC 3(II)/e p167, 168

239. **Ans. (b)** Fascia transversalis
Ref: BDC 3(II)/e p177

240. **Ans. (b)** Anterior division of internal iliac artery
Ref: IB Singh's Anatomy 6(II)/e p292

241. **Ans. (b)** Medial compartment of thigh
Ref: BDC 3(II)/e p54

242. **Ans. (b)** Left 1/3rd of transverse colon
Ref: BDC 3(II)/e p232

243. **Ans. (a)** Superficial fascia of urogenital region
Ref: BDC 3(II)/e p289

244. **Ans. (d)** Inferior mesenteric vein
Ref: BDC 3(II)/e p204

245. **Ans. (d) Gastroduodenal artery**
Ref: BDC 3(II)/e p209

246. **Ans. (c) 4th part of duodenum**
Ref: BDC 3(II)/e p200

247. **Ans. (b) Duodenum**
Ref: BDC 3(II)/e p245

HEAD, NECK AND CRANIAL NERVES

248. **Ans. (c) Trigeminal nerve**
Ref: IB Singh's Anatomy, 6/e Vol: III, p-32

249. **Ans. (c) Temporal bone**
Ref: IB Singh's Anatomy, 6/e Vol: III, p-299

250. **Ans. (c) Cranial nerve V**
Ref: IB Singh's Anatomy 6(III)/e p290

251. **Ans. (a) Ophthalmic nerve**
Ref: BDC 3(III)/e p73

252. **Ans. (d) All of the above**
Ref: IB Singh's Anatomy 6(III)/e p18

253. **Ans. (d) Palatoglossus**
Ref: IB Singh's Anatomy 6(III)/e p311

254. **Ans. (d) Glossopharyngeal**
Ref: IB Singh's Anatomy 6(III)/e p307

255. **Ans. (b) Inferior thyroid artery**
Ref: IB Singh's Anatomy 6(III)/e p249

256. **Ans. (b) 2nd pharyngeal arch**
Ref: IB Singh's Embryology 7/e p115t

257. **Ans. (a) Tensor veli palati**
Ref: IB Singh's Anatomy 6(III)/e p310

258. **Ans. (b) Superior petrosal sinus**
Ref: IB Singh's Anatomy 6(III)/e p268

259. **Ans. (a) Masseter**
Ref: BDC 3(III)/e p110

260. **Ans. (d) 12th**
Ref: IB Singh's Anatomy 6(III)/e p24

261. **Ans. (b) Spinal cord**
Ref: BDC 3(III)/e p24

262. **Ans. (b) Hypoglossal nerve**
Ref: BDC 3(III)/e p181

263. **Ans. (d) Postauricular nodes**
Ref: IB Singh's Anatomy 6(III)/e p173

264. **Ans. (b) Facial artery**
Ref: IB Singh's Anatomy 6(III)/e p59

265. **Ans. (d) Buccal branch of facial nerve**
Ref: Internet resources

266. **Ans. (c) Pretracheal nodes**
Ref: Internet resources

267. **Ans. (d) Equilibrium**
Ref: IB Singh's Anatomy 6(III)/e p304

268. **Ans. (a) Parotid gland**
Ref: IB Singh's Anatomy 6(III)/e p300

269. **Ans. (c) Mandibular**
Ref: IB Singh's Anatomy 6(III)/e p299

270. **Ans. (d) Maxillary**
Ref: BDC 3(III)/e p178

271. **Ans. (a) Palatoglossus**
Ref: IB Singh's Anatomy 6(III)/e p92

272. **Ans. (d) Anterior ethmoidal artery**
Ref: BDC 3(III)/e p87

273. **Ans. (b) Tracheal rings 2 and 3**
Ref: Internet resources

274. **Ans. (a) C2, C3**
Ref: BDC 3(III)/e p43t

275. **Ans. (c) Recurrent laryngeal nerve**
Ref: BDC 3(III)/e p208

276. **Ans. (a) Lateral pterygoid**
Ref: IB Singh's Anatomy 6(III)/e p80

277. **Ans. (d) Posterior cricoarytenoid**
Ref: BDC 3(III)/e p208

278. **Ans. (b) Stylopharyngeus**
Ref: IB Singh's Anatomy 6(III)/e p306

279. **Ans. (d) VI cranial nerve**
Ref: IB Singh's Anatomy 6(III)/e p188

280. **Ans. (c) Levator palpebrae superioris**
Ref: BDC 3(III)/e p86

281. **Ans. (c) Change in shape of lens**
Ref: BDC 3(III)/e p231

282. **Ans. (c) Adduction and intortion**
Ref: IB Singh's Anatomy 6(III)/e p190

283. **Ans. (a) C1**
Ref: BDC 3(III)/e p60

284. **Ans. (b) IV cranial nerve**
Ref: IB Singh's Anatomy 6(III)/e p288

285. **Ans. (c) Orbital**
Ref: IB Singh's Anatomy 6(III)/e p291

286. **Ans. (c) Opposite upper second molar tooth**
Ref: BDC 3(III)/e p110

287. **Ans. (a)** Posterior to inferior nasal concha
Ref: BDC 3(III)/e p183

288. **Ans. (a)** Maxillary processes
Ref: BDC 3(III)/e p113

289. **Ans. (b)** Superior orbital fissure
Ref: BDC 3(III)/e p25

290. **Ans. (d)** Cranial nerve VIII
Ref: IB Singh's Anatomy 6(III)/e p379

291. **Ans. (c)** Posterior cricoarytenoid
Ref: BDC 3(III)/e p208

292. **Ans. (c)** Sphenoid
Ref: IB Singh's Anatomy 6(III)/e p33

293. **Ans. (b)** Cranial nerve VII
Ref: IB Singh's Anatomy 6(III)/e p302

294. **Ans. (b)** Sphenoid sinus
Ref: BDC 3(III)/e p16

295. **Ans. (c)** Cranial nerve VII
Ref: IB Singh's Anatomy 6(III)/e p302

296. **Ans. (c)** Facial nerve
Ref: IB Singh's Anatomy 6(III)/e p121

297. **Ans. (c)** Condylar joint
Ref: IB Singh's Anatomy 6(III)/e p79

298. **Ans. (a)** Great auricular nerve
Ref: IB Singh's Anatomy 6(III)/e p278

299. **Ans. (c)** External carotid artery
Ref: IB Singh's Anatomy 6(III)/e p250

BRAIN AND SPINAL CORD

300. **Ans. (c)** Peripheral ganglia
Ref: IB Singh's Anatomy, 6/e Vol: III, p-341

301. **Ans. (c)** Tractus solitarius
Ref: IB Singh's Anatomy 6(III)/e p303

302. **Ans. (a)** 1400–1500 ml/day
Ref: IB Singh's Anatomy 6(III)/e p435

303. **Ans. (b)** Involuntary movements
Ref: IB Singh's Anatomy 6(III)/e p351

304. **Ans. (d)** Foramen of Monro
Ref: BDC 3(III)/e p246

305. **Ans. (c)** Medulla
Ref: BDC 3(III)/e p253

306. **Ans. (d)** Sensory fibers from thalamus to brain
Ref: IB Singh's Anatomy 6(III)/e p422

307. **Ans. (c)** Thalamus
Ref: IB Singh's Anatomy 6(III)/e p424

308. **Ans. (c)** Rate of CSF absorption
Ref: Internet resources

309. **Ans. (d)** Dorsal nucleus of vagus
Ref: IB Singh's Anatomy 6(III)/e p309

310. **Ans. (c)** Nucleus ambiguus
Ref: IB Singh's Anatomy 6(III)/e p380

311. **Ans. (a)** Pontocerebellar tracts
Ref: IB Singh's Anatomy 6(III)/e p397

312. **Ans. (a)** Choroid plexus
Ref: Internet resources

313. **Ans. (b)** Superior temporal cortex
Ref: IB Singh's Anatomy 6(III)/e p410

314. **Ans. (d)** Left optic radiation
Ref: IB Singh's Anatomy 6(III)/e p439

315. **Ans. (c)** Middle cerebral artery
Ref: BDC 3(III)/e p304

316. **Ans. (b)** Arcuate nucleus
Ref: BDC 3(III)/e p269

317. **Ans. (b)** Corpus callosum
Ref: BDC 3(III)/e p285

318. **Ans. (c)** L3
Ref: Internet resources

JOINTS AND OSTEOLOGY

319. **Ans. (d)** Malleomandibular
Ref: IB Singh's Anatomy, 6/e Vol: III, p-79

320. **Ans. (b)** Maxilla
Ref: GP Pal's General Anatomy 1/e p35

321. **Ans. (b)** Deltoid
Ref: IB Singh's Anatomy 6(I)/e p27

322. **Ans. (d)** Clavicle
Ref: BDC 3(I)/e p7

323. **Ans. (b)** Pivot joint
Ref: IB Singh's Anatomy 6(I)/e p49

324. **Ans. (b)** Talocalcaneal
Ref: BDC 3(II)/e p136

325. **Ans. (d)** Rotation
Ref: BDC 3(I)/e p179

326. **Ans. (b)** Parietal
Ref: IB Singh's Anatomy 6(I)/e p36

327. **Ans. (c) Flexor carpi ulnaris**
Ref: BDC 3(I)/e p96

328. **Ans. (c) Clavicle**
Ref: BDC 3(I)/e p7

329. **Ans. (d) Clavicle**
Ref: IB Singh's Anatomy 6(I)/e p39

330. **Ans. (a) Mandible**
Ref: IB Singh's Anatomy 6(I)/e p36

331. **Ans. (c) Covered by thick periosteum**
Ref: GP Pal's General Anatomy 1/e p35

332. **Ans. (d) 40 years**
Ref: BDC 3(I)/e p172

333. **Ans. (b) Sternum**
Ref: GP Pal's General Anatomy 1/e p31

334. **Ans. (d) Talus**
Ref: BDC 3(II)/e p28

335. **Ans. (c) Schindylesis**
Ref: IB Singh's Anatomy 6(I)/e p45

336. **Ans. (c) Joint between epiphysis and diaphysis**
Ref: GP Pal's General Anatomy 1/e p51

337. **Ans. (b) Hip**
Ref: BDC 3(II)/e p120

338. **Ans. (c) Ball and socket**
Ref: GP Pal's General Anatomy 1/e p57t

339. **Ans. (a) Calcaneum**
Ref: BDC 3(II)/e p30

MISCELLANEOUS

340. **Ans. (b) Elastic**
Ref: IB Singh's Anatomy, 6/e Vol: III, p-214

341. **Ans. (d) Femoral**
Ref: BDC 3(II)/e p49

PRACTICE QUESTIONS

EMBRYOLOGY

1. **Platysma is derived from which pharyngeal arch:**
   a. 1st b. 2nd
   c. 3rd d. 4th
2. **Malleus is a derivative of which pharyngeal arch:**
   a. 1st b. 2nd
   c. 3rd d. 4th
3. **Outer membrane of fetus in amniotic cavity:**
   a. Chorion frondosum
   b. Decidua basalis
   c. Amnion
   d. Decidua capsularis
4. **Horse shoe kidney lies at the level of:**
   a. Aorta
   b. Inferior vena cava
   c. Superior mesenteric artery
   d. Inferior mesenteric artery
5. **Skin is derived from all of the following except:**
   a. Ectoderm
   b. Endoderm
   c. Mesenchyme
   d. Neural crest
6. **Anterior belly of digastric is a derivative of:**
   a. 1st branchial arch b. 2nd branchial arch
   c. 3rd branchial arch d. 4th branchial arch
7. **Adrenal medulla is a derivative of:**
   a. Surface ectoderm b. Endoderm
   c. Neural crest d. Mesoderm
8. **Which of the following is a true statement regarding spermatogenesis:**
   a. Takes around 74 days
   b. Occurs in spermatic cord
   c. Meiosis occurs only after secondary spermatocyte stage
   d. Spermatozoa forms spermatids
9. **Sperm fertilizes egg cell in what form:**
   a. Spermatogonia
   b. Primary spermatid
   c. Secondary spermatid
   d. Spermatozoon
10. **Embryonic period extends from:**
    a. 0–3 weeks b. 3–8 weeks
    c. 8–10 weeks d. 10–15 weeks
11. **Tertiary villi is seen on which day:**
    a. 6th b. 16th
    c. 26th d. 36th
12. **The following are derived from first branchial *except:***
    a. Anterior malleolar ligament
    b. Posterior malleolar ligament
    c. Sphenomandibular ligament
    d. Mandible
13. **Renal agenesis is because of all except:**
    a. Defective development of nephritic tissue
    b. Failure of ureteric bud with metanephros
    c. Failure of ascent of primitive
    d. All of the above
14. **Regarding zona pellucida, which is WRONG:**
    a. Cellular
    b. Contains glycoprotein
    c. Surrounds morula
    d. Surrounds ovum
15. **All of the following are derivative of ectoderm *except:***
    a. Lens
    b. Extraembryonic mesoderm
    c. Chorion
    d. Allantoic diverticulum
16. **All of the following are endodermal in origin *except:***
    a. Hepatocyte b. Odontoblast
    c. Alveolar lining cells d. None
17. **All are mesodermal in origin except:**
    a. Iris stroma b. Ciliary body
    c. Dilator pupillae d. Vitreous
18. **Which bone is NOT present at birth:**
    a. Malleus b. Incus
    c. Stapes d. Petrous temporal
19. **Following are derived from II arch except:**
    a. Malleus/incus
    b. Stylohyoid ligament
    c. Stapes
    d. Smaller cornua of hyoid

Ans.

1. **b.** 2nd	2. **a.** 1st	3. **d.** Decidua capsularis	4. **d.** Inferior mesenteric...
5. **b.** Endoderm	6. **a.** 1st branchial arch	7. **c.** Neural crest	8. **a.** Takes around 74 days
9. **d.** Spermatozoon	10. **b.** 3–8 weeks	11. **b.** 16th	12. **b.** Posterior malleolar...
13. **c.** Failure of...	14. **a.** Cellular	15. **d.** Allantoic...	16. **b.** Odontoblast
17. **c.** Dilator...	18. **d.** Petrous temporal	19. **a.** Malleus/incus	

20. FALSE regarding tongue are all except:
a. Parathyroid gland develops from 3rd and 4th branchial arch
b. Tongue muscles develop from occipital myotomes
c. Superior parathyroid gland develops from 4th branchial arch
d. Inferior parathyroid gland develops from 2nd branchial arch

21. Spleen develops from:
a. Ventral mesogastrium
b. Dorsal mesogastrium
c. Both
d. None

22. Umbilical artery is transformed into:
a. Medial umbilical ligaments
b. Ligamentum teres
c. Ligamentum venosum
d. Ligamentum arteriosus

HISTOLOGY

23. MC type of cartilage covering articular surfaces:
a. Hyaline b. Elastic
c. Fibrous d. All

24. How many layers in tympanic membrane:
a. 1 b. 2
c. 3 d. 4

25. Crypt is a histological feature of:
a. Adenoids b. Thymus
c. Tonsil d. Appendix

26. Goblet cells are seen in:
a. Vagina b. Cornea
c. Trachea d. Esophagus

27. Sinusoids are NOT seen in:
a. Kidney b. Spleen
c. Endocrine glands d. Heart

28. Which is NOT a feature of skeletal muscles:
a. Spindle-shaped fibers
b. Syncytium
c. Striations
d. Peripheral nucleus

29. Which of the following shows membranous ossification:
a. Femur
b. Scapula
c. Radius
d. Parietal bone

30. Which type of epithelium is present in anal canal:
a. Squamous
b. Columnar
c. Both
d. None

31. Which of the following is NOT a muscular artery:
a. Aorta
b. Femoral artery
c. Popliteal artery
d. Splenic artery

32. Which of the following is NOT a MALT tissue:
a. Jejunum
b. Ileum
c. Palatine tonsils
d. Appendix

33. All have NO lymphatics except:
a. Brain
b. Internal ear
c. Dermis
d. Eye

34. The following glands contain the myoepithelial cells except:
a. Mammary glands
b. Salivary glands
c. Sebaceous glands
d. Sweat glands

35. All of the following physiological processes occur during the growth at the epiphyseal plate except:
a. Proliferation and hypertrophy
b. Calcification and ossification
c. Vasculogenesis and erosion
d. Replacement of red bone marrow with yellow marrow

SUPERIOR EXTREMITY

36. Nerve supply of lumbricals:
a. Median nerve
b. Ulnar nerve
c. Both
d. None

37. Cubital tunnel syndrome is compression of:
a. Median nerve at elbow
b. Ulnar nerve at elbow
c. Ulnar nerve at wrist
d. Median nerve at wrist

Ans. **20. b.** Tongue muscles... **21. b.** Dorsal mesog... **22. a.** Medial umbilical... **23. a.** Hyaline
24. c. 3 **25. c.** Tonsil **26. c.** Trachea **27. d.** Heart
28. a. Spindle-shaped fibers **29. d.** Parietal bone **30. c.** Both
31. a. Aorta **32. a.** Jejunum **33. c.** Dermis **34. c.** Sebaceous glands
35. d. Replacement of red... **36. c.** Both **37. b.** Ulnar nerve at elbow

38. Which of the following nerves passes behind medial epicondyle:
a. Ulnar
b. Radial
c. Median
d. Posterior interosseous

39. Each of the following has an attachment to scapula except:
a. Pectoralis major
b. Pectoralis minor
c. Biceps brachii
d. Triceps

40. Following muscle causes retraction of the shoulder except:
a. Trapezius
b. Serratus anterior
c. Rhomboid major
d. Rhomboid minor

41. The quadrilateral space is bounded by the following except:
a. Surgical neck of the humerus
b. Long head of the triceps
c. Deltoid
d. Teres major

42. Which of the following does NOT form the proximal row of carpal bones:
a. Scaphoid
b. Lunate
c. Triquetral
d. Capitate

43. Medial cord of the brachial plexus gives rise to all except:
a. Nerve to supraspinatus
b. Ulnar nerve
c. Medial cutaneous nerve of arm
d. Medial cutaneous nerve of forearm

THORAX

44. Superior epigastric artery is a branch of:
a. Subclavian artery
b. Musculophrenic artery
c. Internal thoracic artery
d. Superior intercostal artery

45. Which of the following is NOT related to the apex of the left lung:
a. Neck of first rib
b. Subclavian artery
c. Sympathetic trunk
d. Brachiocephalic trunk

46. Which of the following does NOT pass through esophageal hiatus:
a. Esophagus
b. Left gastric nerve
c. Right gastric nerve
d. Thoracic duct

47. First branch of arch of aorta:
a. Brachiocephalic artery
b. Right carotid artery
c. Left carotid artery
d. Subclavian artery

48. Apex of right lung is related to:
a. Esophagus
b. Thoracic duct
c. Arch of aorta
d. Subclavian artery

49. Which of the following structures does NOT form right border of heart:
a. Superior vena cava
b. Inferior vena cava
c. Right atrium
d. Right ventricle

50. Which of the following does NOT drain into azygos vein:
a. Hemiazygos vein
b. Posterior intercostal vein
c. Left superior intercostal vein
d. Right superior intercostal vein

51. Which of the following is chiefly responsible for respiration (75%):
a. Diaphragm
b. Internal intercostals
c. External intercostals
d. Serratus anterior

52. Which of the following is NOT an accessory muscle of respiration:
a. Sternocleidomastoid
b. Scalenus
c. Erector spinae
d. None

53. Intercostal vein drains into which of the following:
a. Left brachiocephalic vein
b. Internal jugular vein
c. External jugular vein
d. Azygos vein

Ans.
38. a. Ulnar | **39. a.** Pectoralis major | **40. b.** Serratus... | **41. c.** Deltoid
42. d. Capitate | **43. a.** Nerve to supras... | **44. c.** Internal thoracic artery | **45. d.** Brachiocephalic trunk
46. d. Thoracic duct | **47. a.** Brachiocephalic artery | **48. a.** Esophagus | **49. d.** Right ventricle
50. c. Left superior... | **51. a.** Diaphragm | **52. d.** None | **53. a.** and d.

54. Esophagus pierces diaphragm at which level:
a. T6
b. T8
c. T10
d. T12

55. Right coronary artery supplies all except:
a. Apex of heart
b. Interventricular septum
c. Interatrial septum
d. SA node

56. Bronchopulmonary segment contains all except:
a. Independent pulmonary artery
b. Independent pulmonary vein
c. Tertiary bronchiole
d. Conical segment

57. All are true about trachea except:
a. 15 cm long
b. Bifurcates at C7
c. Lined by pseudostratified columnar epithelium
d. Tracheal cartilage is C-shaped

58. All are direct articulations of a true rib except:
a. Costosternal joint
b. Costochondral joint
c. Costotransverse joint
d. Costovertebral joint

INFERIOR EXTREMITY

59. Area between 1st and 2nd metatarsal is supplied by:
a. Superficial peroneal nerve
b. Deep peroneal nerve
c. Saphenous nerve
d. Sural nerve

60. Positive Trendelenburg test indicates palsy of which group of gluteus muscles:
a. Gluteus medius and Gluteus minimus
b. Gluteus maximus and Gluteus miniumus
c. Gluteus maximus and Gluteus medius
d. Gluteus maximus, Gluteus medius and Gluteus minimus

61. The following structure pass through the subsartorial canal except:
a. Posterior division of the obturator nerve
b. Saphenous nerve
c. Femoral artery
d. Nerve to vastus medialis

62. Femoral nerve does NOT supply:
a. Sartorius
b. Rectus femoris
c. Tensor fascia latae
d. Articularis genu

63. Floor of the femoral triangle is formed by all of the following except:
a. Pectineus
b. Adductor longus
c. Iliacus
d. Adductor magnus

64. Lateral rotators of the hip are all except:
a. Piriformis
b. Quadratus femoris
c. Obturator internus
d. Psoas major

65. Medial longitudinal arch is NOT formed by:
a. Cuboid
b. Calcaneus
c. Talus
d. Navicular

ABDOMEN

66. Which of the following set of structures form boundaries of Calot triangle:
a. Cystic artery, liver and right hepatic duct
b. Cystic duct, liver and common hepatic duct
c. Cystic duct, liver and cystic artery
d. Common bile duct, liver and cystic duct

HEAD AND NECK

67. Nerve to pterygoid canal/vidian nerve is formed by:
a. Deep petrosal nerve + greater petrosal nerve
b. Facial nerve
c. Lesser superficial petrosal nerve
d. Lesser petrosal nerve

68. Right recurrent laryngeal nerve supplies all of the following except:
a. Posterior cricoarytenoid
b. Lateral cricoarytenoid
c. Transverse arytenoid
d. Cricothyroid

69. Which of the following does NOT pass through superior orbital fissure:
a. Mandibular nerve
b. Abducent nerve
c. Trochlear nerve
d. Oculomotor nerve

Ans.
54. c. T10 **55. a.** Apex of heart **56. b.** Independent... **57. b.** Bifurcates at C7
58. a. Costosternal joint **59. b.** Deep peroneal nerve **60. a.** Gluteus medi... **61. a.** Posterior division...
62. c. Tensor fascia latae **63. d.** Adductor magnus **64. d.** Psoas major **65. a.** Cuboid \
66. b. Cystic duct, liver... **67. a.** Deep petrosal nerve... **68. d.** Cricothyroid **69. a.** Mandibular nerve

BRAIN AND SPINAL CORD

70. Corticospinal tract decussates at:
a. Corpus callosum
b. Midbrain
c. Pons
d. Medulla oblongata

71. All of the following are nuclei of basal ganglia except:
a. Caudate nuclei
b. Thalamus
c. Lenticularis nuclei
d. Globus pallidus

72. NOT a nuclei of cerebellum:
a. Dentate
b. Emboliform
c. Globose
d. Dendritic

MISCELLANEOUS

73. Center region of a long bone is known as:
a. Epiphysis
b. Metaphysis
c. Diaphysis
d. Physeal plate

Ans. **70. d.** Medulla oblongata **71. b.** Thalamus
72. d. Dendritic **73. c.** Diaphysis

IMAGE-BASED QUESTIONS

1. Nerve supply of muscle marked as G:

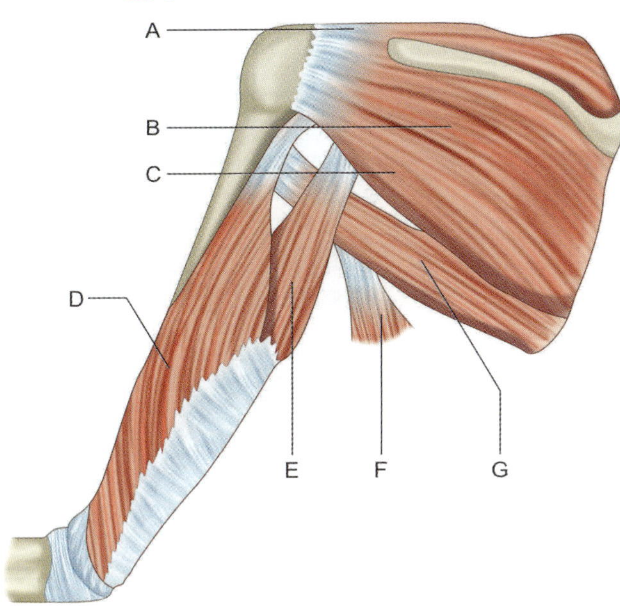

a. Suprascapular nerve
b. Axillary nerve
c. Lower subscapular nerve
d. Radial nerve

Muscle marked as G is teres major, supplied by lower subscapular nerve.

2. Innervation of muscle passing behind structure 11:

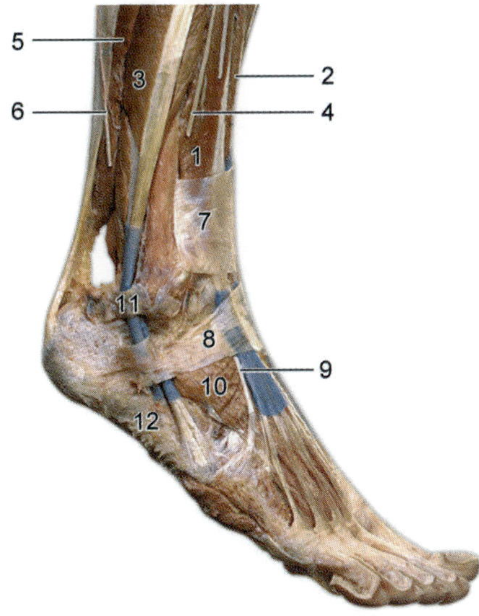

a. Deep peroneal nerve
b. Superficial peroneal nerve
c. Tibial nerve
d. Sural nerve

Peroneus longus and peroneus brevis passes beneath superior peroneal retinacula (marked as 11) and are supplied by superficial peroneal nerve.

3. Identify the bone:

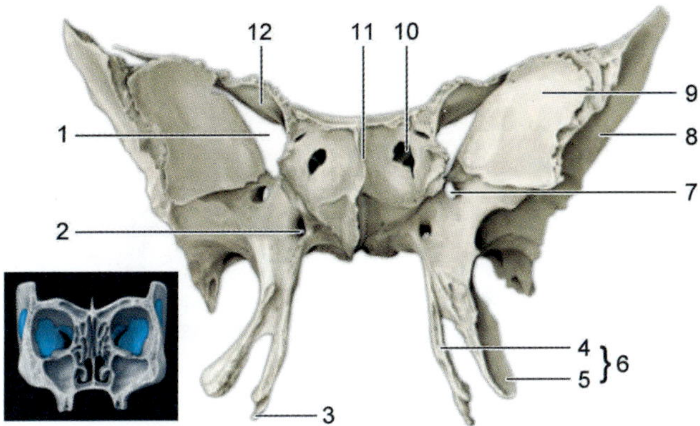

a. Ethmoid
b. Maxilla
c. Sphenoid
d. Vomer

This is sphenoid with greater (marked as 8 and 9) and lesser wings (marked as 12), body (marked as 11) and pterygoid plates (marked as 6).

4. Muscle supplied by the nerve marked as P:

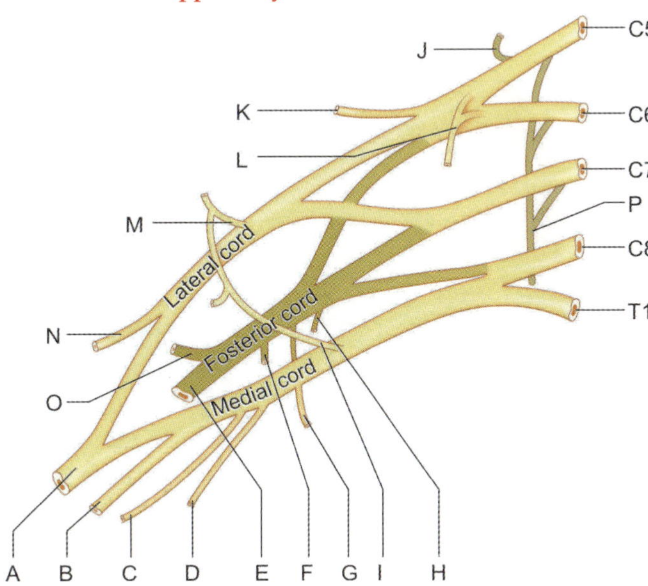

a. Subclavius
b. Serratus anterior
c. Infraspinatus
d. Supraspinatus

The nerve marked as P is long thoracic nerve of Bell, which supplies serratus anterior.

5. Function of area marked as 1:

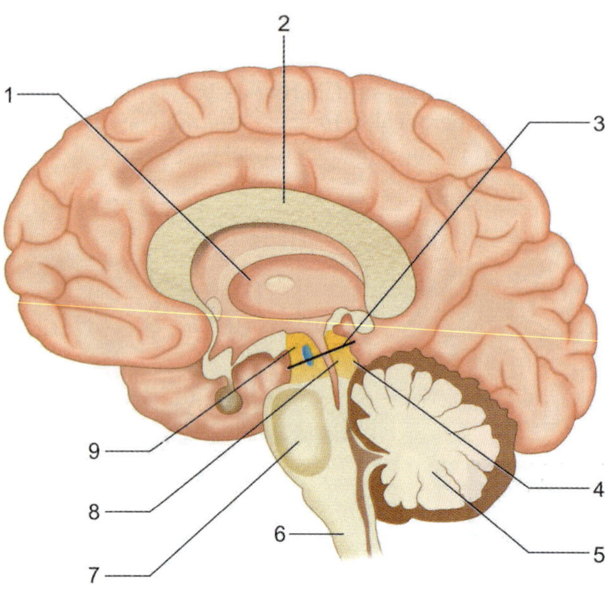

a. Control of voluntary movements
b. Control of involuntary movements
c. Olfaction
d. Sensory integration

Area marked as 1 is thalamus, which is an area of sensory integration and relay station of all the sensory pathways except for the olfactory pathway.

6. Identify the bone marked as 1:

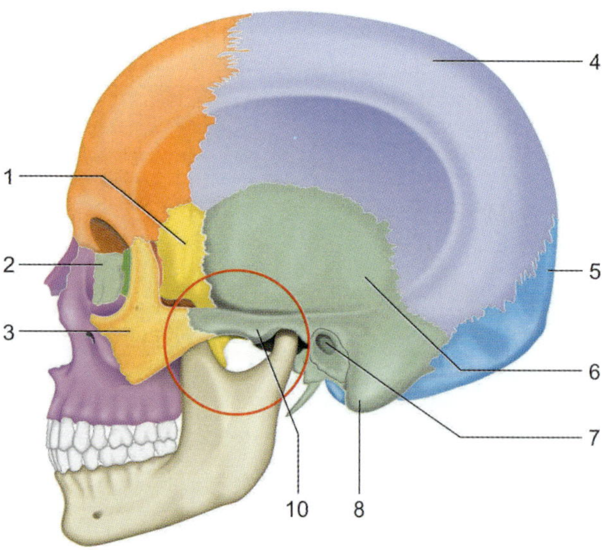

a. Greater wing of sphenoid
b. Lesser wing of sphenoid
c. Temporal
d. Ethmoid

Area marked as 1 is greater wing of sphenoid.

7. Structures passing through area marked as 6:

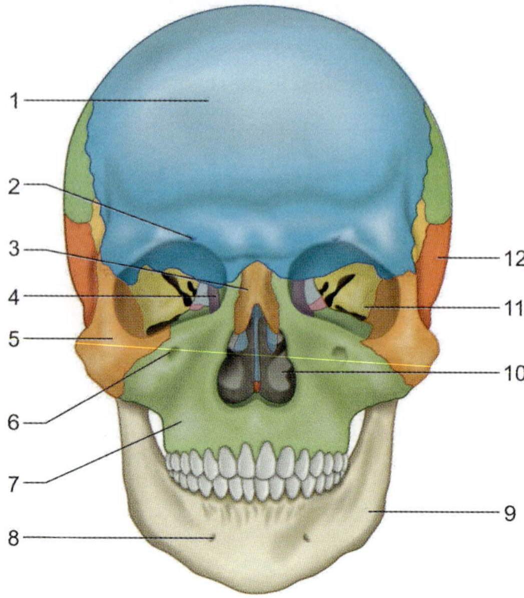

a. Supraorbital nerve and vessels
b. Infraorbital nerve and vessels
c. Zygomaticofacial nerve and vessels
d. Mental nerve and vessels

Area marked as 6 is infraorbital foramen, through which infraorbital vessels and nerve pass.

8. Nerve supply of muscle marked as D:

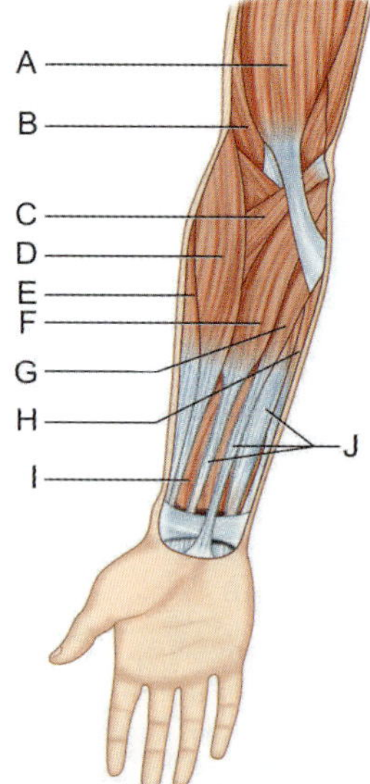

a. Radial nerve
b. Posterior interosseous nerve
c. Ulnar nerve
d. Median nerve

Muscle marked as D is pronator teres, which is innervated by median nerve.

9. Which of the following is NOT an action of muscle marked as 2:

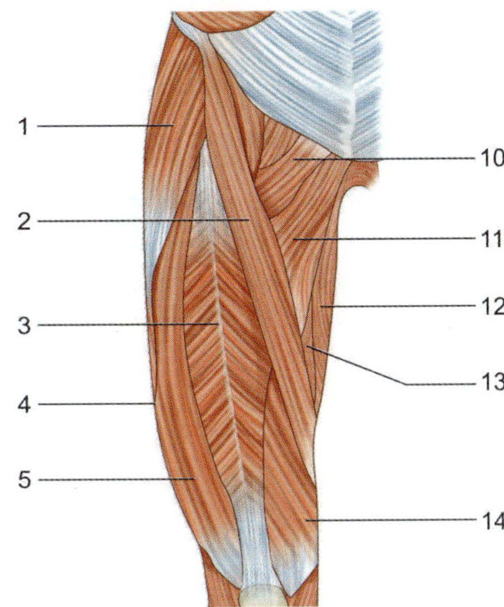

a. Medial rotation of thigh
b. Flexion of thigh
c. Abduction of thigh
d. Lateral rotation of thigh

Muscle marked as 2 is Sartorius, which is also known as tailors muscle. Action includes flexion of leg (at knee), flexion of thigh (at hip), abduction of thigh and lateral rotation of thigh.

10. Action of muscle marked as 10:

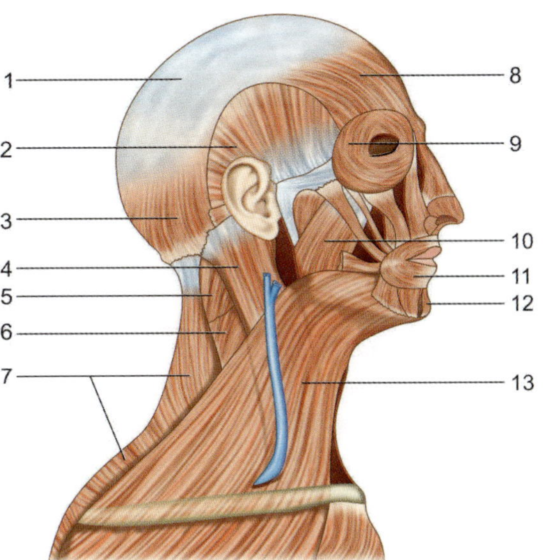

a. Retracts mandible
b. Elevates mandible
c. Depresses mandible
d. Side to side chewing action

Muscle marked as 10 is masseter, which elevates the mandible and closes the mouth. It also protracts the jaw.

MCQ POINTS

S. No.	Question statements	Answers
1.	Porter's tip deformity is a feature of:	***Erb's palsy***
2.	Weight of upper limb is transferred to trunk by which ligament	***Coracoclavicular ligament***
3.	Insertion of pectoralis major	***Lateral lip of bicipital groove on humerus***
4.	Nerve related to spiral groove of humerus	***Radial nerve***
5.	Action of coracobrachialis	***Flexion and medial rotation of arm***
6.	Action of anconeus	***Screwing action***
7.	Structure passing through cubital tunnel	***Ulnar nerve***
8.	Nerve passing through flexor retinaculum	***Media nerve***
9.	Structure passing through Guyon's canal	***Ulnar nerve***
10.	Action of lumbricals	***Flexion at metacarpophalangeal joint, extension at interphalangeal joint***
11.	Muscles supplied by axillary nerve	***Deltoid and teres minor***
12.	Froment's sign tests which nerve	***Ulnar nerve***
13.	Hypothenar muscles are supplied by	***Ulnar nerve***
14.	Complete claw hand is due to injury to which nerve	***Both ulnar and median nerve***
15.	Epithelial lining of true vocal cord	***Stratified squamous nonkeratinized***
16.	Ape thumb deformity suggests injury to	***Median nerve***
17.	Nerve supply of 1st and 2nd lumbricals	***Median nerve***
18.	Loss of opposition is seen in injury to which nerve	***Median nerve***
19.	Injury to lower trunk of brachial plexus is known as	***Klumpke's palsy***
20.	Clinical test which checks adductor pollicis muscle	***Froments sign/ book test***
21.	Nerve supply of pronator teres	***Median nerve***
22.	Nail bed of thumb is supplied by which nerve	***Median nerve***
23.	Posterior interosseous nerve is a branch of	***Radial nerve***
24.	Root value of radial nerve	***C5, 6, 7, 8, T1***
25.	Artery in anatomical snuff box	***Radial artery***
26.	Anterior cardiac vein drains into	***Right atrium***
27.	IVC pierces the central tendon of diaphragm at the level of	***T8***
28.	Tracheal bifurcation is at the level of	***T4***
29.	Flexor of trunk	***Rectus abdominis***
30.	Aortic hiatus contains	***Aorta, azygos vein and thoracic duct***
31.	Lingula is a part of .... lobe of ....lung	***Upper lobe, left lung***
32.	If the circumflex artery gives off posterior interventricular artery, then it is ...... Dominance	***Left dominance***
33.	Location of middle cardiac vein is in ...... sulcus	***Posterior interventricular sulcus***
34.	Right costophrenic recess extends up to the level of which rib in the midaxillary line	***10th rib***
35.	Azygos veins drain into	***Superior vena cava***
36.	Esophagus commences at the	***Lower end of cricoid cartilage***
37.	Right phrenic nerve passes through which hiatus	***Vena cava***
38.	Esophagus enters through which part of diaphragm	***Muscular part***
39.	While doing thoracocentesis, it is advisable to introduce needel along	***Along the upper border of rib***

S. No.	Question statements	Answers
40.	Superior border of heart is formed by	***Both atrium***
41.	Length of an adult trachea	***10 cm***
42.	SA node is supplied by	***Right coronary artery (60%)***
43.	Bronchial veins of the right side opens into .... vein	***azygos vein***
44.	Arch of aorta is at which vertebral level	***T4***
45.	Superior vena cava is formed by the union of .... veins	***Right and left brachiocephalic veins***
46.	Arch of aorta lies in .... mediastinum	***Superior mediastinum***
47.	Base of heart is principally formed by which chamber	***Left atrium***
48.	Vein arching over hilum of right lung	***azygos vein***
49.	Terminal branches of internal mammary artery	***Superior epigastric artery and musculophrenic artery***
50.	Anterior interventricular artery is a branch of	***Left coronary artery***
51.	Insertion of peroneus brevis	***Base of 5th metatarsal***
52.	Abduction and adduction of foot occurs at which joint	***Midtarsal and metatarsophalangeal joint***
53.	Action of popliteus muscle	***Unlocking of knee***
54.	Arterial supply of anterior compartment of thigh	***Femoral artery***
55.	Flexors of the hip joint	***Iliopsoas***
56.	Artery in adductor canal	***Femoral artery***
57.	Extension at the hip is restricted by	***Ileofemoral/ Bigelow ligament***
58.	Short saphenous vein is continuation of	***Lateral marginal vein (from dorsal venous arch)***
59.	Location of saphenous opening with respect to pubic tubercle	***Below and lateral***
60.	While flexing knee, femoral condyles are prevented from rolling backwards by which ligament	***Cruciate ligament***
61.	In femoral triangle, Femoral vein lies ...... to femoral artery	***Medial***
62.	Attachment of anterior cruciate ligament on femur	***Medial surface of lateral femoral condyle***
63.	Major function of gluteus medius and minimus	***Abduction at hip joint***
64.	Nerve supply of popliteus muscle	***Tibial nerve***
65.	Eversion of foot is produced by which muscle	***Peroneus longus and peroneus tertius***
66.	In foreceful inversion of foot, fracture of tuberosity of the 5th metatarsal is due to pull exerted by which tendon	***Peroneus brevis***
67.	Structure medial most in femoral sheath	***Femoral canal***
68.	Superficial inguinal ring is a defect in the	***External oblique aponeurosis***
69.	Medial meniscus is more liable to injured because of	***Fixity to tibial collateral ligament***
70.	Course of great saphenous vein in relation to the malleous	***Front of medial malleolus***
71.	Content of femoral canal	***Deep inguinal lymph node (Cloquet-Rosenmuller)***
72.	Site of injection in gluteal region	***Upper and outer quadrant***
73.	Foot drop occurs as a result of injury to which nerve	***Deep peroneal nerve***
74.	First web-space of the toe is supplied by which nerve	***Deep peroneal nerve***
75.	Flexion of the knee is caused by which muscle	***Hamstrings***
76.	Corresponding to the vas deferens in males, which structures passes through inguinal ring in females	***Round ligament***
77.	Superior rectal artery is a branch of	***Inferior mesenteric artery***
78.	Middle rectal artery arises from the	***Anterior division of internal iliac artery***
79.	Blood supply of jejunum is through the	***Superior mesenteric artery***
80.	Appendicular artery is a branch of the	***Iliocolic artery***

S. No.	Question statements	Answers
81.	Fascia of Denonvillier's lies between	***Rectum and prostate***
82.	Irritation of diaphragm radiates to which spinal nerve segments	***C3, 4, 5***
83.	Normal portal venous pressure	***5-10 mm Hg***
84.	Renal collar is formed by splitting and encircling of the aorta by	***Renal vein***
85.	Least dilatable part of urethra	***Membranous urethra***
86.	During abdominal surgery, under local anesthesia, patient suddenly felt sharp pain. Structure likely to be involved	***Parietal peritoneum***
87.	Superficial fascia between umbilicus and pubis symphysis is known as	***Campers fascia***
88.	Superior mesenteric artery arises opposite which vertebrae	***L1***
89.	Coeliac axis arises from the arch of aorta opposite which vertebrae	***T12-L1***
90.	Deep inguinal ring is a defect in the	***Fascia transversalis***
91.	Carcinoma prostate commonly occurs in which lobe	***Posterior***
92.	Right adrenal vein drains into the	***Inferior vena cava***
93.	Shortest part of colon	***Ascending colon***
94.	Parasympathetic supply to rectum and anal canal	***S2, 3, 4***
95.	Lymphatic drainage of umbilicus is to	***Axillary and inguinal***
96.	Uterine artery is a branch of	***Anterior division of internal iliac artery***
97.	Left testicular vein drains into	***Left renal vein***
98.	Length of inguinal canal is	***3.75 cm***
99.	Pouch of Douglas is situated between	***Uterus and rectum***
100.	Splenic artery is a branch of	***Coelaic axis***
101.	Fascia of Gerota is	***Renal fascia***
102.	Part of GIT supplied by superior mesenteric artery	***Derivative of midgut (from duodenum 2nd part; opening of common bile duct to junction of right 2/3rd and left 1/3rd of transverse colon)***
103.	Left gastroepiploic artery is a branch of	***Splenic artery***
104.	Flexor of the lumbar vertebral column	***Rectus abdominis***
105.	Policeman of the abdomen is	***Greater omentum***
106.	Embryonic ventral mesogastrium gives rise to which structure	***Lesser omentum***
107.	Duodenum develops from	***Foregut and midgut***
108.	Internal pudendal artery is a branch of	***Anterior division of internal iliac artery***
109.	Motor nerve supply to detrusor of the bladder is	***S2, 3, 4***
110.	Length of female urethra is	***4 cm***
111.	Lymphatics from the ovary drains into	***Preaortic and para-aortic nodes***
112.	Main lymphatic drainage of the testis	***Preaortic and para-aortic nodes***
113.	Superficial inguinal ring is a defect in	***External oblique aponeurosis***
114.	Bile duct opens into the	***2nd part of duodenum***
115.	Functional unit of the kidney is known as	***Nephron***
116.	Cremasteric reflex is governed by which nerve root	***L1***
117.	Deep circumflex iliac artery is a branch of	***External iliac artery***
118.	Pancreaticosplenic nodes drains which part of stomach	***Fundus***
119.	Blood supply of the uterus is by	***Uterine and ovarian arteries***
120.	If a missile enters the body just above the pubic ramus through the anterior abdominal wall, it will most likely pierce which viscera	***Urinary bladder***
121.	Nerve supply to the skin around umbilicus	***T10***

S. No.	Question statements	Answers
122.	Iliac crest is at the level of which vertebrae	*L4*
123.	Ligament which provides maximum support to the uterus	*Transverse cervical/Mackenrodt's/cardinal ligament*
124.	Superior gluteal artery arises from	*Posterior division of internal iliac artery*
125.	Ligation of coeliac artery will maximally affect which part of GIT	*Stomach*
126.	One bone forms the axis along which another bone rotates. This is which type of joint	*Pivot joint*
127.	Nerve supply of buccinator	*Facial nerve*
128.	Nasal glands are supplied by	*Facial nerve*
129.	All pharyngeal muscles are supplied by accessory nerve except	*Stylopharyngeus (supplied by glossopharyngeal nerve)*
130.	Thoracic duct passes through … hiatus	*Aortic hiatus*
131.	Source of bleeding in subdural hemorrhage	*Bridging veins*
132.	Histological feature of compact bone	*Haversian canal*
133.	Level of carina of trachea	*T4*
134.	2nd polar body is extruded at the time of	*Fertilization*
135.	Remnant of vitello-intestinal duct	*Meckel's diverticulum*
136.	Schwann cells are derived from	*Neural crest*
137.	Anterior belly of digastric develop from … pharyngeal arch	*First pharyngeal arch*
138.	Safety muscle of larynx	*Posterior cricoarytenoid*
139.	General sensation from anterior 2/3rd of tongue is carried by	*Chorda tympani*
140.	Epithelial lining of true vocal cord	*Stratified squamous nonkeratinized*
141.	Pleural cavity is lined by	*Simple squamous*
142.	Histological feature of cardiac myocytes	*Intercalated disc*
143.	Policeman tips hand is a feature of	*Erb's palsy*
144.	Injury to lower trunk of brachial plexus is known as	*Klumpke's palsy*
145.	Clinical test which checks adductor pollicis muscle	*Froments sign/ Book test*
146.	Axillary nerve supplies which muscle	*Deltoid and teres minor*
147.	Nerve supply of gluteus minimus	*Superior gluteal nerve*
148.	Ligament which prevents falling of trunk backward	*Ileofemoral/ Bigelow ligament*
149.	Dorsiflexion and plantarflexion occurs at … joint	*Ankle*
150.	Brunner glands are present in	*Duodenum*
151.	Vessels in umbilical cord	*2 arteries and 1 vein*
152.	Ligamentum arteriosum is derived from	*Ductus arteriosus*
153.	Artery present in anatomical snuff box	*Radial artery*
154.	Sperm attains motility in	*Epididymis*
155.	Hassal's corpuscles is seen in	*Thymus*
156.	Peyer's patches are present in	*Ileum*
157.	Nerve supply to hypothenar muscle is from	*Median nerve*
158.	Nerve passing superficial to flexor retinaculum at wrist	*Ulnar nerve*
159.	Nerve related to spiral groove of humerus	*Radial nerve*
160.	Azygos veins drain into	*Superior vena cava*
161.	Housemaids knee is inflammation of …. bursa	*Prepatellar bursa*
162.	Superficial inguinal ring is a defect in the	*External oblique aponeurosis*
163.	Left testicular vein drains into	*Left renal vein*
164.	Uterine artery is a branch of	*Anterior division of internal iliac artery*

S. No.	Question statements	Answers
165.	MC position of appendix	***Retrocecal***
166.	Nasolacrimal duct opens into … meatus	***Inferior meatus***
167.	Parasympathetic secretomotor fibers to submandibular gland is through	***Facial nerve***
168.	Opening of parotid duct	***In oral cavity, opposite upper second molar***
169.	Abductor of vocal cord	***Posterior cricoarytenoid***
170.	In adults spinal cord ends at the lower border of … vertebra	***L1***
171.	Muscles supplied by spinal part of accessory nerve	***Trapezius and sternocleidomastoid***
172.	Unlocking of knee is done by	***Popliteus***
173.	Type of cartilage in auricle of ear	***Elastic***
174.	Nerve supply of superior oblique muscle	***Trochlear***
175.	Muscle producing abduction, intorsion and depression of eyeball	***Superior oblique***

CHAPTER

2

PHYSIOLOGY

KEY POINTS

Normal Values

- Normal blood volume: 5–5.5 liters (3 liters plasma + 2 liters of cell volume)
- Intracellular fluid—55 percent
- Extracellular fluid—45 percent
- Total plasma protein in blood is 6.4–8.3 gm/dL
- Normal albumin: globulin ratio is 1.8:1–2:1
- Na^+: 135–145 mEq/L
- K^+: 3.5–5.5 mEq/L
- Ca^{++}: 9–11 mEq/L
- pH: 7.35–7.45
- PCO_2: 34–45 Hg
- PO_2: 85–100 mm Hg
- HCO_3: 25–28 mEq/L
- O_2 saturation: 92–96 percent
- Normal anion gap: 8–16 mEq/L
- Normal glomerular filtration rate—125 mL
- Renal blood flow—1200 mL/min
- Renal threshold for glucose—180 mg/dL
- Tubular maximum for glucose—320 mg/min

Half Lives of Proteins

- Albumin: 2-3 weeks
- Transferrin: 1 week
- Prealbumin, retinol binding protein, fibronectin: 2 days

Function of Cell Organelles

- Mitochondria: Production of energy
- Rough endoplasmic reticulum: Packaging of proteins
- Smooth endoplasmic reticulum: Lipid synthesis
- Ribosomes: Protein synthesis
- Golgi apparatus: Concentration of proteins and poly-saccharides
- Centriole: Initiate the process of cell division
- Lysosome: Break down bacteria and debris from dead tissue cells
- Peroxisomes: Destroy harmful substances

Types of Cell Transport

- Passive diffusion (simple passive+ facilitated diffusions): Transport of a substance along the gradient, energy is not required
- Simple passive diffusion: Diffusion along the gradient, without the requirement of carrier. Not rate limiting. doesn't follow saturation kinetics
- Primary active transport: Transport against gradient. Energy is obtained by breakdown of ATP. Requires transport protein. Rate limiting and saturable
- Secondary active transport: Energy for transport is derived from sodium gradient. Transport against gradient requires transport protein. Rate limiting and saturable

Rheobase and Chronaxie

- Rheobase: The least strength or current which excites the excitable tissue
- Chronaxie: Minimum time required to stmulate the excitable tissue when strength of the current used is double the rheobase

Reflexes/Law's/Rule's in Physiology

- Cushing's reflex: The reflex that tends to restore the blood flow to medulla by causing rise in systemic arterial pressure, slowing of respiration and reflex bradycardia in case of raised intracranial pressure.
- Bainbridge reflex: A true reflex rather than local response to stretch, causes receptor mediated increase in heart rate, is abolished by bilateral Vagotomy
- Starling's law: Within physiological limits, force of contraction is directly proportional to the initial length of the muscle fibres, provided conditions remain the same.
- Bezold-Jarisch reflex: Is a coronary chemoreflex mediated by left ventricular stretch receptors that are C fibers endings, it causes a fall in systemic arterial pressure and heart rate and apnoea followed rapid breathing.

- Bohr effect-effect of CO_2 in the affinity of Hemoglobin for O_2: Shift of oxygen hemoglobin dissociation curve by change in the blood in the blood CO_2, and hydrogen ions to enhance oxygenation of blood in lungs and to enhance release of oxygen from blood in the tissue.
- Haldane effect: Binding of oxygen with hemoglobin tends to displace CO_2 from blood; Important in promoting carbon dioxide transport.
- Herring-Breurer reflex: The stretch receptors in bronchi and bronchioles send inhibitory signals through vagi to inspiratory centre when the lung is overinflated.
- Cushing's response: Onset of irregular respiration, bradycardia and final increased blood pressure with increasing intracranial tension due to brain stem compression.
- Landsteiner's law: States that if an agglutinogen is present in the red cells of the blood, the corresponding agglutinin must be absent from the plasma, if the agglutiongen is absent, corresponding agglutinin must be present in the plasma.
- Sham rage behavior: Physical and motor manifestation of anger seen in destruction of ventromedial hypothalamic nuclei and septal nuclei.
- Muller's doctrine of specific nerve energies: When the nerve pathways from particular sense organs are stimulated, the sensation evoked is that for which the receptor is specialized no matter how or where along the pathway the activity is initiated.
- Weber-Fechner law: Interpreted signal strength = Log × stimulus intensity + constant.

Volumes related to Cardiophysiology

- Stroke volume: Volume of blood that is ejected by each ventricle with each beat. It is normally 70 mL.
- Ventricular end diastolic volume: Volume of blood in the ventricle just prior to the onset of ventricular contraction. Normal 110–120 mL
- Ventricular end systolic volume: Volume of blood remaining in the ventricle at the end of ejection. Normally 40–50 mL

Ecg (Parameters and Coinciding Event)

- P wave (0.08): Atrial depolarization
- PR interval (0.12–0.20 sec): Atrial depolarization and conduction through AV node measured from beginning of QRS complex.
- QRS duration (0.08–0.10 sec): Ventricular depolarization and atrial repolarization
- T wave: Ventricular repolarization
- U wave: Slow repolarization of papillary muscles.

O_2 Dissociation Curve

- Shift to left: Increased pH, Decreased temperature, Fetal hemoglobin
- Shift to right:Decreased pH, Increased temperature, Increased 2,3, DPG

Respiratory Capacities and Volumes

- Tidal volume: Air that is taken in or given out during normal quiet respiration
- Inspiratory reserve volume: Air that can be taken in over and above the tidal volume
- Expiratory reserve volume: Maximum volume of air that can be expired over and above the tidal volume
- Residual volume: Volume of air that remains in the lungs after forceful expiration
- Inspiratory capacity: Maximum volume of air that can be inspired after normal tidal expiration (IC = IRV + TV)
- Vital capacity: Maximum volume of air that can be expired after deepest possible inspiration (VC = IRV +TV + ERV)
- Total lung capacity: Sum of vital capacity and residual volume

Gastric Acid Secretion

- Excitatory: Acetylcholine, Gastrin, Histamine
- Inhibitory: Enterogastric reflex, Enterogastrone, Somatostatin

Hepatic Cells

- Ito cells are fat containing lipocytes in the space of Disse of the liver
- Kupffer cells are phagocytic cells, part of monocyte and macrophage cells.

Hormone Receptors

- Cell membrane receptors:
  - cAMP pathway: Adrenaline, Calcitonin, Glucagon, TSH, FSH, LH, ACTH, PTH.
  - IP3-DAG: Vasopressin, Oxytocin
  - Tyrosine- kinase: Insulin, Growth hormone.
- Cytoplasmic receptors: Steroids (Glucocorticoids, Mineralocorticoids), Estrogen, Progesterone
- Nuclear receptors: Thyroxine

Zones of Adrenal Cortex and Hormones Secreted (GFR)

- Zona Glomerulosa: Aldosterone
- Zona Fasciculate: Cortisol
- Zona Reticularis: Androgens

Juxtaglomerular Apparatus

- Macula densa: Epithelial cells of the initial part of distal tubule, lying in the angle between afferent and efferent arteriole of the glomerulus

- Juxtaglomerular cells/Granular cells: Smooth muscle cells of afferent and efferent arterioles containing dark granules, coming in contact with macula densa.

Hormones and their Effects

- Prolactin: Promote breast development in pregnancy and lactation
- FSH: Stimulate ovarian follicle growth in female and spermatogenesis in male
- LH: Stimulates ovulation and luteinization of ovarian follicles in female and testosterone secretion in male
- Estrogen: Responsible for maintenance of oogenesis, development of sex organs and secondary sexual characters in females at puberty
- Progesterone: Prepares the endometrium for implantation of the fertilized ovum and promotes the growth and development of the breast
- Testosterone: Responsible for maintenance of spermatogenesis, development of sex organs and secondary sexual characters in males at puberty
- Oxytocin: Uterine contraction during labour and promotes milk ejection during breast feeding

Cells of Nervous System

- Macroglia: CNS macrophages
- Astrocytes: Maintain blood-brain barrier. Repair and scar formation
- Oligodendrocytes: Formation of myelin in CNS
- Ependymal cells: Line the ventricular system.

Route of CSF Flow

- Choroid plexus–Lateral ventricle–Foramen of Monro–Third ventricle–Aqueduct of Sylvius–Fourth ventricle–Foramina of Luschka and Magendie–Subarachnoid space–Venous outflow

Nuclei of Hypothalamus

- Lateral nucles: Feeding centre
- Ventromedial nucleus: Satiety centre

Reflexes and Root Values

- Ankle: S1 S2
- Knee jerk: L3, 4
- Biceps reflex: C5, 6
- Triceps jerk: C7, 8
- Radial jerk: C6
- Plantar reflex: S1,S2
- Abdominal reflex: T7, T11
- Cremasteric reflex: L1

Receptors

- Free nerve endings: Detect touch and pressure
- Meissner's corpuscles: Detect movement of light touch
- Merkel's disc: Localizing touch sensations and determining texture
- Hair end organs: Detect the movement of objects on the surface of body
- Ruffini's end organs: Detect degree of joint movement
- Paccinian corpuscles: Detect tissue vibration, extremely rapid changes in mechanical state of tissue.

MCQs WITH SHORT EXPLANATIONS

HAEMATOLOGY AND BODY FLUIDS

1. **Which of the following is true regarding HbF?**
   a. Alpha 2, delta 2
   b. At 20 weeks intrauterine life, there is 90% HbF
   c. 10% persist in adults
   d. Shifts oxygen dissociation curve to right

Fetal hemoglobin/Hemoglobin F/HbF/alpha 2-gamma 2

- It is the main oxygen transport protein in the human fetus during the last seven months of development in the uterus and persists in the newborn until roughly 6 months old.
- Functionally, fetal hemoglobin differs most from adult hemoglobin in that it is able to bind oxygen with greater affinity than the adult form, giving the developing fetus better access to oxygen from the mother's bloodstream.
- In newborns, fetal hemoglobin is nearly completely replaced by adult hemoglobin by approximately 6 months postnatally, except in a few thalassemia cases in which there may be a delay in cessation of HbF production until 3-5 years of age.

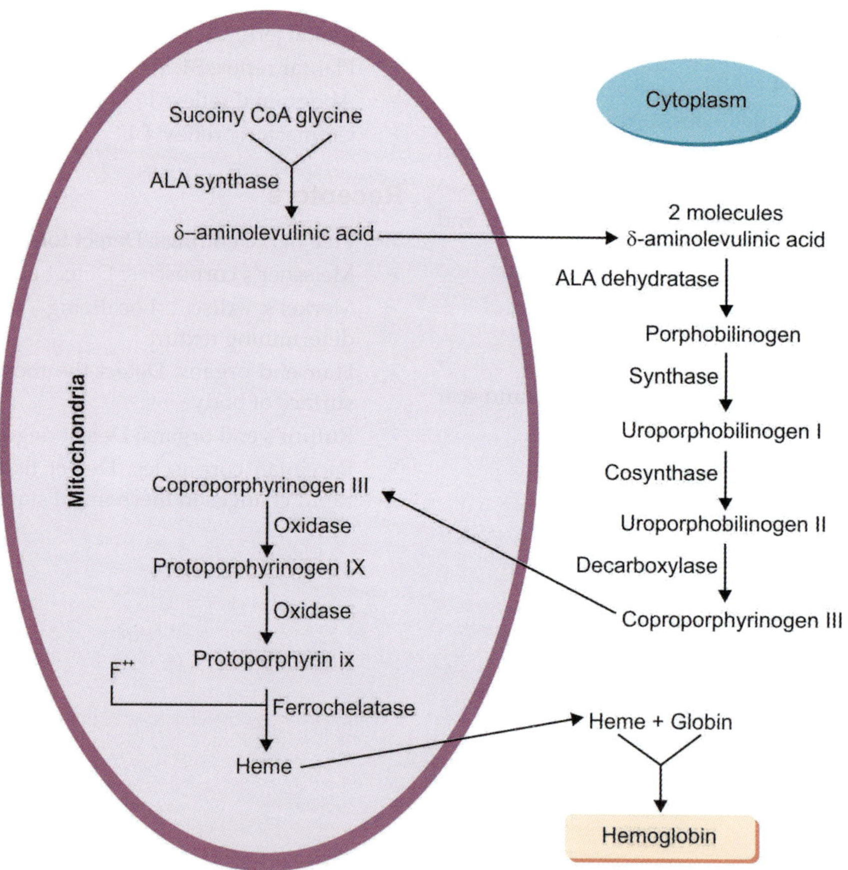

Synthesis of hemoglobin.

2. **Most useful method of estimating total iron content of blood:**
   a. Ferritin
   b. Transferrin
   c. Erythropoietin
   d. Lactoferrin

Plasma ferritin is also an indirect marker of the total amount of iron stored in the body, hence serum ferritin is used as a diagnostic test for iron deficiency anemia.

3. **Substance present in both serum and plasma:**
   a. Fibrinogen
   b. Factor II
   c. Factor VII
   d. Factor V

Factor VII (*blood-coagulation factor VIIa, activated blood coagulation factor VII,* formerly known as **proconvertin**) is **present in both plasma** and **serum** and is essential only for the extrinsic **clotting.**

Ans. 1. **b.** At 20 weeks... 2. **a.** Ferritin 3. **c.** Factor VII

4. **Hemophilia B is deficiency of which factor?**
   a. IX b. XII
   c. VIII d. X

   Haemophilia B (or **hemophilia B**) is caused by a mutation of the factor IX gene, leading to a deficiency of factor IX. It is the second most common form of haemophilia, rarer than haemophilia A. It is sometimes called **Christmas disease**, named after Stephen Christmas, the first patient described with this disease.

5. **Endothelial cells synthesize which of the following?**
   a. Factor XII b. Factor X
   c. vW factor d. Fibrinogen

   vWF is a large multimeric glycoprotein present in blood plasma and produced constitutively as ultra-large vWF in endothelium (in the Weibel-Palade bodies), megakaryocytes (α-granules of platelets), and subendothelial connective tissue.

6. **Normal pH of blood is:**
   a. 7.30 b. 7.20
   c. 7.70 d. 7.40

Constitution of normal blood

Parameter	Value
Hematocrit	45 ± 7 (38–52%) for males 42 ± 5 (37–47%) for females
pH	7.35–7.45
Base excess	−3 to +3
PO_2	10–13 kPa (80–100 mm Hg)
PCO_2	4.8–5.8 kPa (35–45 mm Hg)
HCO_3^-	21–27 mM
Oxygen saturation	Oxygenated: 98–99% Deoxygenated: 75%

7. **Most abundant buffer in blood:**
   a. Phosphate b. Protein
   c. Hemoglobin d. Bicarbonate

   The **bicarbonate buffering system** is an important buffer system in the acid-base homeostasis. As a buffer, it tends to maintain a relatively constant plasma pH and counteract any force that would alter. In this system, carbon dioxide (CO_2) combines with water (H_2O) to form carbonic acid (H_2CO_3), which in turn rapidly dissociates to form hydrogen ions (H^+) and bicarbonate (HCO_3^-).

8. **1 gm hemoglobin binds with:**
   a. 1.22 ml O_2 b. 1.33 ml O_2
   c. 1.44 ml O_2 d. 1.55 ml O_2

   Hemoglobin makes up about 96% of the red blood cells' dry content (by weight), and around 35% of the total content (including water). Hemoglobin has an oxygen-binding capacity of 1.34 mL O_2 per gram, which increases the total blood oxygen capacity seventy-fold compared to dissolved oxygen in blood. The hemoglobin molecule can bind (carry) up to four oxygen molecules.

9. **Plasma makes:**
   a. 20% of body weight b. 15% of body weight
   c. 10% of body weight d. 5% of body weight

   A normal individual weighs 70 kg. Plasma is about 2.75 L.

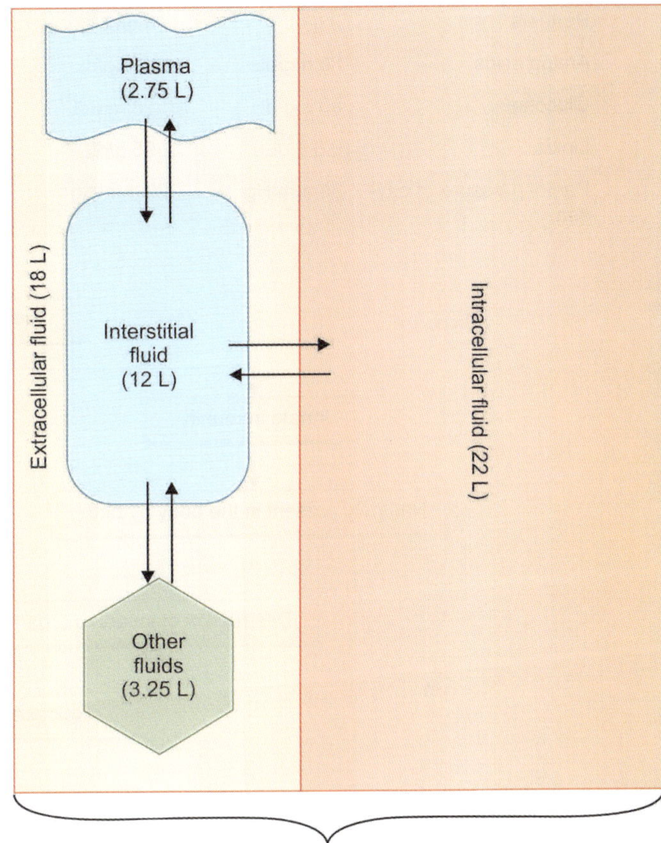

Body fluid compartments and movement of fluid between different compartments. Other fluids = Transcellular fluid, fluid in bones and fluid in connective tissue.

10. **Extracellularly, which ion is found in greatest amount:**
    a. Sodium b. Potassium
    c. Chloride d. Calcium

    Sodium is dominant in ECF whereas potassium in ICF.

Differences between extracellular fluid (ECF) and intracellular fluid (ICF)

Substance	ECF	ICF
Sodium	142 mEq/L	10 mEq/L
Calcium	5 mEq/L	1 mEq/L
Potassium	4 mEq/L	140 mEq/L
Magnesium	3 mEq/L	28 mEq/L
Chloride	103 mEq/L	4 mEq/L
Bicarbonate	28 mEq/L	10 mEq/L

Contd...

Ans. 4. **a.** IX 5. **c.** vW factor 6. **d.** 7.40 7. **d.** Bicarbonate
8. **b.** 1.33 ml O_2 9. **d.** 5% of body weight 10. **a.** Sodium

Contd...

Substance	*ECF*	*ICF*
Phosphate	4 mEq/L	75 mEq/L
Sulfate	1 mEq/L	2 mEq/L
Proteins	2 g/dL	16 g/dL
Amino acids	30 mg/dL	200 mg/dL
Glucose	90 mg/dL	0-20 mg/dL
Lipids	0.5 g/dL	2-95 g/dL
Partial pressure of oxygen	35 mm Hg	20 mm Hg

Contd...

Substance	*ECF*	*ICF*
Partial pressure of carbon dioxide	46 mm Hg	50 mm Hg
Water	15 to 20 L (18)	20 to 25 L (22)
pH	7.4	7.0

11. Source of gamma-globulins:

a. Liver
b. Spleen
c. T-cells
d. Plasma cells

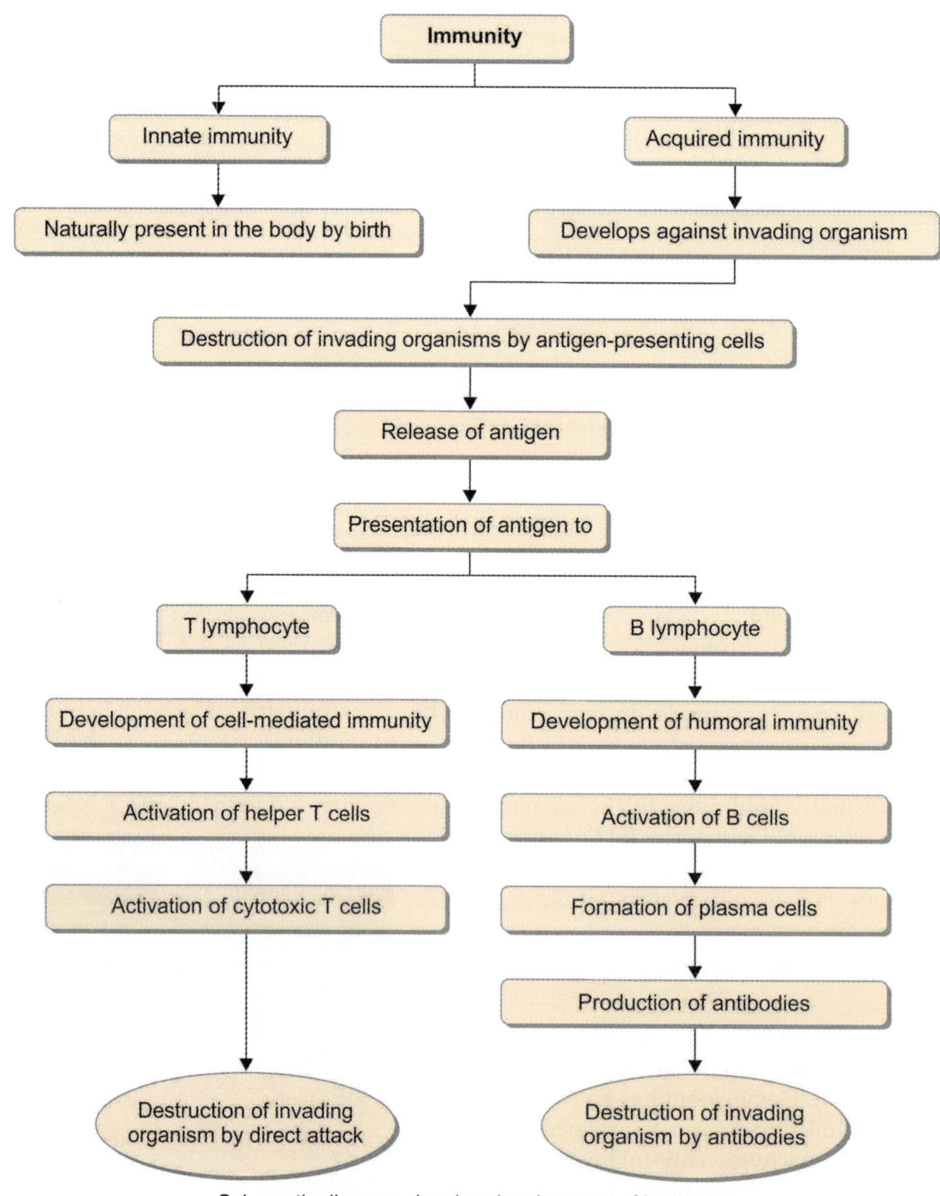

Schematic diagram showing development of immunity.

Ans. **11. d.** Plasma cells

Plasma cells, also called **plasma B cells**, **plasmocytes**, **plasmacytes**, or **effector B cells**, are white blood cells that secrete large volumes of antibodies. The most significant gamma globulins are immunoglobulins ("Igs"), a subclass of which are antibodies, although some Igs are not gamma globulins, and some gamma globulins are not Igs.

12. The following factors are derived from the endothelial cell except:

a. Thrombomodulin
b. Protein S
c. Prostacyclin
d. Thromboxane A2

Thromboxane A2 (TXA2) is a type of thromboxane that is produced by activated platelets and has prothrombotic properties: it stimulates activation of new platelets as well as increases platelet aggregation.

13. Respiratory burst is related to:

a. Hyperventilation after a period of apnea
b. Apnea after a period of hyperventilation
c. Sharp increase in O_2 uptake and metabolism in neutrophils
d. None of the above

Respiratory burst (sometimes called **oxidative burst**) is the rapid release of reactive oxygen species (superoxide radical and hydrogen peroxide) from different types of cells. Usually, it denotes the release of these chemicals from immune cells, e.g. neutrophils and monocytes, as they come into contact with different bacteria or fungi.

14. Monocytes remain in the circulation for:

a. 1-3 days
b. 24 hours
c. 12 hours
d. 6 hours

Monocytes are produced by the bone marrow from precursors called monoblasts, bipotent cells that differentiated from hematopoietic stem cells. Monocytes circulate in the bloodstream for about one to three days and then typically move into tissues throughout the body. They constitute between three to eight percent of the leukocytes in the blood. Half of them are stored as a reserve in the spleen in clusters in the red pulp's Cords of Billroth.

Diameter and lifespan of WBCs

WBC	Diameter (μ)	Lifespan (days)
Neutrophils	10 to 12	2 to 5
Eosinophils	10 to 14	7 to 12
Basophils	8 to 10	12 to 15
Monocytes	14 to 18	2 to 5
Lymphocytes	7 to 12	½ to 1

15. Most common hemoglobin in normal adult is:

a. HbA
b. HbF
c. HbS
d. HbA2

Hemoglobin A (HbA), also known as **adult hemoglobin** or $\alpha_2\beta_2$, is the most common human hemoglobin tetramer, comprising over 97% of the total red blood cell hemoglobin.

16. Reticulocytosis is NOT seen in:

a. Chronic renal failure
b. Hemorrhage
c. Hereditary spherocytosis
d. Paroxysmal nocturnal hemoglobinuria

Patients with severe chronic renal failure almost develop anemia. The most important cause of this is decreased renal secretion of erythropoietin, which stimulates the bone marrow to produce red blood cells.

17. Need of vitamin B12 and folate in formation of red blood cells is primarily due to their effects on:

a. Hemoglobin formation
b. DNA synthesis in the bone marrow
c. Absorption of iron from the gut
d. Synthesis and release of erythropoietin from the kidney

The best-known "function" of B12 (that which is involved with DNA synthesis, cell-division, and anemia) is actually a facultative function which is mediated by B12-conservation of an active form of folate which is needed for efficient DNA production.

18. Hageman factor is involved in:

a. Extrinsic pathway
b. Intrinsic pathway
c. Fibrinolysis
d. None

Factor XII (Hageman factor) is part of the coagulation cascade and activates factor XI and prekallikrein in vitro. Factor XII itself is activated to factor XIIa by negatively charged surfaces, such as glass. This is the starting point of the intrinsic pathway.

Ans. 12. **d.** Thromboxane A2 13. **c.** Sharp increase... 14. **a.** 1-3 days 15. **a.** HbA
16. **a.** Chronic renal... 17. **b.** DNA synthesis... 18. **b.** Intrinsic pathway

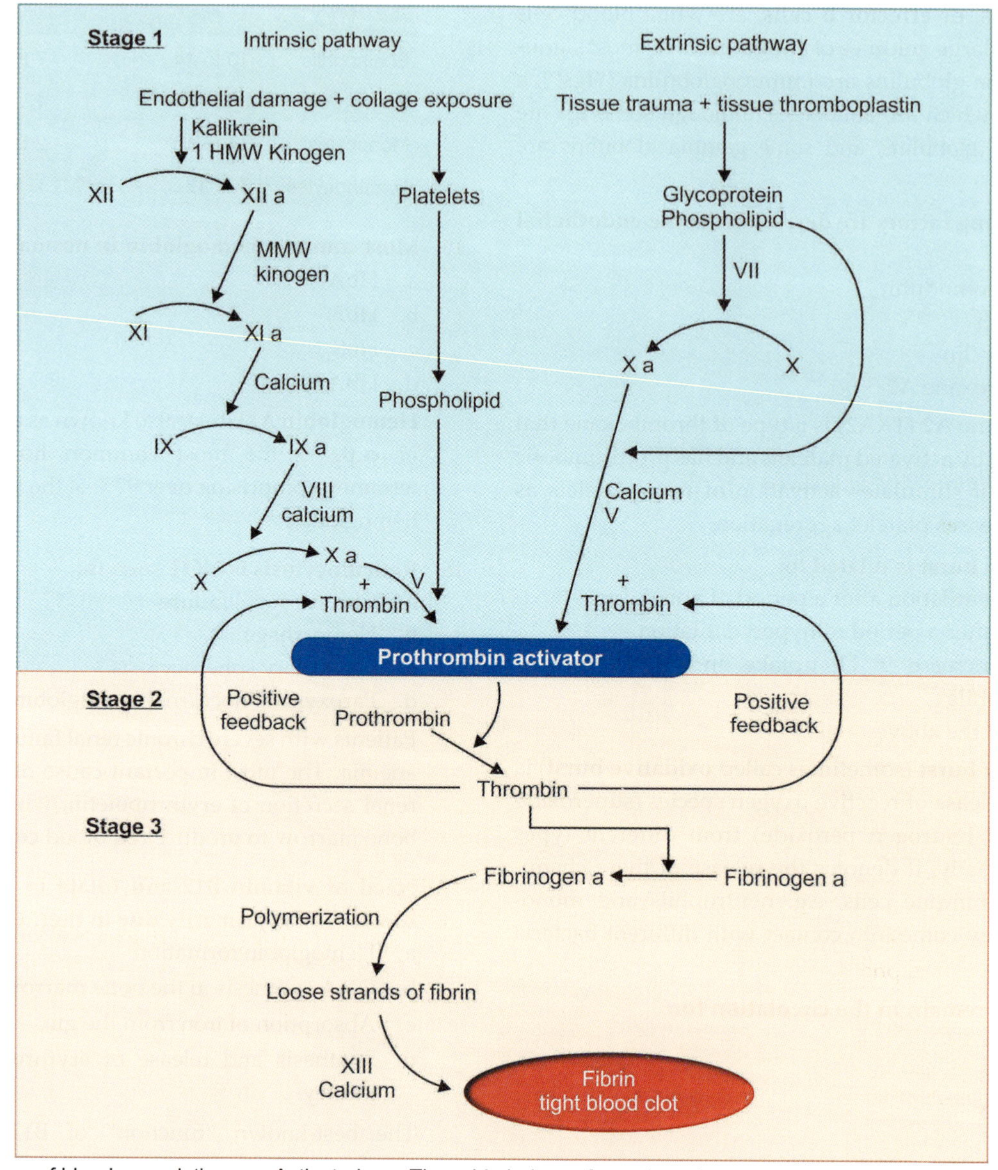

Stages of blood coagulation. a = Activated, + = Thrombin induces formation of more thrombin (positive feedback); HMW = High molecular weight.

19. When aPTT is prolonged, factor unaffected is:

a. XII
b. XI
c. VII
d. IX

Normal PTT times require the presence of the following coagulation factors: I, II, V, VIII, IX, X, XI, and XII. Notably, deficiencies in factors VII or XIII will not be detected with the PTT test.

20. Heparin inhibits the active form of the following factors except:

a. V
b. X
c. XI
d. XII

Heparin binds to the enzyme inhibitor antithrombin III (AT), causing a conformational change that results in its activation through an increase in the flexibility of its reactive site loop. The activated AT then inactivates thrombin and other proteases involved in blood clotting, most notably factor Xa.

Ans. **19. c.** VII **20. a.** V

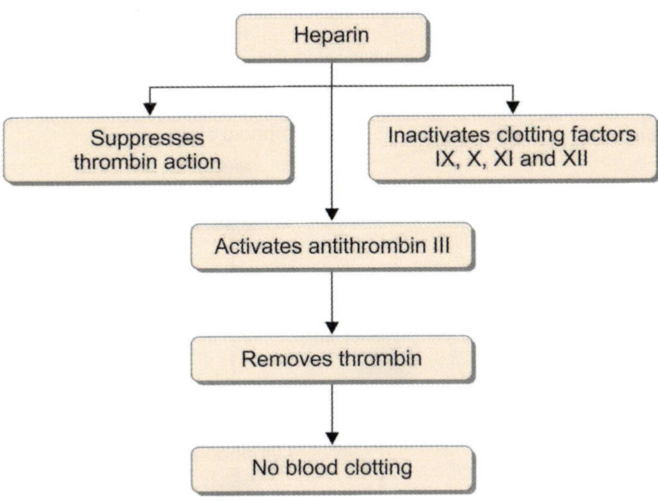

Mechanism of action of heparin

21. Hemoglobin with molecular weight of 64,458:
a. HbA
b. HbF
c. HbS
d. HbA2

Hemoglobin A has a molecular weight of 64,458.

22. Most abundant buffering agent seen in blood:
a. Phosphates
b. Protein
c. Hemoglobin
d. Bicarbonate

Buffering agents in humans, functioning in acid base homeostasis, are extracellular agents (e.g. bicarbonate, ammonia) as well as intracellular agents (including proteins and phosphate).

23. Osmolality of plasma in normal adult:
a. 250-260 mOsm/L
b. 280-290 mOsm/L
c. 310-320 mOsm/L
d. 340-350 mOsm/L

Normal human plasma has an osmolality in the range of 285-295 milliosmol/kg. Agents which have an osmolality higher than 600 cause crenation (shrivelling up) of red blood cells and significant pain. Solutions which have an osmolality less than about 150 milliosmol/kg cause haemolysis (rupture of the red blood cells) and pain at the site of injection.

24. NOT a vitamin K dependent clotting factor (hepatic origin):
a. X
b. VIII
c. VII
d. II

Factor VIII (FVIII) is an essential blood-clotting protein, also known as anti-hemophilic factor (AHF). FVIII is a glycoprotein procofactor. Although the primary site of release in humans is ambiguous, it is synthesized and released into the bloodstream by the vascular, glomerular, and tubular endothelium, and the sinusoidal cells of the liver.

25. Most abundant ion in ICF:
a. Sodium
b. Potassium
c. Chloride
d. Bicarbonate

Potassium is most dominant cation in ICF whereas sodium is most dominant in ECF.

26. Major contributor to plasma osmolality:
a. Sodium ions
b. Potassium ions
c. Chloride ions
d. Calcium ions

Osmolality is a variation of molality that takes into account only solutes that contribute to a solution's osmotic pressure. It is measured in osmoles of the solute per kilogram of water.

27. Prothrombin to thrombin conversion need:
a. Calcium
b. Magnesium
c. Potassium
d. Sodium

Thrombin is produced by the enzymatic cleavage of two sites on prothrombin by activated Factor X (Xa). Prothrombin is produced in the liver and is post-translationally modified in a vitamin K-dependent reaction that converts ten glutamic acids on prothrombin to gamma-carboxyglutamic acid (Gla). In the presence of calcium, the Gla residues promote the binding of prothrombin to phospholipid bilayers.

28. Clotting factor NOT affected in liver disorders:
a. Factor VIII
b. Factor IX
c. Factor IV
d. Factor II

FVIII is a glycoprotein procofactor. Although the primary site of release in humans is ambiguous, it is synthesized and released into the bloodstream by the vascular, glomerular, and tubular endothelium, and the sinusoidal cells of the liver.

29. Iron binding protein:
a. Hephaestin
b. Transferrin
c. Ferroportin-1
d. Ferritin

Transferrins are iron-binding blood plasma glycoproteins that control the level of free iron in biological fluids. Human transferrin is encoded by the *TF* gene.

30. First site for hematopoiesis in fetus:
a. Spleen
b. Liver
c. Yolk sac
d. Bone marrow

Ans. 21. a. HbA 22. d. Bicarbonate 23. b. 280-290 mOsm/L 24. b. VIII
25. b. Potassium 26. a. Sodium ions 27. a. Calcium 28. a. Factor VIII
29. b. Transferrin 30. c. Yolk sac

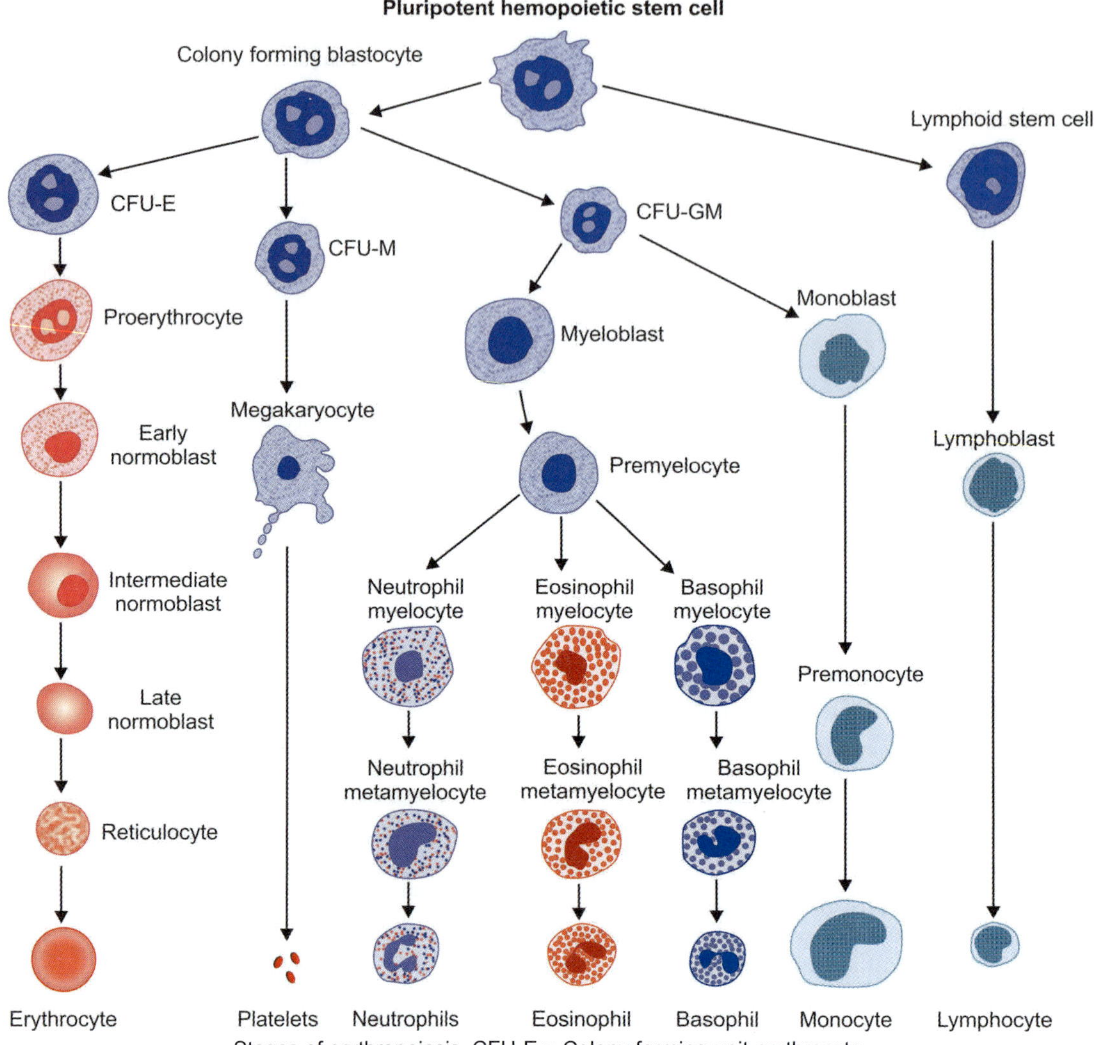

Stages of erythropoiesis. CFU-E = Colony forming unit-erythrocyte, CFU-M = Colony forming unit-megakaryocyte, CFU-GM = Colony forming unit-granulocyte/monocyte.

In developing embryos, blood formation occurs in aggregates of blood cells in the yolk sac, called blood islands. As development progresses, blood formation occurs in the spleen, liver and lymph nodes. When bone marrow develops, it eventually assumes the task of forming most of the blood cells for the entire organism.

31. FALSE statement:

a. HCO_3^- is predominantly seen in ICF
b. Mg^{2+} is one of the major cations of ICF (after K^+)
c. Na^+ is major cation in plasma
d. Cl^- is major anion in interstitial fluid

Bicarbonate levels in ECF is 28 mEq/L whereas in ICF, it is 10 mEq/L.

32. Chief site of hematopoiesis in 2nd trimester of life:

a. Yolk sac b. Liver
c. Spleen d. Bone marrow

During the middle trimester of gestation, the liver is the main organ for production of red blood cells, although reasonable numbers of red blood cells are also produced in the spleen and lymph nodes.

33. Cation more dominant in ICF:

a. Sodium b. Potassium
c. Calcium d. Magnesium

Potassium is more dominant in ICF whereas sodium is more dominant in ECF.

34. Half life of albumin:

a. 7 days b. 14 days
c. 21 days d. 28 days

The reference range for albumin concentrations in serum is approximately 35–50 g/L (3.5-5.0 g/dL). It has a serum half-life of approximately 20 days. It has a molecular mass of 66.5 kDa.

Ans. **31. a.** HCO_3^- is predominantly seen in ICF **32. b.** Liver **33. b.** Potassium **34. c.** 21 days

35. Warm periphery is noticed in which type of shock?

a. Cardiogenic shock b. Septic shock
c. Hemorrhagic shock d. Traumatic shock

Early sepsis is accompanied by a decrease in systemic vascular resistance and a metabolic acidosis. The clinical picture includes fever, tachycardia, tachypnoea, respiratory alkalosis and an increased cardiac output with warm, dry peripheries and a bounding pulse. Advanced sepsis involves varying degrees of venous and myocardial contractile failure, and is characterised by progressive acidaemia, respiratory failure and marked sympathetic adrenergic activation.

36. Anticoagulant secreted by endothelium:

a. Heparin
b. Alpha 2 macroglobulin
c. Thrombomodulin
d. All of the above

Thrombomodulin (**TM**), CD141 or BDCA-3 is an integral membrane protein expressed on the surface of endothelial cells and serves as a cofactor for thrombin. It reduces blood coagulation by converting thrombin to an anticoagulant enzyme from a procoagulant enzyme. Thrombomodulin is also expressed on human mesothelial cell, monocyte and a dendritic cell subset.

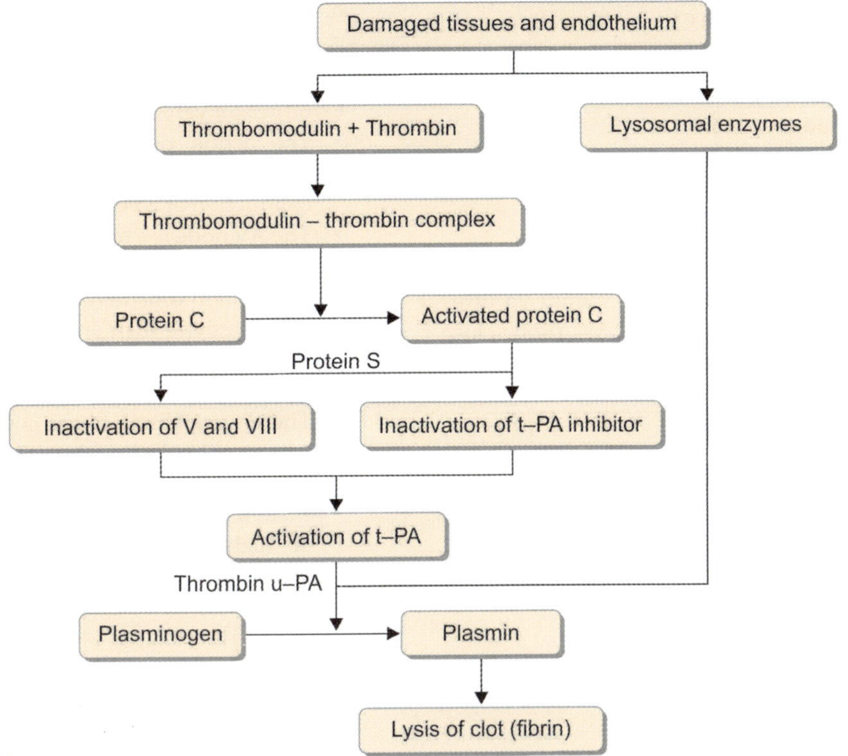

Fibrinolysis. t-PA = Tissue plasminogen activator, u-PA = Urokinase plasminogen activator.

37. Phagocytosis is done by:

a. Eosinophil b. Basophil
c. Neutrophil d. Lymphocyte

Neutrophils are a type of phagocyte and are normally found in the bloodstream. During the begi-nning (acute) phase of inflammation, particularly as a result of bacterial infection, environmental exposure, and some cancers, neutrophils are one of the first-responders of inflammatory cells to migrate towards the site of inflammation.

38. Best for ECF volume measurement:

a. Tritium oxide
b. Evans blue
c. Inulin
d. Antipyrine

Marker substances used to measure body fluid compartments

Fluid compartment	*Marker substances*
Total body water	1. Deuterium oxide (D_2O) 2. Tritium oxide (T_2O) 3. Antipyrine
Extracellular fluid	1. Radioactive sodium, chloride, bromide, sulfate and thiosulfate. 2. Non-metabolizable saccharides like inulin, mannitol, raffinose and sucrose
Plasma	1. Radioactive iodine (^{131}I) 2. Evans blue (T-1824)

39. Total plasma volume is measured by:

a. Mannitol b. Evans blue
c. Inulin d. Sucrose

Ans. 35. **b.** Septic shock 36. **c.** Thrombomodulin 37. **c.** Neutrophil 38. **c.** Inulin 39. **b.** Evans blue

T-1824 or **Evans Blue**, often incorrectly rendered as **Evan's Blue**, is an azo dye which has a very high affinity for serum albumin. Because of this, it can be useful in physiology in estimating the proportion of body water contained in blood plasma.

40. T cells mature in:

a. Thyroid
b. Tongue
c. Thymus
d. Trachea

T-cell can be distinguished from other lymphocytes, such as B cells and natural killer cells (NK cells), by the presence of a T-cell receptor (TCR) on the cell surface. They are called T cells because they mature in the thymus (although some also mature in the tonsils.

41. Major portion of body water is:

a. Intracellular
b. Extracellular
c. Both the compartments
d. Variable

In a body containing 40 litres of fluid, about 25 litres is intracellular, which amounts to 62.5% (5/8), close enough to the 2/3 rule of thumb.

CARDIOVASCULAR SYSTEM

42. Which of the following is NOT a true statement for Stroke volume?

a. Reduced because of an increase in heart rate
b. Depends on after load
c. Depends on pre-diastolic volume
d. Directly proportional to heart rate

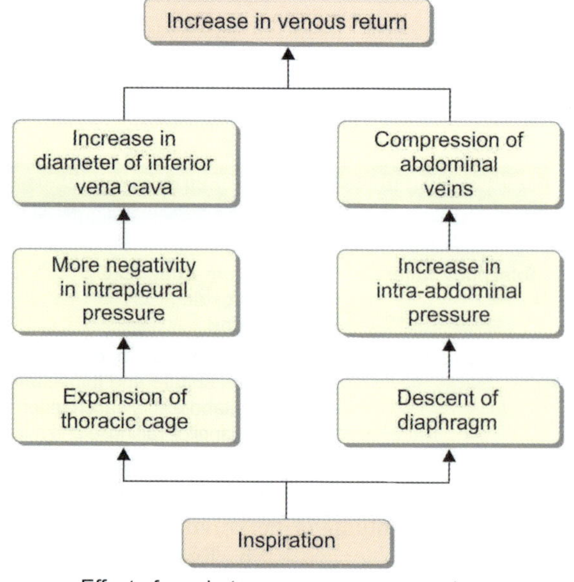

Effect of respiratory pump on venous return.

Increase in heart rate gives less time for ventricles to fill and hence less end diastolic volume so a fall in stroke volume.

Stroke volume

- Prolonged aerobic exercise training may also increase stroke volume, which frequently results in a lower (resting) heart rate.
- Reduced heart rate prolongs ventricular diastole (filling), increasing end-diastolic volume, and ultimately allowing more blood to be ejected.

43. Slowest conduction is observed in:

a. Bundle of His
b. Purkinje fibres
c. AV node
d. SA node

Conduction velocity

- The action potentials generated by the *SA node* spread throughout the atria primarily by cell-to-cell conduction at a velocity of about 0.5 m/sec.
- The AV node is a highly specialized conducting tissue (cardiac, not neural in origin) that slows the impulse conduction considerably (to about 0.05 m/sec).
- The impulses then enter the base of the ventricle at the **Bundle of His** and then follow the **left and right bundle branches** along the interventricular septum. These specialized fibers conduct the impulses at a very rapid velocity (about 2 m/sec).
- The bundle branches then divide into an extensive system of **Purkinje fibers** that conduct the impulses at high velocity (about 4 m/sec) throughout the ventricles.

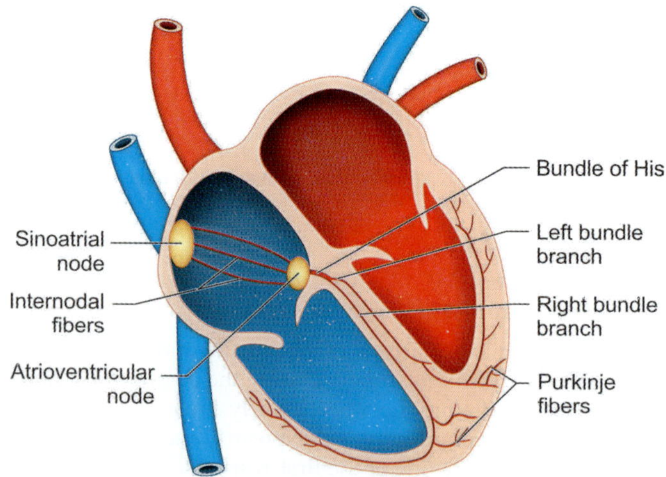

Sinoatrial node and conductive system of the heart.

44. Cardiac event at the end of isometric relaxation phase:

a. Atrioventricular valves open
b. Atrioventricular valves closes
c. Corresponds to peak of C wave in JVP
d. Corresponds to T wave in ECG

Ans. 40. **c.** Thymus 41. **a.** Intracellular 42. **a.** Reduced because of an increase in heart rate
43. **c.** AV node 44. **a.** Atrioventricular valves open

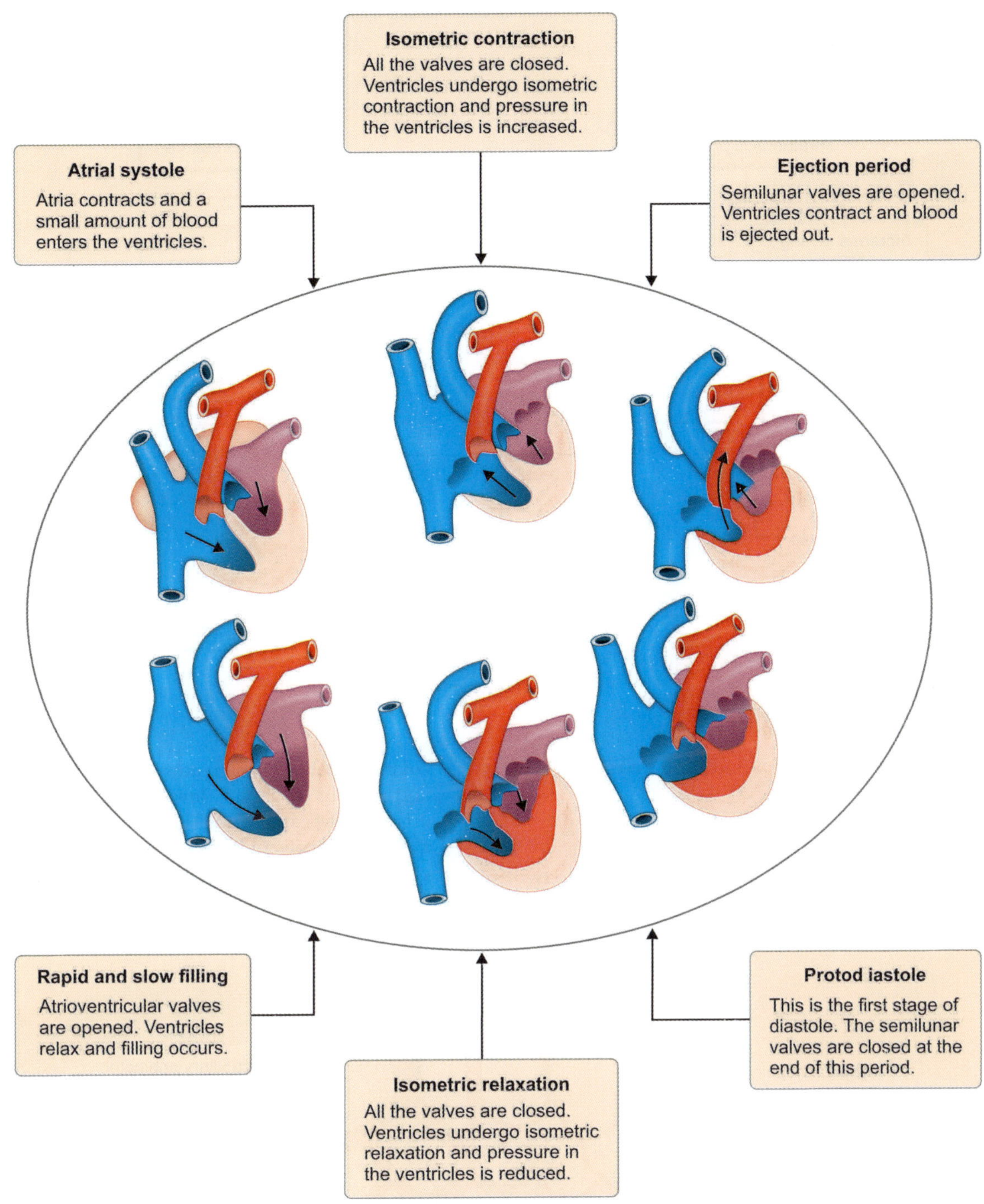

Events of the cardiac cycle.

The isovolumic relaxation time (IVRT) is the interval from the aortic component of the second heart sound (that is, closure of the aortic valve), to onset of filling by opening of the mitral valve.

45. Bainbridge reflex causes:

a. Decreased distension of large somatic veins
b. Decreased BP
c. Decreased HR
d. Increased HR

The **Bainbridge reflex**, also called the **atrial reflex**, is an increase in heart rate due to an increase in central venous pressure. Increased blood volume is detected by stretch receptors (baroreceptors) located in both atria at the venoatrial junctions.

Ans. **45. d.** Increased HR

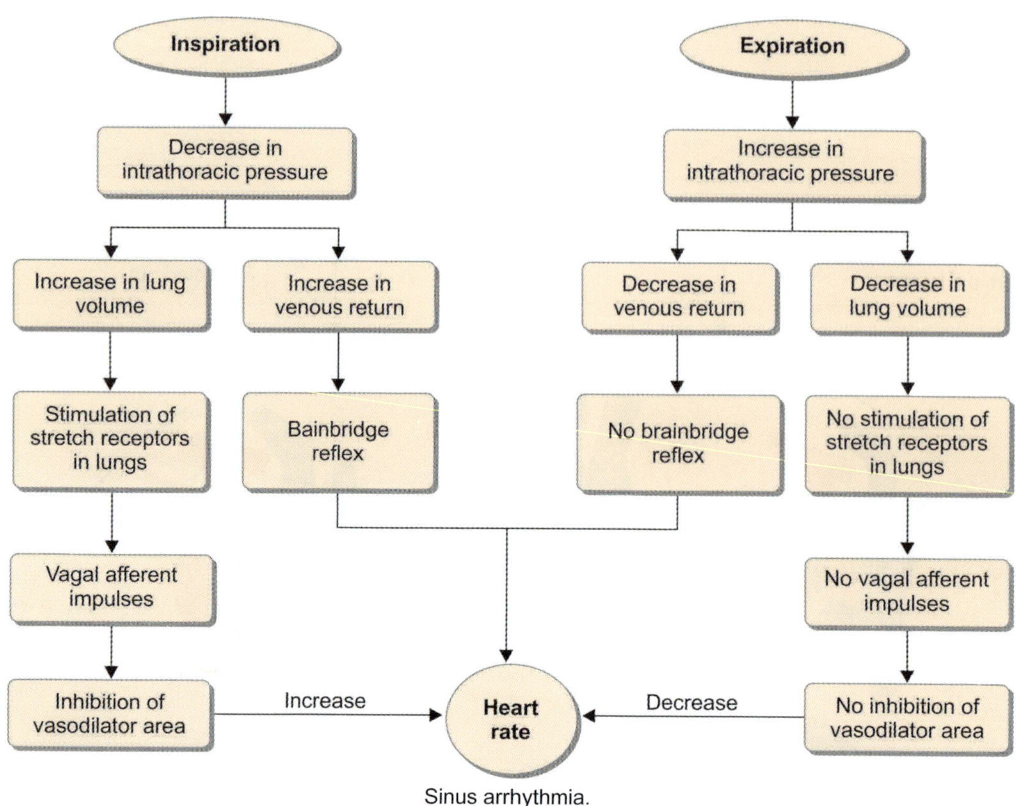

Sinus arrhythmia.

46. Greatest resistance in peripheral blood circulation is due to:

a. Capillaries
b. Veins
c. Arterioles
d. Arteries

Arterioles have muscular walls (usually only one to two layers of smooth muscle) and are the primary site of vascular resistance. The greatest change in blood pressure and velocity of blood flow occurs at the transition of arterioles to capillaries. The decreased velocity of flow in the capillaries reduces the pressure and increases exchange of gas and nutrients.

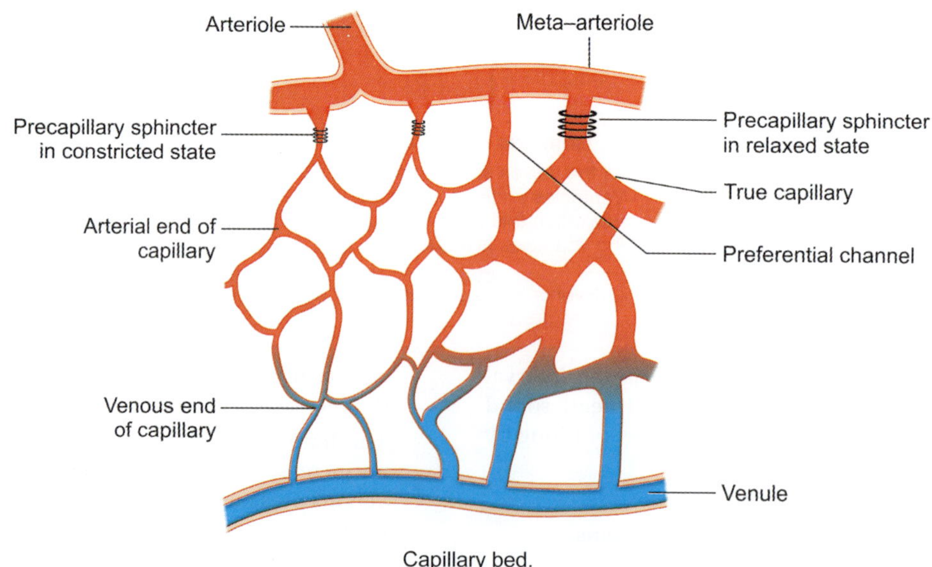

Capillary bed.

Ans. 46. c. Arterioles

47. **Single most important factor controlling contractility of heart:**
   a. Myocardial wall thickness
   b. Right atrial volume
   c. SA node pacemaker potential
   d. Sympathetic stimulation

Sympathetic system stimulation increases rate and force of contraction.

48. **During flight or fight reaction, factor responsible for increase in local blood flow:**
   a. Sympathetic system mediated cholinergic release
   b. Local hormones
   c. Parasympathetic cholinergic
   d. Endocrine factors only

The **fight-or-flight response** (also called the **fight, flight, freeze, or fawn response**, **hyperarousal**, or the **acute stress response**) is a physiological reaction that occurs in response to a perceived harmful event, attack, or threat to survival. It was first described by Walter Bradford Cannon. His theory states that animals react to threats with a general discharge of the sympathetic nervous system, priming the animal for fighting or fleeing. More specifically, the adrenal medulla produces a hormonal cascade that results in the secretion of catecholamines, especially norepinephrine and epinephrine. The hormones estrogen, testosterone and cortisol, and the neurotransmitters dopamine and serotonin, also affect how organisms react to stress.

49. **An afferent arteriolar dilator:**
   a. Antihistaminic
   b. Aspirin
   c. Propranolol
   d. Prostacyclin

Prostacyclin (also called **prostaglandin I2** or **PGI_2**) is a prostaglandin member of the family of lipid molecules known as eicosanoids. It inhibits platelet activation and is also an effective vasodilator.

50. **NOT characteristic of cardiac muscle:**
   a. Pacemaker potential
   b. Tetany
   c. Length-tension relationship
   d. All or none phenomenon

Tetany is characterized by contraction of distal muscles of the hands (carpal spasm with extension of interphalangeal joints and adduction and flexion of the metacarpophalangeal joints) and feet (pedal spasm) and is associated with tingling around the mouth and distally in the limbs.

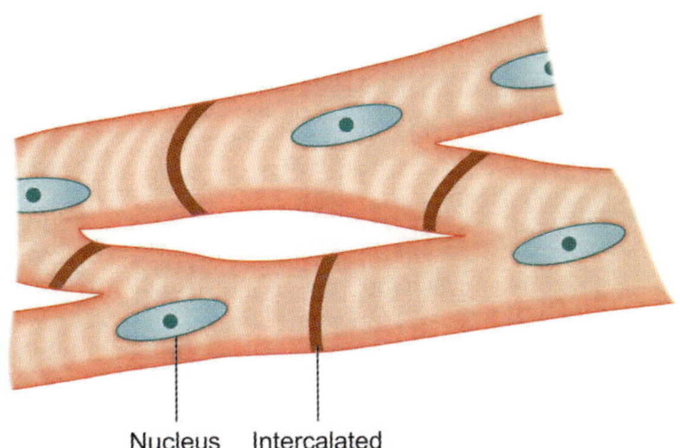

Cardiac muscle fibers.

51. **The coronary blood flow (mL/min) is:**
   a. 250 mL/min
   b. 500 mL/min
   c. 750 mL/min
   d. 850 mL/min

Resting coronary blood flow is roughly 225 ml/min which results in 4–5% of the total cardiac output. The coronary circulation is in place as only 1/10 mm of the endocardial heart layer is supplied by blood from the chambers.

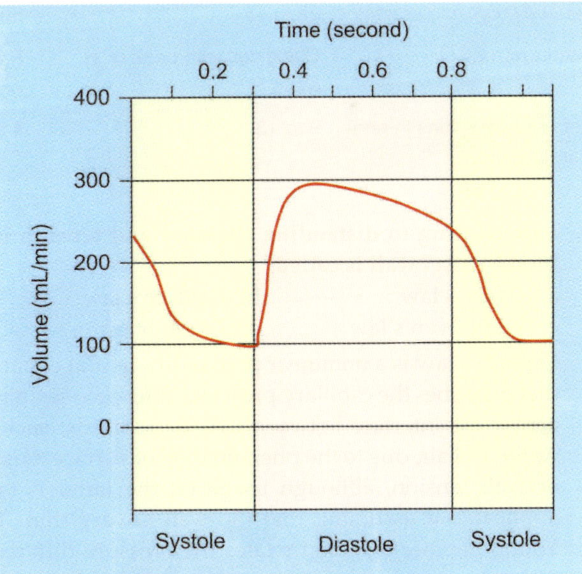

Phasic changes in coronary blood flow.

52. **Splanchnic vessels and venules contain:**
   a. 10-20% of blood volume
   b. 20-30% of blood volume
   c. 40-50% of blood volume
   d. 60-70% of blood volume

The **splanchnic** bed (blood flow through the gut itself plus blood flow through the spleen, pancreas, and liver) **contains** a little more than one-fifth of the total **blood volume**.

Ans. 47. **d.** Sympathetic... 48. **a.** Sympathetic... 49. **d.** Prostacyclin 50. **b.** Tetany
51. **a.** 250 mL/min 52. **b.** 20–30% of blood volume

Distribution of blood pumped out of left ventricle		
Organ	*Amount of blood (mL/minute)*	*Percentage*
Liver	1,500	30
Kidney	1,300	26
Skeletal muscles	900	18
Brain	800	16
Skin, bone and GI tract	300	6
Heart	200	4
Total	5,000	100

53. First heart sound indicates onset of:

a. Ventricular diastole
b. Ventricular systole
c. Atrial systole
d. Atrial diastole

The first heart sound, or S_1, forms the "lub" of "lub-dub" and is composed of components M_1 and T_1. Normally M_1 precedes T_1 slightly. It is caused by the sudden block of reverse blood flow due to closure of the atrioventricular valves, i.e. tricuspid and mitral (bicuspid), at the beginning of ventricular contraction, or systole.

Heart sounds				
Features	*First heart sound*	*Second heart sound*	*Third heart sound*	*Fourth heart sound*
Occurs during	Isometric contraction period and part of ejection period	Protodiastole and part of isometric relaxation	Rapid filling phase	Atrial systole
Characteristics	Long, soft and low pitched Resembles the word 'LUBB'	Short, sharp and high pitched Resembles the word 'DUP'	Low pitched	Inaudible sound
Cause	Closure of atrioventricular valves	Closure of semilunar valves	Rushing of blood into ventricle	Contraction of atrial musculature
Duration (sec)	0.10 to 0.17	0.10 to 0.14	0.07 to 0.10	0.02 to 0.04
Frequency (cycles per sec)	25 to 45	50	1 to 6	1 to 4
Relation with ECG	Coincides with peak of 'R' wave	Precedes or appears 0.09 second after peak of 'T' wave	Between 'T' wave and 'P' wave	Between 'P' wave and 'Q' wave
Number of vibrations in phonocardiogram	9 to 13	4 to 6	1 to 4	1 to 2

54. Law relating to distending pressure and tension in a blood vessel wall is called:

a. Mary's law
b. LaPlace's law
c. Einthoven's law
d. Frank-Starling's law

Laplace's law is a nonlinear partial differential equation that describes the capillary pressure difference sustained across the interface between two static fluids, such as water and air, due to the phenomenon of surface tension or wall tension, although usage on the latter is only applicable if assuming that the wall is very thin. The Young-Laplace equation relates the pressure difference to the shape of the surface or wall and it is fundamentally important in the study of static capillary surfaces.

55. Mediator of 'Flare' in triple response:

a. Axon reflex
b. Arteriolar dilation
c. Histamine release
d. Local hormones

An **axon reflex** (also referred to as the flare response) is a response brought on by peripheral nerve stimulation. Examples include vasodilation originally described by Lewis as the "hunter's response" or autonomic reaction to loss of body heat in the extremities (also known as "Lewis wave" and "Lewis reaction").

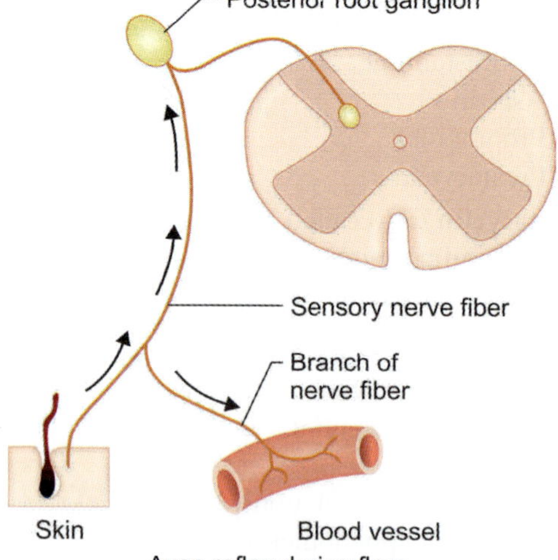

Axon reflex during flare.

56. Ion responsible for plateau phase of action potential in myocardium:

a. Closure of voltage gated potassium channels
b. Influx of potassium
c. Influx of calcium
d. Efflux of sodium

Ans. 53. **b.** Ventricular systole
54. **b.** LaPlace's law
55. **a.** Axon reflex
56. **c.** Influx of calcium

The "plateau" phase of the cardiac action potential (absent in pacemaker cells), is sustained by a balance between inward movement of Ca^{2+} (I_{Ca}) through L-type calcium channels (opened in response to large depolarization), and outward movement of K^+ through the slow delayed rectifier K channel, I_{Ks}. The influx of calcium into the cell is balanced by in the efflux of potassium out of the cell, which results in the plateau in action potential graph.

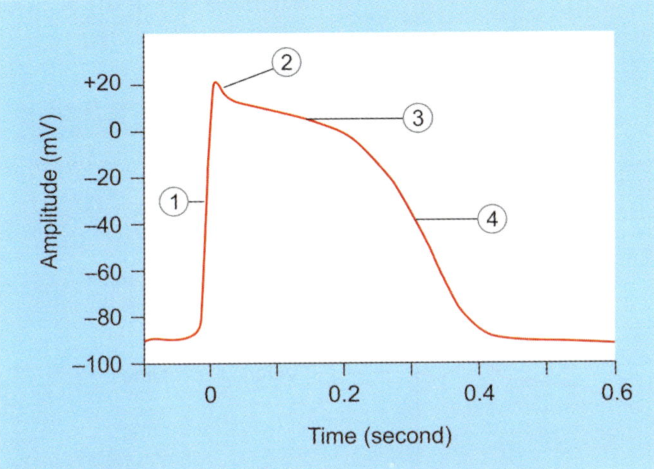

Action potential in ventricular muscle. 1 = Depolarization, 2 = Initial rapid repolarization, 3 = Plateau, 4 = Final repolarization.

57. Structure responsible for peripheral vascular resistance:

a. Aorta b. Venules
c. Capillaries d. Arterioles

The major regulator of vascular resistance in the body is regulation of vessel radius. In humans, there is very little pressure change as blood flows from the aorta to the large arteries, but the small arteries and arterioles are the site of about 70% of the pressure drop, and are the main regulators of SVR.

58. Organ receiving maximum blood flow (ml/kg minute):

a. Lungs b. Brain
c. Liver d. Kidney

Blood flow to kidney under basal conditions

- 22% of cardiac output
- 1100 ml/min
- 360 ml/min/100 gram

59. Law which relates to preload?

a. Mary's law b. LaPlace law
c. Einthoven's law d. Frank-starling's law

The **Frank-Starling law** of the heart (also known as **Starling's law** or the **Frank-Starling mechanism** or **Maestrini heart's law**) states that the stroke volume of the heart increases in response to an increase in the volume of blood filling the heart (the end diastolic volume) when all other factors remain constant.

60. Which of the following does NOT increase length of cardiac muscle fibre:

a. Increased venous tone
b. Increased total blood volume
c. Increased negative intrathoracic pressure
d. Lying to standing change in posture

The effects of gravity on venous return seem paradoxical because when a person stands up, hydrostatic forces cause the right atrial pressure to decrease and the venous pressure in the dependent limbs to increase. This increases the pressure gradient for venous return from the dependent limbs to the right atrium; however, venous return actually decreases. The reason for this is when a person initially stands, cardiac output and arterial pressure decrease (because right atrial pressure falls). The flow through the entire systemic circulation falls because arterial pressure falls more than right atrial pressure; therefore, the pressure gradient driving flow throughout the entire circulatory system is decreased.

61. During the cardiac cycle, opening of aortic valve occurs at:

a. Beginning of systole
b. End of isovolumetric contraction
c. End of diastole
d. End of diastasis

At the end of isovolumetric contraction, when the pressure within the ventricle is more than large vessels, aortic and pulmonary valves open.

(See Diagram on next page)

62. Mean pulmonary artery pressure:

a. 25 mm Hg b. 20 mm Hg
c. 15 mm Hg d. 10 mm Hg

Pulmonary artery pressure: Diastolic is 4-12 mm Hg and systolic is 15-30 mm Hg. The mean pressure is typically 11-18 mm Hg, and the *wedge pressure* measured in the left atrium may be 6-12 mm Hg.

63. SA node is known as pacemaker because it:

a. Has rich sympathetic innervation
b. Has rich cholinergic innervation
c. Generates impulses at a highest rate
d. Generates impulses spontaneously

Although some of the heart's cells have the ability to generate the electrical impulses (or action potentials) that trigger cardiac contraction, the sinoatrial node normally initiates it, simply because it generates impulses slightly faster than the other areas with pacemaker potential.

64. Effect of vagal stimulation on heart:

a. Increased force of contraction
b. Increased cardiac output
c. Increased heart rate
d. Increased R-R interval

Ans. 57. **d.** Arterioles 58. **d.** Kidney 59. **d.** Frank-Starling's law 60. **d.** Lying to standing..
61. **b.** End of isovo... 62. **c.** 15 mm Hg 63. **c.** Generates impulses... 64. **d.** Increased R-R interval

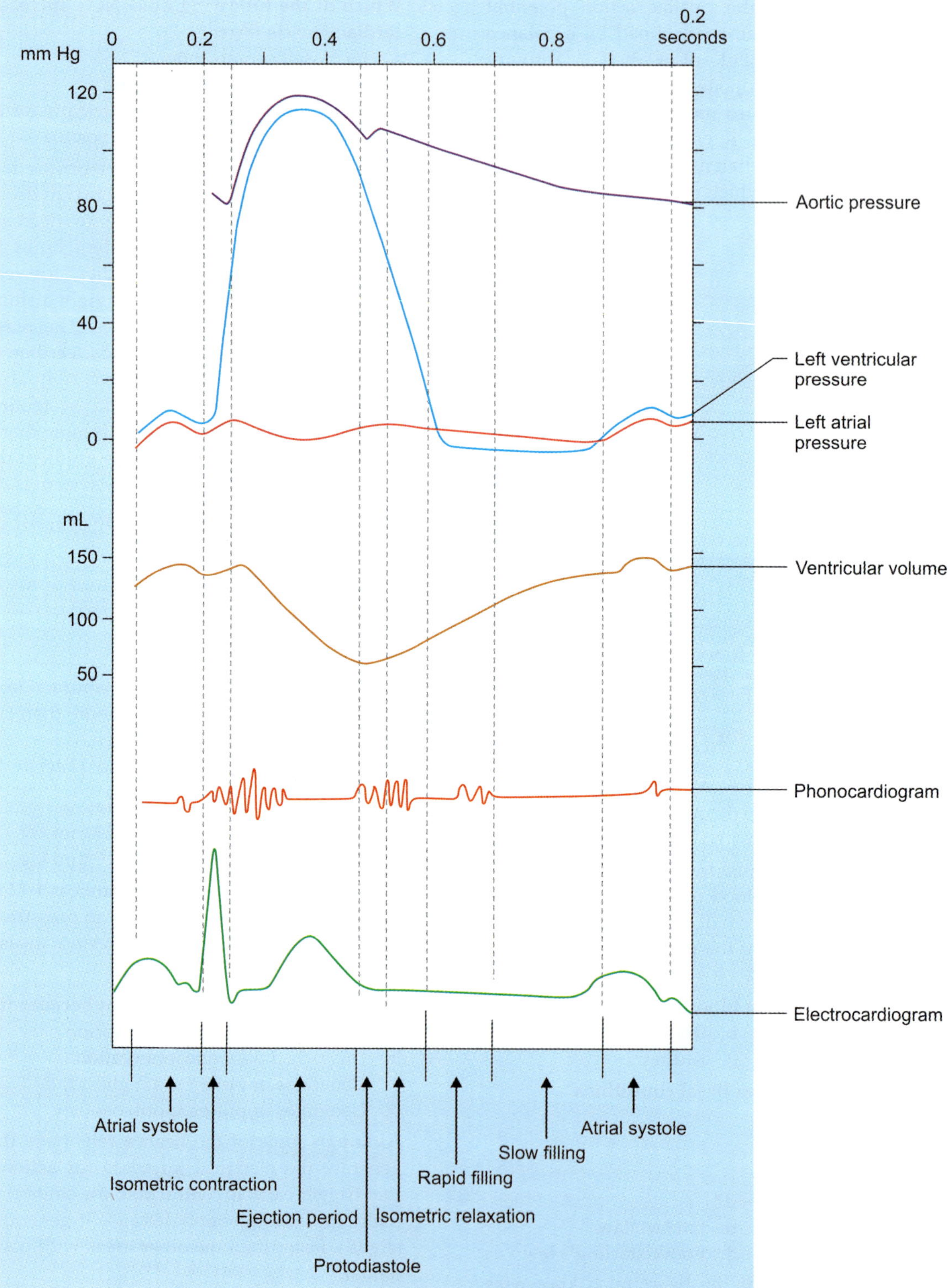

Comprehensive diagram showing ECG, phonocardiogram, pressure changes and volume changes during cardiac cycle.

The vagus nerve of the parasympathetic nervous system acts to decrease the heart rate (prolongation of R-R interval), and nerves from the sympathetic trunk act to increase the heart rate.

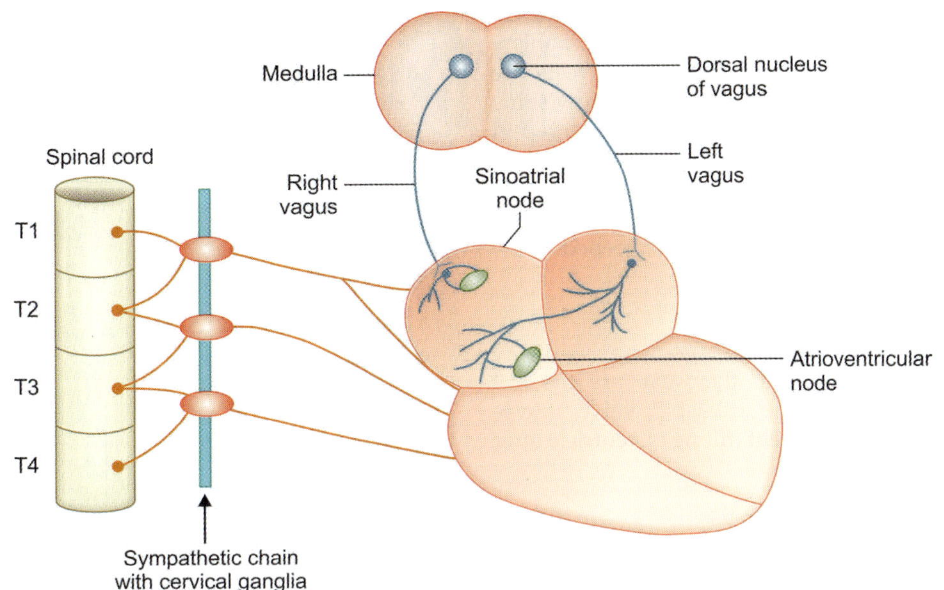

Nerve supply to heart.

65. QRS complex is mainly due to:
a. Atrial depolarization
b. Atrial repolarization
c. Ventricular depolarization
d. Ventricular repolarization

QRS complex corresponds to the depolarization of the right and left ventricles of the human heart. In adults, it normally lasts 0.06–0.10s; in children and during physical activity, it may be shorter.

Waves of normal ECG

Wave/segment	*From – To*	*Cause*	*Duration (second)*	*Amplitude (mV)*
P wave	–	Atrial depolarization	0.1	0.1 to 0.12
QRS complex	Onset of Q wave to the end of S wave	Ventricular depolarization and atrial repolarization	0.08 to 0.10	Q = 0.1 to 0.2 R = I S = 0.4
T wave	–	Ventricular repolarization	0.2	0.3
P-R interval	Onset of P wave to onset of Q wave	Atrial depolarization and conduction through AV node	0.18 (0.12 to 0.2)	–
Q-T interval	Onset of Q wave and end of T wave	Ventricular depolarization and ventricular repolarization	0.4 to 0.42	–
S-T segment	End of S wave and onset of T wave	Isoelectric	0.08	–

66. Preload measures:
a. Stroke volume
b. Peripheral resistance
c. End diastolic volume
d. End systolic volume

Preload is the end diastolic volume that stretches the right or left ventricle of the heart to its greatest geometric dimensions under variable physiologic demand. In other words, it is the initial stretching of the cardiomyocytes prior to contraction; therefore, it is related to the sarcomere length at the end of diastole.

67. Largest pool of blood is in:
a. Venules
b. Veins
c. Arteries
d. Capillaries

Veins serve to return blood from organs to the heart. Veins are also called "capacitance vessels" because most of the blood volume (60%) is contained within veins.

68. Autoregulation is observed in:
a. Muscles
b. Brain
c. Kidney
d. All of the above

Ans. **65. c.** ventricular... **66. c.** End diastolic volume **67. b.** Veins **68. d.** All of the above

Autoregulation is a process within many biological systems, resulting from an internal adaptive mechanism that works to adjust (or mitigate) that system's response to stimuli. While most systems of the body show some degree of autoregulation, it is most clearly observed in the kidney, the heart, mesentery, skeletal muscle, liver and the brain. Perfusion of these organs is essential for life, and through autoregulation the body can divert blood (and thus, oxygen) where it is most needed.

69. Negative wave in jugular venous pulse:

a. a wave b. v wave
c. c wave d. x wave

The downward deflections of the wave are the "x" (the atrium relaxes and the tricuspid valve moves downward) and the "y" descent (filling of ventricle after tricuspid opening).

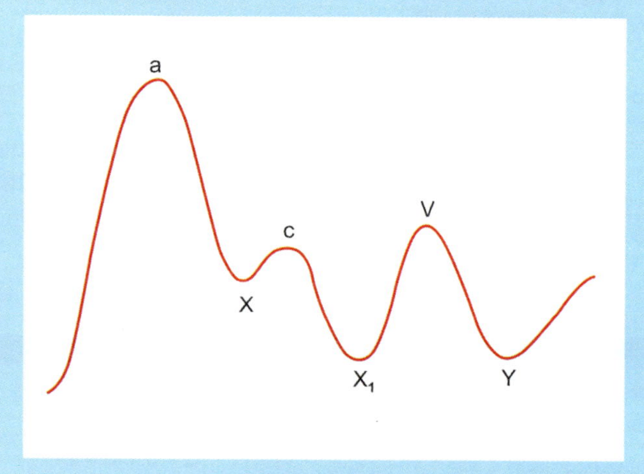

Phlebogram.

70. Cause of 'red reaction' in triple response:

a. Decreased capillary permeability
b. Axon reflex
c. Capillary dilation
d. Local edema

Triple response

- Red spot: Due to capillary dilatation
- Flare: Redness in the surrounding area due to arteriolar dilatation mediated by axon reflex.
- Wheal: Due to exudation of fluid from capillaries and venules

71. Maximum filling of ventricles is observed in:

a. Atrial contraction b. Ventricular diastole
c. Isovolumetric relaxation d. Protodiastole

During ventricular diastole, the pressure in the (left and right) ventricles drops from the peak that it reaches in systole. When the pressure in the left ventricle drops to below the pressure in the left atrium, the mitral valve opens, causing accumulated blood from the atrium to flow into the ventricle.

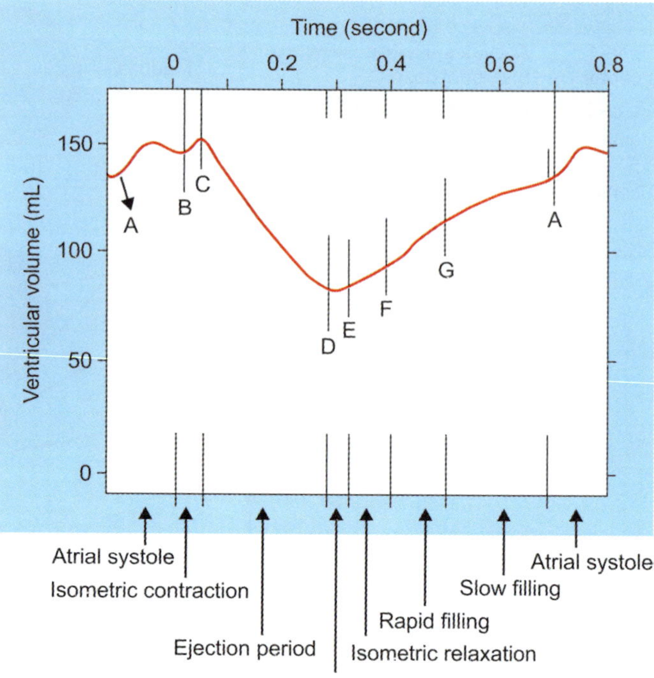

Ventricular volume changes during cardiac cycle.

72. Heart musculature is perfused during:

a. Isovolumetric contraction phase
b. Protodiastole
c. Ventricular diastole
d. Maximum ejection phase

During contraction of the ventricular myocardium (systole), the subendocardial coronary vessels (the vessels that enter the myocardium) are compressed due to the high ventricular pressures. However, the epicardial coronary vessels (the vessels that run along the outer surface of the heart) remain patent, or open and unobstructed. Because of this, blood flow in the subendocardium stops during ventricular contraction. As a result, most myocardial perfusion occurs during heart relaxation (diastole) when the subendocardial coronary vessels are open and under low pressure. Flow never comes to zero in the right coronary artery, since the right ventricular pressure is less than the left ventricular pressure.

73. Effect of norepinephrine mainly due to excitation of:

a. Alpha receptors
b. Beta receptors
c. Both are stimulated equally
d. None is stimulated

The **alpha-1** (α_1) **adrenergic receptor** is a G protein-coupled receptor (GPCR) associated with the G_q heterotrimeric G-protein. It consists of three highly homologous subtypes, including α_{1A}-, α_{1B}-, and α_{1D}-adrenergic. Catecholamines like norepinephrine (noradrenaline) and epinephrine (adrenaline) signal through the α_1-adrenergic receptor in the central and peripheral nervous systems.

Ans. 69. **d.** x wave 70. **c.** Capillary dilation 71. **b.** Ventricular diastole 72. **c.** Ventricular diastole 73. **a.** Alpha receptors

Receptor	Mode of action	Response
Alpha-1 receptor	Activates IP_3 through phospholipase C	Mediates more of noradrenaline actions than adrenaline actions
Alpha-2 receptor	Inhibits adenyl cyclase and cAMP	
Beta-1 receptor	Activates adenyl cyclase and cAMP	Mediates actions of adrenaline and noradrenaline equally
Beta-2 receptor	Activates adenyl cyclase and cAMP	Mediates more of adrenaline actions than noradrenaline actions

74. Precapillary resistance vessels are:

a. Arteries b. Veins
c. Arterioles d. Venules

The **precapillary resistance vessels** (**arterioles**) provide the majority of the systemic vascular resistance.

75. Marey's law denotes relationship between:

a. Heart rate and cardiac output
b. Heart rate and BP
c. Heart rate and stroke volume
d. Heart rate and presystolic volume

Marey's law

- The pulse rate varies inversely with the blood pressure; that is, the pulse is slow when the pressure is high; an expression of baroreceptor reflex influences on heart rate.

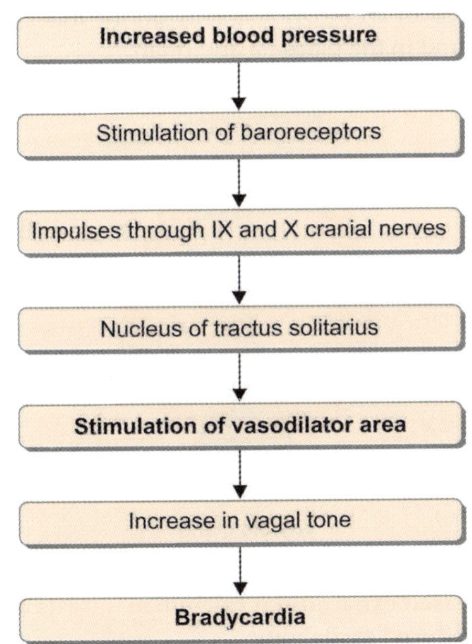

Marey (cardioinhibitory) reflex.

76. Prepotential in SA node is due to all except:

a. Calcium spark
b. Leakiness of the membrane to sodium
c. Increase in potassium permeability
d. Transient calcium channel opening

The influx of calcium and sodium ions through the calcium-sodium channels ceases, while at the same time larger quantities of positive potassium ions diffuse out of the fiber, thus reducing the intracellular potential back to its negative level and therefore terminating the action potential.

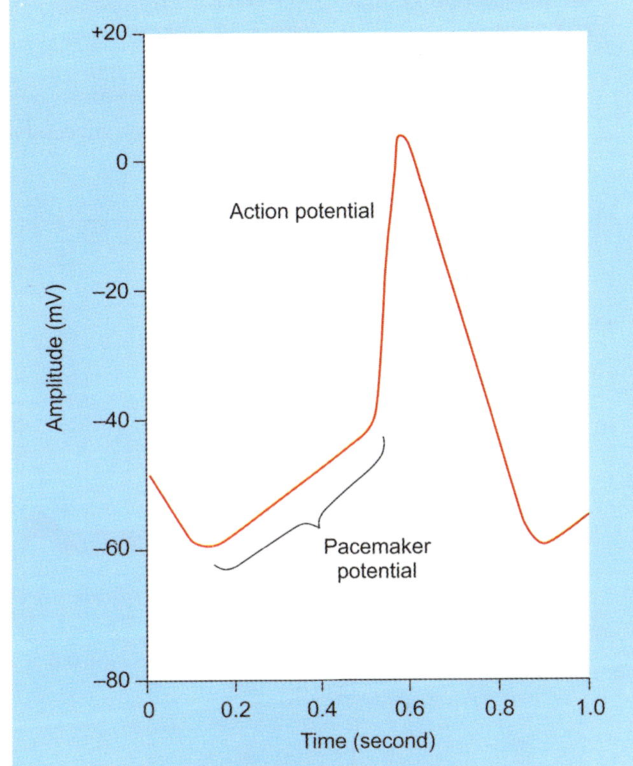

Pacemaker potential.

77. Baroreceptors respond well to changes in:

a. Sustained pressure b. Pulse pressure
c. Both of the above d. None of the above

The carotid receptors respond both to sustained pressure and to pulse pressure. The aortic receptors have not been studied in such great detail, but there is no reason to believe that their responses differ significantly from those of the receptors in the carotid sinus.

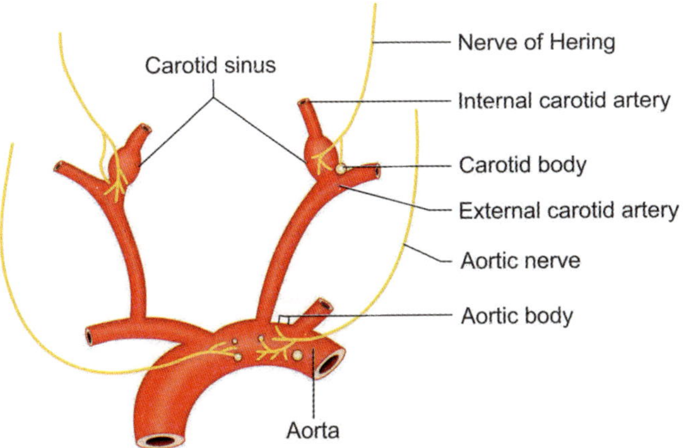

Nerve supply to baroreceptors and chemoreceptors.

MCQs with Short Explanations

Ans. 74. c. Arterioles 75. b. Heart rate and BP 76. c. Increase in... 77. c. Both of the above

78. From an ECG tracing, heart rate can be calculated as:

a. 60/R-R interval (in seconds)
b. 150/R-R interval (in seconds)
c. 600/R-R interval (in seconds)
d. 1500/R-R interval (in seconds)

Calculation of heart rate (HR) from ECG

- HR = 1500/RR in mm
- HR = 60/RR interval in seconds
- HR = 300/number of large squares between successive R waves

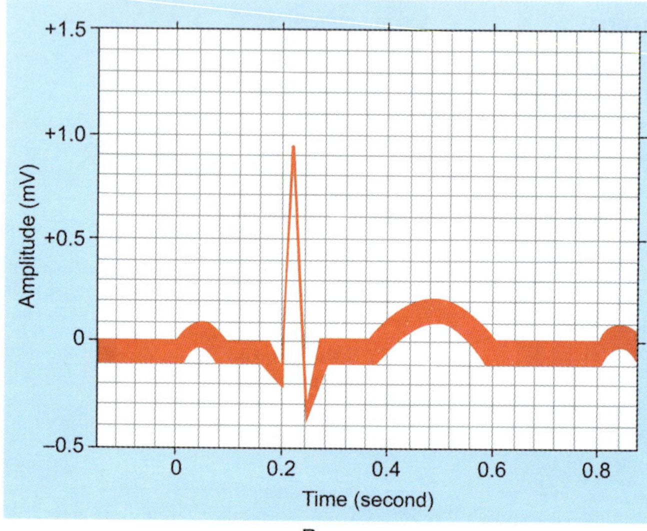

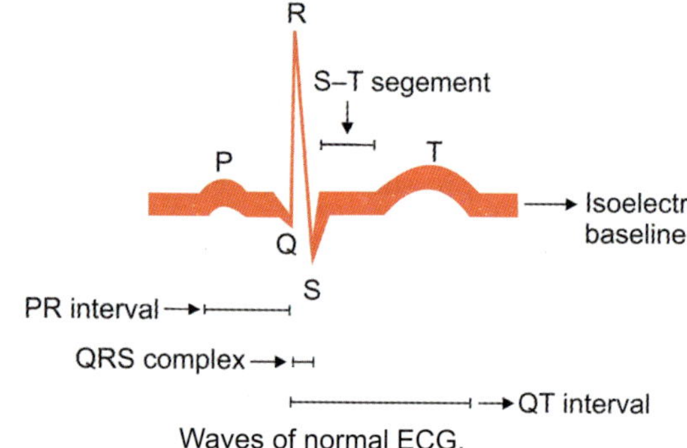

Waves of normal ECG.

79. 'a' wave in JVP is due to:

a. Atrial contraction
b. Atrial relaxation
c. Ventricular contraction
d. Ventricular relaxation

The upward deflections of JVP are the "a" (atrial contraction), "c" (ventricular contraction and resulting bulging of tricuspid into the right atrium during isovolumetric systole) and "v" = atrial venous filling.

80. At rest, blood flow is maximum in:

a. Heart
b. Kidney
c. Brain
d. Skin

The **renal circulation** receives around 20% of the cardiac output, whereas liver receives 27% (maximum).

81. Mediator of 'Flare' in triple response:

a. Axon reflex
b. Arteriolar dilation
c. Histamine release
d. Local hormones

Flare is redness in the surrounding area due to arteriolar dilatation mediated by axon reflex.

ENDOCRINOLOGY

82. Which of the following enzyme is required to convert T_4 to T_3 in kidney?

a. Type I iodothyronine deiodinase
b. Type II iodothyronine deiodinase
c. Type III iodothyronine deiodinase
d. Phenylethanolamine N methyltransferase

DI/Iodothyronine deiodinase

- DI in liver and kidney mirosomes (Type I DI/5′-DI) catalyzes both the outer ring deiodination of T_4 to form T_3, and conversion of RT_3 to 3′,5′-di-iodoyjronine. 5′-DI is unique in that it contains the rare amino acid selenocysteine
- Type II DI (5′-DII), which has similar actions, is found in the brain, the pituitary, and brown fat
- Type III DI (5-DI) acts only on the inner ring and is found in the placenta and brain.

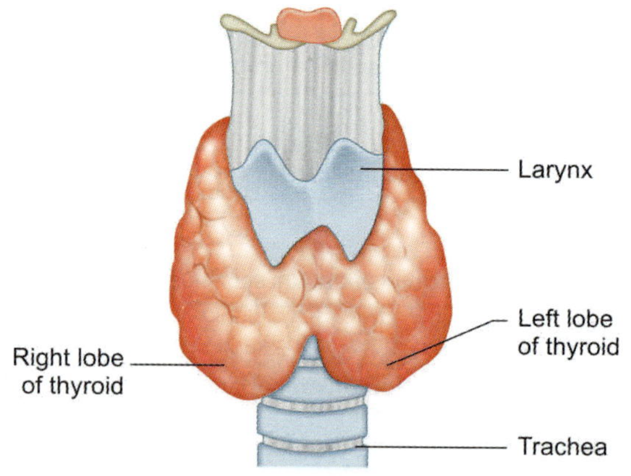

Thyroid gland.

83. Decreased extracellular calcium manifests as:

a. Reduced excitability
b. Reduced membrane stability
c. Reduces neuromuscular irritability
d. No change in amount of depolarization needed to produce action potential

Hypocalcemia

- The neuromuscular symptoms of hypocalcemia are caused by a positive bathmotropic effect due to the decreased interaction of calcium with sodium channels.

Ans. **78. a.** 60/R-R interval (in seconds) **79. a.** Atrial contraction
80. b. Kidney **81. a.** Axon reflex
82. a. Type I iodothyronine deiodinase **83. b.** Reduced membrane stability

- Since calcium blocks sodium channels and inhibits depolarization of nerve and muscle fibers, diminished calcium lowers the threshold for depolarization.
- The symptoms can be recalled by the mnemonic "CATS go numb"- Convulsions, Arrhythmias, Tetany and numbness/parasthesias in hands, feet, around mouth and lips.

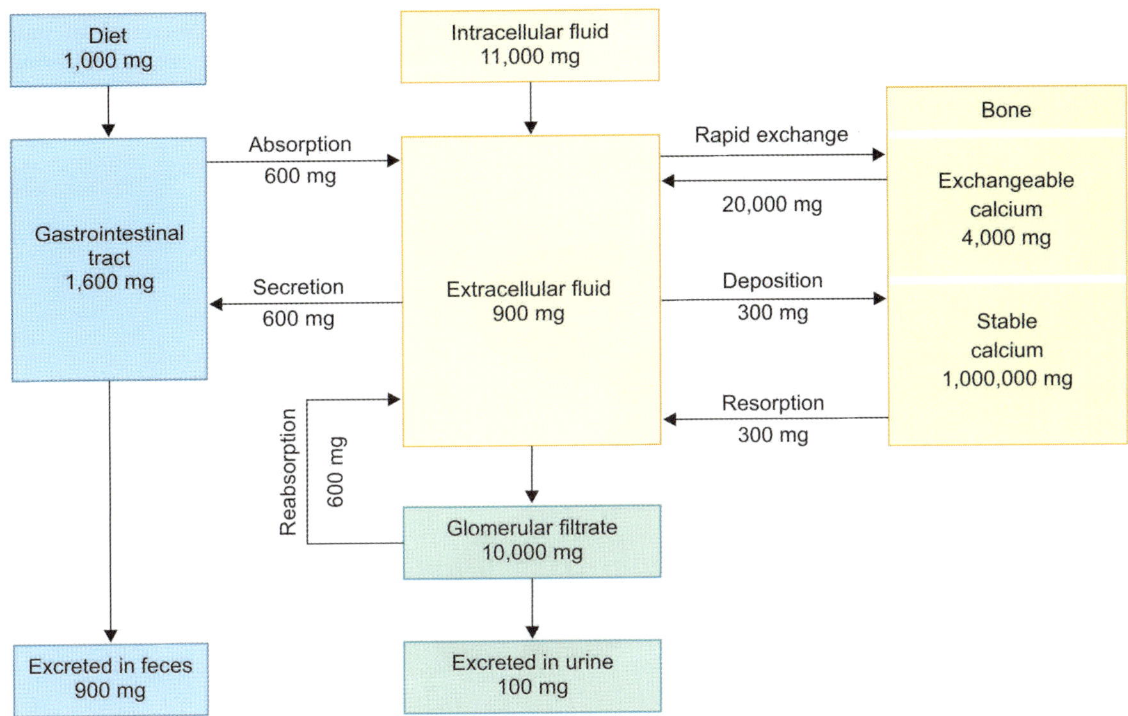

Schematic diagram showing calcium metabolism. Values belong to adults.

84. Which of the following is a non-glycoprotein hormone?

a. HCG b. Progesterone
c. TSH d. FSH

Progesterone is a C_{21} steroid

Gonadotropins (or glycoprotein hormones)

- They are protein hormones secreted by gonadotrope cells of the anterior pituitary of vertebrates.
- This is a family of proteins, which include the mammalian hormones follicle stimulating hormones (FSH), luteinizing hormone (LH), placental chorionic gonadotropin hCG and chorionic gonadotropin (CG)
- These hormones are central to the complex endocrine system that regulates normal growth, sexual development, and reproductive function.
- The hormones LH and FSH are secreted by the anterior pituitary gland, while hCG is secreted by the placenta

Classification of hormones depending upon chemical nature

Steroids	*Proteins*	*Derivatives of tyrosine*
Aldosterone 11-deoxycorticosterone Cortisol Corticosterone Testosterone Dihydrotestosterone Dehydroepiandrosterone Androstenedione Estrogen Progesterone	Growth hormone (GH) Thyroid-stimulating hormone (TSH) Adrenocorticotropic hormone (ACTH) Follicle-stimulating hormone (FSH) Luteinizing hormone (LH) Prolactin Antidiuretic hormone (ADH) Oxytocin Parathormone Calcitonin Insulin Glucagon Somatostatin Pancreatic polypeptide Human chorionic gonadotropin (HCG) Human chorionic somatomammotropin.	Thyroxine (T_4) Triiodothyronine (T_3) Adrenaline (Epinephrine) Noradrenaline (Norepinephrine) Dopamine.

Ans. **84. b.** Progesterone

85. Hormone related to breast milk feeding:

a. Prolactin
b. Oxytocin
c. Galactogen
d. Growth hormone

Letdown reflex: In lactating (breastfeeding) mothers, oxytocin acts at the mammary glands, causing milk to be 'let down' into subareolar sinuses, from where it can be excreted via the nipple. Suckling by the infant at the nipple is relayed by spinal nerves to the hypothalamus. The stimulation causes neurons that make oxytocin to fire action potentials in intermittent bursts; these bursts result in the secretion of pulses of oxytocin from the neurosecretory nerve terminals of the pituitary gland.

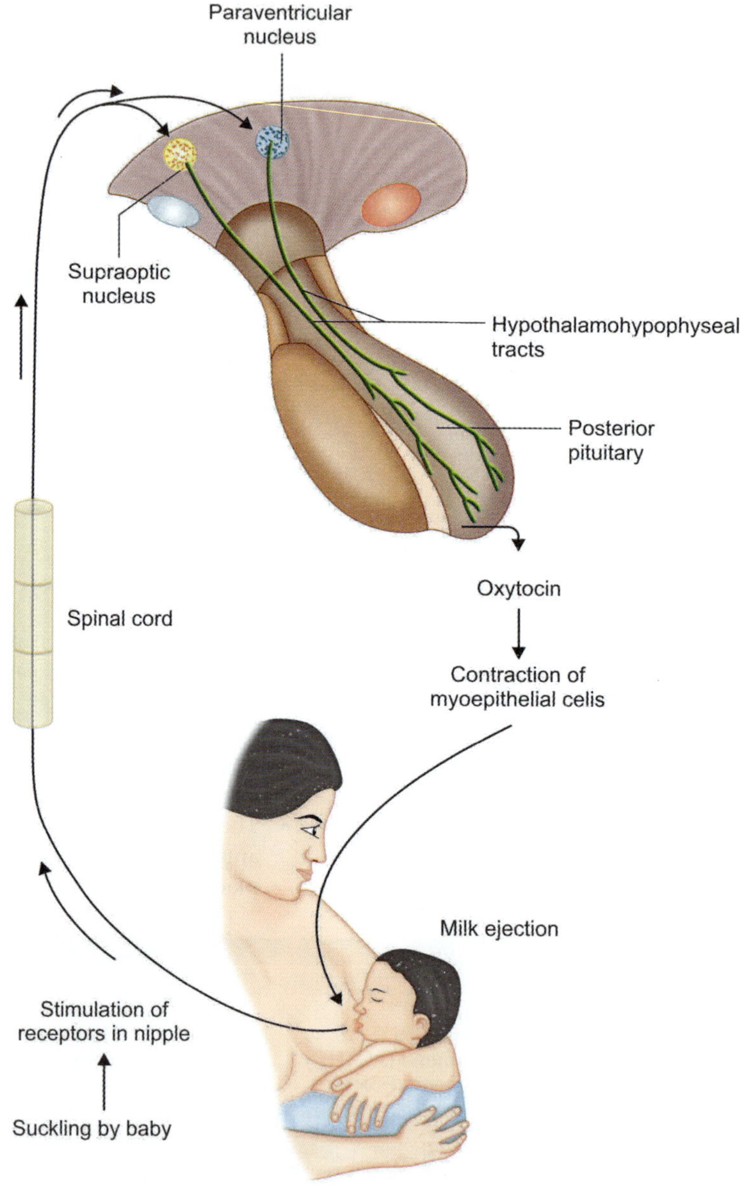

Milk ejection reflex.

86. Regarding thyroid hormone, FALSE is:

a. T3 is more avidly bound to nuclear receptors than T4
b. T4 has the maximum plasma concentration
c. T3 is more active than T4
d. T4 has shorter half life than T3

The major form of thyroid hormone in the blood is thyroxine (T_4), which has a longer half-life than T_3.

Ans. **85. b.** Oxytocin **86. d.** T4 has shorter half life than T3

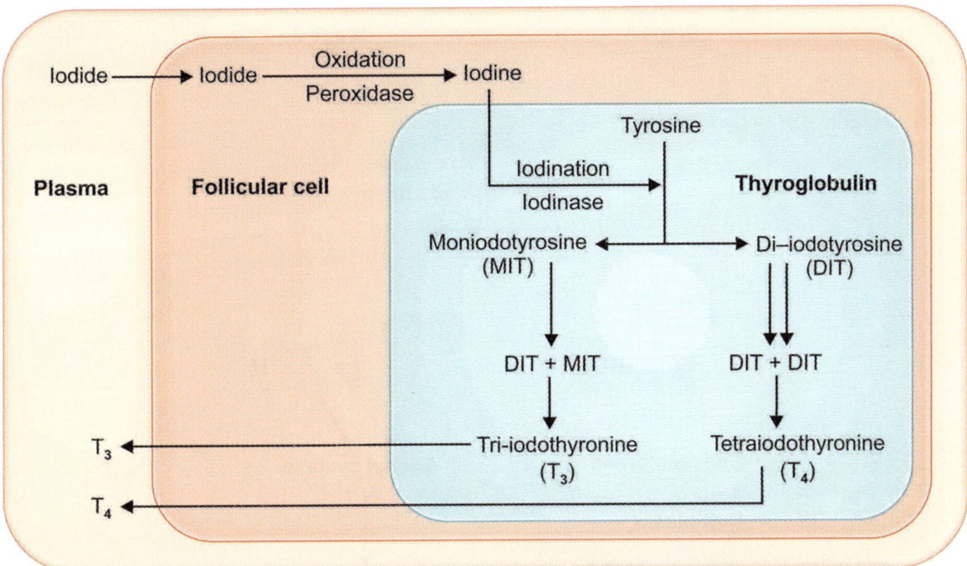

Synthesis of thyroid hormones.

87. Calcitonin is produced by:

a. Thyroid gland
b. Parathyroid gland
c. Adrenal cortex
d. Pituitary gland

Calcitonin (also known as **thyrocalcitonin**) is a 32-amino acid linear polypeptide hormone that is produced primarily by the parafollicular cells (also known as C-cells) of the thyroid, and in many other animals in the ultimobranchial body. It acts to reduce blood calcium (Ca^{2+}), opposing the effects of parathyroid hormone (PTH).

Increased by

Parathormone from parathyroid
Calcitriol from kidneys
Growth hormone from anterior pituitary

Blood calcium level

Calcitonin from thyroid gland
Cortisol from adrenal cortex

Decreased by

Effect of hormones on blood calcium level.

88. Sudden decrease in serum calcium is associated with:

a. Increased thyroxine and PTH secretion
b. Increased phosphate
c. Increased excitability of muscles and nerves
d. Cardiac conduction abnormalities

The neuromuscular symptoms of hypocalcemia are caused by a positive bathmotropic effect due to the decreased interaction of calcium with sodium channels. Since calcium blocks sodium channels and inhibits depolarization of nerve and muscle fibers, diminished calcium lowers the threshold for depolarization.

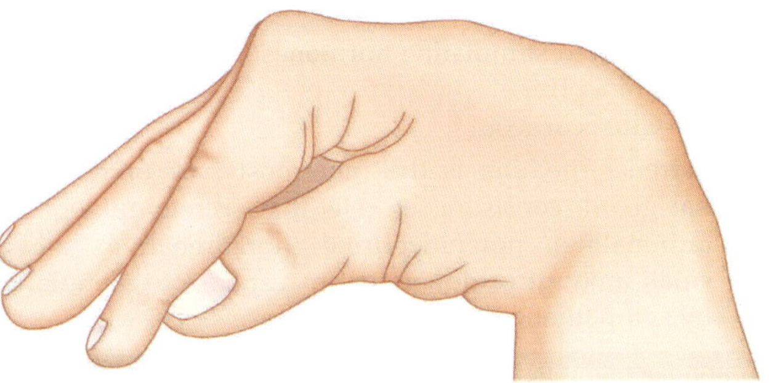

Carpopedal spasm.

89. c-AMP is a second messenger for all of the following except:

a. Glucagon
b. LH
c. FSH
d. GH

cAMP is a second messenger, used for intracellular signal transduction, such as transferring into cells the effects of hormones like glucagon and adrenaline, which cannot pass through the plasma membrane. It is involved in the activation of protein kinases and regulates the effects of adrenaline and glucagon. cAMP also binds to and regulates the function of ion channels such as the HCN channels and a few other cyclic nucleotide-binding proteins such as Epac1 and RAPGEF2.

Ans. **87. a.** Thyroid gland **88. c.** Increased excitability... **89. d.** GH

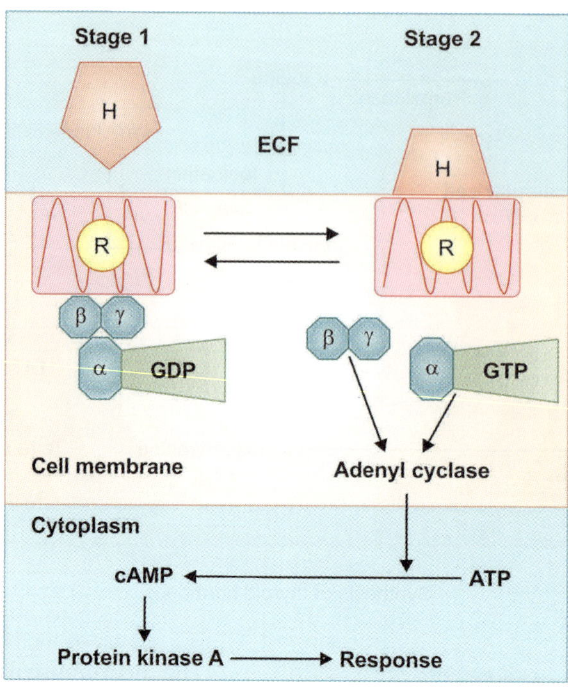

Mode of action of protein hormones and catecholamines. H = Hormone. R = Receptor, α, β, γ = G protein, GDP = Guanosine diphosphate, GTP = Guanosine triphosphate, ECF = Extracellular fluid, cAMP = Cyclic adenosine 3'5'-monophosphate, ATP = Adenosine triphosphate.

90. Adrenal medulla secretes:

a. Sex hormon es
b. Thyroid stimulating hormones
c. Epinephrine
d. Glucocorticoid

Adrenal medulla is the innermost part of the adrenal gland, consisting of cells that secrete epinephrine (adrenaline), norepinephrine (noradrenaline), and a small amount of dopamine in response to stimulation by sympathetic preganglionic neurons.

Hormones secreted by major endocrine glands			
Anterior pituitary	1. Growth hormone (GH) 2. Thyroid-stimulating hormone (TSH) 3. Adrenocorticotropic hormone (ACTH) 4. Follicle stimulating hormone (FSH) 5. Luteinizing hormone (LH) 6. Prolactin	Adrenal cortex	*Mineralocorticoids* 1. Aldosterone 2. 11-deoxycorticosterone *Glucocorticoids* 1. Cortisol 2. Corticosterone *Sex hormones* 1. Androgens 2. Estrogen 3. Progesterone
Posterior pituitary	1. Antidiuretic hormone (ADH) 2. Oxytocin		

Hormones secreted by major endocrine glands			
Thyroid gland	1. Thyroxine (T_4) 2. Triiodothyronine (T_3) 3. Calcitonin		
Parathyroid gland	Parathormone	Adrenal medulla	1. Catecholamines 2. Adrenaline (epinephrine) 3. Noradrenaline (norepinephrine) 4. Dopamine
Pancreas – Islets of Langerhans	1. Insulin 2. Glucagon 3. Somatostatin 4. Pancreatic polypeptide		

91. Inhibitor of glucagon secretion:

a. Exercise
b. Beta-2 adrenergic agonist
c. Secretin
d. Amino acids

Secretion of glucagon is **stimulated** by:

- Hypoglycemia
- Epinephrine (via β2, α2, and α1 adrenergic receptors)
- Arginine
- Alanine (often from muscle-derived pyruvate/glutamate transamination)
- Acetylcholine
- Cholecystokinin
- Exercise

Ans. **90. c.** Epinephrine **91. c.** Secretin

Differences between insulin and glucagon		
Features	*Insulin*	*Glucagon*
Source of secretion	β-cells of islets of langerhans	α-cells of islets of langerhans
Action on carbohydrate metabolism	*Decreases blood glucose level by:* 1. Facilitating transport and uptake of glucose by all cells except liver cells 2. Increasing peripheral utilization of glucose 3. Increasing glycogenesis in liver and muscle 4. Preventing glycogenolysis 5. Preventing gluconeogenesis	*Increases blood glucose level by:* 1. Facilitating glucose transport into liver cells 2. Increasing glycogenolysis 3. Increasing gluconeogenesis
Action on protein metabolism	1. Facilitates amino acid transport 2. Accelerates protein synthesis 3. Prevents protein catabolism 4. Prevents conversion of proteins into glucose	1. Increases transport of amino acids into liver cells 2. Increases utilization of amino acids for gluconeogenesis
Action on fat metabolism	1. Increases synthesis and storage of fat 2. No ketogenic effect	1. Increases lipolysis 2. Promotes ketogenesis
Blood fatty acids	Decreases	Increases
Hypersecretion leads to	Hypoglycemia	Hyperglycemia
Hyposecretion leads to	Diabetes mellitus	Hypoglycemia

92. Normal value for fasting blood sugar:

a. 140-160 mg/100 ml
b. 120-140 mg/100 ml
c. 100-120 mg/100 ml
d. 80-100 mg/100 ml

A range of blood sugar of 4 to 5.5 mmol/l (70 to 99 mg/dl) before a meal is normal. Continual fasting levels of 5.5 to 7 mmol/l (101–125 mg/dl) causes concern of possible prediabetes and may be worth monitoring. 7 mmol/l (126 mg/dl) and above means a risk of diabetes.

93. Long-term status of blood sugar can be ascertained by:

a. HbA1c
b. HbA
c. Serial measurement of fasting blood sugar
d. Oral GTT

Long-term glucose control is judged by glycosylated hemoglobin whereas short-term glucose control is assessed by serum fructosamine.

94. cAMP does NOT mediate action of:

a. Estrogen
b. Luteinizing hormone
c. Follicle stimulating hormone
d. Glucagon

The actions of estrogen are mediated by the estrogen receptor (ER), a dimeric nuclear protein that binds to DNA and controls gene expression. Like other steroid hormones, estrogen enters passively into the cell where it binds to and activates the estrogen receptor. The estrogen:ER complex binds to specific DNA sequences called a hormone response element to activate the transcription of target genes (in a study using an estrogen-dependent breast cancer cell line as model, 89 such genes were identified). Since estrogen enters all cells, its actions are dependent on the presence of the ER in the cell. The ER is expressed in specific tissues including the ovary, uterus and breast.

95. TRH control release of:

a. Prolactin
b. TSH
c. Both of the above
d. None of the above

Thyrotropin-releasing hormone (**TRH**), also called **thyrotropin-releasing factor** (**TRF**), **thyroliberin** or **protirelin**, is a tropic, tripeptidal hormone, produced by the hypothalamus, that stimulates the release of TSH (thyroid-stimulating hormone) and prolactin from the anterior pituitary.

Ans. **92. d.** 80-100 mg/100 ml **93. a.** HbA1c **94. a.** Estrogen **95. c.** Both of the above

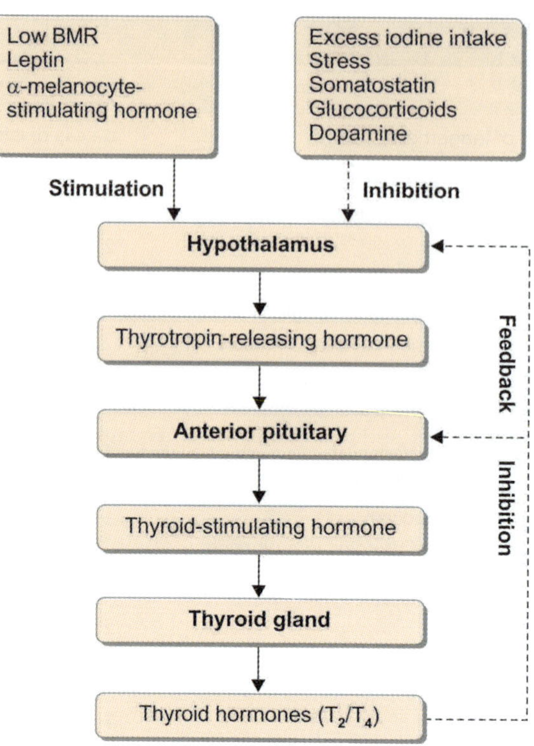

Regulation of secretion of thyroid hormones.

96. Growth hormone secretion is stimulated by:

a. Glucose
b. Cortisol
c. Methyl-prednisolone
d. Hypoglycemia

Stimulators of growth hormone (GH) secretion

- Peptide hormones
  - GHRH (*somatocrinin*) through binding to the growth hormone-releasing hormone receptor (GHRHR)
  - Ghrelin through binding to growth hormone secretagogue receptors (GHSR)
- Sex hormones
  - Increased androgen secretion during puberty (in males from testis and in females from adrenal cortex)
  - Estrogen
- Clonidine and L-DOPA by stimulating GHRH release
- Alpha4β2 nicotinic agonists, including nicotine, which also act synergistically with clonidine.
- Hypoglycemia, arginine and propranolol by inhibiting somatostatin release
- Deep sleep
- Niacin as nicotinic acid (vitamin B3)
- Fasting
- Vigorous exercise

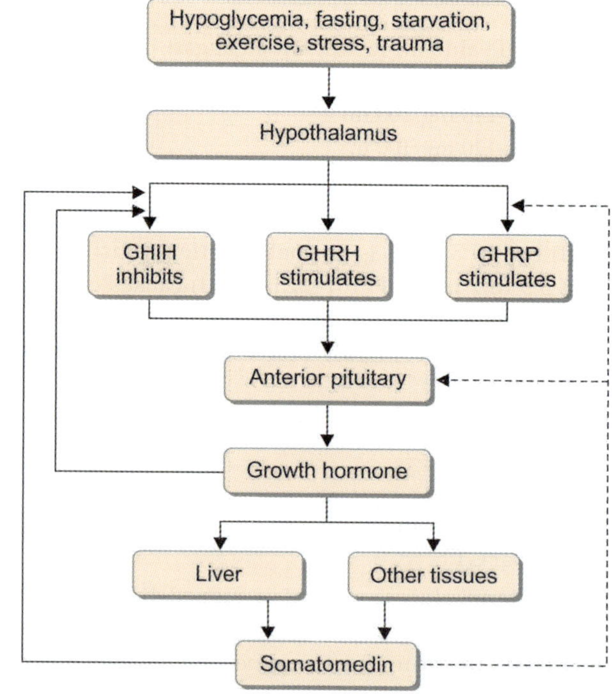

Regulation of GH secretion. GHIH = Growth hormone-inhibi-ting hormone, GHRH = Growth hormone-releasing hormone, GHRP = Growth hormone-releasing polypeptide. Growth hormone and somatomedin stimulate hypothalamus to release GHIH. Somatomedin inhibits anterior pituitary directly. Solid green line = Stimulation/secretion, Dashed red line = Inhibition.

Ans. **96. d.** Hypoglycemia

97. NOT increased during surgical stress:

a. ACTH b. Insulin
c. Norepinephrine d. GH

Release of insulin is strongly inhibited by the stress hormone norepinephrine (noradrenaline), which leads to increased blood glucose levels during stress. It appears that release of catecholamines by the sympathetic nervous system has conflicting influences on insulin release by beta cells, because insulin release is inhibited by α_2-adrenergic receptors and stimulated by β_2-adrenergic receptors.

98. Fall in extracellular calcium leads to:

a. Reduced membrane stability
b. Reduced excitability
c. Decrease in irritability of nerves
d. All of the above

Since calcium blocks sodium channels and inhibits depolarization of nerve and muscle fibers, diminished calcium lowers the threshold for depolarization. The symptoms can be recalled by the mnemonic "CATS go numb" Convulsions, Arrhythmias, Tetany and numbness/paresthesia in hands, feet, around mouth and lips.

99. Iodine uptake in thyroid gland is:

a. Endocytosis
b. Facilitated diffusion
c. Primary active transport
d. Secondary active transport

Secondary active transport makes use of potential energy, which are usually derived through exploitation of an electrochemical gradient. This involves pore-forming proteins that form channels across the cell membrane.

100. D cells of pancreas secrete:

a. Glucagon b. Insulin
c. Somatostatin d. Pancreatic polypeptide

Delta cells (δ-cells or D cells) are somatostatin-producing cells. They can be found in the stomach, intestine and the islets of langerhans in the pancreas.

101. A neurotransmitter and a hormone as well:

a. ACTH b. Cortisol
c. GABA d. Somatostatin

Somatostatin (also known as **growth hormone-inhibiting hormone** (**GHIH**) or **somatotropin release-inhibiting factor** (**SRIF**)) or **somatotropin release-inhibiting hormone** is a peptide hormone that regulates the endocrine system and affects neurotransmission and cell proliferation via interaction with G protein-coupled somatostatin receptors and inhibition of the release of numerous secondary hormones. Somatostatin inhibits insulin and glucagon secretion.

102. Thyroid hormones in plasma are bound mainly to:

a. Globulin b. Prealbumin
c. Albumin d. Preglobulin

Thyroxine-binding globulin (TBG) binds thyroid hormone in circulation. It is one of three proteins (along with transthyretin and albumin) responsible for carrying the thyroid hormones thyroxine (T4) and 3,5,3′-triiodothyronine (T3) in the bloodstream.

103. Hypocalcemia may be associated with all except:

a. Increased calcitonin
b. Increased PTH
c. Decreased absorption of calcium from gut
d. Decreased vitamin D

Parathyroid hormone (**PTH**), **parathormone** or **parathyrin**, is secreted by the chief cells of the parathyroid glands as a polypeptide containing 84 amino acids, yet effective hormone-receptor interaction requires solely the 34-N-terminal amino acids. While PTH acts to increase the concentration of ionic calcium (Ca^{2+}) in the blood, calcitonin, a hormone produced by the parafollicular cells (C cells) of the thyroid gland, acts to decrease ionic calcium concentration.

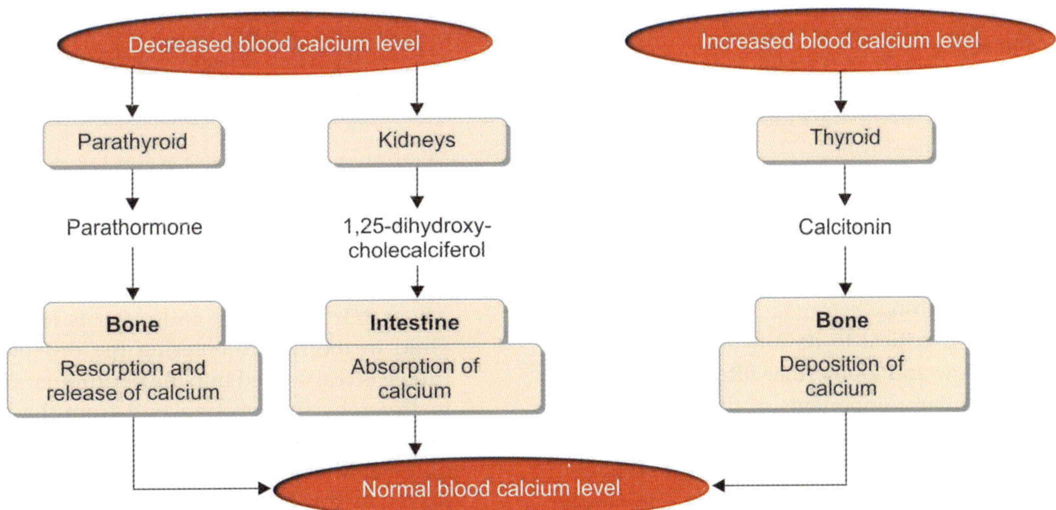

Schematic diagram showing regulation of blood calcium level.

Ans. 97. b. Insulin 98. a. Reduced membrane... 99. d. Secondary active... 100. c. Somatostatin
101. d. Somatostatin 102. a. Globulin 103. b. Increased PTH

104. Wolff-Chaikoff effect is due to:

a. Inhibition of iodide trapping
b. Inhibition of iodide-organic binding
c. Inhibition of cAMP response of TSH
d. Inhibition of thyroglobulin proteolysis

The **Wolff-Chaikoff effect** discovered by Drs. Jan Wolff and Israel Lyon Chaikoff at the University of California, is a reduction in thyroid hormone levels caused by ingestion of a large amount of iodine. In 1948, Wolff and Chaikoff reported that injection of iodine in rats almost completely inhibited organification (thyroglobulin iodination) in the thyroid gland.

105. Most important stimulus for thyrocalcitonin/calcitonin secretion is:

a. Increase in serum calcium levels
b. Decrease in serum calcium levels
c. Decrease in serum phosphorous
d. Increase in serum phosphorous

Secretion of calcitonin is stimulated by

- An increase in serum [Ca^{2+}]
- Gastrin and pentagastrin.

106. All of the following hormones are increased during stress except:

a. Cortisol
b. Insulin
c. Adrenaline
d. Noradrenaline

Stress can lead to changes in the serum level of many hormones including glucocorticoids, catecholamines, growth hormone and prolactin.

EXCRETORY SYSTEM

107. Afferent arteriole of kidney contains:

a. Lacis cells
b. Macula densa
c. JG cells
d. All of the above

Juxtaglomerular apparatus

- Microscopic structure in the kidney that regulates the function of each nephron.
- The juxtaglomerular apparatus is named for its proximity to the glomerulus.
- It is found between the vascular pole of the renal corpuscle and the returning distal convoluted tubule of the same nephron.
- This location is critical to its function in regulating renal blood flow and glomerular filtration rate.
- The three cellular components of the apparatus are the macula densa of the distal convoluted tubule, smooth muscle cells of the afferent arteriole known as juxtaglomerular cells, and extraglomerular mesangial cells.

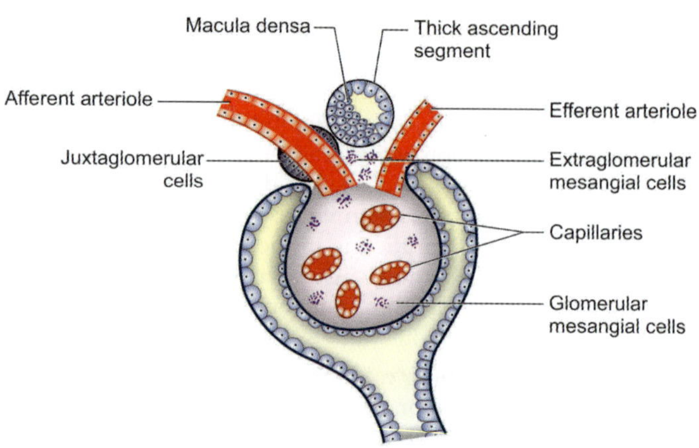

Juxtaglomerular apparatus.

108. Transport maximum of glucose in a nephron is:

a. 120 mg
b. 150 mg
c. 180 mg
d. 320 mg

Transport maximum for glucose tubular transport system in adult humans is about 320 mg/min. Normally, filtered glucose is about 125 mg/min.

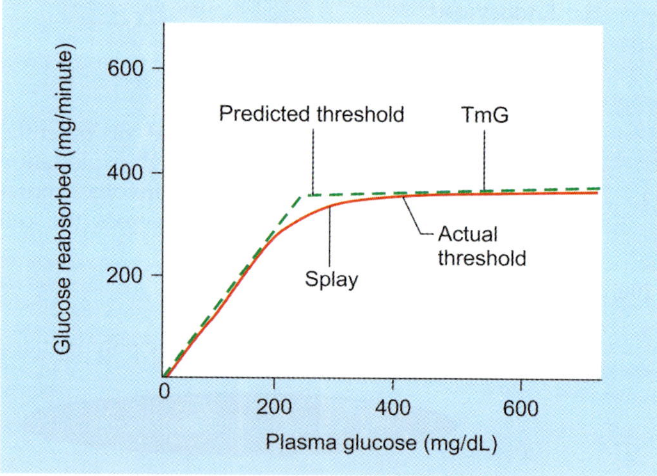

Splay in renal threshold curve for glucose.

109. Maximum absorption of water takes place in:

a. PCT
b. DCT
c. Collecting duct
d. Loop of Henle

About 2/3rd of sodium and water is reabsorbed in PCT. Fluid in the filtrate entering the proximal convoluted tubule is reabsorbed into the peritubular capillaries. This is driven by sodium transport from the lumen into the blood by the Na^+/K^+ ATPase in the basolateral membrane of the epithelial cells. Sodium reabsorption is primarily driven by this P-type ATPase. This is the most important transport mechanism in the PCT.

Ans. 104. b. Inhibition of... 105. a. Increase in... 106. b. Insulin 107. c. JG cells
108. d. 320 mg 109. a. PCT

110. Deficiency of vasopressin leads to:

a. Decreased urine output
b. Hyperkalemia
c. Increased sodium loss
d. Inability of the kidney to concentrating urine

ADH/Vasopressin/AVP regulates the body's retention of water by acting to increase water reabsorption in the kidney's collecting ducts, the tubules which receive the very dilute urine produced by the functional unit of the kidney, the nephrons. Decreased AVP release (neurogenic, i.e. due to alcohol intoxication or tumour) or decreased renal sensitivity to AVP (nephrogenic, i.e. by mutation of V2 receptor or AQP) leads to diabetes insipidus, a condition featuring hypernatremia (increased blood sodium concentration), polyuria (excess urine production), and polydipsia (thirst).

Hormones regulating tubular reabsorption

Hormone	*Action*
Aldosterone	Increases sodium reabsorption in ascending limb, distal convoluted tubule and collecting duct
Angiotensin II	Increases sodium reabsorption in proximal tubule, thick ascending limb, distal tubule and collecting duct (mainly in proximal convoluted tubule)
Antidiuretic hormone	Increases water reabsorption in distal convoluted tubule and collecting duct
Atrial natriuretic factor	Decreases sodium reabsorption
Brain natriuretic factor	Decreases sodium reabsorption
Parathormone	Increases reabsorption of calcium, magnesium and hydrogen Decreases phosphate reabsorption
Calcitonin	Decreases calcium reabsorption

111. Renin is secreted by:

a. Tubular cells
b. Macula densa
c. JG cells
d. All of the above

The enzyme renin is secreted by the afferent arterioles of the kidney from specialized cells called granular cells of the juxtaglomerular apparatus. It mediates extracellular volume (i.e., that of the blood plasma, lymph and interstitial fluid), and arterial vasoconstriction. Thus, it regulates the body's mean arterial blood pressure.

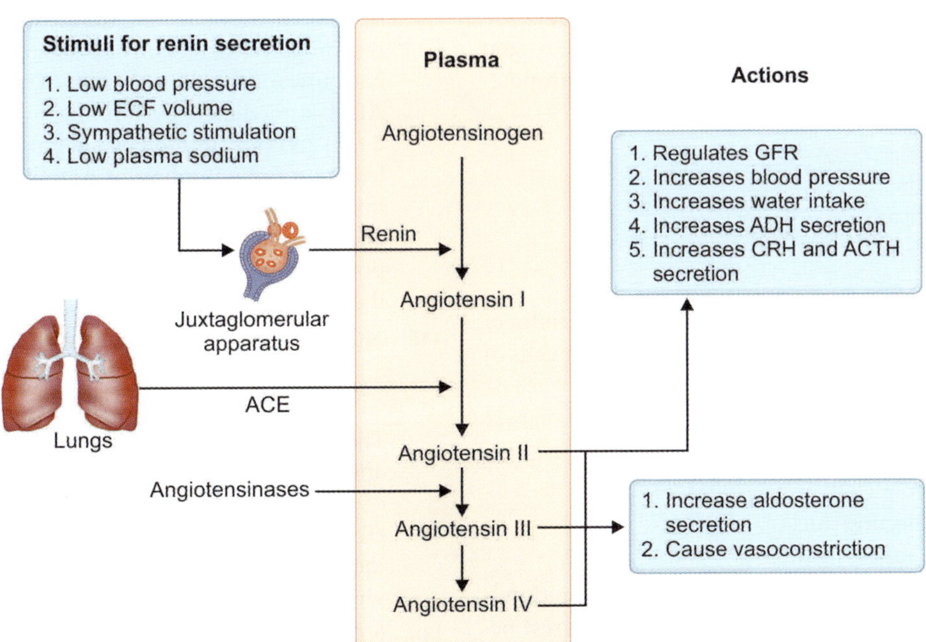

Reninangiotensin system. ECF = Extracellular fluid, ACE = Angiotensin-converting enzyme, GFR = Glomerular filtration rate, ADH = Antidiuretic hormone, CRH = Corticotropin-releasing hormone, ACTH = Adrenocorticotropic hormone.

Ans. **110. d.** Inability of the... **111. c.** JG cells

112. Under effect of vasopressin, greatest fraction of filtered water is reabsorbed in:

a. PCT
b. DCT
c. Loop of Henle
d. Collecting duct

Water is maximally reabsorbed from PCT (whether under influence of vasopressin or not)

113. Inulin clearance closely resembles:

a. PAH clearance
b. Creatinine clearance
c. Renal plasma flow
d. GFR

Inulin is uniquely treated by nephrons in that it is completely filtered at the glomerulus but neither secreted nor reabsorbed by the tubules. This property of inulin allows the clearance of inulin to be used clinically as a highly accurate measure of glomerular filtration rate (GFR) — the rate of plasma from the afferent arteriole that is filtered into Bowman's capsule measured in mL/min.

114. Erythropoietin is secreted by:

a. Interstitial cells of kidney
b. Extraglomerular mesangial cells
c. Macula densa
d. Renal tubular epithelial cells

It is not known exactly where in the kidneys the erythropoietin is formed. One likely possibility is that the renal tubular epithelial cells secrete the erythropoietin because anemic blood is unable to deliver enough oxygen from the peritubular capillaries to the highly oxygen consuming tubular cells, thus stimulating erythropoietin production.

115. Secretion of renin is by:

a. Tubular cells
b. Macula densa
c. JG cells
d. None of the above

The enzyme renin is secreted by the afferent arterioles of the kidney from specialized cells called granular cells of the juxtaglomerular apparatus.

116. Main site of bicarbonate reabsorption is:

a. PCT
b. Loop of Henle
c. Cortical collecting duct
d. Medullary collecting duct

The process of bicarbonate reabsorption occur predominantly in the proximal tubule (about 90%). The rest occur in the thick ascending limb and in the collecting tubule. All involve **hydrogen ion secretion.**

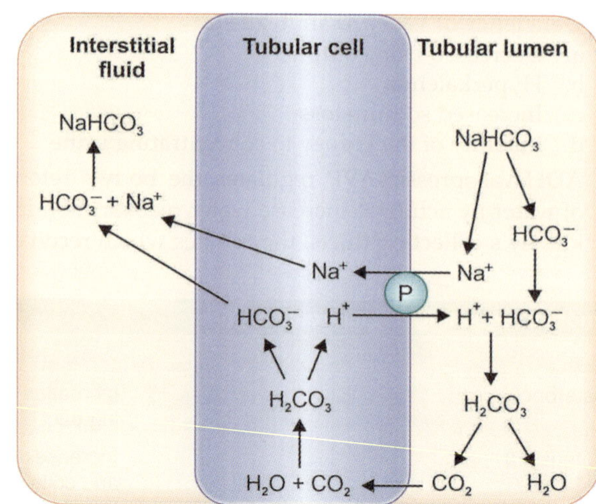

Reabsorption of bicarbonate ions by secretion of hydrogen ions in renal tubule. P = sodium-hydrogen antiport pump.

117. Factor which increases renal urinary concentrating ability:

a. Increase in GFR
b. Increase in RBF
c. Contraction in ECF volume
d. Reduction in medullary hyperosmolarity

Alterations in arterial blood pressure and plasma osmolality are the main physiologic signals regulating ADH secretion. As plasma water decreases, increases in plasma sodium concentration and osmolality are sensed by nuclei in the hypothalamus, with a resultant increase in production of ADH by the supraoptic and paraventricular nuclei. ADH acts to increase renal free water reabsorption in the collecting tubule to restore plasma water, resulting in a correction of plasma sodium concentration back toward the normal range. The antidiuretic effect of ADH is mediated by binding to the vasopressin type 2 (V_2) receptor in the basolateral membrane of the collecting tubule. Binding of ADH leads to an increase in intracellular cyclic adenosine monophosphate (cAMP) and ultimately to the insertion of a water channel (aquaporin 2) into the luminal membrane and an increase in the aquaporin 2 mRNA level.

118. NOT absorbed in early part of DCT:

a. Chloride b. Water
c. Sodium d. Potassium

The early part of the distal tubule is highly convoluted and has many of the same absorptive characteristics of the thick segment of the ascending limb of loop of Henle. That is, it avidly reabsorbs most of the ions, including sodium, potassium, and chloride, but is virtually impermeable to water and urea.

119. NOT absorbed in PCT:

a. Hydrogen ions b. Sodium
c. Amino acids d. Glucose

Ans. **112. a.** PCT **113. d.** GFR **114. d.** Renal tubular epithelial cells
115. c. JG cells **116. a.** PCT **117. c.** Contraction in ECF volume
118. b. Water **119. a.** Hydrogen ions

Functions of PCT

- PCT reabsorbs 2/3 of the filtered Na or (65–80% of Na) and H_2O
- It reabsorbs **all** of the **glucose**, and **amino acids**
- Glucose is reabsorbed via **Na-Glucotransporter**
- It also reabsorbs a fraction of the bicarbonate, potassium, phosphate and calcium
- It secretes ammonia, which functions as a buffer for secreted H^+. It also secretes creatine, which is used to access the function of the kidney.

120. NOT present in renal medulla:

a. Collecting duct b. Vasa recta
c. Loop of Henle d. JG apparatus

The **juxtaglomerular apparatus** is a microscopic structure in the kidney that regulates the function of each nephron, the functional units of the kidney. The juxtaglomerular apparatus is named because it is next to (juxta-) the glomerulus (in cortex).

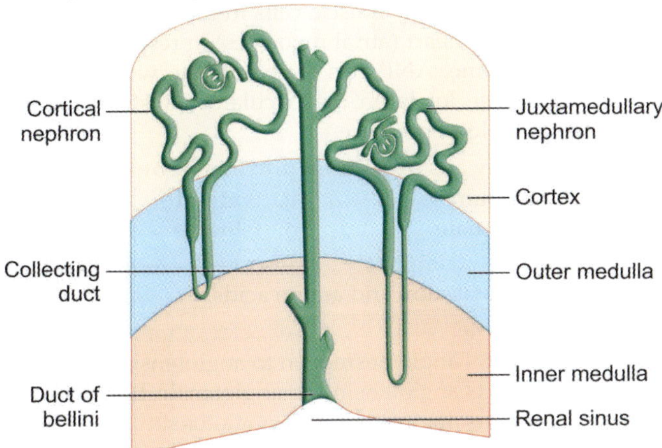

Types of nephron.

121. Ureteric peristalsis is as a result of:

a. Parasympathetic activity
b. Sympathetic activity
c. Both parasympathetic and sympathetic activity
d. Pacemaker activity of the smooth muscle cells in renal pelvis

Urine flowing from the collecting ducts into the renal calices and increases their inherent pacemaker activity, which in turn initiates peristaltic contractions that spread to the renal pelvis and then downward along the length of the ureter, thereby forcing urine from the renal pelvis toward the bladder.

122. 100% filtration coefficient is seen in:

a. Inulin
b. Creatinine
c. Albumin
d. Urea

Inulin and its analog sinistrin are used to help measure kidney function by determining the glomerular filtration rate (GFR), which is the volume of fluid filtered from the renal (kidney) glomerular capillaries into the Bowman's capsule per unit time. Inulin is of particular use as it is not secreted or reabsorbed in any appreciable amount at the nephron, allowing GFR to be calculated.

123. Maximum absorption of water occurs in:

a. PCT b. DCT
c. Collecting duct d. Loop of Henle

Fluid (about 2/3rd) in the filtrate entering the proximal convoluted tubule is reabsorbed into the peritubular capillaries. This is driven by sodium transport from the lumen into the blood by the Na^+/K^+ ATPase in the basolateral membrane of the epithelial cells. Sodium reabsorption is primarily driven by this P-type ATPase. This is the most important transport mechanism in the PCT.

124. True regarding chemical structure of ADH:

a. Octapeptide
b. Nonapeptide
c. Hexapeptide
d. Pentapeptide

The vasopressins are peptides consisting of nine amino acids (nonapeptides).

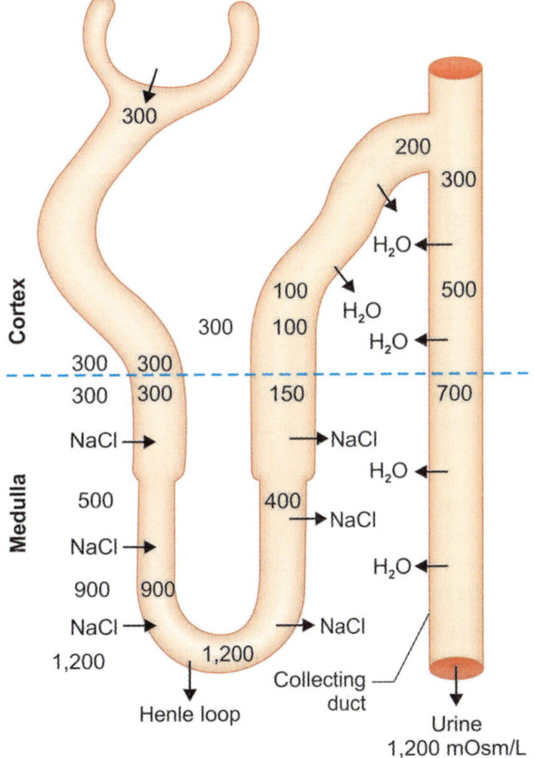

Role of ADH in the formation of concentrated urine. ADH increases the permeability for water in distal convoluted tubule and collecting duct. Numerical indicate osmolarity (mOsm/L).

125. Part of nephron impermeable to water:

a. PCT
b. Thick ascending loop of Henle
c. Thin descending loop of Henle
d. Collecting ducts

Ans. 120. **d.** JG apparatus 121. **d.** Pacemaker activity.. 122. **a.** Inulin 123. **a.** PCT
124. **b.** Nonapeptide 125. **b.** Thick ascending loop of Henle

Thick ascending limb of loop of Henle

- Sodium (Na^+), potassium (K^+) and chloride (Cl^-) ions are reabsorbed from the urine by secon-dary active transport by a Na-K-Cl cotranspor-ter (NKCC2).
- The electrical and concentration gradient drives more reabsorption of Na^+, as well as other cations such as magnesium (Mg^{2+}) and calcium (Ca^{2+}).

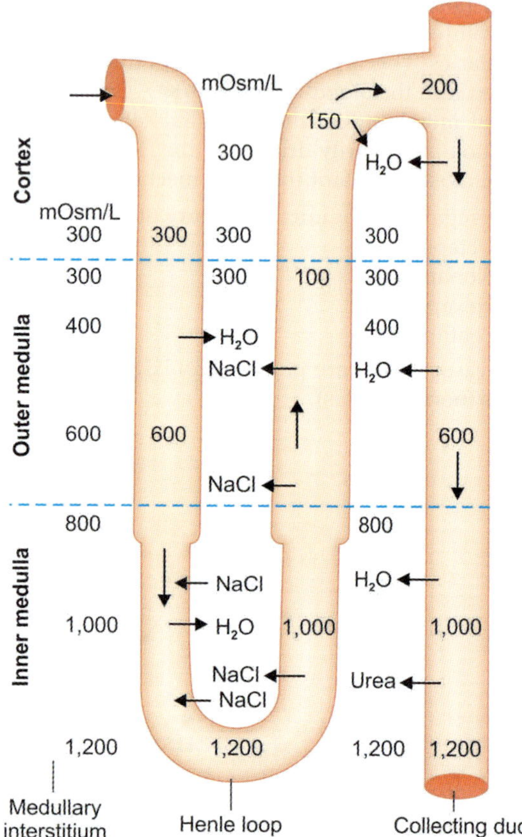

Countercurrent multiplier. Numerical indicate osmolarity (mOsm/L).

126. Renin secretion is increased in all except:
a. Sympathetic stimulation
b. Low sodium in DCT
c. Low afferent arteriolar low pressure
d. High sodium in PCT

Stimuli for rennin release

- A decrease in arterial blood pressure (that could be related to a decrease in blood volume) as detected by baroreceptors (pressure-sensitive cells). This is the most direct causal link between blood pressure and renin secretion (the other two methods operate via longer pathways).
- A decrease in sodium levels in the ultrafiltrate of the nephron. This flow is measured by the macula densa of the juxtaglomerular apparatus.
- Sympathetic nervous system activity, which also controls blood pressure, acting through the β_1 adrenergic receptors.

127. Secreted actively in collecting duct:
a. Potassium ion b. Hydrogen ion
c. Sodium ion d. Magnesium ion

Intercalated cells (of collecting duct system)

Type of cell	Secretes	Reabsorbs
α-intercalated cells	Acid (via an apical H^+-ATPase and H^+/K^+ exchanger) in the form of hydrogen ions	Bicarbonate (via band 3, a basolate-ral Cl^-/HCO_3^- exchanger)
β-intercalated cells	Bicarbonate (via pendrin a specia-lised apical Cl^-/HCO_3^-)	Acid (via a basal H^+-ATPase)

128. True for atrial natriuretic peptide is:
a. Increases blood volume
b. Inhibit reabsorption of sodium by the collecting ducts
c. Secreted by kidneys
d. All of the above

ANP is released by muscle cells in the upper chambers (atria) of the heart (atrial myocytes) in response to high blood volume. ANP acts to reduce the water, sodium and adipose loads on the circulatory system, thereby reducing blood pressure.

129. Completely absorbed from proximal tubules:
a. Potassium b. Sodium
c. Bicarbonate d. Glucose

Substances completely reabsorbed from PCT are glucose, potassium and amino acids.

130. Renin action:
a. Converts angiotensinogen to angiotensin-I
b. Converts angiotensin-I to angiotensin-II
c. Converts angiotensin-II to angiotensin-III
d. All of the above

Renin also known as an **angiotensinogenase**, is an enzyme that participates in the body's renin-angiotensin aldosterone system (RAAS)—also known as the renin-angiotensin-aldosterone axis—that mediates extracellular volume (i.e. that of the blood plasma, lymph and interstitial fluid), and arterial vasoconstriction. Renin is often improperly referred to as a hormone even though it has no peripheral receptors and rather has an enzymatic activity with which it hydrolyses angiotensinogen to angiotensin I.

131. ANP acts at:
a. PCT b. Collecting duct
c. DCT d. Loop of Henle

ANP decreases sodium reabsorption in the distal convo-luted tubule (interaction with NCC) and cortical collecting duct of the nephron via guanosine 3′,5′-cyclic monophos-phate (cGMP) dependent phosphorylation of ENaC.

132. Renin secretion is inhibited by:
a. Cardiac failure b. Hemorrhage
c. ANP d. Diuretics

ANP Inhibits renin secretion, thereby inhibiting the renin-angiotensin-aldosterone system.

Ans. 126. **d.** High sodium... 127. **b.** Hydrogen ion 128. **b.** Inhibit... 129. **d.** Glucose
130. **a.** Converts ang... 131. **b.** Distension of stomach 132. **c.** ANP

DIGESTIVE SYSTEM

133. Which of the following is true regarding different phases of gastric juice secretion?

a. Cephalic phase – 30% of total secretion
b. Gastric phase – 20% of total secretion
c. Intestinal phase – 20% of total secretion
d. Intestinal phase – 70% of total secretion

Phases of gastric acid secretion

- The cephalic phase:
  - Thirty percent of the total gastric acid secretions to be produced is stimulated by anticipation of eating and the smell or taste of food.
  - This signalling occurs from higher centres in the brain through the vagus nerve.
  - It activates parietal cells to release acid and ECL cells to release histamine.
  - The vagus nerve also releases gastrin releasing peptide onto G cells. Finally, it also inhibits somatostatin release from D cells.
- The gastric phase:
  - About fifty percent of the total acid for a meal is secreted in this phase.
  - Acid secretion is stimulated by distension of the stomach and by amino acids present in the food.
- The intestinal phase:
  - The remaining 10% of acid is secreted when chyme enters the small intestine, and is stimulated by small intestine distension and by amino acids.
  - The duodenal cells release entero-oxyntin which acts on parietal cells without affecting gastrin.

Digestive enzymes of gastric juice

Enzyme	*Activator*	*Substrate*	*End products*
Pepsin	Hydrochloric acid	Proteins	Proteoses, peptones and polypeptides
Gastric lipase	Acid medium	Triglycerides of butter	Fatty acids and glycerols
Gastric amylase	Acid medium	Starch	Dextrin and maltose (negligible action)
Gelatinase	Acid medium	Gelatin and collagen of meat	Peptides
Urase	Acid medium	Urea	Ammonia

134. As compared to bile of liver, bile of gall bladder is more:

a. Acidic
b. Alkaline
c. Hypotonic
d. Hypertonic

Acidification of the bile is one important function of gallbladder.

Gallbladder Bile

- The bile that is secreted by the liver and stored in the gallbladder is not the same as the bile that is secreted by the gallbladder.
- During gallbladder storage of bile, it is concentrated by removal of some water and electrolytes.
- This is through the active transport of sodium ions across the epithelia of the gallbladder, which creates an osmotic pressure that also causes water and other electrolytes such as chlorine to be reabsorbed.

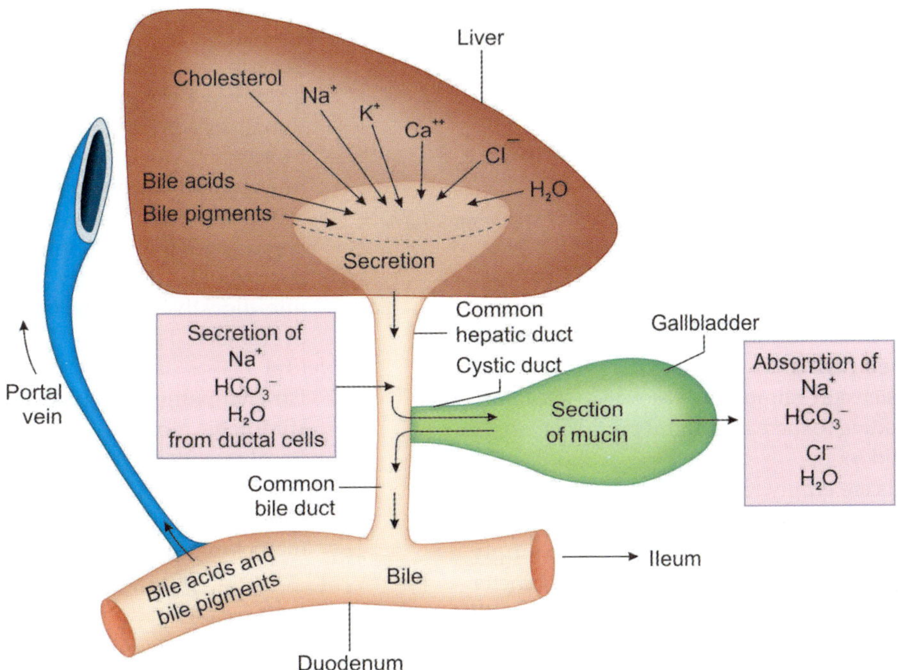

Diagram showing the formation of bile from liver and changes taking place in the composition of gallbladder bile.

Ans. **133. a.** Cephalic phase – 30% of total secretion **134. a.** Acidic

135. Secretin release is best stimulated by:

a. Water
b. Food carbohydrate
c. Fatty acids
d. Acid and protein

Secretin is released into circulation and/or intestinal lumen in response to low duodenal pH that ranges between 2 and 4.5 (depending on species). Also, the secretion of secretin is increased by the products of protein digestion bathing the mucosa of the upper small intestine.

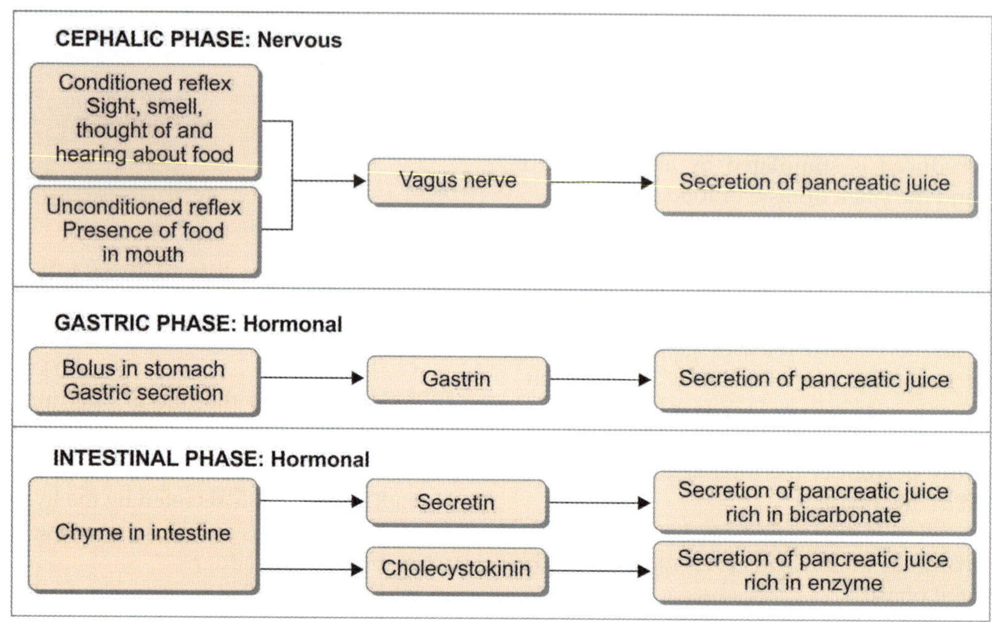

Schematic diagram showing the regulation of pancreatic secretion.

136. Bicarbonate is highest in:

a. Bile
b. Saliva
c. Pancreatic secretions
d. Succus entericus

Pancreatic secretions from ductal cells contain bicarbonate ions and are alkaline in order to neutralize the acidic chyme that the stomach churns out.

137. Gastric motility is increased in:

a. Fatty food in stomach
b. Distension of stomach
c. Tryptophan in duodenum
d. Acid in duodenum

Factors Promoting stomach emptying

- Gastric volume
  - Increased food volume in stomach promotes increased emptying
  - Antral distension stimulates vasovagal excitatory reflexes leading to increased antral pump activity
- Liquid vs solid food
  - Clear fluids are empty rapidly (T1/2 of 30 minutes). Solids stay in stomach longer (T1/2 of 1-2 hours)
  - Pylorus is open enough for H_2O/fluids to empty with ease. Constriction of the pyloric sphincter to solids until chyme is broken down into small particles and mixed to almost fluid consistency.
- Types of food
  - Protein empties fastest, followed by carbohydrates. Fats take longest to empty
  - Note: High protein food especially meat stimulate release of gastrin from antral mucosa
- Hormonal factors
  - Gastrin has mild to moderate stimulatory effects on motor functions in the body of the stomach. Enhances activity of pyloric pump
  - Motilin released by epithelium of the small intestine enhances the strength of the migrating motor complex which is a peristaltic wave that begins within the oesophagus and travels through the whole GIT every 60-90 mins during the interdigestive period. Help empty remaining food in stomach.
- Neural
  - Parasympathetic innervation (via vagus) stimulates motility
  - Local myenteric reflex
- Drugs
  - Prokinetics, e.g. cisapride, erythromycin metoclopramide

138. Acid secretion in stomach is increased in all of the following except:

a. Gastrin
b. Food in stomach
c. Secretin
d. Histamine

Ans. 135. **d.** Acid and protein 136. **c.** Pancreatic secretions 137. **b.** Distension of... 138. **c.** Secretin

Gastric acid production is regulated by both the autonomic nervous system and several hormones. The parasympathetic nervous system, via the vagus nerve, and the hormone gastrin stimulate the parietal cell to produce gastric acid, both directly acting on parietal cells and indirectly, through the stimulation of the secretion of the hormone histamine from enterochromaffin-like cells (ECL). Vasoactive intestinal peptide, cholecystokinin, and secretin all inhibit production.

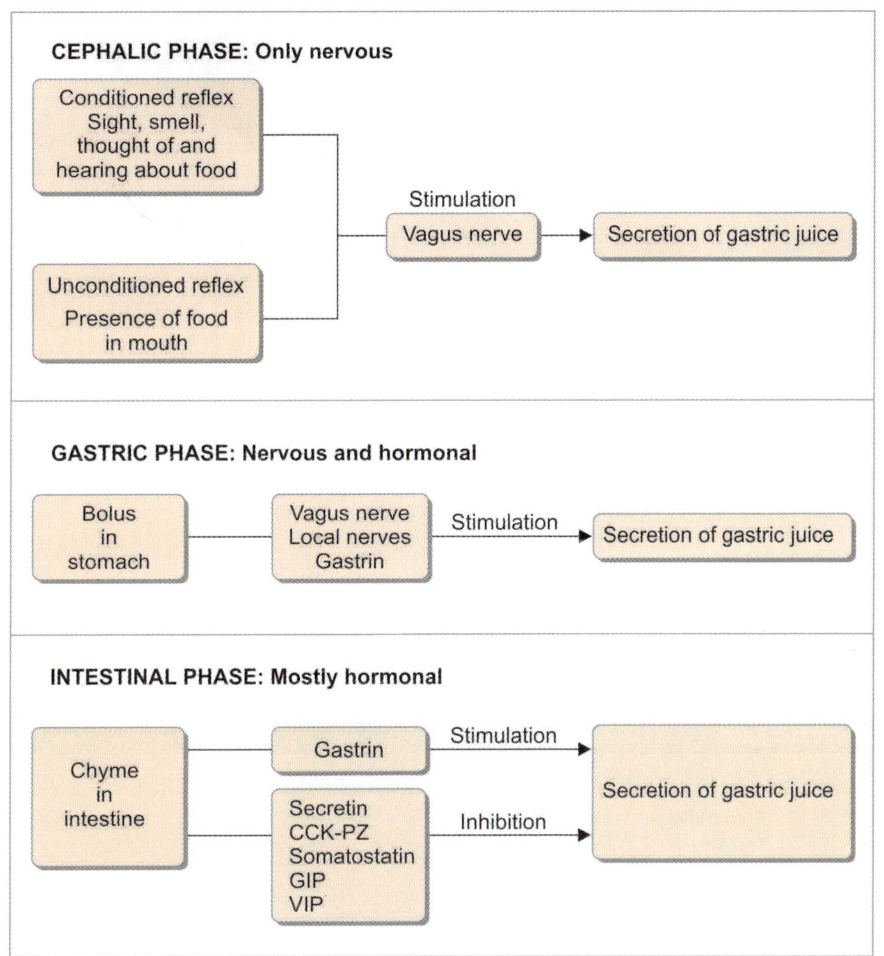

Schematic diagram showing the regulation of gastric secretion CCK-PZ = Cholecystokinin-pancreozymin, GIP = Gastric inhibitory peptide, VIP = Vasoactive intestinal peptide.

139. Factor increasing gastric motility:

a. Presence of fatty food in stomach
b. Distension of stomach
c. Presence of tryptophan in stomach
d. Presence of acid in stomach

Antral distension stimulates vasovagal excitatory reflexes leading to increased antral pump activity.

140. NOT produced by hepatocytes:

a. Prothrombin
b. Fibrinogen
c. Albumin
d. Gamma-globulin

An **antibody** (AB), also known as an **immunoglobulin** (Ig)/gamma globulin, is a large, Y-shape protein produced by plasma cells that is used by the immune system to identify and neutralize pathogens such as bacteria and viruses.

141. Site of formation of urobilinogen:

a. Spleen b. Kidney
c. Liver d. Intestine

Urobilinogen is a colourless by-product of bilirubin reduction. It is formed in the intestines by bacterial action on bilirubin. About half of the urobilinogen formed is reabsorbed and taken up via the portal vein to the liver, enters circulation and is excreted by the kidney.

Ans. **139. b.** Distension of... **140. d.** Gamma-globulin **141. d.** Intestine

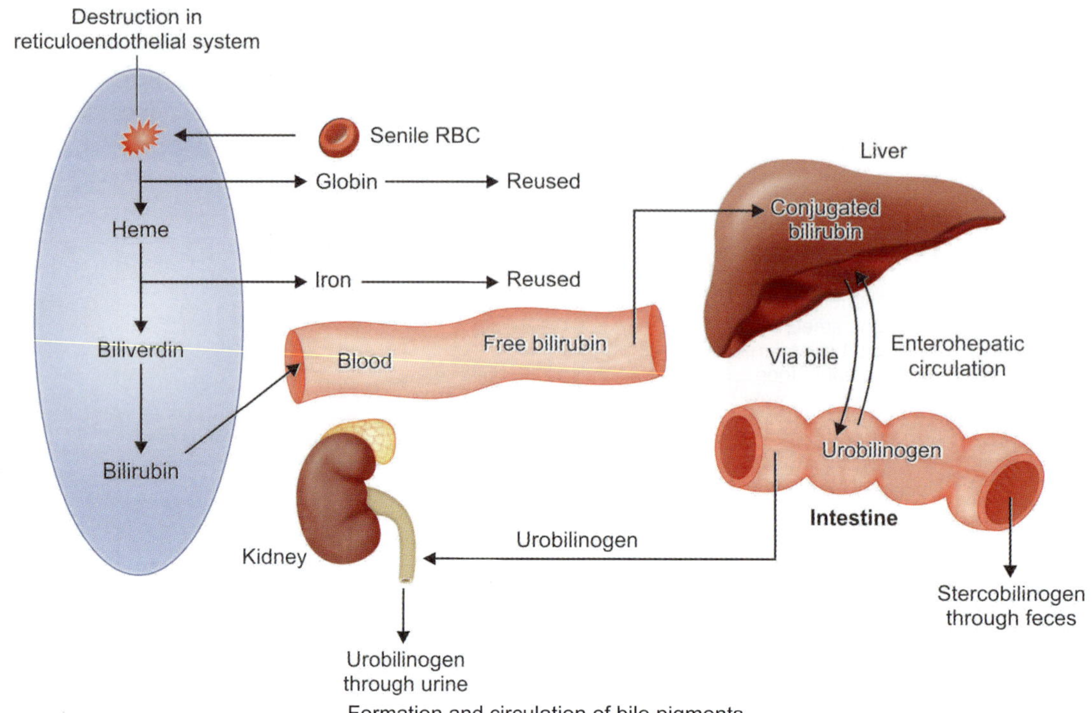

Formation and circulation of bile pigments.

142. Activation of chymotrypsinogen to chymotrypsin is done by:

a. Trypsin
b. Pepsin
c. Renin
d. HCl

Chymotrypsinogens are activated to chymotrypsins by trypsin.

Digestive enzymes of pancreatic juice

Enzyme	*Activator*	*Acts on (substrate)*	*End products*
Trypsin	Enterokinase Trypsin	Proteins	Proteoses and polypeptides
Chymotrypsin	Trypsin	Proteins	Polypeptides
Carboxypeptidases	Trypsin	Polypeptides	Amino acids
Nucleases	Trypsin	RNA and DNA	Mononucleotides
Elastase	Trypsin	Elastin	Amino acids
Collagenase	Trypsin	Collagen	Amino acids
Pancreatic lipase	Alkaline medium	Triglycerides	Monoglycerides and fatty acids
Cholesterol ester hydrolase	Alkaline medium	Cholesterol ester	Cholesterol and fatty acids
Phospholipase A	Trypsin	Phospholipids	Lysophospholipids
Phospholipase B	Trypsin	Lysophospholipids	Phosphoryl choline and free fatty acids
Colipase	Trypsin	Facilitates action of pancreatic lipase	–
Bile-salt-activated lipase	Trypsin	Phospholipids	Lysophospholipids
		Cholesterol esters	Cholesterol and fatty acids
		Triglycerides	Monoglycerides and fatty acids
Pancreatic amylase	–	Starch	Dextrin and maltose

Ans. 142. a. Trypsin

143. True regarding physiological gastrectomy:

a. Ligation of only 4 arteries
b. Resection of upper 1/3rd of stomach
c. Antrectomy
d. Ligation of all major arteries

Physiological gastrectomy is the operation of ligature of the arteries of the stomach to relieve hyperacidity and to prevent recurrent ulceration after gastroenterostomy.

144. Gastrocolic reflex is related to:

a. Colonic disorders b. Pendular movements
c. Segmental movements d. Mass peristalsis

The **gastrocolic reflex** or **gastrocolic response** is one of a number of physiological reflexes controlling the motility, or peristalsis, of the gastrointestinal tract. It involves an increase in motility of the colon in response to stretch in the stomach and byproducts of digestion in the small intestine. Thus, this reflex is responsible for the urge to defecate following a meal. The small intestine also shows a similar motility response. The gastrocolic reflex helps make room for more food.

145. Cause of refeeding edema:

a. Increased release of growth hormone
b. Increased release of glucocorticoids
c. Increased release of insulin
d. Increased release of thyroxine

During refeeding, insulin secretion resumes in response to increased blood sugar; resulting in increased glycogen, fat and protein synthesis. This process requires phosphates, magnesium and potassium which are already depleted and the stores rapidly become used up. Formation of phosphorylated carbohydrate compounds in the liver and skeletal muscle depletes intracellular ATP and 2,3-diphosphoglycerate in red blood cells, leading to cellular dysfunction and inadequate oxygen delivery to the body's organs. Refeeding increases the basal metabolic rate. Intracellular movement of electrolytes occurs along with a fall in the serum electrolytes, including phosphate, potassium and magnesium.

146. In stomach, H+ is secreted, in exchange for:

a. Chloride b. Calcium
c. Potassium d. Sodium

Water becomes dissociated into hydrogen ions and hydroxyl ions in the parietal cell cytoplasm. The hydrogen ions are then actively secreted into the canaliculus in exchange for potassium ions; this active exchange process is catalyzed by H^+K^+ATPase.

147. Action of ghrelin:

a. Suppression of sleep b. Stimulation of sleep
c. Suppression of appetite d. Stimulation of appetite

Ghrelin, the "hunger hormone", also known as **lenomorelin** (INN), is a peptide hormone produced by ghrelinergic cells in the gastrointestinal tract which functions as a neuropeptide in the central nervous system. Besides regulating appetite, ghrelin also plays a significant role in regulating the distribution and rate of use of energy.

148. Maximal post-prandial motility is observed in:

a. Transverse colon b. Sigmoid colon
c. Descending colon d. Ascending colon

Force and **motility** increase up to **sigmoid colon**.

149. Gastric secretion, when compared to blood, contains more of:

a. Na^+ b. K^+
c. HCO_3^- d. Cl^-

Parietal cell secretion may well be an isotonic solution of essentially pure HCl that contains 150 mEq of Cl^- and 150 mEq of H^+ per litre. The comparable concentrations per litre of plasma are about 100 mEq of Cl^- and 0.00004 mEq of H^+.

150. Main site of vitamin B12 absorption:

a. Colon b. Ileum
c. Duodenum d. Stomach

The function of the ileum is mainly to absorb vitamin B_{12} and bile salts and whatever products of digestion were not absorbed by the jejunum.

151. Amount of bile produced (ml/day):

a. 100-500 b. 500-1000
c. 1000-1500 d. 1500-2000

Humans normally produce 0.5-1 litre of hepatic bile per day with bile salts, lecithin, cholesterol and 1.5 g of bile pigments.

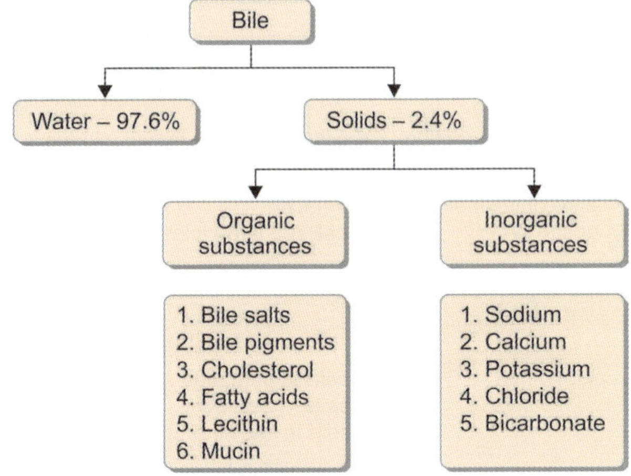

Composition of bile.

152. Form in which small intestine absorbs majority of carbohydrates:

a. Polysaccharide b. Disaccharide
c. Monosaccharide d. Pentose sugars

All carbohydrates absorbed in the small intestine must be hydrolyzed to monosaccharides prior to absorption.

Ans. 143. **d.** Ligation of all major arteries 144. **d.** Mass peristalsis 145. **c.** Increased release... 146. **c.** Potassium 147. **d.** Stimulation... 148. **c.** Descending colon 149. **d.** Cl^- 150. **b.** Ileum 151. **b.** 500-1000 152. **c.** Monosaccharide

153. Emptying of stomach is facilitated by:

a. Secretin
b. CCK-PZ
c. GIP
d. Gastrin

Functions of gastrin

- The presence of gastrin stimulates parietal cells of the stomach to secrete hydrochloric acid (HCl)/gastric acid.
- Stimulates parietal cell maturation and fundal growth.
- Causes chief cells to secrete pepsinogen, the zymogen (inactive) form of the digestive enzyme pepsin.
- Increases antral muscle mobility and promotes stomach contractions.
- Strengthens antral contractions against the pylorus, and constricts the pyloric sphincter, which diminishes the rate of gastric emptying.
- Plays a role in the relaxation of the ileocecal valve.
- Induces pancreatic secretions and gallbladder emptying.
- May impact lower esophageal sphincter (LES) tone, causing it to contract, although pentagastrin, rather than endogenous gastrin, may be the cause

154. Effect of secretin:

a. Reduces secretion of alkaline pancreatic juice
b. Reduces gastric acid secretion
c. Relaxation of sphincter
d. Reduces insulin secretion

Secretin also helps regulate the pH of the duodenum by: inhibiting the secretion of gastric acid from the parietal cells of the stomach; and stimulating the production of bicarbonate from the centroacinar cells and intercalated ducts of the pancreas.

Gastrointestinal hormones

Hormone	*Source of secretion*	*Actions*
Gastrin	G cells in stomach TG cells in GI tract Islets in fetal pancreas Anterior pituitary Brain	Stimulates gastric secretion and motility Promotes growth of gastric mucosa Stimulates release of pancreatic hormones Stimulates secretion of pancreatic juice Stimulates secretion of pancreatic hormones
Secretin	S cells of small intestine	Stimulates secretion of watery and alkaline pancreatic secretion Inhibits gastric secretion and motility Constricts pyloric sphincter Increases potency of cholecystokinin action
Cholecystokinin	I cells of small intestine	Contracts gallbladder Stimulates pancreatic secretion with enzymes Accelerates secretin activity Increases enterokinase secretion Inhibits gastric motility Increases intestinal motility Augments contraction of pyloric sphincter Suppresses hunger Induces drug tolerance to opioids
Gastric inhibitory peptide (GIP)	K cells in duodenum and jejunum Antrum of stomach	Stimulates insulin secretion Inhibits gastric secretion and motility
Vasoactive intestinal polypeptide (VIP)	Stomach Small and large intestines	Dilates splanchnic (peripheral) blood vessels Inhibits HCl secretion in gastric juice Stimulates secretion of succus entericus Relaxes smooth muscles of intestine Augments acetylcholine action on salivary glands Stimulates insulin secretion
Glucagon	α-cells in pancreas A cells in stomach L cells in intestine	Increases blood sugar level
Glicentin	L cells in duodenum and jejunum	Increases blood sugar level
Glucagon-like polypeptide-1 (GLP-1)	α-cells in pancreas Brain	Stimulates insulin secretion Inhibits gastric motility
GLP-2	L cells in ileum and colon	Suppresses appetite
Somatostatin	Hypothalamus D cells in pancreas D cells in stomach and small intestine	Inhibits secretion of growth hormone Inhibits gastric secretion and motility Inhibits secretion of pancreatic juice Inhibits secretion of GI hormones

Ans. **153. d.** Gastrin **154. b.** Reduces gastric acid secretion

Hormone	Source of secretion	Actions
Pancreatic polypeptide	PP cells in pancreas Small intestine	Increases secretion of glucagons Decreases pancreatic secretion
Peptide YY	L cells of ileum and colon	Inhibits gastric secretion and motility Reduces secretion of pancreatic juice Inhibits intestinal motility and bowel passage Suppresses appetite and food intake
Neuropeptide Y	Ileum and colon Brain and autonomic nervous system (ANS)	Increases blood flow in enteric blood vessels
Motilin	Mo cells in stomach and intestine Enterochromaffin cells in intestine	Accelerates gastric emptying Increases movements of small intestine Increases peristalsis in colon
Substance P	Brain Small intestine	Increases movements of small intestine
Ghrelin	Stomach Hypothalamus Pituitary Kidney Placenta	Promotes growth hormone (GH) release Induces appetite and food intake Stimulates gastric emptying

155. Extrinsic factor is another name for:

a. Vitamin B_{12} b. Folate
c. Pyridoxine d. Thiamine

Castle factors

- **Extrinsic factor**, much more commonly known as vitamin B_{12}
- **Intrinsic factor**, a glycoprotein produced by the parietal cells of the stomach, which is necessary for the absorption of vitamin B_{12}

156. Vitamin synthesized by enteric bacteria:

a. Vitamin A b. Vitamin D
c. Vitamin K d. Vitamin B_{12}

Because vitamin K is synthesized by bacteria in the colon, it is rare when a person has a bleeding tendency because of vitamin K deficiency in the diet.

157. Difference between hepatic and gallbladder bile:

a. More solid in hepatic bile
b. Less water in gallbladder bile
c. Less bile salt in gallbladder bile
d. Hepatic bile is more viscous

Bile is produced continuously by the liver (liver bile), and stored and concentrated in the gallbladder (gallbladder bile). After eating, this stored bile is discharged into the duodenum. The composition of gallbladder bile is 97% water, 0.7% bile salts, 0.2% bilirubin, 0.51% fats (cholesterol, fatty acids and lecithin), and 200 mEq/l inorganic salts.

Differences between liver bile and gallbladder bile

Types of entities	Liver bile	Gallbladder bile
pH	8 to 8.6	7 to 7.6
Specific gravity	1010 to 1011	1026 to 1032
Water content	97.6%	89%
Solids	2.4%	11%
Organic substances		
Bile salts	0.5 g/dL	6.0 g/dL
Bile pigments	0.05 g/dL	0.3 g/dL
Cholesterol	0.1 g/dL	0.5 g/dL
Fatty acids	0.2 g/dL	1.2 g/dL
Lecithin	0.05 g/dL	0.4 g/dL
Mucin	Absent	Present
Inorganic substances		
Sodium	150 mEq/L	135 mEq/L
Calcium	4 mEq/L	22 mEq/L
Potassium	5 mEq/L	12 mEq/L
Chloride	100 mEq/L	10 mEq/L
Bicarbonate	30 mEq/L	10 mEq/L

Contd...

Contd...

158. It is abnormal, if there is no air in rectum (in a neonate) by:

a. 6 hours b. 12 hours
c. 24 hours d. 48 hours

The intestinal pneumatization process follows neonatal swallowing of air. This air will go through the bowel loops to reach caecum around the 6th hour, the sigmoid colon in the 11th hour, and the rectum in the 12th to 24th hour of life.

159. Iron is absorbed in:

a. Stomach
b. Duodenum
c. Ileum
d. Duodenum + Jejunum

Ans. 155. a. Vitamin B_{12} 156. c. Vitamin K 157. b. Less water in... 158. b. 12 hours
159. d. Duodenum + Jejunum

Only about 10% of dietary **iron** is **absorbed** (1–2 mg/day). **Iron absorption**. **Iron** is mainly **absorbed** in the **duodenum** and upper jejunum.

160. Bulk mass contraction is seen in:

a. Stomach
b. Duodenum
c. Ileum
d. Colon

The **mass** movements force the faecal material rapidly in **mass** down the **colon**.

NERVOUS SYSTEM

161. Flight or fight response is mediated by:

a. Parasympathetic system
b. Sympathetic system
c. Pyramidal system
d. Extrapyramidal system

Noradrenergic discharge

- This division discharges as a unit in emergency situation
- The effects of this discharge are of considerable value in preparing the individual to cope with the emergency. For example, noradrenergic discharge:
  - Relaxes accommodation and dilates the pupil (letting more light into the eyes)
  - Accelerates the heartbeat and raises the blood pressure (providing better perfusion of the vital organs and muscles)
  - Constricts the blood vessels of the skin (which limits bleeding from wounds)
  - Lower thresholds in the reticular formation (reinforcing the alert, aroused state)
  - Elevate plasma glucose and free fatty acid levels (supplying more energy)
- On the basis of effects like these, Cannon called the emergency induced discharge of the noradrenergic nervous system the 'preparation for flight or fight.'

Actions of sympathetic and parasympathetic divisions of autonomic nervous system

Effector organ		*Sympathetic division*	*Parasympathetic division*
1. Eye	Ciliary muscle	Relaxation	Contraction
	Pupil	Dilatation	Constriction
2. Lacrimal glands		Decrease in secretion	Increase in secretion
3. Salivary glands		Decrease in secretion and vasoconstriction	Increase in secretion and vasodilatation
4. Gastrointestinal tract	Motility	Inhibition	Acceleration
	Secretion	Decrease	Increase
	Sphincters	Constriction	Relaxation
	Smooth muscles	Relaxation	Contraction
5. Gallbladder		Relaxation	Contraction
6. Urinary bladder	Detrusor muscle	Relaxation	Contraction
	Internal sphincter	Constriction	Relaxation
7. Sweat glands		Increase in secretion	–
8. Heart – rate and force		Increase	Decrease
9. Blood vessels		Constriction of all blood vessels, except those in heart and skeletal muscle	Dilatation
10. Bronchioles		Dilatation	Constriction

162. All of the following cells are present in cerebral cortex EXCEPT:

a. Fusiform cells
b. Pyramidal cells
c. Stellate cells
d. Bipolar cells

Bipolar cell

- It is a type of neuron which has two extensions.
- Bipolar cells are specialized sensory neurons for the transmission of special senses. As such, they are part of the sensory pathways for smell, sight, taste, hearing and vestibular functions.
- Common examples are the bipolar cells of the retina, the ganglia of the vestibulocochlear nerve, and the extensive use of bipolar cells to transmit efferent (motor) signals to control muscles.

Ans. **160. d.** Colon **161. b.** Sympathetic system **162. d.** Bipolar cells

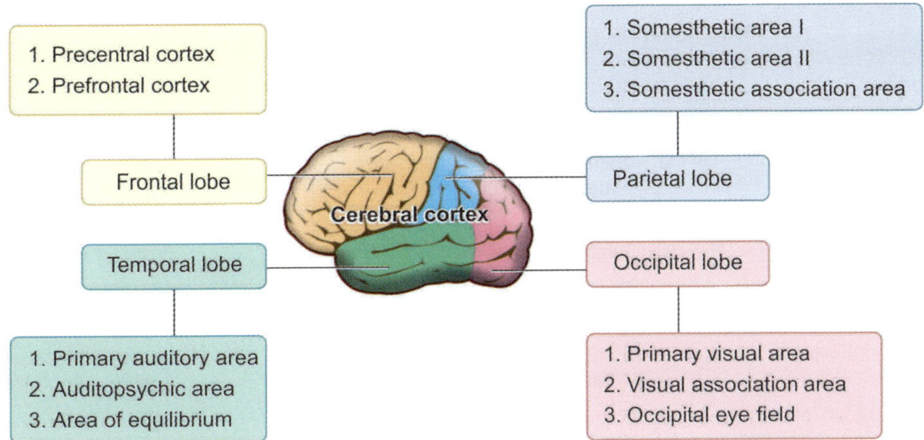

Parts of cerebral cortex.

163. Mediator of auditory pathway:
a. Medial geniculate body
b. Lateral geniculate body
c. Medial lemniscus
d. Lateral lemniscus

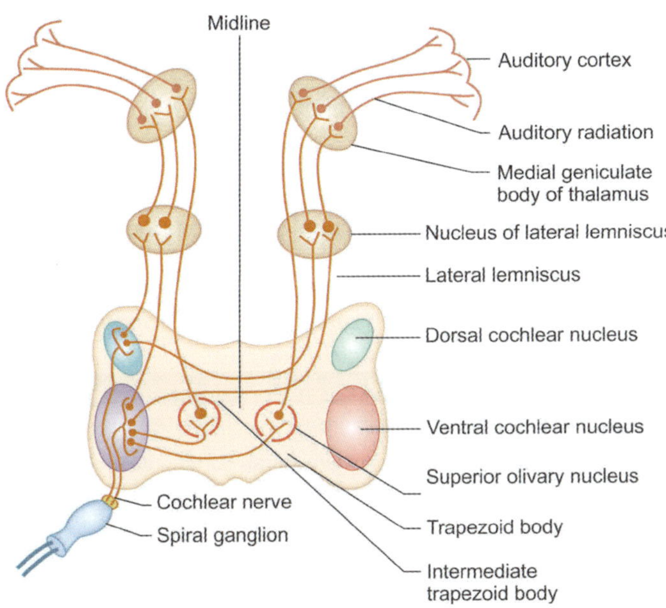

Auditory pathway. Blue = First order neuron, Red = Second order neuron, Green = Third order neuron, Black = Auditory radiation.

The Medial Geniculate Body has three major divisions; ventral (VMGB), dorsal (DMGB) and medial (MMGB). Whilst the VMGB is specific to auditory information processing, the DMGB and MMGB also receive information from nonauditory pathways.

164. Effect of fever:
a. Resetting of skin temperature
b. Thermoregulatory centre to shift to new level
c. Both of the above
d. None of the above

In many respects, the hypothalamus works like a thermostat. Temperature is ultimately regulated in the hypothalamus. A trigger of the fever, called a pyrogen, causes a release of prostaglandin E2 (PGE2). PGE2 then in turn acts on the hypothalamus, which generates a systemic response back to the rest of the body, causing heat-creating effects to match a new temperature level.

165. NOT a function of hypothalamus:
a. Temperature regulation
b. Increase in heart rate with exercise
c. Food intake
d. Hypophyseal control

Mass sympathetic discharge occurs during exercise. Sympathetic stimulation causes the release of the neurotransmitter norepinephrine (also known as noradrenaline) at the neuromuscular junction of the cardiac nerves. This shortens the repolarization period, thus speeding the rate of depolarization and contraction, which results in an increased heart rate. It opens chemical or ligand-gated sodium and calcium ion channels, allowing an influx of positively charged ions.

Functions of hypothalamus

Functions	*Action/Center*	*Nuclei/Parts involved*
1. Control of anterior pituitary	Releasing hormones Inhibiting hormones	Discrete areas
2. Secretion of posterior pituitary hormones	Oxytocin Antidiuretic hormone (ADH)	Paraventricular nucleus Supraoptic nucleus

Contd...

Ans. **163. a.** Medial geniculate body **164. b.** Thermoregulatory centre to shift to new level
165. b. Increase in heart rate with exercise

Contd...

Functions	Action/Center	Nuclei/Parts involved
3. Control of adrenal cortex	Corticotropin-releasing hormone (CRH)	Paraventricular nucleus
4. Control of adrenal medulla	Catecholamines during emotion	Posterior and dorsomedial nuclei
5. Regulation of autonomic nervous system (ANS)	Sympathetic Parasympathetic	Posterior and lateral nuclei Anterior nuclei
6. Regulation of heart rate	Acceleration Inhibition	Posterior and lateral nuclei Preoptic and anterior nuclei
7. Regulation of blood pressure	Pressor effect Depressor effect	Posterior and lateral nuclei Preoptic area
8. Regulation of body temperature	Heat gain center Heat loss center	Posterior hypothalamus Anterior hypothalamus
9. Regulation of hunger and food intake	Feeding center Satiety center	Lateral nucleus Ventromedial nucleus
10. Regulation of water intake	Thirst center Water retention by ADH	Lateral nucleus Supraoptic nucleus
11. Regulation of sleep and wakefulness	Sleep Wakefulness	Anterior hypothalamus Mammillary body
12. Regulation of behavior and emotion	Reward center Punishment center	Ventromedial nucleus Posterior and lateral nuclei
13. Regulation of sexual function	Sexual cycle	Arcuate and posterior nuclei
14. Regulation of response to smell	Autonomic responses	Posterior hypothalamus
15. Role in circadian rhythm	Rhythmic changes	Suprachiasmatic nucleus

166. A lesion of ventrolateral part of spinal cord will lead to loss (below the level of lesion) of:

a. Pain sensation on same side
b. Proprioception on opposite side
c. Pain sensation on opposite side
d. Proprioception on same side

Hemisection of spinal cord

- On the ipsilateral side of the injury (same side), there is a loss of motor function, proprioception, vibration, and light touch.
- Contralaterally (opposite side of injury), there is a loss of pain, temperature, and crude touch sensations.

Ascending tracts of spinal cord

Situation	Tract	Origin	Course	Termination	Function
Anterior white column	1. Anterior spinothalamic tract	Chief sensory nucleus	Crossing in spinal cord Forms spinal lemniscus	Ventral posterolateral nucleus of thalamus	Crude touch sensation
Lateral white column	1. Lateral spinothalamic tract	Substantia gelatinosa	Crossing in spinal cord Forms spinal lemniscus	Ventral posterolateral nucleus of thalamus	Pain and temperature sensations
	2. Ventral spinocerebellar tract	Marginal nucleus	Crossing in spinal cord	Anterior lobe of cerebellum	Subconscious kinesthetic sensations
	3. Dorsal spinocerebellar tract	Clarke nucleus	Uncrossed fibers	Anterior lobe of cerebellum	Subconscious kinesthetic sensations
	4. Spinotectal tract	Chief sensory nucleus	Crossing in spinal cord	Superior colliculus	Spinovisual reflex
	5. Fasiculus dorsolateralis	Posterior nerve root ganglion	Component of lateral spinothalamic tract	Substantia gelatinosa	Pain and temperature sensations
	6. Spinoreticular tract	Intermediolateral cells	Crossed and uncrossed fibers	Reticular formation of brainstem	Consciousness and awareness

Contd...

Ans. 166. c. Pain sensation on opposite side

Contd...

Situation	*Tract*	*Origin*	*Course*	*Termination*	*Function*
	7. Spino-olivary tract	Nonspecific	Uncrossed fibers	Olivary nucleus	Proprioception
	8. Spinovestibular tract	Nonspecific	Crossed and uncrossed fibers	Lateral vestibular nucleus	Proprioception
Posterior white column	1. Fasciculus gracilis	Posterior nerve root ganglia	Uncrossed fibers No synapse in spinal cord	Nucleus gracilis in medulla	Tactile sensation Tactile localization Tactile discrimination Vibratory sensation Conscious kinesthetic sensation Stereognosis
	2. Fasciculus cuneatus	Posterior nerve root ganglia	Uncrossed fibers No synapse in spinal cord	Nucleus cuneatus in medulla	

167. In adults, nonshivering thermogenesis is due to:

a. Pancreatic hormones
b. Yellow fat between the shoulders
c. Noradrenaline
d. Muscle metabolism

Nonshivering thermogenesis occurs in brown adipose tissue. Nonshivering thermogenesis is regulated mainly by sympathetic nervous system. Some hormones, such as norepinephrine, may stimulate thermogenesis by activating the sympathetic nervous system.

168. Sensation lost on same side in Brown Sequard syndrome:

a. Proprioception b. Touch
c. Temperature d. Pain

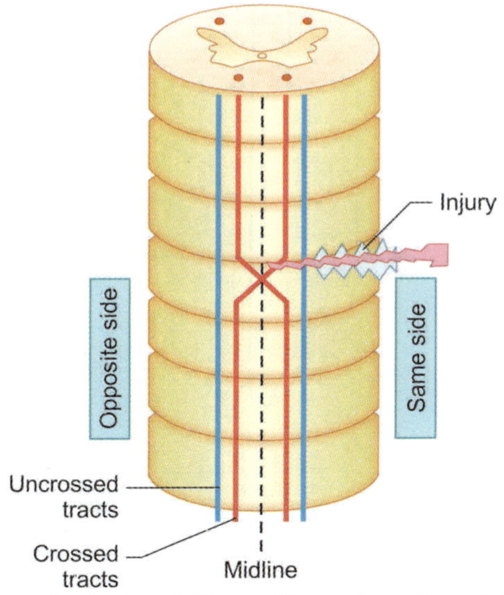

Hemisection of spinal cord (Brown-Séquard syndrome). Below the level of lesion: same side = loss of sensations carried by uncrossed fibers, opposite side = loss of sensations carried by crossed fibers. At the level of lesion: same side = complete anesthesia, opposite side = loss of sensations carried by crossed fibers.

Brown-Séquard syndrome (also known as **Brown-Séquard's hemiplegia, Brown-Séquard's paralysis, hemiparaplegic syndrome, hemiplegia et hemiparaplegia spinalis,** or **spinal hemiparaplegia**) is caused by damage to one half of the spinal cord, resulting in paralysis and loss of proprioception on the same (or ipsilateral) side as the injury or lesion, and loss of pain and temperature sensation on the opposite (or contralateral) side as the lesion.

169. Nightmare is seen in:

a. REM sleep b. Stage I NREM sleep
c. Stage II NREM sleep d. Stage IV NREM sleep

Rapid eye movement sleep (REM sleep, REMS) is a unique phase of mammalian sleep characterized by random movement of the eyes, low muscle tone throughout the body, and the propensity of the sleeper to dream vividly. This phase is also known as **paradoxical sleep** (PS) and sometimes **desynchronized sleep** because of physiological similarities to waking states, including rapid, low-voltage desynchronized brain waves.

Rapid eye movement (REM) sleep and non-rapid eye movement (NREM) sleep

Characteristics	*REM sleep*	*Non-REM sleep*
1. Rapid eye movement (REM)	Present	Absent
2. Dreams	Present	Absent
3. Muscle twitching	Present	Absent
4. Heart rate	Fluctuating	Stable
5. Blood pressure	Fluctuating	Stable
6. Respiration	Fluctuating	Stable
7. Body temperature	Fluctuating	Stable
8. Neurotransmitter	Noradrenaline	Serotonin

170. Satiety centre is located in:

a. Frontal lobe
b. Supraoptic nucleus
c. Ventro-medial nucleus
d. Lateral hypothalamus

The extreme lateral part of the ventromedial nucleus of the hypothalamus is responsible for the control of food intake. Stimulation of this area causes increased food intake. Bilateral lesion of this area causes complete cessation of food intake.

Ans. **167. c.** Noradrenaline **168. a.** Proprioception **169. a.** REM sleep
170. c. Ventro-medial nucleus

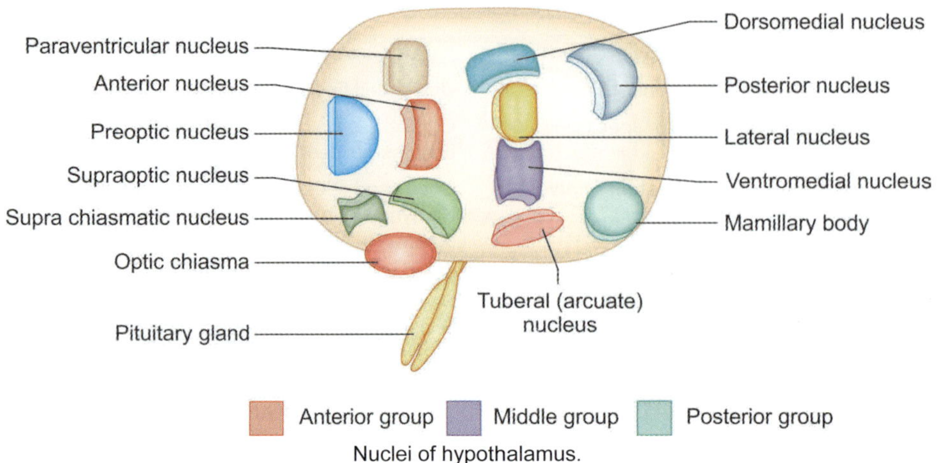

Nuclei of hypothalamus.

171. Chemoreceptor trigger zone is located in:

a. Lateral hypothalamus b. Ventral hypothalamus
c. Pons d. Area postrema

The CTZ is located within the area postrema, which is on the floor of the fourth ventricle and is outside of the blood-brain barrier. It is also part of the vomiting center itself.

172. Location of hunger centre:

a. Ventromedial nucleus b. Supraoptic nucelus
c. Frontal lobe d. Lateral hypothalamus

The extreme lateral part of the ventromedial nucleus of the hypothalamus is responsible for the control of food intake (satiety) and lateral hypothalamic area controls thirst and hunger.

Anterior or Preoptic group	Middle or Tuberal group	Posterior or Mamillary group
1. Preoptic nucleus 2. Paraventricular nucleus 3. Anterior nucleus 4. Supraoptic nucleus 5. Suprachiasmatic nucleus	1. Dorsomedial nucleus 2. Ventromedial nucleus 3. Lateral nucleus 4. Arcuate (tuberal) nucleus	1. Posterior nucleus 2. Mamillary body

173. NOT carried by anterolateral system:

a. Crude touch b. Pain
c. Temperature d. Proprioception

Proprioception

- Conscious proprioception is communicated by the posterior column-medial lemniscus pathway to the cerebrum.
- Unconscious proprioception is communicated primarily via the dorsal spinocerebellar tract and ventral spinocerebellar tract, to the cerebellum.

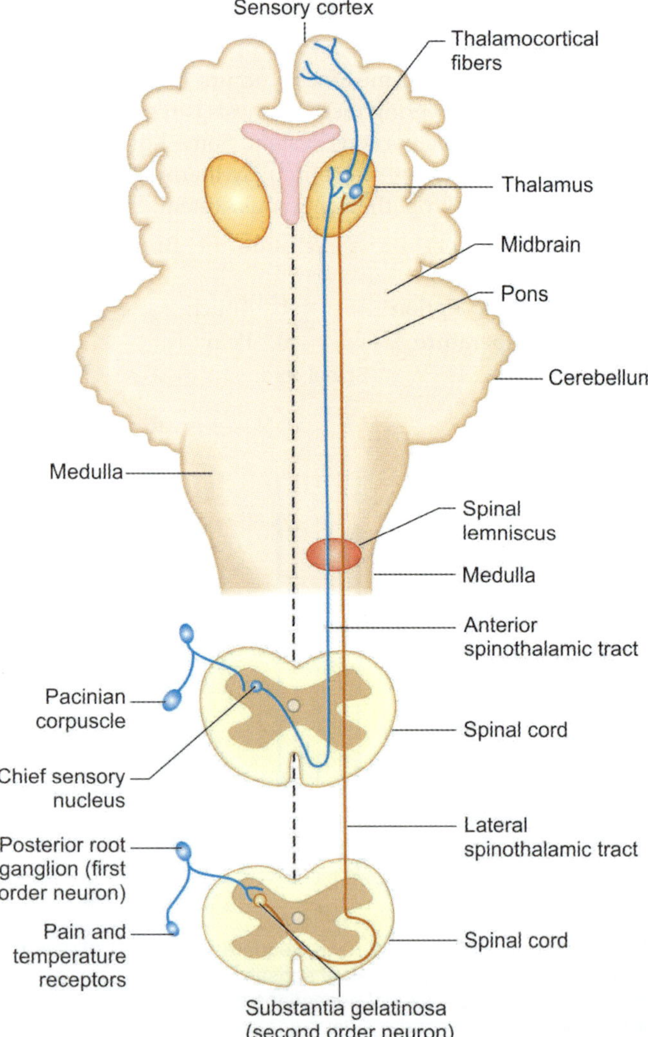

Spinothalamic tracts and pathways for crude touch, pain and temperature sensations. Anterior spinothalamic tract (red) carries crude touch sensation. Lateral spinothalamic tract (blue) carries pain and temperature sensations.

Ans. **171. d.** Area postrema **172. d.** Lateral hypothalamus **173. d.** Proprioception

174. Positive supporting reaction is integrated at:

a. Medulla b. Midbrain
c. Spinal cord d. Vestibular nucleus

Stretch reflex, positive and negative supporting reaction is integrated at spinal cord.

175. Sensation lost on the same side in Brown-Sequard syndrome:

a. Proprioception b. Temperature
c. Touch d. Pain

Brown-sequard syndrome is caused by damage to one half of the spinal cord, resulting in paralysis and loss of proprioception on the same (or ipsilateral) side as the injury or lesion, and loss of pain and temperature sensation on the opposite (or contralateral) side as the lesion.

Descending tracts of spinal cord

	Tract	Situation	Origin	Course	Function
Pyramidal Tracts	1. Anterior corticospinal tract	Anterior white column	Betz cells and other cells of motor area	Uncrossed fibers	i. Control of voluntary movements ii. Form upper motor neurons
	2. Lateral corticospinal tract	Lateral white column	Betz cells and other cells of motor area	Crossed fibers	
Extrapyramidal tracts	1. Medial longitudinal fasciculus	Anterior white column	Vestibular nucleus Reticular formation Superior colliculus and cells of Cajal	Uncrossed fibers Extend up to upper cervical segments	i Coordination of reflex ocular movements ii. Integration of movements of eyes and neck
	2. Anterior vestibulospinal tract	Anterior white column	Medial vestibular nucleus	Uncrossed fibers Extend up to upper thoracic segments	i. Maintenance of muscle tone and posture ii. Maintenance of position of head and body during acceleration
	3. Lateral vestibulospinal tract	Lateral white column	Lateral vestibular nucleus	Mostly uncrossed Extend to all segments	
	4. Reticulospinal tract	Lateral white fasciculus	Reticular formation of pons and medulla	Mostly uncrossed Extend up to thoracic segments	i. Coordination of voluntary and reflex movements ii. Control of muscle tone iii. Control of respiration and diameter of blood vessels
	5. Tectospinal tract	Anterior white column	Superior colliculus	Crossed fibers Extend up to lower cervical segments	Control of movement of head in response to visual and auditory impulses
	6 Rubrospinal tract	Lateral white column	Red nucleus	Crossed fibers Extend up to thoracic segments	Facilitatory influence on flexor muscle tone
	7. Olivospinal tract	Lateral white column	Inferior olivary nucleus	Mostly crossed Extent – not clear	Control of movements due to proprioception

176. The main excitatory neurotransmitter in the CNS is:

a. Glycine b. Acetylcholine
c. Aspartate d. Glutamate

Glutamate is an important excitatory neurotransmitter that plays the principal role in neural activation.

Neurotransmitters

Group	Name	Site of secretion	Action
Amino acids	GABA	Cerebral cortex, cerebellum, basal ganglia, retina and spinal cord	Inhibitory
	Glycine	Forebrain, brainstem, spinal cord and retina	Inhibitory
	Glutamate	Cerebral cortex, brainstem and cerebellum	Excitatory
	Aspartate	Cerebellum, spinal cord and retina	Excitatory
Amines	Noradrenaline	Postganglionic adrenergic sympathetic nerve endings, cerebral cortex, hypothalamus, basal ganglia, brainstem, locus coeruleus and spinal cord	Excitatory and inhibitory
	Adrenaline	Hypothalamus, thalamus and spinal cord	Excitatory and inhibitory
	Dopamine	Basal ganglia, hypothalamus, limbic system, neocortex, retina and sympathetic ganglia	Inhibitory
	Serotonin	Hypothalamus, limbic system, cerebellum, spinal cord, retina, gastrointestinal (GI) tract, lungs and platelets	Inhibitory
	Histamine	Hypothalamus, cerebral cortex, GI tract and mast cells	Excitatory

Contd...

Ans. 174. **c.** Spinal cord 175. **d.** Pain 176. **d.** Glutamate

Contd...

Group	Name	Site of secretion	Action
Others	Nitric oxide	Many parts of CNS, neuromuscular junction and GI tract	Excitatory
	Acetylcholine	Preganglionic parasympathetic nerve endings Postganglionic parasympathetic nerve endings Preganglionic sympathetic nerve endings Postganglionic sympathetic cholinergic nerve endings Neuromuscular junction, cerebral cortex, hypothalamus, basal ganglia, thalamus, hippocampus and amacrine cells of retina	Excitatory

177. In adults, nonshivering thermogenesis, is due to:

a. Brown fat between the shoulders
b. Norepinephrine
c. Metabolism in muscles
d. Thyroid hormone

Nonshivering thermogenesis can also produce heat in response to cold stress. This type of thermogenesis is stimulated by sympathetic nervous system activation, which releases norepinephrine and epinephrine that in turn increase metabolic activity and heat generation

178. Blind spot of Mariotte:

a. Ora serrata
b. Macula lutea
c. Optic disc
d. Fovea centralis

Blind spot known as the *physiological blind spot*, "blind point", or *punctum caecum*, is the place in the visual field that corresponds to the lack of light-detecting photoreceptor cells on the optic disc of the retina where the optic nerve passes through the optic disc. Because there are no cells to detect light on the optic disc, the corresponding part of the field of vision is invisible.

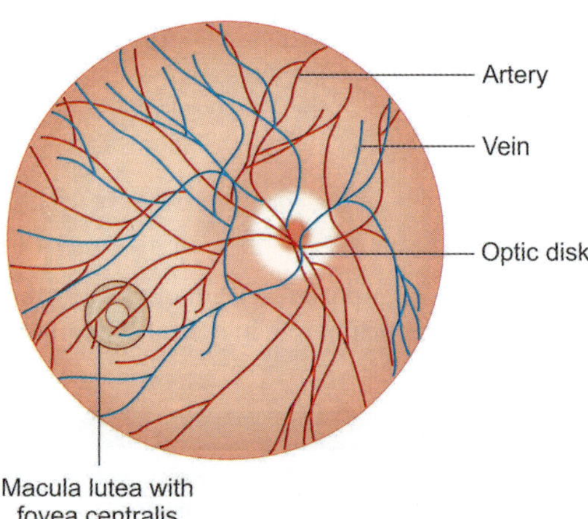

Fundus oculi.

179. Hemitransection of spinal cord above the pyramidal tract decussation results in:

a. Contralateral loss of vibration and joint position
b. Ipsilateral loss of pain and temperature
c. Contralateral loss of proprioception
d. UMN features opposite half of the body

If fibres of the *corticospinal* tracts are damaged anywhere along their course from the cerebral cortex to the lower end of the spinal cord, this will give rise to an upper motor neuron syndrome. A few days after the injury to the upper motor neurons, a pattern of motor signs and symptoms appears, including spasticity, hyperactive reflexes, a loss of the ability to perform fine movements, and an extensor plantar response known as the Babinski sign.

180. Law explaining phantom limb:

a. Pascal law
b. Fechner law of degeneration
c. Law of projection
d. Weber law

Each locality sends sensory impulses to the brain via a specific sensory pathway. Stimulation of any point along the course of this pathway produces a sensation felt at this specific locality. So, the locality of the stimulus is also coded by the specific sensory pathway which serves this locality. This is called the "law of projection". It explains the phantom limb phenomenon which occurs in amputees.

181. Temperature regulation is done by:

a. Midbrain
b. Pons
c. Medulla
d. Hypothalamus

The hormones from the hypothalamus govern physiologic functions such as temperature regulation, thirst, hunger, sleep, mood, sex drive, and the release of other hormones within the body.

182. NOT a neuroglial cell of CNS:

a. Astrocytes
b. Kupffer cells
c. Microglia
d. Oligodendrocytes

Kupffer cells (KC) constitute 80-90% of the tissue macrophages present in the body. They reside within the lumen of the liver sinusoids, and are therefore constantly exposed to gut-derived bacteria, microbial debris and bacterial endotoxins, known to activate macrophages.

Ans. 177. **b.** Norepinephrine 178. **c.** Optic disc 179. **d.** UMN features... 180. **c.** Law of projection 181. **d.** Hypothalamus 182. **b.** Kupffer cells

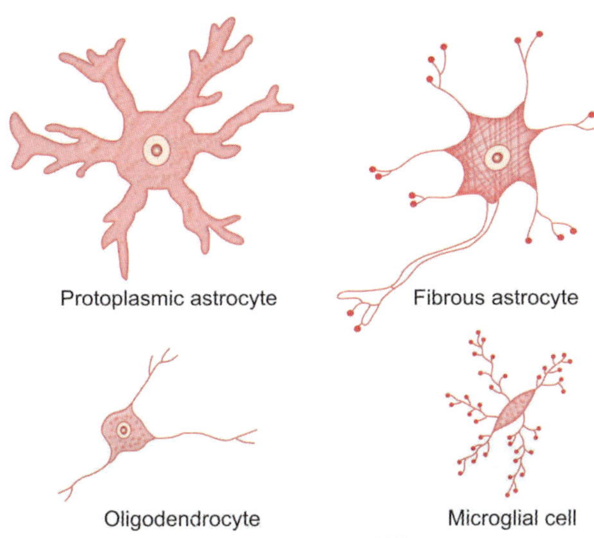

Neuroglial cells in CNS.

183. Circadian rhythm is under control of:
a. Supraoptic nuclei
b. Median eminence
c. Paramedian nuclei
d. Suprachiasmatic nuclei

The **suprachiasmatic nucleus** or **nuclei** (**SCN**) is a tiny region located in the hypothalamus, situated directly above the optic chiasm. It is responsible for controlling circadian rhythms. The neuronal and hormonal activities it generates regulate many different body functions in a 24-hour cycle, using around 20,000 neurons.

184. Pretectal area is related to:
a. Doll's eye movements
b. Auditory reflex
c. Light reflex
d. Stapedial reflex

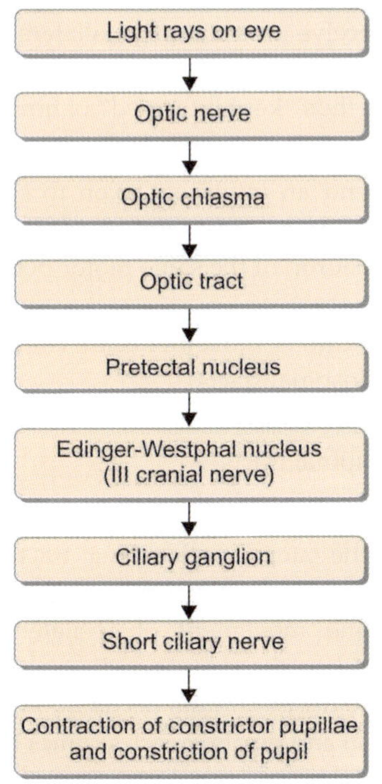

Pathway for light reflex.

The **pretectal area**, or **pretectum**, is a midbrain structure composed of seven nuclei and comprises part of the subcortical visual system. Through reciprocal bilateral projections from the retina, it is involved primarily in mediating behavioral responses to acute changes in ambient light such as the pupillary light reflex, the optokinetic reflex, and temporary changes to the circadian rhythm.

185. Function of neocerebellum:
a. Motor activity execution
b. Equilibrium
c. Ocular movements
d. Motor planning

The **neocerebellum** is part of the large network for timing, motor, cognitive functions, and social contact. It might improve movement timing or enhance **motor planning**.

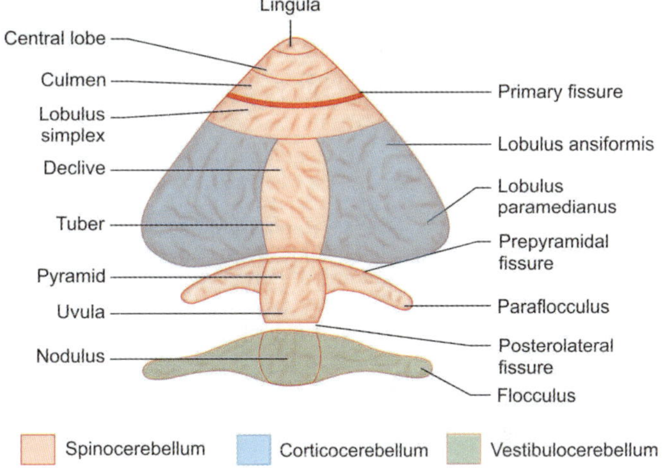

Parts and functional divisions of cerebellum.

186. Last to be affected in central transection of spinal cord:
a. Pain
b. Temperature
c. Proprioception
d. Pinprick

CCS/central cord syndrome is characterized by disproportionately greater motor impairment in upper compared to lower extremities, and variable degree of sensory loss below the level of injury in combination with bladder dysfunction and urinary retention. This syndrome differs from that of a complete lesion, which is characterized by total loss of all sensation and movement below the level of the injury.

187. Neural tube defects in newborn may be associated with maternal deficiency of:
a. Cyanocobalamin
b. Folate
c. Pyridoxine
d. Thiamine

Folate (vitamin B_9) and vitamin B_{12} are very important in reducing the occurrences of NTDs. Folate is required for the production and maintenance of new cells, for DNA synthesis and RNA synthesis. Folate is needed to carry one carbon groups for methylation and nucleic acid synthesis. It has been hypothesized that the early human embryo may be particularly vulnerable to folate

Ans. 183. **d.** Suprachiasmatic 184. **c.** Light reflex 185. **d.** Motor planning 186. **c.** Proprioception 187. **b.** Folate deficiency due to differences of the functional enzymes in this pathway during embryogenesis combined with high demand for post-translational methylations of the cytoskeleton in neural cells during neural tube closure.

188. All are seen in REM sleep except:
a. Active dreaming
b. Decreased muscle tone
c. Threshold for arousal by sensory stimuli is lowered
d. Bruxism

The threshold for arousal by sensory stimuli and by stimulation of the reticular formation is sometimes elevated in REM sleep.

189. MC cause of hemiplegia:
a. Occlusion of middle cerebral artery
b. Occlusion of vertebral artery
c. Occlusion of basilar artery
d. Occlusion of anterior cerebral artery

Contralateral hemiparesis and hemisensory loss of the face, upper and lower extremities is the most common presentation of MCA syndrome. Lower extremity function is more spared than that of the faciobrachial region. The majority of the primary motor and somatosensory cortices are supplied by the MCA and the cortical homunculus can, therefore, be used to localize the defects more precisely.

Types of paralysis

Paralysis	*Parts of the body affected*	*Causes*
Monoplegia	Paralysis of one limb	Isolated damage of central nervous system or peripheral nervous system
Diplegia	Paralysis of both the upper limbs or both the lower limbs	Isolated damage of brain
Hemiplegia	Paralysis of upper limb and lower limb on one side of the body	Lesion in motor cortex and corticospinal tracts in posterior limb of internal capsule on the side opposite to the paralysis
Paraplegia	Paralysis of lower half of the body	Injury to lower part of spinal cord
Quadriplegia or tetraplegia	Paralysis of all the four limbs	Injury to upper part of spinal cord (shoulder level or above, at which the motor nerves of upper limbs leave the spinal cord)

190. Renshaw inhibitory interneurons are seen in:
a. White matter of spinal cord
b. Gray matter of spinal cord
c. Gray matter of brain
d. White matter of brain

Renshaw cells are inhibitory interneurons found in the gray matter of the spinal cord, and are associated in two ways with an alpha motor neuron.

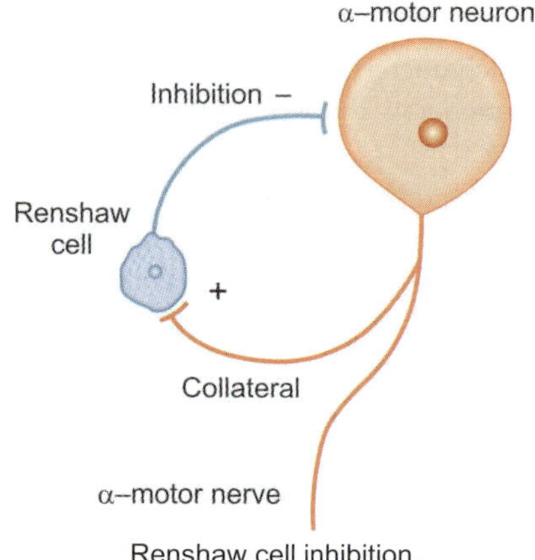

Renshaw cell inhibition.

- They receive an excitatory collateral from the alpha neuron's axon as they emerge from the motor root, and are thus "kept informed" of how vigorously that neuron is firing.
- They send an inhibitory axon to synapse with the cell body of the initial alpha neuron and/or an alpha motor neuron of the same motor pool.

191. Skilled voluntary movements are controlled by:
a. Reticulospinal tracts
b. Tectospinal tracts
c. Rubrospinal tracts
d. Lateral corticospinal tract

Axons in the lateral corticospinal tract leave out of the tract and into the anterior horns of the spinal cord. It controls fine movement of ipsilateral limbs (albeit contralateral to the corresponding motor cortex) as it lies distal to the pyramidal decussation. Control of more central axial and girdle muscles comes from the anterior corticospinal tract.

Ans. **188. c.** Threshold for... **189. a.** Occlusion of middle... **190. b.** Gray matter... **191. d.** Lateral corticospinal tract

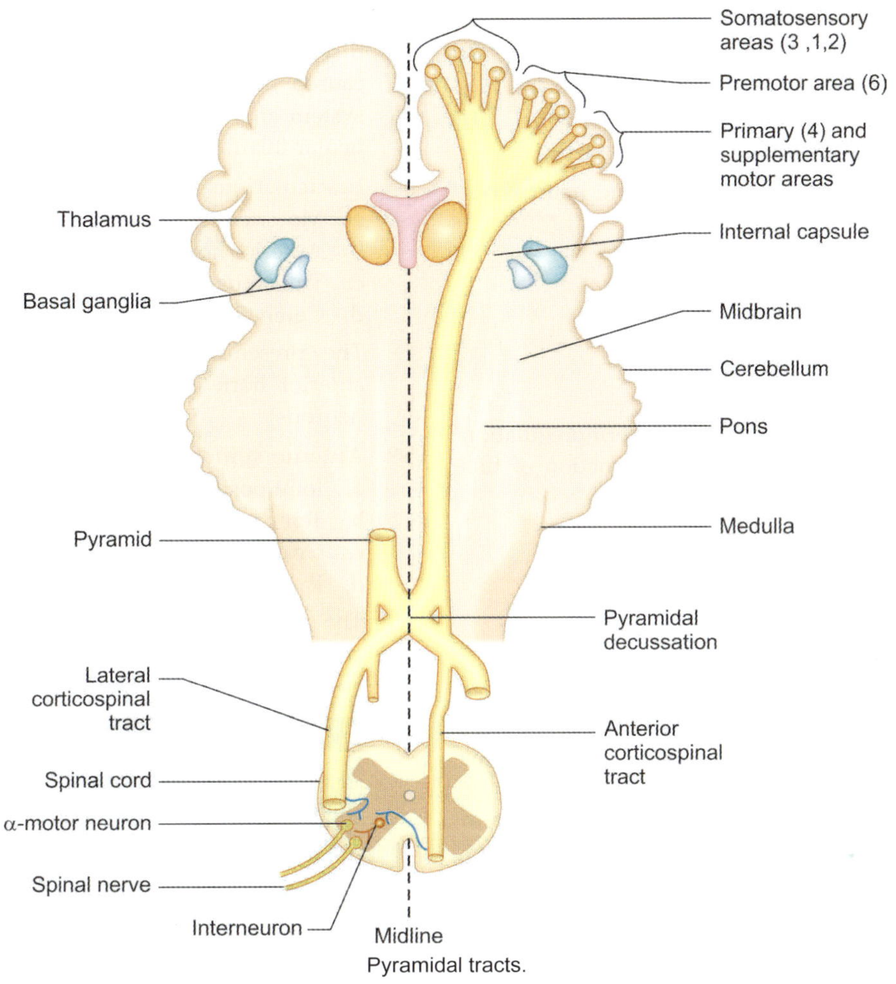

Pyramidal tracts.

192. Transducin is seen in:

a. Adrenal medulla
b. Skeletal muscle
c. Retina
d. Glomerulus

Transducin (G_t) is naturally expressed invertebrate retina rods and cones, with different α subunits in rod and cone photoreceptors.

193. In eyes, Acetylcholine is secreted by:

a. Amacrine cells
b. Ganglion cells
c. Horizontal cells
d. Bipolar cells

Amacrine cells operate at the inner plexiform layer (IPL), the second synaptic retinal layer where bipolar cells and retinal ganglion cells form synapses. Each type of amacrine cell releases one or several neurotransmitters (GABA, glycine, dopamine, acetylcholine and indolamine) where it connects with other cells.

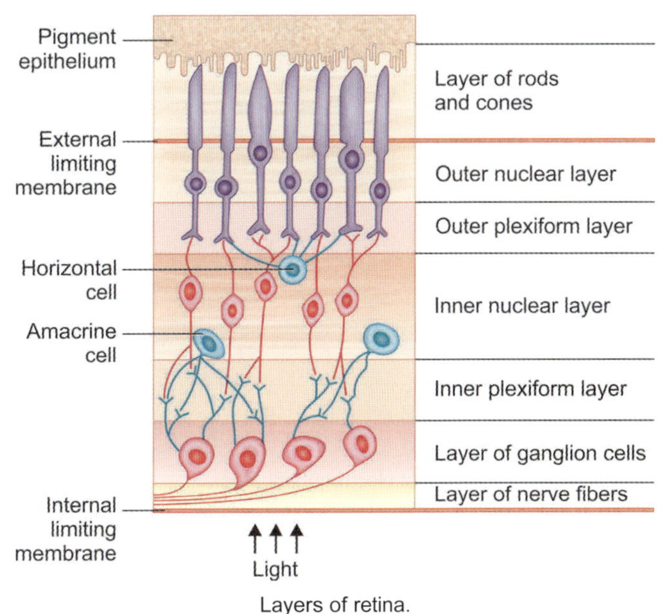

Layers of retina.

Ans. **192. c.** Retina **193. a.** Amacrine cells

194. Location of satiety centre:

a. Preoptic nucleus
b. Supramedian nucleus
c. Lateral hypothalamus
d. Ventromedial nucleus

Ventromedial nucleus controls satiety and neuroendocrine control

195. Shivering is controlled by:

a. Dorsomedial nucleus
b. Posterior hypothalamus
c. Perifornical nucleus
d. Lateral hypothalamic area

Posterior hypothalamus function is thermoregulation (heating) of the body. Damage or destruction of this nucleus causes hypothermia.

196. True for alpha waves are all except:

a. Amplitude of 5-10 microvolts
b. Awake state, eyes closed
c. Frequency of 8-13 cycles/sec
d. Predominantly recorded from occipital region

Alpha waves are neural oscillations in the frequency range of 7.5–12.5 Hz (and amplitude of around 50 mV) arising from synchronous and coherent (in phase or constructive) electrical activity of thalamic pacemaker cells in humans. They are also called Berger's wave in memory of the founder of EEG.

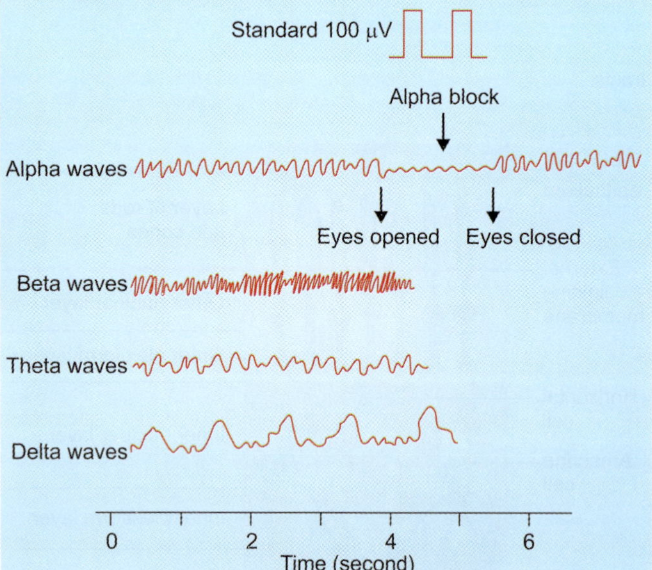

Waves of electroencephalogram.

197. Wernicke's encephalopathy is seen in deficiency of:

a. Vitamin B_1
b. Vitamin B_2
c. Vitamin B_3
d. Vitamin B_{12}

Wernicke's encephalopathy or now often **Wernicke's disease** refers to the presence of neurological symptoms caused by biochemical lesions of the central nervous system after exhaustion of B-vitamin reserves, in particular thiamine (vitamin B1).

198. Fasciculations are seen in lesions of:

a. Motor cortex
b. Anterior horn cells
c. Thalamus
d. Cerebellum

The presence of fasciculation suggests damage to anterior horn cells or motor axons (i.e. lower motor neurons).

199. Anterior spinothalamic tract carries:

a. Joint position sense
b. Temperature
c. Crude touch
d. Pain

The anterior spinothalamic tract carries information about crude touch. The lateral spinothalamic tract conveys pain and temperature.

List of ascending tracts of spinal cord.

White column	*Tract*
Anterior white column	1. Anterior spinothalamic tract
Lateral white column	1. Lateral spinothalamic tract 2. Ventral spinocerebellar tract 3. Dorsal spinocerebellar tract 4. Spinotectal tract 5. Fasiculus dorsolateralis 6. Spinoreticular tract 7. Spino-olivary tract 8. Spinovestibular tract
Posterior white column	1. Fasciculus gracilis 2. Fasciculus cuneatus 3. Comma tract of Schulze

200. Intensity of sensory stimulus is directly related to:

a. Frequency of action potential
b. Amplitude of action potential
c. Duration of action potential
d. All of the above

The amplitude of an action potential is independent of the amount of current that produced it. In other words, larger currents do not create larger action potentials. Therefore, action potentials are said to be all-or-none signals, since either they occur fully or they do not occur at all. This is in contrast to receptor potentials, whose amplitudes are dependent on the intensity of a stimulus. In both cases, the frequency of action potentials is correlated with the intensity of a stimulus.

201. Sweat glands of palms are supplied by:

Ans. **194. d.** Ventromedial... **195. b.** Posterior... **196. a.** Amplitude of... **197. a.** Vitamin B_1
198. b. Anterior horn... **199. c.** Crude touch **200. a.** Frequency... **201. d.** Sympathetic...

a. Sympathetic adrenergic
b. Sympathetic non-adrenergic
c. Parasympathetic-cholinergic
d. Sympathetic cholinergic

When **sympathetic** postganglionic neurons innervate **sweat glands** they secrete acetylcholine and hence are termed **sympathetic "cholinergic"** neurons.

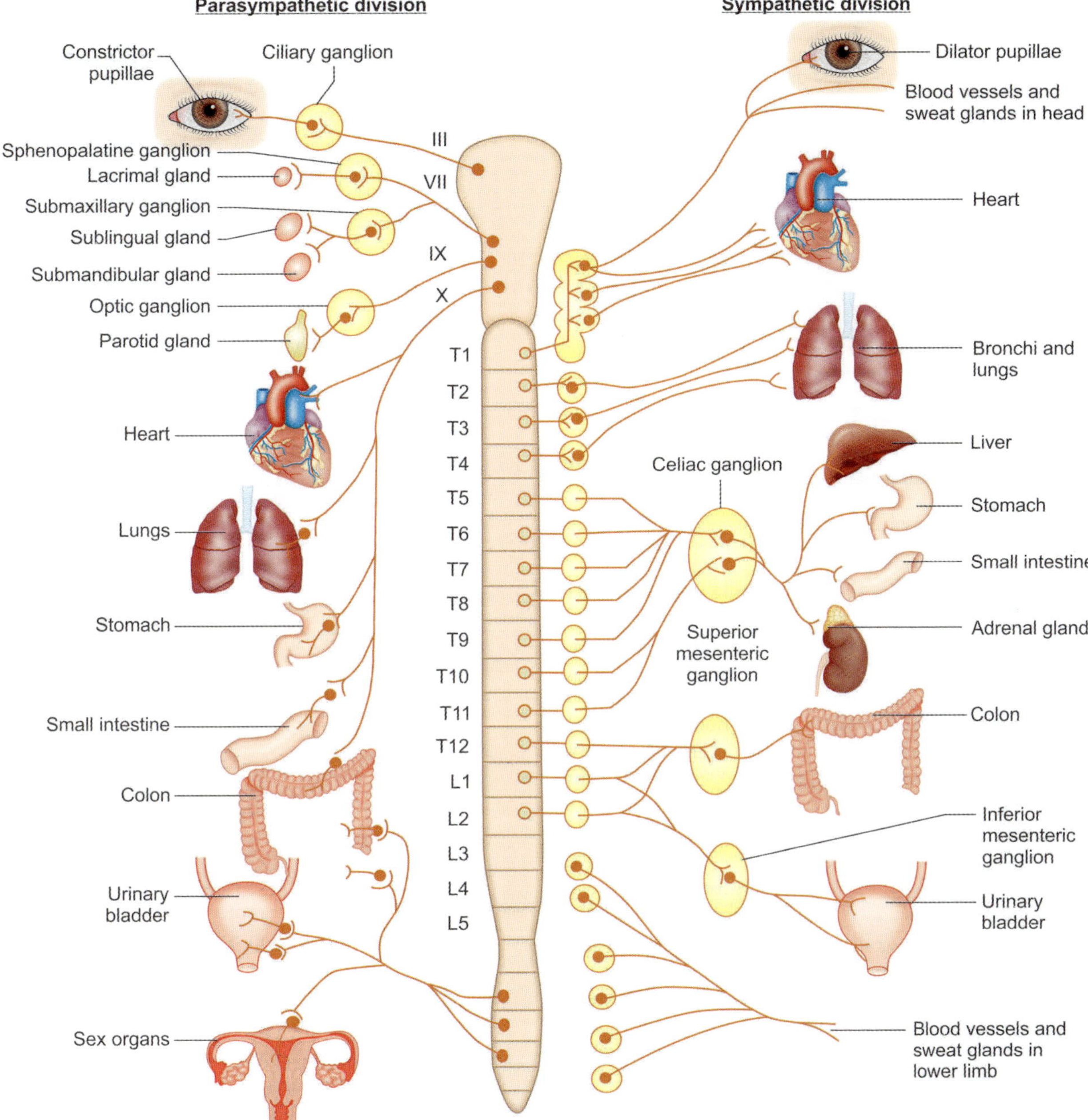

Autonomic nervous system.

202. Thirst centre is located in:
a. Supraoptic nucleus
b. Lateral hypothalamus
c. Dorsomedial nucleus
d. Ventromedial nucleus

The thirst centre is located in the lateral hypothalamus. It receives input from osmoreceptors in the AV3V region and from the subfornical organ and the organum vasculosum of the lamina terminalis (OVLT) which are sites for angiotensin II action. The OVLT is in the AV3V region.

Ans. 202. **b.** Lateral hypothalamus

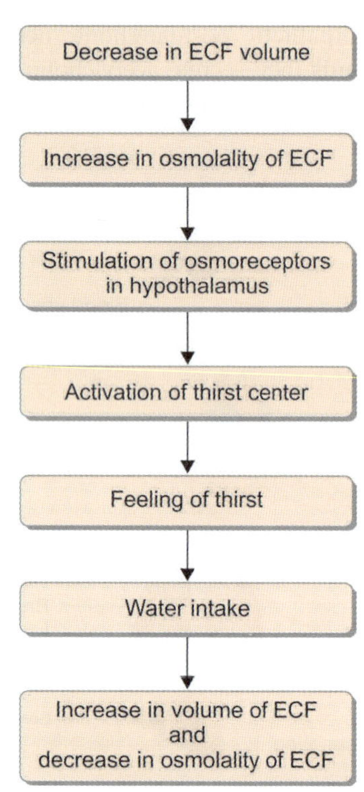

Thirst mechanism. ECF = Extracellular fluid.

203. Receptor for leptin is present in:

a. Thalamus b. Medulla
c. Hypothalamus d. Midbrain

Leptin, the "satiety hormone," is a hormone made by adipose cells that helps to regulate energy balance by inhibiting hunger. Leptin is opposed by the actions of the hormone ghrelin, the "hunger hormone". Both/ hormones act on receptors in the arcuate nucleus of the hypothalamus to regulate appetite to achieve energy homeostasis.

204. Prolactin-inhibiting factor secreted by hypotha-lamus is:

a. Adrenaline b. Noradrenaline
c. Dopamine d. Dobutamine

The arcuate nucleus (cell group A12) and periventricular nucleus (cell group A14) of the hypothalamus is a dopaminergic area. An important projection from these dopaminergic neurons, termed the *tuberoinfundibular pathway*, goes to the pituitary gland, where it influences the secretion of the hormone prolactin. Dopamine is the primary neuroendocrine inhibitor of the secretion of prolactin from the anterior pituitary gland.

Neurotransmitter	*Released by*	*Action*
1. Dopamine	Fibers from substantia nigra to corpus striatum	Inhibition
2. Gamma aminobutyric acid	Intrinsic fibers of corpus striatum and substantia nigra	Inhibition
3. Acetylcholine	Fibers from cerebral cortex to caudate nucleus and putamen	Excitation
4. Substance P	Fibers from globus pallidus reaching substantia nigra	Excitation
5. Enkephalins	Fibers from globus pallidus reaching substantia nigra	Excitation
6. Noradrenaline	Fibers between basal ganglia and reticular formation	Excitation
7. Glutamic acid	Fibers from subthalamic nucleus to globus pallidus and substantia nigra	Excitation

205. Degenerative changes of putamen manifests as:

a. Chorea b. Athetosis
c. Ballism d. All of the above

Chorea is a primary feature of Huntington's disease, a progressive neurological disorder. The most prominent early effects of HD are in a part of the basal ganglia called the neostriatum, which is composed of the caudate nucleus and putamen.

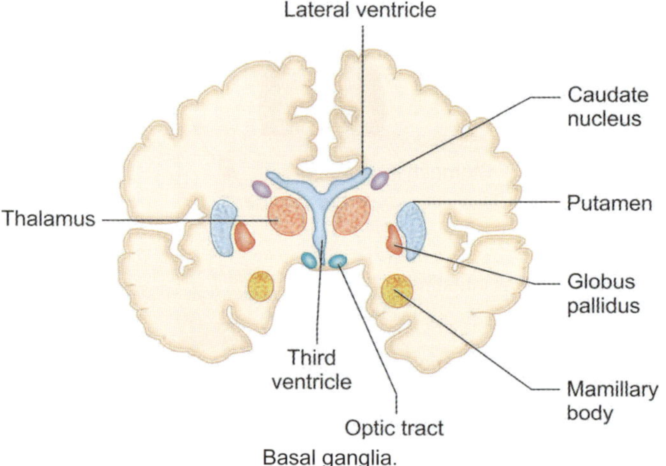

Basal ganglia.

206. NOT a sign of upper motor neuron lesion:

a. Exaggerated tendon reflexes
b. Spastic paralysis
c. Babinski sign
d. Denervated muscular EMG

Electromyography (EMG) is an electrodiagnostic medicine technique for evaluating and recording the electrical activity produced by skeletal muscles. EMG is performed using an instrument called an **electromyograph**, to produce a record called an **electromyogram**. An electromyograph detects the electrical potential generated by muscle cells when these cells are electrically or neurologically activated. The signals can be analyzed to detect medical abnormalities, activation level, or recruitment order or to analyze the biomechanics of human or animal movement.

Ans. 203. c. Hypothalamus 204. c. Dopamine 205. a. Chorea 206. d. Denervated muscular...

Effects of upper motor neuron lesion and lower motor neuron lesion

	Effects	Upper motor neuron lesion	Lower motor neuron lesion
Clinical observation	Muscle tone	Hypertonia	Hypotonia
	Paralysis	Spastic type of paralysis	Flaccid type of paralysis
	Wastage of muscle	Wastage of muscle occurs	Wastage of muscle occurs
	Superficial reflexes	Lost	Lost
	Plantar reflex	Abnormal plantar reflex – Babinski sign	Absent
	Deep reflexes	Exaggerated	Lost
	Clonus	Present	Absent
Clinical confir-mation	Electrical activity	Normal	Absent
	Muscles affected	Groups of muscles are affected	Individual muscles are affected
	10. Fascicular twitch in EMG	Absent	Present

207. Intention tremors are seen in lesion of:

a. Basal ganglia
b. Temporal lobe
c. Frontal lobe
d. Cerebellum

Intention tremor, also known as **cerebellar tremor**, is a dyskinetic disorder characterized by a broad, coarse, and low frequency (below 5 Hz) tremor. The amplitude of an intention tremor increases as an extremity approaches the endpoint of deliberate and visually guided movement (hence the name intention tremor).

208. Neurotransmitter present in nigro-striatal pathway is:

a. Acetylcholine
b. Dopamine
c. Epinephrine
d. GABA

The nigrostriatal pathway, or the nigrostriatal bundle (NSB), is a dopaminergic pathway that connects the substantia nigra with the striatum. It is one of the four major dopamine pathways in the brain, and is particularly involved in the production of movement, as part of a system called the basal ganglia motor loop.

209. Neural tube defect is due to deficiency of:

a. Vitamin B_{12}
b. Thiamine
c. Folic acid
d. Riboflavin

Folate (vitamin B_9) and vitamin B_{12} are very important in reducing the occurrences of NTDs.

210. In adults, non shivering thermogenesis is due to:

a. Thyroid hormones
b. Yellow fat
c. Noradrenaline
d. Muscle metabolism

Nonshivering thermogenesis was originally defined as a cold-induced increase in heat production not associated with the muscle activity of shivering. Recent research shows it to be a metabolic process located primarily in brown adipose tissue and controlled by the activity of the sympathetic nervous supply of this tissue.

211. Pain is carried by:

a. A-delta nerve fibres
b. A-gamma nerve fibres
c. A-beta nerve fibres
d. A-alpha nerve fibres

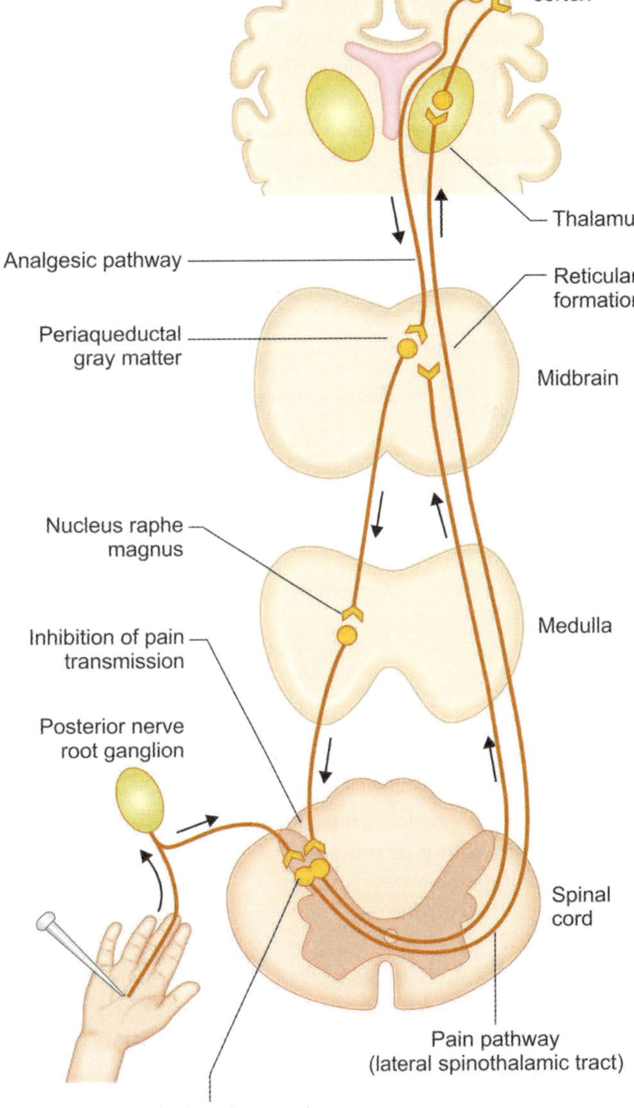

Pain pathway and analgesic pathway.

Ans. 207. **d.** Cerebellum 208. **b.** Dopamine 209. **c.** Folic acid 210. **c.** Noradrenaline 211. **a.** A-delta nerve fibres

Nociceptors have two different types of axons. The first are the Aδ fiber axons. They are myelinated and can allow an action potential to travel at a rate of about 20 meters/second toward the CNS. The other type is the more slowly conducting C fiber axons. These only conduct at speeds of around 2 meters/second. This is due to the light or nonmyelination of the axon. As a result, pain comes in two phases.

212. MC type of synapse is:

a. Axoaxonal
b. Axodendritic
c. Axosomatic
d. Dendrodendritic

Synapses can be classified by the type of cellular structures serving as the pre- and post-synaptic components. The vast majority of synapses in the mammalian nervous system are classical axodendritic synapses (axon synapsing upon a dendrite), however a variety of other arrangements exist. These include but are not limited to axo-axonic, dendrodendritic, axosecretory, somato-dendritic, dendrosomatic, and somatosomatic synapses.

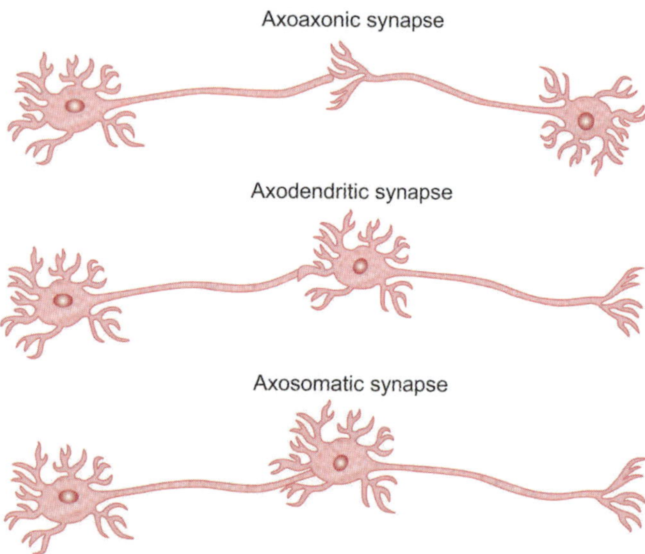

Anatomical synapses.

213. Synaptic potential can be recorded by:

a. Patch clamp technique
b. Voltage clamp technique
c. Microelectrode
d. EEG

There are two types of electrical signals that **can be recorded by** microelectrodes: fast, large action potentials, and slow, small **synaptic potentials**.

214. The intrafusal fibres of the striated skeletal muscles are innervated by one of the following type of motor neurons. Choose the correct answer:

a. Alpha
b. Gamma
c. Beta
d. Delta

The motor component of muscle spindle is provided by up to a dozen gamma motoneurons and to a lesser extent by one or two beta motoneurons. Gamma and beta motoneurons are called fusimotor neurons, because they activate the intrafusal muscle fibers. Gamma motoneurons innervate only intrafusal muscle fibers, whereas beta motoneurons innervate both extrafusal and intrafusal muscle fibers and so are referred to as skeletofusimotor neurons.

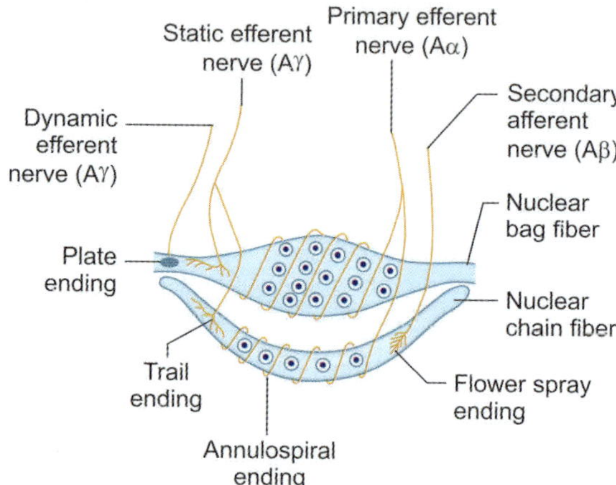

Nerve supply to muscle spindle. Red = Afferent (sensory) nerve fibers, Blue = Efferent (motor) nerve fibers. Letters in parenthesis indicate the type of nerve fibers.

215. Golgi tendon organ detects:

a. Static muscle length
b. Muscle tension
c. Muscle action
d. Dynamic muscle length

The **Golgi organ** (also called **Golgi tendon organ**, GTO, tendon organ, neurotendinous organ or neurotendinous spindle) senses changes in muscle tension. It is a proprioceptive sensory receptor organ that is at the origins and insertion of skeletal muscle fibers into the tendons of skeletal muscle. It provides the sensory component of the Golgi tendon reflex.

216. Change observed during repolarization:

a. Increased permeability to sodium
b. Increased permeability to potassium
c. Increased permeability to calcium
d. Increased permeability to magnesium

Repolarization refers to the change in membrane potential that returns it to a negative value just after the depolarization phase of an action potential has changed the membrane potential to a positive value. The repolarization phase usually returns the membrane potential back to the resting membrane potential. The efflux of K^+ ions

Ans. 212. **b.** Axodendritic 213. **c.** Microelectrode 214. **b.** Gamma 215. **b.** Muscle tension
216. **b.** Increased permeability to potassium

results in the falling phase of an action potential. The ions pass through the selectivity filter of the K^+ channel pore. There are several K^+ channels that contribute to repolarization, including A-type channels, delayed rectifiers, and Ca^{2+}-activated K^+ channels

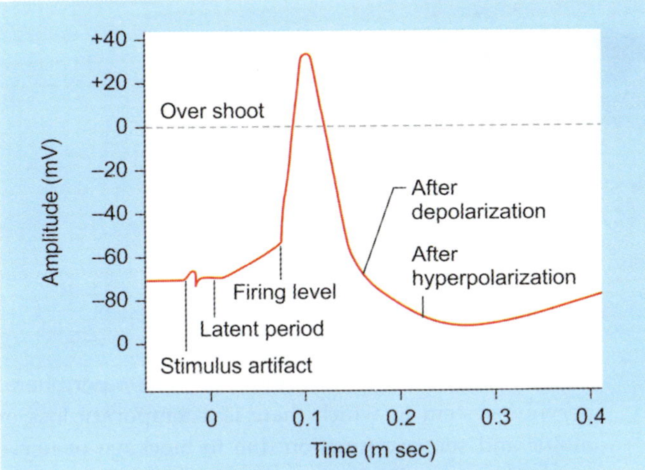

Action potential in nerve fiber.

217. Nerve fibres most susceptible to local anaesthetic:

a. A
b. B
c. C
d. All of the above are equally sensitive

All nerve fibers are sensitive to local anesthetics, but due to a combination of diameter and myelination, fibers have different sensitivities to local anesthetic blockade, termed "Differential Blockade." Type C fibers are the most sensitive followed by Type B, Type A delta (temperature), Type A gamma (proprioception), Type A beta (sensory touch and pressure) and Type A alpha (motor).

218. Inverse stretch reflex is due to:

a. Muscle spindle
b. Tail fibre ending
c. Golgi tendon
d. Trail fibre ending

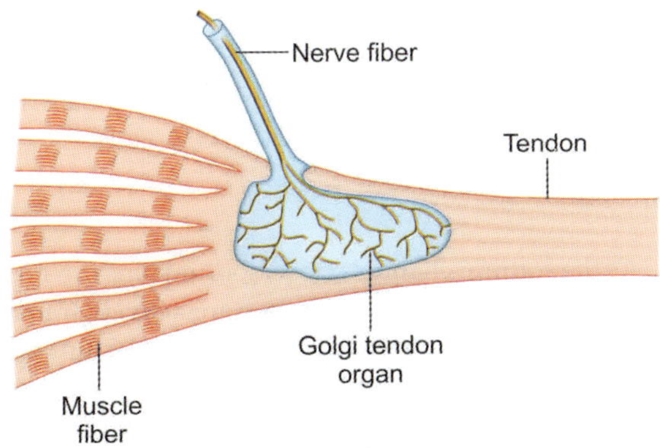

Golgi tendon apparatus.

In a Golgi tendon reflex, skeletal muscle contraction causes the agonist muscle to simultaneously lengthen and relax. This reflex is also called the **inverse myotatic reflex**, because it is the inverse of the stretch reflex. Though muscle tension is increasing during the contraction, alpha motor neurons in the spinal cord supplying the muscle are inhibited. However, antagonistic muscles are activated.

219. Sensory fibre with LEAST conduction velocity:

a. Gamma fibre
b. Beta fibre
c. Alpha fibre
d. C-fibre

C-fibres has a conduction velocity of 0.5-2 m/s

Types of nerve fibers		
Type	*Diameter (μ)*	*Velocity of conduction (meter/second)*
A alpha	12 to 24	70 to 120
A beta	6 to 12	30 to 70
A gamma	5 to 6	15 to 30
A delta	2 to 5	12 to 15
B	1 to 2	3 to 10
C	< 1.5	0.5 to 2

220. Resting membrane potential is due to:

a. Sodium ion
b. Chloride ion
c. Potassium ion
d. Calcium ion

The typical resting membrane potential of a cell arises from the separation of potassium ions from intracellular, relatively immobile anions across the membrane of the cell. Because the membrane permeability for potassium is much higher than that for other ions (disregarding voltage-gated channels at this stage), and because of the strong chemical gradient for potassium, potassium ions flow from the cytosol into the extracellular space carrying out positive charge, until their movement is balanced by build-up of negative charge on the inner surface of the membrane. Again, because of the high relative permeability for potassium, the resulting membrane potential is almost always close to the potassium reversal potential.

Ans. **217. c.** C **218. c.** Golgi tendon **219. d.** C-fibre **220. c.** Potassium ion

Ionic basis of the resting membrane potential

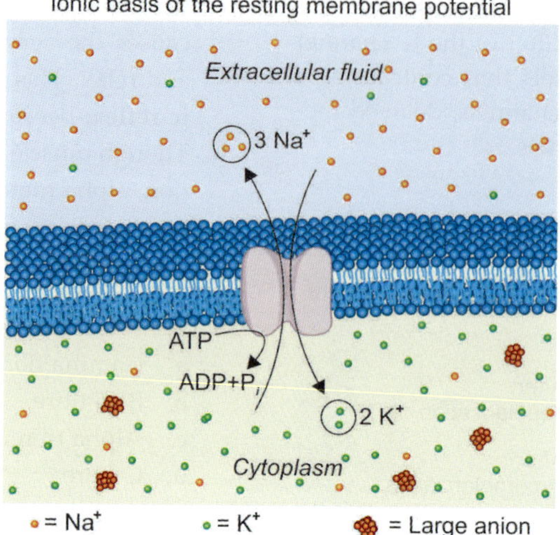

221. Magnitude of action potential depends on:

a. Sodium ion b. Chloride ion
c. Potassium ion d. Calcium ion

Increasing the concentration of extracellular sodium (Na_o) increases the sodium current during the action potential which increases the rate of depolarization of the action potential and increases the magnitude of the action potential.

222. Neuronal degeneration is NOT seen in:

a. Crush nerve injury b. Fetal development
c. Senescence d. Neurapraxia

Neurapraxia is a disorder of the peripheral nervous system in which there is a temporary loss of motor and sensory function due to blockage of nerve conduction, usually lasting an average of six to eight weeks before full recovery.

223. Synaptic conduction is mostly orthodromic because:

a. Dendrites cannot be depolarized
b. Once repolarized, an area cannot be depolarized
c. The strength of antidromic impulse is less
d. Chemical mediator is localized only in the presynaptic terminal

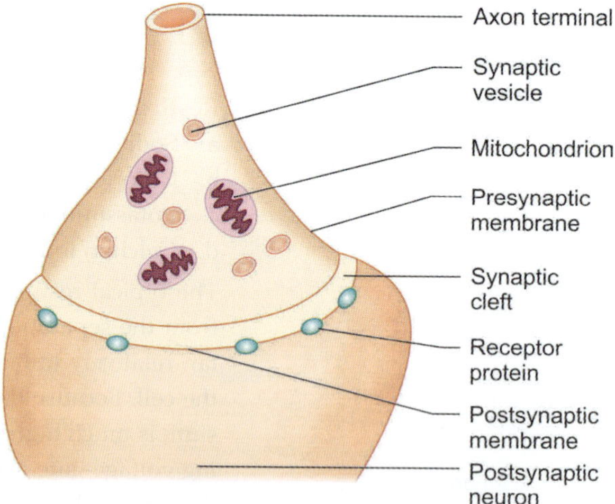

Structure of chemical synapse.

Synaptic vesicles (or **neurotransmitter vesicles**) in presynaptic terminal store various neurotransmitters that are released at the synapse.

224. Repolarization of a nerve fibre is due to:

a. Sodium ions b. Potassium ions
c. Chloride ions d. Calcium ions

As the sodium channels close, sodium ions can no longer enter the neuron, and then they are actively transported back out of the plasma membrane. Potassium channels are then activated, and there is an outward current of potassium ions, returning the electrochemical gradient to the resting state (repolarization).

Ans. **221. a.** Sodium ion **222. d.** Neurapraxia **223. d.** Chemical mediator... **224. b.** Potassium ions

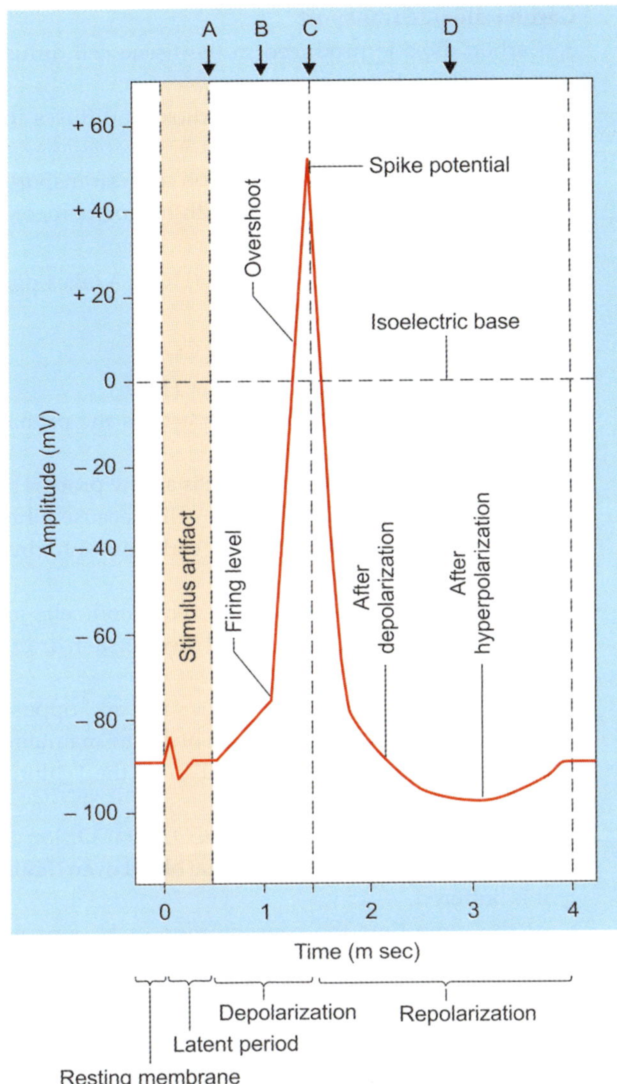

Action potential in a skeletal muscle

A = Opening of few Na^+ channels

B = Opening of many Na^+ channels

C = Closure of Na^+ channels and opening of K^+ channels

D = Closure of K^+ channels

225. All or none law is related to:

a. Membrane potential b. Resting potential
c. Action potential d. Rheobase and chronaxie

The magnitude of the action potential set up in any single nerve fiber is independent of the strength of the exciting stimulus, provided the latter is adequate. An electrical stimulus below threshold strength fails to elicit a propagated spike potential. If it is of threshold strength or over, a spike (a nervous impulse) of maximum magnitude is set up. Either the single fiber does not respond with spike production, or it responds to the utmost of its ability under the conditions at the moment. This property of the single nerve fiber is termed the all-or-none relationship.

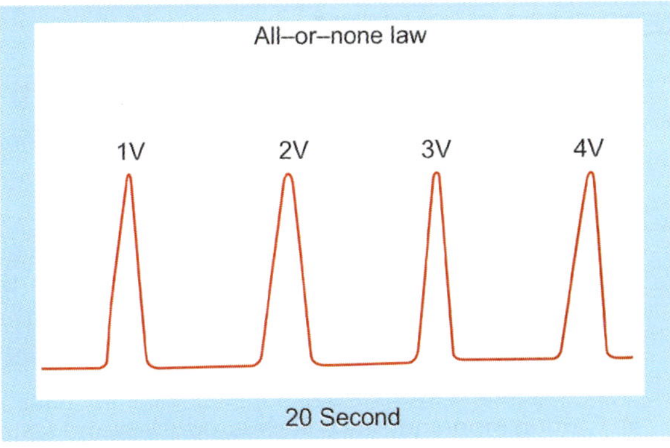

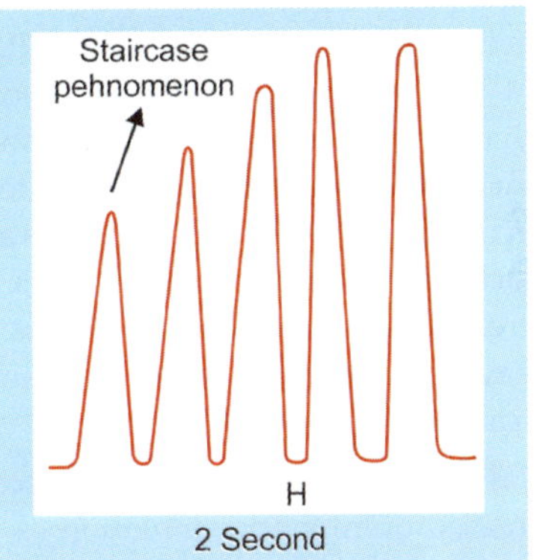

All-or-none law and staircase phenomenon in cardiac muscle

226. How to assess the function of nerve after injury:

a. Nervography
b. Open dissection
c. Nerve conduction study
d. Muscle biopsy

Nerve conduction studies along with needle electromyography measure nerve and muscle function, and may be indicated when there is pain in the limbs, weakness from spinal nerve compression, or con cern about some other neurologic injury or disorder.

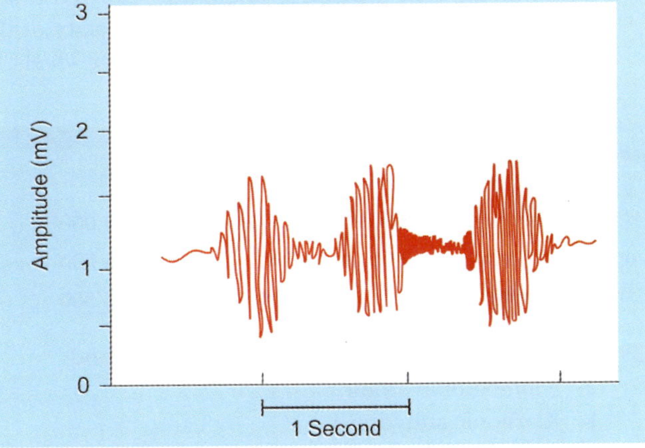

Electromyogram during alternate contraction and relaxation of biceps muscle.

Ans. 225. c. Action potential **226. c.** Nerve conduction study

RESPIRATORY SYSTEM

227. Which of the following gas has high affinity for haemoglobin?

a. Oxygen
b. Nitrogen
c. Carbon dioxide
d. Carbon monoxide

Affinity of gases to hemoglobin

- Hemoglobin binding affinity for CO is 250 times greater than its affinity for oxygen, meaning that small amounts of CO dramatically reduce hemoglobin's ability to transport oxygen.
- Carbon monoxide is a colorless, odorless and tasteless gas, and poses a potentially fatal threat.
- When hemoglobin combines with CO, it forms a very bright red compound called carboxyhemoglobin, which may cause the skin of CO poisoning victims to appear pink in death, instead of white or blue.
- When inspired air contains CO levels as low as 0.02%, headache and nausea occur; if the CO concentration is increased to 0.1%, unconsciousness will follow.
- In heavy smokers, up to 20% of the oxygen-active sites can be blocked by CO.

228. At high altitudes, acclimatization is because of:

a. Decreased pulmonary ventilation
b. Reduced ability of tissues to utilize oxygen
c. Increased RBC/Hemoglobin
d. Reduced diffusing capacity of lungs

Hypoxia is the principal stimulus for causing an increase in red blood cell production.

Acclimatization to high altitude

- It continues for months or even years after initial ascent, and ultimately enables humans to survive in an environment that, without acclimatization, would kill them.
- Humans who migrate permanently to a higher altitude naturally acclimatize to their new environment by developing an increase in the number of red blood cells to increase the oxygen carrying capacity of the blood, in order to compensate for lower levels of oxygen in the air.

Different altitudes		
Altitude	*Feet*	*Meter*
High altitude	8,000 to 13,000	2,500 to 4,000
Very high altitude	13,000 to 18,000	4,000 to 5,500
Extreme altitude	> 18,000	> 5,500

229. Mainly responsible for CO_2 transport in blood:

a. Hemoglobin affinity
b. Carbonic anhydrase
c. Attachment to proteins
d. None of the above

Carbon dioxide transport

- Carbon dioxide produced in the tissue cell diffuses into the blood plasma.
- The largest fraction of carbon dioxide diffuses into the red blood cells.
- The carbon dioxide in the red blood cells is transported as: dissolved CO_2, combined with hemoglobin, or as bicarbonate (largest fraction).

The formation of bicarbonate ions (HCO_3^-) takes place by the following reactions:

Hydration of CO_2: $CO_2 + HOH = H_2CO_3$

Dissociation of H_2CO_3: $H_2CO_3 = H^+ + HCO_3^-$

- The H_2CO_3/HCO_3^- combination acts as the primary buffer of the blood.
- The hydration of carbon dioxide is a slow process but occurs rapidly in the red blood cells because a high concentration of the enzyme carbonic anhydrase catalyzes the reaction.
- Bicarbonate diffuses out of the red blood cells into the plasma in venous blood and vise versa in arterial blood.
- Chloride ion always diffuses in an opposite direction of bicarbonate ion in order to maintain a charge balance. This is referred to as the "chloride shift".
- The changes in concentration of CO_2 or HCO_3^- ion can influence slight pH changes in the blood even though it is buffered.
- At the same time the concentration of H^+ ions will influence the concentrations of CO_2 and HCO_3^- ions.

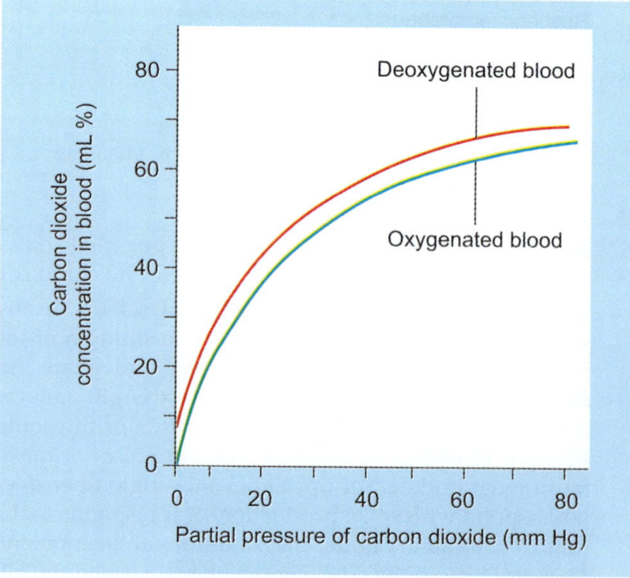

Carbon dioxide dissociation curve.

Ans. **227. d.** Carbon... **228. c.** Increased RBC... **229. b.** Carbonic anhydrase

230. **In bronchial muscles, sympathetic system acts on which receptors?**
a. Alpha1 adrenergic
b. Beta1 adrenergic
c. Beta2 adrenergic
d. Alpha2 adrenergic

Beta2 receptor location
- Smooth muscle relaxation, e.g. in bronchi, GI tract (decreased motility).
- Lipolysis in adipose tissue
- Anabolsim in skeletal muscle
- Relax non-pregnant uterus
- Relax detrusor urinae muscle of bladder wall
- Dilate arteries to skeletal muscle
- Glycogenolysis and gluconeogenesis
- Stimulates insulin secretion
- Contract sphincters of GI tract
- Thickened secretions from salivary glands
- Inhibit histamine-release from mast cells
- Increase renin secretion from kidney
- Relaxation of Bronchioles (salbutamol, a beta2 agonist relieves bronchiole constriction)
- Involved in brain - immune communication

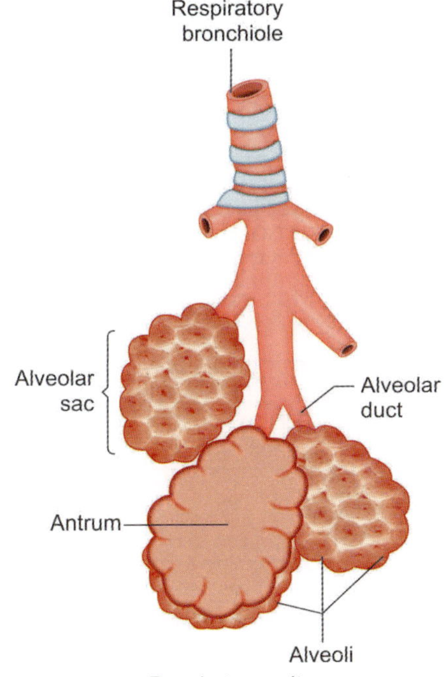

Respiratory unit.

231. **Cyanosis with normal arterial oxygen content is NEVER seen in:**
a. Hypoxic hypoxia
b. Histotoxic hypoxia
c. Stagnant hypoxia
d. Anemia hypoxia

A person with anemia almost never becomes cyanotic as there is not enough hemoglobin for 5 grams to be deoxygenated in 100 milliliters of arterial blood.

Characteristic features of different types of hypoxia

Features	Hypoxic hypoxia	Anemic hypoxia	Stagnant hypoxia	Histotoxic hypoxia
1. pO_2 in arterial blood	Reduced	Normal	Normal	Normal
2. Oxygen carrying capacity of blood	Normal	Reduced	Normal	Normal
3. Velocity of blood flow	Normal	Normal	Reduced	Normal
4. Utilization of oxygen by tissues	Normal	Normal	Normal	Reduced
5. Efficacy of oxygen therapy	100%	75%	< 50%	Not useful

232. **FALSE for type-II penumocytes:**
a. Appear at 5th month intrauterine life
b. Forms blood-air barrier
c. Mesodermal
d. Secrete surfactant

Type II pneumocytes cover a minority of the alveolar surface. Their function is to secrete surfactant, which decreases surface tension within the alveoli.

233. **Tidal volume is:**
a. Inspiratory capacity minus the inspiratory reserve volume
b. Total lung capacity minus the reserve volume
c. Functional residual capacity minus residual volume
d. Vital capacity minus expiratory reserve volumes

Lung volumes
- **Tidal volume/TV** is the lung volume representing the normal volume of air displaced between normal inhalation and exhalation when extra effort is not applied. In a healthy, young human adult, tidal volume is approximately 500 mL per inspiration or 7 mL/kg of body mass.
- Inspiratory reserve volume/IRV: The maximal volume that can be inhaled from the end-inspiratory level
- Inspiratory capacity: IRV + TV

MCQs with Short Explanations

Ans. 230. **c.** Beta2 adrenergic 231. **d.** Anemia hypoxia 232. **b.** Forms blood... 233. **a.** Inspiratory capacity...

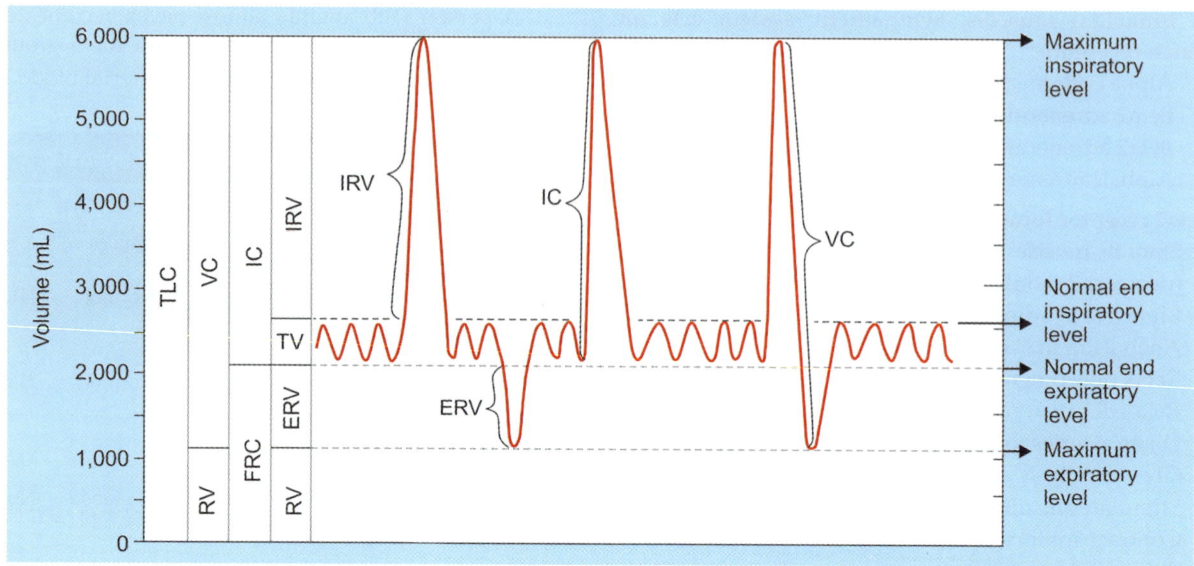

Spirogram. TV = Tidal volume, IRV = Inspiratory reserve volume, ERV = Expiratory reserve volume, RV = Residual volume, IC = Inspiratory capacity, FRC = Functional residual capacity, VC = Vital capacity, TLC = Total lung capacity.

234. Most important stimulator of respiratory centre/RC:

a. Decreased pH b. Hypocapnia
c. Hypercapnia d. Decreased PaO_2

In healthy individuals the presence of elevated carbon dioxide levels in the blood is the stimulant that the RC responds to in order to signal the respiratory muscles to breathe. Chemoreceptors found in carotid bodies and aortic bodies are responsible for detecting decrease in blood pH by this carbon dioxide.

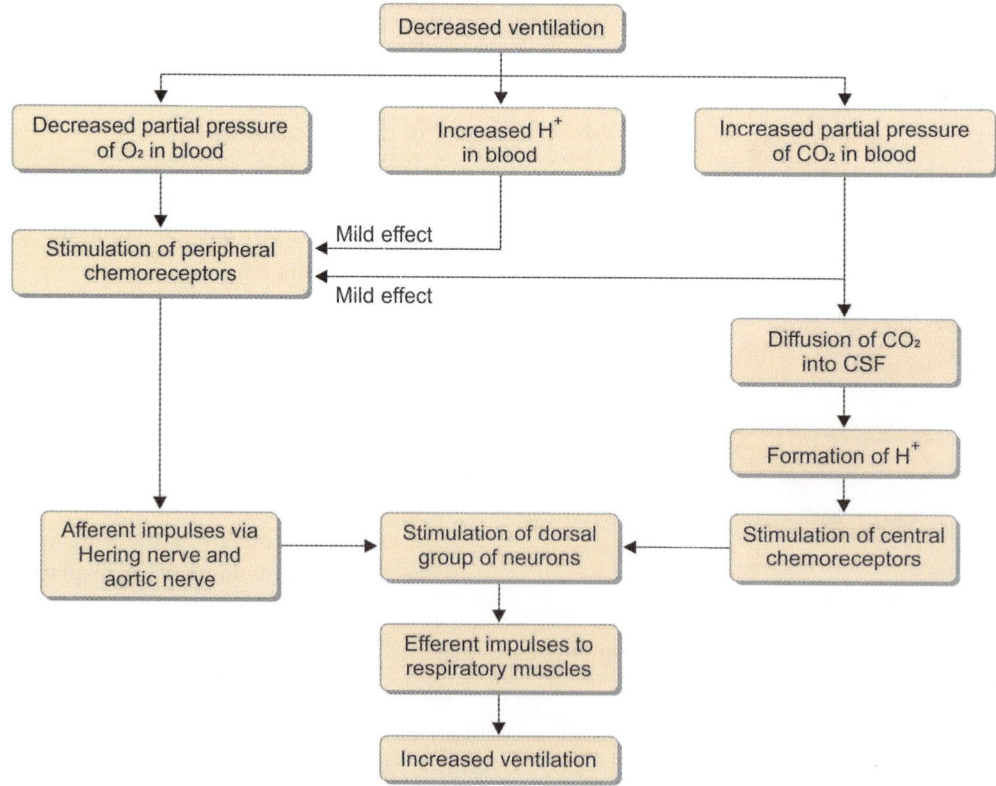

Chemical regulation of respiration. CSF = Cerebrospinal fluid.

Ans. **234.** **c.** Hypercapnia

235. Increase in which of the following will shift the oxygen dissociation curve to left:
a. Temperature
b. Partial pressure of carbon dioxide
c. 2, 3 DPG concentration
d. Oxygen affinity for hemoglobin

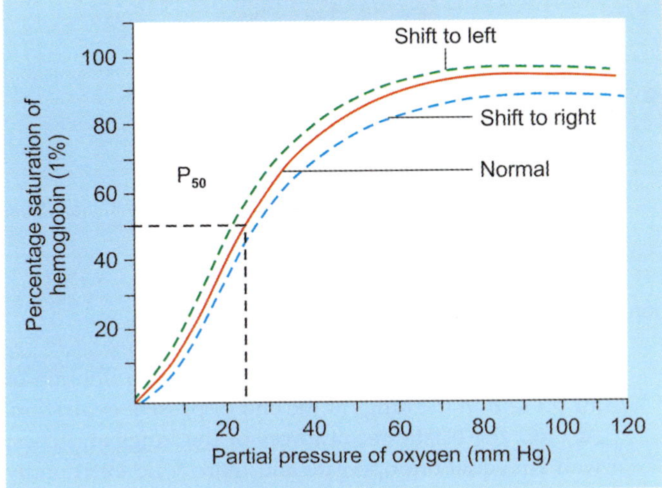

Oxygen-hemoglobin dissociation curve.

The P_{50} is a conventional measure of hemoglobin affinity for oxygen. An increased P_{50} indicates a rightward shift of the standard curve, which means that a larger partial pressure is necessary to maintain a 50% oxygen saturation. This indicates a decreased affinity. Conversely, a lower P_{50} indicates a leftward shift and a higher affinity.

236. Ratio of physiological to anatomical dead space, in a normal adult, is:
a. 1:1
b. 2:1
c. 1:2
d. 2:2

Alveolar dead space is negligible in healthy individuals, but can increase dramatically in some lung diseases due to ventilation-perfusion mismatch. So in normal individuals, physiological dead space equals anatomical dead space.

237. Tidal volume at rest, in a normal man at rest:
a. 0.5 L
b. 1.2 L
c. 3.3 L
d. 4.8 L

Tidal volume is the lung volume representing the normal volume of air displaced between normal inhalation and exhalation when extra effort is not applied. In a healthy, young human adult, tidal volume is approximately 500 mL per inspiration or 7 mL/kg of body mass.

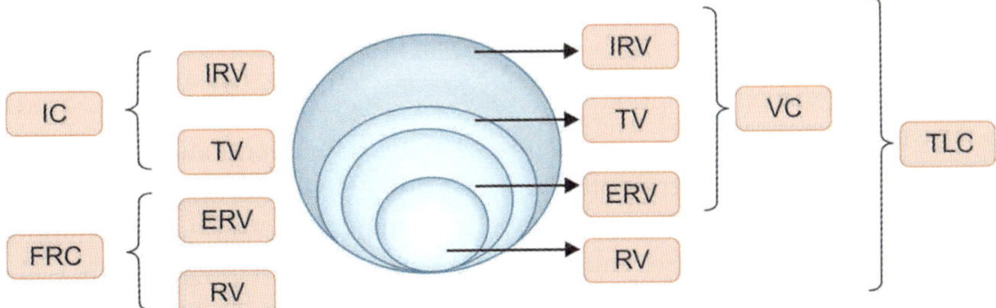

Lung volumes and capacities. TV = Tidal volume, IRV = Inspiratory reserve volume, ERV = Expiratory reserve volume, RV = Residual volume, IC = Inspiratory capacity, FRC = Functional residual capacity, VC = Vital capacity, TLC = Total lung capacity.

238. Oxygen dissociation curve shifts to right in:
a. Anemia
b. Metabolic alkalosis
c. Hypokalemia
d. Hyperkalemia

The causes of shift to right can be remembered using the mnemonic, "**CADET**, face Right!" for **C**O_2, **A**cid/**A**nemia, 2,3-**D**PG, **E**xercise and **T**emperature.

239. Carbon-dioxide is transported in plasma as:
a. Dissolved form
b. Carbamino compounds
c. Bicarbonate
d. All of the above

CO_2 transport

- Most of it (about 70% to 80%) is converted to bicarbonate ions/HCO_3^- by the enzyme carbonic anhydrase in the red blood cells, by the reaction $CO_2 + H_2O \rightarrow H_2CO_3 \rightarrow H^+ + HCO_3^-$.
- 5% – 10% is dissolved in the plasma
- 5% – 10% is bound to hemoglobin as carbamino compounds

Ans. **235. d.** Oxygen affinity for hemoglobin
236. a. 1: 1
237. a. 0.5 L
238. a. Anemia
239. d. All of the above

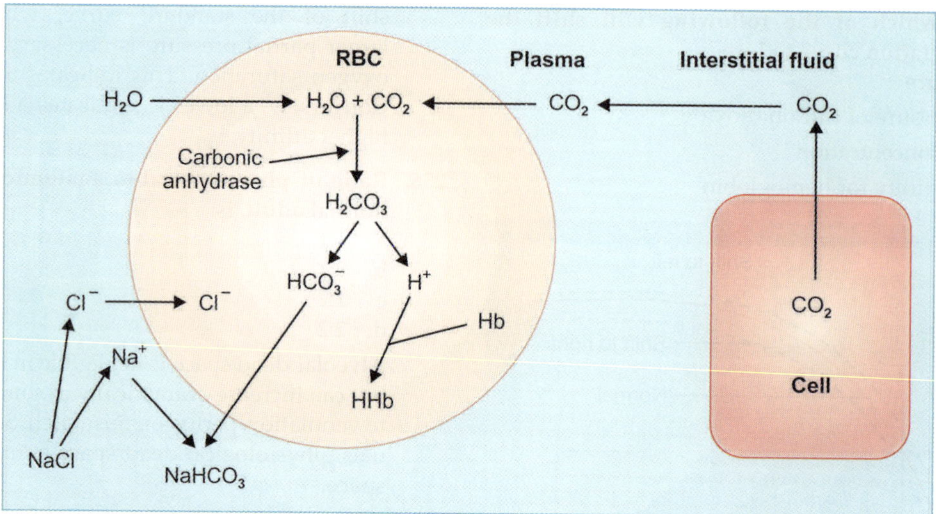

Transport of carbon dioxide in blood in the form of bicarbonate and chloride shift.

240. Surfactant is produced by:

a. Type II pneumocytes b. Type I pneumocytes
c. Macrophages d. Endothelial cells

Type II cells are responsible for the production and secretion of surfactant (the majority of which are dipalmitoylphosphatidylcholine), a group of phospholipids that reduce the alveolar surface tension.

241. Which does NOT increase oxygen supply to muscles during exercise:

a. Oxygen dissociation curve shift to left
b. Increased stroke volume
c. Increased extraction of oxygen from the blood
d. Increased blood flow to muscles

Factors that move the oxygen dissociation curve to the right are those physiological states where tissues need more oxygen. For example during exercise, muscles have a higher metabolic rate, and consequently need more oxygen, produce more carbon dioxide and lactic acid, and their temperature rises.

242. Spirometry can measure all of the following except:

a. Vital capacity b. FEV
c. Tidal volume d. None of the above

The spirometer cannot be used in a direct way to measure the functional residual capacity because the air in the residual volume of the lungs cannot be expired into the spirometer, and this volume constitutes about one half of the functional residual capacity.

243. FRC is combination of:

a. Residual volume and expiratory reserve volume
b. Inspiratory reserve volume and tidal volume
c. Tidal volume and expiratory reserve volume
d. Tidal volume and residual volume

Functional Residual Capacity (**FRC**) is the volume of air present in the lungs at the end of passive expiration. At FRC, the elastic recoil forces of the lungs and chest wall are equal but opposite and there is no exertion by the diaphragm or other respiratory muscles.

FRC is the sum of Expiratory Reserve Volume (ERV) and Residual Volume (RV) and measures approximately 2400 mL in an 80 kg, average-sized male. It can not be estimated through spirometry, since it includes the residual volume.

244. Oxygen therapy is of no use in:

a. Anemic hypoxia
b. Hypoxic hypoxia
c. Hypoventilation hypoxia
d. Histotoxic hypoxia

In the different types of hypoxia caused by inade-quate tissue use of oxygen, there is abnormality neither of oxygen pickup by the lungs nor of transport to the tissues. Instead the tissue metabolic enzyme system is simply incapable of using the oxygen that is delivered. Therefore, oxygen therapy is of hardly any measurable benefit.

245. FALSE regarding type II pneumocytes:

a. Mesodermal in origin
b. Appears at 5th month of intrauterine life
c. Secretes surfactant
d. Forms air-blood barrier

Type I pneumocyte cells (also called **type I alveolar cells** or **squamous alveolar cells**) are extremely attenuated cells that line the alveolar surfaces of the lungs. They cover 97% of the alveolar surface, with type II pneumocytes covering the remainder. These cells are so thin (sometimes only 25 nm) that the electron microscope was needed to prove that all alveoli are covered with an epithelial lining. It is important that

Ans. **240. a.** Type II pneum... **241. a.** Oxygen... **242. d.** None of the above **243. a.** Residual... **244. d.** Histotoxic... **245. d.** Forms air...

these cells are thin so that gas exchange between the alveoli and blood can occur easily. Their main role is to provide a barrier of minimal thickness that is readily permeable to gases such as oxygen and carbon dioxide.

246. True regarding high altitude:

a. Reduced RBC count
b. Percentage of oxygen is less in air
c. pCO_2 is more
d. pO_2 is less

Hypoxic hypoxia is a result of insufficient oxygen available to the lungs. A blocked airway, a drowning or a reduction in partial pressure (high altitude above 10,000 feet) are examples of how lungs can be deprived of oxygen.

Barometric pressure, partial pressure of oxygen and common effects at different altitudes

Altitude (feet)	*Barometric pressure (mm Hg)*	*Partial pressure of oxygen (mm Hg)*	*Common effects*
Sea level	760	159	–
5,000	600	132	No hypoxia
10,000	523	110	Mild symptoms of hypoxia start appearing
15,000	400	90	Moderate hypoxia develops with following symptoms: Reduction in visual acuity Effects on mental functions: – Improper judgment and – Feeling of over confidence
20,000	349	73	Severe hypoxia appears with cardiorespiratory symptoms such as: Increase in heart rate and cardiac output Increase in respiratory rate and respiratory minute volume This is the highest level for permanent inhabitants
25,000	250	62	This is the critical altitude for survival Hypoxia becomes severe Breathing oxygen becomes essential
29,628	235	49	This is the height of Mount Everest
30,000	226	47	Symptoms become severe even with oxygen
50,000	87	18	Hypoxia becomes more severe even with pure oxygen

247. Most important stimulus for respiratory centre:

a. Reduced pH
b. Hypocapnia
c. Hypercapnia
d. Reduced PaO_2

Hypercapnia normally triggers a reflex which increases breathing and access to oxygen, such as arousal and turning the head during sleep. A failure of this reflex can be fatal, for example as a contributory factor in sudden infant death syndrome.

248. FALSE for Hering-Breuer inflation reflex:

a. Protects against under-inflation of lungs
b. Involves inhibition of inspiratory centre
c. Involve pulmonary stretch receptors
d. A protective reflex

The **Hering–Breuer inflation reflex**, named for Josef Breuer and Ewald Hering, is a reflex triggered to prevent over-inflation of the lung. Pulmonary stretch receptors present in the smooth muscle of the airways respond to excessive stretching of the lung during large inspirations. Once activated, they send action potentials through large myelinated fibers of the vagus nerve to the inspiratory area in the medulla and pneumotaxic center of the pons. In response, the inspiratory area is inhibited directly and the apneustic center is inhibited from activating the inspiratory area. This inhibits inspiration, allowing expiration to occur.

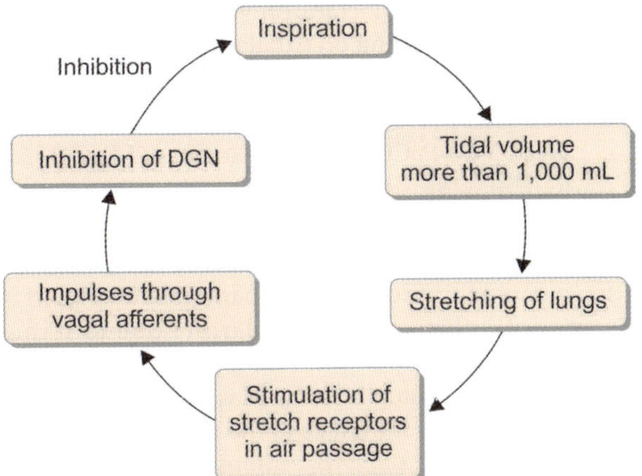

Hering-Breuer inflation reflex. DGN = Dorsal respiratory group of neurons. Dashed red arrow indicates inhibition.

Ans. **246. d.** pO_2 is less **247. c.** Hypercapnia **248. a.** Protects against under-inflation of lungs

249. In which of the following, a reduction in arterial oxygen tension occurs:

a. Anemia b. CO poisoning
c. Moderate exercise d. Hypoventilation

- Hypoventilation (low alveolar ventilation)
- P(A-a) O_2 is normal
- $PaCO_2$ is elevated (hypercapnia)
- Increasing the fraction of inspired oxygen (FIO_2) can alleviate the hypoxemia and the hypercapnia can be corrected by mechanically ventilating the patient to eliminate CO_2

250. NOT seen during acclimatization to high altitudes:

a. Increase in minute ventilation
b. Increase in sensitivity of central chemoreceptors
c. Increase in sensitivity of the carotid body to hypoxia
d. Shift in the oxygen dissociation curve to the left

Factors that move the oxygen dissociation curve to the right are those physiological states where tissues need more oxygen. For example during exercise, muscles have a higher metabolic rate, and consequently need more oxygen, produce more carbon dioxide and lactic acid, and their temperature rises. Increase in 2,3 DPG is also associated with right shift. Conditions of low tissue oxygen concentration such as high altitude (2,3-BPG levels are higher in those acclimated to high altitudes), airway obstruction, or congestive heart failure will tend to cause RBCs to generate more 2,3-BPG in their effort to generate energy by allowing more oxygen to be released in tissues deprived of oxygen.

251. True for surfactant:

a. Produced in the basement membrane of lungs
b. Of little value in adults
c. Prevents collapse of alveoli
d. All of the above

The surfactant is packaged by the cell in structures called lamellar bodies, and extruded into the air-spaces. The lamellar bodies then unfold into a complex lining of the air-space. This layer reduces the surface tension of the fluid that lines the alveolar air-space. By reducing surface tension, surfactant prevents the air-spaces from completely collapsing on exhalation.

252. Does NOT shift the oxygen dissociation curve to right:

a. Reduced pH b. Increased 2,3-DPG
c. Decreased $PaCO_2$ d. Increased $PaCO_2$

Carbon dioxide affects the curve in two ways: First, CO_2 accumulation causes carbamino compounds to be generated through chemical interactions, which bind to hemoglobin forming carbaminohemoglobin and, second it influences intracellular pH due to formation of bicarbonate ion. The formation of a bicarbonate ion will release a proton into the plasma, increasing acidity which also shifts the curve to the right.

253. HbF shifts the oxygen dissociation curve to:

a. Neutral b. Right
c. Left d. None

Fetal hemoglobin (HbF) is structurally different from normal adult hemoglobin (HbA), giving HbF a higher affinity for oxygen than HbA. HbF is composed of two alpha and two gamma chains whereas HbA is composed of two alpha and two beta chains. The fetal dissociation curve is shifted to the left relative to the curve for the normal adult.

254. Vagal stimulation causes:

a. Decreased depth of respiration
b. Bronchodilation
c. Increased depth of respiration
d. Increased rate of respiration

Vagus nerve stimulation causes an increase in respiratory rate, decrease in respiratory amplitude, decrease in tidal volume, and decrease in oxygen saturation during periods of device activation.

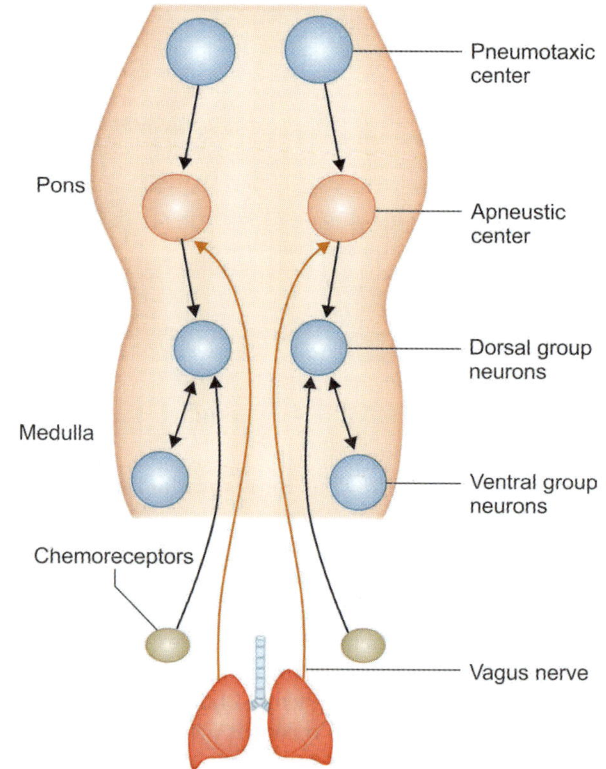

Nervous regulation of respiration. Solid green line = Stimulation, Dotted red line = Inhibition.

255. True for anatomical dead space:

a. 15 ml/kg BW
b. 10 ml/kg BW
c. 1/3rd of tidal volume
d. 2/5th of tidal volume

The normal value for dead space volume (in mL) is approximately the lean mass of the body (in pounds), and averages about a third of the resting tidal volume (450-500 mL).

Ans. **249.** **d.** Hypoventilation **250.** **d.** Shift in the oxygen... **251.** **c.** Prevents collapse... **252.** **c.** Decreased $PaCO_2$ **253.** **c.** Left **254.** **a.** Decreased depth of... **255.** **c.** 1/3rd of tidal volume

256. Transpulmonary pressure:
a. Difference between bronchus and atmospheric pressure
b. Difference between intra-alveolar and atmospheric pressure
c. Difference between intra-pleural and atmospheric pressure
d. Difference between pressure in alveoli and intra-pleural pressure

Transpulmonary pressure is the difference between the alveolar pressure and the intra-pleural pressure in the lungs. During human ventilation, air flows because of pressure gradients. $P_{tp} = P_{alv} - P_{ip}$. Where P_{tp} is transpulmonary pressure, P_{alv} is alveolar pressure, and P_{ip} is intrapleural pressure.

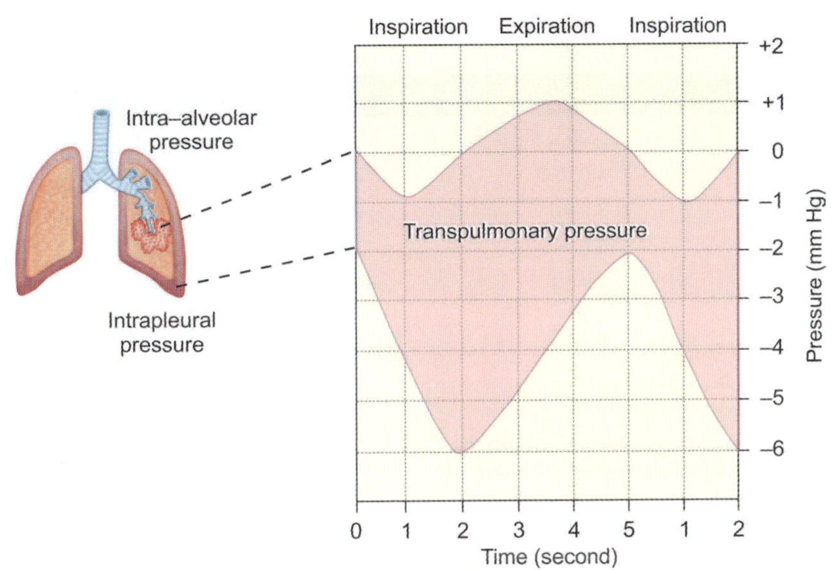

Changes in respiratory pressures during inspiration and expiration. '0' indicates the normal atmospheric pressure (760 mm Hg).

257. Source of surfactant:
a. Type I alveolar cells b. Type II alveolar cells
c. Alveolar macrophages d. Alveolar lymphocytes

Type II cells are responsible for the production and secretion of surfactant (the majority of which are dipalmitoylphosphatidylcholine), a group of phospholipids that reduce the alveolar surface tension.

258. Transection at which level will result in complete apneusis:
a. Cerebellum b. Midbrain
c. Lower pons d. Medulla

Apneustic respiration (**apneusis**) is an abnormal pattern of breathing characterized by deep, gasping inspiration with a pause at full inspiration followed by a brief, insufficient release. It is caused by damage to the pons or upper medulla caused by strokes or trauma. Specifically, concurrent removal of input from the vagus nerve and the pneumotaxic center causes this pattern of breathing. It is an ominous sign, with a generally poor prognosis.

259. Central and peripheral chemoreceptors respond to:
a. Decreased arterial CO_2 b. Increased arterial CO_2
c. Decreased arterial O_2 d. Increased arterial O_2

Chemoreceptors

- Central chemoreceptors are located on the ventrolateral surface of medulla oblongata and detect changes in pH of cerebrospinal fluid. They have also been shown experimentally to respond to hypercapnic hypoxia (elevated CO_2, decreased O_2), and eventually desensitize. These are sensitive to pH and CO_2.
- Peripheral chemoreceptors: Consists of aortic and carotid bodies. Aortic body detects changes in blood oxygen and carbon dioxide, but not pH, while carotid body detects all three. They do not desensitize. Their effect on breathing rate is less than that of the central chemoreceptors.

260. Effect of bilateral vagotomy and mid-pontine section on respiration:
a. Rate of respiration will be increased
b. Respiration will be shallow and rapid
c. Prolonged inspiratory spasms
d. No effect

Mid-pontine transection with the vagi cut, removes all inhibitory influences of pneumotaxic centre and vagi on apneustic centre and results in apneusis (sustained gasping inspiration followed by short, inefficient expiration).

261. Total amount of new air moved into the respiratory passages per minute is known as:
a. Tidal volume
b. Minute respiratory volume
c. Vital capacity
d. Inspiratory reserve volume

Ans. 256. **d.** Difference... 257. **b.** Type II alveolar cells 258. **c.** Lower pons 259. **b.** Increased arterial CO_2
260. **c.** Prolonged... 261. **b.** Minute respiratory volume

Respiratory minute volume (or **minute ventilation** or **expired minute volume**) is the volume of gas inhaled (inhaled minute volume) or exhaled (exhaled minute volume) from a person's lungs per minute. It is an important parameter in respiratory medicine due to its relationship with blood carbon dioxide levels.

262. Effect of sympathetic impulses on bronchus:
a. Increased bronchial secretion
b. Bronchodilation
c. Bronchoconstriction
d. None of the above

Sympathetic system dilates bronchioles via circulating adrenaline.

263. pO2 in venous blood (mm Hg) of systemic capillary:
a. 35
b. 45
c. 55
d. 65

Reference ranges for pO_2 and pCO_2

	Unit	*Arterial blood gas*	*Venous blood gas*	*Cerebrospinal fluid*	*Alveolar pulmonary gas pressures*
pO_2	kPa	11–13	4.0–5.3	5.3–5.9	14.2
	mmHg	75–100	30–40	40–44	107
pCO_2	kPa	4.7–6.0	5.5–6.8	5.9–6.7	4.8
	mmHg	35–45	41–51	44–50	36

264. Physiological dead space of lung:
a. 100 ml
b. 150 ml
c. 200 ml
d. 250 ml

In humans, about a third of every resting breath has no change in O_2 and CO_2 levels. In adults, it is usually in the range of 150 mL. Normally, anatomical is equal to physiological dead space as normally alveolar dead space is zero.

265. A fall in pH reduces the binding capacity of oxygen to hemoglobin. This is known as:
a. Head paradoxical reflex
b. Chloride shift
c. Haldane effect
d. Bohr effect

The **Bohr effect** is a physiological phenomenon first described in 1904 by the Danish physiologist Christian Bohr, stating that *hemoglobin's oxygen binding affinity is inversely related both to acidity and to the concentration of carbon dioxide.* Increase in blood CO_2 concentration which leads to a decrease in blood pH will result in hemoglobin proteins releasing their load of oxygen.

266. Centre of respiration is:
a. Dorsal respiratory group
b. Pneumotaxic centre
c. Ventral respiratory group
d. Pre-Botzinger complex

The **pneumotaxic center**, also known as the **pontine respiratory group (PRG)**, is a network of neurons in the rostral dorsal lateral pons. It consists of the Kölliker-Fuse nucleus and the medial parabrachial nucleus. It is considered an antagonist to the apneustic center, which produces abnormal breathing during inhalation.

Medullary centers

Features	*Dorsal group*	*Ventral group*
Situation	Diffusely situated in nucleus of tractus solitarius	In nucleus ambiguous and nucleus retroambiguous
Type of neurons	Inspiratory neurons	Inspiratory and expiratory neurons
Function	Always active Generate inspiratory ramp Has autorhythmic property	Inactive during quiet breathing Active during forced breathing

267. In RBC, 2, 3-DPG is involved in:
a. O_2 binding to hemoglobin
b. O_2 delivery to tissues
c. CO_2 binding to hemoglobin
d. CO_2 delivery to tissues

2, 3-DPG interacts with deoxygenated hemoglobin beta subunits by decreasing their affinity for oxygen, so it allosterically promotes the release of the remaining oxygen molecules bound to the hemoglobin, thus enhancing the ability of RBCs to release oxygen near tissues that need it most. 2,3-BPG is thus an allosteric effector.

268. FALSE statement regarding difference between apex and base of lung, in erect posture is:
a. V/Q is low at the apex of lung
b. V/Q is high at the apex of lung
c. V/Q remain same at both apex and base
d. None of the above

Because the lung is centered vertically around the heart, part of the lung is superior to the heart, and part is inferior. This has a major impact on the V/Q ratio:
- Apex of lung – higher
- Base of lung – lower

Ans. **262. b.** Bronchodilation **263. b.** 45 **264. b.** 150 ml **265. d.** Bohr effect
266. b. Pneumotaxic ... **267. b.** O_2 delivery to tissues **268. c.** V/Q remain same at both apex and base

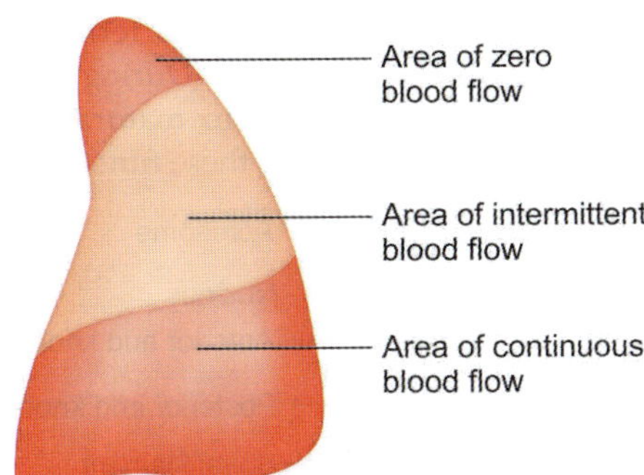

Pattern of blood flow in various areas of lungs.

269. **Surfactant is produced by:**
   a. Type II pneumocytes
   b. Type I pneumocytes
   c. Macrophages
   d. Endothelial cells

Type II pneumocytes also called alveolar type II cells, **great alveolar cells** or **septal cells** are granular and roughly cuboidal in shape. Type II pneumocytes are typically found at the alveolar-septal junction. Type II cells are responsible for the production and secretion of surfactant (the majority of which are dipalmitoylphosphatidylcholine), a group of phospholipids that reduce the alveolar surface tension.

270. **Which does NOT increase oxygen supply to muscles during exercise:**
   a. Oxygen dissociation curve shifts to left
   b. Increased stroke volume
   c. Increased extraction of oxygen from the blood
   d. Increased blood flow to muscles

In exercise, several factors shift the dissociation curve considerably to the right, thus delivering extra amounts of oxygen to the active, exercising muscle fibers.

REPRODUCTIVE SYSTEM

271. **Which of the following is FALSE regarding capacitation?**
   a. Sperms loses its cholesterol content in process
   b. Occurs in epididymis
   c. Makes sperm capable of fertilizing egg
   d. Membrane of the head becomes more weaker

Capacitation

- It is the penultimate step in the maturation of mammalian spermatozoa and is required to render them competent to fertilize an oocyte.
- This step is a biochemical event; the sperm move normally and look mature prior to capacitation.
- In vivo this step typically occurs after ejaculation, in the female reproductive tract (isthmus part of fallopian tubes).
- In vitro, capacitation can occur by incubating sperms that have either undergone ejaculation or have been extracted from the epididymis in a defined medium for several hours.
- The uterus aids in the steps of capacitation by secreting sterol-binding albumin, lipoproteins, proteolytic and glycosidasic enzymes such as heparin.

272. **Inhibin inhibits:**
   a. FSH
   b. Estrogen and progesterone
   c. LH
   d. LHRH

Inhibin downregulates FSH synthesis and inhibits FSH secretion.

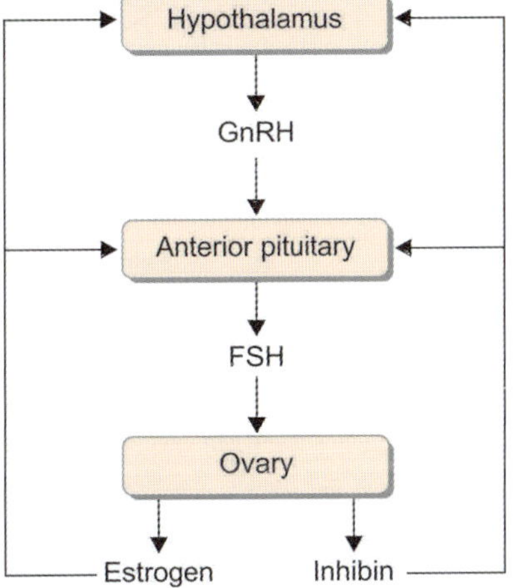

Regulation of estrogen secretion. Red dotted lines indicate inhibition.

273. **Asthenospermia is:**
   a. Absence of semen
   b. Absence of sperms
   c. Reduction in motility of sperms
   d. Reduction in number of sperms

Terms ending with 'spermia'

(A) spermia - complete lack of semen
(Asthenozoo) spermia - reduced sperm motility
(Azoo) spermia - absence of sperm cells in semen
(Hyper) spermia - large semen volume
(Hypo) spermia - small semen volume
(Oligozoo) spermia - few spermatozoa in semen
(Necrozoo) spermia - dead or immobile sperms
(Teratozoo) spermia - sperm with abnormal morphology

274. **Term period for embryonic life:**
   a. 0-14 days of gestation
   b. 14 days-9 weeks of gestation
   c. 9 weeks-birth
   d. 22 weeks-7 days after birth

Embryonic stage extends from beginning of 2nd week to 8th weeks of pregnancy.

Ans. 269. **a.** Type II pneu... 270. **a.** Oxygen... 271. **b.** Occurs in epidi... 272. **a.** FSH
273. **c.** Reduction in... 274. **b.** 14 days-9 weeks of gestation

275. Ovulation is due to ... surge:

a. TSH b. Prolactin
c. FSH d. LH

Estrogen levels peak towards the end of the follicular phase. This causes a surge in levels of luteinizing hormone (LH) and follicle-stimulating hormone (FSH). This lasts from 24 to 36 hours, and results in the rupture of the ovarian follicles, causing the oocyte to be released from the ovary via the oviduct.

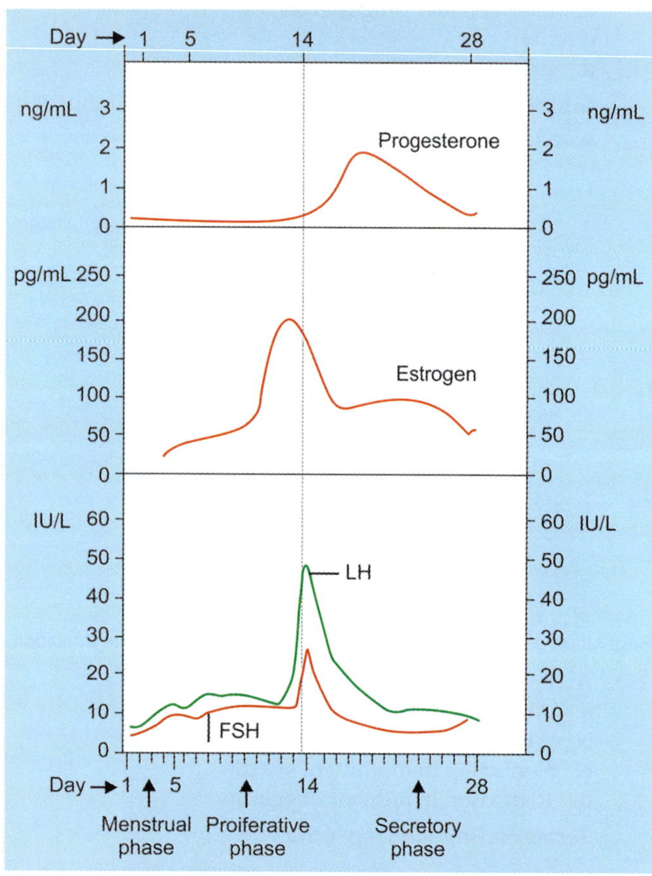

Hormonal level during menstrual cycle. LH = Luteinizing hormones, FSH = Follicle-stimulating hormone.

276. Fertilization occurs in:

a. Interstitial b. Ampulla
c. Isthmus d. Fimbria

Ampulla averages 5 to 8 cm in length. It is within this highly ciliated portion of the oviduct that fertilization and early embryo development occur. The ampulla is most often the site for ectopic implantation.

277. Sperms attain motility in:

a. Vas deferens b. Testis
c. Epididymis d. Prostatic urethra

Spermatozoa formed in the testis enter the caput epididymis, progress to the corpus, and finally reach the cauda region, where they are stored. Sperm entering the caput epididymis are incomplete—they lack the ability to swim forward (motility) and to fertilize an egg. It stores the sperm for 2–3 months. During their transit in the epididymis, sperm undergo maturation processes necessary for them to acquire these functions.

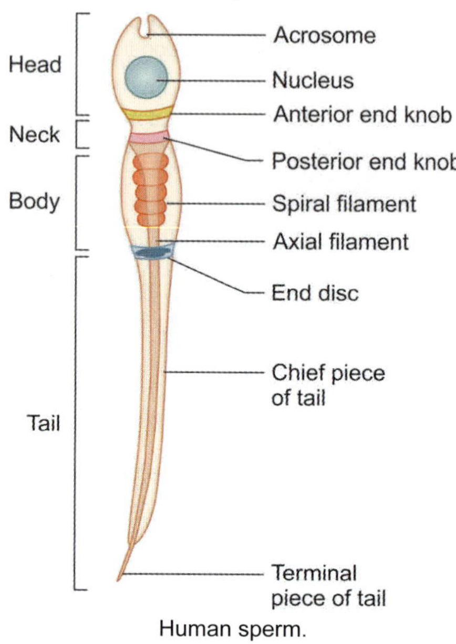

Human sperm.

278. hCG is seceretd by:

a. Liver b. Yolk sac
c. Syncytiotrophoblast d. Chorionic membrane

Human chorionic gonadotropin (**hCG**) is a hormone produced by the Syncytiotrophoblast, a portion of the placenta following implantation. The presence of hCG is detected in pregnancy tests.

279. Estrogen secretion is maximum:

a. Before ovulation b. At menstruation
c. At puberty d. Just before menopause

Estrogen levels vary through the menstrual cycle, with levels highest near the end of the follicular phase just before ovulation.

280. In female genital tract, sperms move at the rate of:

a. 1-3 mm/day b. 4-6 mm/day
c. 6-8 mm/day d. 8-10 mm/day

Sperm transport

- Motility of spermatozoa – they move at the speed of 2-3 mm/hour
- Contractions in the female genital tract

281. Source of androgen binding protein:

a. Leydig cells b. Sertoli cells
c. Liver d. Pituitary

Androgen-binding protein (**ABP**) is a glycoprotein (beta-globulin) produced by the Sertoli cells in the seminiferous tubules of the testis that binds specifically to testosterone (T), dihydrotestosterone (DHT), and 17-beta-estradiol.

Ans. 275. **d.** LH 276. **b.** Ampulla 277. **c.** Epididymis 278. **c.** Syncytiotrophoblast
279. **a.** Before ovulation 280. **a.** 1-3 mm/day 281. **b.** Sertoli cells

282. During ejaculation, sperms are released from:

a. Prostate
b. Vas deferens
c. Epididymis
d. Seminal vesicle

Vas (ductus) deferens serves as a secondary storehouse for spermatozoa which will be released at the time of ejaculation.

283. Interstitial cell of Leydig secretes:

a. Aromatase
b. Testosterone
c. Anti-mullerian hormone
d. Inhibin

Leydig cells, also known as **interstitial cells of Leydig**, are found adjacent to the seminiferous tubules in the testicle. They produce testosterone in the presence of luteinizing hormone (LH).

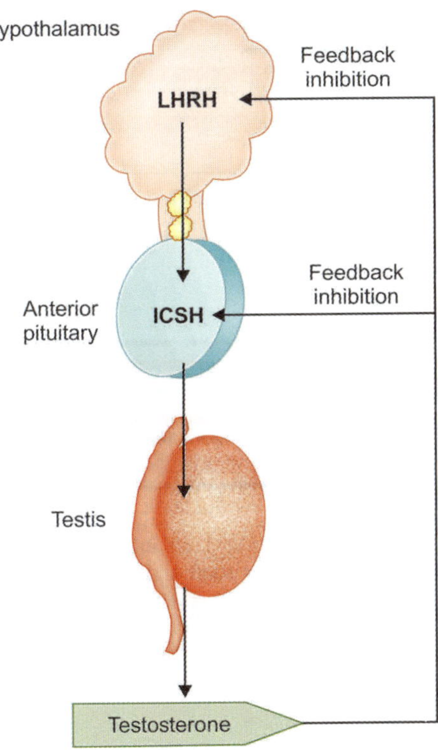

Regulation of testosterone secretion. LHRH = Luteinizing hormone-releasing hormone, ICSH = Interstitial cell-stimulating hormone.

284. Fertilized ovum reaches uterine cavity by:

a. 3-4 days
b. 5-6 days
c. 7-8 days
d. 10-11 days

The fertilized egg reaches uterine cavity by 3-4 days and process of implantation occurs within 6-9 days.

285. Hormone level raised in post-menopausal women:

a. FSH
b. Estrogen
c. Androgen
d. Progesterone

Natural or physiological menopause occurs as a part of a woman's normal aging process. It is the result of the eventual depletion of almost all of the oocytes and ovarian follicles in the ovaries. This causes an increase in circulating follicle stimulating hormone (FSH) and luteinizing hormone (LH) levels because there are a decreased number of oocytes and follicles responding to these hormones and producing estrogen.

286. NOT a function of estrogen:

a. Breast enlargement during puberty
b. Secondary sexual character development in female
c. Secretory effect on endometrium
d. Proliferative effect on endometrium

Progesterone converts the endometrium to its secretory stage to prepare the uterus for implantation. At the same time, progesterone affects the vaginal epithelium and cervical mucus, making it thick and impenetrable to sperm.

287. FALSE for seminal vesicles:

a. Contains large amount of fructose
b. Stores sperms
c. Situated on either side near prostate
d. Secretion of seminal vesicle gives mucoid consistency to semen

Sperms are stored in epididymis

288. Hormone NOT needed in spermatogenesis:

a. Testosterone
b. FSH
c. LH
d. Oxytocin

Stage of spermatogenesis	Hormones necessary
Stage of proliferation	*Follicle-stimulating hormone* *Growth hormone*
Stage of growth	*Testosterone* *Growth hormone*
Stage of maturation	*Testosterone* *Growth hormone*
Stage of transformation	*Testosterone* *Estrogen*

Male reproductive system and other organs of pelvis

Oxytocin plays a role in intimacy, sexual reproduction of both sexes, and during and after childbirth as well as social bonding. It is released in large amounts after distension of the cervix and uterus during labor and with stimulation of the nipples following childbirth. This helps with birth, maternal bonding, and lactation.

289. Penile erection mechanism:

a. Constriction of arterioles
b. Dilatation of arterioles
c. Constriction of venules
d. Dilatation of venules

An erection occurs when two tubular structures, called the corpora cavernosa, that run the length of the penis, become engorged with venous blood. This may result from any of various physiological stimuli, also known as sexual stimulation and sexual arousal. The corpus spongiosum is a single tubular structure located just below the corpora cavernosa, which contains the urethra, through which urine and semen pass during urination and ejaculation respectively. This may also become slightly engorged with blood, but less so than the corpora cavernosa.

Ans. 282. **b.** Vas deferens 283. **b.** Testosterone 284. **a.** 3-4 days 285. **a.** FSH
286. **c.** Secretory effect... 287. **b.** Stores sperms 288. **d.** Oxytocin 289. **b.** Dilatation of arterioles

MUSCLE PHYSIOLOGY

290. Which protein prevents contraction by covering binding sites on actin and myosin:

a. Troponin b. Calmodulin
c. Thymosin d. Tropomyosin

Muscle tropomyosin isoforms are involved in regulating interactions between actin and myosin in the muscle sarcomere and play a pivotal role in regulated muscle contraction. X-ray diffraction and cryoelectron microscopy suggest that tropomyosin sterically blocks the access of myosin to the actin filament.

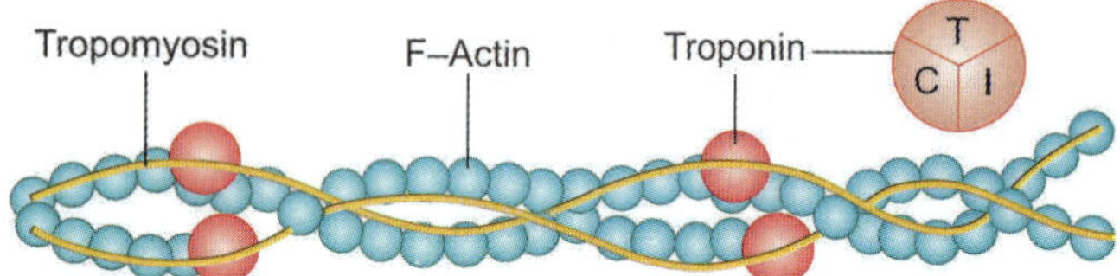

Part of actin filament. Troponin has three subunits, T, C and I.

291. A twitch of a single motor unit is known as:

a. Myoclonic jerk b. Fasciculation
c. Tremor d. Chorea

A **fasciculation** or **muscle twitch** is a small, local, involuntary muscle contraction and relaxation which may be visible under the skin. Deeper areas can be detected by EMG testing, though they can happen in any skeletal muscle in the body. Fasciculations arise as a result of *spontaneous depolarization* of a lower motor neuron leading to the synchronous contraction of all the skeletal muscle fibers within a single motor unit.

292. Contractile unit of muscle:

a. Sarcotubular system b. Myofibril
c. Sarcolemma d. Sarcomere

A **sarcomere** (Greek *sarx* "flesh", *meros*"part") is the basic unit of a muscle. Muscles are composed of tubular muscle cells (myocytes or myofibers), which are formed in a process known as myogenesis. Muscle cells are composed of tubular myofibrils. Myofibrils are composed of repeating sections of sarcomeres, which appear under the microscope as dark and light bands. Sarcomeres are composed of long, fibrous proteins that slide past each other when the muscles contract and relax.

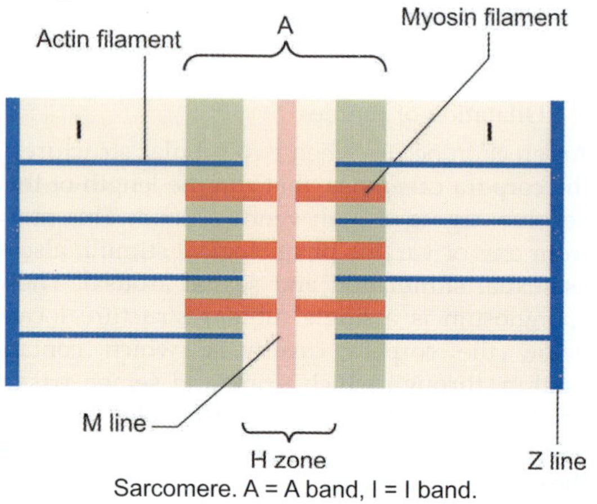

Sarcomere. A = A band, I = I band.

293. Physiological change during muscle contraction:

a. Shortening of A band
b. Shortening of A and H bands
c. Shortening of A and I bands
d. Shortening of H and I bands

Upon muscle contraction, the A-bands do not change their length (1.85 micrometer in mammalian skeletal muscle), whereas the I-bands and the H-zone shorten. This causes the Z lines to come closer together.

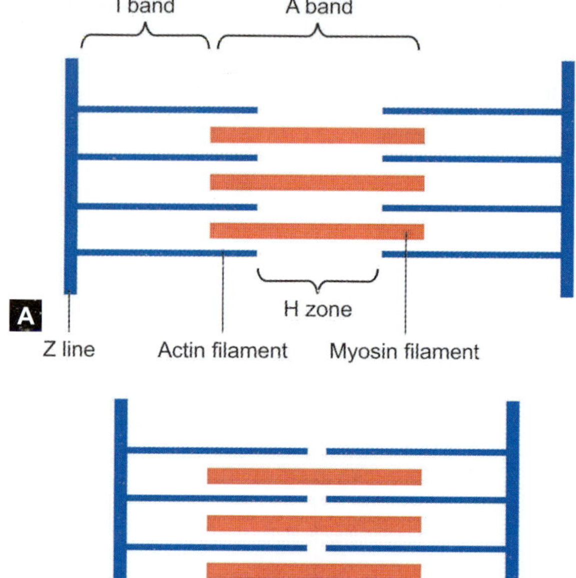

Sarcomere in resting muscle (A) Contracted muscle; (B) During contraction; Z lines come close, H zone and I band are reduced and no change in A band.

294. Feature of denervation of smooth muscle:

a. Reduced neurotransmitter release at neuromuscular junction
b. Increased sensitivity to chemical mediators
c. Reduced receptors for neurotransmitters
d. Muscular atrophy

Autonomic effector organs (smooth muscles) deprived of their nerve supply show a phenomenon seen to a very limited extent in skeletal muscle: they become hypersensitive to chemical agents. This phenomenon of denervation hypersensitivity sometimes has the paradoxical result of increasing the type of activity for which autonomic nerve section has been carried out. For example, there is a distressing disease called Raynaud's disease in which paroxysms of cutaneous vasospasm in the fingers give rise to intense pain. If the vasoconstrictor autonomic fibers which supply the hand are out, the resulting denervation hypersensitivity may make the attacks even more severe than they were.

Ans. 290. **d.** Tropomyosin 291. **b.** Fasciculation 292. **d.** Sarcomere 293. **d.** Shortening of H... 294. **b.** Increased sensitivity to chemical mediators

295. NOT a cause of skeletal muscle fibrillation:
a. Strong stimulus
b. Abundance of receptors on entire muscle membrane
c. Hypersensitivity to acetylcholine
d. Long time after denervation

Strong stimulus will result in muscle contraction proper. Fibrillation is a feature of lower motor neuron lesion.

296. Time taken to generate an action potential:
a. Refractory period b. Rheobase
c. Chronaxie d. Threshold

Rheobase is a measure of membrane excitability. Rheobase is the minimal current amplitude of infinite duration (in a practical sense, about 300 milliseconds) that results in the depolarization threshold of the cell membranes being reached, such as an action potential or the contraction of a muscle.

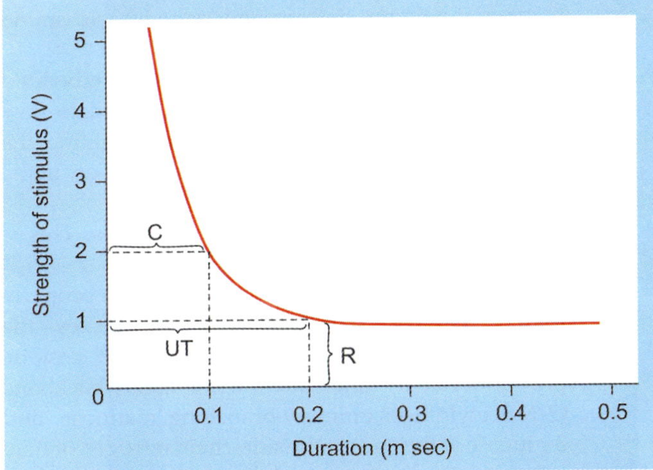

Strength–duration curve. R = Rheobase, UT = Utilization time, C = Chronaxie.

297. Band uncovered by actin:
a. Z band b. I band
c. M band d. H band

Within the A-band (because of myosin filaments) is a paler region called the **H-zone** (from the German "heller", *brighter*). Named for their lighter appearance under a polarization microscope. H-band is the zone of the thick filaments that is not superimposed by the thin (actin) filaments.

298. True for action potential:
a. Does NOT follow all or none principle
b. Potassium moves from ECF to ICF
c. Decremental phenomenon
d. Threshold stimulus is required

Action potentials are generated by special types of voltage-gated ion channels embedded in a cell's plasma membrane. These channels are shut when the membrane potential is near the resting potential of the cell, but they rapidly begin to open, if the membrane potential increases to a precisely defined threshold value.

299. The site where myosin heads bind to actin in skeletal muscles is covered by:
a. Calcium b. Troponin
c. Tropomyosin d. All of the above

Tropomyosins are a large family of integral components of actin filaments that play a critical role in regulating the function of actin filaments in both muscle and nonmuscle cells. These proteins consist of rod-shaped coiled-coil hetero- or homodimers that lie along the α-helical groove of most actin filaments.

300. Chronaxie is shortest in:
a. Cardiac muscle b. Nerve fibre
c. Skeletal muscle d. Equal in all

The chronaxie values for human arm sensory nerves range from 0.35 to 1.17 ms, a ratio of 3.3.

301. Chronaxie is maximum in:
a. Cardiac muscle b. Nerve fibre
c. Skeletal muscle d. Equal in all

The chronaxie of excitable tissues varies; it is less prolonged in nerves than inskeletal muscles. Among the different types of muscle tissue, skeletal striated muscles have the briefest chronaxie. The chronaxie of the heart muscle is more prolonged, and that of the smooth muscles is the most prolonged.

302. Essential for muscle contraction:
a. Sodium entry b. Potassium entry
c. Magnesium entry d. Calcium entry

Two of the important proteins are myosin, which forms the thick filament, and actin, which forms the thin filament. Myosin has a long, fibrous tail and a globular head, which binds to action. The myosin head also binds to ATP, which is the source of energy for muscle movement. Myosin can only bind to actin when the binding sites on actin are exposed by calcium ions.

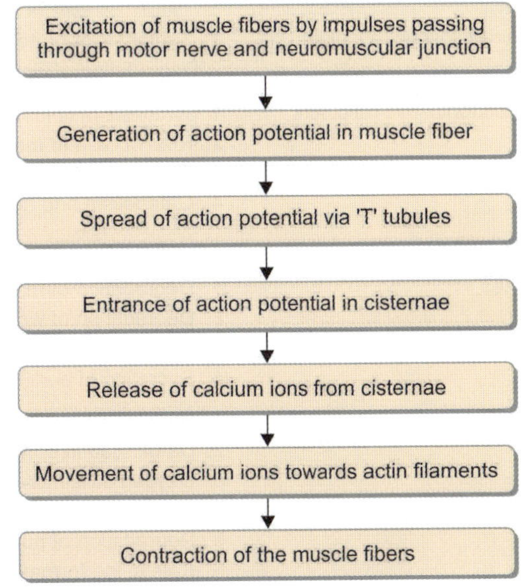

Excitation-contraction coupling.

Ans. 295. **a.** Strong stimulus 296. **b.** Rheobase 297. **d.** H band 298. **d.** Threshold stimulus is...
299. **c.** Tropomyosin 300. **b.** Nerve fibre 301. **a.** Cardiac muscle 302. **d.** Calcium entry

303. Elasticity and extensibility of the myofibril is due to:

a. Myomesin
b. Titin
c. Dystrophin
d. All of the above

Titin is important in the contraction of striated muscle tissues. It connects the Z line to the M line in the sarcomere. The protein contributes to force transmission at the Z line and resting tension in the I band region. It contains two kinds of folded domains, and these provide muscle with its elasticity.

GENERAL PHYSIOLOGY

304. Membrane contains protein and lipid in the ratio of (on weight basis):

a. 4:1
b. 2:1
c. 1:1
d. 1:2

The cell membrane has large content of proteins, typically around 55% of membrane volume. 25% is phospholipids; cholesterol is 13% and other lipids 4%.

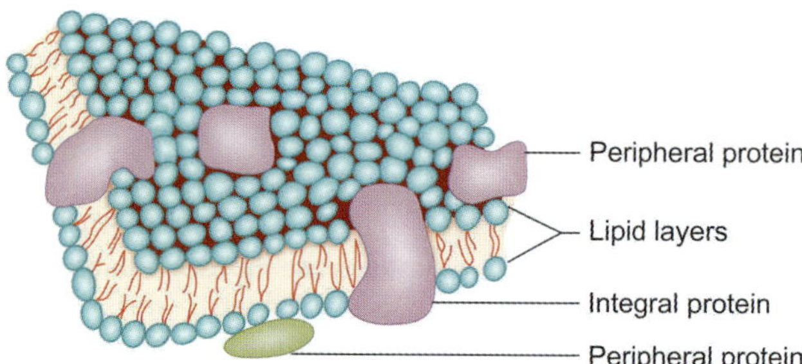

Diagram of the cell membrane.

305. Does NOT undergo cell division:

a. Satellite cell of skeletal muscle
b. Smooth muscle cell
c. Cardiac muscle cell
d. Pericyte

The **heart muscle** cells **can**'t **divide**.

306. Protein synthesis occurs in:

a. Smooth endoplasmic reticulum
b. Rough endoplasmic reticulum
c. Golgi bodies
d. Nucleus

Function of rough endoplasmic reticulum

- Manufacture of lysosomal enzymes with a mannose-6-phosphate marker added in the *cis*-Golgi network
- Manufacture of secreted proteins, either secreted constitutively with no tag or secreted in a regulatory manner involving clathrin and paired basic amino acids in the signal peptide.
- Integral membrane proteins that stay embedded in the membrane as vesicles exit and bind to new membranes. Rab proteins are key in targeting the membrane; SNAP and SNARE proteins are key in the fusion event.
- Initial glycosylation as assembly continues. This is N-linked (O-linking occurs in the Golgi).
- N-linked glycosylation: If the protein is properly folded, Oligosaccharyltransferase recognizes the AA sequence NXS or NXT (with the S/T residue phosphorylated) and adds a 14-sugar backbone (2-*N*-acetylglucosamine, 9-branching mannose, and 3-glucose at the end) to the side-chain nitrogen of Asn.

Functions of cytoplasmic organelles

Organelles	*Functions*
Rough endoplasmic reticulum	1. Synthesis of proteins 2. Degradation of worn-out organelles
Smooth endoplasmic reticulum	1. Synthesis of lipids and steroids 2. Role in cellular metabolism 3. Storage and metabolism of calcium 4. Catabolism and detoxification of toxic substances
Golgi apparatus	1. Processing, packaging, labeling and delivery of proteins and lipids
Lysosomes	1. Degradation of macromolecules 2. Degradation of worn-out organelles 3. Removal of excess of secretory products 4. Secretion of perforin, granzymes, melanin and serotonin
Peroxisomes	1. Breakdown of excess fatty acids 2. Detoxification of hydrogen peroxide and other metabolic products 3. Oxygen utilization 4. Acceleration of gluconeogenesis 5. Degradation of purine to uric acid 6. Role in the formation of myelin 7. Role in the formation of bile acids

Ans. 303. **b.** Titin 304. **b.** 2:1 305. **c.** Cardiac muscle cell 306. **b.** Rough endoplasmic...

Organelles	Functions
Centrosome	1. Movement of chromosomes during cell division
Mitochondria	1. Production of energy 2. Synthesis of ATP 3. Initiation of apoptosis
Ribosomes	1. Synthesis of proteins
Cytoskeleton	1. Determination of shape of the cell 2. Stability of cell shape 3. Cellular movements
Nucleus	1. Control of all activities of the cell 2. Synthesis of RNA 3. Sending genetic instruction to cytoplasm for protein synthesis 4. Formation of subunits of ribosomes 5. Control of cell division 6. Storage of hereditary information in genes (DNA)

307. Non-membrane bound cell organelle:

a. Mitochondria
b. Nucleolus
c. Nucleus
d. Endoplasmic reticulum

The **nucleolus** is a round body located inside the nucleus of a eukaryotic cell. It is not surrounded by a membrane but sits in the nucleus. The nucleolus makes ribosomal subunits from proteins and ribosomal RNA, also known as rRNA. It then sends the subunits out to the rest of the cell where they combine into complete ribosomes. Ribosomes make proteins; therefore, the nucleolus plays a vital role in making proteins in the cell.

Cytoplasmic organelles
Organelles with limiting membrane
1. Endoplasmic reticulum 2. Golgi apparatus 3. Lysosome 4. Peroxisome 5. Centrosome and centrioles 6. Secretory vesicles 7. Mitochondria 8. Nucleus
1. Ribosomes 2. Cytoskeleton

308. Amoeboid motility of cell is because of:

a. Nucleus
b. Ribosome
c. Lysosome
d. Actin

Actin is a globular multi-functional protein that forms microfilaments. It is found in essentially all eukaryotic cells (the only known exception being nematode sperm). It can be present as either a free monomer called **G-actin** (globular) or as part of a linear polymer **microfilament** called **F-actin** (filamentous), both of which are essential for such important cellular functions as the mobility and contraction of cells during cell division.

309. Mitochondrial DNA is:

a. Linear
b. Nicked circular
c. Closed circular
d. Open circular

In most multicellular organisms, the mtDNA is organized as a circular, covalently closed, double-stranded DNA.

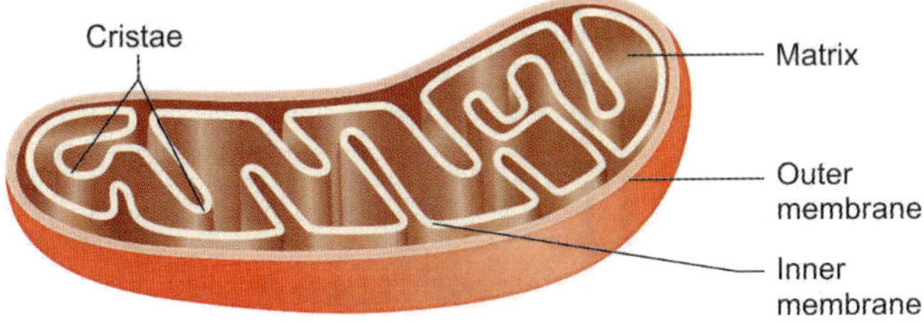

Structure of mitochondrion.

310. NOT an adhesion molecule:

a. Integrin
b. Selectin
c. Cadherin
d. Transferrin

Transferrins are iron-binding blood plasma glycoproteins that control the level of free iron in biological fluids.

Ans. **307. b.** Nucleolus **308. d.** Actin **309. c.** Closed circular **310. d.** Transferrin

Cell junctions			
Junction type	*Proteins involved*	*Function*	*Example*
Tight junction	Occludin Claudin JAMs Cingulin Symplekin ZO-1, 2, 3	Strength and stability to tissues Selective permeability Fencing function Maintenance of cell polarity Formation of blood-brain barrier	Epithelial lining of intestinal mucosa and renal tubule Endothelium in capillary wall and choroid plexus
Gap junction	Connexins	Allows passage of small molecules, ions and chemical messengers Propagation of action potential	Epithelial lining Heart Intestine
Adherens junction	Cadherins	Cell to cell attachment	Epithelial lining Heart Epidermis
Focal adhesions	Integrins	Cell attachment to Basal lamina Extracellular matrix	Epithelial lining
Desmosome	Cadherins	Cell to cell attachment	Epithelial lining Skin
Hemidesmosome	Integrins	Cell attachment to Basal lamina Extracellular matrix	Epithelial lining

311. Melanocytes are present in:

a. St. corneum b. St. basale
c. St. granulosum d. Dermis

Melanocytes are melanin-producing cells located in the bottom layer (the stratum basale) of the skin's epidermis, the middle layer of the eye (the uvea), the inner ear, meninges, bones, and heart. Melanin is the pigment primarily responsible for skin color. Once synthesised, melanin is contained in a special organelle called a melanosome and moved along arm-like structures called dendrites, so as to reach the keratinocytes.

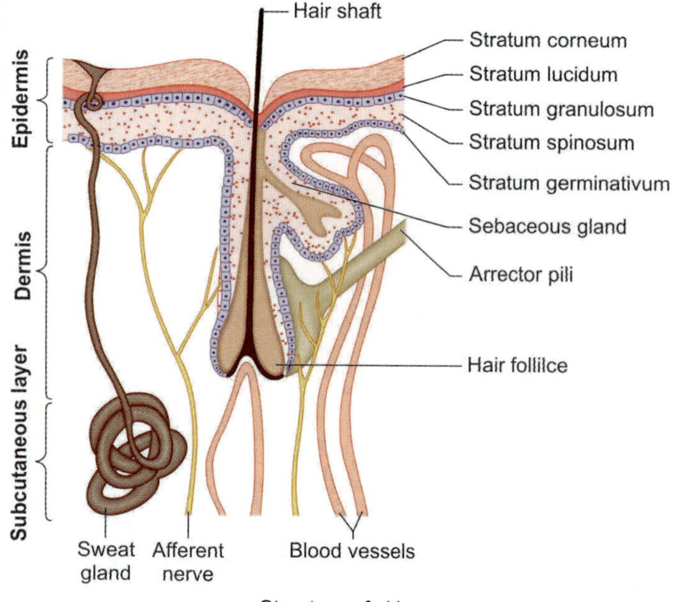

Structure of skin.

MISCELLANEOUS

312. Which band is NOT covered by actin filament in a sarcomere?

a. A
b. H
c. I
d. Z

The sarcomeres are what give skeletal and cardiac muscles their striated appearance.

- A sarcomere is defined as the segment between two neighbouring Z-lines (or Z-discs, or Z bodies). In electron micrographs of cross-striated muscle, the **Z-line** (from the German "Zwischenscheibe", the disc in between the I bands) appears as a series of dark lines.
- Surrounding the Z-line is the region of the **I-band** (for isotropic). I-band is the zone of thin filaments that is not superimposed by thick filaments.
- Following the I-band is the **A-band** (for anisotropic). Named for their properties under a polarizing microscope. An A-band contains the entire length of a single thick filament.
- Within the A-band is a paler region called the **H-zone** (from the German "heller", brighter). Named for their lighter appearance under a polarization microscope. H-band is the zone of the thick filaments that is not superimposed by the thin filaments.
- Inside the H-zone is a thin **M-line** (from the German "Mittelscheibe", the disc in the middle of the sarcomere) formed of cross-connecting elements of the cytoskeleton.

Ans. 311. b. St. basale **312. b.** H

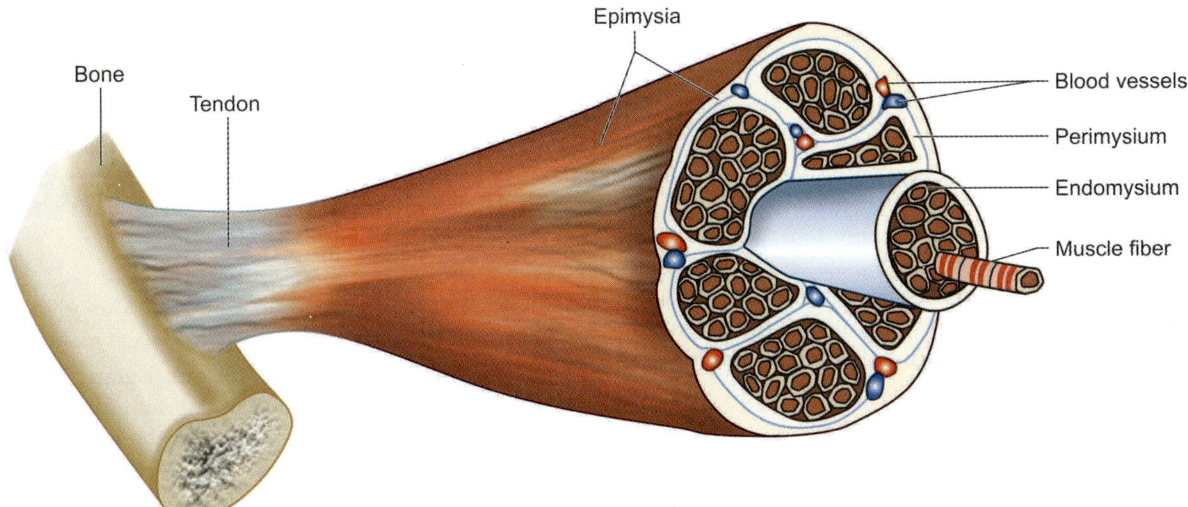

Structure of a skeletal muscle.

313. Which of the following event causes after hyperpolarization?

a. Potassium efflux
b. Sodium efflux
c. Calcium efflux
d. Magnesium efflux

Afterhyperpolarization/AHPs

- It describes the hyperpolarizing phase of a neuron's action potential where the cell's membrane potential falls below the normal resting potential.
- This is also commonly referred to as an action potential's **undershoot phase**.
- Fast and medium AHPs can be generated by single action potentials.
- Slow AHPs generally develop only during trains of multiple action potentials.
- During single action potentials, transient depolarization of the membrane opens more voltage gated K^+ channels than are open in the resting state, many of which do not close immediately when the membrane returns to its normal resting voltage.
- This can lead to an "undershoot" of the membrane potential to values that are more polarized ("hyperpolarized") than was the original resting membrane potential.
- Ca^{2+} activated K^+ channels that open in response to the influx of Ca^{2+} during the action potential carry much of the K^+ current as the membrane potential becomes more negative.
- The K^+ permeability of the membrane is transiently unusually high, driving the membrane voltage V_M even closer to the K^+ equilibrium voltage E_K.
- Hence, hyperpolarization persists until the membrane K^+ permeability returns to its usual value.

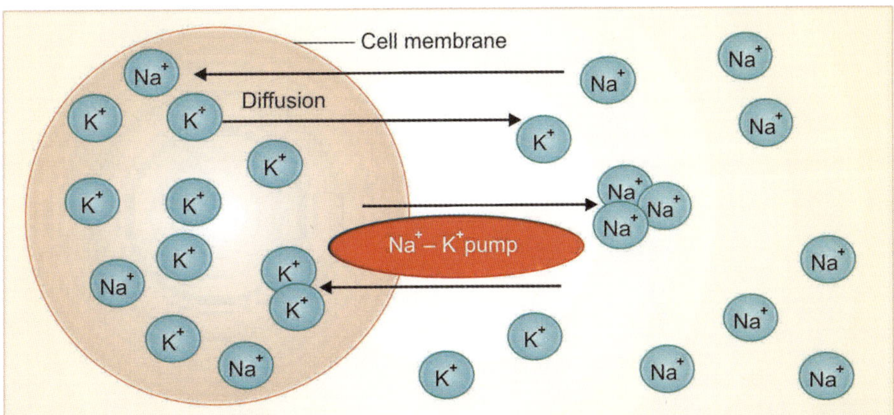

Development of resting membrane potential by sodium-potassium (Na^+-K^+) pump and diffusion of ions. Na^+-K^+ pump actively pumps three Na^+ outside and two K^+ into the cell. However, the diffusion of K^+ out of the cell is many times greater than the diffusion of Na^+ inside the cell because many of the K^+ leak channels are opened and many of the Na^+ leak channels are closed.

Ans. 313. a. Potassium efflux

314. Serotonin is secreted by:
a. Thyroid gland
b. Adrenal cortex
c. Adrenal medulla
d. Argentaffin cells

Serotonin or **5-hydroxytryptamine (5-HT)** is a monoamine neurotransmitter. Biochemically derived from tryptophan, serotonin is primarily found in the gastrointestinal tract (GI tract), blood platelets, and the central nervous system (CNS). Approximately 90% of the human body's total serotonin is located in the enterochromaffin/argentaffin cells in the GI tract, where it is used to regulate intestinal movements.

315. Molecule used for cell signalling:
a. N_2
b. NO
c. CO_2
d. O_2

NO is one of the few gaseous signalling molecules known and is additionally exceptional due to the fact that it is a radical gas. The endothelium (inner lining) of blood vessels uses nitric oxide to signal the surrounding smooth muscle to relax, thus resulting in vasodilation and increasing blood flow.

316. Respiratory quotient of proteins is:
a. 1 b. 0.8
c. 0.75 d. 0.5

Respiratory quotient

Name of the substance	Respiratory Quotient
Carbohydrates	1
Proteins	0.8-0.9
Ketones (eucaloric)	0.73
Ketones (hypocaloric)	0.66
Triolein (fat)	0.7

317. All are in excess in colostrums (as compared to milk) except:
a. Immunoglobulins b. Protein
c. Fat d. Mineral

Colostrum contains essentially the same concentrations of proteins and lactose as milk but almost no fat, and its maximum rate of production is about 1/100 the subsequent rate of milk production.

318. Gland which secretes oily substance:
a. Lacrimal gland b. Salivary gland
c. Meibomian gland d. Sweat gland

The **meibomian glands** (or **tarsal glands**) are a special kind of sebaceous gland at the rim of the eyelids inside the tarsal plate, responsible for the supply of meibum, an oily substance that prevents evaporation of the eye's tear film. Meibum prevents tear spillage onto the cheek, trapping tears between the oiled edge and the eyeball, and makes the closed lids airtight. There are approximately 50 glands on the upper eyelids and 25 glands on the lower eyelids.

319. Ratio of arginine to lysine in total serum proteins is:
a. 10:14 b. 10:18
c. 10:24 d. 10:36

In plasma proteins, ratio of arginine to lysine is 10:18

320. Maximum sweat rate in a normal, unacclimatized person:
a. 1 litre/hour b. 2 litre/hour
c. 3 litre/hour d. 4.5 litre/hour

A **normal**, unacclimatized **person** seldom produces more than about **1 liter** of **sweat per hour.** Sweating is primarily a means of thermoregulation which is achieved by the water-rich secretion of the eccrine glands. Maximum sweat rates of an adult can be up to 2–4 liters per hour or 10–14 liters per day (10–15 g/min · m^2), but is less in children prior to puberty.

Ans. **314. d.** Argentaffin cells **315. b.** NO **316. b.** 0.8 **317. c.** Fat
318. c. Meibomian... **319. b.** 10:18 **320. a.** 1 litre/hour

ANSWERS WITH REFERENCES

HAEMATOLOGY AND BODY FLUIDS

1. **Ans. (b) At 20 weeks intrauterine life, there is 90% HbF**
Ref: Sembulingam's Physiology, 6/e p81

2. **Ans. (a) Ferritin**
Ref: Guyton and Hall 10/e p387

3. **Ans. (c) Factor VII**
Ref: Internet resources

4. **Ans. (a) IX**
Ref: Guyton and Hall 10/e p426

5. **Ans. (c) vW factor**
Ref: Sembulingam 6/e p124

6. **Ans. (d) 7.40**
Ref: Guyton and Hall 10/e p347

7. **Ans. (d) Bicarbonate**
Ref: Guyton and Hall 10/e p348

8. **Ans. (b) 1.33 ml O_2**
Ref: Guyton and Hall 10/e p466

9. **Ans. (d) 5% of body weight**
Ref: Sembulingam 6/e p52

10. **Ans. (a) Sodium**
Ref: Sembulingam 6/e p53

11. **Ans. (d) Plasma cells**
Ref: Sembulingam 6/e p109

12. **Ans. (d) Thromboxane A2**
Ref: Guyton and Hall 10/e p419

13. **Ans. (c) Sharp increase in O_2 uptake and metabolism in neutrophils**
Ref: Sembulingam 6/e p102

14. **Ans. (a) 1-3 days**
Ref: Sembulingam 6/e p98

15. **Ans. (a) HbA**
Ref: Guyton and Hall 10/e p387

16. **Ans. (a) Chronic renal failure**
Ref: Guyton and Hall 10/e p376

17. **Ans. (b) DNA synthesis in the bone marrow**
Ref: Guyton and Hall 10/e p386

18. **Ans. (b) Intrinsic pathway**
Ref: Sembulingam 6/e p131

19. **Ans. (c) VII**
Ref: Harrison/ 18th / 974t

20. **Ans. (a) V**
Ref: Sembulingam 6/e p134

21. **Ans. (a) HbA**
Ref: Internet resources

22. **Ans. (d) Bicarbonate**
Ref: Guyton and Hall 10/e p348

23. **Ans. (b) 280-290 mOsm/ L**
Ref: Guyton and Hall 10/e p267t

24. **Ans. (b) VIII**
Ref: Ganong 20/e p526

25. **Ans. (b) Potassium**
Ref: Guyton and Hall 10/e p2

26. **Ans. (a) Sodium ions**
Ref: Internet resources

27. **Ans. (a) Calcium**
Ref: Guyton and Hall 10/e p421

28. **Ans. (a) Factor VIII**
Ref: Internet resources

29. **Ans. (b) Transferrin**
Ref: Ganong 20/e p462

30. **Ans. (c) Yolk sac**
Ref: Sembulingam 6/e p73

31. **Ans. (a) HCO_3^- is predominantly seen in ICF**
Ref: Guyton and Hall 10/e p2

32. **Ans. (b) Liver**
Ref: Guyton and Hall 10/e p382

33. **Ans. (b) Potassium**
Ref: Guyton and Hall 10/e p2

34. **Ans. (c) 21 days**
Ref: Internet resources

35. **Ans. (b) Septic shock**
Ref: Internet resources

36. **Ans. (c) Thrombomodulin**
Ref: Sembulingam 6/e p132

37. **Ans. (c) Neutrophil**
Ref: Guyton and Hall 10/e p394

38. **Ans. (c) Inulin**
Ref: Sembulingam 6/e p54

39. **Ans. (b) Evans blue**
Ref: Guyton and Hall 10/e p269

40. **Ans. (c) Thymus**
Ref: Guyton and Hall 10/e p403

41. **Ans. (a) Intracellular**
Ref: Guyton and Hall 10/e p273

CARDIOVASCULAR SYSTEM

42. **Ans. (a) Reduced because of an increase in heart rate**
Ref: Sembulingum's Physiology, 6/e p573

43. **Ans. (c) AV node**
Ref: Sembulingam 6/e p529

44. **Ans. (a) Atrioventricular valves open**
Ref: Sembulingam 6/e p537

45. **Ans. (d) Increased HR**
Ref: Sembulingam 6/e p563

46. **Ans. (c) Arterioles**
Ref: Sembulingam 6/e p642

47. **Ans. (d) Sympathetic stimulation**
Ref: Guyton and Hall 10/e p219

48. **Ans. (a) Sympathetic system mediated cholinergic release**
Ref: Guyton and Hall 10/e p706

49. **Ans. (d) Prostacyclin**
Ref: Guyton and Hall 10/e p290

50. **Ans. (b) Tetany**
Ref: Sembulingam 6/e p521

51. **Ans. (a) 250 mL/min**
Ref: Sembulingam 6/e p631

52. **Ans. (b) 20-30% of blood volume**
Ref: Sembulingam 6/e p574

53. **Ans. (b) Ventricular systole**
Ref: Sembulingam 6/e p545

54. **Ans. (b) Laplace's law**
Ref: Internet resources

55. **Ans. (a) Axon reflex**
Ref: Sembulingam 6/e p647

56. **Ans. (c) Influx of calcium**
Ref: Sembulingam 6/e p526

57. **Ans. (d) Arterioles**
Ref: Guyton and Hall 10/e p150

58. **Ans. (d) Kidney**
Ref: Guyton and Hall 10/e p176

59. **Ans. (d) Frank-Starling's law**
Ref: Ganong 20/e p552

60. **Ans. (d) Lying to standing change in posture**
Ref: Ganong 20/e p552t

61. **Ans. (b) End of isovolumetric contraction**
Ref: Sembulingam 6/e p541

62. **Ans. (c) 15 mm Hg**
Ref: Ganong 20/e p639

63. **Ans. (c) Generates impulses at a highest rate**
Ref: Guyton and Hall 10/e p111

64. **Ans. (d) Increased R-R interval**
Ref: Sembulingam 6/e p589

65. **Ans. (c) Ventricular depolarization**
Ref: Sembulingam 6/e p554

66. **Ans. (c) End diastolic volume**
Ref: Guyton and Hall 10/e p103

67. **Ans. (b) Veins**
Ref: Guyton and Hall 10/e p160

68. **Ans. (d) All of the above**
Ref: Ganong 20/e p574

69. **Ans. (d) x wave**
Ref: Sembulingam 6/e p628

70. **Ans. (c) Capillary dilation**
Ref: Sembulingam 6/e p647

71. **Ans. (b) Ventricular diastole**
Ref: Sembulingam 6/e p542

72. **Ans. (c) Ventricular diastole**
Ref: Guyton and Hall 10/e p227

73. **Ans. (a) Alpha receptors**
Ref: Sembulingam 6/e p441

74. **Ans. (c) Arterioles**
Ref: Guyton and Hall 10/e p150

75. **Ans. (b) Heart rate and BP**
Ref: Sembulingam 6/e p592

76. **Ans. (c) Increase in potassium permeability**
Ref: Sembulingam 6/e p528

77. **Ans. (c) Both of the above**
Ref: Sembulingam 6/e p592

78. **Ans. (a) 60/R-R interval (in seconds)**
Ref: Sembulingam 6/e p555

79. **Ans. (a) Atrial contraction**
Ref: Guyton and Hall 10/e p100

80. **Ans. (b) Kidney**
Ref: Guyton and Hall 10/e p176t

81. **Ans. (a) Axon reflex**
Ref: Sembulingam 6/e p647

ENDOCRINOLOGY

82. **Ans. (a) Type I iodothyronine deiodinase**
Ref: Sembulingam's Physiology, 6/e p388

83. **Ans. (b) Reduced membrane stability**
Ref: Sembulingam's Physiology, 6/e p406

84. **Ans. (b) Progesterone**
Ref: Sembulingam's Physiology, 6/e p371

85. **Ans. (b) Oxytocin**
Ref: Sembulingam 6/e p383

86. **Ans. (d) T4 has shorter half life than T3**
Ref: Sembulingam 6/e p390

87. **Ans. (a) Thyroid gland**
Ref: Sembulingam 6/e p407

88. **Ans. (c) Increased excitability of muscles and nerves**
Ref: Sembulingam 6/e p403

89. **Ans. (d) GH**
Ref: Sembulingam 6/e p373

90. **Ans. (c) Epinephrine**
Ref: Sembulingam 6/e p369

91. **Ans. (c) Secretin**
Ref: Sembulingam 6/e p419

92. **Ans. (d) 80-100 mg/ 100 ml**
Ref: Ganong 20/e p283

93. **Ans. (a) HbA1c**
Ref: Sembulingam 6/e p424

94. **Ans. (a) Estrogen**
Ref: Guyton and Hall 10/e p842t

95. **Ans. (c) Both of the above**
Ref: Sembulingam 6/e p395

96. **Ans. (d) Hypoglycemia**
Ref: Sembulingam 6/e p380

97. **Ans. (b) Insulin**
Ref: Internet resources

98. **Ans. (a) Reduced membrane stability**
Ref: Guyton and Hall 10/e p342

99. **Ans. (d) Secondary active transport**
Ref: Guyton and Hall 10/e p49

100. **Ans. (c) Somatostatin**
Ref: Guyton and Hall 10/e p893

101. **Ans. (d) Somatostatin**
Ref: Guyton and Hall 10/e p848

102. **Ans. (a) Globulin**
Ref: Guyton and Hall 10/e p860

103. **Ans. (b) Increased PTH**
Ref: Sembulingam 6/e p407

104. **Ans. (b) Inhibition of iodide-organic binding**
Ref: Internet resources

105. **Ans. (a) Increase in serum calcium levels**
Ref: Ganong/ 20th/ 381

106. **Ans. (b) Insulin**
Ref: Internet resources

EXCRETORY SYSTEM

107. **Ans. (c) JG cells**
Ref: Sembulingam's Physiology, 6/e p309

108. **Ans. (d) 320 mg**
Ref: Sembulingam 6/e p323

109. **Ans. (a) PCT**
Ref: Guyton and Hall 10/e p300

110. **Ans. (d) Inability of the kidney to concentrating urine**
Ref: Sembulingam 6/e p321

111. **Ans. (c) JG cells**
Ref: Sembulingam 6/e p311

112. **Ans. (a) PCT**
Ref: Guyton and Hall 10/e p300

113. **Ans. (d)** GFR
Ref: Guyton and Hall 10/e p310

114. **Ans. (d)** Renal tubular epithelial cells
Ref: Guyton and Hall 10/e p385

115. **Ans. (c)** JG cells
Ref: Ganong 20/e p442

116. **Ans. (a)** PCT
Ref: Sembulingam 6/e p331

117. **Ans. (c)** Contraction in ECF volume
Ref: Guyton and Hall 10/e p313

118. **Ans. (b)** Water
Ref: Guyton and Hall 10/e p

119. **Ans. (a)** Hydrogen ions
Ref: Guyton and Hall 10/e p300

120. **Ans. (d)** JG apparatus
Ref: Sembulingam 6/e p305

121. **Ans. (d)** Pacemaker activity of the smooth muscle cells in renal pelvis
Ref: Guyton and Hall 10/e p365

122. **Ans. (a)** Inulin
Ref: Ganong 20/e p681

123. **Ans. (a)** PCT
Ref: Guyton and Hall 10/e p300

124. **Ans. (b)** Nonapeptide
Ref: Sembulingam 6/e p328

125. **Ans. (b)** Thick ascending loop of Henle
Ref: Sembulingam 6/e p326

126. **Ans. (d)** High Sodium in PCT
Ref: Guyton and Hall 10/e p292

127. **Ans. (b)** Hydrogen ion
Ref: Sembulingam 6/e p332

128. **Ans. (b)** Inhibit reabsorption of sodium by the collecting ducts
Ref: Guyton and Hall 10/e p838t

129. **Ans. (d)** Glucose
Ref: Guyton and Hall 10/e p305

130. **Ans. (a)** Converts angiotensinogen to angiotensin-I
Ref: Ganong/ 20th/ 439

131. **Ans. (b)** Collecting duct
Ref: Guyton and Hall 10/e p335

132. **Ans. (c)** ANP
Ref: Internet resources

DIGESTIVE SYSTEM

133. **Ans. (a)** Cephalic phase – 30%
Ref: Sembulingam's Physiology, 6/e p233

134. **Ans. (a)** Acidic
Ref: Sembulingam's Physiology, 6/e p257

135. **Ans. (d)** Acid and protein
Ref: Sembulingam 6/e p246

136. **Ans. (c)** Pancreatic secretions
Ref: Guyton and Hall 10/e p746

137. **Ans. (b)** Distension of stomach
Ref: Guyton and Hall 10/e p732

138. **Ans. (c)** Secretin
Ref: Sembulingam 6/e p236

139. **Ans. (b)** Distension of stomach
Ref: Guyton and Hall 10/e p732

140. **Ans. (d)** Gamma-globulin
Ref: Ganong 20/e p522

141. **Ans. (d)** Intestine
Ref: Sembulingam 6/e p254

142. **Ans. (a)** Trypsin
Ref: Sembulingam 6/e p245

143. **Ans. (d)** Ligation of all major arteries
Ref: Internet resources

144. **Ans. (d)** Mass peristalsis
Ref: Guyton and Hall 10/e p736

145. **Ans. (c)** Increased release of insulin
Ref: Internet resources

146. **Ans. (c)** Potassium
Ref: Guyton and Hall 10/e p743

147. **Ans. (d)** Stimulation of appetite
Ref: Sembulingam 6/e p286

148. **Ans. (c)** Descending colon
Ref: Internet resources

149. **Ans. (d)** Cl^-
Ref: Ganong 20/e p477

150. **Ans. (b)** Ileum
Ref: Ganong 20/e p462

151. **Ans. (b)** 500-1000
Ref: Sembulingam 6/e p252

152. **Ans. (c) Monosaccharide**
Ref: Guyton and Hall 10/e p755

153. **Ans. (d) Gastrin**
Ref: Guyton and Hall 10/e p732

154. **Ans. (b) Reduces gastric acid secretion**
Ref: Sembulingam 6/e p282

155. **Ans. (a) Vitamin B_{12}**
Ref: Internet resources

156. **Ans. (c) Vitamin K**
Ref: Guyton and Hall 10/e p812

157. **Ans. (b) Less water in gallbladder bile**
Ref: Sembulingam 6/e p252

158. **Ans. (b) 12 hours**
Ref: Internet resources

159. **Ans. (d) Duodenum + Jejunum**
Ref: Guyton and Hall 10/e p388

160. **Ans. (d) Colon**
Ref: Guyton and Hall 10/e p735

NERVOUS SYSTEM

161. **Ans. (b) Sympathetic system**
Ref: Sembulingam's Physiology, 6/e p955

162. **Ans. (d) Bipolar cells**
Ref: Sembulingam's Physiology, 6/e p885

163. **Ans. (a) Medial geniculate body**
Ref: Sembulingam 6/e p1014

164. **Ans. (b) Thermoregulatory centre to shift to new level**
Ref: Guyton and Hall 10/e p830

165. **Ans. (b) Increase in heart rate with exercise**
Ref: Sembulingam 6/e p858

166. **Ans. (c) Pain sensation on opposite side**
Ref: Sembulingam 6/e p808

167. **Ans. (c) Noradrenaline**
Ref: Guyton and Hall 10/e p821

168. **Ans. (a) Proprioception**
Ref: Sembulingam 6/e p823

169. **Ans. (a) REM sleep**
Ref: Sembulingam 6/e p932

170. **Ans. (c) Ventro-medial nucleus**
Ref: Sembulingam 6/e p856

171. **Ans. (d) Area postrema**
Ref: Guyton and Hall 10/e p768

172. **Ans. (d) Lateral hypothalamus**
Ref: Sembulingam 6/e p856

173. **Ans. (d) Proprioception**
Ref: Sembulingam 6/e p810

174. **Ans. (c) Spinal cord**
Ref: Guyton and Hall 10/e p630

175. **Ans. (d) Pain**
Ref: Sembulingam 6/e p824

176. **Ans. (d) Glutamate**
Ref: Sembulingam 6/e p788

177. **Ans. (b) Norepinephrine**
Ref: Guyton and Hall 10/e p821

178. **Ans. (c) Optic disc**
Ref: Sembulingam 6/e p971

179. **Ans. (d) UMN features opposite half of the body**
Ref: Sembulingam 6/e p816

180. **Ans. (c) Law of projection**
Ref: Internet resources

181. **Ans. (d) Hypothalamus**
Ref: Guyton and Hall 10/e p826

182. **Ans. (b) Kupffer cells**
Ref: Sembulingam 6/e p774

183. **Ans. (d) Suprachiasmatic nuclei**
Ref: Guyton and Hall 10/e p690

184. **Ans. (c) Light reflex**
Ref: Sembulingam 6/e p995

185. **Ans. (d) Motor planning**
Ref: Sembulingam 6/e p864

186. **Ans. (c) Proprioception**
Ref: Internet resources

187. **Ans. (b) Folate**
Ref: Ganong 20/e p305t

188. **Ans. (c) Threshold for arousal by sensory stimuli is lowered**
Ref: Ganong 20/e p190, 194

189. **Ans. (a) Occlusion of middle cerebral artery**
Ref: Sembulingam 6/e p837

190. **Ans. (b) Gray matter of spinal cord**
Ref: Sembulingam 6/e p784

191. **Ans. (d) Lateral corticospinal tract**
Ref: Sembulingam 6/e p815

192. **Ans. (c) Retina**
Ref: Guyton and Hall 10/e p582

193. **Ans. (a) Amacrine cells**
Ref: Sembulingam 6/e p970

194. **Ans. (d) Ventromedial nucleus**
Ref: Guyton and Hall 10/e p683f

195. **Ans. (b) Posterior hypothalamus**
Ref: Guyton and Hall 10/e p683

196. **Ans. (a) Amplitude of 5-10 microvolts**
Ref: Sembulingam 6/e p930

197. **Ans. (a) Vitamin B_1**
Ref: Guyton and Hall 10/e p810

198. **Ans. (b) Anterior horn cells**
Ref: Internet resources

199. **Ans. (c) Crude touch**
Ref: Sembulingam 6/e p807

200. **Ans. (a) Frequency of action potential**
Ref: Internet resources

201. **Ans. (d) Sympathetic cholinergic**
Ref: Sembulingam 6/e p956

202. **Ans. (b) Lateral hypothalamus**
Ref: Sembulingam 6/e p861

203. **Ans. (c) Hypothalamus**
Ref: Guyton and Hall 10/e p807

204. **Ans. (c) Dopamine**
Ref: Sembulingam 6/e p881

205. **Ans. (a) Chorea**
Ref: Sembulingam 6/e p879

206. **Ans. (d) Denervated muscular EMG**
Ref: Sembulingam 6/e p836

207. **Ans. (d) Cerebellum**
Ref: Guyton and Hall 10/e p655

208. **Ans. (b) Dopamine**
Ref: Guyton and Hall 10/e p680

209. **Ans. (c) Folic acid**
Ref: Internet resources

210. **Ans. (c) Noradrenaline**
Ref: Guyton and Hall 10/e p821

211. **Ans. (a) A-delta nerve fibres**
Ref: Sembulingam 6/e p841

212. **Ans. (b) Axodendritic**
Ref: Sembulingam 6/e p781

213. **Ans. (c) Microelectrode**
Ref: Internet resources

214. **Ans. (b) Gamma**
Ref: Sembulingam 6/e p909

215. **Ans. (b) Muscle tension**
Ref: Guyton and Hall 10/e p628

216. **Ans. (b) Increased permeability to potassium**
Ref: Sembulingam 6/e p767

217. **Ans. (c) C**
Ref: Ganong 20/e p59

218. **Ans. (c) Golgi tendon**
Ref: Sembulingam 6/e p911

219. **Ans. (d) C-fibre**
Ref: Sembulingam 6/e p765

220. **Ans. (c) Potassium ion**
Ref: Sembulingam 6/e p190

221. **Ans. (a) Sodium ion**
Ref: Guyton and Hall 10/e p56

222. **Ans. (d) Neurapraxia**
Ref: Internet resources

223. **Ans. (d) Chemical mediator is localized only in the presynaptic terminal**
Ref: Sembulingam 6/e p781

224. **Ans. (b) Potassium ions**
Ref: Sembulingam 6/e p191

225. **Ans. (c) Action potential**
Ref: Sembulingam 6/e p530

226. **Ans. (c) Nerve conduction study**
Ref: Sembulingam 6/e p210

RESPIRATORY SYSTEM

227. **Ans. (d) Carbon monoxide**
Ref: Ganong's Physiology, 23rd ed., p-621

228. **Ans. (c) Increased RBC/Hemoglobin**
Ref: Sembulingam's Physiology, 6/e p737

229. **Ans. (b) Carbonic anhydrase**
Ref: Sembulingam's Physiology, 6/e p715

230. **Ans. (c) Beta2 adrenergic**
Ref: Sembulingam's Physiology, 6/e p675

231. **Ans. (d) Anemia hypoxia**
Ref: Sembulingam 6/e p727

232. **Ans. (b) Forms blood-air barrier**
Ref: Guyton and Hall 10/e p434

233. **Ans. (a) Inspiratory capacity minus the inspiratory reserve volume**
Ref: Sembulingam 6/e p693

234. **Ans. (c) Hypercapnia**
Ref: Sembulingam 6/e p722

235. **Ans. (d) Oxygen affinity for hemoglobin**
Ref: Sembulingam 6/e p712

236. **Ans. (a) 1:1**
Ref: Guyton and Hall 10/e p439

237. **Ans. (a) 0.5 L**
Ref: Sembulingam 6/e p691

238. **Ans. (a) Anemia**
Ref: Sembulingam 6/e p713

239. **Ans. (d) All of the above**
Ref: Sembulingam 6/e p714

240. **Ans. (a) Type II pneumocytes**
Ref: Guyton and Hall 10/e p434

241. **Ans. (a) Oxygen dissociation curve shift to left**
Ref: Guyton and Hall 10/e p468

242. **Ans. (d) None of the above**
Ref: Guyton and Hall 10/e p437

243. **Ans. (a) Residual volume and expiratory reserve volume**
Ref: Guyton and Hall 10/e p437

244. **Ans. (d) Histotoxic hypoxia**
Ref: Guyton and Hall 10/e p491

245. **Ans. (d) Forms air-blood barrier**
Ref: Guyton and Hall 10/e p434

246. **Ans. (d) pO_2 is less**
Ref: Sembulingam 6/e p738

247. **Ans. (c) Hypercapnia**
Ref: Ganong 20/e p654

248. **Ans. (a) Protects against under-inflation of lungs**
Ref: Sembulingam 6/e p719

249. **Ans. (d) Hypoventilation**
Ref: Ganong 20/e p664

250. **Ans. (d) Shift in the oxygen dissociation curve to the left**
Ref: Ganong 20/e p663

251. **Ans. (c) Prevents collapse of alveoli**
Ref: Guyton and Hall 10/e p435

252. **Ans. (c) Decreased $PaCO_2$**
Ref: Guyton and Hall 10/e p468

253. **Ans. (c) Left**
Ref: Guyton and Hall 10/e p947

254. **Ans. (a) Decreased depth of respiration**
Ref: Sembulingam 6/e p717

255. **Ans. (c) 1/3rd of tidal volume**
Ref: Guyton and Hall 10/e p437, 439

256. **Ans. (d) Difference between pressure in alveoli and intra-pleural pressure**
Ref: Sembulingam 6/e p686

257. **Ans. (b) Type II alveolar cells**
Ref: Ganong 20/e p634

258. **Ans. (c) Lower pons**
Ref: Internet resources

259. **Ans. (b) Increased arterial CO_2**
Ref: Guyton and Hall 10/e p478

260. **Ans. (c) Prolonged inspiratory spasms**
Ref: Internet resources

261. **Ans. (b) Minute respiratory volume**
Ref: Guyton and Hall 10/e p438

262. **Ans. (b) Bronchodilation**
Ref: Guyton and Hall 10/e p440

263. **Ans. (b) 45**
Ref: Sembulingam 6/e p708

264. **Ans. (b) 150 ml**
Ref: Guyton and Hall 10/e p439

265. **Ans. (d) Bohr effect**
Ref: Ganong/ 20th/ 645

266. **Ans. (b) Pneumotaxic centre**
Ref: Sembulingam 6/e p717

267. **Ans. (b) O_2 delivery to tissues**
Ref: Guyton and Hall 10/e p468

268. **Ans. (c) V/Q remain same at both apex and base**
Ref: Sembulingam 6/e p680

269. **Ans. (a)** Type II pneumocytes
Ref: Guyton and Hall 10/e p434

270. **Ans. (a)** Oxygen dissociation curve shifts to left
Ref: Guyton and Hall 10/e p468

REPRODUCTIVE SYSTEM

271. **Ans. (b)** Occurs in epididymis
Ref: Guyton & Hall's Physiology, South Asian ed., p-627

272. **Ans. (a)** FSH
Ref: Sembulingam 6/e p479

273. **Ans. (c)** Reduction in motility of sperms
Ref: Internet resources

274. **Ans. (b)** 14 days-9 weeks of gestation
Ref: Internet resources

275. **Ans. (d)** LH
Ref: Sembulingam 6/e p489

276. **Ans. (b)** Ampulla
Ref: Guyton and Hall 10/e p944

277. **Ans. (c)** Epididymis
Ref: Sembulingam 6/e p471

278. **Ans. (c)** Syncytiotrophoblast
Ref: Guyton and Hall 10/e p948

279. **Ans. (a)** Before ovulation
Ref: Ganong 20/e p426

280. **Ans. (a)** 1-3 mm/day
Ref: Ganong 20/e p413

281. **Ans. (b)** Sertoli cells
Ref: Ganong 20/e p412

282. **Ans. (b)** Vas deferens
Ref: AK Jain/ 1st / 767

283. **Ans. (b)** Testosterone
Ref: Sembulingam 6/e p465

284. **Ans. (a)** 3-4 days
Ref: Guyton and Hall 10/e p945

285. **Ans. (a)** FSH
Ref: Guyton and Hall 10/e p940

286. **Ans. (c)** Secretory effect on endometrium
Ref: Guyton and Hall 10/e p936

287. **Ans. (b)** Stores sperms
Ref: Guyton and Hall 10/e p918

288. **Ans. (d)** Oxytocin
Ref: Sembulingam 6/e p460

289. **Ans. (b)** Dilatation of arterioles
Ref: Ganong/ 20th/ 414

MUSCLE PHYSIOLOGY

290. **Ans. (d)** Tropomyosin
Ref: Sembulingam 6/e p173

291. **Ans. (b)** Fasciculation
Ref: Guyton and Hall 10/e p75

292. **Ans. (d)** Sarcomere
Ref: Sembulingam 6/e p171

293. **Ans. (d)** Shortening of H and I bands
Ref: Sembulingam 6/e p172

294. **Ans. (b)** Increased sensitivity to chemical mediators
Ref: Sembulingam 6/e p771

295. **Ans. (a)** Strong stimulus
Ref: Internet resources

296. **Ans. (b)** Rheobase
Ref: Sembulingam 6/e p177

297. **Ans. (d)** H band
Ref: Guyton and Hall 10/e p68f

298. **Ans. (d)** Threshold stimulus is required
Ref: Guyton and Hall 10/e p64

299. **Ans. (c)** Tropomyosin
Ref: Guyton and Hall 10/e p71

300. **Ans. (b)** Nerve fibre
Ref: Internet resources

301. **Ans. (a)** Cardiac muscle
Ref: Internet resources

302. **Ans. (d)** Calcium entry
Ref: Sembulingam 6/e p195

303. **Ans. (b)** Titin
Ref: Ganong/ 20th/ 64

GENERAL PHYSIOLOGY

304. **Ans. (b)** 2:1
Ref: Sembulingam 6/e p4

305. **Ans. (c)** Cardiac muscle cell
Ref: Internet resources

306. **Ans. (b) Rough endoplasmic reticulum**
Ref: Sembulingam 6/e p7

307. **Ans. (b) Nucleolus**
Ref: Sembulingam 6/e p7 (Box 1.1)

308. **Ans. (d) Actin**
Ref: Guyton and Hall 10/e p21

309. **Ans. (c) Closed circular**
Ref: Sembulingam 6/e p11

310. **Ans. (d) Transferrin**
Ref: Sembulingam 6/e p25

311. **Ans. (b) St. basale**
Ref: Sembulingam 6/e p352

MISCELLANEOUS

312. **Ans. (b) H**
Ref: Sembulingam's Physiology, 6/e p170

313. **Ans. (a) Potassium efflux**
Ref: Sembulingam's Physiology, 6/e p190

314. **Ans. (d) Argentaffin cells**
Ref: Internet resources

315. **Ans. (b) NO**
Ref: Guyton and Hall 10/e p179

316. **Ans. (b) 0.8**
Ref: Guyton and Hall 10/e p804

317. **Ans. (c) Fat**
Ref: Guyton and Hall 10/e p955

318. **Ans. (c) Meibomian gland**
Ref: Internet resources

319. **Ans. (b) 10:18**
Ref: Internet resources

320. **Ans. (a) 1 litre/hour**
Ref: Guyton and Hall/ 10th/826

PRACTICE QUESTIONS

BLOOD

1. **If both mother and father are Rh-ve then:**
   a. All children will be Rh+ve
   b. All children will be Rh-ve
   c. 50% children will be Rh-ve
   d. 25% children will be Rh-ve
2. **Oxygen carrying capacity of haemoglobin is:**
   a. 1.24 mL/g b. 1.34 mL/g
   c. 1.44 mL/g d. 1.54 mL/g
3. **FALSE for fetal hemoglobin:**
   a. Adult haemoglobin is replaced by fetal haemoglobin by 10-12th weeks of life
   b. Alpha2, epsilon2
   c. Shifts the oxygen dissociation curve to right
   d. Functionally different from adult hemoglobin

CIRCULATORY

4. **Capacitance vessels are:**
   a. Arteries b. Venules
   c. Capillaries d. Arterioles
5. **3rd heart sound is heard in:**
   a. Isometric contraction phase
   b. Rapid filling phase
   c. Atrial systole
   d. Isometric relaxation
6. **A subject changed his position from lying down to standing erect. What will be the effect on BP of this postural change:**
   a. No change b. BP will increase
   c. BP will decrease d. Variable
7. **Total cross-sectional area is maximum for:**
   a. Artery b. Arteriole
   c. Veins d. Capillaries
8. **Continuous murmur is heard in:**
   a. Mitral stenosis
   b. Aortic stenosis
   c. Patent ductus arteriosus
   d. Coarctation of aorta
9. **Cut-off value of systolic BP for hypertension:**
   a. >140 b. >150
   c. >160 d. >170
10. **Event at the end of isovolumetric relaxation:**
    a. Closure of AV valves
    b. Closure of semilunar valves
    c. Opening of AV valves
    d. Opening of semilunar valves

ENDOCRINO

11. **FALSE regarding insulin:**
    a. Increased glycogenesis
    b. Increased protein synthesis
    c. Increased lipogenesis d. Increased ketogenesis
12. **Which type of GLUT receptors are present on adipose cells?**
    a. GLUT I b. GLUT II
    c. GLUT III d. GLUT IV
13. **GH formation is promoted by which of the following:**
    a. Cortisol b. REM phase of sleep
    c. Glucose d. Glucagon
14. **Which of the following does NOT stimulate prolactin secretion?**
    a. Dopamine b. Sleep
    c. Estrogen d. Pregnancy
15. **Conversion of 25-dihydroxycholecalciferol to 1,25-dihydroxycholecalciferol occurs in:**
    a. Skin b. Lung
    c. Liver d. Kidney
16. **Cortisol is produced in:**
    a. Zona glomerulosa b. Zona reticularis
    c. Zona fasciculata d. Adrenal medulla
17. **Which substance maintains potassium balance in the body?**
    a. Cortisol b. Renin
    c. Aldosterone d. Rennin
18. **Insulin action involves activation of:**
    a. Nuclear receptors b. Protein kinase
    c. Calmodulin d. Inositol triphosphate

EXCRETORY

19. **Bicarbonate is MC absorbed from:**
    a. DCT
    b. Collecting duct
    c. PCT
    d. Ascending loop of Henle

Ans. 1. **b.** All childrens... 2. **b.** 1.34 mL/g 3. **b.** Alpha2, epsilon2 4. **b.** Venules
5. **b.** Rapid filling... 6. **b.** BP will increase 7. **d.** Capillaries 8. **c.** Patent ductus arteriosus
9. **b.** >150 10. **c.** Opening of AV valves 11. **d.** Increased... 12. **d.** GLUT IV
13. **d.** Glucagon 14. **a.** Dopamine 15. **d.** Kidney 16. **c.** Zona fasciculata
17. **c.** Aldosterone 18. **b.** Protein kinase 19. **c.** PCT

20. **Which of the following is important for maintenance of osmotic gradient in renal calyx?**
 a. Water
 b. Sodium
 c. Bicarbonate
 d. Ammonia

21. **Which of the following regulates Renin-Aldosterone-Angiotensin system mechanism?**
 a. Losartan
 b. Alpha blockers
 c. Aldosterone antagonists
 d. Sodium potassium antagonist

22. **Which of the following is FALSE regarding GFR?**
 a. Fall in GFR by 30-40% after the age of 70 years
 b. GFR is best estimated by creatinine clearance
 c. GFR has no effect on urine formation
 d. In children, GFR depends on height

GIT

23. **Which of the following is LEAST concerned with digestion of carbohydrates?**
 a. Small intestine
 b. Pancreas
 c. Stomach
 d. Mouth

24. **Which stimuli helps in secretion of gastric acid?**
 a. Secretin
 b. Somatostatin
 c. Vagus
 d. VIP

25. **Parietal cell secretes:**
 a. Renin
 b. Mucin
 c. Histamine
 d. Intrinsic factor of Castle

26. **Which is WRONG for iron absorption?**
 a. Absorbed in ferrous form
 b. 1 glass milk contains sufficient quantity of milk needed per day
 c. HCl needed for absorption
 d. Absorbed from small intestine

27. **Carbohydrates are absorbed from GIT in the form of:**
 a. Disaccharide
 b. Monosaccharide
 c. Polysaccharide
 d. Lactose

28. **Substance necessary to absorb iron from intestine:**
 a. Tannic acid
 b. Bile
 c. Phytates
 d. Vitamin C

29. **Factor responsible for absorption of fat soluble vitamin:**
 a. Pancreatic amylase
 b. Pancreatic lipase
 c. Chymotrypsin
 d. Trypsin

NERVOUS SYSTEM

30. **Dopamine is NOT secreted from:**
 a. Basal ganglia
 b. Hypothalamus
 c. Thalamus
 d. Retina

31. **Which of the following is the fastest conducting nerve fibre?**
 a. A-Alpha
 b. A-Beta
 c. A-Gamma
 d. A-Delta

32. **Bruxism is seen in which phase of NREM sleep:**
 a. I
 b. II
 c. III
 d. IV

33. **Which of the following is NOT a part of basal ganglia?**
 a. Caudate nucleus
 b. Thalamus
 c. Globus pallidus
 d. Putamen

34. **Which phase of NREM sleep is of longest duration:**
 a. I
 b. II
 c. III
 d. IV

35. **A coneurotransmitter at presynaptic region:**
 a. ATP
 b. Epinephrine
 c. Norepinephrine
 d. Acetylcholine

36. **Tickling and itching sensation is carried by which pathway?**
 a. Lateral spinothalamic tract
 b. Anterior spinothalamic tract
 c. Dorsal column
 d. Anterior horn cells

Ans. 20. **b.** Sodium 21. **a.** Losartan 22. **c.** GFR has no effect... 23. **c.** Stomach 24. **c.** Vagus 25. **d.** Intrinsic factor... 26. **b.** 1 glass milk contains... 27. **b.** Monosaccharide 28. **b.** Bile 29. **a.** Pancreatic amylase 30. **c.** Thalamus 31. **a.** A-Alpha 32. **d.** IV 33. **b.** Thalamus 34. **b.** II 35. **d.** Acetylcholine 36. **c.** Dorsal column

RESPIRATORY SYSTEM

37. Lung surfactant is chemically:
a. Glycoprotein
b. Proteoglycans
c. Lipopolysaccharide
d. Phospholipids

38. Exchange of gases between lung capillaries and alveoli is which type of transport:
a. Facilitated diffusion
b. Passive diffusion
c. Filtration
d. Active transport

39. Protective reflex which prevents over-inflation of lungs:
a. Chemoreceptor reflex
b. Hering-Breuer reflex
c. Baroreflex
d. Juxtacapillary reflex

REPRODUCTIVE

40. Which hormone is responsible for initiation of spermatogenesis?
a. LH
b. FSH
c. GH
d. ACTH

MISCELLANEOUS

41. Glucose is transported along with:
a. Potassium
b. Magnesium
c. Sodium
d. Manganese

42. Which is more abundant in microfilament:
a. Myosin
b. Actin
c. Tubulin
d. Keratin

43. LEAST sodium content is in:
a. Sweat
b. Saliva
c. Urine
d. Stool

Ans. **37. d.** Phospholipids **38. b.** Passive diffusion **39. b.** Hering-Breuer reflux **40. b.** FSH
41. c. Sodium **42. b.** Actin **43. d.** Stool

IMAGE-BASED QUESTIONS

1. **Study the action potential of a ventricular muscle. Phase marked 3 is because of:**

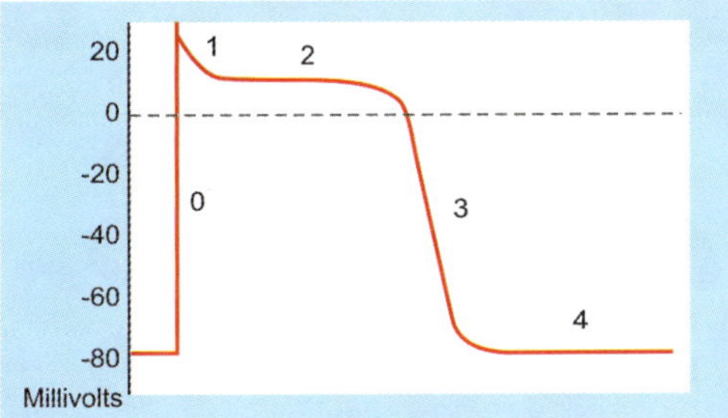

a. Efflux of potassium ions
b. Slow opening of calcium channels
c. Fast opening of calcium channels
d. Rapid influx of sodium ions

Phase marked 3 is final repolarization phase which is due to efflux of potassium ions.

2. **Study the tracts of spinal cord. Sensation carried by tract marked as 1:**

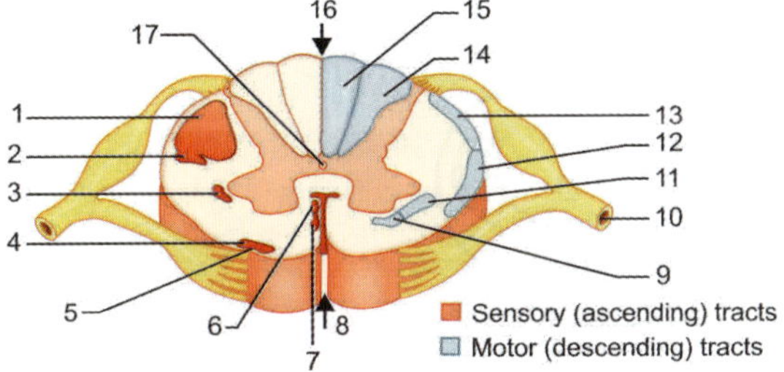

a. Subconscious kinaesthetic sensations
b. Crude touch
c. Proprioception
d. Pain and temperature

Tract marked as 1 is lateral spinothalamic tract, which carries pain and temperature sensations.

3. **Study the image of hypothalamo-hypophyseal tract. Identify structure 2:**

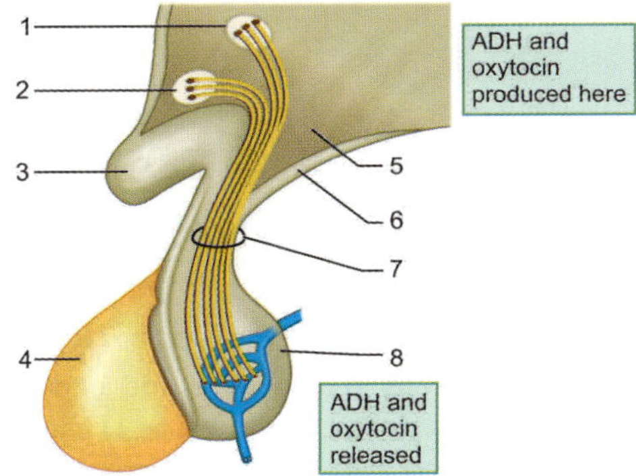

a. Paraventricular nuclei
b. Suprachiasmatic nuclei
c. Supraoptic nuclei
d. Mammillary body

Structure labelled as 2 is supraoptic nuclei.

4. **Study the following image of events in cardiac cycle. Duration of phase N is:**

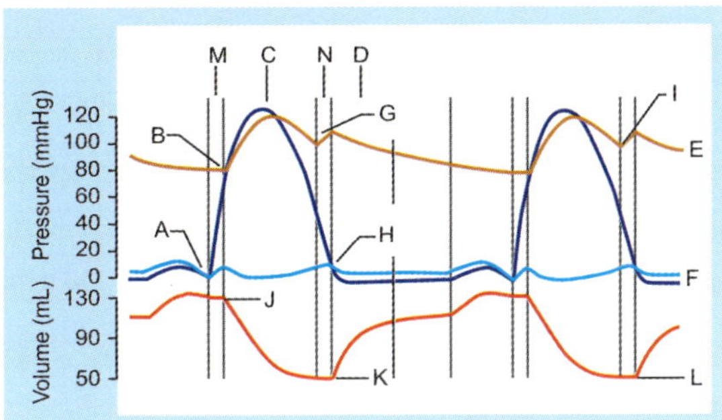

a. 0.04 sec
b. 0.08 sec
c. 0.12 sec
d. 0.16 sec

Phase N is protodiastole, which lasts for 0.04 seconds.

5. **Study the following image. This illustrates what type of transport?**

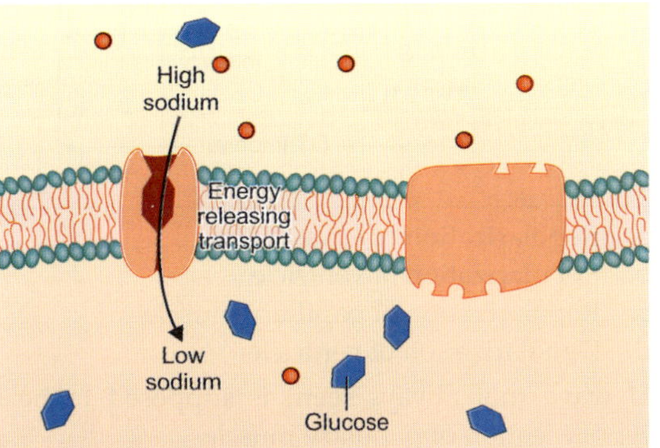

a. Primary active transport
b. Primary passive transport
c. Secondary active transport
d. Secondary passive transport

Sodium cotransport is an example of secondary active transport, the energy for movement of sodium is obtained by breakdown of ATP.

6. **Study the following image. Which type of haemoglobin is formed because of mutation:**

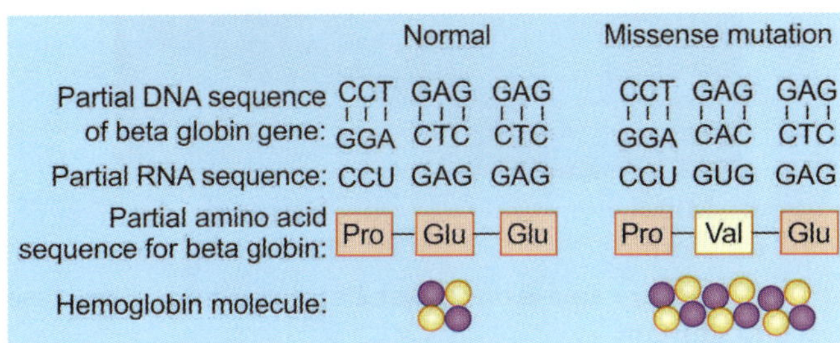

a. HbF
b. COHb
c. HbS
d. HbA2

The image shows replacement of glutamate by valine at beta-6 resulting in formation of HbS (sickle cell anemia).

7. Study the ECG. Wave U is formed because of:

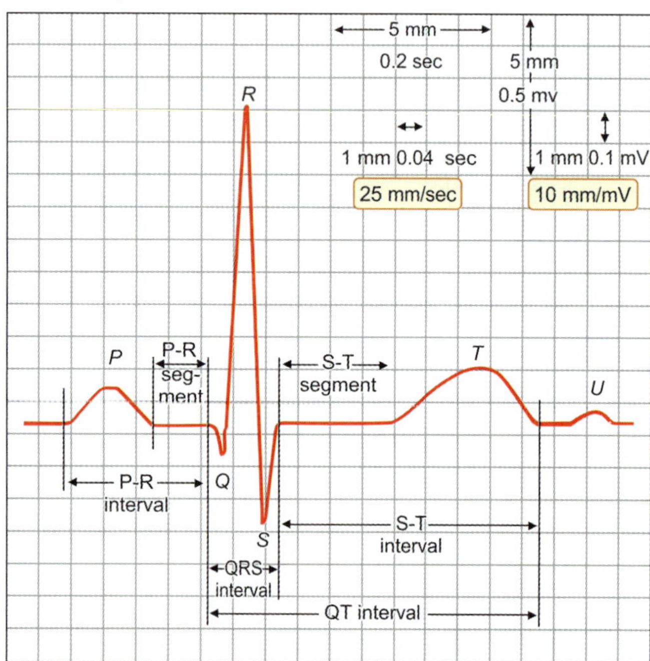

a. Repolarization of atria
b. Repolarization of ventricle
c. Repolarization of papillary muscle
d. Depolarization of ventricle

U wave (not always seen) is supposed to be due to repolarization of papillary muscle.

8. Study the image. Which valvular area is being auscultated?

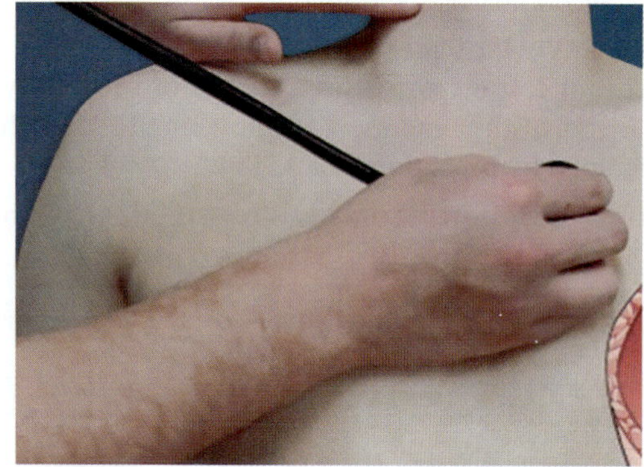

a. Mitral
b. Tricuspid
c. Aortic
d. Pulmonary

Pulmonary area is on the left 2nd intercostals space, close to sternum.

9. Study the peripheral smear. Cells marked as 'd' are decreased in which conditions:

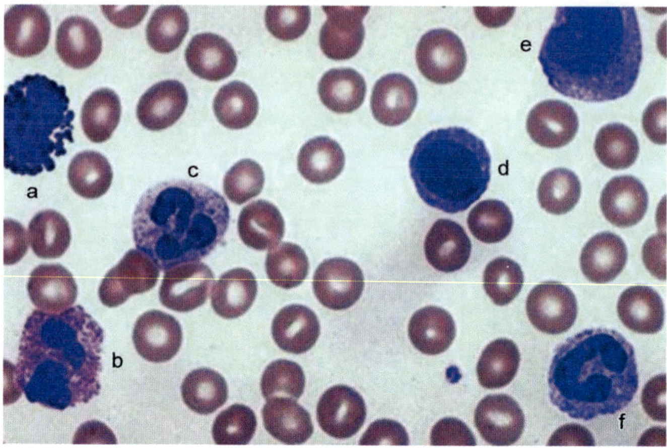

a. AIDS
b. Diphtheria
c. TB
d. Syphilis

Cells marked as 'd' are lymphocytes (clear cytoplasm and nucleus occupying whole of cytoplasm). They are decreased in AIDS, Hodgkins, etc.

10. Study the histological slide of kidney. Area marked as 1 is:

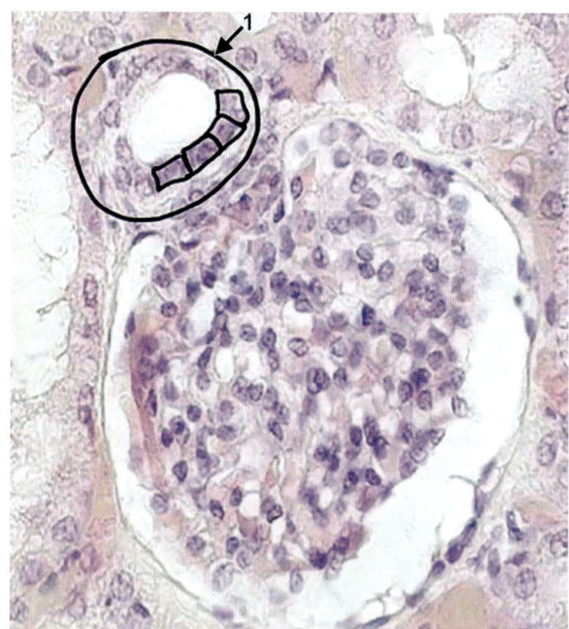

a. Glomerulus
b. PCT
c. DCT
d. Thick ascending segment of loop of Henle

Macula densa (cells redrawn) is the end portion of thick ascending segment (encircled as 1) before it opens into DCT, situated between the afferent and efferent arterioles of the same nephron. It is very close to afferent arteriole.

MCQ POINTS

S. No.	Question statements	Answers
1.	Gatekeeper of the heart is	***AV node***
2.	SA node acts as a pacemaker of the heart because of the fact that it	***It generates impulses at fastest rate***
3.	Einthoven's triangle, what is the value of lead III when lead I = 2 mV and Lead II = 1 mV	***Lead I + Lead III = Lead II***
4.	What is Einthoven's law?	***Lead I + Lead III = Lead II***
5.	QRS complex indicates which process of cardiac cycle	***Ventricular depolarization***
6.	What is the order of activation after stimulation of Purkinje fibres	***Endocardium to epicardium***
7.	During the cardiac cycle, the opening of the aortic valve takes place at the end of	***Isometric ventricular contraction***
8.	Which valvular event occurs at the end of isometric relaxation phase	***Opening of AV valves***
9.	Isometric relaxation is defined as	***Relaxation of ventricle with both AV and semilunar valves closed***
10.	Preload leads to	***Ventricular systole***
11.	Duration of second heart sound is	***0.12 sec***
12.	S_3 is produced due to	***Ventricular wall turbulence due to mid dia-stolic filling***
13.	Cardiac output (L/min)/heart rate is equal to	***Stroke volume***
14.	Ejection fraction is calculated as	***Stroke volume/end diastolic volume***
15.	Normal value of cardiac index is (L/min/m^2)	***3.2***
16.	What happens to cardiac output when a subject stands up from lying position	***Decreased venous return will result in decreased end diastolic volume and a re-duction in cardiac output***
17.	Effect of increased blood volume on preload	***Increase in preload***
18.	Increased VR leads to increased CO. This is which law	***Frank starlings law***
19.	Mean arterial BP is calculated as	***1/3 (pulse pressure) + diastolic blood pressure***
20.	Mean arterial pressure is calculated as	***Mean arterial pressure depends on car-diac output and peripheral resistance***
21.	SI unit for measuring BP is	***kPa***
22.	During diastole, the arterial pressure is maintained by	***Elastic recoil of aorta***
23.	BP measured by a sphygmomanometer is ...... than the intra-arterial pressure	***More***
24.	Basis of Korotkoff's sound	***Turbulent blood flow in artery***
25.	Effect of vagal stimulation on R-R interval	***Increased***
26.	Effect of parasympathetic denervation on heart	***Increase in heart rate***
27.	Single most important factor which controls myocardial contractility	***Sympathetic control***
28.	Effect of inhibition of vasomotor centre on BP	***Decrease***
29.	Effect of Clamping of the carotid arteries above/distal the carotid sinus, on BP	***Occlusion of common carotid artery on both sides above the carotid sinus will lead to decrease in heart rate and BP***
30.	When a person changes position from standing to lying down, what happens to venous return	***Increase in venous return***
31.	Baroreceptor reflex causes a .... in HR when BP increases	***Decrease***
32.	Second messenger for Nitric oxide	***cGMP***
33.	NO is synthesized from	***Arginine***
34.	Vasodilatation produced by CO_2 is maximum in which organ	***Brain***
35.	Relationship of diameter of vessel with turbulence of blood flow	***Indirect (more the diameter, less will be the turbulence)***
36.	Main site of peripheral vascular resistance	***Arterioles***

S. No.	Question statements	Answers
37.	Windkessel effect is seen in	***Elastic arteries***
38.	In which part of vessels, velocity of blood is maximum	***Elastic arteries***
39.	Distribution of blood flow is mainly regulated by which vessels	***Arterioles***
40.	Microcirculation consist of which vessels	***Arteriole + capillaries + venules***
41.	Capillaries contains ..... % of total blood volume	***5%***
42.	.... in hydrostatic pressure of capillaries favours filtration at the arteriolar end of capillary bed	***Increase***
43.	Which vessels are maximum reservoir of blood	***Veins***
44.	Arterioles are also known as .... vessels	***Resistance***
45.	Perfusion pressure is calculated as	***Difference in pressure on the arterial and venular end of capillaries***
46.	Blood supply to brain is	***55 ml/100 m/minute***
47.	Effect of hypoxia on pulmonary circulation	***Vasoconstriction***
48.	Blood in splanchnic circulation is decreased during exercise because of	***Venoconstriction***
49.	Lewis triple response is mediated by which hormone	***Histamine***
50.	Flare in triple response is mediated by	***Axon reflex***
51.	Regulation of coronary circulation is by	***Autoregulation***
52.	Orthopnoea in heart failure develops due to reservoir function of	***Large veins of leg***
53.	Site of RBC production in a 20-year-old healthy male	***Flat bones***
54.	Type of hemoglobin which has LEAST affinity for 2, 3 DPG	***HbF (fetal)***
55.	2nd MC hemoglobin in adults is written as $alpha_2$ and $...._2$	***Alpha2, delta2***
56.	Heme is converted to bilirubin mainly in which organ	***Spleen***
57.	Metalloporphyrins help in jaundice by what mechanism	***Inhibiting heme oxygenase***
58.	Proteins which prevent loss of hemoglobin from plasma	***Hemopexin***
59.	G-CSF and GM-CSF in haematopoiesis will result in production of which blood cells	***WBC***
60.	Vitamin K dependent clotting factors	***II, VII, IX and X***
61.	Prothrombin is clotting factor number	***Factor II***
62.	Fibrinogen to fibrin conversion is catalyzed by	***Thrombin***
63.	Which clotting factor helps in bridging the fibrin in a clot and stabilizes the clot	***Factor XIII***
64.	The blood in the vessels normally does not clot because the vascular endothelium is lined by	***Glycocalyx***
65.	Thromboxane A_2 is produced mainly by	***Platelets***
66.	Thrombosthenin is a contractile protein found in which blood cells	***Platelets***
67.	von-Willebrand factor is produced by	***Endothelial cells***
68.	Absolute refractory period of heart is the gap of time in which	***Heart does not respond to any strength of stimulus***
69.	At what stage of erythropoiesis, does hemoglobin appear	***Intermediate normoblast***
70.	Earliest change in iron deficiency anemia	***Decrease serum ferritin***
71.	Left ventricular failure is indicated if pulmonary artery wedge pressure is more than .... mm Hg	***25 mm Hg***
72.	The coronary artery most commonly involved in atherosclerosis is	***Left anterior descending***
73.	Normal blood pH is	***7.4***
74.	Half life of transfused platelets is	***3-6 days***
75.	P-R interval in ECG corresponds to	***Beginning of atrial depolarization to beginning of ventricular depolarization***
76.	The first reactionary change to occur after hemorrhage is	***Vasoconstriction***
77.	Normal hepatic blood flow per minute is	***50 cc/100 gm of liver tissue***
78.	Arterial oxygen content is reduced in which type of hypoxia	***Anemic***

S. No.	Question statements	Answers
79.	Distribution of blood flow is mainly regulated by which vessels	***Arterioles***
80.	Fetal hemoglobin has higher affinity for oxygen due to decreased	***2, 3 DPG***
81.	ECG changes in hyperkalemia	***Tall tented T waves***
82.	Which is a potent stimulus for the production of erythropoietin	***Hypoxia***
83.	Mean life of RBCs in transfused blood is	***60 days***
84.	Normal QRS interval is	***0.12 sec***
85.	Liver has maximum oxygen consumption. The next organ to have the maximum oxygen consumption is	***Skeletal muscle***
86.	Effect of a decrease in the velocity of impulse conduction through the AV node, on PQ interval	***Increase PQ interval***
87.	Arneth count is	***Counting lobes of neutrophils***
88.	Preservative used for storing blood for transfusion is	***CDP-A***
89.	Relationship of myocardial oxygen demand with heart rate	***Direct relationship (more the heart rate, more the oxygen demand)***
90.	Conduction velocity is LEAST in	***AV node***
91.	Under normal resting condition, the cardiac output is	***5.25 L/min***
92.	Which one of the following is released by blood platelets during hemorrhage to produce vasoconstriction	***Serotonin***
93.	Macrophages are the mature form of	***Monocyte***
94.	First component of first heart sound is usually clearly heard on the ventral surface of chest at ...... intercostal space and to the .... of sternum	***5th intercostal space, left***
95.	The average coronary blood flow in human being at rest is .... % of the cardiac output	***4-5%***
96.	...... heart sound heard immediately before the first heart sound when atrial pressure is high	***Fourth***
97.	Coronary blood flow stops during the phase of	***Isometric contraction***
98.	Calculate the peripheral resistance if the CO is 5.4 L and the BP is 90 mm Hg	***16 (mean arterial pressure = CO × PR)***
99.	Ejection fraction of the ventricle refers to the ratio of	***Stroke volume/end diastolic volume***
100.	Arrange liver, kidney, brain and heart in descending order in terms of blood flow	***Liver, kidney, brain and heart***
101.	FSH level after menopause	***Increase***
102.	Oxytocin is secreted by	***Posterior pituitary (synthesized in hypothalamus)***
103.	Tapping of facial nerve results in contraction of facial muscles. This is which sign	***Chvostek sign***
104.	Effect of calcitonin on calcium metabolism	***Decrease serum calcium***
105.	Delta cells of pancreas secretes which hormone	***Somatostatin***
106.	Hormone not released in stressful conditions	***Insulin***
107.	Site of absorption of iron	***Duodenum***
108.	Effect of secretin	***Promotes secretion of alkaline, watery media from pancreas***
109.	Site of absorption of calcium	***Proximal intestine***
110.	Substance transported with sodium	***Glucose***
111.	Major part of glomerular filtrate is absorbed in	***Proximal convoluted tubule***
112.	Increase in temperature shifts the oxygen dissociation curve to	***Right***
113.	Which centre is present in dorsal pons	***Pneumotaxic centre***
114.	Pulmonary surfactant is produced by	***Type II pneumocytes***
115.	Amount of blood at the end of relaxation phase is known as	***End diastolic volume***
116.	Carbon dioxide is primarily transported in arterial blood as bicarbonate. Which enzyme is involved	***Carbonic anhydrase***
117.	Law of projection explains which phenomenon	***Phantom limb***
118.	Maturation of sperm takes place in	***Epididymis***

S. No.	Question statements	Answers
119.	Capacity of the sperm to fertilize ovum is known as	***Capacitation***
120.	Volume of blood ejected with each heart beat is known as	***Stroke volume***
121.	Inhibin is secreted by	***Sertoli cells***
122.	Active sites of actin are covered by tropomyosin. Which substance is necessary to remove it	***Calcium***
123.	Intracellular fluid is similar in composition to which inner ear fluid	***Endolymph***
124.	Power house of cells are	***Mitochondria***
125.	Function of microtubules	***Shape and motility***
126.	Size of action potential depends upon which ion	***Sodium***
127.	Repolarization of a nerve is due to which ion	***Potassium***
128.	Most abundant cation in intracellular fluid	***Potassium***
129.	Fertilization takes place in which part of fallopian tube	***Ampulla***
130.	Separation of 1st polar body occurs at the time of	***Ovulation***
131.	Milk ejection is controlled by	***Oxytocin***
132.	Ovulation is due to surge of	***LH***
133.	Gas, responsible for respiratory drive	CO_2
134.	Temperature regulation is done by	***Hypothalamus***
135.	Inhibitory post-synaptic potential is due to which ion:	***Chloride***
136.	Function of muscle spindle:	***Detects muscle length***
137.	Dreaming is commoner in which phase of sleep	***Rapid eye movement/REM***
138.	Neurotransmitter depleted in Parkinson's disease	***Dopamine***
139.	Law explaining phantom limb	***Law of projection***
140.	Action potential obeys which law	***All or none***
141.	Function of Kupffer cells in liver:	***Phagocytosis***
142.	Chymotrypsinogen is activated into chymotrypsin by	***Trypsin***
143.	Site of action of antidiuretic hormone/ADH	***Collecting duct and DCT***
144.	Normal GFR is … ml/min	***125 ml/min***
145.	Reabsorption of water is maximum in	***Proximal convoluted tubules***
146.	Effect of parathormone on calcium levels	***Increase in serum calcium***
147.	Aortic valve closure marks the beginning of which phase of cardiac cycle	***Isovolumic relaxation***
148.	QRS complex is due to which electrophysiological event	***Ventricular depolarization***
149.	1st heart sound is due to	***Closure of AV valves***
150.	Most useful parameter for estimating total iron content of blood	***Serum ferritin***

CHAPTER

3

BIOCHEMISTRY

KEY POINTS

Respiratory Quotient

- Carbohydrates: 1
- Protein: 0.8
- Fat: 0.7

Cells and Their Fuels

- Muscle cells: Can utilize glucose, fatty acids and ketone bodies
- Brain: Can utilize ketone bodies and glucose
- Hepatocytes: Cannot utilize ketone bodies (As it lack the enzyme necessary to convert acetoacetate to acetoacety CoA)

Must Know Facts

- Ubiquitin: Eukaryotic protein for degradation of intracellular proteins
- Chaperones: Proteins which play a role in the assembly or proper folding of other proteins without themselves being components of the latter.
- Shine-Dalgarno sequence: A polypurine sequence in bacterial m RNA, 7 nucleotides in front of initiation codon AUG. It is involved in binding of mRNA to ribosome, and hence initiation of protein synthesis.
- HbS: Substitution of glutamate by valine in B chain in the 6th position

Isoenzymes of Lactate Dehydrogenase

- LDH1: Heart and RBC
- LDH2: Heart and RBC
- LDH3: Brain and kidney
- LDH4: Liver and skeletal muscle
- LDH5: Skeletal muscle and liver

Types of Enzyme Inhibition

- Uncompetitive inhibition: Inhibitor doesn't bind with enzyme, but only binds with the enzyme-substrate complex
- Competitive inhibition: Inhibitor competes with the substrate and binds to the active site of the enzyme but doesn't undergo any catalysis
- Non-competitive inhibition: The inhibitor has no structural resemblance with substrate and binds at a site other than the active site on the enzyme surface and thus impairs enzyme function
- Allosteric inhibition: The allosteric modulator binds to the allosteric site and regulates enzyme activity.

Enzyme Deficiency Diseases/Syndromes

- Acute Intermittent Porphyria: Uroporphyrinogen -1 synthase
- Congenital erythropoeitic porphyria: Uroporphyrinogen -3 cosynthase
- Porphyria cutanea tarda: Uroporphyrinogen decaboxylase
- Erythropoeitic porphyria: Ferrochelatase
- Criggler-Najjar: UDP- glucuronyl transferase
- Von Gierke's: Glucose-6-phosphatase
- Pompe's: Acid maltase (Acid alpha glucosidase)
- McArdle's: Muscle glycogen phosphorylase
- Niemann-Pick's: Sphingomyelinase
- Faber's: Ceramidase
- Gaucher's: Beta-glucosidase
- Krabbe's: Beta -galactosidase
- Tay-Sach's: Hexosaminidase –A
- Phenylketonuria: Phenylalanine hydroxylase
- Alkaptonuria: Homogentisate oxidase
- Albinism: Tyrosinase
- Metachromatic leucodystrophy: Arylsulphatase A
- Lesch-Nyhan syndrome: HGPRT
- Xeroderma pigmentosa: DNA exinuclease
- Maple syrup urine: Branched chain alpha-ketoacid dehydrogenase complex (BCKDC)
- MPS-1/Hurler's syndrome: Alpha-L- iduronidase
- MPS-2: L-iduronosulphate

Commonly Asked Rate Limiting Steps

- Urea synthesis: Carbamoy1 phosphate synthase I
- Glycolysis: Phosphofructokinase
- Bile acid synthesis: 7- alpha hydroxylase
- Cholesterol synthesis: HMG-CoA reductase

Commonly Asked Rate Limiting Enzymes

- Uric acid synthesis: Xanthine oxidase
- Denovo purine biosynthesis: PRPP synthetase
- Porphyrin synthesis: ALA synthetase
- Fatty acid synthesis: Acetyl CoA carboxylase

Phenylketonuria

- Autosomal recessive inheritance
- Deficiency of: Phenylalanine hydroxylase
- Cause of neurological signs and mental retardation: As brain cell are deprive of essential amino acids
- High phenylalanine concentration results in: Competitive inhibition of tyrosine leading to:
  - Blonde hair
  - Blue eyes
  - Fair skin
- Accessory metabolic pathway leads to: Accumulation of phenylacetic acid and other metabolites leading to mousy odour
- Diagnosis: Provocative protein meal test; A plasma phenylalanine level >20 mg/dl; A normal plasma tyrosine level
- Screening tests: Guthrie's test ferric chloride solution-green colour; 2,4 dinitrophenol hydrazine -Yellow precipitate
- Treatment: Low phenylalanine levels, however it should not be completely eliminated; Tyrosine becomes essential, hence adequate intake should be ensured

Hartnup's Disease

- Hereditary disorder of tryptophan metabolism
- Clinical symptoms include dermatitis, ataxia, and mental retardation
- Characterised by low plasma levels of tryptophan and their elevated urinary excretion.

Essential Amino Acids (Mnemonic: MATTVILPhly)

- Methionine
- Arginine
- Threonine
- Tryptophan
- Valine
- Isoleucine
- Leucine
- Phenylalanine
- Lysine

Semi-Essential Amino Acids

- Histidine
- Arginine

Protein Structure (Bonds and Detection)

- Primary: Linear sequence of amino acids, consisting of peptide bonds; Edman's degeneration technique
- Secondary: Special structure of proteins, by twisting of polypeptide chains, consisting of alpha helix and beta pleated sheets (Hydrogen bonds); X-ray diffraction, crystallography and nuclear magnetic resonance
- Tertiary: Three dimensional structure of functional proteins (Disulfide bonds); X-ray diffraction, crystallography and nuclear magnetic resonance
- Quaternary: Three dimensional structure of functional proteins; Detected by X-ray diffraction, crystallography and nuclear magnetic resonance

Some Important Proteins and Their Functions

- Haptoglobin: Binds with free hemoglobin
- Ceruloplasmin: Transports copper
- Alpha 1 antitrypsin: Inhibitor of trypsin
- Alpha 1 lipoprotein: Transport of cholesterol and phospholipids

Vitamins as Coenzymes

- Thiamine: TPP, TDP
- Riboflavin: FAD, FMN
- Niacin: NAD, NADP
- Pantothenic acid: CoA, Acyl carrier protein
- Pyridoxine: Pyridoxal phosphate
- Folic acid: Tetrahydrofolate

Markers for Vitamin Deficiencies

- B1: RBC transketolase
- B2: RBC glutathione peroxidase
- B6: Urine xanthurenic acid
- Folic acid: Urine FIGLU
- B12: Urine methylmalonic acid

Glycolysis

- Location: Cytosol
- Substrate level phosphorylation: Phosphoglycerate kinase, Pyruvate kinase

- Inhibitors:
  - Fluoride: Enolase
  - Oxamate: Glyceraldehyde-3-phosphate dehydrogenase
  - Bromohydroxyacetone phosphate: Phosphate isomerase
- Irreversible steps: Hexokinase, Phosphofructokinase, Pyruvate kinase

Uncouplers of Electron Transport Chain are:

- 2,4 dinitrophenol
- Dinitrocresol
- Pentachlorophenol
- Triflurocarbonyl
- Long chain free fatty acids
- Unconjugated bilirubin

Apolipoproteins

- Chylomicron: AI, A II, B 48
- VLDL: B100, CI, C II, C III, E
- LDL: B 100
- HDL: AI, AII, CI, C II, C III D, E.

Functions of:

- Chylomicron: Transport exogenous triglycerides
- VLDL: Transports endogenous triglyceride
- LDL: Transports cholesterol to peripheral tissues
- HDL: Transports cholesterol from peripheral tissues to liver for degradation.

MCQs WITH SHORT EXPLANATIONS

ENZYMES

1. Which of the following is true for non-competitive inhibition:

a. Low Km, high Vmax
b. High Km, high Vmax
c. Normal Km, low Vmax
d. Normal Km, high Vmax

Enzyme inhibition

- Competitive: High Km, normal Vmax
- Non-competitive: Normal Km, low Vmax

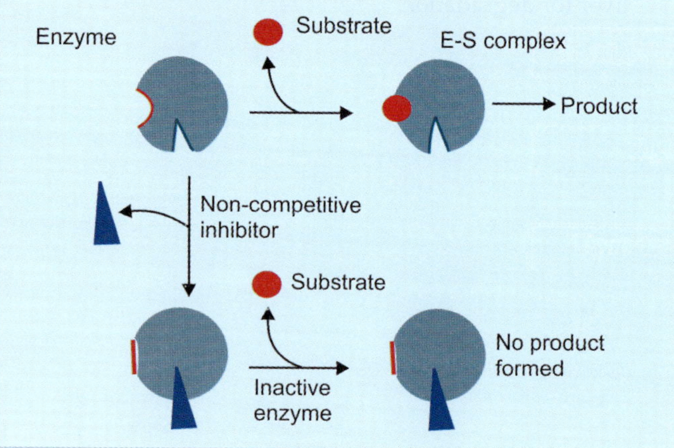

Non-competitive inhibition.

2. Kinases require:

a. Mn^{2+} b. Cu^{2+}
c. Mg^{2+} d. Inorganic phosphate

All known protein kinases, except CASK [calcium/calmodulin (CaM)-activated serine-threonine kinase], require magnesium ions (Mg^{2+}) to stimulate the transfer of a phosphate from adenosine 5′-triphosphate (ATP) to a protein substrate.

Metallo-enzymes	
Metal	*Enzymes containing metals*
Zinc	Carbonic anhydrase, carboxy peptidase, alcohol dehydrogenase
Magnesium	Hexokinase, phosphofructokinase, enolase, glucose-6-phosphatase
Manganese	Phosphoglucomutase, hexokinase, enolase, glycosyl transferases
Copper	Tyrosinase, cytochrome oxidase, lysyl oxidase, superoxide dismutase
Iron	Cytochrome oxidase, catalase, peroxidase, xanthine oxidase
Calcium	Lecithinase, lipase
Molybdenum	Xanthine oxidase

3. The combination of coenzyme and apoenzyme is called:

a. Apoenzyme b. Coenzyme
c. Holoenzyme d. Constitutive enzyme

Enzymes that require a cofactor but do not have one bound are called *apoenzymes* or *apoproteins*. An enzyme together with the cofactor(s) required for activity is called a *holoenzyme* (or haloenzyme). The term *holoenzyme* can also be applied to enzymes that contain multiple protein subunits, such as the DNA polymerases; here the holoenzyme is the complete complex containing all the subunits needed for activity.

4. K_m increases, but V_{max} remains same. This is .... inhibition:

a. Competitive
b. Non-competitive
c. Irreversible
d. Uncompetitive

In competitive inhibition, the maximum velocity (V_{max}) of the reaction is unchanged, while the apparent affinity of the substrate to the binding site is decreased (the K_d dissociation constant is apparently increased). The change in K_m (Michaelis-Menten constant) is parallel to the alteration in K_d. Any given competitive inhibitor concentration can be overcome by increasing the substrate concentration in which case the substrate will outcompete the inhibitor in binding to the enzyme.

Comparison of two types of inhibition		
	Competitive inhibition	*Non-competitive inhibition*
Acting on	Active site	May or may not
Structure of inhibitor	Substrate analog	Unrelated molecule
Inhibition is	Reversible	Generally irreversible
Excess substrate	Inhibition relieved	No effect
K_m	Increased	No change
V_{max}	No change	Decreased
Significance	Drug action	Toxicological

5. K_m of an enzyme is:

a. Dissociation constant
b. The normal physiological substrate concentration
c. The substrate concentration at half maximum velocity
d. Numerically identical for all isozymes that catalyze a given reaction

Ans. **1. c.** Normal Km, low **2. c.** Mg^{2+} **3. c.** Holoenzyme **4. a.** Competitive **5. c.** The substrate...

The Michaelis constant K_m is the substrate concentration at which the reaction rate is at half-maximum, and is an inverse measure of the substrate's affinity for the enzyme—as a small K_m indicates high affinity, meaning that the rate will approach V_{max} more quickly. The value of K_m is dependent on both the enzyme and the substrate, as well as conditions such as temperature and pH.

6. **Carbamoyl phosphate synthetase-I is:**
   a. Lysosolic enzyme b. Cytosolic enzyme
   c. Mitochondrial enzyme d. All of the above

Carbamoyl Phosphate Synthetase I is a ligase enzyme located in the mitochondria involved in the production of urea. Carbamoyl Phosphate Synthetase I (CPSI) transfers an ammonia molecule from glutamine or glutamate to a molecule of bicarbonate that has been phosphorylated by a molecule of ATP. The resulting carbamate is then phosphorylated with another molecule ATP.

Comparison, CPS I and II enzymes

	CPS-I	*CPS-II*
1. Site	Mitochondria	Cytosol
2. Pathway of	Urea	Pyrimidine
3. Positive effector	NAG	Nil
4. Source for N	Ammonia	Glutamine
5. Inhibitor	Nil	CTP

7. **Enzyme helping in catalyzing conversion of aldose sugars to ketose sugars:**
   a. Oxidoreductase
   b. Phosphotriose isomerase
   c. Decarboxylase
   d. Aldolase

Triose-phosphate isomerase (TPI or TIM) is an enzyme that catalyzes the reversible interconversion of the triose phosphate isomers dihydroxyacetone phosphate and D-glyceraldehyde 3-phosphate.

8. **Enzymes are usually:**
   a. Lipid b. Nucleic acids
   c. Carbohydrates d. Protein

Most enzymes are proteins, although a few are catalytic RNA molecules.

9. **Other name of AST:**
   a. SGOT b. SGPT
   c. Alkaline phosphatase d. Acid phosphatase

Aspartate transaminase (AST) or **aspartate aminotransferase**, also known as **AspAT/ASAT/AAT** or **serum glutamic oxaloacetic transaminase (SGOT)**, is a pyridoxal phosphate (PLP)-dependent transaminase enzyme. AST catalyzes the reversible transfer of an α-amino group between aspartate and glutamate and, as such, is an important enzyme in amino acid metabolism.

10. **Enzyme primarily responsible for protein degradation in stomach is:**
   a. Trypsin b. Pepsin
   c. Chymotrypsin d. Endopeptidase

Pepsin is an enzyme whose zymogen (pepsinogen) is released by the chief cells in the stomach and that degrades food proteins into peptides.

11. **Cytochrome oxidase contains:**
   a. Copper b. Iron
   c. Both d. None

The cytochrome oxidase complex is a large integral membrane protein composed of several metal prosthetic sites and 14 protein subunits in mammals. In mammals, eleven subunits are nuclear in origin, and three are synthesized in the mitochondria. The complex contains two hemes, a cytochrome a and cytochrome a3, and two copper centers, the Cu_A and Cu_B centers.

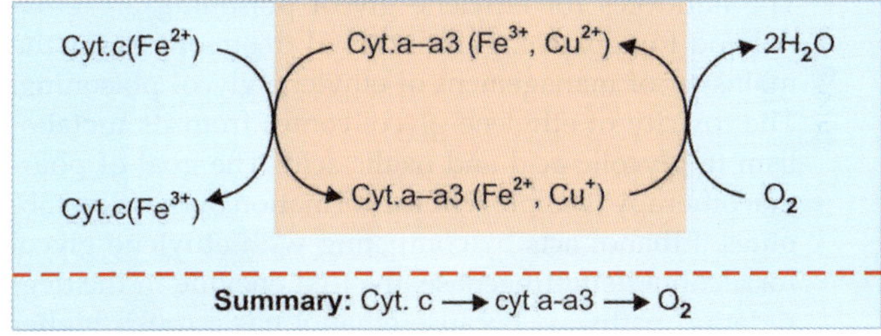

Complex IV (cytochrome oxidase) of respiratory chain.

12. **Enzyme involved in respiratory burst:**
   a. Catalase b. Peroxidase
   c. Dehydrogenase d. Oxidase

Respiratory burst (sometimes called **oxidative burst**) is the rapid release of reactive oxygen species (superoxide radical and hydrogen peroxide) from different types of cells. NADPH oxidase, an enzyme family in the vasculature (in particular, in vascular disease), produces superoxide, which spontaneously recombines with other molecules to produce reactive free radicals.

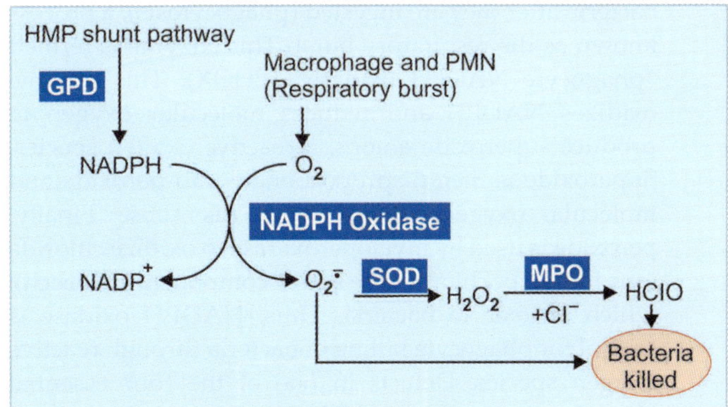

Generation of ROS in macrophages.

13. **A functional plasma enzyme:**
   a. Prostatic specific phosphatase
   b. Alkaline phosphatase
   c. Lactate dehydrogenase
   d. Lipoprotein lipase

Ans. 6. **c.** Mitochondrial... 7. **b.** Phosphotriose... 8. **d.** Protein 9. **a.** SGOT 10. **b.** Pepsin 11. **c.** Both 12. **d.** Oxidase 13. **d.** Lipoprotein lipase

Lipoprotein lipase (LPL) is a member of the lipase gene family, which includes pancreatic lipase, hepatic lipase, and endothelial lipase. It is a water-soluble enzyme that hydrolyzes triglycerides in lipoproteins, such as those found in chylomicrons and very low-density lipoproteins (VLDL), into two free fatty acids and one monoacylglycerol molecule. It is also involved in promoting the cellular uptake of chylomicron remnants, cholesterol-rich lipoproteins, and free fatty acids.

14. Ethanol is used in ethylene glycol poisoning as it is:

a. Non-competitive inhibitor of aldehyde dehydrogenase
b. Competitive inhibitor of aldehyde dehydrogenase
c. Competitive inhibitor of alcohol dehydrogenase
d. Competitive inhibitor of NADPH oxidase

The antidotes for ethylene glycol poisoning are ethanol and fomepizole. This antidotal treatment forms the mainstay of management of ethylene glycol poisoning. The toxicity of ethylene glycol comes from its metabolism to glycolic acid and oxalic acid. The goal of pharmacotherapy is to prevent the formation of these metabolites. Ethanol acts by competing with ethylene glycol for alcohol dehydrogenase, the first enzyme in the degradation pathway. Because ethanol has a much higher affinity for alcohol dehydrogenase, about a 100-time greater affinity, it successfully blocks the breakdown of ethylene glycol into glycoaldehyde, which prevents the further degradation.

15. Deficiency of NADPH oxidase causes:

a. Leucocyte adhesion defect-II
b. Leucocyte adhesion defect-I
c. Chediak-Higashi syndrome
d. Chronic granulomatous disease

Phagocytes (i.e., neutrophils and macrophages) require an enzyme to produce reactive oxygen species to destroy bacteria after they are ingested (phagocytosis), a process known as the respiratory burst. This enzyme is termed "phagocyte NADPH oxidase" (PHOX). This enzyme oxidizes NADPH and reduces molecular oxygen to produce superoxide anions, a reactive oxygen species. Superoxide is then disproportionate into peroxide and molecular oxygen by superoxide dismutase. Finally, peroxide is used by myeloperoxidase to oxidize chloride ions into hypochlorite (the active component of bleach), which is toxic to bacteria. Thus, NADPH oxidase is critical for phagocyte killing of bacteria through reactive oxygen species. Defects in one of the four essential subunits of phagocyte NADPH oxidase (PHOX) can all cause CGD of varying severity, dependent on the defect.

16. Peptidyl transferase is:

a. Elongation factor b. Enzyme
c. Catalyst d. Ribozyme

Peptidyl transferase activity is carried out by the ribosome. Peptidyl transferase activity is not mediated by any ribosomal proteins but by ribosomal RNA (rRNA), a ribozyme. Ribozymes are the only enzymes which are not made up of proteins, but ribonucleotides. All other enzymes are made up of proteins.

17. Cofactor for xanthine oxidase:

a. Zinc b. Copper
c. Molybdenum d. Selenium

Xanthine oxidase

- The protein is large, having a molecular weight of 270 kDa, and has 2 flavin molecules (bound as FAD), 2 molybdenum atoms, and 8 iron atoms bound per enzymatic unit.
- The molybdenum atoms are contained as molybdopterin cofactors and are the active sites of the enzyme.
- The iron atoms are part of [2Fe-2S] ferredoxin iron-sulfur clusters and participate in electron transfer reactions.

18. Nor-epinephrine to epinephrine conversion requires:

a. Transaldolase
b. Tyrosine hydroxylase
c. Alpha ketoglutarate
d. Phenylethanolamine-N-methyltrasferase

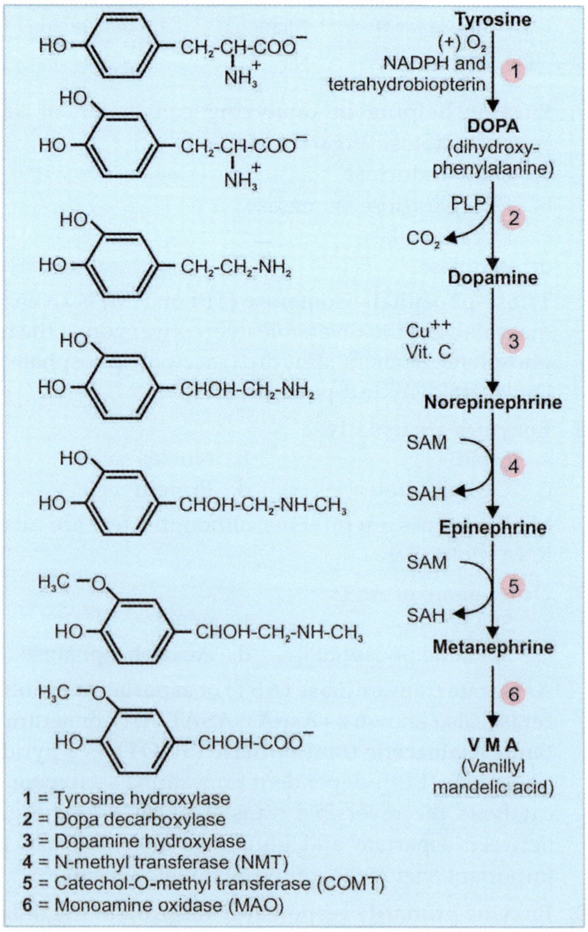

Tyrosine → (1; (+) O_2, NADPH and tetrahydrobiopterin) → DOPA (dihydroxy-phenylalanine) → (2; PLP, CO_2) → Dopamine → (3; Cu^{++}, Vit. C) → Norepinephrine → (4; SAM → SAH) → Epinephrine → (5; SAM → SAH) → Metanephrine → (6) → VMA (Vanillyl mandelic acid)

1 = Tyrosine hydroxylase
2 = Dopa decarboxylase
3 = Dopamine hydroxylase
4 = N-methyl transferase (NMT)
5 = Catechol-O-methyl transferase (COMT)
6 = Monoamine oxidase (MAO)

Metabolism of catecholamines.

Ans. 14. **c.** Competitive... 15. **d.** Chronic granu... 16. **d.** Ribozyme 17. **c.** Molybdenum 18. **d.** Phenylethan...

Phenylethanolamine N-methyltransferase (PNMT) is an enzyme found in the adrenal medulla that converts norepinephrine (noradrenaline) to epinephrine (adrenaline).

19. **Isozymes:**
    a. Forms of different enzyme that catalyzes different reaction
    b. Forms of different enzyme that catalyzes same reaction
    c. Forms of same enzyme that catalyzes different reaction
    d. Forms of same enzyme that catalyzes same reaction

Isozymes (also known as **isoenzymes** or more generally as **Multiple forms of enzymes**) are enzymes that differ in amino acid sequence but catalyze the same chemical reaction. These enzymes usually display different kinetic parameters (e.g. different K_M values), or different regulatory properties.

20. **In competitive inhibition:**
    a. V_{max} unchanged
    b. Apparent K_m unchanged
    c. Apparent K_m decreased
    d. V_{max} decreased

In competitive inhibition, the maximum velocity (V_{max}) of the reaction is unchanged, while the apparent affinity of the substrate to the binding site is decreased (the K_d dissociation constant is apparently increased).

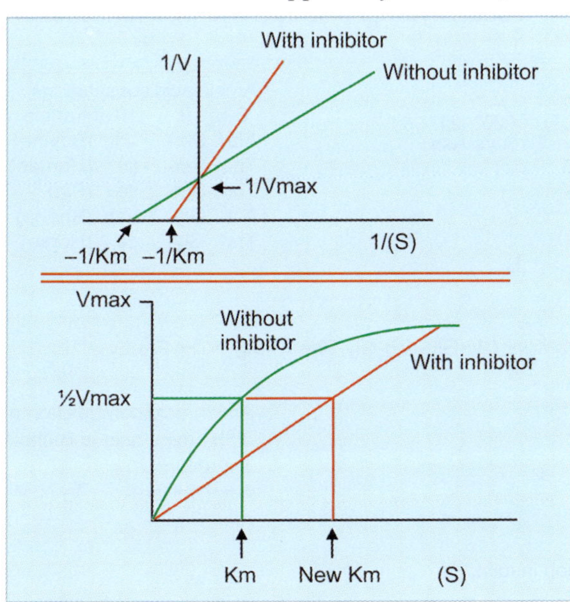

Substrate saturation curve in presence and absence of competitive inhibitor.

21. **A functional enzyme:**
    a. Acid phosphatase
    b. Prothrombin
    c. Amylase
    d. LDH

Clotting factors, e.g. prothrombin, lipoprotein lipase and pseudocholinesterase comes under functional enzymes.

22. **Activator of sulfite oxidase:**
    a. Iron
    b. Copper
    c. Molybdenum
    d. Zinc

Sulfite oxidase is a metallo-enzyme that utilizes a molybdopterin cofactor and a heme group. It is one of the cytochromes b5 and belongs to the enzyme super-family of molybdenum oxotransferases that also includes DMSO reductase, xanthine oxidase, and nitrite reductase.

23. **Molybdenum is a constituent of:**
    a. Xanthine oxidase
    b. Cytochrome oxidase
    c. Phosphofructokinase
    d. Carbonic anhydrase

At least 50 molybdenum-containing enzymes were known by 2002, mostly in bacteria, and their number is increasing with every year; those enzymes include aldehyde oxidase, sulfite oxidase and xanthine oxidase.

24. **Selenocysteine is an important component of:**
    a. Carbonic anhydrase
    b. Glutathione peroxidase
    c. Phosphofructokinase
    d. Hexokinase

The main reaction that glutathione peroxidase catalyzes is:

$$2GSH + H_2O_2 \rightarrow GS\text{–}SG + 2H_2O$$

where GSH represents reduced monomeric glutathione, and GS–SG represents glutathione disulfide. The mechanism involves oxidation of the selenol of a selenocysteine residue by hydrogen peroxide.

25. **Butyrylcholinesterase degrades:**
    a. Allopurinol
    b. Ephedrine
    c. Succinylcholine
    d. Lovastatin

Suxamethonium is quickly degraded by plasma butyrylcholinesterase and the duration of effect is usually in the range of a few minutes. When plasma levels of butyrylcholinesterase are greatly diminished or an atypical form is present (an otherwise harmless inherited disorder), paralysis may last much longer, as is this the case in liver failure or in neonates.

26. **Rennin is:**
    a. A proteolytic enzyme liberated by kidneys
    b. Proteolytic enzyme in gastric juice of infants
    c. Stimulates synthesis of hemoglobin
    d. All of the above

Chymosin or **rennin** is a protease found in rennet. It is produced by newborn ruminant animals in the lining

Ans. 19. **d.** Forms of same... 20. **a.** V_{max} unchanged 21. **b.** Prothrombin 22. **c.** Molybdenum 23. **a.** Xanthine oxidase 24. **b.** Glutathione... 25. **c.** Succinylcholine 26. **b.** Proteolytic....

of the fourth stomach to curdle the milk they ingest, allowing a longer residence in the bowels and better absorption.

27. True regarding isozymes is:

a. Forms of the same enzymes that catalyze different reaction
b. Forms of the same enzymes that catalyze same reaction
c. Forms of the different enzymes that catalyze different reaction
d. Forms of the different enzymes that catalyze same reaction

Isozymes were first described by R.L. Hunter and Clement Markert (1957) who defined them as *different variants of the same enzyme having identical functions and present in the same individual*. This definition encompasses (1) enzyme variants that are the product of different genes and thus represent different loci (described as *isozymes*) and (2) enzymes that are the product of different alleles of the same gene (described as *allozymes*)

28. Norepinephrine to epinephrine conversion requires which enzyme:

a. Phenylethanolamine-N-methyltransferase
b. Transaldolase
c. Tyrosine hydroxylase
d. Alpha ketoglutarate

Norepinephrine itself can further be converted into epinephrine by the enzyme phenylethanolamine N-methyltransferase with S-adenosyl-L-methionine as cofactor.

29. Red blood cell transketolase level is a marker for deficiency of:

a. Vitamin B1 b. Vitamin B2
c. Vitamin B6 d. Vitamin B12

Red blood cell transketolase activity is reduced in deficiency of thiamine (vitamin B1), and may be used in the diagnosis of Wernicke's encephalopathy and other B1-deficiency syndromes if the diagnosis is in doubt.

AMINO ACIDS AND PROTEIN METABOLISM

30. Which of the following is the main bond in primary structure of protein:

a. Hydrogen bond
b. Hydrophobic interaction
c. Ionic bonds d. Covalent peptide bonds

Proteins structure

- Amino acids (in primary structure) are held together by covalent peptide bonds/ linkages
- Secondary
  - Alpha helix is stabilized by extensive hydrogen bonding
  - Beta pleated sheet is composed of two or more segments of fully extended polypeptide chains (hydrogen bonds)
- Tertiary and quaternary structures of protein are stabilized by non-covalent bonds such as hydrogen bonds, hydrophobic interactions, ionic bonds

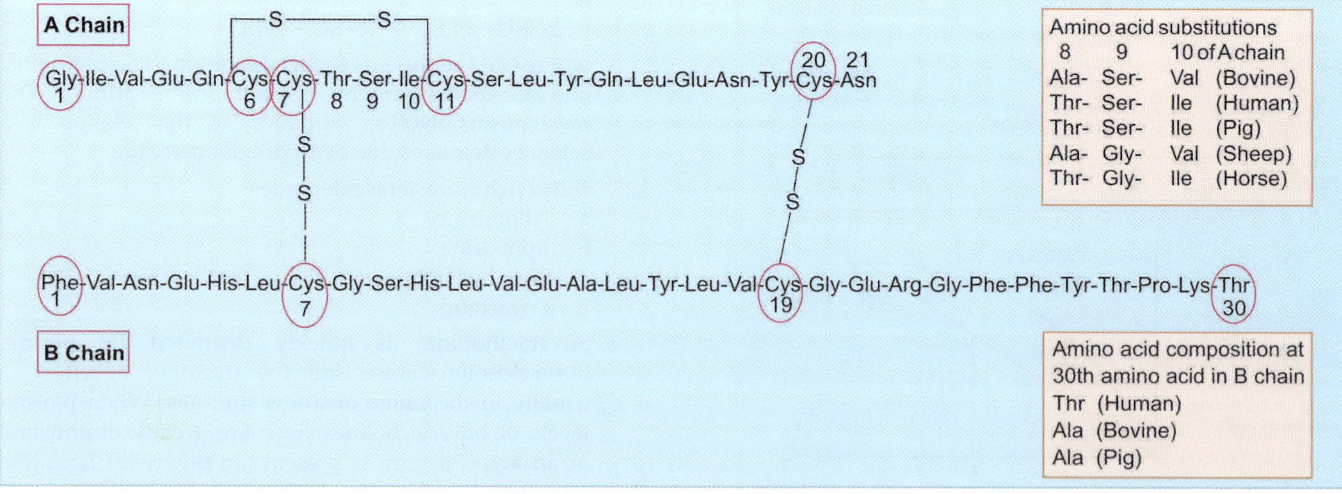

Primary structure of human insulin.

31. First product of tryptophan metabolism:

a. Xantheurenic acid b. Bradykinin
c. Leucotriene d. Kynerunine

Tryptophan as a biochemical precursor:

- Serotonin (a neurotransmitter), synthesized via tryptophan hydroxylase. Serotonin, in turn, can be converted to melatonin (a neurohormone), via N-acetyltransferase and 5-hydroxyindole-O-methyltransferase activities.
- Niacin is synthesized from tryptophan via kynurenine and quinolic acids as key biosynthetic intermediates.
- Auxin (a phytohormone) when sieve tube elements undergo apoptosis tryptophan is converted to auxins.

Ans. 27. **b.** Forms... 28. **a.** Phenylethano... 29. **a.** Vitamin B1 30. **d.** Covalent peptide bonds
31. **d.** Kynurenine

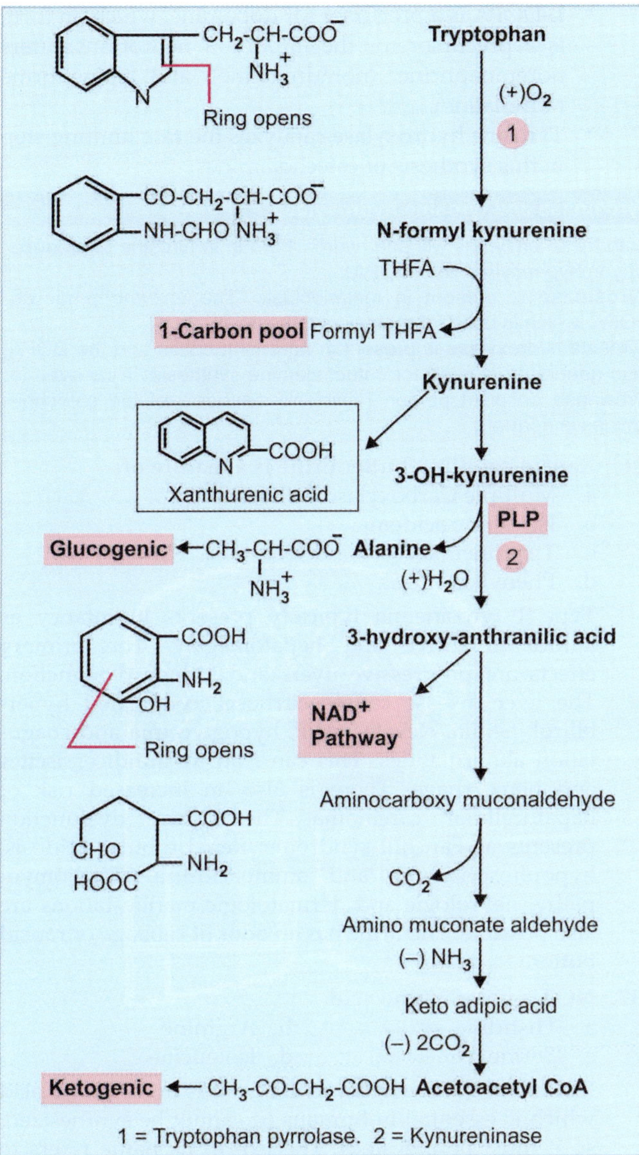

Metabolism of tryptophan.

32. Protein denaturation does NOT affect:

a. Primary structure
b. Secondary structure
c. Tertiary structure
d. Quaternary structure

Protein structure

- In **quaternary structure** denaturation, protein subunits are dissociated and/or the spatial arrangement of protein subunits is disrupted.
- **Tertiary structure** denaturation involves the disruption of:
  - Covalent interactions between amino acid side chains (such as disulfide bridges between cysteine groups)
  - Non-covalent dipole-dipole interactions between polar amino acid side-chains (and the surrounding solvent)
  - Van der Waals (induced dipole) interactions between nonpolar amino acid side-chain
- In **secondary structure** denaturation, proteins lose all regular repeating patterns such as alpha helices and beta-pleated sheets, and adopt a random coil configuration.
- Primary structure, such as the sequence of amino acids held together by covalent peptide bonds, is not disrupted by denaturation

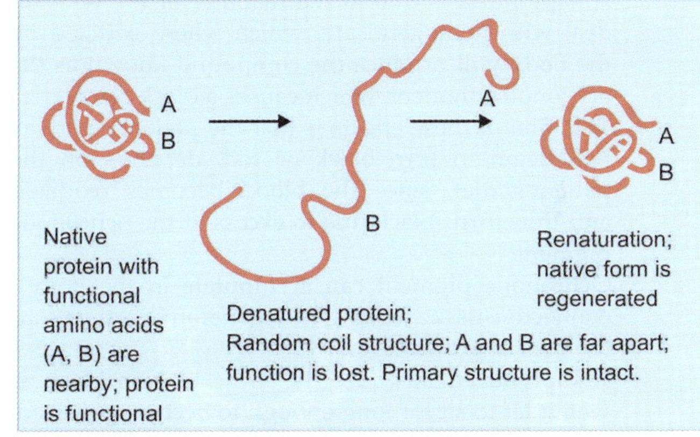

Denaturation of protein.

33. Below isoelectric pH, amino acids exists as:

a. Zwitter ion
b. Anion
c. Cation
d. Dipolar

Isoelectric point, sometimes abbreviated IEP

- It is the pH at which a particular molecule carries no net electrical charge.
- Standard nomenclature of isoelectric point is pH(I), although pI is also commonly seen
- The net charge on the molecule is affected by pH of its surrounding environment and can become more positively or negatively charged due to the gain or loss, respectively, of protons (H^+).

Significance of isoelectric pH (pI)
1. The amino acid composition will determine the isoelectric pH (pI) of protein. The alpha amino group and carboxyl group are utilized for peptide bond formation, and hence are not ionizable. All other ionizable groups present in the protein will influence the pI of the protein.
2. At the isoelectric point, the number of anions and cations present on the protein molecule will be equal and the **net charge is zero**.
3. At the pI value, the proteins **will not migrate** in an electrical field. At the pI, solubility, buffering capacity and viscosity will be minimum; and **precipitation** will be maximum.
4. On the acidic side of pI, the proteins are cations and on alkaline side, they are anions in nature.
5. The pI of pepsin is 1.1; casein 4.6; human albumin 4.7; human insulin 5.4; human globulins 6.4; human hemoglobin 6.7; myoglobin 7; and lysozyme 11.

Contd...

Ans. 32. **a.** Primary structure 33. **c.** Cation

Contd...

6. **Acidic dyes** such as eosin will dissociate into H^+ + dye which will then attach with protein–NH_3^+ (proteincations). **Basic dyes** such as hematoxylin and methylene blue are dissociated to OH^- + dye+, which will then stain Protein-COO^- (anions). Thus, the staining characteristic of a protein is determined by the pI of that protein.

34. Which of the following enzyme is deficient in alkaptonuria:

a. Xanthine oxidase b. HMG CoA reductase
c. Homogentisate oxidase d. Tyrosinase

Homegentisate 1,2 dioxygenase

- Deficiency leads to alkaptonuria.
- Alkaptonuria is due to the inability of the body to deal with homogentisate, which when oxidized by the body will produce the compound known as the ochronotic pigment, which causes a black color
- This first of these effects is that the patient's earwax will begin to turn black or red, depends on the patient's diet, since the blood becomes oxidized and thus turns black due to excess of the ochronotic pigment.
- Ochronotic pigment can accumulate in the body's connective tissue leading to degenerative arthritis, as the person grows older.
- Alkaptonuria can cause the urine to turn black as well if let to sit for long enough to become oxidized, though is this often a method for testing for the genetic defect.
- The metabolic disease is autosomal recessive, such that both parents must pass the gene on to their children in order for child to have the defect

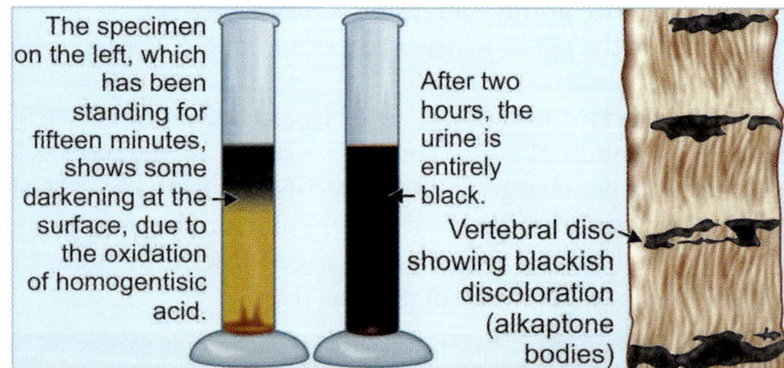

Left side, urine of alkaptonuria; Right side alkatone bodies deposited in vertebral disc of patient.

35. Which of the following is the rate limiting step in catecholamine synthesis:

a. Tryptophan decarboxylase
b. Dopa decarboxylase
c. Tyrosine hydroxylase
d. Phenylethanolamine N-methyltransferase

Tyrosine hydroxylase or tyrosine 3-monooxygenase

- It is the enzyme responsible for catalyzing the conversion of the amino acid L-tyrosine to L-3,4 dihydroxy-phenylalanine (L-DOPA).
- It does so using molecular oxygen (O_2), as well as iron (Fe^{2+}) and tetrahydrobiopterin as cofactors.
- L-DOPA is a precursor for dopamine, which, in turn, is a precursor for the important neurotransmitters norepinephrine (noradrenaline) and epinephrine (adrenaline).
- Tyrosine hydroxylase catalyzes the rate limiting step in this synthesis of catecholamines.

Tyrosinase and tyrosine hydroxylase

Both these enzymes will add hydroxyl group to tyrosine to produce dihydroxyphenylalanine **(DOPA).**
Tyrosinase is present in melanoblasts. The enzyme produces DOPA, which is used for melanin synthesis.
Tyrosine hydroxylase is present in adrenal medulla and the DOPA thus generated is used for catecholamine synthesis. Thus even in tyrosinase deficient person (albinism) synthesis of the catecholamines is normal.

36. Rancid smelling butter urine is a feature of:

a. Multiple Carboxylase deficiency
b. Isovaleric acidemia
c. Tyrosinemia
d. Phenylketonuria

Type 1 tyrosinemia typically presents in infancy as failure to thrive and hepatomegaly. The primary effects are progressive livers and kidney dysfunction. The liver disease causes cirrhosis, conjugated hyperbilirubinemia, elevated AFP, hypoglycemia and coagulation abnormalities. This can lead to jaundice, ascites and hemorrhage. There is also an increased risk of hepatocellular carcinoma. The kidney dysfunction presents as Fanconi syndrome: Renal tubular acidosis, hypophosphatemia and aminoaciduria. Cardiomyopathy, neurologic and dermatologic manifestations are also possible. The urine has an odor of cabbage or rancid butter.

37. NOT a polar amino acid:

a. Histidine b. Arginine
c. Serine d. Isoleucine

Isoleucine (abbreviated as **Ile** or **I**) is an α-amino acid which is essential in humans (it cannot be synthesized, so it must be ingested). The iso- in its name refers to it being an isomer of leucine. Its chemical formula is $HO_2CCH(NH_2)CH\ (CH_3)CH_2CH_3$. Its codons are AUU, AUC and AUA. With a hydrocarbon side chain, isoleucine is classified as a hydrophobic amino acid. Together with threonine, isoleucine is one of two common amino acids that have a chiral side chain.

38. Histidine to histamine conversion is what type of reaction:

a. Transmination b. Decarboxylation
c. Both d. None

Decarboxylation is a chemical reaction that removes a carboxyl group and releasescarbon dioxide (CO_2). Usually, decarboxylation refers to a reaction of carboxylic acids, removing a carbon atom from a carbon chain. The reverse process, which is the first chemical step in photosynthesis, is called carboxylation, the addition of CO_2 to a compound.

Ans. **34. c.** Homogentisate... **35. c.** Tyrosine hydroxylase **36. c.** Tyrosinemia **37. d.** Isoleucine **38. b.** Decarboxylation

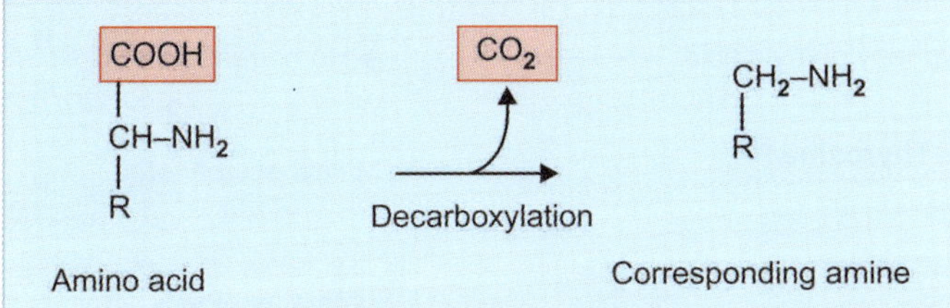

Decarboxylation of amino acid.

39. In Maple syrup urine disease, amino acid NOT excreted in urine is:
a. Phenylalanine
b. Isoleucine
c. Leucine
d. Valine

MSUD is a metabolic disorder caused by a deficiency of the branched-chain alpha-keto acid dehydrogenase complex (BCKDC), leading to a buildup of the branched-chain amino acids (leucine, isoleucine, and valine) and their toxic by-products (ketoacids) in the blood and urine.

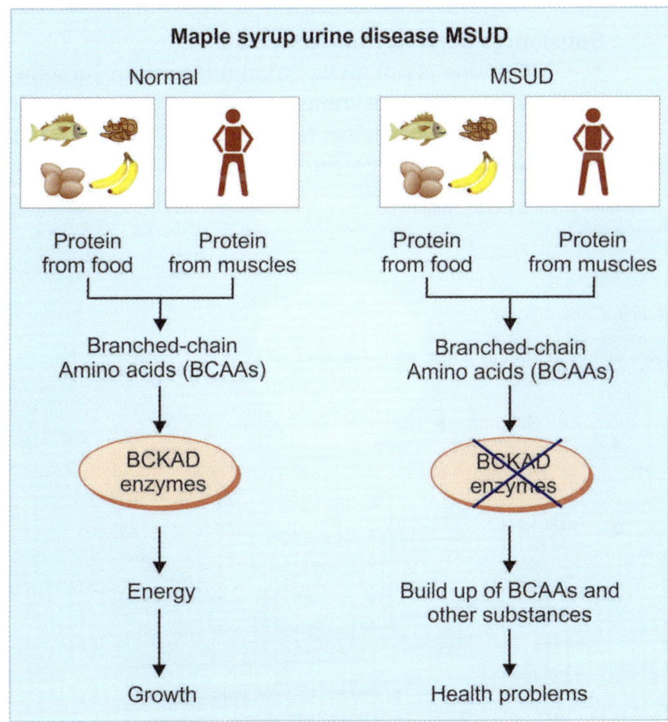

Pathology of maple syrup urine disease.

40. Glycine is NOT useful in:
a. Synthesis of spermine
b. Heme synthesis
c. Creatine synthesis
d. Purine synthesis

Spermine is a polyamine involved in cellular metabolism found in all eukaryotic cells. The precursor for synthesis of spermine is the amino acid ornithine.

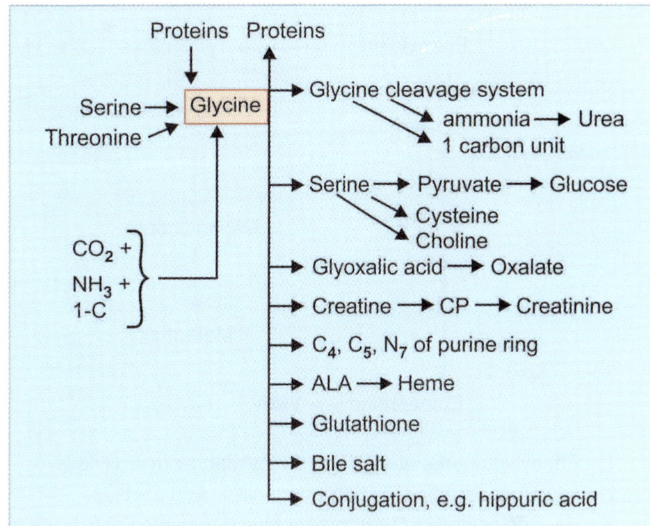

Overview of glycine metabolism.

41. Ammonia is detoxified in brain by:
a. Creatinine
b. Uric acid
c. Glutamine
d. Urea

Glutamine synthetase (GS) in brain is located mainly in astrocytes. One of the primary roles of astrocytes is to protect neurons against excitotoxicity by taking up excess ammonia and glutamate and converting it into glutamine via the enzyme GS.

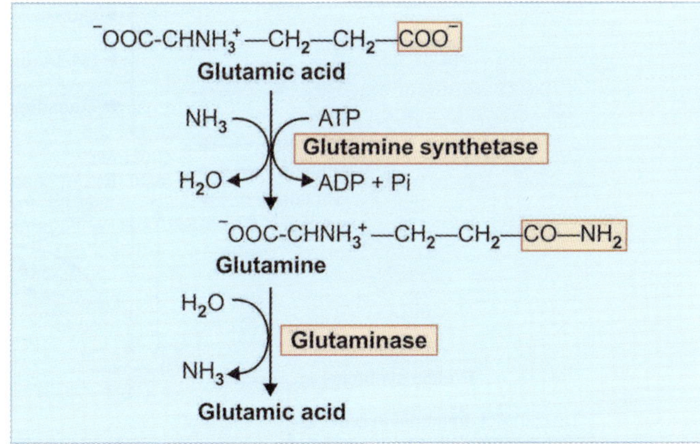

Ammonia trapping as glutamine.

42. Thyroxine is synthesized from:
a. Phenylalanine
b. Tryptophan
c. Tyrosine
d. None of the above

The thyroid hormones triiodothyronine (T_3) and thyroxine (T_4) in the colloid of the thyroid also are derived from tyrosine.

Ans. **39. a.** Phenylalanine **40. a.** Synthesis of spermine **41. c.** Glutamine **42. c.** Tyrosine

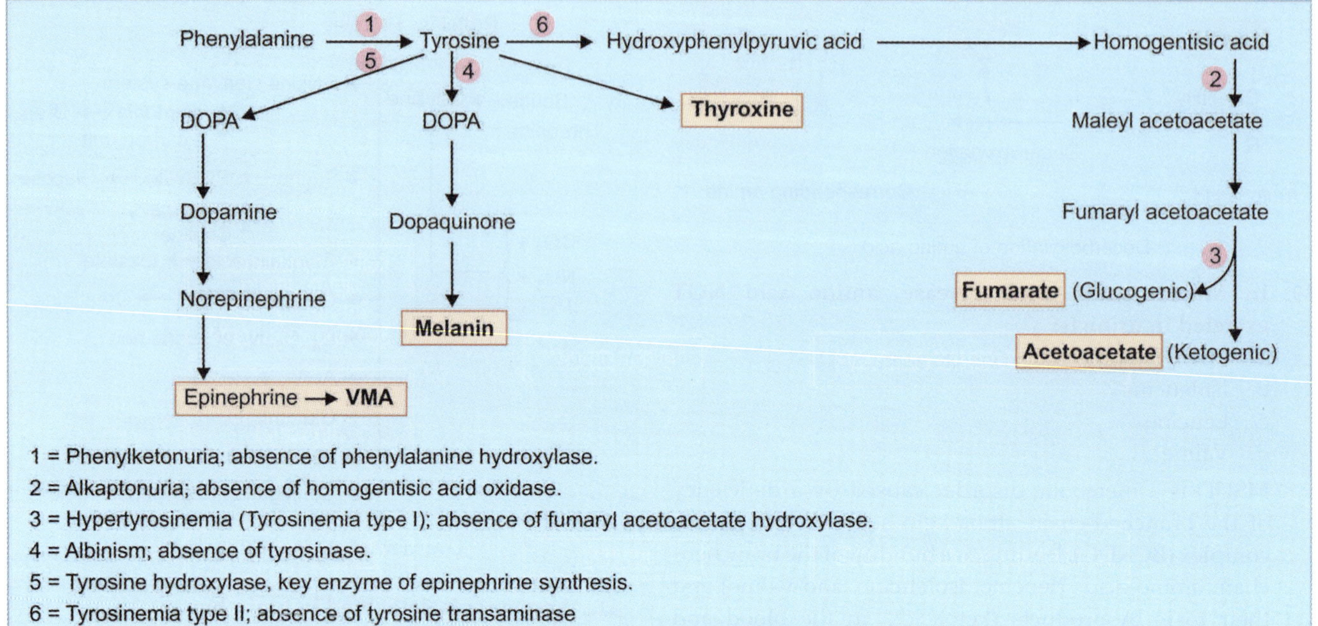

Summary of tyrosine metabolism.

43. Glutamate is NOT a precursor of:
a. GABA
b. Alpha ketoglutarate
c. Glutathione
d. Histidine

Substances derived from glutamate
- Glutathione is not an essential nutrient for humans, since it can be biosynthesized in the body from the amino acids L-cysteine, L-glutamic acid, and glycine.
- Glutamic acid is decarboxylated to GABA

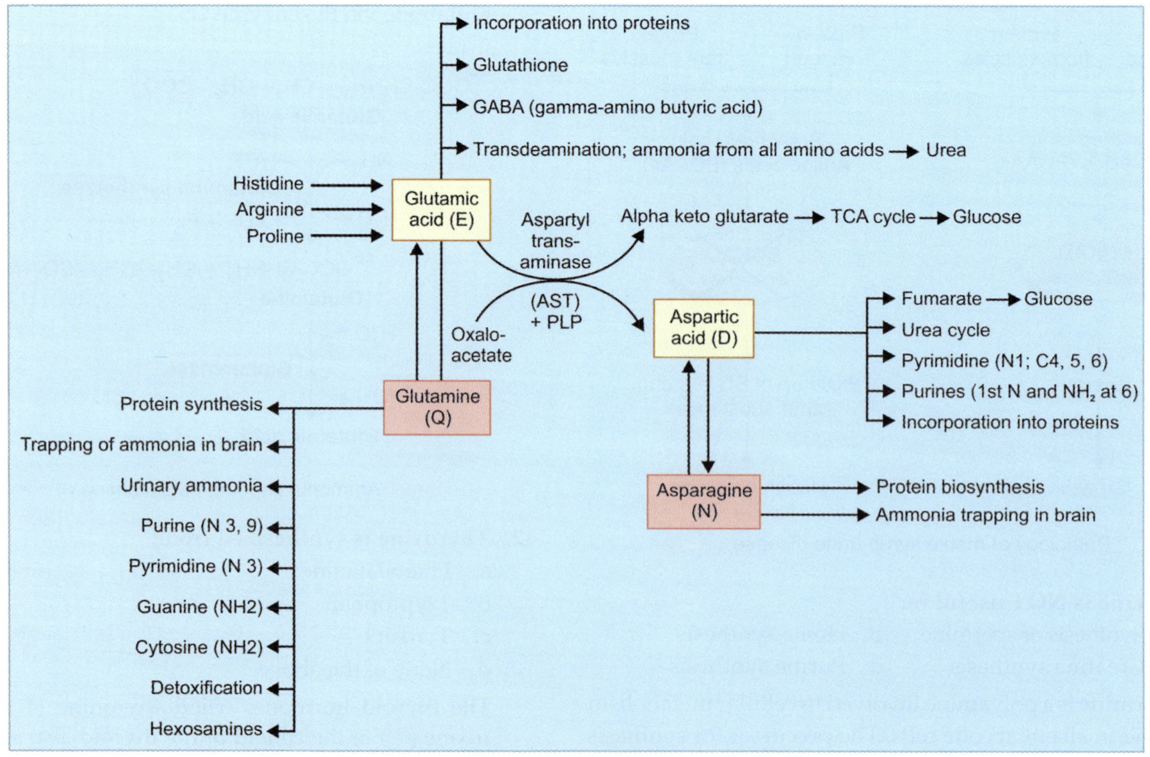

Summary metabolisms of aspartic acid, asparagine, glutamic acid, and glutamine.

Ans. **43. d.** Histidine

44. Melatonin is synthesized from:

a. Tryptophan
b. Serotonin
c. Phenylalanine
d. Histidine

In animal cells melatonin is directly synthesised from the essential amino acid tryptophan, but in other organisms through the shikimic acid pathway.

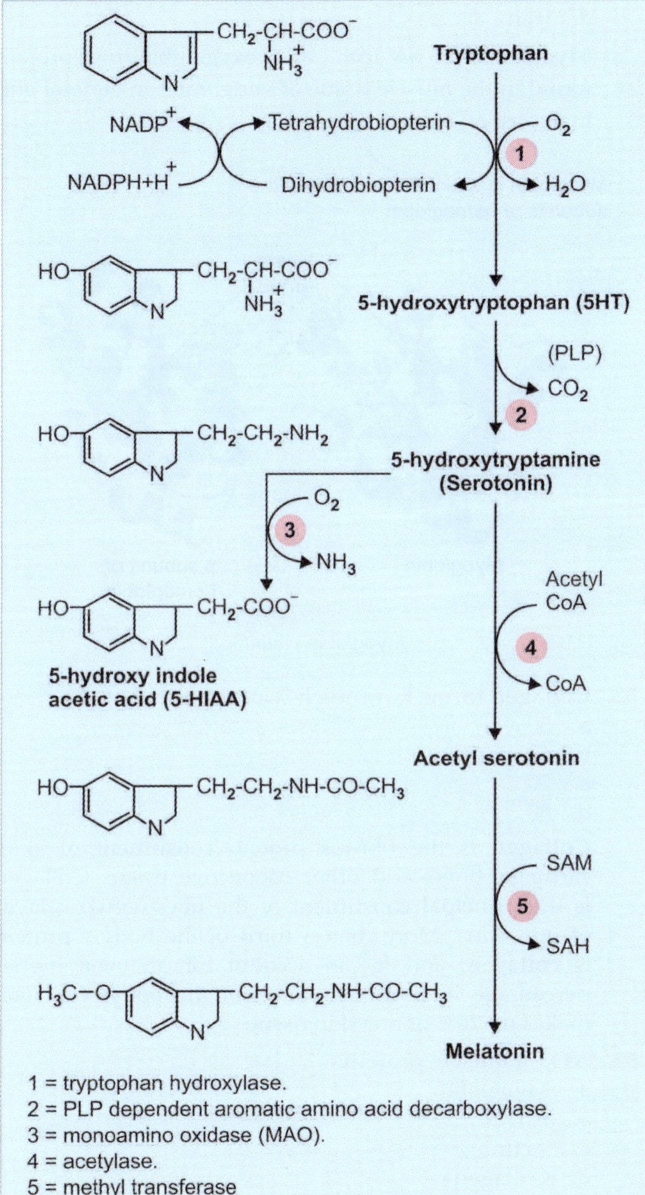

Serotonin and melatonin synthesis.

Melatonin biosynthesis in humans and some other organisms involves four enzymatic steps from the essential dietary amino acid tryptophan, which follows a serotonin pathway.

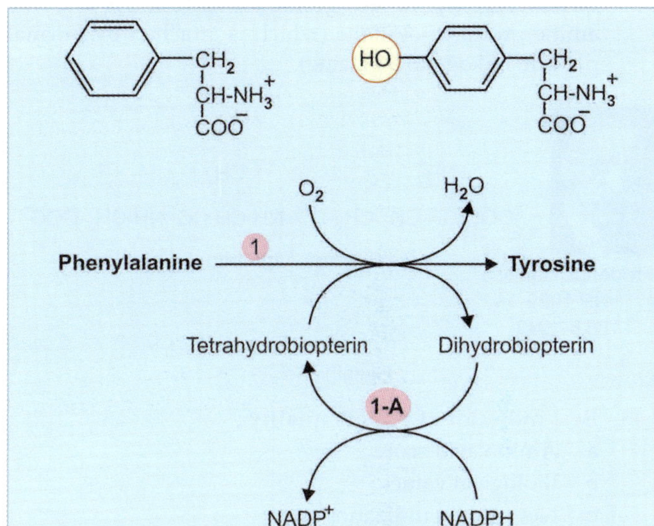

Phenylalanine catabolism; 1 = Phenylalanine hydroxylase; 1-A = NADPH dependent reductase.

45. Phenyl-alanine is NOT a precursor of:

a. Tyrosine
b. Epinephrine
c. Thyroxine
d. Melatonin

46. Leucine is an amino acid with a:

a. Non-polar side chain
b. Polar side chain
c. Negatively charged side-chain
d. Positively charged side-chain

The non-polar amino acids include: alanine, cysteine, glycine, isoleucine, leucine, methionine, phenylalanine, proline, tryptophan.

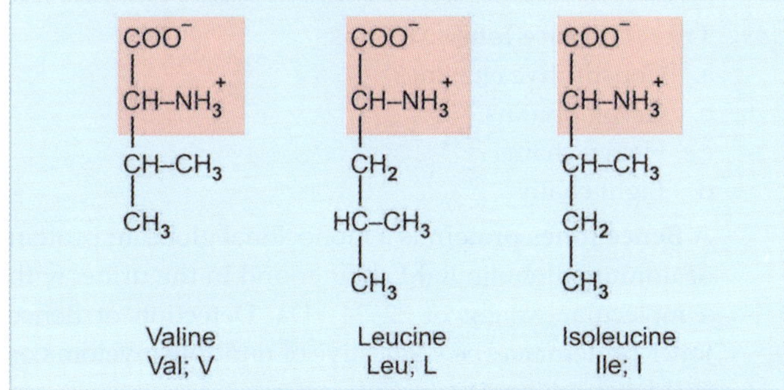

Branched chain amino acids.

47. Glutathione is:

a. Dipeptide
b. Oligopeptide
c. Tripeptide
d. Polypeptide

Glutathione (GSH) is an important antioxidant in plants, animals, fungi, and some bacteria and archaea,

Ans. **44. a.** Tryptophan **45. d.** Melatonin **46. a.** Non-polar... **47. c.** Tripeptide

preventing damage to important cellular components caused by reactive oxygen species such as free radicals, peroxides, lipid peroxides and heavy metals. It is a tripeptide with a gamma peptide linkage between the carboxyl group of the glutamate side-chain and the amine group of cysteine (which is attached by normal peptide linkage to a glycine).

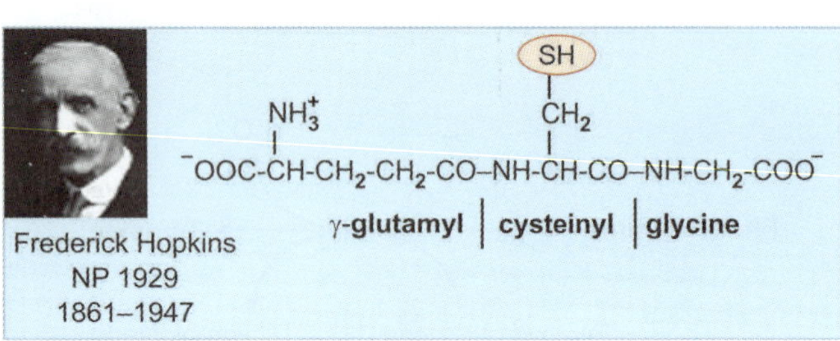

Glutathione.

48. Best indicator of protein quality:

a. Amino acid score
b. Biological value
c. Net protein utilization
d. Digestibility coefficient

The **net protein utilization**, or NPU, is the ratio of amino acid converted to proteins to the ratio of amino acids supplied. This figure is somewhat affected by the salvage of essential amino acids within the body, but is profoundly affected by the level of limiting amino acids within a foodstuff.

Experimentally, this value can be determined by determining dietary protein intake and then measuring nitrogen excretion. NPU is a better index than biological value to denote nutritional quality and availability of a protein.

49. True for Bence Jones proteins:

a. Constitutive enzymes
b. Cryoglobulins
c. Heavy chains
d. Light chains

A **Bence Jones protein** is a monoclonal globulin protein or immunoglobulin light chain found in the urine, with a molecular weight of 22–24 kDa. Detection of Bence Jones protein may be suggestive of multiple myeloma or Waldenström's macroglobulinemia.

50. Unstable amino acid in Alpa-helix:

a. Tryptophan
b. Glutamine
c. Alanine
d. Proline

Proline acts as a structural disruptor in the middle of regular secondary structure elements such as alpha helices and beta sheets; however, proline is commonly found as the first residue of an alpha helix and also in the edge strands of beta sheets. Proline is also commonly found in turns (another kind of secondary structure), and aids in the formation of beta turns.

51. Myoglobin contains:

a. Calcium
b. Sulphur
c. Lead
d. Iron

Myoglobin is an iron- and oxygen-binding protein found in the muscle tissue of vertebrates in general and in almost all mammals.

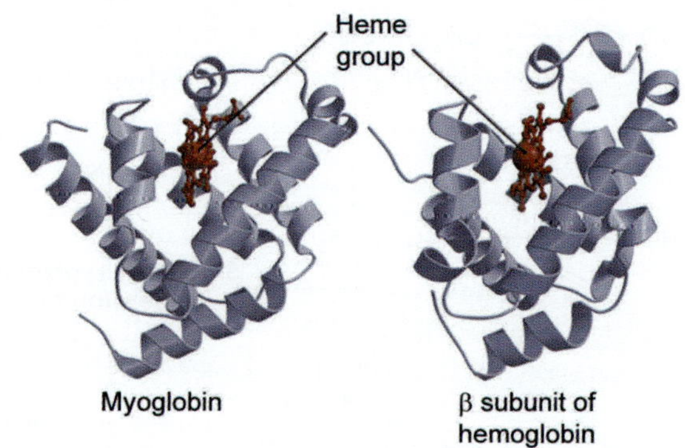

Myoglobin chain.

52. Collagen forms how much % of the skin:

a. 50
b. 60
c. 70
d. 80

Collagen is the fibrous protein constituent of skin, cartilage, bone, and other connective tissue. Collagen is the principal constituent of the fiber-network layer of our skin. More than a third of the body›s protein is **collagen**, and it can account for an even higher percentage in particular parts of the body. Collagen makes up 70% of our skin tissue.

53. NOT a muscle protein:

a. Myoglobin
b. Ferritin
c. Actin
d. Collagen

Ferritin is a ubiquitous intracellular protein that stores iron and releases it in a controlled fashion.

54. Atherosclerosis is associated with:

a. Lysine
b. Histidine
c. Homocysteine
d. Leucine

Ans. **48. c.** Net protein... **49. d.** Light chains **50. d.** Proline **51. d.** Iron **52. c.** 70 **53. b.** Ferritin **54. c.** Homocysteine

A high level of homocysteine in the blood (hyperhomocysteinemia) makes a person more prone to endothelial cell injury, which leads to inflammation in the blood vessels, which in turn may lead to atherogenesis, which can result in ischemic injury. Hyperhomocysteinemia is therefore a possible risk factor for coronary artery disease.

CARBOHYDRATE METABOLISM

55. Sodium fluoride is used for in-vitro preservation of glucose in blood samples. Which of the following enzyme is inhibited by sodium fluoride:

a. Malonate
b. Aconitase
c. Enolase
d. Hexokinase

Enolase

- It is also known as phosphopyruvate hydratase
- It is a metalloenzyme responsible for the catalysis of the conversion of 2-phosphoglycerate (2-PG) to phosphoenolpyruvate (PEP), the ninth and penultimate step of glycoslysis.
- Enolase belongs to the class Lyase.
- Enolase can also catalyze the reverse reaction, depending on environmental concentrations of substrates.
- The optimum pH for this enzyme is 6.5.
- Enolase is present in all tissues and organisms capable of glycolysis or fermentation.
- The enzyme was discovered by Lohmann and Meyerhof in 1934
- In humans, deficiency of ENO1 is linked to hereditary haemolytic anemia while ENO3 deficiency is linked to glycogen storage disease XIII.

Key enzymes	
Irreversible steps in glycolysis	Corresponding key gluconeogenic enzymes
Pyruvate kinase (step 9)	Pyruvate carboxylase; Phosphoenol pyruvate-carboxy kinase
Phosphofructokinase (step 3)	Fructose-1,6- bisphosphatase
Hexokinase (step 1)	Glucose-6-phosphatase

56. Which of the following metabolic pathway occur in more than one organ:

a. Lipogenesis
b. Oxidation of fatty acids
c. Gluconeogenesis
d. Glycolysis

Lactate, glycerol, propionate and some amino acids are good precursors for glucose synthesis (gluconeogenesis) that actively occurs in liver and kidney

Gluconeogenesis (GNG)

- It results in the generation of glucose from non-carbohydrate carbon substrates such as pyruvate, lactate, glycerol, and glucogenic amino acids.
- It is one of the two main mechanisms humans and many other animals use to keep blood glucose levels from dropping too low (hypoglycemia).
- The other means of maintaining blood glucose levels is through the degradation of glycogen (glycogenolysis)
- Gluconeogenesis is a ubiquitous process, present in plants, animals, fungi, bacteria, and other microorganisms.
- In vertebrates, gluconeogenesis takes place mainly in the liver and, to a lesser extent, in the cortex of kidneys.
- The process is highly endergonic until it is coupled to the hydrolysis of ATP or GTP, effectively making the process exoergic.
- For example, the pathway leading from pyruvate to glucose-6-phosphate requires 4 molecules of ATP and 2 molecules of GTP to proceed spontaneously.
- Gluconeogenesis is often associated with ketosis.
- Gluconeogenesis is also a target of therapy for type II diabetes, such as metformin, which inhibits glucose formation and stimulates glucose uptake by cells.

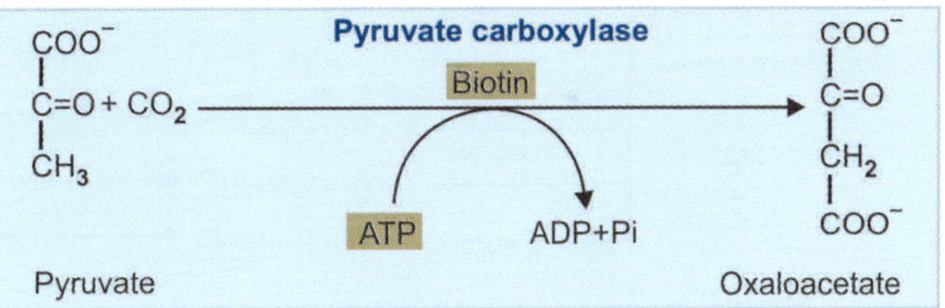

First step in gluconeogenesis.

57. Which of the following is produced in HMP shunt:

a. ATP
b. FMN
c. NADPH
d. NADP+

The **pentose phosphate pathway** (also called the **phosphogluconate pathway** and the **hexose monophosphate shunt**)

- It is parallel to glycolysis, and generates NADPH and pentoses (5-carbon sugars).
- While it does involve oxidation of glucose, its primary role is anabolic rather than catabolic.
- There are two distinct phases in the pathway.
  - The first is the oxidative phase, in which NADPH is generated, and
  - The second is the non-oxidative synthesis of 5-carbon sugars.
- For most organisms, the pentose phosphate pathway takes place in the cytosol; in plants, most steps take place in plastids.

Ans. 55. c. Enolase 56. c. Gluconeogenesis 57. c. NADPH

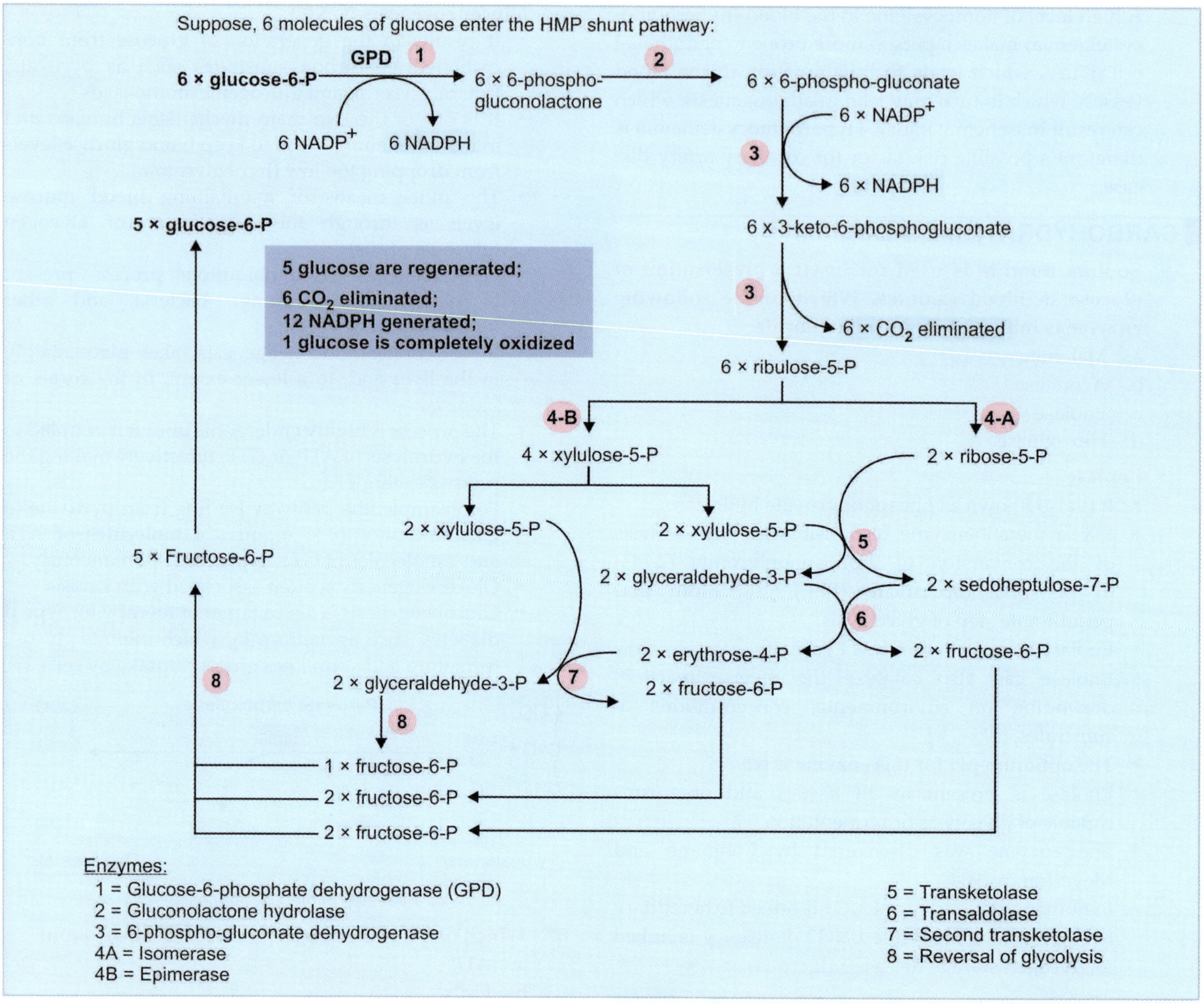

Suppose, 6 molecules of glucose enter the HMP shunt pathway:

GPD (1): 6 × glucose-6-P → 6 × 6-phospho-gluconolactone (6 $NADP^+$ → 6 NADPH)

(2): 6 × 6-phospho-gluconolactone → 6 × 6-phospho-gluconate

(3): 6 × 6-phospho-gluconate → 6 x 3-keto-6-phosphogluconate (6 × $NADP^+$ → 6 × NADPH)

(3): 6 x 3-keto-6-phosphogluconate → 6 × ribulose-5-P (6 × CO_2 eliminated)

(4-B): 4 × xylulose-5-P; (4-A): 2 × ribose-5-P

4 × xylulose-5-P → 2 × xylulose-5-P + 2 × xylulose-5-P

(5): 2 × xylulose-5-P + 2 × ribose-5-P → 2 × glyceraldehyde-3-P + 2 × sedoheptulose-7-P

(6): 2 × glyceraldehyde-3-P + 2 × sedoheptulose-7-P → 2 × erythrose-4-P + 2 × fructose-6-P

(7): 2 × xylulose-5-P + 2 × erythrose-4-P → 2 × glyceraldehyde-3-P + 2 × fructose-6-P

(8): 2 × glyceraldehyde-3-P → 1 × fructose-6-P

1 × fructose-6-P + 2 × fructose-6-P + 2 × fructose-6-P → 5 × Fructose-6-P → 5 × glucose-6-P (8)

5 glucose are regenerated;
6 CO_2 eliminated;
12 NADPH generated;
1 glucose is completely oxidized

Enzymes:
1 = Glucose-6-phosphate dehydrogenase (GPD)
2 = Gluconolactone hydrolase
3 = 6-phospho-gluconate dehydrogenase
4A = Isomerase
4B = Epimerase
5 = Transketolase
6 = Transaldolase
7 = Second transketolase
8 = Reversal of glycolysis

Summary of shunt pathway; numbers shows the steps referred in the text.

58. Oxidative phosphorylation leads to formation of:

a. ADP b. ATP
c. Phosphate d. Oxygen

Oxidative phosphorylation (or OXPHOS in short)

- It is the metabolic pathway in which the mitochondrial in cells use their structure, enzymes, and energy released by the oxidation of nutrients to reform ATP.
- ATP is the molecule that supplies energy to metabolism.
- Almost all aerobic organism carry out oxidative phosphorylation.
- During oxidative phosphorylation, electrons are transferred from electron donors to electron acceptors such as oxygen, in redox reactions.
- These redox reactions release energy, which is used to form ATP.

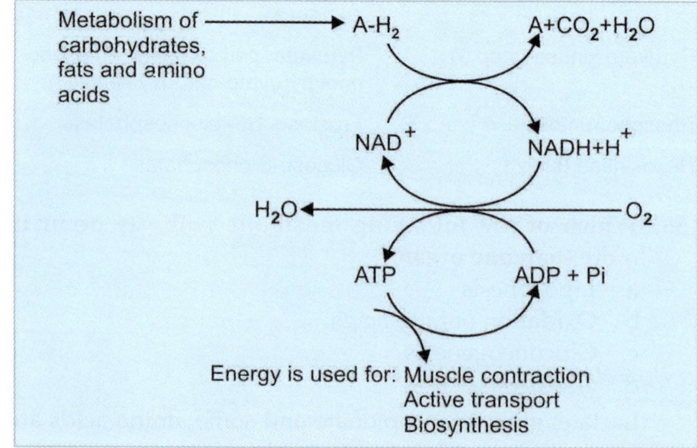

ATP generation. Food is catabolized; energy from food is trapped as ATP; it is then used for anabolic reactions.

Ans. **58. b. ATP**

59. Which of the following releases carbon dioxide:
a. Glycolysis
b. HMP pathway
c. Amino acid synthesis
d. All of the above

The overall reaction for oxidative process of HMP shunt is:

Glucose 6-phosphate + 2 $NADP^+$ + H_2O → ribulose 5-phosphate + 2 NADPH + 2 H^+ + CO_2

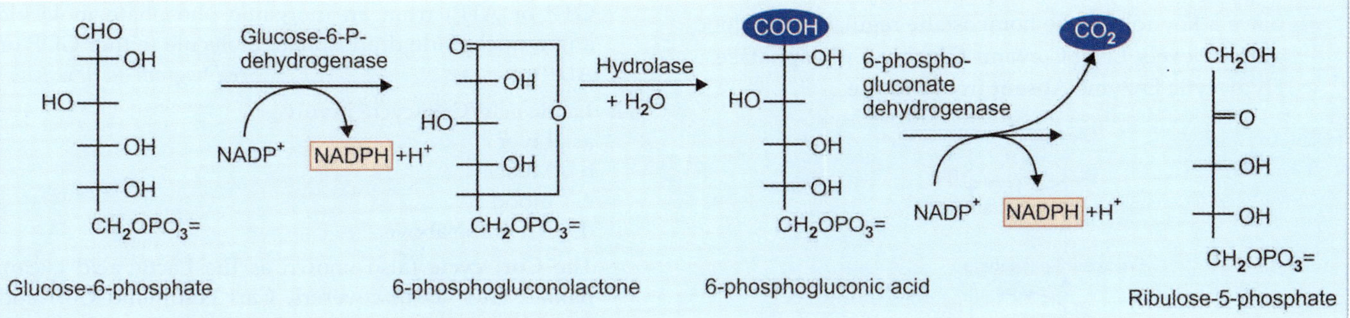

Oxidative phase of HMP shunt pathway; Steps 1, 2 and 3.

60. First product of glycogenolysis:
a. Fructose-1-phosphate
b. Glucose-1-phosphate
c. Glucose-1,6-diphosphate
d. Glucose-6-phosphate

The overall reaction for the breakdown of glycogen to glucose-1-phosphate is:

glycogen (**n residues**) + Pi ⇌ glycogen (**n-1 residues**) + glucose-1-phosphate

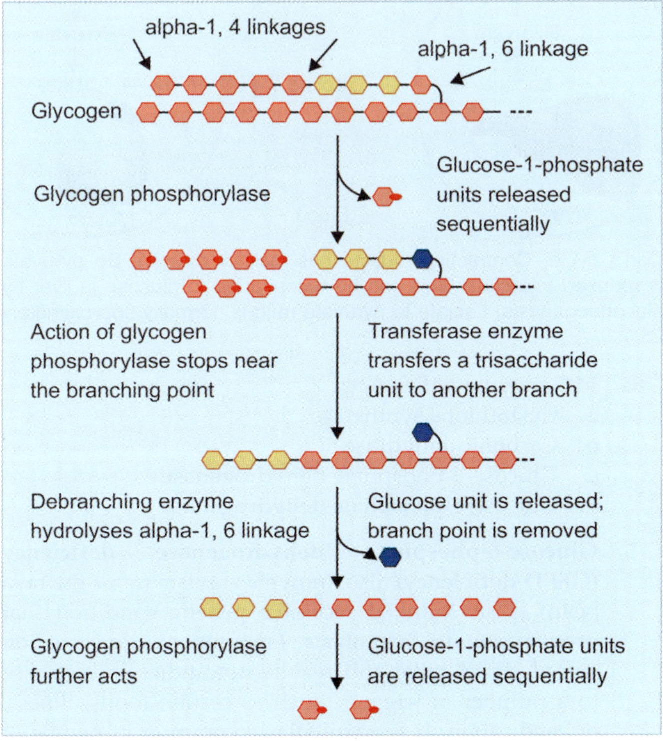

Glycogenolysis.

61. End product of anaerobic glycolysis:
a. Pyruvate
b. Lactate
c. Ethanol
d. Cholesterol

Anaerobic glycolysis is only an effective means of energy production during short, intense exercise, providing energy for a period ranging from 10 seconds to 2 minutes. The anaerobic glycolysis (lactic acid) system is dominant from about 10–30 seconds during a maximal effort. It replenishes very quickly over this period and produces 2 ATP molecules per glucose molecule, or about 5% of glucose's energy potential.

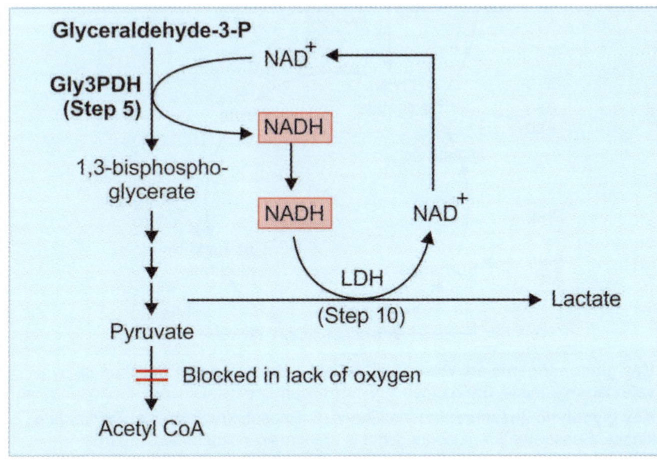

Lactate formation is necessary for reconversion of NADH to NAD+ during anaerobiasis.

62. Blood glucose levels cannot be augmented by mobilization of muscle glycogen due to lack of:
a. G-6-P dehydrogenase
b. G-6-phosphatase
c. Aldolase
d. Glucokinase

Ans. **59. b.** HMP pathway **60. b.** Glucose-1-phosphate **61. b.** Lactate **62. b.** G-6-phosphatase

Glucose 6-phosphatase (G6Pase) is an enzyme that hydrolyzes glucose-6-phosphate, resulting in the creation of a phosphate group and free glucose. Glucose is then exported from the cell via glucose transporter membrane proteins. This catalysis completes the final step in gluconeogenesis and glycogenolysis and therefore plays a key role in the homeostatic regulation of blood glucose levels. Liver Contains **Glucose 6-phosphatase**, a Hydrolytic Enzyme **Absent** from **Muscle**.

Key gluconeogenic enzymes: 1=Pyruvate carboxylase; 2=Phosphoenol pyruvate carboxykinase; 3=Fructose-1, 6-bisphosphatase; 4=Glucose-6-phosphatase
Key glycolytic enzymes: 5=Hexokinase; 6=Phosphofructokinase; 7=Pyruvate kinase. Substrates for gluconeogenesis are shown inside brown squares.

Gluconeogenic pathway.

63. In TCA cycle, substrate level phosphorylation occurs at:

a. Succinate dehydrogenase
b. Malonate reduction
c. Thiokinase
d. Fructase

Succinyl coenzyme A synthetase (**SCS**, also known as **succinyl-CoA synthetase** or **succinate thiokinase** or **succinate-CoA ligase**) is an enzyme that catalyzes the reversible reaction of succinyl-CoA to succinate. The enzyme facilitates the coupling of this reaction to the formation of a nucleoside triphosphate molecule (either GTP or ATP) from an inorganic phosphate molecule and a nucleoside diphosphate molecule (either GDP or ADP). *(See Diagram on next page)*

64. Lactic acid/Cori cycle involves:

a. Liver
b. Muscle
c. Blood
d. All of the above

The **Cori cycle** (also known as the Lactic acid cycle), named after its discoverers, Carl Ferdinand Cori and Gerty Cori, refers to the metabolic pathway in which lactate produced by anaerobic glycolysis in the muscles moves to the liver and is converted to glucose, which then returns to the muscles and is metabolized back to lactate.

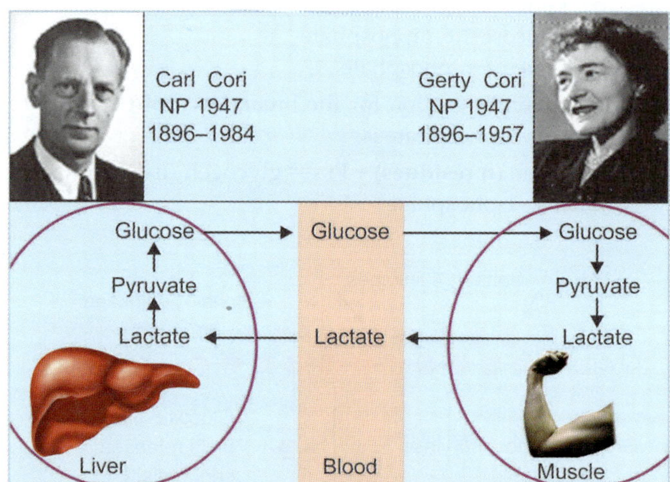

Cori's cycle. Contracting muscle has lack of oxygen. So pyruvate is reduced to lactate. This can be reconverted to glucose in liver by gluconeogenesis. Lactate to pyruvate ratio is normally approximately 25:1.

65. MC enzyme deficiency:

a. Cystathione synthetase
b. Carbonic anhydrase
c. Glucose-6-phosphate dehydrogenase
d. Glucose-1-phosphate dehydrogenase

Glucose-6-phosphate dehydrogenase deficiency (G6PD deficiency) also known as favism (after the fava bean) is an X-linked recessive genetic condition that predisposes to hemolysis (spontaneous destruction of red blood cells) and resultant jaundice in response to a number of triggers, such as certain foods, illness, or medication. It is parti-cularly common in people of Mediterranean and African origin.

Ans. **63. c.** Thiokinase **64. d.** All of the above **65. c.** Glucose...

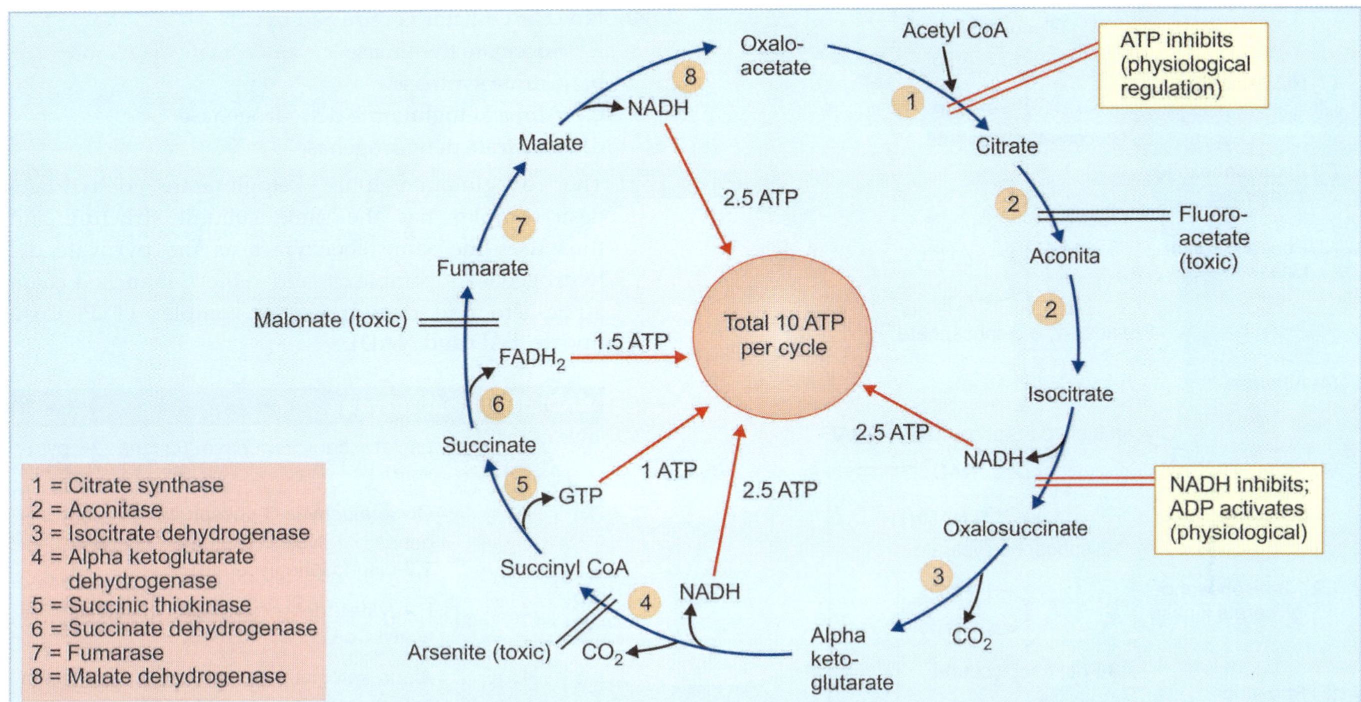

Summary of Krebs citric acid cycle. Enzymes are numbered. Reactions number 3 and 4 are carbon dioxide elimination steps. Physiological regulatory steps are: Step No.1(citrate synthase) is physiologically inhibited by ATP. Step No.3 (ICDH) is inhibited by NADH and activated by ADP. Steps where energy is trapped are marked with the co-enzyme and the number of ATP generated during that reaction. A total of 10 ATPs are generated during one cycle. Recent work shows that in the electron transport chain, NADH may produce only 2 ½ ATPs and FADH only 1 ½ ATPs.

66. By which of the following anticoagulants, used in estimating blood glucose, glycolysis is prevented:

a. EDTA
b. Heparin
c. Sodium fluoride
d. Sodium citrate

Fluoride is a known competitor of enolase's substrate 2-PG. The fluoride is part of a complex with magnesium and phosphate, which binds in the active site instead of 2-PG. As such, drinking fluoridated water provides fluoride at a level that inhibits oral bacteria enolase activity. Disruption of the bacteria's glycolytic pathway—and, thus, its normal metabolic functioning—prevents dental caries from forming.

67. Phosphofructokinase is the key enzyme of:

a. TCA cycle
b. Beta oxidation
c. Gluconeogenesis
d. Glycolysis

Phosphofructokinase is a kinase enzyme that phosphorylates fructose 6-phosphate in glycolysis.

(See Diagram on next page)

68. Mucopolysacchridoses results in accumulation of:

a. Acetyl CoA
b. Glycogen
c. Glycosaminoglycans
d. Sorbitol

Mucopolysaccharidoses are a group of metabolic disorders caused by the absence or malfunctioning of lysosomal enzymes needed to break down molecules called glycosaminoglyc

Features of mucopolysaccharidoses

Type	*Eponym*	*Deficient enzyme*	*Clinical findings*
I	Hurler's	L-Iduronidase	MR^{+++}; Skeletal deformity^{++}; Corneal opacity^{++}; DS and HS in urine
II	Hunter's	Iduronate sulfatase	MR^{+}; Skeletal deformity^{++}; deafness; no corneal clouding; DS and HS in urine
III	Sanfilippo's	N-Acetyl glucosaminidase, Heparan sulfatase	MR^{++}; Skeletal deformity^{+}; corneal clouding^{+}; HS in urine; 3 different types are reported
IV	Morquio's	Galactosamine sulfatase, β-D-galactosidase	MR^{+}; Skeletal deformity^{+}; epiphyseal dysplasia^{+}; Corneal opacity^{+}; KS and CS in urine; 2 types reported
V	Scheie's	L-Iduronidase	No MR; Mild skeletal changes; corneal opacity^{++}; DS in urine
VI	Maroteaux-Lamy's	N-Acetyl-β-D-Galactosamino-4-Sulfatase	Skeletal deformity^{+++}; corneal opacity^{++}; No MR; DS in urine
VII	Sly's	β-Glucuronidase	MR^{+}; DS and HS in urine

MR = mental retardation; CS = chondroitin sulfate;
KS = keratan sulfate; HS = heparan sulfate;
DS = dermatan sulfate.

Ans. **66. c.** Sodium fluoride **67. d.** Glycolysis **68. c.** Glycosaminoglycans

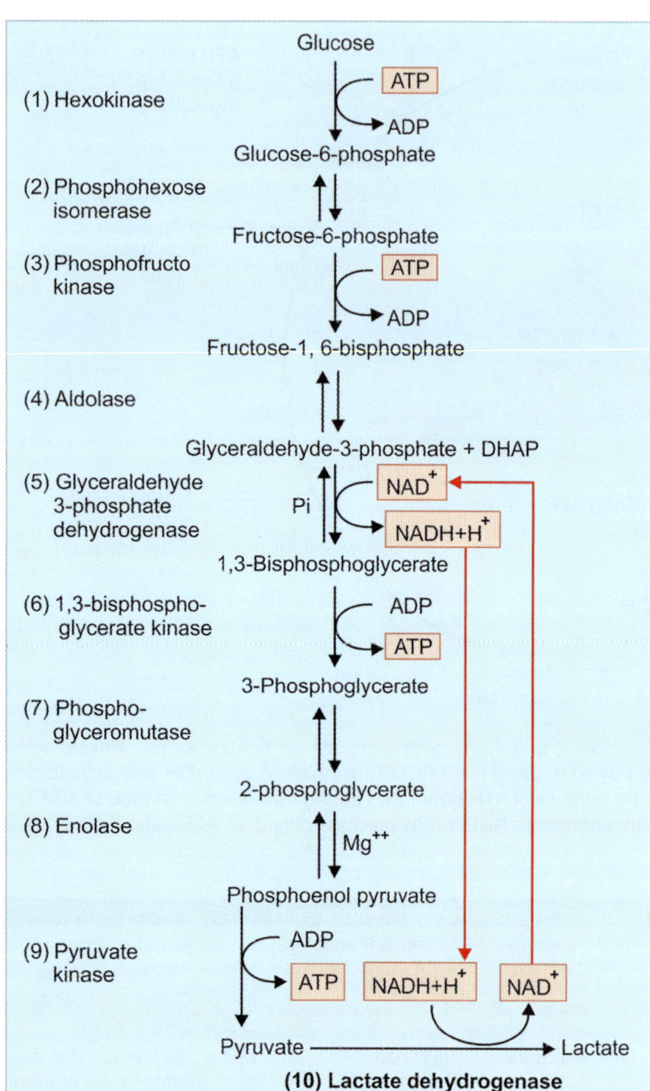

Summary of glycolysis (Embden-Meyerhof - Parnas pathway). Steps 1, 3 and 9 are key enzyems; these reactions are irreversible. Steps 6 and 9 produce energy. Steps 5 and 10 are coupled for regeneration of NAD+.

69. Oxidation may lead to hemolysis in:

a. Hemophilics
b. Sickle cell anemia
c. Hereditary spherocytosis
d. G-6-PD deficients

G6PD converts glucose-6-phophate into 6-phosphoglucono-δ-lactone and is the rate-limiting enzyme of this metabolic pathway that supplies reducing energy to cells by maintaining the level of the reduced form of the co-enzyme nicotinamide adenine dinucleotide phosphate (NADPH). The NADPH in turn maintains the supply of reduced glutathione in the cells that is used to mop up free radicals that cause oxidative damage.

70. NAD as cofactor is required by:

a. Succinate thiokinase
b. Citrate synthase
c. Alpha ketoglutarate dehydrogenase
d. Isocitrate dehydrogenase

The oxoglutarate/alpha ketoglutarate dehydrogenase complex has the same subunit structure and thus uses the same coenzymes as the pyruvate dehydrogenase complex and the branched-chain alpha-keto acid dehydrogenase complex (TTP, CoA, lipoate, FAD and NAD).

NAD⁺ dependent enzymes	
1.	Lactate dehydrogenase (lactate → pyruvate)
2.	Glyceraldehyde-3-phosphate dehydrogenase (glyceraldehyde-3-phosphate → 1,3-bisphosphoglycerate)
3.	Pyruvate dehydrogenase (pyruvate → acetyl CoA)
4.	Alpha ketoglutarate dehydrogenase (alpha ketoglutarate → succinyl CoA)
5.	Beta hydroxyacyl CoA dehydrogenase (beta hydroxyacyl CoA → beta ketoacyl CoA
6.	Glutamate dehydrogenase (Glutamate → alpha ketoglutarate

71. Glucose can be synthesized from all EXCEPT:

a. Amino acids
b. Glycerol
c. Acetoacetate
d. Lactic acid

Gluconeogenesis (GNG) is a metabolic pathway that results in the generation of glucose from non-carbohydrate carbon substrates such as pyruvate, lactate, glycerol, and glucogenic amino acids. While primarily odd-chain fatty acids can be converted into glucose, it is possible for at least some even-chain fatty acids.

72. All increase serum glucose EXCEPT:

a. Glucagon
b. Epinephrine
c. Cortisol
d. Vasopressin

Vasopressin is a peptide hormone that increases water permeability of the kidney's collecting duct and distal convoluted tubule by inducing translocation of aquaporin-CD water channels in the plasma membrane of collecting duct cells. It also increases peripheral vascular resistance, which in turn increases arterial blood pressure.

Ans. 69. d. G-6-PD deficients **70. c.** Alpha ketoglut... **71. c.** Acetoacetate **72. d.** Vasopressin

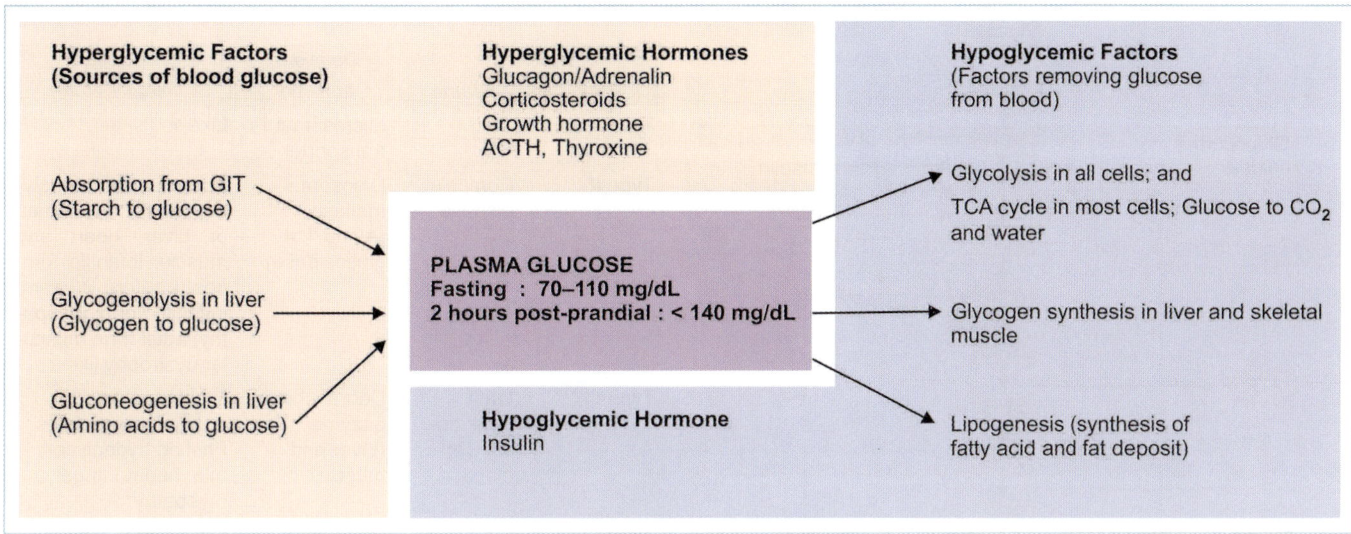

Overview of regulation of blood sugar.

73. All are common in diabetes and starvation EXCEPT:
a. Increased gluconeogenesis
b. Increased glycogen degradation
c. Increased fatty acid mobilization from adipose tissue
d. Cholesterol synthesis

Fasting suppressed cholesterol synthesis by 90%. **Insulin** leads to a decrease in cAMP, which in turn activates **cholesterol synthesis**.

74. Mature RBC contains all EXCEPT:
a. Enzyme of HMP shunt pathway
b. Enzyme of TCA cycle
c. Glycolytic enzymes
d. Pyridine molecules

RBC lacks mitochondria, which is the site of TCA cycle

75. Increased glycosaminoglycans in urine is pathognomic of:
a. Maple syrup urine disease
b. Tyrosinemia
c. Mucopolysaccharidosis
d. Cushing's disease

Mucopolysaccharidosis are a group of metabolic disorders caused by the absence or malfunctioning of lysosomal enzymes needed to break down molecules called glycosaminoglycans—long chains of sugar carbohydrates in each of our cells that help build bone, cartilage, tendons, corneas, skin and connective tissue. Glycosaminoglycans (formerly called mucopolysaccharides) are also found in the fluid that lubricates our joints.

76. Hexose sugar is NOT present in:
a. Ribose
b. Glucose
c. Fructose
d. Galactose

Ribose is an organic compound with the formula $C_5H_{10}O_5$; specifically, a pentose monosaccharide (simple sugar) with linear form H–(C=O)–$(CHOH)_4$–H, which has all the hydroxyl groups on the same side in the Fischer projection.

Common monosaccharides

No. of carbon atoms	*Generic name*	*Aldoses (with aldehyde group)*	*Ketoses (with keto group)*
3	Triose	Glyceraldehyde	Dihydroxyacetone
4	Tetrose	Erythrose	Erythrulose
5	Pentose	Arabinose, Xylose, Ribose	Xylulose, Ribulose
6	Hexose	Glucose, Galactose, Mannose	Fructose
7	Heptose		Sedoheptulose

77. Key glycolytic enzymes in glycolysis are all EXCEPT:
a. Phosphofructokinase
b. Hexokinase
c. Pyruvate kinase
d. Glucose 1,6,diphosphate synthase

Glucose-1,6-bisphosphate synthase is a type of enzyme called a phosphotransferase and is involved in mammalian starch and sucrose metabolism. It catalyzes the transfer of a phosphate group from 1,3-bisphosphoglycerate to glucose-1-phosphate, yielding 3-phosphoglycerate and glucose-1,6-bisphosphate.

Ans. 73. **d.** Cholesterol... 74. **b.** Enzyme of TCA cycle 75. **c.** Mucopoly... 76. **a.** Ribose 77. **d.** Glucose 1,6,...

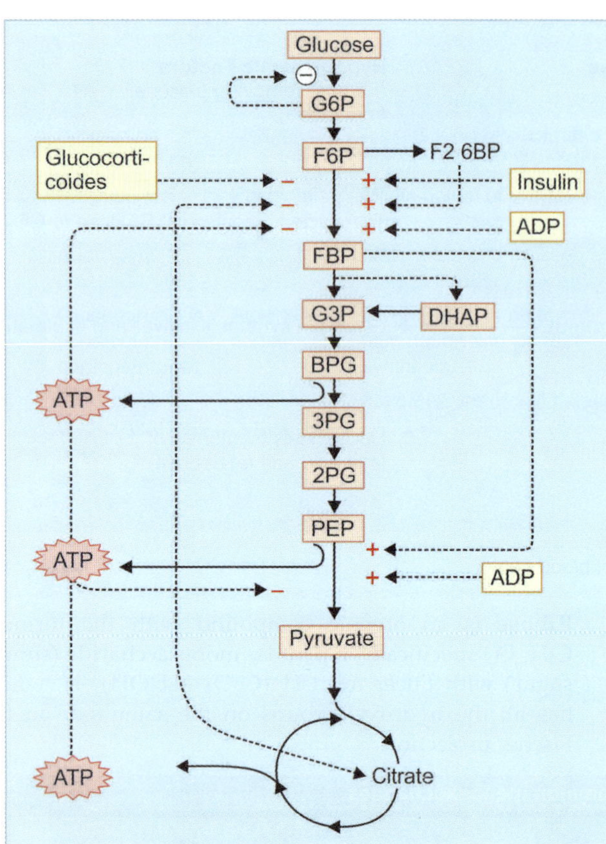

Summary of regulation of glycosis.

78. Andersen disease is due to lack of:

a. Branching enzyme
b. Debranching enzyme
c. Acid maltase
d. Myophosphorylase

Glycogen storage disease type IV is a rare hereditary metabolic disorder. It is the result of a mutation in GBE1 gene, which causes a defect in the glycogen branching enzyme. Therefore, glycogen is not made properly and abnormal glycogen cells accumulate in cells; most severely in cardiac and muscle cells.

Glycogen storage diseases

Type	*Name*	*Deficient enzyme*	*Clinical features*
Type 0a		Glycogen synthase 2 (Liver)	Hypoglycemia, hyperketonemia, early death
Type Ia	von Gierke's disease	Glucose-6-phosphatase	Fasting hypoglycemia; hepatomegaly, thrombocyte dysfunction
Type Ib		Microsomal glucose 6 phosphate translocase	Same as above, plus neutropenia and recurrent infections
Type Ic		Microsomal Pi transporter	Like 1
Type II	Pompe's disease	Lysosomal maltase (Alpha 1, 4 glucosidase)	Accumulation of glycogen in lysosomes of Liver, heart and muscle; infantile form death before 2 years; juvenile form myopathy; adult form muscular dystrophy like
Type III	Limit dextrinosis Cori's disease	Debranching enzyme (Liver and muscle)	Highly branched dextrin accumulates; Fasting hypoglycemia; hepatomegaly, myopathy
Type IV	Amylopectinosis Anderson's disease	Branching enzyme (Liver and muscle)	Glycogen with few branches; hepatospleno- megaly, cirrhosis; death before age of 5
Type V	McArdle's disease	Muscle phosphorylase (Skeletal muscle)	Excercise intolerance; accumulation of glycogen in muscles, myoglobinuria
Type VI	Hers' disease	Liver phosphorylase	Mild hypoglycemia; hepatomegaly; hyperlipidemia, ketosis; better prognosis than other types
Type VII	Tarui's disease	Muscle PFK-1 Muscle, RBCs)	Glycogen accumulates in muscles; exercise intolerance; hemolytic anemia
Type VIII		Liver phosphorylase kinase	Mild hypoglycemia; better prognosis
Type IXa, b		Muscle phosphorylase kinase (liver, leukocytes, muscle)	Like VI
Fanconi Bickel hepatorenal glycogenosis		GLUT-2	Failure to thrive, hepatomegaly, rickets, proximal renal tubular dysnfunction

79. Which is debranching enzyme:

a. Glycogen synthetase
b. Glucose-6-phosphatase
c. Amylo-1, 6-glucosidase
d. Amylo-1, 4-1, 6-transglycoslase

Glucosyltransferase and glucosidase are performed by a single enzyme in mammals, yeast, and some bacteria, but by two distinct enzymes in E. coli and other bacteria, complicating nomenclature. Proteins that catalyze both functions are referred to as glycogen debranching enzymes (GDEs). When glucosyltransferase and

Ans. **78. a.** Branching... **79. c.** Amylo...

glucosidase are catalyzed by distinct enzymes, "glycogen debranching enzyme" usually refers to the glucosidase enzyme.

80. Required by phosphofructokinase:

a. Copper
b. Magnesium
c. Manganese
d. Inorganic phosphate

PFK is about 300 amino acids in length, and structural studies of the bacterial enzyme have shown it comprises two similar (alpha/beta) lobes: one involved in ATP binding and the other housing both the substrate-binding site and the allosteric site (a regulatory binding site distinct from the active site, but that affects enzyme activity). The identical tetramer subunits adopt 2 different conformations: in a 'closed' state, the bound magnesium ion bridges the phosphoryl groups of the enzyme products (ADP and fructose-1,6-bisphosphate); and in an 'open' state, the magnesium ion binds only the ADP, as the 2 products are now further apart.

81. Major fate of glucose-6-phosphate in tissues in a well fed state:

a. Hydrolysis to glucose
b. Conversion to glycogen
c. Isomerization to fructose-6-phosphatase
d. Conversion to ribulose-5-phosphate

Because of its prominent position in cellular chemistry, glucose 6-phosphate has many possible fates within the cell. It lies at the start of two major metabolic pathways: glycolysis and the pentose phosphate pathway. In addition to these metabolic pathways, glucose 6-phosphate may also be converted to glycogen or starch for storage. This storage is in the liver and muscles in the form of glycogen for most multicellular animals, and in intracellular starch or glycogen granules for most other organisms.

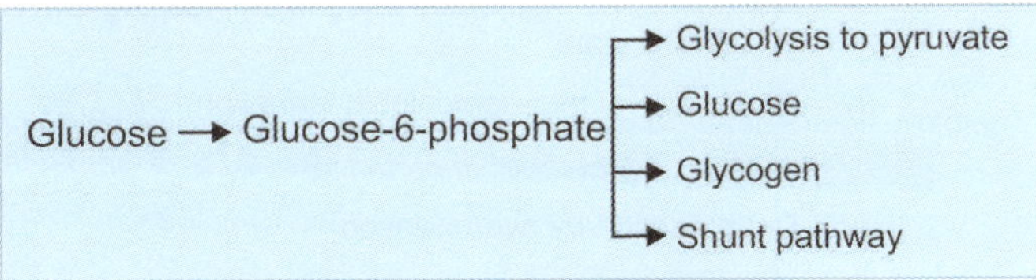

Fate of glucose-6-phosphate.

82. L or D form of a sugar is based on:

a. Glucose
b. Glycogen
c. Glyceraldehyde
d. Fructose

In the D/L system, glyceraldehyde is used as the configurational standard for carbohydrates. Monosaccharides with an absolute configuration identical to (*R*)-glyceraldehyde at the last stereocentre, for example C5 in glucose, are assigned the stereo-descriptor D-. Those similar to (*S*)-glyceraldehyde are assigned an L-.

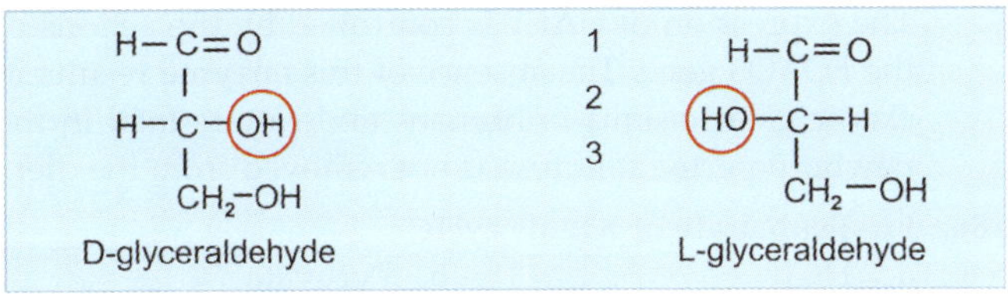

Stereoisomers.

83. Stimulation to increase diphosphoglycerate content in RBC:

a. Hypoxia
b. Chronic anemia
c. Both
d. None

Conditions of low tissue oxygen concentration such as high altitude (2,3-BPG levels are higher in those acclimated to high altitudes), airway obstruction, or congestive heart failure will tend to cause RBCs to generate more 2,3-BPG in their effort to generate energy by allowing more oxygen to be released in tissues deprived of oxygen.

84. Phase of Kreb cycle blocked by succinyl CoA:

a. Succinate dehydrogenase
b. Isocitrate dehydrogenase
c. Alpha ketoglutarate dehydrogenase
d. Malate dehydrogenase

Oxoglutarate/alpha ketoglutarate dehydrogenase is a key control point in the citric acid cycle. It is inhibited by its products, succinyl CoA and NADH. A high energy charge in the cell will also be inhibitive. ADP and calcium ions are allosteric activators of the enzyme.

85. MC enzyme deficient in galactosemics:

a. Galactose-1-phosphate uridyl transferase/ GALT
b. Galactosidase
c. UDP galactose epimerase
d. Galactokinase

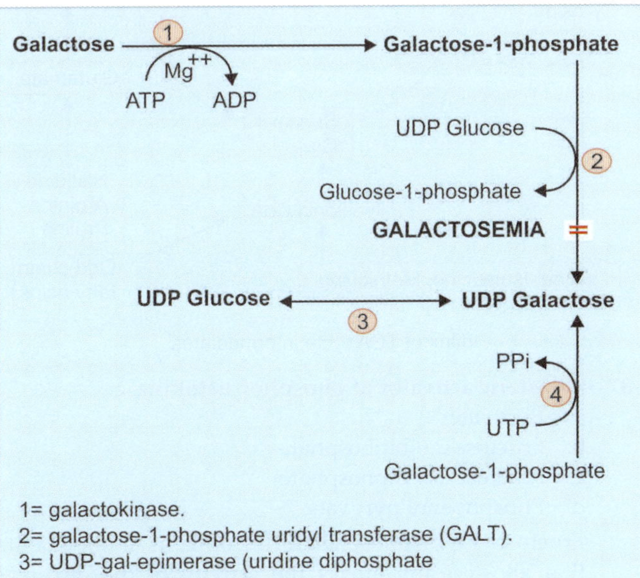

Summary of galactose metabolism.

Ans. 80. **b.** Magnesium 81. **b.** Conversion... 82. **c.** Glyceraldehyde 83. **c.** Both
84. **c.** Alpha ketogl... 85. **a.** Galactose...

The expression of GALT is controlled by the actions of the FOXO3 gene. The absence of this enzyme results in classic galactosemia in humans and can be fatal in the newborn period if lactose is not removed from the diet.

86. First substrate of Kreb's cycle:

a. HCl b. Pyruvate
c. Lipoprotein d. Glycine

The citric acid cycle is a key metabolic pathway that unifies carbohydrate, fat, and protein metabolism. The reactions of the cycle are carried out by 8 enzymes that completely oxidize acetate, in the form of acetyl-CoA, into two molecules each of carbon dioxide and water. Through catabolism of sugars, fats, and proteins, a two-carbon organic product acetate in the form of acetyl-CoA is produced which enters the citric acid cycle.

One of the primary sources of acetyl-CoA is from the breakdown of sugars by glycolysis which yield pyruvate that in turn is decarboxylated by the enzyme pyruvate dehydrogenase generating acetyl-CoA.

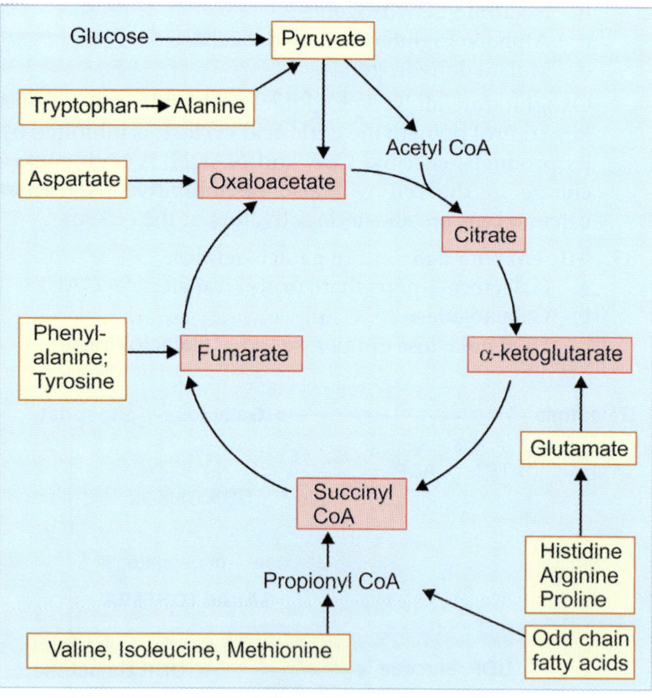

Influx of TCA cycle intermediates.

87. Allosteric activator of phosphofructokinase:

a. Pyruvate
b. Fructose-2,6-biphosphate
c. Fructose-1,6-biphosphate
d. Phosphoenol pyruvate

Fructose 2,6-bisphosphate/Fru-2,6-P2, is a metabolite that allosterically affects the activity of the enzymes phosphofructokinase 1 (PFK-1) and fructose 1,6-bisphosphatase (FBPase-1) to regulate glycolysis and gluconeogenesis.

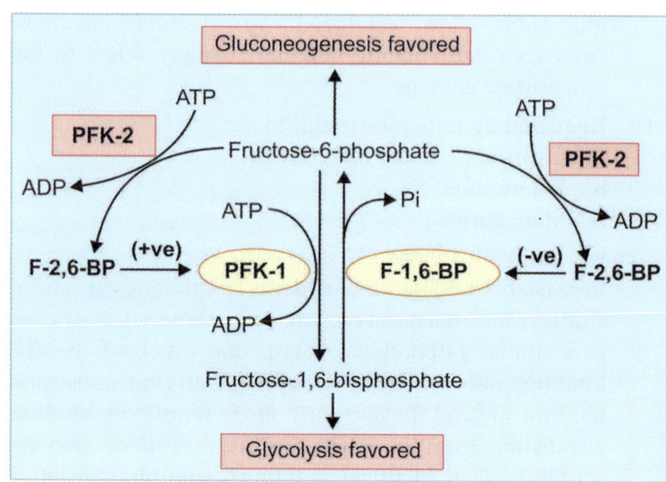

Reciprocal regulation of PFK-2 and fructose-2,6-bisphosphatase by phosphorylation.

88. Product of pentose phosphate pathway:

a. ATP
b. Pyruvate
c. NADPH
d. Lactate

The **pentose phosphate pathway** (also called the **phosphogluconate pathway** and the **hexose monophosphate shunt**) is a metabolic pathway parallel to glycolysis that generates NADPH and pentoses (5-carbon sugars). While it does involve oxidation of glucose, its primary role is anabolic rather than catabolic.

Significance of HMP shunt pathway
Metabolic importance:
1. To produce NADPH and pentose phosphates
NADPH is required for
i. Reductive biosynthesis—fatty acids, cholesterol and steroid hormones
ii. Free radical scavenging
iii. Maintain RBC membrane integrity by keeping GSH in reduced state
iv. Prevention of met-hemoglobin formation
Metabolic importance:
v. Detoxification by hydroxylation
vi. Maintain the transparency of lens
vii. Bactericidal activity of macrophages
2. Ribose-5-phosphate is required for nucleic acid synthesis Clinical Importance
i. Glucose-6-phosphate dehydrogenase deficiency
ii. Drug induced hemolytic anemia
iii. Met-hemoglobinemia
iv. Thiamine deficiency leads to reduced transketolase activity

Ans. 86. **b.** Pyruvate 87. **b.** Fructose-2,6... 88. **c.** NADPH

89. Adipocyte use:
a. GLUT4 b. GLUT3
c. GLUT2 d. GLUT1

GLUT4 is primarily found in
- Skeletal muscle
- Cardiac muscle
- Adipose tissue

Glucose transporters		
Transporter	*Present in*	*Properties*
GluT1	RBC, brain, kidney, colon, retina, placenta	Glucose uptake in most of cells
GluT2	Serosal surface of intestinal cells, liver, beta cells of pancreas	Low affinity; glucose uptake in liver; glucose sensor in beta cells
GluT3	Neurons, brain	High affinity; glucose into brain cells
GluT4	Skeletal, heart muscle, adipose tissue	Insulin-mediated glucose uptake
GluT5	Small intestine, testis, sperms, kidney	Fructose transporter; poor ability to transport glucose
GluT7	Liver endoplasmic reticulum	Glucose from ER to cytoplasm
SGluT	Intestine, kidney	Cotransport; from lumen into cell

90. C peptide is part of:
a. Pro-insulin b. Insulin
c. ACTH d. Growth hormone

The **connecting peptide**, or **C-peptide**, is a short 31-amino-acid polypeptide that connects insulin's A-chain to its B-chain in the proinsulin molecule.

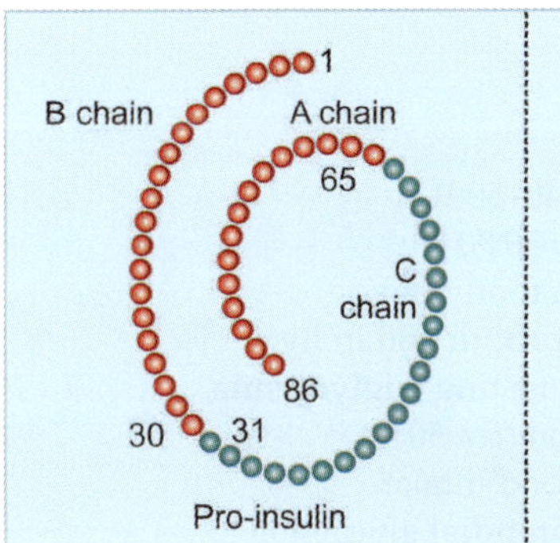

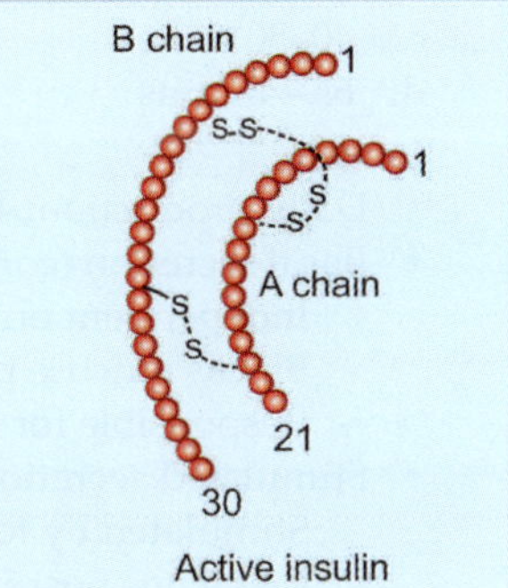

Insulin biosynthesis.

91. Insulin is NOT required for glucose transport in:
a. Heart muscle b. Adipose tissue
c. Skeletal muscle d. RBC

GLUT4 is the insulin-regulated glucose transporter found primarily in adipose tissues and striated muscle (skeletal and cardiac).

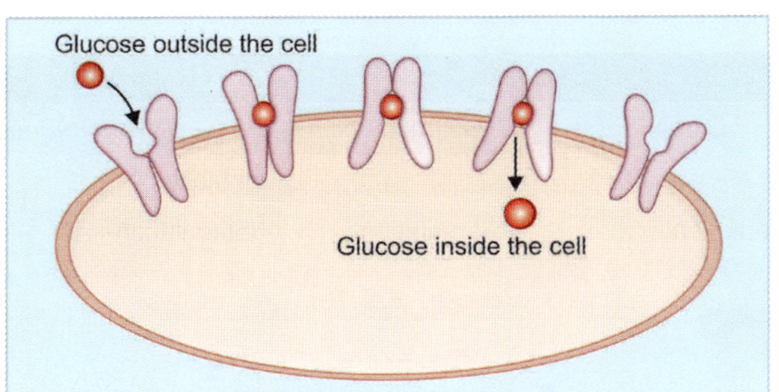

GluT-Glucose transport in cells.

92. Insulin stimulates glucose uptake by:
a. GLUT4 b. GLUT3
c. GLUT2 d. GLUT1

Under conditions of low insulin, Most GLUT4 is sequestered in intracellular vesicles in muscle and fat cells. Insulin induces a rapid increase in the uptake of glucose by inducing the translocation of GLUT4 from these vesicles to the plasma membrane.

93. True regarding insulin receptor:
a. Trimeric structure
b. Tyrosine kinase activity
c. 3 subunits
d. Subnuits held together by glycosidic linkages

The **insulin receptor (IR)** is a transmembrane receptor that is activated by insulin, IGF-I, IGF-II and belongs to the large class of tyrosine kinase receptors.

Protein kinases (Phosphorylated proteins)				
Signal molecule	*Second messenger*	*Protein kinase*	*Type*	*Substrates*
Hormones (glucagon, epinephrine, HSL, ADH, glycogen, ACTH, PTH, etc.	cAMP	Protein kinase A	Ser/Thr	Enzymes like phosphorylase, PFK2, CREBs, etc.
Nitric oxide, AMP	cGMP	Protein kinase G	Ser.Thr	Myosin, transducin
Serotonin, TRH	Calcium, IP3	Cam kinase	Ser/Thr	Exocytosis, smooth muscle contraction
Oxytocin, PDGF	DAG	Protein kinase C	Ser/Thr	Transcription factors, ion channel transporters

Contd...

Ans. 89. **a.** GLUT4 90. **a.** Pro-insulin 91. **d.** RBC 92. **a.** GLUT4
93. **b.** Tyrosine kinase..

Contd...

Signal molecule	*Second messenger*	*Protein kinase*	*Type*	*Substrates*
Growth factors, cytokines	PIP3	Protein kinase B	Ser/Thr	Glycogen metabolism, glucose transport, death signals like BAD
Insulin and insulin like growth factors	RTK in receptor	Tyrosine kinase	Tyr	IRS-1 (Insulin response substrate 1), IRS-2, MAP kinase, PDK
GH, prolactin, cytokines	RTK in receptor	Janus kinase (JAK)	Tyr	STAT (Signal transducers and activators of transcription)

94. Insulin stimulates glucose entry into:

a. Brain b. Cardiac muscle
c. Kidney d. Retina

GLUT4 is the insulin-regulated glucose transporter found primarily in adipose tissues and striated muscle (skeletal and cardiac).

95. Insulin secretion is inhibited by:

a. Glucose
b. Amino acid
c. Gastrointestinal hormones
d. Norpinephrine

Release of insulin is strongly inhibited by the stress hormone norepinephrine (noradrenaline), which leads to increased blood glucose levels during stress. It appears that release of catecholamines by the sympathetic nervous system has conflicting influences on insulin release by beta cells, because insulin release is inhibited by α_2-adrenergic receptors and stimulated by β_2-adrenergic receptors.

Effects of hormones on glucose level in blood
A. Effect of insulin (hypoglycemic hormone) 1. Lowers blood glucose 2. Favors glycogen synthesis 3. Promotes glycolysis 4. Inhibits gluconeogenesis
B. Glucagon (hyperglycemic hormone) 1. Increases blood glucose 2. Promotes glycogenolysis 3. Enhances gluconeogenesis 4. Depresses glycogen synthesis 5. Inhibits glycolysis (Details given below)
C. Cortisol (hyperglycemic hormone) 1. Increases blood sugar level 2. Increases gluconeogenesis 3. Releases amino acids from the muscle
D. Epinephrine or Adrenaline (hyperglycemic) 1. Increases blood sugar level 2. Promotes glycogenolysis 3. Increases gluconeogenesis 4. Favors uptake of amino acids
E. Growth hormone (hyperglycemic) 1. Increases blood sugar level 2. Decreases glycolysis 3. Mobilizes fatty acids from adipose tissue

96. Daily insulin secretion:

a. 10–15 units
b. 25–30 units
c. 40–50 units
d. 65–75 units

Insulin

- Daily production: 40–50 IU
- Basal secretion *(cca 50%)*
  - Independent on food intake
  - Blocks glucose production in liver
  - Responsible for fasting euglycaemia
- Stimulated secretion *(cca 50%)*
  - Stimulated by food intake
  - Regulates postprandial glycaemia

97. Effect of glucagon:

a. Retard glycogenolysis
b. Retards ketogenesis
c. Promote gluconeogenesis
d. Increases plasma amino acids

Glucagon generally elevates the concentration of glucose in the blood by promoting gluconeogenesis and glycogenolysis.

Comparison of action of insulin and anti-insulin hormones

Metabolism	*Key enzymes*	*Insulin*	*Glucagon*	*Glucocorticoids*	*Growth hormone*
Glycolysis	GK, PFK and PK	Stimulation			Inhibition
Gluconeogenesis	PEPCK, G6 Pase, F-bisphosphatase	Inhibition	Stimulation	Stimulation	Stimulation
Glycogen synthesis	Glycogen synthase	Activation	Inhibition		

Contd...

Ans. **94. b.** Cardiac muscle **95. d.** Norpinephrine **96. c.** 40–50 units **97. c.** Promote...

Contd...

Metabolism	*Key enzymes*	*Insulin*	*Glucagon*	*Glucocorticoids*	*Growth hormone*
Glycogenolysis	Phosphorylase	Inactivation	Activation		
Lipolysis	Hormone sensitive lipase	Inhibition	Stimulation	Stimulation	Stimulation
Ketogenesis	Carnitine acyl transferase	Inhibition	Stimulation		Stimulation
Protein breakdown	Transaminases	Inhibition		Stimulation	
Protein synthesis		Anabolism		Catabolism	Anabolism
Blood sugar level		Decreases	Increases	Increases	Increases

98. Insulin resistance in diabetes is due to reduction in:

a. GLUT-1
b. GLUT-2
c. GLUT-3
d. GLUT-4

Many stressing factors may lead to increased cortisol in the bloodstream. Cortisol counteracts insulin, contributes to hyperglycemia-causing hepatic gluconeogenesis, and inhibits the peripheral utilization of glucose, which eventually leads to insulin resistance. It does this by decreasing the translocation of glucose transporters (especially GLUT4) to the cell membrane.

99. Muscle glycogen stores cannot be used to provide glucose into the circulation due to lack of:

a. Glucose-6-phosphate dehydrogenase
b. Glutamate dehydrogenase
c. Glucose-6-phosphatase
d. Glucokinase

Genes coding for the Glucose-6-Phosphatase enzyme are primarily expressed in the liver, in the kidney cortex and (to a lesser extent) in the β-cells of the pancreatic islets and intestinal mucosa (especially during times of starvation).

100. Alternative oxidative pathway for glucose:

a. Glycogenolysis
b. Gluconeogenesis
c. Glycogenesis
d. Glucuronic acid pathway

Glucuronic acid pathway It is a quantitatively minor route of glucose metabolism. it involves the conversion of gl-6-phosphate into glucuronic acid. Liver is the major tissue performing this function. The enzymes involved are located in the cytosol. Glucouronic acid is a component of glycosaminoglycans and it is used for detoxification of non-polar toxic compounds (examples: bilirubin and steroid hormones).

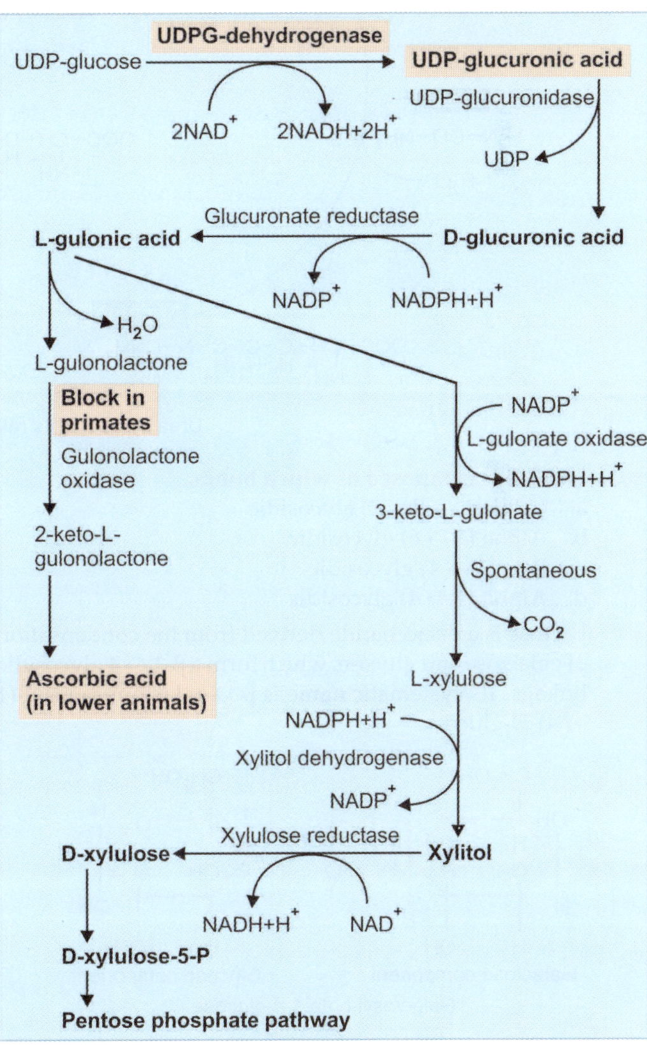

Glucuronic acid pathway.

101. ATP saved, when TCA cycle is linked with urea cycle:

a. 2
b. 4
c. 6
d. 8

10 ATPs are generated in TCA cycle whereas 4 ATPS are consumed in Urea cycle.

Ans. 98. d. GLUT-4 99. c. Glucose-6... 100. d. Glucuronic... 101. c. 6

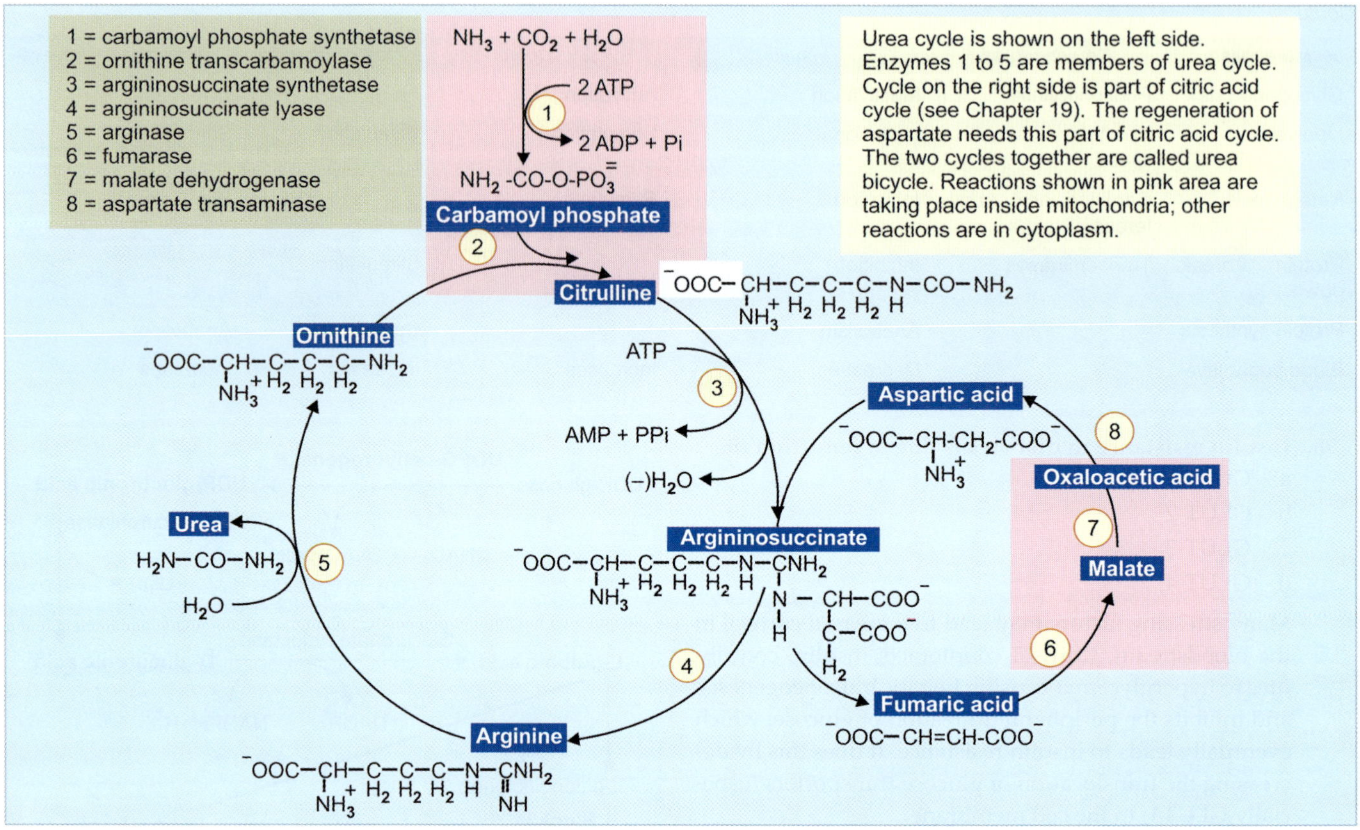

1 = carbamoyl phosphate synthetase
2 = ornithine transcarbamoylase
3 = argininosuccinate synthetase
4 = argininosuccinate lyase
5 = arginase
6 = fumarase
7 = malate dehydrogenase
8 = aspartate transaminase

Urea cycle is shown on the left side. Enzymes 1 to 5 are members of urea cycle. Cycle on the right side is part of citric acid cycle (see Chapter 19). The regeneration of aspartate needs this part of citric acid cycle. The two cycles together are called urea bicycle. Reactions shown in pink area are taking place inside mitochondria; other reactions are in cytoplasm.

$NH_3 + CO_2 + H_2O$ → (1; 2 ATP → 2 ADP + Pi) → NH_2-CO-O-$PO_3^=$ Carbamoyl phosphate → (2) → Citrulline $^-OOC-CH(NH_3^+)-CH_2-CH_2-CH_2-NH-CO-NH_2$ → (3; ATP → AMP + PPi, (–)H_2O; Aspartic acid) → Argininosuccinate → (4) → Arginine + Fumaric acid; Arginine → (5; H_2O → Urea $H_2N-CO-NH_2$) → Ornithine $^-OOC-CH(NH_3^+)-CH_2-CH_2-CH_2-NH_2$; Fumaric acid $^-OOC-CH=CH-COO^-$ → (6) → Malate → (7) → Oxaloacetic acid → (8) → Aspartic acid $^-OOC-CH(NH_3^+)-CH_2-COO^-$

Urea cycle and its relation with citric acid cycle.

102. Lactose is composed of which bonds:

a. (Alpha1 → Beta2) glycosidic
b. Alpha (1 → 6) glycosidic
c. Beta (1 → 4) glycosidic
d. Alpha (1 → 4) glycosidic

Lactose is a disaccharide derived from the condensation of galactose and glucose, which form a β-1 → 4 glycosidic linkage. Its systematic name is β-D-galactopyranosyl-(1 → 4)-D-glucose.

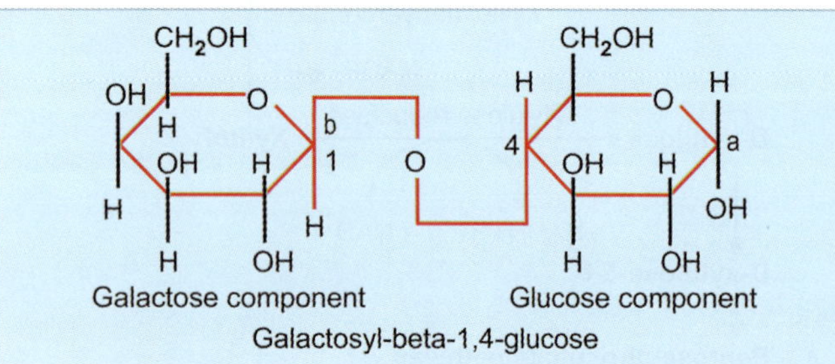

Lactose.

103. Substrate level phosphorylation in glycolysis is mediated by:

a. Phosphoglycerate kinase/PGK
b. Enolase
c. Malonate
d. Lactate dehydrogenase

PGK is a major enzyme used in glycolysis, in the first ATP-generating step of the glycolytic pathway.

Energy yield (number of ATP generated) per molecule of glucose in the glycolytic pathway, under aerobic conditions (oxygen is available)

Step	*Enzyme*	*Source*	*No. of ATPs gained per glucose mol*
1	Hexokinase	-	Minus 1
3	Phosphofructokinase	-	Minus 1
5	Glyceraldehyde-3-phosphate dehydrogenase	NADH	2.5 × 2 = 5
6	l,3-bisphosphogly-cerate kinase	ATP	1 × 2 = 2
9	Pyruvate kinase	ATP	1 × 2 = 2
		Total = 9 minus 2 = 7	

104. Essential fructosuria is due to deficiency of:

a. Fructokinase
b. L-iodouronidase
c. Aldolase B deficiency
d. Beta-glucuronidase

Essential fructosuria caused by a deficiency of the enzyme hepatic fructokinase is a clinically benign condition characterized by the incomplete metabolism of fructose in the liver, leading to its excretion in urine.

Ans. 102. c. Beta (1 → 4)... **103. a.** Phosphoglycerate... **104. a.** Fructokinase

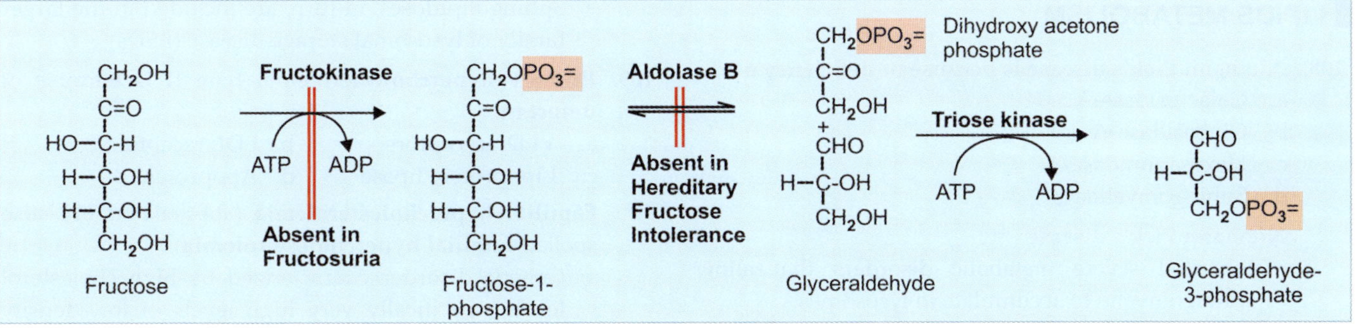

Fructose entering glycolysis.

105. Flouride ion inhibits:

a. Enolase
b. Phosphofructokinase
c. Lactate dehydrogenase
d. Pyruvate kinase

Fluoride is a known competitor of enolase's substrate 2-PG. The fluoride is part of a complex with magnesium and phosphate, which binds in the active site instead of 2-PG. As such, drinking fluoridated water provides fluoride at a level that inhibits oral bacteria enolase activity.

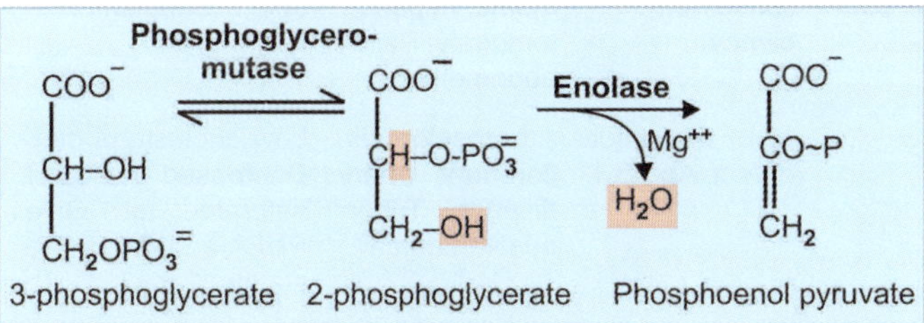

Steps 7 and 8 of glycolysis.

106. In glycolysis, insulin affects all of the following enzymes EXCEPT:

a. Phosphofructokinase
b. Pyruvate kinase
c. Glucokinase
d. Hexokinase

A **hexokinase** is an enzyme that phosphorylates hexoses (six-carbon sugars), forming hexose phosphate. In most organisms, glucose is the most important substrate of hexokinases, and glucose-6-phosphate the most important product.

Comparison of hexokinase and glucokinase

	Hexokinase	*Glucokinase*
Occurrence	In all tissues	Only in liver
Km value	10^{-2} mmol/L	20 mmol/L
Affinity to substrate	High	Low
Specificity	Acts on glucose, fructose and mannose	Acts only on glucose
Induction	Not induced	Induced by insulin and glucose
Function	Even when blood sugar level is low, glucose is utilized by body cells	Acts only when blood glucose level is more than 100 mg/dL; then glucose is taken up by liver cells for glycogen synthesis

107. Insulin is required for glucose transport in all of the following EXCEPT:

a. RBC
b. Skeletal muscles
c. Adipose tissue
d. Heart muscles

An elevated blood glucose concentration results in the secretion of insulin: glucose is transported into body cells. The uptake of glucose by liver, kidney and brain cells is by diffusion and does not require insulin.

Glucose transporters

Transporter	*Present in*	*Properties*
GluT1	RBC, brain, kidney, colon, retina, placenta	Glucose uptake in most of cells
GluT2	Serosal surface of intestinal cells, liver, beta cells of pancreas	Low affinity; glucose uptake in liver; glucose sensor in beta cells
GluT3	Neurons, brain	High affinity; glucose into brain cells
GluT4	Skeletal, heart muscle, adipose tissue	Insulin-mediated glucose uptake
GluT5	Small intestine, testis, sperms, kidney	Fructose transporter; poor ability to transport glucose
GluT7	Liver endoplasmic reticulum	Glucose from ER to cytoplasm
SGluT	Intestine, kidney	Cotransport; from lumen into cell

Ans. 105. a. Enolase **106. d.** Hexokinase **107. a.** RBC

LIPIDS METABOLISM

108. Niemann Pick's disease is because of deficiency of:

a. Galactosidase-A
b. Glucosidase-A
c. Hexosaminidase-A
d. Sphingomyelinase

Niemann Pick's disease

- Inherited severe metabolic disorders that allow sphingomyelin to accumulate in lysosomes.
- The severe form is fatal in toddlerhood; people with milder forms may live into their teens or young adulthood.
- This disease involves dysfunctional metabolism of sphingolipids, which are fats found in cell membranes, so it is a kind of sphingolipidosis.
- Sphingolipidoses, in turn, are included in the larger family of lysosomal storage disease (LSDs)

109. Primary hypercholesterolemia type II is because of defect in:

a. VLDL receptors
b. LDL receptors
c. Lipoprotein lipase
d. Apoprotein B

Familial hypercholesterolemia (abbreviated **FH**, also spelled **familial hypercholesterolemia**)

- Genetic disorder characterized by high cholesterol levels, specifically very high levels of low-density lipoprotein (LDL, "bad cholesterol")
- Many patients have mutations in the LDLR gene that encodes the LDL receptor protein, which normally removes LDL from the circulation, or apolipoprotein B (ApoB), which is the part of LDL that binds with the receptor; mutations in other genes are rare.

Frederickson's classification of hyperlipoproteinemias (N = Normal; ↑ = Increased)

Type	*Lipoprotein fraction elevated*	*Cholesterol level*	*TAG level*	*Appearance of plasma after 24 hr*	*Metabolic defect*	*Features*	*Management*
Type I	Chylomicrons	N	↑↑	Creamy layer over clear plasma	Lipoprotein lipase deficiency	Eruptive xanthoma; hepatomegaly; Pain abdomen.	Restriction of fat intake. Supplementation with MCT
Type II A	LDL	↑↑	N	Clear	LDL Receptor defect; Apo B ↑	Atherosclerosis, coronary artery disease, Tuberous xanthoma	Low cholesterol diet. Decreased intake of saturated fat. Give PUFA and drugs like statins.
Type II B	LDL and VLDL	↑↑	↑	Slightly cloudy	Apo B ↑ Apo CII	Corneal arcus	Do
Type III	Broad beta-VLDL and Chylomicrons	↑↑	↑	Cloudy	Abnormal apo-E; Apo CII ↑	Palmar xanthoma. High incidence of vascular disease	Reduction of weight, restriction of fat and chol. Give PUFA and drugs
Type IV	VLDL	↑	↑↑	Cloudy or milky	Over production of VLDL; Apo CII ↑	Associated with diabetes, heart disease, obesity.	Reduction of body weight. Restrict carbohydrate and cholesterol
Type V	VLDL Chylomicrons	N	↑↑	Creamy layer over milky plasma	Secondary to other causes	Chronic pancreatitis	High PUFA intake, hypocholipidemic drug

110. Which of the following is an example of omega-3 fatty acid:

a. Arachidonic acid
b. Oleic acid
c. Linoleic acid
d. Alpha linolenic acid

Omega-3 fatty acids (also called ω-3 fatty acids or n-3 fatty acids)

- They are polyunsaturated fatty acids (PUFAs) with a double bond (C=C) at the third carbon atom from the end of the carbon chain.
- The fatty acids have two ends, the carboxylic acid (-COOH) end, which is considered the beginning of the chain, thus "alpha", and the methyl (CH_3) end, which is considered the "tail" of the chain, thus "omega."

Ans. 108. **d.** Sphingomyelinase 109. **b.** LDL receptors 110. **d.** Alpha linolenic acid

- The nomenclature of the fatty acid is taken from the location of the first double bond, counted from the methyl end, that is, the omega (ω-) or the n- end.
- Mammals have a limited ability to synthesize omega-3 fats when the diet includes the shorter-chain omega-3 fatty acid ALA (alpha linolenic acid, 18 carbons and 3 double bonds) to form the more important long-chain omega-3 fatty acids, EPA (eicosapentaenoic acid, 20 carbons and 5 double bonds) and then from EPA, the most crucial, DHA (docosahexanoic acid, 22 carbons and 6 double bonds) with even greater inefficiency.
- Unsaturated fatty acids are vulnerable to oxidation and rancidity.

Characteristics of common fatty acids

Common name	No. of carbon atoms	Chemical nature	Occurrence
A. Even chain, saturated fatty acids			
Acetic	2	Saturated; small chain	Vinegar
Butyric	4	do	Butter
Caproic	6	do	Butter
Capric	10	do	Coconut oil
Lauric	12	do	Coconut oil
Myristic	14	do	Coconut oil
Palmitic	16	Saturated; long chain	Body fat
Stearic	18	do	do
Arachidic	20	do	Peanut oil (Arachis oil)
B. Odd-chain fatty acids			
Propionic	3	Saturated; odd chain	Metabolism
C. Even chain, unsaturated fatty acids			
Palmitoleic	16	Monounsaturated (ω7)	Body fat
Oleic	18	do (ω9)	do
Erucic	22	do (ω9)	Mustard oil
Nervonic	24	do (ω9)	Brain lipids
Linoleic	18	2 double bonds (ω6)	Vegetable oils
Linolenic	18	3 double bonds (ω3)	do
Arachidonic	20	4 double bonds (ω6)	Vegetable oils
Timnodonic	20	Eicosapentaenoic (ω3)	Fish oils, brain
Clupanodonic	22	Docosapentaenoic (ω3)	Fish oils, brain
Cervonic	22	Docosahexaenoic (ω3)	Fish oils, brain
D. Branched fatty acids			
Isovaleric acid	5	Branched	Metabolic intermediate
E. Hydroxy fatty acids			
Cerebronic acid	24	Hydroxy acid	Brain lipids

111. Enzyme deficient in Tay-Sachs disease:

a. Galactosidase-A b. Glucosidase-A
c. Hexosaminidase-A d. Galactosidase-B

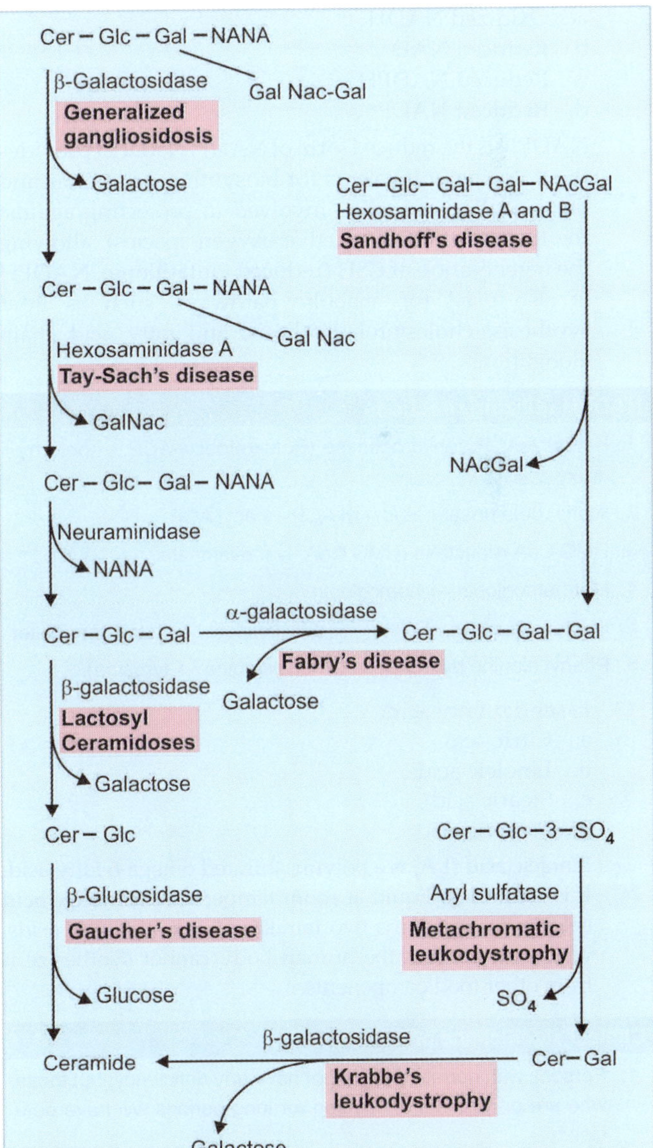

Summary of lipid storage diseases; Cer = ceramide; Glc = glucose; Gal = galactose; NAc = N-acetyl; NANA = N-acetyl neuraminic acid.

Ans. 111. c. Hexosaminidase-A

Hexosaminidase-A

- It is an enzyme involved in the hydrolysis of terminal N-acetyl-D-hexosamine residues in N-acetyl-β-D-hexosaminides.
- There are numerous mutations that lead to hexosaminidase deficiency including gene deletions, nonsense mutations, and missense mutations.
- Tay-Sachs disease occurs when hexosaminidase A loses its ability to function.
- People with Tay-Sachs disease are unable to remove the GalNAc residue from the G_{M2} ganglioside, and as a result, they end up storing 100 to 1000 times more G_{M2} gangliosides in the brain than the normal person.

112. 'Reducing power' is basically due to:

a. Oxidized NADH
b. Reduced NAD
c. Reduced NADPH
d. Reduced $NADP^+$

NADPH is the reduced form of NADP. NADPH provides the reducing equivalents for biosynthetic reactions and the oxidation-reduction involved in protecting against the toxicity of ROS (reactive oxygen species), allowing the regeneration of GSH (reduced glutathione). NADPH is also used for anabolic pathways, such as lipid synthesis, cholesterol synthesis, and fatty acid chain elongation.

NADPH utilizing reactions
1. Ketoacyl-ACP dehydrogenase (Beta-ketoacyl-ACP → beta hydroxy acyl ACP)
2. Alpha, beta unsaturated acyl ACP → acyl ACP
3. HMG CoA reductase (HMG CoA → mevalonate
4. Met-hemoglobin → hemoglobin
5. Folate reductase (Folate → dihydrofolate → tetrahydrofolate)
6. Phenyl alanine hydroxylase (Phenylalanine → tyrosine).

113. Essential fatty acid:

a. Citric acid
b. Linoleic acid
c. Stearic acid
d. Palmitic acid

Linoleic acid (LA) is a polyunsaturated omega-6 fatty acid. It is a colorless liquid at room temperature. **Linoleic acid** belongs to one of the two families of essential fatty acids, which means that the human body cannot synthesize it from other food components.

Clinical significance of PUFA and EFA
1. Persons with normal diet will not have any deficiency; but those who are on parenteral nutrition for long periods will have deficiency.
2. PUFAs are used for esterification and excretion of cholesterol. PUFA will reduce serum cholesterol level
3. Deficiency of EFA causes acanthocytosis, hyperkeratosis, acrodermatitis and hypercholesterolemia.
4. EFA deficiency is connected with acrodermatitis enteropathica, hepatorenal syndrome and CNS manifestations.
5. Elevated PUFA levels are seen in Zellweger's syndrome.
6. DHA levels in blood are low in patients with retinitis pigmentosa.
7. Trans fatty acids will compete with EFAs, and may increase the EFA deficiency and decrease fluidity of membranes.
8. Trans fatty acids decrease HDL-cholesterol and may cause atherosclerosis.

114. NOT a product of oxygenase pathway:

a. LT6
b. PGF2
c. PGD2
d. PGE2

Leukotrienes are a family of eicosanoid inflammatory mediators produced in leukocytes by the oxidation of arachidonic acid by the enzyme arachidonate 5-lipoxygenase. **Leukotriene** production is usually accompanied by the production of histamine and prostaglandins, which also act as inflammatory mediators. LTC4, LTD4, LTE4 and LTF4 are often called **cysteinyl leukotrienes** due to the presence of the amino acid cysteine in their structure.

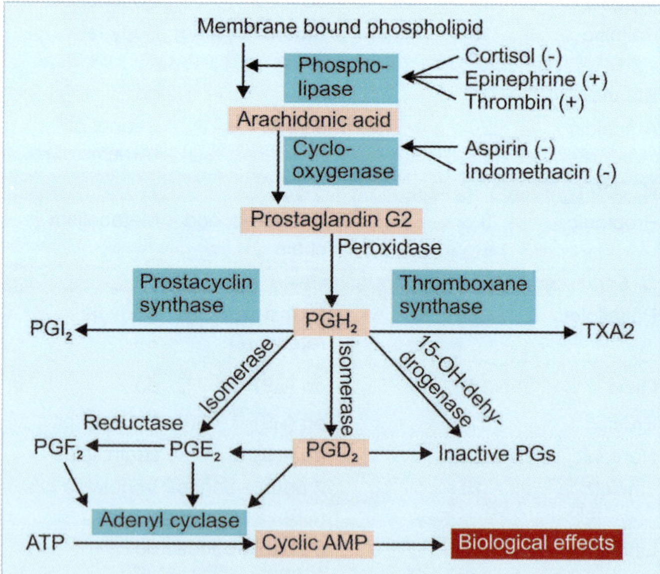

Synthesis and action of prostaglandins.

115. Accumulation of increased amount of sphingomyelin in spleen and liver is found in:

a. Goucher's disease
b. Obstructive jaundice
c. Von Gierke's disease
d. Niemann-Pick's disease

Mutations in the *SMPD1* gene cause Niemann-Pick disease types A and B. They stop the body from making an enzyme, acid sphingomyelinase, that breaks down lipids.

Ans. **112. d.** Reduced $NADP^+$ **113. b.** Linoleic acid **114. a.** LT6 **115. d.** Niemann-Pick's disease

Sphingolipidoses or lipid storage diseases				
No	*Disease*	*Enzyme defect*	*Lipid accumulating*	*Salient features*
1.	Gaucher's disease	β-glucosidase	Glucocerebroside	3 types—adult, infantile, juvenile hepatosplenomegaly, erosion of bone, moderate anemia
2.	Niemann-Pick disease	Sphingomyeli-nase	Sphingomyelin	Severe CNS damage, mental retardation, hepatosplenomegaly Cherry red spot in macula. Death occurs by 2 years of age
3.	Krabbe's leukod-ystrophy	β-galactosidase	Galactocerebroside	Severe mental retardation. Total absence of myelin in CNS Glo-boid bodies in white matter
4.	Metachromatic leukodystrophy	Sulfatidesulfatase	Sulfogalactocerebroside	Accumulates in most tissues. Neurological deficit, difficulty in speech and optic atrophy. Demyelination is also seen
5.	Fabry's disease	α-galactosidase	Ceramide trihexoside	Kidney is the site of accumulation. Progressive renal failure Death by 5 years of age. Purplish papules appear. 'X' linked in-heritence
6.	Tay Sach's disease	Hexosaminidase A	Ganglioside (GM2)	Incidence 1 in 6000 births. Mental retardation. Cherry red spot in the macula. Progressive deterioration. Death by 3–4 years
7.	Generalized gangliosidoses	β-galactosidase	Ganglioside (GM1)	Mental retardation, hepatomegaly, skeletal deformities. Foam cells in bone marrow. Cherry red spot in the retina
8.	Lactosyl cerami-doses	β-galactosidase	Lactosyl ceramide	Mainly CNS and reticuloendothelial system affected
9.	Sandhoff's disease	Hexosaminidase A and B	Globoside	Neurological deficit, mental retardation

116. Saturated fatty acid is maximum in:

a. Sunflower oil
b. Coconut oil
c. Soyabean
d. Safflower oil

Examples of foods containing a high proportion of saturated fat include animal fat products such as cream, cheese, butter, ghee, suet, tallow, lard, and fatty meats. Certain vegetable products have high saturated fat content, such as coconut oil and palm kernel oil. Many prepared foods are high in saturated fat content, such as pizza, dairy desserts, and sausage.

Composition of oils and fats			
Name	*Saturated fatty acids (%)*	*Mono-unsaturated fatty acids (%)*	*PUFA (%)*
Coconut oil	(*) 86	12	2
Groundnut oil	18	46	36
Gingelly oil (Til oil)	13	50	37
Palm oil	42	52	6
Corn oil	13	25	62
Cotton seed oil	26	19	55
Seasame oil	12	48	40
Mustard oil (rape-seed)	34(**)	48	18
Safflower oil (Kar-di)	9	12	79
Sunflower oil	12	24	64
Butter	75	20	5
Ox (Tallow)	53	42	5
Pig (Lard)	42	46	12
Fish oil	30	13	57

Contd...

Contd...

(*) these saturated fatty acids are medium chain fatty acids.
(**) contains erucic acid, 22 C, 1 double bond.

117. The major fuel for brain after several weeks of starvation:

a. Glucose
b. Fatty acids
c. Beta hydroxy butyrate
d. Glycerol

When food intake ceases, the body enters the starvation response. Initially, the body's glycogen stores are used up in about 24 hours. The level of insulin in circulation is low and the level of glucagon is very high. The main means of energy production is lipolysis. Gluconeogenesis converts glycerol into glucose and the Cori cycle converts lactate into usable glucose. Two systems of energy enter the gluconeogenesis: proteolysis provides alanine and lactate produced from pyruvate, while acetyl CoA produces dissolved nutrients (ketone bodies), which can be detected in urine and are used by the brain as a source of energy.

Ans. 116. b. Coconut oil **117. c.** Beta hydroxy butyrate

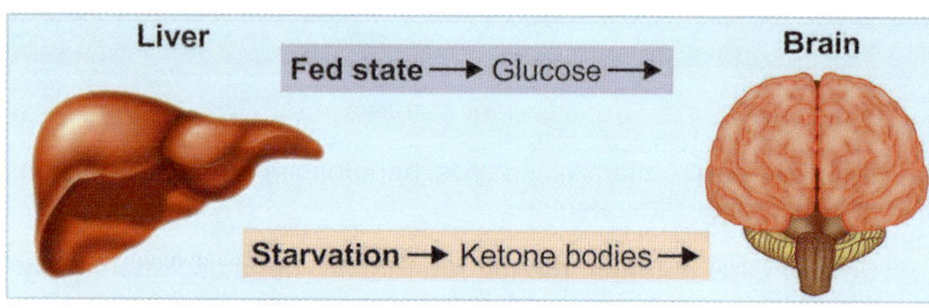

Metabolic alterations in brain.

118. The following is a ketone body:

a. Oxaloacetate
b. Pyruvate
c. Acetyl CoA
d. Acetoacetate

The three endogenous ketone bodies are acetone, acetoacetic acid, and beta-hydroxybutyric acid.

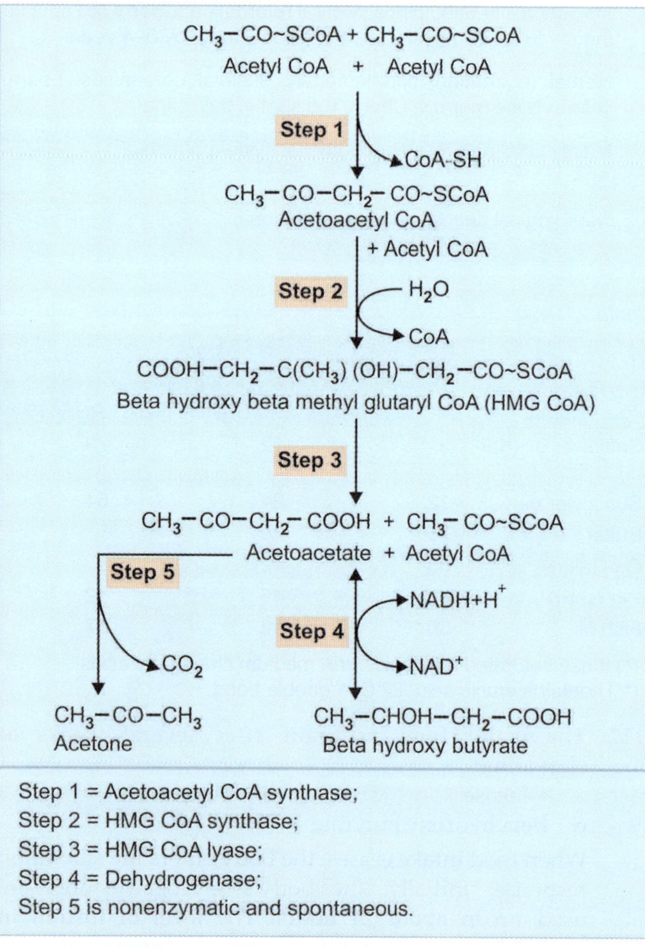

Ketone body formation (Ketogenesis).

119. The precursor of steroid is:

a. Amino acids
b. Fatty acids
c. Cholesterol
d. All of the above

In addition to its importance within cells, cholesterol also serves as a precursor for the biosynthesis of steroid hormones, bile acids, and vitamin D. Cholesterol is the principal sterol synthesized by animals.

Functions of cholesterol	
1.	**Cell membranes:** Cholesterol is a component of membranes and has a modulating effect on the fluid state of the membrane.
2.	**Nerve conduction:** Cholesterol is used to insulate nerve fibers.
3.	Bile acids and bile salts are derived from cholesterol. Bile salts are important for fat absorption.
4.	**Steroid hormones:** Glucocorticoids, androgens and estrogens are from cholesterol.
5.	Vitamin D3 is from 7-dehydro-cholesterol.
6.	**Esterification:** The OH group of cholesterol is esterified to fatty acids to form cholesterol esters. This esterification occurs in the body by transfer of a PUFA moiety by lecithin cholesterol acyl transferase.

120. Gerhardt's test is positive in significant degree of:

a. Hematuria
b. Ketosis
c. Bilirubinemia
d. Pancreatitis

Gerhardt's test is based on reaction of FeCl3 with diacetic acid to form a port wine or Bordeaux red colour. Neither acetone nor hydroxyl-butyric acid can be detected by this test.

121. Myocardium normally utilizes:

a. Glucose
b. Lactose
c. Fatty acid
d. Glycogen

Many cell types can use either glucose or fatty acids for this purpose. In particular, heart and skeletal muscle prefer fatty acids.

Adaptations during starvation

Fed state	*Skeletal muscle*	*Cardiac muscle*
Preferred fuel at rest	Fatty acids	FFA, ketone bodies, lactate
Exercise	Glycogen to lactate	Fatty acids
Starvation Adaptations	Protein breakdown; release of amino acids; FFA, ketone bodies and bran-ched chain amino acids utilized	Fatty acids, branched chain amino acids and ketone bodies utilized

122. Rate limiting step in cholesterol synthesis:

a. HMG CoA synthetase
b. HMG CoA lyase
c. HMG CoA reductase
d. Mevalinate synthetase

HMG-CoA reductase (3-hydroxy-3-methyl-glutaryl-CoA reductase HMGCR is the rate-controlling enzyme; NADPH-dependent, of the mevalonate pathway, the metabolic pathway that produces cholesterol and other isoprenoids.

Ans. **118. d.** Acetoacetate **119. c.** Cholesterol **120. b.** Ketosis **121. c.** Fatty acid **122. c.** HMG CoA reductase

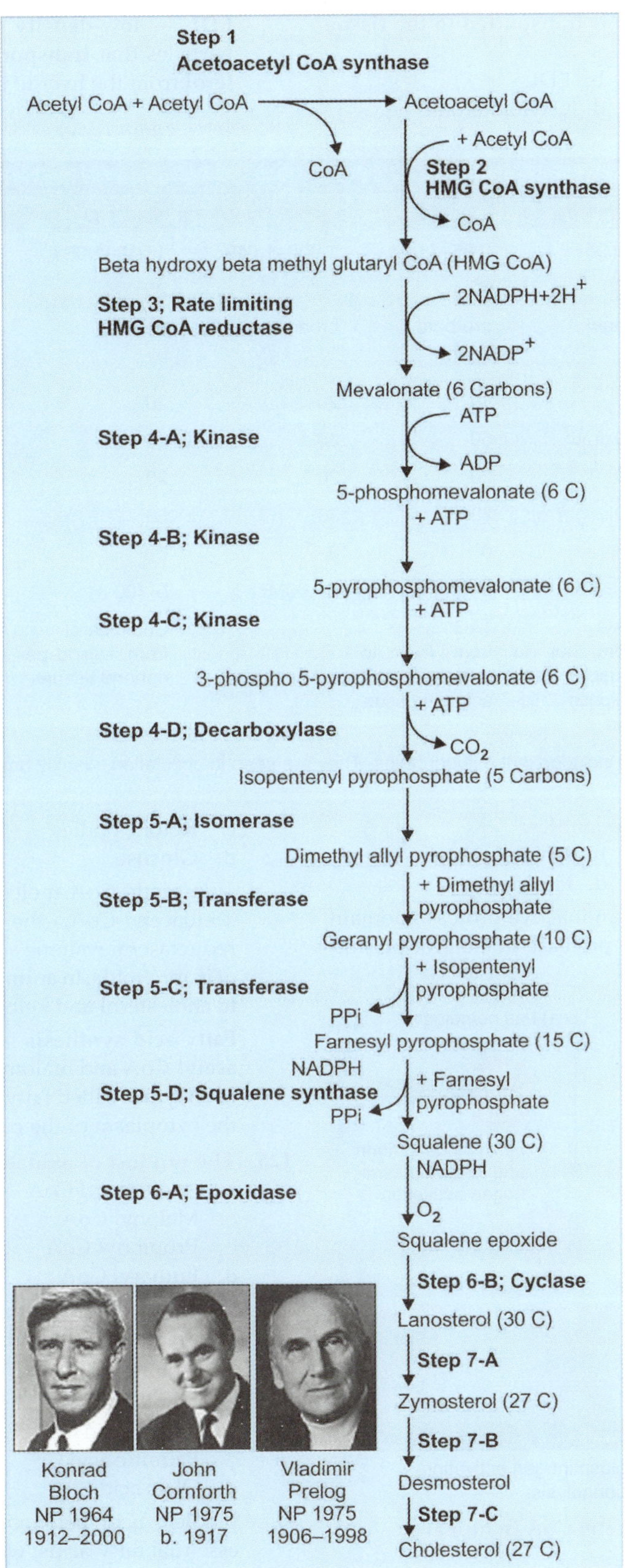

Cholesterol biosynthesis.

123. Cholesterol from the liver is transported to the tissue mainly by:

a. HDL
b. LDL
c. VLDL
d. Chylomicrons

LDL — **low-density lipoprotein:** A group of related particles that **transport** endogenous TAGs and **cholesterol** from the liver to the **tissues**.

Characteristics of different classes of lipoproteins						
	Chylomicron	*VLDL*	*IDL*	*LDL*	*HDL*	*FFA (*)*
Density g/L	<0.95	0.95–1.006	1.006–1.019	1.019–1.063	1.063–1.121	1.28–1.3
Diameter (nm)	500	70	30	25	15	-
Electrophoretic mobility	origin	pre-beta	broad beta	beta	alpha	albumin
% Composition						
Protein	2	10	20	20	30-60	99
TAG	80	50	30	10	10	0
Phospholipids	10	20	20	20	20-30	0
Cholesterol	10	20	30	50	10-30	0
FFA	0	0	0	0	0	1
Apoproteins	A,B-48,C-II,E	B-100, C-II,E	B-100, E	B-100	A-I, C, E	Albumin
Transport function	TAG from gut to muscle and adipose tissue	TAG from liver to muscle and adipose tissue		Cholesterol from liver to peripheral tissues	Cholesterol from peripheral tissues to liver	FFA from adipose T to muscle and liver

(*) Free fatty acids are not generally included in the lipoproteins. They are seen in circulation, weakly bound to albumin.

124. Domain of plasminogen resembles:

a. Prothrombin
b. Apolipoprotein A
c. LDL receptor
d. Fibrinogen

The apo (a) gene contains an inactive protease domain with 94% homology to the protease domain of plasminogen.

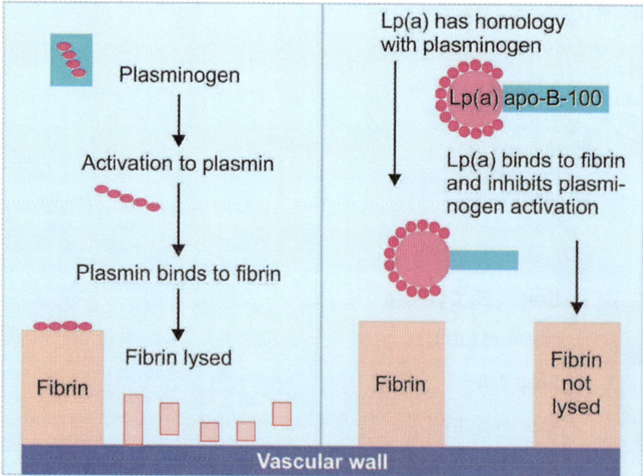

Lp(a) competitively inhibits plasminogen activation; and so inhibits fibrinolysis.

125. NOT a direct product of acetyl CoA in humans:

a. Cholesterol
b. Fatty acids
c. Ketone bodies
d. Glucose

Two acetyl-CoA molecules can be condensed to create acetoacetyl-CoA, the first step in the HMG-CoA reductase/mevalonic acid pathway, leading to synthesis of isoprenoids. In animals, HMG-CoA is a vital precursor to cholesterol and ketone body synthesis.

Fatty acid synthesis is the creation of fatty acids from acetyl-CoA and malonyl-CoA precursors through action of enzymes called fatty acid synthases that takes place in the cytoplasm of the cell.

126. The product of oxidation of odd chain fatty acids is:

a. Acetoacetyl CoA
b. Malonyl CoA
c. Propionyl CoA
d. Fumaryl CoA

Propionyl CoA is formed as a product of beta-oxidation of odd-chain fatty acids.

127. Which fatty acid is NOT synthesized by man?

a. Linoleic acid
b. Stearic acid
c. Palmitic acid
d. Oleic acid

Linoleic acid belongs to one of the two families of essential fatty acids, which means that the human body cannot synthesize it from other food components.

Ans. 123. **b.** LDL 124. **b.** Apolipoprotein A 125. **d.** Glucose 126. **c.** Propionyl CoA 127. **a.** Linoleic acid

Clinical significance of PUFA
1. Linoleic and linolenic acids are polyunsaturated fatty acids.
2. They are called essential fatty acids, because they cannot be synthesized by the body and have to be supplied in the diet.
3. Unsaturated fatty acids are also designated as
ω3 family — Linolenic acids
ω6 family — Linoleic and Arachidonic acids
ω9 family — Oleic acid
4. Arachidonic acid is the precursor of prostaglandins. Arachidonic acid can be synthesized in the body, if the essential fatty acids are supplied in the diet.
5. The penta-enoic acid present in fish oils is of great nutritional importance (w3 unsaturated fatty acid).
6. Eicosanoids (eicosa = twenty) are derived from 20 C arachidonic acid. They are poly-enoic fatty acids. They are prostanoids (prostaglandins, prostacyclins, thromboxanes) and leukotrienes.

128. Stored tri-acyl-glycerol and cholesterol are released by:

a. Lysosomal lipase
b. Lipoprotein lipase
c. LCAT
d. Hormone sensitive lipase/HSL

HSL is an intracellular neutral lipase that is capable of hydrolyzing a variety of esters. The enzyme has a long and a short form. The long form is expressed in steroidogenic tissues such as testis, where it converts cholesteryl esters to free cholesterol for steroid hormone production. The short form is expressed in adipose tissue, among others, where it hydrolyzes stored triglycerides to free fatty acids.

Physiologically important lipases

Lipase	*Site of action*	*Preferred substrate*	*Product(s)*
Lingual/acid-stable lipase	Mouth, stomach	TAGs with short and medium chain FAs	FFA+DAG
Pancreatic lipase + co-lipase	small intestine	TAGs with long-chain FAs	FFA+2MAG
Intestinal lipase with bile acids	small intestine	TAGs with medium chain FAs	3 FFA+ glycerol
Phospholipase A_2 + bile acids	small intestine	PLs with unsat. FA on position 2	Unsat FFA Lysolecithin
Lipoprotein lipase	capillary walls	TAGs in chylomicron or VLDL	FFA+ glycerol
Hormone sensitive lipase	adipocytes	TAG stored in adipose tissue	FFA+ DAG

129. NOT a bad cholesterol:

a. IDL
b. LDL
c. VLDL
d. HDL

HDL particles, unlike the larger particles, transfer fats away from cells, artery walls and tissues (around the body, body wide) through the bloodstream, back to both (a) LDL particles and (b) back to the liver for other disposition.

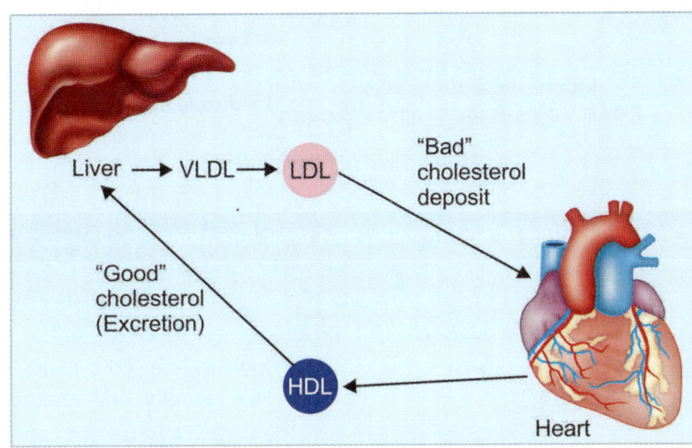

Forward and reverse transport of cholesterol.

130. Opposite biological activity is exhibited by:

a. Acteone and beta-hydroxy-butyrate
b. Thromboxane A2 and prostacyclin (PGI-2)
c. Cholic acid and Lithocholic acid
d. 5-HPETE and leukotriene D4

Thromboxane A2 (TXA2) is a type of thromboxane that is produced by activated platelets and has prothrombotic properties: it stimulates activation of new platelets as well as increases platelet aggregation. It is a vasoconstrictor.

Prostacyclin (also called **prostaglandin** I2 or **PGI$_2$**) is a prostaglandin member of the family of lipid molecules known as eicosanoids. It inhibits platelet activation and is also an effective vasodilator.

Prostacyclins and thromboxane

	PGI_2	*TXA_2*
Structure	Cyclopentane ring	Oxane ring
Site of formation	Endothelium	Platelets
Cyclic AMP level	Increased	Decreased
Platelet aggregation	Inhibited	Enhanced
Blood vessel	Vasodilatation	Constriction
Bronchioles	Relaxation	Constriction

131. NOT a product of lipo-oxygenase pathway:

a. Histamine
b. PGF2
c. PGD2
d. PGE2

Ans. 128. **d.** Hormone... 129. **d.** HDL 130. **b.** Thromboxane... 131. **a.** Histamine

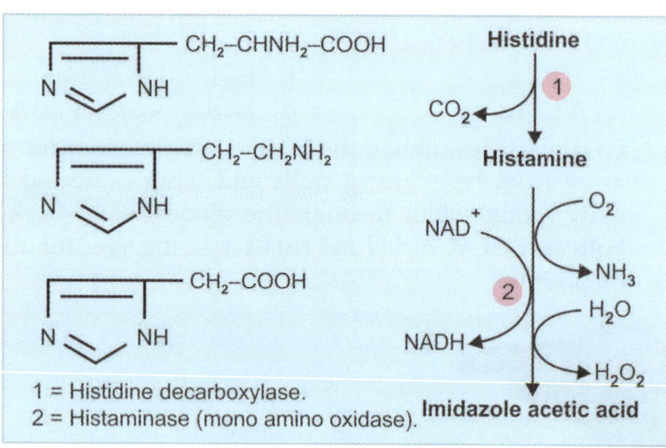

Metabolism of histamine.

Histamine is derived from the decarboxylation of the amino acid histidine, a reaction catalyzed by the enzyme L-histidine decarboxylase.

132. Apoprotein for cholesterol:

a. ApoE
b. ApoC1
c. ApoA2
d. ApoA1

APOE transports lipoproteins, fat-soluble vitamins, and cholesterol into the lymph system and then into the blood. It is synthesized principally in the liver, but has also been found in other tissues such as the brain, kidneys, and spleen.

Characteristics of apoproteins and their functions

Apoprotein	*Component of*	*Functions*	*Molecular weight*	*Blood level mg/dL*	*Site of production*
apo A-I	HDL	Activation of LCAT; ligand for HDL receptor; Anti-atherogenic	28,000	150	Intestine; liver
apo A-II	HDL	Inhibits LCAT; stimulates lipase	17,000	30	Intestine; liver
apo B-100	LDL; VLDL	Binds LDL receptor	550,000	100	Liver
apo B-48	Chylomicrons	48% size of B-100. Major structural apoprotein of chylomicrons	250,000	–	Intestine
apo C-I	Chylo; VLDL	Activation of LCAT; anti atherogenic	7,000	10	Liver
apo E	LDL; VLDL; chylomicron	Arginine rich; ligand for hepatic uptake	30,000	2	Liver
apo Lp(a)	Lp(a)	Attached to B-100; impairs fibrinolysis; highly atherogenic		< 30	Liver

133. L-CAT activator lipoprotein is:

a. ApoE
b. ApoC3
c. ApoC2
d. ApoA1

ApoA1 is a cofactor for lecithin cholesterolacyltransferase (LCAT) which is responsible for the formation of most plasma cholesteryl esters.

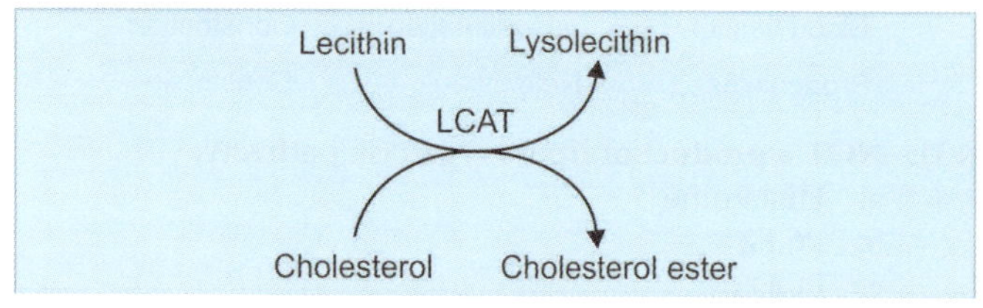

Lecithin cholesterol acyl transferase (LCAT).

134. NOT seen in starvation:

a. Ketoacidosis
b. Lipolysis
c. Hypercholesterolemia
d. Hypoglycemia

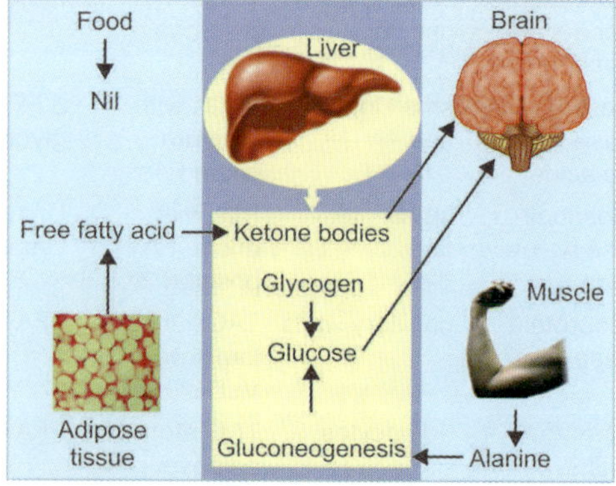

Metabolism in fasting state.

Ans. **132. a.** ApoE **133. d.** ApoA1 **134. c.** Hypercholes...

When food intake ceases, the body enters the starvation response. Initially, the body's glycogen stores are used up in about 24 hours. The level of insulin in circulation is low and the level of glucagon is very high. The main means of energy production is lipolysis. Gluconeogenesis converts glycerol into glucose and the Cori cycle converts lactate into usable glucose. Two systems of energy enter the gluconeogenesis: proteolysis provides alanine and lactate produced from pyruvate, while acetyl CoA produces dissolved nutrients (ketone bodies), which can be detected in urine and are used by the brain as a source of energy.

In terms of insulin resistance, starvation conditions make more glucose available to the brain.

135. Carrier of dietary cholesterol from intestine to liver:

a. Apo-E
b. Apo-C
c. Apo-A
d. Apo-B

Nascent chylomicrons are composed primarily of triglycerides (85%) and contain some cholesterol and cholesteryl esters. The main apolipoprotein component is apolipoprotein B-48 (apo B-48). They transport dietary lipids from the intestines to other locations in the body.

136. Lipoproteins elevated in a person, who is growing obese as a result of fat free, carbohydrate rich diet:

a. HDL
b. LDL
c. VLDL
d. Chylomicrons

If a **person** on **fat free carbohydrate rich diet** continues to **grow obese**, **VLDL** is **elevated**.

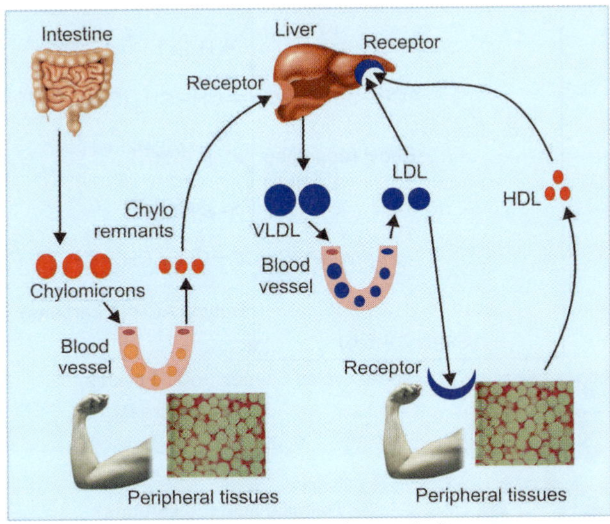

Summary of lipoprotein metabolism.

137. Beta-oxidation of odd chain fatty acids will yield:

a. Malonyl CoA
b. Acetyl CoA
c. Propionyl CoA
d. Succinyl CoA

There are several different ways in which propionyl CoA is formed:

- It is formed as a product of beta-oxidation of odd-chain fatty acids.
- It is also a product of metabolism of isoleucine and valine.
- It is a product of alpha-ketobutyric acid, which in turn is a product of digestion of threonine and methionine.
- It is formed as a by-product during the conversion of cholesterol to bile acids.

Difference in the two pathways

	Beta-oxidation	*Fatty acid synthesis*
Site	Mitochondria	Cytoplasm
Intermediates	Present as CoA derivatives	Covalently linked to SH group of ACP
Enzymes	Present as independent proteins	Multi-enzyme complex
Sequential units	Two carbon units split off as acetyl CoA	Two carbon units added, as 3 carbon malonyl CoA
Co-enzymes	NAD^+ and FAD are reduced	NADPH used as reducing power
Carrier	Carnitine	Citrate
Regulation	Insuliun ↓ Glucagon ↑	Insuliun ↑ Glucagon ↓

138. Lipoxin belongs to:

a. Arachidonic acid metabolites
b. Chemokines
c. Cytokines
d. Kinin system

Lipoxins/LXA4 are members of the family of bioactive products generated from Arachidonic Acid (AA). They have a number of immunomodulatory and anti-inflammatory actions.

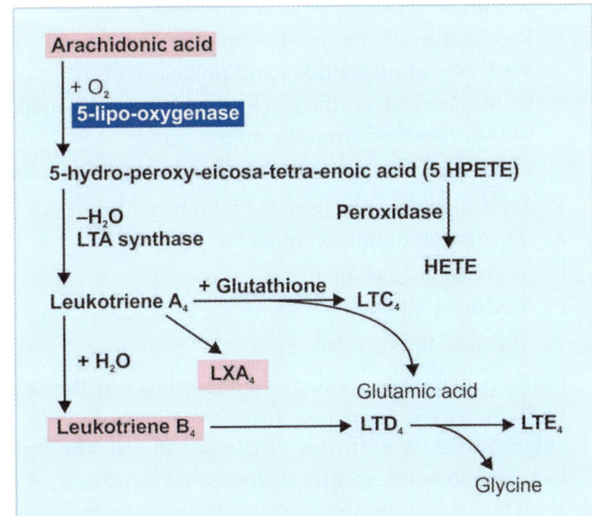

Synthesis of leukotrienes. LT = leukotriene; LXA = lipoxin; HETE = hydroxy eicosatetraenoic acid.

139. Ketone bodies are synthesized in:

a. Liver
b. Muscle
c. Kidney
d. Brain

Ans. 135. **d.** Apo-B 136. **c.** VLDL 137. **c.** Propionyl... 138. **a.** Arachidonic... 139. **a.** Liver

Ketone bodies are produced from acetyl-CoA mainly in the mitochondrial matrix of hepatocytes (liver tissue) when carbohydrates are so scarce that energy must be obtained from breaking down fatty acids.

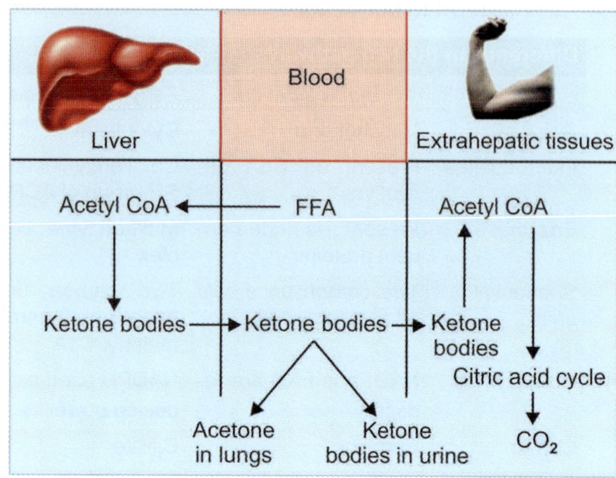

Formation, utilization and excretion of ketone bodies.

140. Source of reducing agent in lipogenesis:

a. Gluconeogenesis
b. TCA cycle
c. Glycolysis
d. Pentose phosphate pathway

The primary results of the pentose phosphate pathway are:

- The generation of reducing equivalents, in the form of NADPH, used in reductive biosynthesis reactions within cells (e.g. fatty acid synthesis).
- Production of ribose 5-phosphate (R5P), used in the synthesis of nucleotides and nucleic acids.
- Production of erythrose 4-phosphate (E4P) used in the synthesis of aromatic amino acids.

(See Diagram on right side colomn)

141. Reduction in atherosclerosis by dietary fibres is due to:

a. Formation of antioxidants
b. Increased fluid retention
c. Reduced VLDL
d. Binding to bile acids

Binding of bile acids to fiber or bacteria in the cecum with increased fecal loss from the entero-hepatic circulation occurs with use of dietary fibers. The enteric loss of bile acids results in increased synthesis of bile acids from cholesterol which in turn reduces body cholesterol.

142. Transporter of free fatty acid:

a. Transthyretin
b. Albumin
c. Pre-albumin
d. Ceruloplasmin

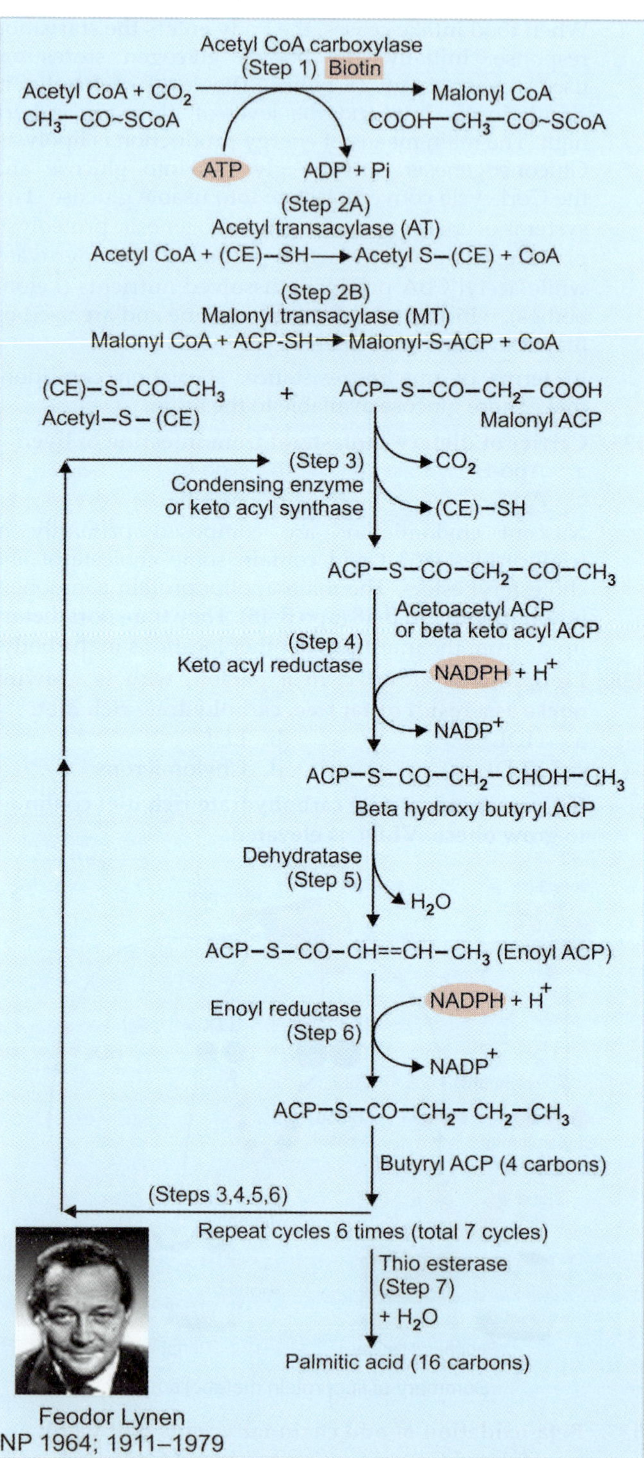

De novo synthesis of fatty acid (Lynen cycle). Steps 4 and 6 utilize NADPH.

Serum albumin is the main protein of human blood plasma. It binds water, cations (such as Ca^{2+}, Na^+ and K^+), fatty acids, hormones, bilirubin, thyroxine (T4) and pharmaceuticals (including barbiturates) — its main function is to regulate the colloidal osmotic pressure

Ans. **140. d.** Pentose... **141. d.** Binding to bile... **142. b.** Albumin

of blood. Alpha-fetoprotein (alpha-fetoglobulin) is a fetal plasma protein that binds various cations, fatty acids and bilirubin. Vitamin D-binding protein binds to vitamin D and its metabolites, as well as to fatty acids.

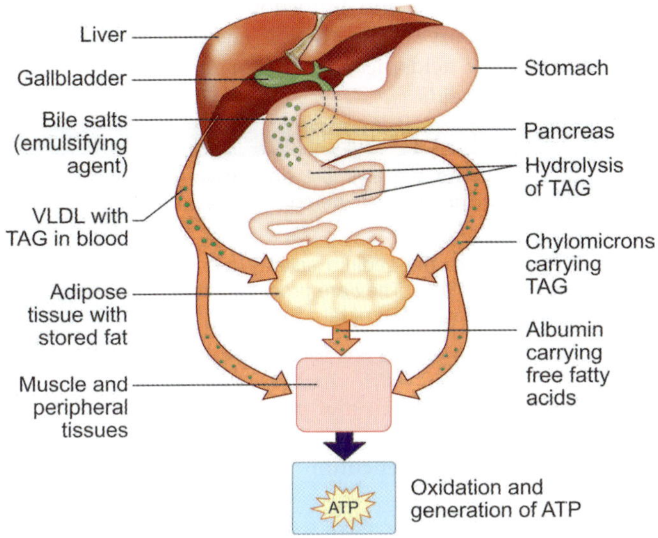

Summary of utilization of fat.

143. Primary ketone body:

a. Acetone b. Beta-hydroxy butyric acid
c. Acetoacetate d. Arachidonic acid

The three endogenous ketone bodies are acetone, acetoacetic acid, and *beta*-hydroxybutyric acid. Ketone bodies are transported from the liver to other tissues, where acetoacetate and *beta*-hydroxybutyrate can be reconverted to acetyl-CoA to produce energy, via the citric acid cycle.

144. Fatty liver results due to accumulation of:

a. VLDL b. LDL
c. Lipoproteins d. Triglycerides

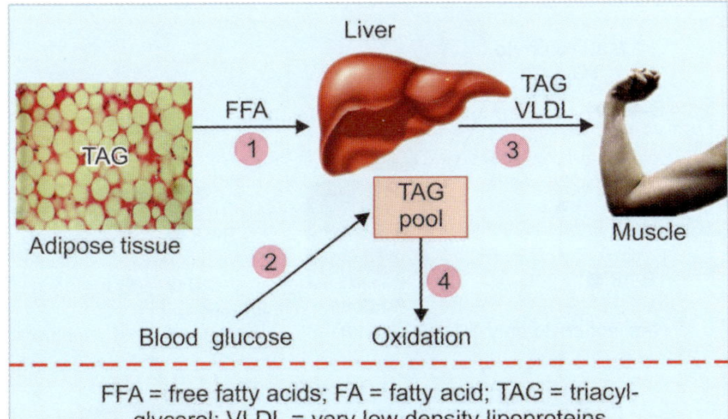

Causes for fatty liver.

Fatty liver, also known as **fatty liver disease (FLD)**, is a reversible condition wherein large vacuoles of triglyceride fat accumulate in liver cells via the process of steatosis (i.e., abnormal retention of lipids within a cell).

145. Source of prostaglandins:

a. Arachidonic acid b. Linoleic acid
c. Oleic acid d. Steroids

Prostaglandins are found in most tissues and organs. They are produced by almost all nucleated cells. They are autocrine and paracrine lipid mediators that act upon platelets, endothelium, uterine and mast cells. They are synthesized in the cell from the essential fatty acids (EFAs).

An intermediate arachidonic acid is created from diacylglycerol via phospholipase-A2, then brought to either the cyclooxygenase pathway or the lipoxygenase pathway to form either prostaglandin and thromboxane or leukotriene respectively.

Salient features of prostaglandins

Name	*Substituent groups*
PGA	Keto group at C9; double bond C10 and 11
PGB	Keto group at C9; double bond C8 and 12
PGD	OH group at C9; keto group at C11
PGE	Keto group at C9; OH group at C11
PGF	OH groups at C9 and C11 (Fig.14.2)
PGG	Two oxygen atoms, interconnected to each other, and bonded at C9 and C11; hydroperoxide group at C15
PGH	Same ring as PGG; but C15 has OH group
PGI	Double ring. Oxygen attached to C6 and C9, to form another 5-membered ring. Hence called prostacyclin.

146. Building block for fatty acid synthesis:

a. Acetate b. Acyl CoA
c. Acetyl CoA d. NADH

Fatty acid synthesis is the creation of fatty acids from acetyl-CoA and malonyl-CoA precursors through action of enzymes called fatty acid synthases that takes place in the cytoplasm of the cell.

147. Involved in transport of long chain acyl CoA in mitochondria:

a. Albumin b. Carnitine
c. Xanthine d. Ornithine

Carnitine is a quaternary ammonium compound biosynthesized from the amino acids lysine and methionine.

In eukaryotic cells, it is required for the transport of fatty acids from the intermembraneous space in the mitochondria, into the mitochondrial matrix during the breakdown of lipids (fats) for the generation of metabolic energy.

Ans. **143. c.** Acetoacetate **144. d.** Triglycerides **145. a.** Arachidonic acid **146. c.** Acetyl CoA
147. b. Carnitine

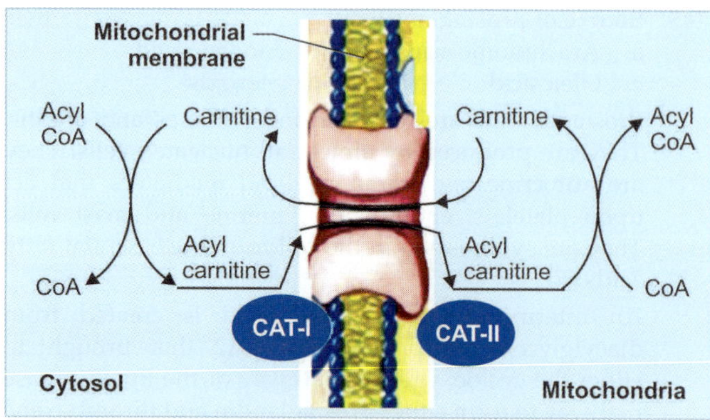

Role of carnitine in transport of acyl groups
CAT = Carnitine acyl transferase.

148. Cholesterol is NOT a precursor of:

a. Sex hormone b. Vitamin D
c. Bile pigment d. Bile acid

Bilins, bilanes or **bile pigments** are biological pigments formed in many organisms as a metabolic product of certain porphyrins.

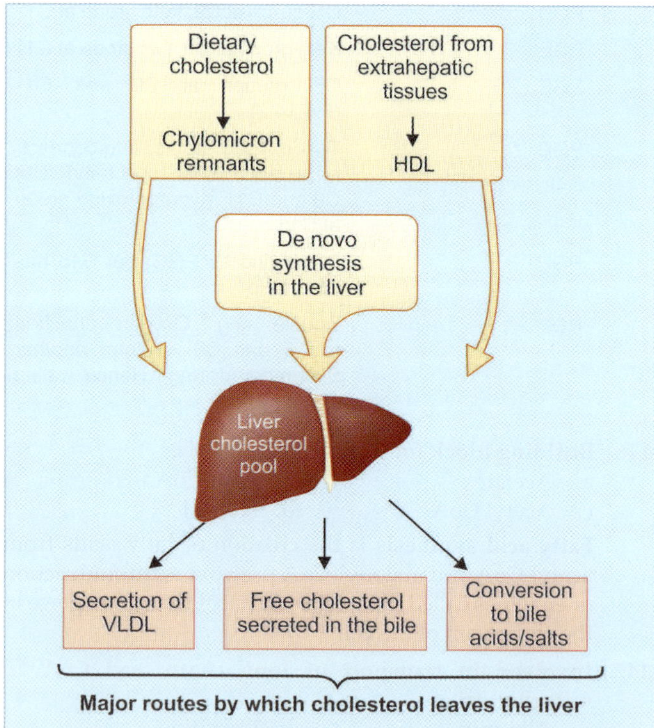

Cholesterol pool in the liver.

149. NOT a constituent of bile acids:

a. Chenodeoxycholic acid
b. Deoxycholic acid
c. Taurocholic acid d. Lithocholic acid

Primary bile acids are those synthesized by the liver. **Secondary bile acids** result from bacterial actions in the colon. In humans, taurocholic acid and glycocholic acid (derivatives of cholic acid) and taurochenodeoxycholic acid and glycochenodeoxycholic acid (derivatives of chenodeoxycholic acid) are the major bile salts in bile and are roughly equal in concentration. The conjugated salts of their 7-alpha-dehydroxylated derivatives, deoxycholic acid and lithocholic acid, are also found, with derivatives of cholic, chenodeoxycholic and deoxycholic acids accounting for over 90% of human biliary bile acids.

Bile pigments and bile salts
Bile pigments are Bilirubin and Biliverdin. They are the breakdown products of heme; they are useless excretory products.
Bile salts are the sodium salts of bile acids (glycocholate and taurocholate). They are produced from cholesterol; they help in the absorption of fat.
Both bile pigments and bile salts are present in the bile.

150. Site of alpha oxidation of phytanic acids:

a. Peroxisomes
b. Endoplasmic reticulum
c. Both d. None

Alpha-oxidation of fatty acids occurs in endoplasmic reticulum, does not require CoA, but does not generate energy. Some fatty acids undergo alpha hydroxylation in peroxisomes also.

151. Chylomicron core is made up of:

a. Free fatty acids b. Triglyceride
c. Triglyceride and cholesterol
d. Triglyceride, phospholipids and cholesterol

Chylomicrons (**chylo**, meaning **juiceor milky fluid**, and **micron**, meaning **small particle**) are lipoprotein particles that consist of triglycerides (85–92%), phospholipids (6–12%), cholesterol (1–3%), and proteins (1–2%). They transport dietary lipids from the intestines to other locations in the body.

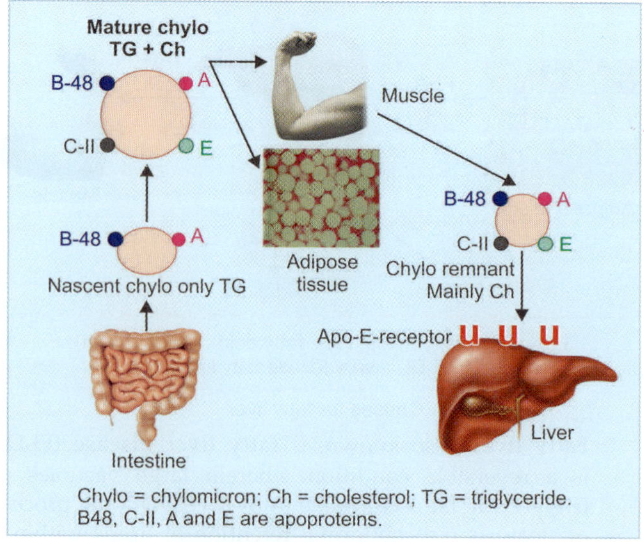

Chylo = chylomicron; Ch = cholesterol; TG = triglyceride.
B48, C-II, A and E are apoproteins.

Metabolism of chylomicrons.

Ans. 148. c. Bile pigment 149. c. Taurocholic acid 150. c. Both 151. c. Triglyceride...

152. NOT seen in starvation:

a. Elevated glycogen degradation
b. Ketone body formation
c. Lipolysis
d. Reduced gluconeogenesis

Gluconeogenesis (GNG) is a metabolic pathway that results in the generation of glucose from non-carbohydrate carbon substrates such as pyruvate, lactate, glycerol, and glucogenic amino acids. The process occurs during periods of fasting, starvation, low-carbohydrate diets, or intense exercise.

Key enzymes under well-fed conditions, fasting and starvation

Enzyme	*Fed*	*Fasting*	*Activator*	*Inhibitor*
Glucokinase	Increase	Decrease	Insulin, glucose	F-6-P
Phosphofructokinase1	Increase	Decrease	F-2,6-bisP, AMP	ATP, Citrate
Fructose 1,6 bisphosphatase	Decrease	Increase	ATP, Citrate	F-2,6-bisP, AMP
Pyruvate carboxylase	Decrease	Increase	Acetyl CoA	
PEPCK	Decrease	Increase	Glucagon, corticoids	Insulin
Glycogen phosphorylase	Decrease	Increase	Glucagon, AMP	Insulin
Glycogen synthase	Increase	Decrease	Insulin, G-6-P	Glucagon
Carnitine acyltransferase		Increase	Glucagon	Malonyl CoA
Acetyl CoA carboxylase	Increase	Decrease	Insulin, citrate	Fatty acyl CoA
Hormone sensitive lipase	Decrease	Increase	Glucagon	Insulin

PEPCK = phosphoenol pyruvate carboxykinase; F-6-P = fructose-6-phosphate; F-2,6-bisP = fructose-2,6-bisphosphate; G-6-P = glucose-6-phosphate

153. Energy reserve of the body is:

a. Carbohydrate
b. Triglyceride
c. Proteins
d. Fibres

When the body requires fatty acids as an energy source, the hormone glucagon signals the breakdown of the triglycerides by hormone-sensitive lipase to release free fatty acids. As the brain cannot utilize fatty acids as an energy source (unless converted to a ketone), the glycerol component of triglycerides can be converted into glucose, via gluconeogenesis by conversion into Dihydroxyacetone phosphate and then into Glyceraldehyde 3-phosphate, for brain fuel when it is broken down. Fat cells may also be broken.

Energy reserves of man

Stored fuel	*Weight (in gram)*	*Energy equivalent (in kilo calories)*
Glycogen in liver	70	280
Glycogen in muscle	120	480
Glucose in body fluids	20	80
Fat in adipose tissue	15,000	135,000
Protein in muscle	6,000	24,000

154. Linoleic acid belongs to:

a. ω3 series
b. ω6 series
c. ω9 series
d. None of the above

Linoleic acid (LA) is a polyunsaturated omega-6 fatty acid. It is a colorless liquid at room temperature. In physiological literature, it has a lipid number of 18:2 *cis,cis*-9,12.

Linoleic **(C_{18})** Δ9, 12 **(two double bonds)** (ω6 family)

$CH_3-(CH_2)4-CH=CH-CH_2-CH=CH-(CH_2)_7-COOH$

18 **ω6** 12 9 1

Linolenic **(C_{18})** Δ9, 12, 15 **(three double bonds)** (ω3 family)

$CH_3-CH_2-CH=CH-CH_2-CH=CH-CH_2-CH=CH-(CH_2)_7-COOH$

18 **ω3** 15 12 9 1

Arachidonic **(C_{20})** Δ5, 8, 11, 14 **(four double bonds)** (ω6 family)

$CH_3-(CH_2)4-CH=CH-CH_2-CH=CH-CH_2-CH=CH-CH_2-CH=CH-(CH_2)_3-COOH$

20 **ω6** 14 11 8 5 1

Polyunsaturated fatty acids (PUFA).

Ans. 152. **d.** Reduced... 153. **b.** Triglyceride 154. **b.** ω6 series

155. In starvation, ketosis is mainly due to:
a. Impaired carbohydrate metabolism
b. Increased fat degradation
c. Decreased fat degradation
d. Increased carbohydrate metabolism

In glycolysis, higher levels of insulin promote storage of body fat and block release of fat from adipose tissues, while in ketosis, fat reserves are readily released and consumed. For this reason, ketosis is sometimes referred to as the body's "fat burning" mode.

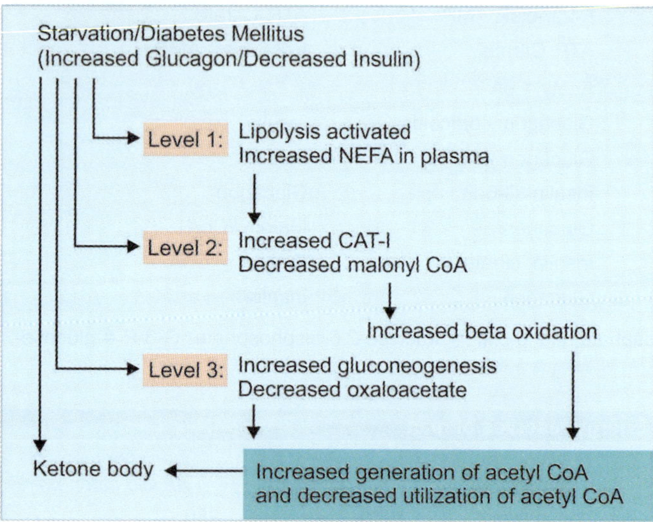

Summary of ketosis.

NUCLEOTIDE METABOLISM

156. Rate limiting enzyme in pyrimidine synthesis:
a. OMP decarboxylase
b. Dihydro-orotase dehydrogenase
c. Carbamoyl phosphate synthase II
d. Acetyl CoA carboxylase

Carbamoyl phosphate synthetase

- It catalyzes the ATP-dependent synthesis of carbamoyl phospshate from glutamine) or ammonia and bicarbonate.
- Carbomoyl phosphate reacts with ammonia to give carbamate.
- In turn, carbamate reacts with a second ATP to give carbamoyl phosphate plus ADP.
- It represents the first committed step in pyrimidine and arginine biosynthesis in prokaryotes and eukaryotes, and in the urea cycle in most terrestrial vertebrates
- There are three different forms that serve very different functions:
  - Carbamoyl phosphate synthetase I (mitochondria, urea cycle)
  - Carbamoyl phosphate synthetase II (cytosol, pyrimidine metabolism).
  - Carbamoyl phosphate synthetase III (found in fish).

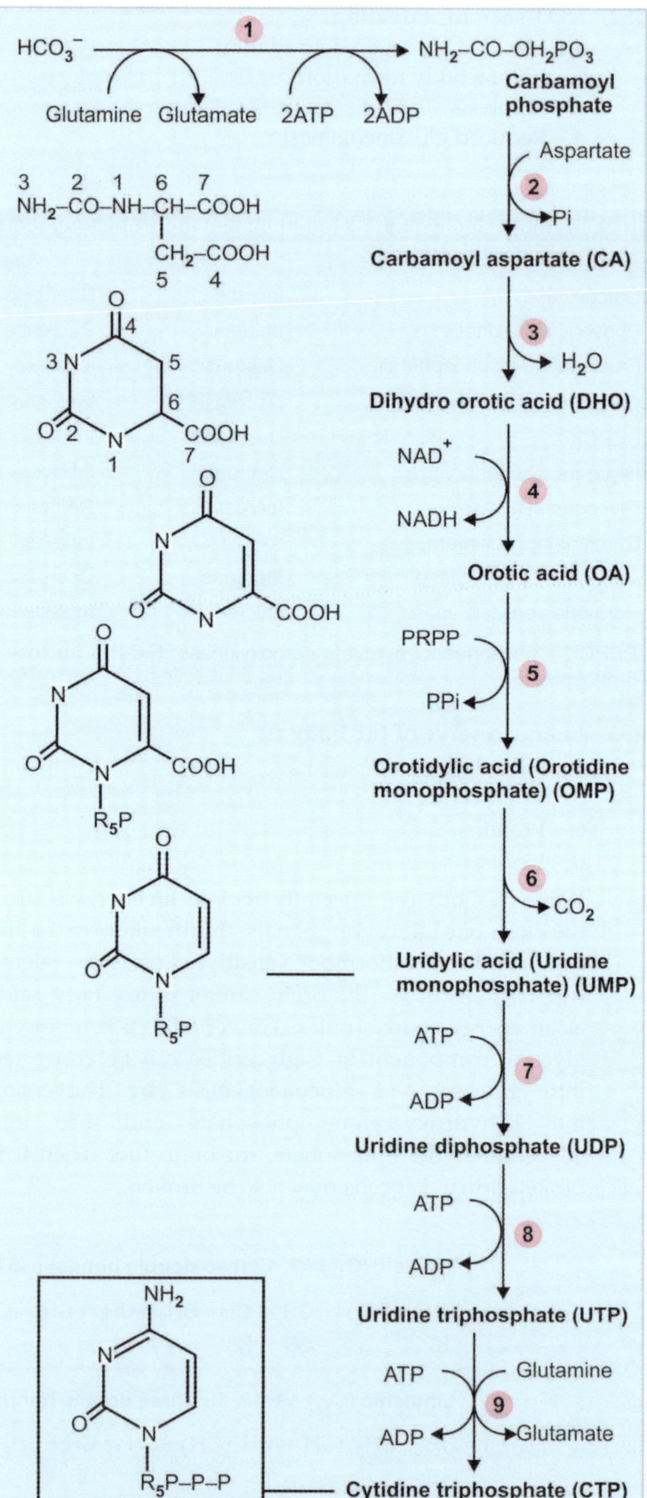

1 = carbamoyl phosphate synthase-II (CPS-II); 2 = aspartyl trans-carbamoylase (ATC); 3 = dihydro orotase (DHOase); 4 = dihydro orotate dehydrogenase (DHODH); 5 = orotate phospho ribosyl transferase (OPRTase); 6 = OMP-decarboxylase (OMPDC); 7 = UMP kinase; 8 = nucleoside diphosphate kinase; 9 = CTP synthetase

Synthesis of pyrimidine nucleotides.

Ans. **155. b.** Increased fat degradation **156. c.** Carbamoyl phosphate synthase II

157. **Location of Carbamoyl phosphate synthetase-II:**

a. Mitochondria b. Nucleus
c. Cytoplasm
d. Both mitochondria and cytoplasm

Carbamoyl phosphate synthetase II

- It is an enzyme that catalyzes the reactions that produce carbamoyl phosphate in the cytosol (as opposed to type I, which functions in the mitochondria).
- Its systemic name is hydrogen-carbonate: L-glutamine amido-ligase (ADP-forming, carbamate-phosphorylating)

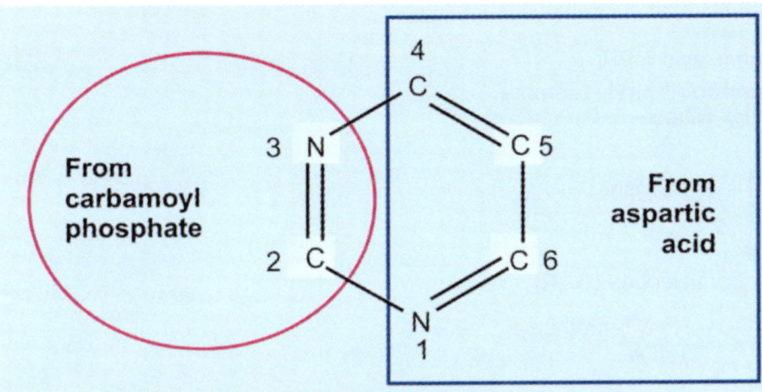

Sources of C and N atoms of pyrimidine.

158. **Lesch-Nyhan syndrome is due to:**

a. Total deficiency of HGPRTase
b. Partial deficiency of HGPRTase
c. Total deficiency of PRPPase
d. Partial deficiency of PRPPase

Lesch–Nyhan syndrome (LNS), also known as **Nyhan's syndrome** and juvenile gout, is a rare inherited disorder caused by a deficiency of the enzyme hypoxanthine-guanine phosphoribosyltransferase (HGPRT), produced by mutations in the HPRT gene located on the X chromosome.

Disorders of purine metabolism

Disorder	*Defect*	*Nature of defect*
Gout	PRPP synthetase, HGPRT, glucose 6 phosphatase	Hyperuricemia
Lesch-Nyhan syndrome	HGPRT	Lack of enzyme
SCID	ADA	Lack of enzyme
Immuno-deficiency	Purine nucleotide phosphorylase	Lack of enzyme
Renal lithiasis	APRT	Dihydroxyadenine, renal lithiasis
Xanthinuria	Xanthine oxidase	hypouricemia, xanthine renal lithiasis
von Gierke disease	Glucose-6-phos-phatase	Lack of enzyme

159. **Nucleotide is composed of:**

a. Nucleobase + sugar b. Nucleobase + phosphate
c. Nucleobase + sugar + phosphate
d. Sugar + phosphate

Nucleotides are organic molecules that serve as the monomers, or subunits, of nucleic acids like DNA and RNA. The building blocks of nucleic acids, nucleotides are composed of a nitrogenous base, a five-carbon sugar (ribose or deoxyribose), and at least one phosphate group. Thus a nucleoside plus a phosphate group yields a nucleotide.

Base + sugar + phosphate = nucleotide		
Ribonucleotides		
Adenosine	+ Pi	→Adenosine monophosphate (AMP) (Adenylic acid)
Guanosine	+ Pi	→Guanosine monophosphate (GMP) (Guanylic acid)
Cytidine	+ Pi	→Cytidine monophosphate (CMP) (Cytidylic acid)
Uridine	+ Pi	→Uridine monophosphate (UMP) (Uridylic acid)
Inosine	+ Pi	→Inosine monophosphate (IMP) (Inosinic acid)
Deoxyribonucleotides		
d-adenosine	+ Pi	→d-AMP (d-adenylic acid)
d-guanosine	+ Pi	→d-GMP (d-guanylic acid)
d-cytidine	+ Pi	→d-CMP (d-cytidylic acid)
d-thymidine	+ Pi	→d-TMP (d-thymidylic acid)

160. **In humans, uric acid is the product of metabolism of:**

a. Proteins b. Carbohydrate
c. Purine d. Pyrimidine

Uric acid is a product of the **metabolic** breakdown of **purine** nucleotides.

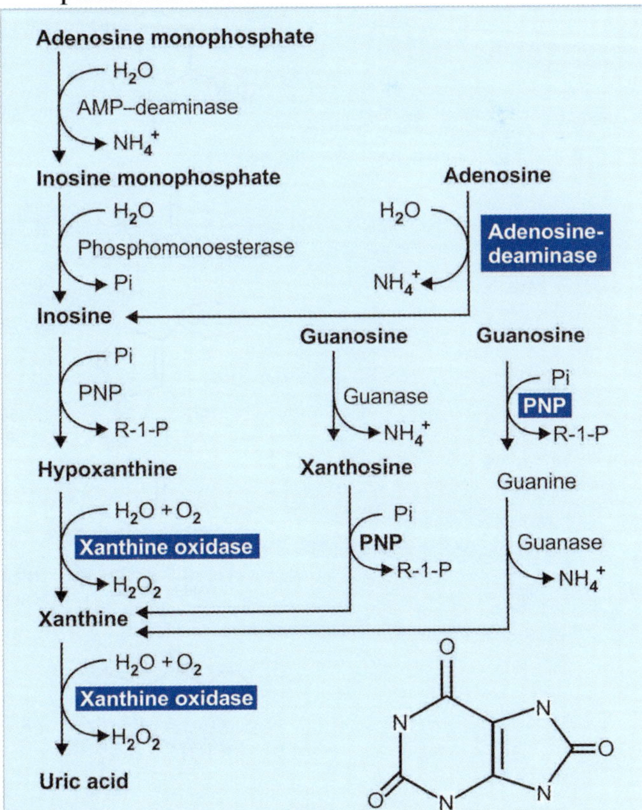

Degradation of purine nucleotides. Main pathway is in red arrows. PNP = purine nucleoside phosphorylase; R-1-P = ribose-1-phosphate.

Ans. 157. c. Cytoplasm 158. a. Total deficiency... 159. c. Nucleobase... 160. c. Purine

161. Disorder of nucleotide metabolism:

a. Von-Gierke's disease b. Gout
c. Niemann-Pick disease d. Atherosclerosis

Gout is a disorder of purine metabolism, and occurs when its final metabolite, uric acid, crystallizes in the form of monosodium urate, precipitating and forming deposits (tophi) in joints, on tendons, and in the surrounding tissues.

162. Enzyme associated with hyperuricemia:

a. Glucose-6-phosphatase
b. PRPP (PhosphoRibosyl PyroPhosphate) glutamylamidotransferase
c. Xanthine oxidase
d. 5-phosphoribosyl amido transferase

Enzmyes related to primary gout

- 5-phosphoribosyl amido transferase
- Abnormal PRPP synthetase
- Deficiency of enzymes of salvage pathway
- Glucose-6-phosphatase deificiency

163. Amino acid which contributes to biosynthesis of purine ribonucleotide are all EXCEPT:

a. Aspartate b. Histidine
c. Glutamine d. Glycine

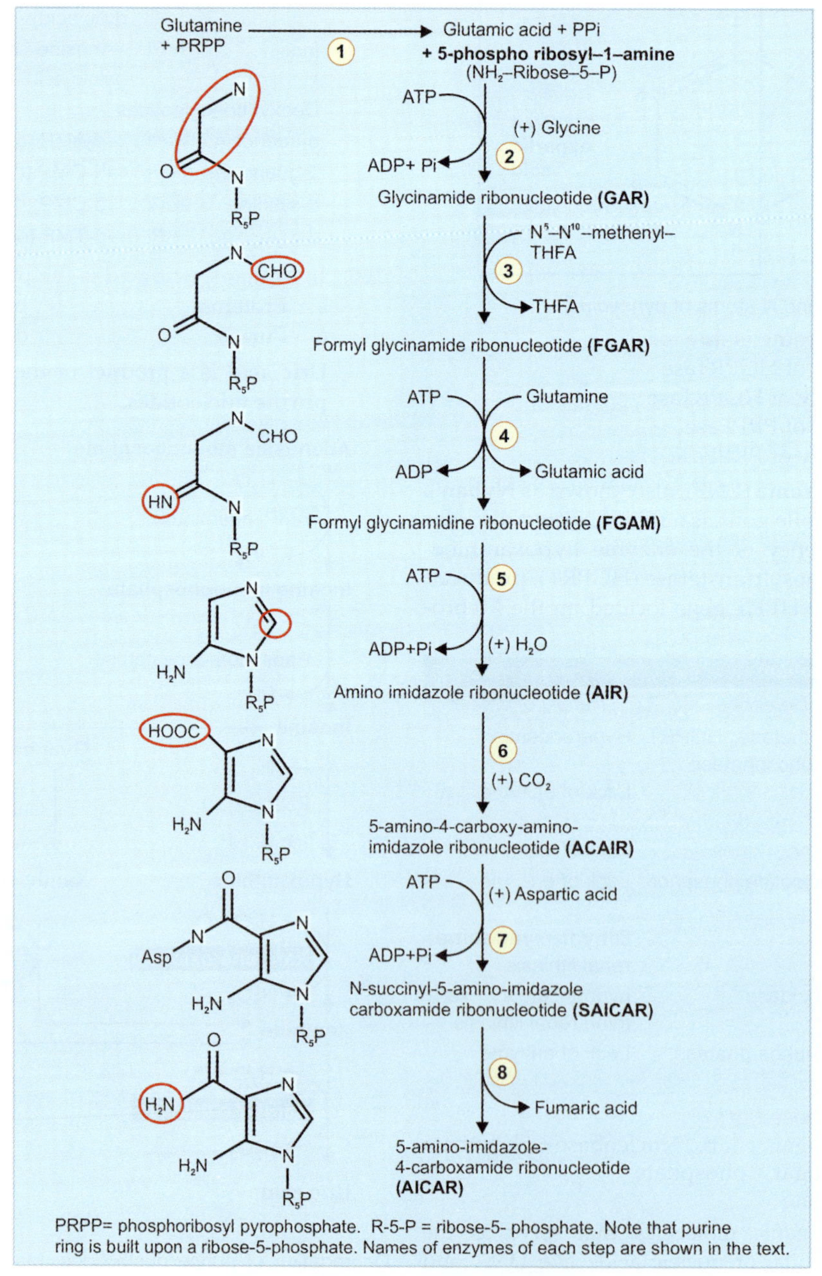

First eight steps of purine synthesis.

Ans. **161. b.** Gout **162. c.** Xanthine oxidase **163. b.** Histidine

Inosine monophosphate is synthesized on a pre-existing ribose-phosphate through a complex pathway. The source of the carbon and nitrogen atoms of the purine ring, 5 and 4 respectively, come from multiple sources. The amino acid glycine contributes all its carbon and nitrogen atoms, with additional nitrogen atoms from glutamine and aspartic acid, and additional carbon atoms from formyl groups, which are transferred from the coenzyme tetrahydrofolate as 10-formyltetrahydrofolate, and a carbon atom from bicarbonate. Formyl groups build carbon-2 and carbon-8 in the purine ring system, which are the ones acting as bridges between two nitrogen atoms.

MISCELLANEOUS

164. NOT included in DNA repair mechanism:

a. Base pair correction
b. Post-replication repair
c. Nucleoside excision repair
d. Mismatch repair

DNA repair mechanism

- When only one of the two strands of a double helix has a defect, the other strand can be used as a template to guide the correction of the damaged strand.
- In order to repair damage to one of the two paired molecules of DNA, there exist a number of excision repair mechanisms that remove the damaged nucleotide and replace it with an undamaged nucleotide complementary to that found in the undamaged DNA strand.
  - Base excision repair (BER), which repairs damage to a single base caused by oxidation, alkylation, hydrolysis, or deamination.
    - The damaged base is removed by a DNA glycosylase.
    - The "missing tooth" is then recognized by an enzyme called AP endonuclease, which cuts the phosphodiester bond.
    - The missing part is then resynthesized by a DNA polymerase, and a DNA ligase performs the final nick-sealing step.
  - Nucleotide excision repair (NER), which recognizes bulky, helix-distorting lesions such as pyrimidine dimmers and 6,4 photoproducts.
    - The A specialized form of NER known as transcription-coupled repair deploys NER enzymes to genes that are being actively transcribed.
  - Mismatch repair (MMR), which corrects errors of DNA replication and recombination that result in mispaired (but undamaged) nucleotides.

DNA repair mechanisms

Mechanism	Defect	Repair
Mismatch repair	Copying error 1–5 bases unpaired	Strand cutting, exonuclease digestion
Nucleotide exicision repair (NER)	Chemical damage to a segment	30 bases removed; then correct bases added
Base excision repair	Chemical damage to single base	Base removed by N-glycosylase; new base added
Double strand break	Free radicals and radiation	Unwinding, alignment, ligation

165. Which of the following ion is used in polymerase chain reaction/ PCR:

a. Manganese
b. Magnesium
c. Molybdenum
d. Iron

The **polymerase chain reaction** (**PCR**)

- It is a biochemical technology in molecular biology used to amplify a single copy or a few copies of a piece of DNA across several orders of magnitude, generating thousands to millions of copies of a particular DNA sequence.
- Developed in 1983 by Kary Mullis, PCR is now a common and often indispensable technique used in medical and biological research labs for a variety of applications.
- These include
  - DNA cloning for sequencing,
  - DNA-based phylogeny, or
  - Functional analysis of genes;
  - The diagnosis of hereditary diseases;
  - The identification of genetic fingerprints (used in forensic sciences and paternity testing); and
  - The detection and diagnosis of infectious diseases.
- The method relies on thermal cycling, consisting of cycles of repeated heating and cooling of the reaction for DNA melting and enzymatic replication of the DNA.
- Primers (short DNA fragments) containing sequences complementary to the target region along with a DNA polymerase (after which the method is named) are key components to enable selective and repeated amplification.
- As PCR progresses, the DNA generated is itself used as a template for replication, setting in motion a chain reaction in which the DNA template is exponentially amplified.
- Almost all PCR applications employ a heat-stable DNA polymerase, such as Taq polymerase (an enzyme originally isolated from the bacterium Thermus aquaticus).
- This DNA polymerase enzymatically assembles a new DNA strand from DNA building-blocks, the nucleotides, by using single-stranded DNA as a

Ans. **164. b.** Post-replication repair **165. b.** Magnesium

template and DNA oligonucleotides (also called DNA primers), which are required for initiation of DNA synthesis.

- The vast majority of PCR methods use thermal cycling, i.e., alternately heating and cooling the PCR sample through a defined series of temperature steps.
  - In the first step, the two strands of the DNA double helix are physically separated at a high temperature in a process called DNA melting.
  - In the second step, the temperature is lowered and the two DNA strands become templates for DNA polymerase to selectively amplify the target DNA.

Applications of PCR

Detection of infectious diseases
AIDS, tuberculosis, CMV, H1N1, hepatitis C, etc.
Lyme disease—joint inflammation from tick bites.
Detect 3 sexually transmitted diseases in one swab—herpes, papillomar virus, Chlamydia.
PCR can diagnosis even one bacteria or virus present in the specimen.
Latent viruses can also be diagnosed.
Detection of variations and mutations in genes
Detects people with inherited disorders and carriers
Track presence or absence of DNA abnormalities characteristic of cancer
Prenatal diagnosis of genetic disorders.
PCR combined with RE cleavage and Southern blotting is used for mutation detection.
PCR and the law
DNA fingerprinting—can multiply small amounts of DNA found in blood samples, hair, semen, and other body fluids

166. Which of the following holds true regarding DNA:
a. Left hand double helix
b. Two strands run in parallel direction
c. Two polynucleotide chains are identical
d. Hydrogen bond is between a purine and a pyrimidine only

Structure of DNA

- Most DNA molecules consist of two bipolymer strands coiled around each other to form a double helix.
- The two DNA strands are known as polynucleotides since they are composed of simpler units called nucleotides.
- Each nucleotide is composed of a nitrogen containing nucleobase—either guanine (G), adenine (A), thymine (T), or cytosine (C)—as well as a monosaccharide sugar called deoxyribose and a phosphate group.
- The nucleotides are joined to one another in a chain by covalent bonds between the sugar of one nucleotide and the phosphate of the next, resulting in an alternating sugar-phosphate backbone.
- According to base pairing rules (A with T and C with G), hydrogen bonds bind the nitrogenous bases of the two separate polynucleotide strands to make double-stranded DNA.

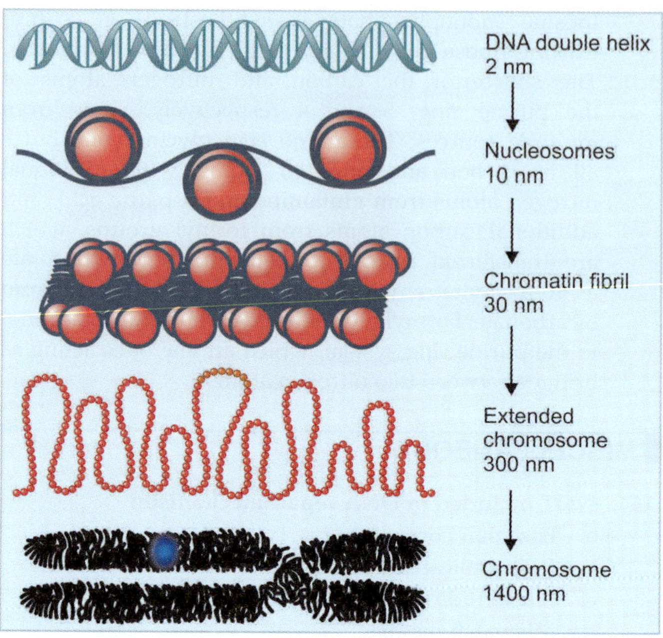

DNA condenses repeatedly to form chromosome.

167. Location of Codons:
a. tRNA
b. mRNA
c. rRNA
d. DNA

Codons

- A series of codons in part of a messenger RNA (mRNA) molecule.
- Each codon consists of three nucleotides, usually corresponding to a single amino acid.
- The nucleotides are abbreviated with the letters A, U, G and C.
- This is mRNA, which uses U (uracil).
- DNA uses T (thymine) instead.
- This mRNA molecule will instruct a ribosome to synthesize a protein according to this code.

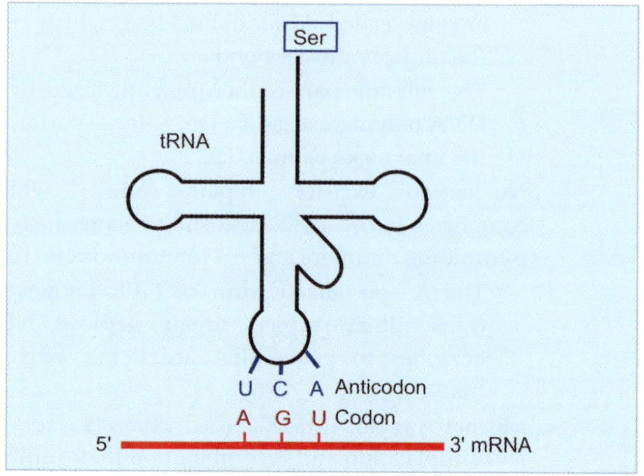

Transfer RNA carrying serine.

Ans. **166. d.** Hydrogen bond... **167. b.** mRNA

168. Menadione is:

a. Vitamin K1
b. Vitamin K2
c. Vitamin K3
d. All of the above

Vitamin K

- All 3 forms of the vitamin are naphthoquinone derivatives
- Vitamin K_1 (phylloquinone)
  - Phylloquinone has a phytyl side chain.
  - Present in plants
- Vitamin K_2 (menaquinone).
  - Side chain is composed of a varying number of isoprenoid residues.
  - The most common number of these residues is four, since animal enzymes normally produce menaquinone-4 from plant phylloquinone.
  - Produced by the intestinal bacteria also found in animals
- Vitamin K_3 (menadione).
  - Synthetic form

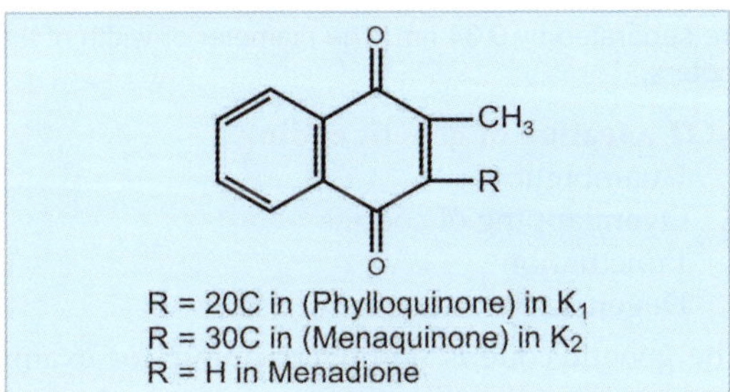

Vitamin K.

169. Vitamin C is necessary for the formation of collagen as it is required for:

a. Conversion of pyridoxine to PLP
b. Conversion of glutamate to gamma-carboxy-glutamate
c. Conversion of methionine to SAM
d. Conversion to proline to hydroxy-proline

Vitamin C

- It acts as an electron donor for eight different enzymes
- Three enzymes (prolyl-3-hydroxylase, prolyl-4-hydroxylase, and lysyl hydroxylase) that are required for the hydroxylation of proline and lysine in the synthesis of collagen
- These reactions add hydroxyl groups to the amino acids proline or lysine in the collagen molecule via prolyl hydroxylase and lysyl hydroxylase, both requiring vitamin C as a cofactor.
- Hydroxylation allows the collagen molecule to assume its triple helix structure, and thus vitamin C is essential to the development and maintenance of scar tissue, blood vessels, and cartilage.
- Two enzymes (epsilon-N-trimethyl-L-lysine hydroxylase and gamma-butyrobetaine hydroxylase) that are necessary for synthesis of carnitine
- Carnitine is essential for the transport of fatty acids into mitochondria for ATP generation.
- The remaining three enzymes have the following functions in common, but have other functions as well:
  - Dopamine beta hydroxylase participates in the biosynthesis of norepinephrine from dopamine
  - Peptidoglycine alpha-amidating monoxygenase amidates peptide hormones by removing the glyoxylate residue from their c-terminal glycine residues.
  - This increases peptide hormone stability and activity.
  - 4-hydroxyphenylpyruvate dioxygenase modulates tyrosine metabolism.

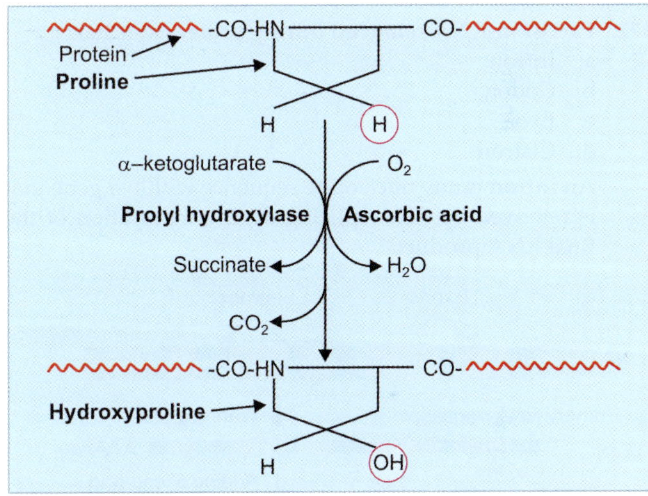

Hydroxylation of proline to hydroxyproline needs ascorbic acid.

170. Chromsomal studies are done in:

a. Anaphase
b. Telophase
c. Metaphase
d. Prophase

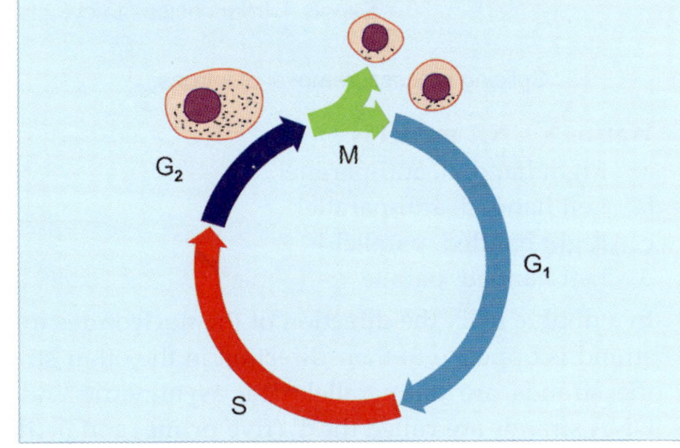

Cell cycle.

The analysis of metaphase chromosomes is one of the main tools of classical cytogenetics and cancer studies. Chromosomes are condensed (thickened) and highly coiled in metaphase, which makes them most suitable

Ans. **168. c.** Vitamin K3 **169. d.** Conversion... **170. c.** Metaphase for visual analysis. Metaphase chromosomes make the classical picture of chromosomes (karyotype).

171. True for ribozyme:

a. They play a key role in RNA synthesis
b. They play a key role in post-transcription conversion of pre-mRNA to mature mRNA
c. They are DNA molecules
d. They are not present in ribosomes

Within the ribosome, ribozymes function as part of the large subunit ribosomal RNA to link amino acids during protein synthesis. They also participate in a variety of RNA processing reactions, including RNA splicing, viral replication, and transfer RNA biosynthesis. Examples of ribozymes include the hammerhead ribozyme, the VS ribozyme, Leadzyme and the hairpin ribozyme.

172. Part of m-RNA removed during protein synthesis:

a. Intron
b. Codon
c. Exon
d. Cistron

An **intron** is any nucleotide sequence within a gene that is removed by RNA splicing during maturation of the final RNA product.

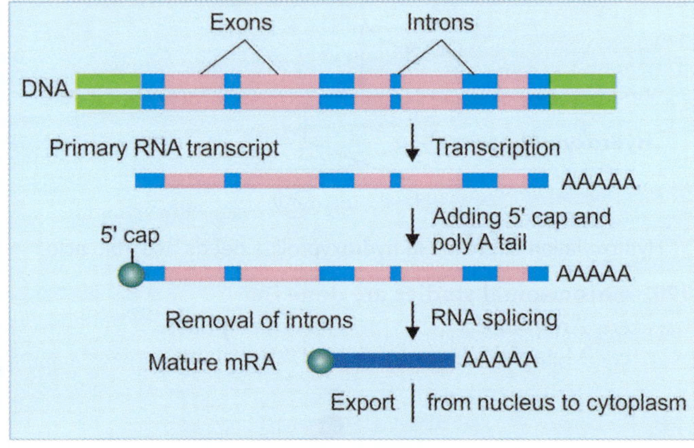

Splicing process; removal of introns.

173. Watson's DNA model is:

a. Right handed, anti-parallel
b. Left handed, anti-parallel
c. Right handed, parallel
d. Left handed, paralle

In a double helix the direction of the nucleotides in one strand is opposite to their direction in the other strand: the strands are antiparallel. The asymmetric ends of DNA strands are called the 5′ (**five prime**) and 3′ (**three prime**) ends, with the 5′ end having a terminal phosphate group and the 3′ end a terminal hydroxyl group. One major difference between DNA and RNA is the sugar, with the 2-deoxyribose in DNA being replaced by the alternative pentose sugar ribose in RNA.

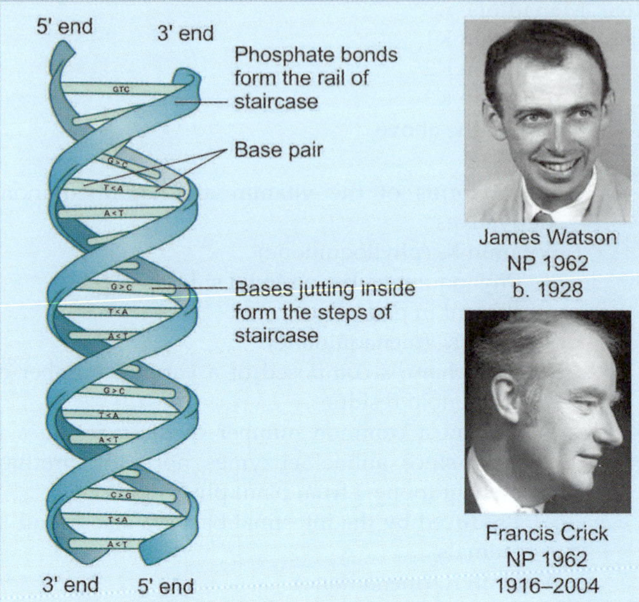

Watson-Crick model of double helical structure of DNA. Adjacent bases are separated by 0.34 nm. The diameter or width of the helix is 2 nanometers.

174. NOT a feature of genetic coding:

a. Unambiguous
b. Overalapping of codons
c. Punctuation
d. Degeneracy

The genetic code is non-overlapping; for example in a sequence of ABCDEF, ABC would code the first amino acid and DEF the second whereas in an overlapping code ABC could code for the first amino acid and BCD the second.

Salient features of genetic code	
1.	Triplet base sequence
2.	Non-overlapping
3.	Non-punctuated
4.	Degenerate
5.	Unambiguous
6.	Universal

175. Base ABSENT in DNA:

a. Thymine
b. Uracil
c. Guanine
d. Adenine

Uracil (U) is one of the four nucleobases in the nucleic acid of RNA that are represented by the letters A, G, C and U. The others are adenine (A), cytosine (C), and guanine (G). In RNA, uracil binds to adenine via two hydrogen bonds. In DNA, the uracil nucleobase is replaced by thymine.

Ans. 171. **b.** They play... 172. **a.** Intron 173. **a.** Right handed... 174. **b.** Overalapping of codons
175. **b.** Uracil

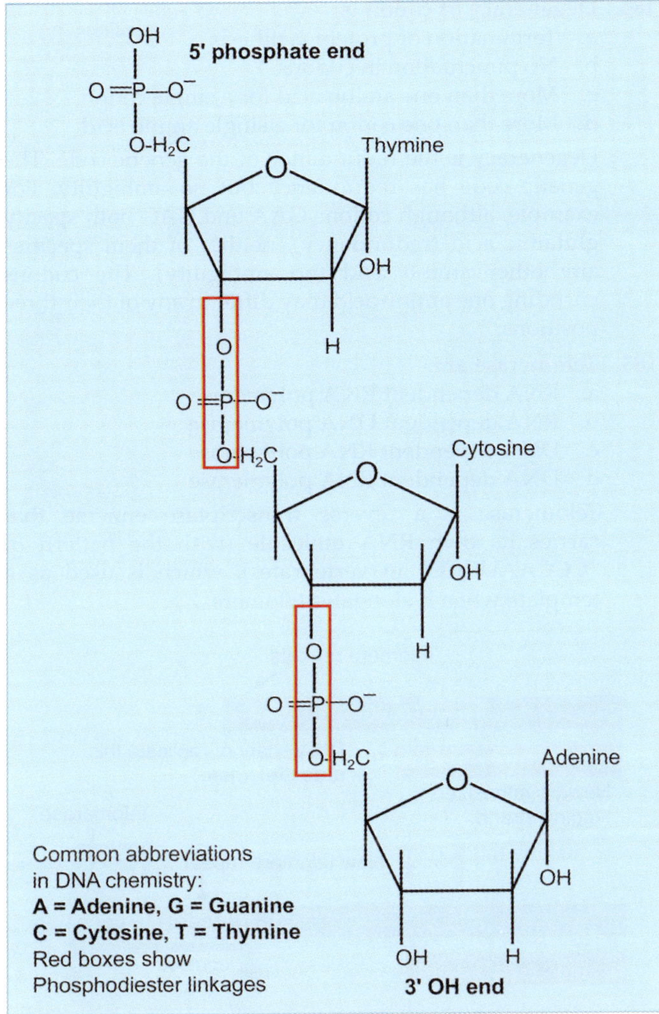

Polynucleotide.

176. Stacking of base pairs in DNA stabilize the double helix by:

a. Hydrophobic effect
b. Hyperchromicity effect
c. Hypochromicity effect
d. Linear dichromacity effect

The stacking of base pairs stabilize the double helix by the hydrophobic effect and confirmation of the ring systems.

177. True for banding:

a. Trypsin and Giemsa is used
b. Chromosome is seen in interphase
c. Fluorescence filters are used
d. Method to detect single gene deletion

Interphase chromosome-specific multicolor **banding** (ICS-MCB) has become the solution providing for studying **interphase** chromosomes in their integrity at molecular resolution.

178. Visualization of specific RNA fragment using RNA probe is:

a. Southern blotting
b. Western blotting
c. Eastern blotting
d. Northern blotting

The **northern blot** is a technique used in molecular biology research to study gene expression by detection of RNA (or isolated mRNA) in a sample.

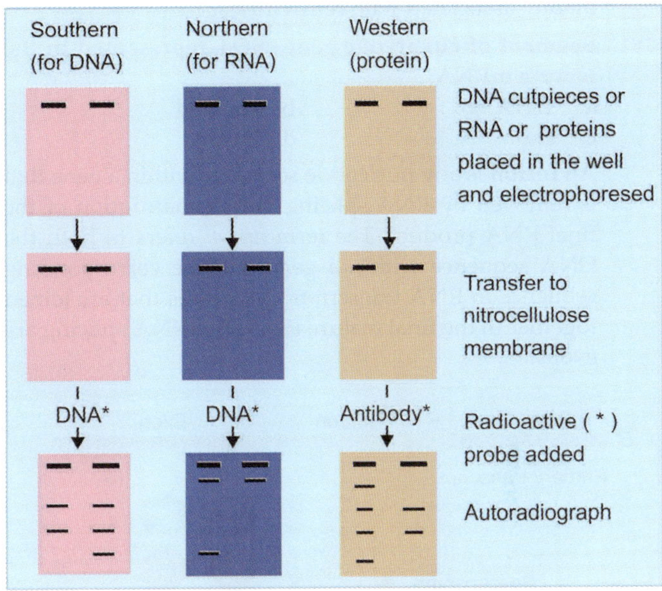

Comparison of blot transfer techniques.

179. On complete hydrolysis of DNA molecule, we will get all of the following EXCEPT:

a. Deoxy pentose sugar
b. Phosphoric acid
c. Adenosine
d. Purine bases

Adenosine is a purine nucleoside composed of a molecule of adenine attached to a ribose sugar molecule (ribofuranose) moiety via a β-N_9-glycosidic bond.

180. An enzyme that makes a double stranded DNA copy from a single stranded RNA template molecule is:

a. DNA polymerase
b. RNA polymerase
c. Reverse transcriptase
d. Phosphokinase

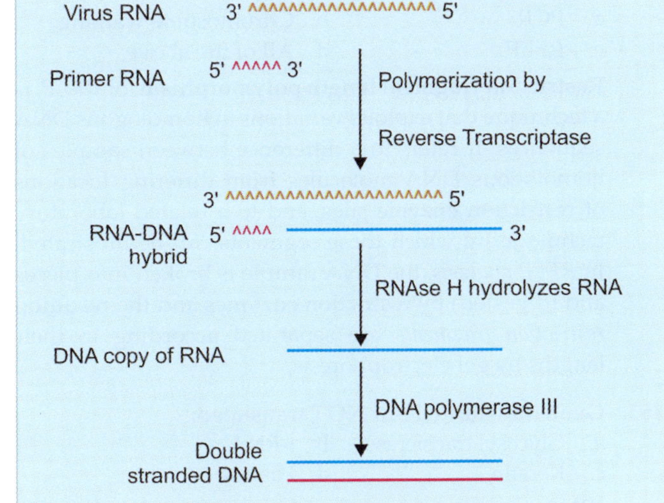

Action of reverse transcriptase.

Ans. 176. **a.** Hydrophobic... 177. **b.** Chromosome... 178. **d.** Northern blotting 179. **c.** Adenosine 180. **c.** Reverse...

A **Reverse transcriptase** (RT) is an enzyme used to generate complementary DNA (cDNA) from an RNA template, a process termed *reverse transcription*. It is mainly associated with retroviruses.

181. Segment of eukaryotic gene, NOT represented in the mature mRNA:

a. TATA box b. Plasmid
c. Exon d. Intron

An **intron** is any nucleotide sequence within a gene that is removed by RNA splicing during maturation of the final RNA product. The term *intron* refers to both the DNA sequence within a gene and the corresponding sequence in RNA transcripts. Sequences that are joined together in the final mature RNA after RNA splicing are exons.

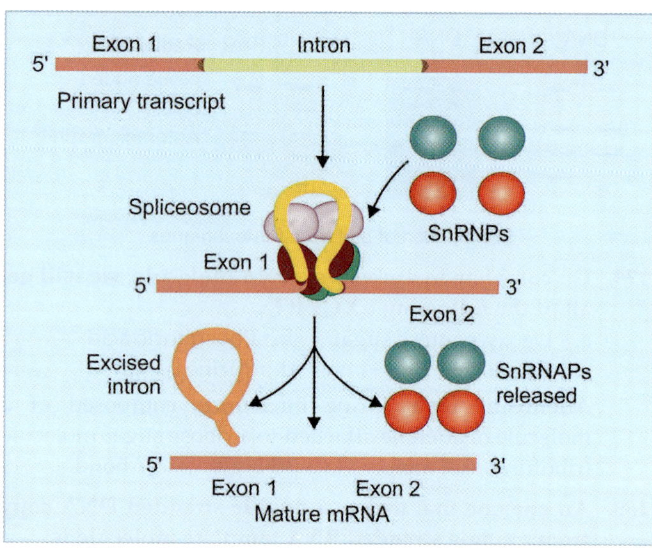

Spliceosome excise intron.

182. Method employed to read large chromosomes of 50-100 base pairs:

a. PCR b. Chromosome walking
c. RFLP d. All of the above

Restriction fragment length polymorphism, or RFLP, is a technique that exploits variations in homologous DNA sequences. It refers to a difference between samples of homologous DNA molecules from differing locations of restriction enzyme sites, and to a related laboratory technique by which these segments can be illustrated. In *RFLP analysis*, the DNA sample is broken into pieces and (digested) by restriction enzymes and the resulting *restriction fragments* are separated according to their lengths by gel electrophoresis.

183. Gene transmitted but NOT translated:

a. Glycosyl transferase b. t-RNA
c. Keratin d. Histone

rRNA**genes** are transcribed **but not translated; genes** for mRNA are both transcribed and **translated**.

184. Degeneracy of codon is:

a. Termination of protein synthesis
b. No punctuation in codons
c. More than one amino acid for a single codon
d. More than one codon for a single amino acid

Degeneracy is the redundancy of the genetic code. The genetic code has redundancy but no ambiguity. For example, although codons GAA and GAG both specify glutamic acid (redundancy), neither of them specifies any other amino acid (no ambiguity). The codons encoding one amino acid may differ in any of their three positions.

185. Telomerase are:

a. RNA dependent RNA polymerase
b. RNA dependent DNA polymerase
c. DNA dependent RNA polymerase
d. DNA dependent RNA polymerase

Telomerase is a reverse transcriptase enzyme that carries its own RNA molecule (with the pattern of "CCCAAUCCC" in vertebrates), which is used as a template when it elongates telomeres.

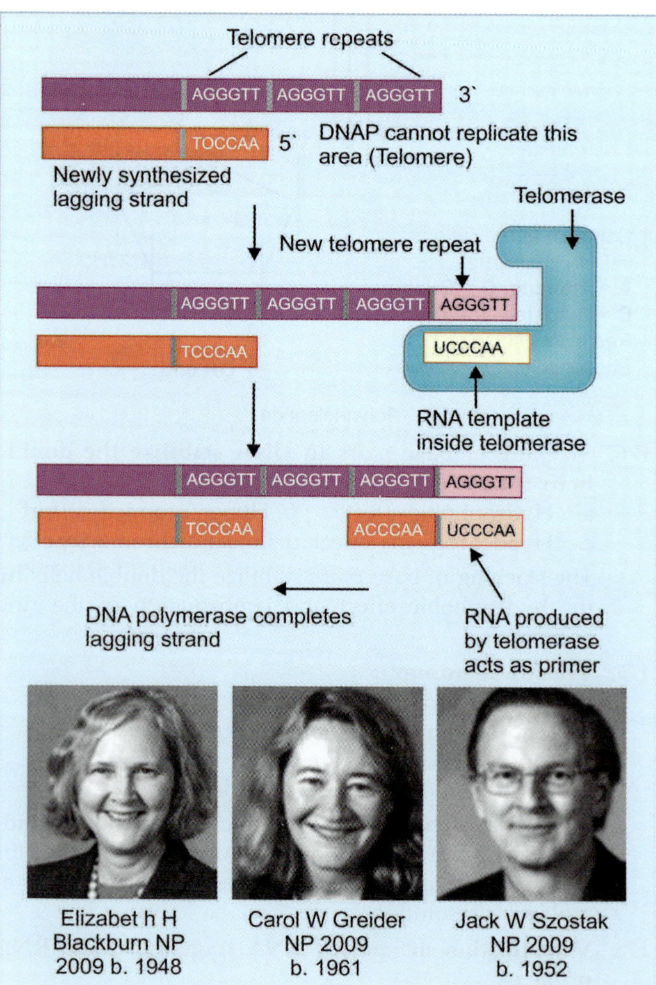

During replication, there will be a gap at the 5' end of new strand. Telomerase is required to fill this gap.

Ans. **181. d.** Intron **182. c.** RFLP **183. b.** t-RNA **184. d.** More than one codon... **185. b.** RNA dependent...

186. **Western blot is done for:**
a. DNA b. RNA
c. Lipid d. Protein

The **western blot** (sometimes called the **protein immunoblot**) is a widely used analytical technique used to detect specific proteins in a sample of tissue homogenate or extract.

187. **RNA polymerase/RNAP recognizes:**
a. Stop site
b. Regulator site
c. Promoter site
d. Initiation site

RNAP can initiate transcription at specific DNA sequences known as promoters. It then produces an RNA chain, which is complementary to the template DNA strand. The process of adding nucleotides to the RNA strand is known as elongation; in eukaryotes, RNAP can build chains as long as 2.4 million nucleotides (the full length of the dystrophin gene). RNAP will preferentially release its RNA transcript at specific DNA sequences encoded at the end of genes, which are known as terminators.

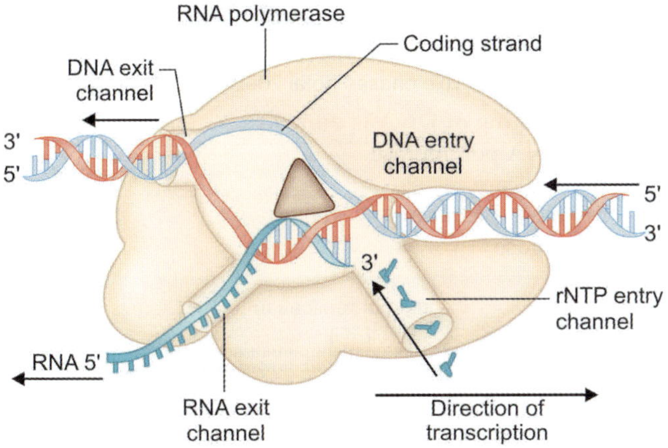

Transcription process.

188. **Shine Dalgarno sequence in prokaryotes is associated with:**
a. Translocation
b. Tramscription
c. Translation
d. Replication

The **Shine-Dalgarno (SD) sequence** is a ribosomal binding site in prokaryotic messenger RNA, generally located around 8 bases upstream of the start codon AUG. The RNA sequence helps recruit the ribosome to the mRNA to initiate protein synthesis by aligning the ribosome with the start codon.

189. **DNA double helix is maintained by:**
a. Covalent bond
b. Disulfide bond
c. Van der Waals forces
d. Hydrogen bond

Highly hydrated B-DNA occurs naturally in living cells in such a paracrystalline state, which is a dynamic one in spite of the relatively rigid DNA double-helix stabilized by parallel hydrogen bonds between the nucleotide base-pairs in the two complementary, helical DNA chains.

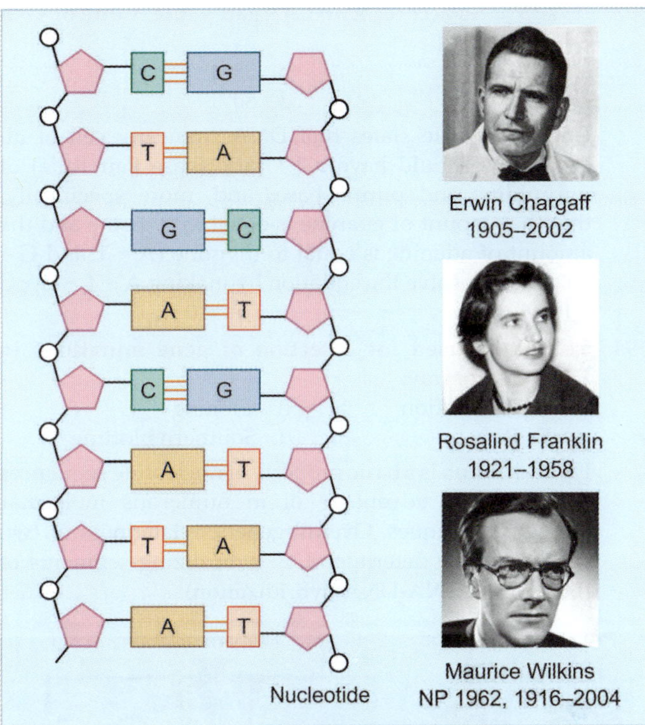

Base pairing rule. Base pairing of A with T and G with C. Hydrogen bonds between bases.

190. **Palindrome is associated with:**
a. Small nuclear RNA
b. Sequence of DNA
c. Extra-chromosmal molecule of DNA
d. Synthesis of DNA

A **palindromic sequence** is a nucleic acid sequence on double-stranded DNA or RNA wherein reading 5′ (five prime) to 3′ (three prime) forward on one strand matches the sequence reading backward 5′ to 3′ on the complementary strand with which it forms a double helix. This definition of palindrome thus depends on complementary strands being palindromic of each other.

191. **Maximum numbers of bond are between:**
a. C-T b. A-G
c. G-C d. A-T

Purines form hydrogen bondsto pyrimidines, with adenine bonding only to thymine in two hydrogen bonds, and cytosine bonding only to guanine in three hydrogen bonds.

192. **NOT a circular DNA:**
a. Yeast b. Plasmid
c. Nuclear d. Mitochondrial

Ans. 186. **d.** Protein 187. **c.** Promoter site 188. **c.** Translation 189. **d.** Hydrogen bond
190. **b.** Sequence... 191. **c.** G-C 192. **c.** Nuclear

Nuclear DNA is a nucleic acid, a complex organic compound, found in the nucleus of eukaryotic organisms. Its structure is a double helix, with two strands wound around each other. This double helix structure was first described by Francis Crick and James D. Watson (1953) using data collected by Rosalind Franklin.

193. A is 15%. So according to Chargaff's rule, value of G in DNA should be:

a. 15% b. 35%
c. 70% d. 80%

Chargaff's rule states that DNA from any cell of all organisms should have a 1:1 ratio (base Pair Rule) of pyrimidine and purine bases and, more specifically, that the amount of guanine is equal to cytosine and the amount of adenine is equal to thymine (A = T and G = C). One can solve the equation by making A + T + G + C = 100%.

194. Technique used for detection of gene mutations in DNA microarray:

a. Hybridization b. Cloning
c. PCR d. Southern blotting

Hybridization is a basic property of nucleotide sequences and is taken advantage of in numerous molecular biology techniques. Overall genetic relatedness of two species can be determined by hybridizing segments of their DNA (DNA-DNA hybridization).

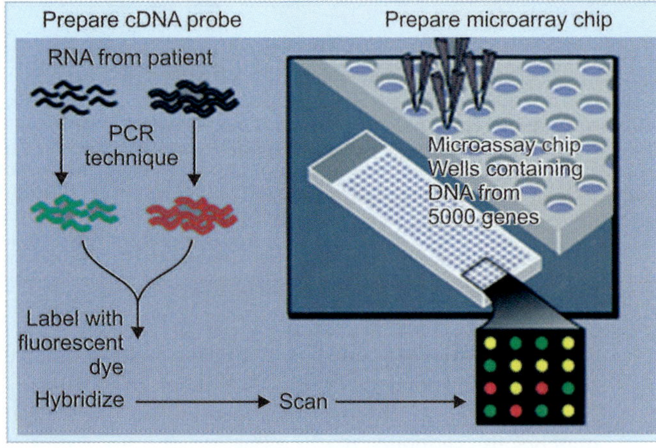

Microarray technology.

195. Technique related to single base pair substitution:

a. Southern blot b. FISH
c. PCR d. RFLP

Restriction fragment length polymorphism, or RFLP, is a technique that exploits variations in homologous DNA sequences. It refers to a difference between samples of homologous DNA molecules from differing locations of restriction enzyme sites, and to a related laboratory technique by which these segments can be illustrated.

196. DNA replication occurs in:

a. G1 phase b. G2 phase
c. S phase d. M phase

Within eukaryotes, DNA replication is controlled within the context of the cell cycle. As the cell grows and divides, it progresses through stages in the cell cycle; DNA replication takes place during the S phase (synthesis phase).

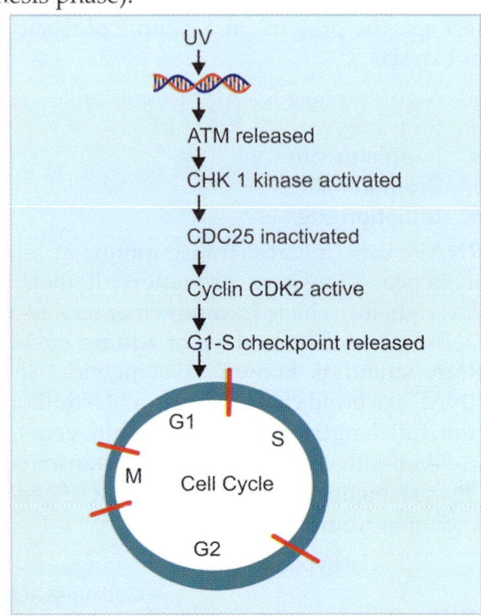

Cell cycle phases (total 20–22 hours).

197. Unwinding of DNA is done by:

a. DNA polymerase
b. Helicase
c. DNA primase
d. Ligase

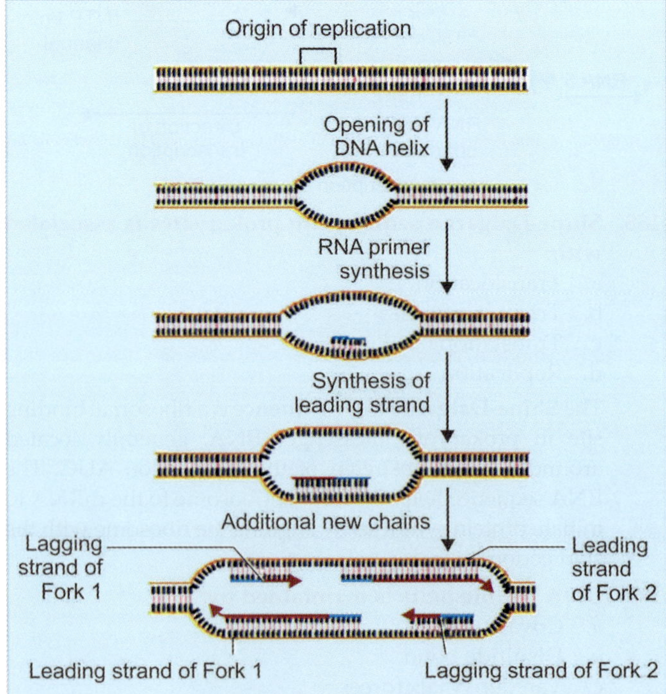

Replication bubble (Replication fork).

Ans. 193. **b.** 35% 194. **a.** Hybridization 195. **d.** RFLP 196. **c.** S phase
197. **b.** Helicase

Helicases are often used to separate strands of a DNA double helix or a self-annealed RNA molecule using the energy from ATP hydrolysis, a process characterized by the breaking of hydrogen bonds between annealed nucleotide bases.

198. Heat stable enzyme obtained from thermophilus aquaticus and used in PCR:

a. DNA gyrase b. Taq polymerase
c. DNA polymerase-III d. Endonuclease

***Taq* polymerase** is a thermostable DNA polymerase named after the thermophilic bacterium **Thermus aquaticus** from which it was originally isolated by Chien et al. in 1976.

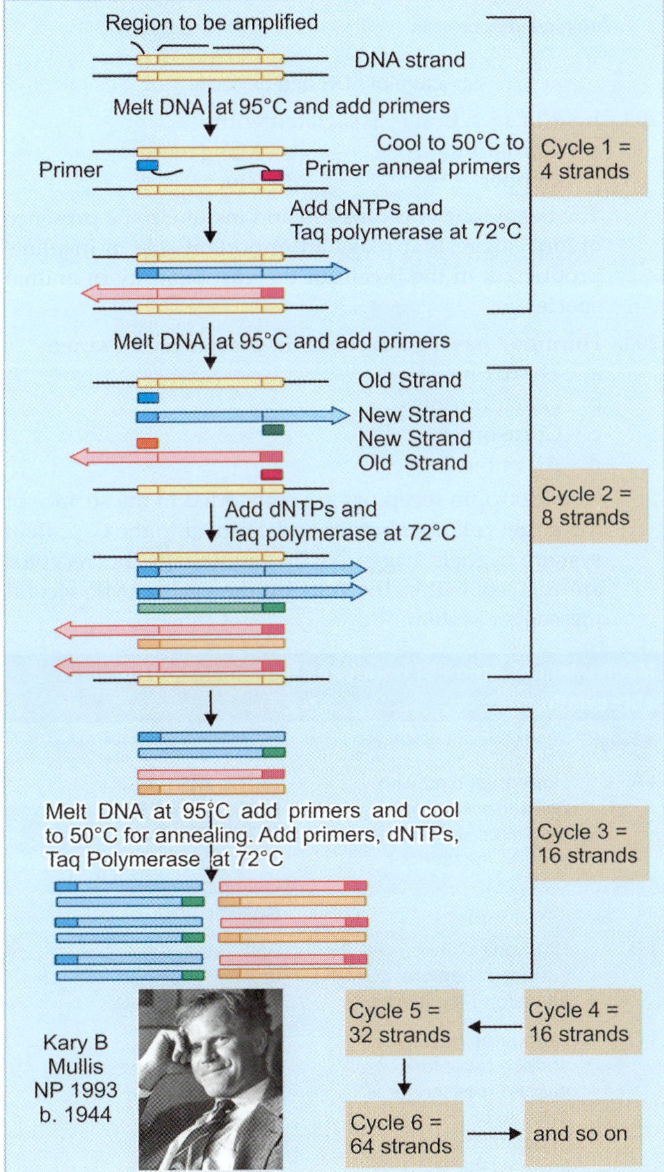

Polymerase chain reaction (PCR).

199. DNA segments are identified by:

a. Polymerase chain reaction
b. Western blotting
c. Northern blotting
d. Dideoxynucleotide method

Dideoxynucleotides are chain-elongating inhibitors of DNA polymerase, used in the Sanger method for DNA sequencing. They are also known as 2′,3′ dideoxynucleotides, and abbreviated as *ddNTPs* (ddGTP, ddATP, ddTTP and ddCTP).

200. TATA box is:

a. Transcription factor b. Enhancer
c. Promoter region d. RNA splicer

The **TATA box** (also called **Goldberg-Hogness box**) is a DNA sequence (cis-regulatory element) found in the promoter region of genes in archaea and eukaryotes; approximately 24% of human genes contain a TATA box within the core promoter.

201. Transport of mitochondrial proteins from cytoplasm to mitochondria is done by:

a. Clathrin b. Ubiquitin
c. Clathrin d. Chaperones

Many chaperones are heat shock proteins, that is, proteins expressed in response to elevated temperatures or other cellular stresses. The reason for this behaviour is that protein folding is severely affected by heat and, therefore, some chaperones act to prevent or correct damage caused by misfolding.

Other types of chaperones are involved in transport across membranes, for example membranes of the mitochondria and endoplasmic reticulum (ER) in eukaryotes. Bacterial translocation-specific chaperone maintains newly synthesized precursor polypeptide chains in a translocation-competent (generally unfolded) state and guides them to the translocon.

202. Primary role of chaperones is to help in:

a. Protein synthesis
b. Protein degradation
c. Protein denaturation
d. Protein folding

Molecular chaperones are proteins that assist the covalent folding or unfolding and the assembly or disassembly of other macromolecular structures. Chaperones are present when the macromolecules perform their normal biological functions and have correctly completed the processes of folding and/or assembly.

203. Chaperones are:

a. Purine metabolism mediators
b. Antigen presenting cells
c. Mediators of post-transitional assembly of protein complexes
d. None of the above

Ans. 198. **b.** Taq polymerase 199. **d.** Dideoxynucleotide... 200. **c.** Promoter... 201. **d.** Chaperones
202. **d.** Protein... 203. **c.** Mediators...

Chaperones are present when the macromolecules perform their normal biological functions and have correctly completed the processes of folding and/or assembly. The chaperones are concerned primarily with protein folding.

204. Structure that wraps histone:

a. Nucleosome　　b. DNA double helix
c. Chromatin　　d. mRNA

Histones are highly alkaline proteins found in eukaryotic cell nuclei that package and order the DNA into structural units called nucleosomes. They are the chief protein components of chromatin, acting as spools around which DNA winds, and playing a role in gene regulation.

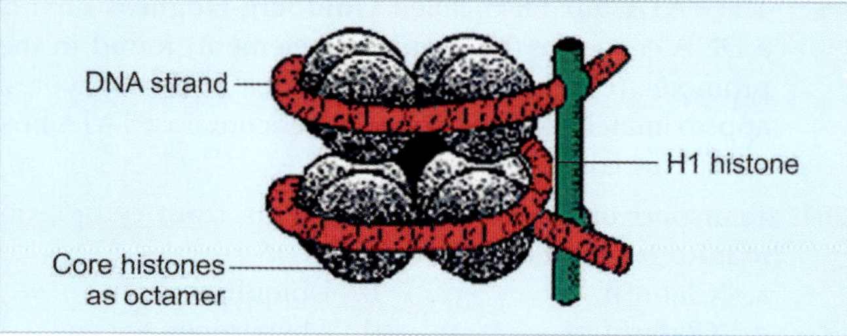

DNA wraps twice around histone octamer to form one nucleosome.

205. All terminator codons begin with:

a. A　　b. T
c. G　　d. U

The three stop/terminator codons have been given names: UAG is **amber**, UGA is **opal** (sometimes also called **umber**), and UAA is **ochre**.

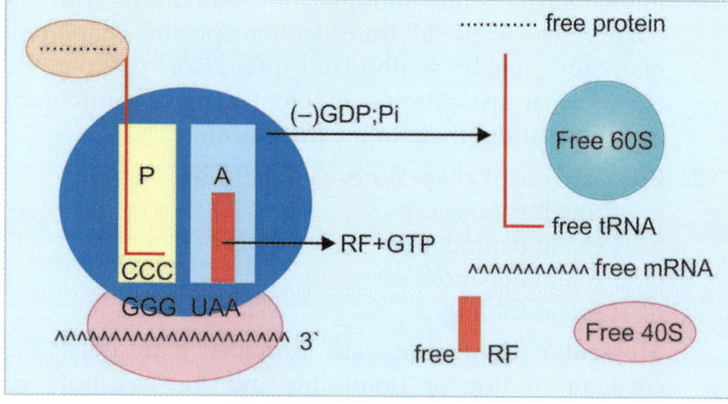

Termination of translation.

206. Thirst is related to:

a. Dopamine　　b. Epinephrine
c. Noradrenalin　　d. ADH

Thirst is "the physiological urge to drink water". In studies, it is recognised when subjects report the conscious sensation of a desire to drink. Under normal conditions, most water intake is due not to thirst but to social and cultural factors (e.g. drinking with meals or at work breaks, water in food). Thirst offers a backup to these behavioural factors and to the ADH response. Both the thirst and the ADH mechanisms are regulated in the hypothalamus. Water intake can be considered to consist of two components: a regulatory component (due to thirst) and a non-regulatory component (all other fluid intake).

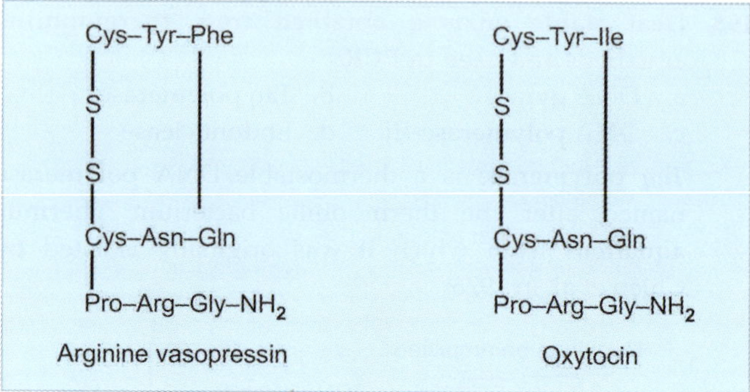

Structure of ADH and oxytocin.

207. Insulin secretion is associated with:

a. Chromium　　b. Manganese
c. Copper　　d. Zinc

The behaviour of proinsulin and insulin in the presence of zinc suggests it plays an important role in insulin's production in the B-cell for the vast majority of animal species.

208. Hormone having a receptor in plasma membrane:

a. Thyroxine
b. Gonadotropins
c. Cortisone
d. All of the above

Gonadotropin receptors are embedded in the surface of the target cell membranes and coupled to the G-protein system. Signals triggered by binding to the receptor are relayed within the cells by the cyclic AMP second messenger system.

Mechanism of action of hormones (for expansions or abbreviations)

Group	*Mechanism of action*	*Examples of hormone*
I A	Hormones bind with cell surface receptors with cAMP as the second messenger	ACTH, ADH, FSH HCG, LH, TSH MSH, PTH, CRH Glucagon, Calcitonin Catecholamines Retinoic acid
I B	Hormones having cell surface receptors; cGMP as second messenger	ANF (atrial natriuretic factor), NO (nitric oxide)
I C	Hormones having cell surface receptors; second messenger is calcium or phosphatidyl inositol (PIP2)	TRH, GnRH catecholamines Acetylcholine CCK, Gastrin Vasopressin Oxytocin, PDGF

Contd…

Ans. 204. b. DNA double... 205. d. U 206. d. ADH 207. d. Zinc 208. b. Gonadotropins

Contd...

Group	*Mechanism of action*	*Examples of hormone*
I D	Hormones having cell surface receptors and mediated through tyrosine kinase	Insulin Somatomedin EGF, FGF PDGF, CGSF NGF, IGF
I E	Hormones having cell surface receptors, but intracellular messenger is a kinase or utilize phosphatase cascade	IL, GH, PRL, TNF, Adiponectin, Leptin, Resistin, Erythropoietin
I I	Hormones that bind to intracellular receptors	Glucocorticoids Mineralocorticoids Estrogens, Progesterone Androgens Calcitriol, Thyroxine

209. 17-hydroxylase deficiency causes:

a. Increased estrogen b. Decreased glucagon
c. Decreased estrogen d. Decreased testosterone

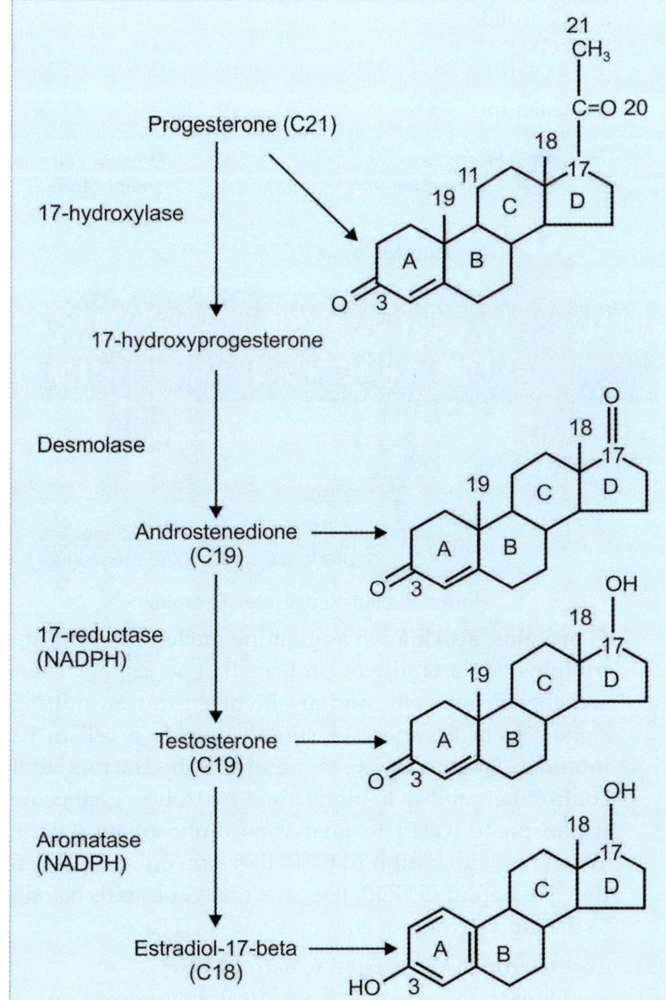

Synthesis of sex hormones.

Congenital adrenal hyperplasia due to 17α-hydroxylase deficiency is an uncommon form of congenital adrenal hyperplasia resulting from a defect in the gene CYP17A1, which encodes for the enzyme 17α-hydroxylase. It produces decreased synthesis of both cortisol and sex steroids, with resulting increase in mineralocorticoid production. Thus, common symptoms include mild hypocortisolism, ambiguous genitalia in genetic males or failure of the ovaries to function at puberty in genetic females, and hypertension (respectively).

210. NOT a glycoprotein:

a. GH b. TSH
c. FSH d. LH

Growth hormone (**GH** or **HGH**), also known as **somatotropin** or **somatropin**, is a peptide hormone that stimulates growth, cell reproduction and regeneration in humans and other animals. It is a type of mitogen which is specific only to certain kinds of cells. Growth hormone is a 191-amino acid, single-chain polypeptide that is synthesized, stored, and secreted bysomatotropic cells within the lateral wings of the anterior pituitary gland.

Functions of glycoprotein

Function	*Example of glycoprotein*
Structural substance	Collagen, bacterial cell walls
Enzymes	Ribonuclease-B, Prothrombin
Transport proteins	Ceruloplasmin, Transferrin
Hormones	Thyroglobulin, Erythropoietin, TSH
Immunity	Immunoglobulins, Blood group
Lubricant	Mucin
Message transfer	Receptor proteins on cell surfaces
Cell adhesion	Selectins and integrins

211. Powerful conservator of sodium:

a. Progesterone b. Testosterone
c. Aldosterone d. Hydrocortisone

Aldosterone is a steroid hormone (mineralocorticoid family) produced by the outer section (zona glomerulosa) of the adrenal cortex in the adrenal gland. It plays a central role in the regulation of blood pressure mainly by acting on the distal tubules and collecting ducts of the nephron, increasing reabsorption of ions and water in the kidney, to cause the conservation of sodium, secretion of potassium, increase in water retention, and increase in blood pressure and blood volume.

Summary of steroid hormones

Hormone	*Tissue of origin*	*Function*
Estrogen (Estradiol)	Ovarian	Maturation and function of female secondary sex organs
Estrogens	Placental	Maintenance of pregnancy

Contd...

Ans. **209. d.** Decreased... **210. a.** GH **211. c.** Aldosterone

Contd...

Hormone	Tissue of origin	Function
Progestins (Progesterone)	Ovarian	Implantation of ovum and maintenance of pregnancy
Progestins	Placental	Mimic action of progester-one
Androgens (Testosterone)	Testicular	Maturation and function of male secondary sex organs
Glucocorticoids (Cortisol and corticosterone)	Adrenal cortex	Diverse effects on in-flammation and protein synthesis
Mineralocorti-coids (Aldoster-one)	Adrenal cortex	Maintenance of salt balance

212. Structurally and genetically similar to alpha feto-protein:

a. Growth hormone b. Fibrinogen
c. Transferrin d. Albumin

There are several striking structural and functional similarities between AFP and albumin, which have led to the suggestion that AFP serves as a fetal albumin, and that their genes arose in evolution as the consequence of a duplication of an ancestral gene, followed by divergence.

Common tumor markers

Name	Serum level increased in
Oncofetal Products Alpha feto-protein (AFP)	Hepatoma, germ cell cancers
Carcinoembryonic antigen (CEA)	Colorectal, gastrointesti-nal, and lung cancer
Carbohydrate Antigens CA-125	Ovarian cancer of epithe-lial origin
Tissue Antigens Tissue polypep-tide antigen	General cancer load
Enzymes Alkaline phosphatase (ALP) Bone secondaries Pla-cental type ALP (Regan)	Lung, seminoma
Prostatic acid phosphatase (PAP)	Prostate cancer
Prostate specific	Prostate cancer Antigen (PSA)
Neuron Specific Enolase	Neuro-endocrine tumors
Hormones and their Metabolites	
Beta-hCG	Choriocarcinoma
Calcitonin	Medullary thyroid carci-noma
Big ACTH	Lung oat cell cancer
Vasoactive intestinal polypep-tide (VIP)	Apudomas (Amine pre-cursor uptake decarbox-ylation-omas)

Contd...

Contd...

Name	Serum level increased in
Vanillyl mandelic acid (VMA)	Pheochromocytoma and neuroblastoma
Hydroxy indole acetic acid	Carcinoid syndrome
Tissue Catabolic Product	
Hydroxy proline	Bone metastasis
Serum Proteins Immunoglobu-lins (Ig)	Multiple myeloma, mac-roglobulinemia
Bence-Jones proteins (in urine)	Multiple myeloma

213. NOT an example of steroid hormone:

a. Cortisol
b. Testosterone
c. Thyroxine
d. Aldosterone

Amino acid derived hormones—examples inc-lude melatonin and thyroxine.

214. Which is NOT a second messenger:

a. G protein
b. cGMP
c. cAMP
d. Calcium

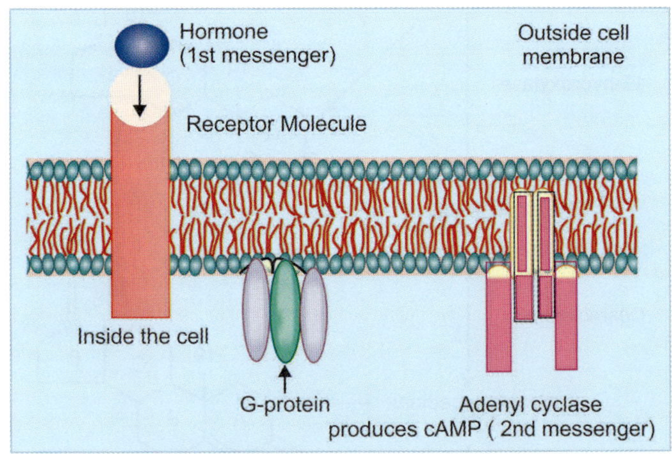

Hormone binding activates G-protein.

G proteins, also known as **guanine nucleotide-binding proteins**, are a family of proteins that act as molecular switches inside cells, and are involved in transmitting signals from a variety of stimuli outside a cell to its interior. Their activity is regulated by factors that control their ability to bind to and hydrolyze guanosine triphosphate (GTP) to guanosine diphosphate (GDP). When they are bound to GTP, they are 'on', and, when they are bound to GDP, they are 'off'. G proteins belong to the larger group of enzymes called GTPases.

215. Testosterone is converted to estrogen by:

a. Dihydrotestosterone b. 16 alpha-hydoxylase
c. Aromatase d. 5 alpha reductase

Ans. 212. **d.** Albumin 213. **c.** Thyroxine 214. **a.** G protein 215. **c.** Aromatase

Aromatase, also called **estrogen synthetase or estrogen synthase**, is an enzyme responsible for a key step in the biosynthesis of estrogens. It is a member of the cytochrome P450 superfamily, which are monooxygenases that catalyze many reactions involved in steroid genesis. In particular, aromatase is responsible for the aromatization of androgens into estrogens.

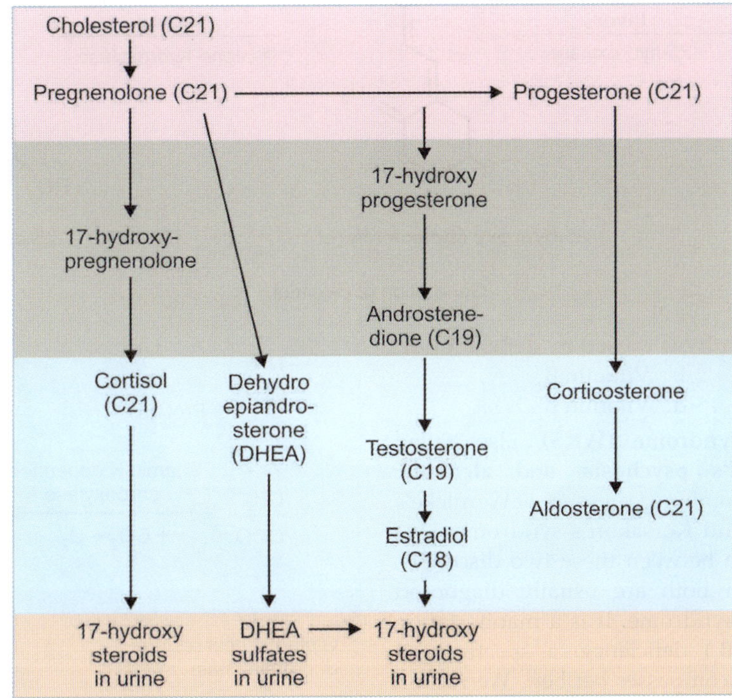

Summary of major pathways for production of glucocorticoids, mineralocorticoids and sex steroids. Precursors in red box; intermediaries in gray box; hormones in blue box; excretory products in brown box.

216. Activated pantothenic acid is found in:
a. G-6-PD dehydrogenase
b. Coenzyme A
c. GMP
d. All of the above

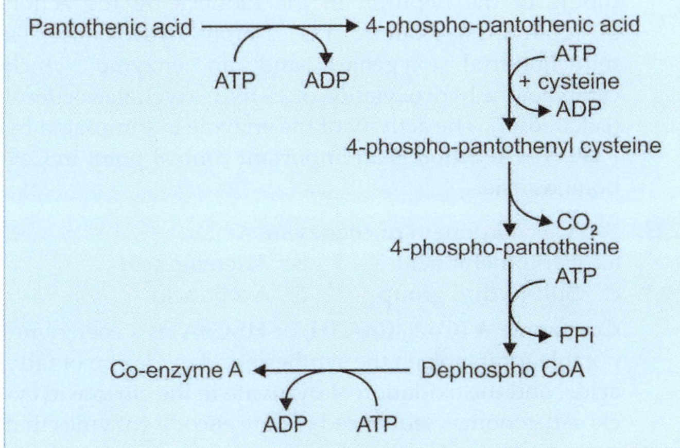

Synthesis of CoA.

Coenzyme A (**CoA**, **CoASH**, or **HSCoA**) is a coenzyme, notable for its role in the synthesis and oxidation of fatty acids, and the oxidation of pyruvate in the citric acid cycle. All genomes sequenced to date encode enzymes that use coenzyme A as a substrate, and around 4% of cellular enzymes use it (or a thioester, such as acetyl-CoA) as a substrate. In humans, CoA biosynthesis requires cysteine, pantothenate, and adenosine triphosphate (ATP).

217. FIGLU is intermediate product of:
a. Methionine
b. Cystine
c. Arginine
d. Histidine

Formiminoglutamic acid (FIGLU) is an intermediate in the metabolism of histidine. The "FIGLU" test is used to identify deficiency of vitamin B_{12} or folate deficiency or liver disease.

218. The most active form of vitamin D is:
a. 25, hydroxycholecalciferol
b. 25, hydroxyergocaliferol
c. 24, 25-dihydroxycholecalciferol
d. 1,25-dihydrocholecalciferol

Calcitriol also called **1,25-dihydroxycholecalciferol** or **1,25-dihydroxyvitamin D_3**, is the hormonally active metabolite of vitamin D with three hydroxyl groups (abbreviated **1,25-$(OH)_2D_3$** or simply **1,25 $(OH)_2D$**).

Ans. **216. b.** Coenzyme A **217. d.** Histidine **218. d.** 1,25-dihydro...

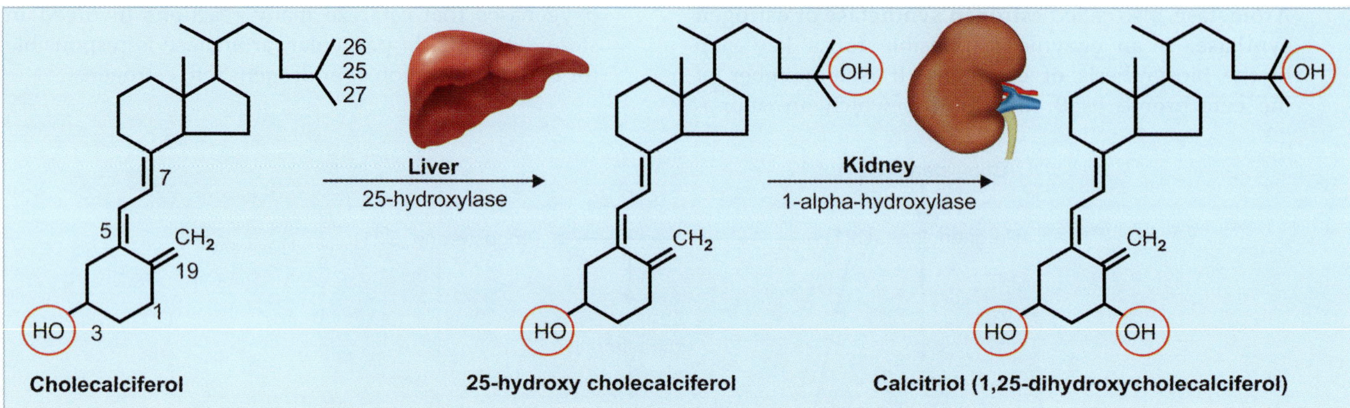

Generation of calcitriol.

219. Wernicke's encephalopathy is caused by deficiency of:

a. Vitamin B_1 b. Vitamin B_2
c. Vitamin B_6 d. Vitamin B_{12}

Wernicke–Korsakoff syndrome (WKS), also called **wet brain**, **Korsakoff's psychosis**, and **alcoholic encephalopathy**, is the combined presence of Wernicke's encephalopathy (WE) and Korsakoff's syndrome. Due to the close relationship between these two disorders, patients suffering from both are usually diagnosed with WKS, as a single syndrome. It is a manifestation of thiamine (vitamin B_1) deficiency, a spectrum of disorders which also encompasses beriberi, Wernicke's encephalopathy, and Korsakoff's psychosis.

Thiamine and thymine are different
THYMINE is the base present in DNA
THIAMINE is vitamin B_1

220. Malonyl aciduria is seen in deficiency of:

a. Pyridoxine b. Vitamin B_{12}
c. Folic acid d. Riboflavin

Diagnosis of vitamin B_{12} is typically based on vitamin B_{12} blood levels below 120–180 picomol/L (170–250 pg/mL) in adults. Elevated methylmalonic acid levels (values >0.4 micromol/L) may also indicated deficiency. A type of low red blood cells known as megaloblastic anemia is often but not always present.

221. Vitamin K is required for:

a. Hydroxylation b. Chelation
c. Transamination d. Carboxylation

Carboxylation is a post-translational modification of glutamate residues, to γ-carboxyglutamate, in proteins. It occurs primarily in proteins involved in the blood clotting cascade, specifically factors II, VII, IX, and X, protein C, and protein S, and also in some bone proteins. This modification is required for these proteins to function. Carboxylation occurs in the liver and is performed by γ-glutamyl carboxylase.

The carboxylase requires vitamin K as a cofactor and performs the reaction in a processive manner

—NH
|
CH-CO-Protein
|
CH_2
|
CH_2
|
COO^-

Vitamin K dependent carboxylase
$+ CO_2 + O_2$

—NH
|
CH-CO-Protein
|
CH_2
|
CH
^-OOC COO^-
Ca^{++}

Glutamic acid residue of protein chain

Gamma carboxy glutamate in protein (GCG)

Vitamin K as co-factor in GCG synthesis.

222. Site of 1,25 hydroxylation of vitamin D in kidney:

a. Distal convoluted tubules
b. Proximal convoluted tubules
c. Glomerulus
d. Collecting ducts

Calcitriol is produced in the cells of the proximal tubule of the nephron in the kidneys by the action of 25-hydroxyvitamin D3 1-alpha-hydroxylase, a mitochondrial oxygenase and an enzyme which catalyzes the hydroxylation of 25-hydroxycholecalciferol (calcifediol). The activity of the enzyme is stimulated by PTH. The reaction is an important control point in Ca^{2+} homeostasis.

223. NOT a component of coenzyme A:

a. Pantothenic acid b. Adenylic acid
c. Sulf-hydryl group d. Acetic acid

Coenzyme A (**CoA, CoASH**, or **HSCoA**) is a coenzyme, notable for its role in the synthesis and oxidation of fatty acids, and the oxidation of pyruvate in the citric acid cycle. All genomes sequenced to date encode enzymes that use coenzyme A as a substrate, and around 4% of cellular enzymes use it (or a thioester, such as acetyl-CoA) as a substrate. In humans, CoA biosynthesis requires cysteine, pantothenate, and adenosine triphosphate (ATP).

Ans. **219. a.** Vitamin B_1 **220. b.** Vitamin B_{12} **221. d.** Carboxylation **222. b.** Proximal convoluted... **223. d.** Acetic acid

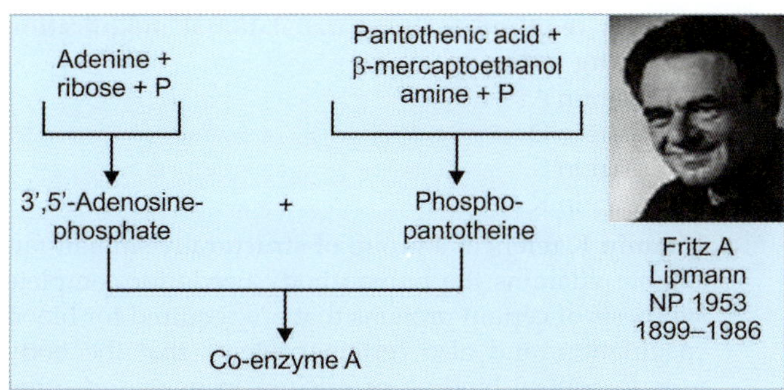

Structure of Co-enzyme A (CoA).

224. Which is an allosteric activator of Acetyl CoA carboxylase:

a. Biotin
b. Citrate
c. Acetyl CoA
d. Malonyl CoA

Acetyl-CoA carboxylase (ACC) is a biotin-dependent enzyme that catalyzes the irreversible carboxylation of acetyl-CoA to produce malonyl-CoA through its two catalytic activities, biotin carboxylase (BC) and carboxyltransferase (CT).

Summary of water soluble vitamins discussed in this chapter

Name	*Co-enzyme form*	*RDA*	*Main reaction using the co-enzyme*	*Deficiency disease*
Thiamine	Thiamine pyrophosphate (TPP)	1–1.5 mg	Oxidative decarboxylation of alpha keto acids	Beriberi
Riboflavin	Flavin adenine dinucleotide (FAD)	1.5 mg	Dehydrogenation, oxidized in ETC (1.5 ATP)	Glossitis, angular stomatitis
Niacin	Nicotinamide adenine dinucleotide (NAD and NADP)	20 mg	Dehydrogenation, oxidized in ETC (2.5 ATP), reductive biosynthetic reactions and hydroxylation	Pellagra
Pyridoxine	Pyridoxal phosphate (PLP)	1–2 mg	Transamination, decarboxylation of amino acids	Seizures, anemia, homocystinuria
Pantothenic acid	Co-enzyme A, ACP	10 mg	CoA derivatives, acyl carrier proteins	Burning foot syndrome
Biotin	Biotin	200–300 mg	Carboxylation	No specific disease

Note: The requirements are significantly higher in pregnancy and lactation.

225. Vitamin synthesized in body:

a. Vitamin B_{12}
b. Vitamin D
c. Nicotininc acid
d. Vitamin C

Cholecalciferol and ergocalciferol can be ingested from the diet and from supplements. Very few foods contain vitamin D; synthesis of vitamin D (specifically cholecalciferol) in the skin is the major natural source of the vitamin. Dermal synthesis of vitamin D from cholesterol is dependent on sun exposure (specifically UVB radiation).

Synthesis of cholecalciferol or vitamin D3.

Ans. **224. a.** Biotin **225. b.** Vitamin D

226. Mediator of CH-2 transfer reaction:

a. Vitamin B_{12}
b. Butyric acid
c. Folic acid
d. All of the above

Methylene-THF (CH_2FH_4) is formed from THF by the addition of a methylene bridge from one of three carbon donors: formate, serine, or glycine. Methyl tetrahydrofolate (CH_3_ THF, or methyl-THF) can be made from methylene-THF by reduction of the methylene group with NADPH.

227. Damaged in case of hypervitaminosis:

a. Lysosome
b. Mitochondria
c. Microtubule
d. Rough endoplasmic reticulum

Acute **hypervitaminosis A** caused instability of liver lysosomes and release of lysosomal enzymes.

228. NOT a source of vitamin A:

a. Tomato
b. Milk
c. Egg
d. Sunflower seeds

In a 100 gram serving, dried whole sunflower seeds provide 584 calories as a nutrient-dense food. The seeds are an excellent source (20% or higher of the Daily Value) of protein, dietary fiber, all B vitamins and vitamin E. The seeds also contain high levels of the dietary minerals, magnesium, manganese, phosphorus, iron and zinc.

Half of a 100 gram serving is fat, mainly monounsaturated and polyunsaturated fats, principally linoleic acid. Additionally, the seeds contain phytosterols which may contribute toward lower levels of blood cholesterol.

229. Coenzyme in carboxylation reactions:

a. Pyridoxine
b. Thiamine
c. Biotin
d. Cyanocobalamin

Biotin is a coenzyme for carboxylase enzymes, involved in the synthesis of fatty acids, isoleucine, and valine, and in gluconeogenesis.

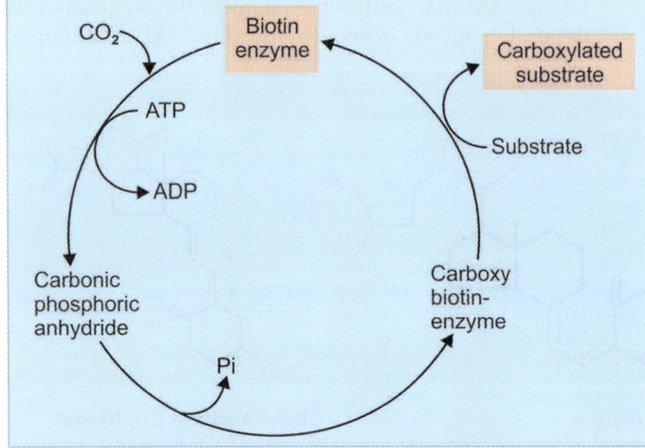

Biotin helps in carboxylation reactions.

230. Vitamin required for post-translational modification of clotting factors:

a. Vitamin A
b. Vitamin D
c. Vitamin E
d. Vitamin K

Vitamin K refers to a group of structurally similar, fat-soluble vitamins the human body needs for complete synthesis of certain proteins that are required for blood coagulation, and also certain proteins that the body uses to control binding of calcium in bone and other tissues.

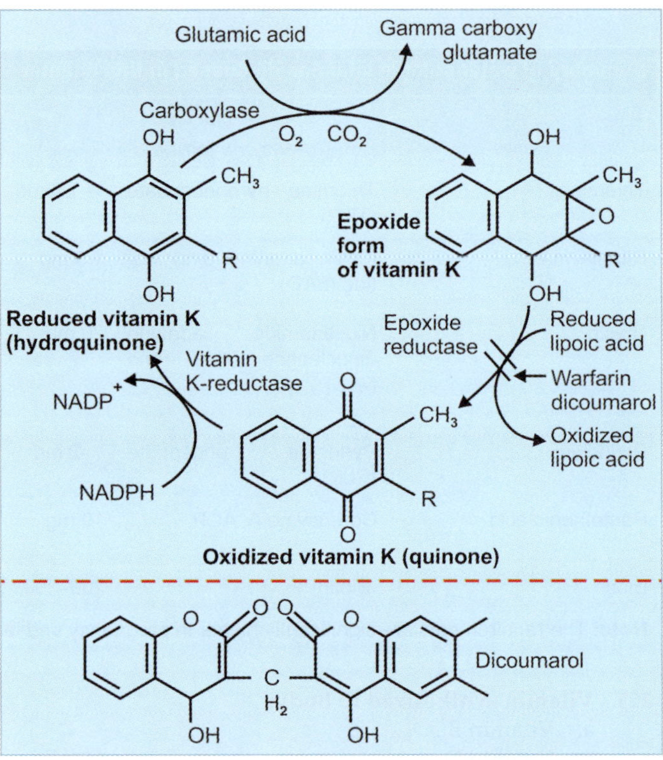

Vitamin K cycle. Dicoumarol, a structural analog inhibits vitamin K reductase.

231. Which vitamin deficiency may be observed in a patient on INH therapy:

a. Thiamine
b. Pyridoxine
c. Folic acid
d. Cyanocobalamin

Use of oral contraceptives and treatment with certain anticonvulsants, isoniazid, cycloserine, penicillamine, and hydrocortisone negatively impact vitamin B6 status. Hemodialysis reduces vitamin B6 plasma levels.

232. A patient on phenytoin therapy needs supplements of:

a. Vitamin B1
b. Vitamin B6
c. Folic acid
d. Vitamin B12

Ans. 226. **c.** Folic acid 227. **a.** Lysosome 228. **d.** Sunflower seeds 229. **c.** Biotin
230. **d.** Vitamin K 231. **b.** Pyridoxine 232. **c.** Folic acid

Anticonvulsant medications (such as phenytoin, primidone, carbamazepine or valproate) result in folic acid deficiency.

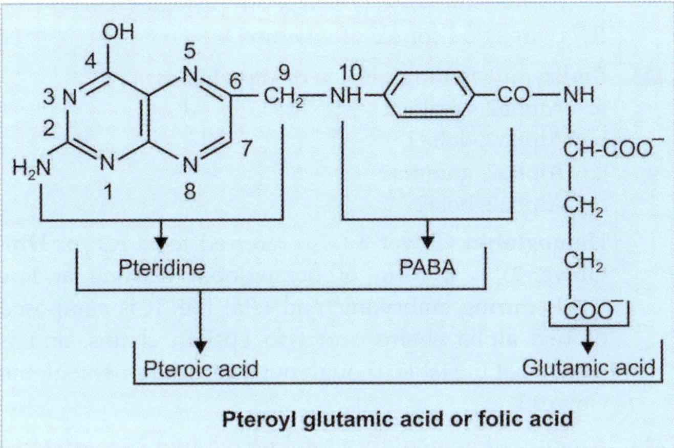

Structure of folic acid.

233. Casal's necklace is seen in deficiency of:

a. Vitamin A deficiency
b. Niacin
c. Vitamin B12 deficiency
d. Iron deficiency anemia

The **Casal collar** or **Casal necklace** is a clinical sign in which there is an erythematous pigmented skin rash in the distribution of a broad collar (dermatomes C3 and C4). It is seen in patients with pellagra.

234. Vitamin used in the treatment of hyperlipoproteinemia:

a. Vitamin B1
b. Vitamin B6
c. Niacin
d. Vitamin B12

Pharmaceutical and supplemental niacin are primarily used to treat hypercholesterolemia (high cholesterol) and pellagra (niacin deficiency).

235. True for hypervitaminosis A EXCEPT:

a. Dermatitis
b. Alopecia
c. Increased synthesis of peroxidases
d. Cell membranes are affected particularly

Symptoms of hypervitaminosis A

- Abnormal softening of the skull bone (craniotabes—infants and children)
- Blurred vision
- Bone pain or swelling
- Bulging fontanelle (infants)
- Changes in consciousness
- Decreased appetite
- Dizziness
- Double vision (young children)
- Drowsiness
- Headache
- Gastric mucosal calcinosis
- Heart valve calcification
- Hypercalcemia
- Increased intracranial pressure manifesting as cerebral edema, papilledema, and headache (may be referred to as Idiopathic intracranial hypertension)
- Irritability
- Liver damage
- Nausea
- Poor weight gain (infants and children)
- Skin and hair changes
- Cracking at corners of the mouth
- Hair loss
- Higher sensitivity to sunlight
- Oily skin and hair (seborrhea)
- Premature epiphyseal closure
- Skin peeling, itching
- Spontaneous fracture

236. Vitamin B_{12} is absorbed in:

a. Stomach
b. Duodenum
c. Ileum
d. Colon

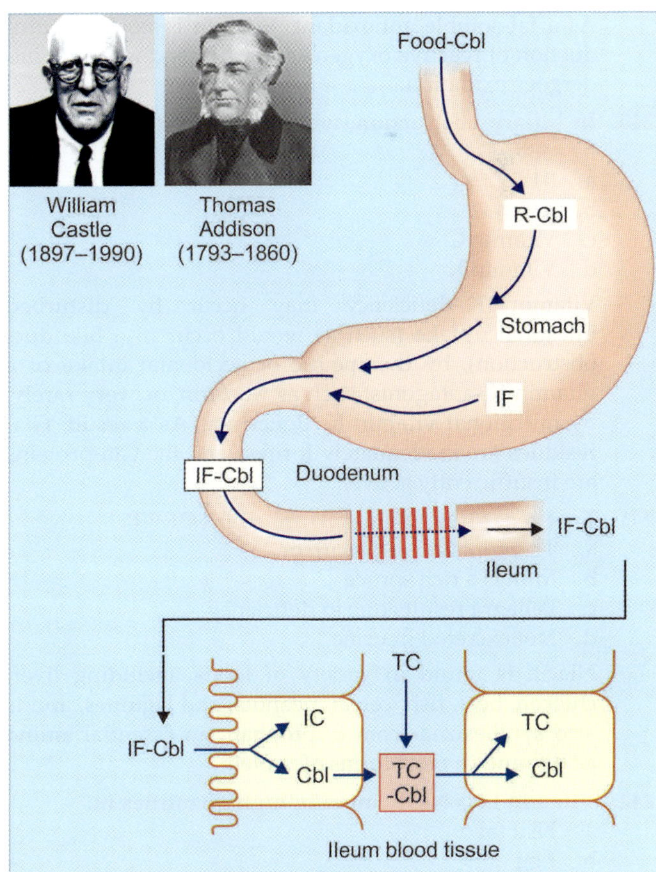

Absorption and storage of vitamin B12. R = cobalophilin; Cbl = cobalamin; IF = intrinsic factor; TC = transcobalamin.

Ans. 233. **b.** Niacin 234. **c.** Niacin 235. **c.** Increased... 236. **c.** Ileum

B_{12} must be attached to IF for it to be absorbed, as receptors on the enterocytes in the terminal ileum of the small bowel only recognize the B_{12}-IF complex; in addition, intrinsic factor protects the vitamin from catabolism by intestinal bacteria.

237. Folic acid requirement during pregnancy is:
a. 200 microgram
b. 300 microgram
c. 400 microgram
d. 500 microgram

Folic acid requirement during pregnancy is 500 and during lactation is 300 microgram/day

238. FIGLU test is done for determining deficiency of:
a. Thiamine
b. Pyridoxine
c. Folic acid
d. Riboflavin

The "FIGLU" test is used to identify deficiency of vitamin B_{12} or folate deficiency or liver disease.

239. Vitamin E function:
a. Post-translation modification
b. Antioxidant
c. Calcium homeostasis
d. Vision

As a fat-soluble antioxidant, Vitamin E stops the production of reactive oxygen species formed when fat undergoes oxidation.

240. In biliary obstruction, which vitamin deficiency will be seen:
a. B1
b. B12
c. Vitamin C
d. Vitamin K

Vitamin K_1-deficiency may occur by disturbed intestinal uptake (such as would occur in a bile duct obstruction), by therapeutic or accidental intake of a vitamin K_1-antagonist such as warfarin, or, very rarely, by nutritional vitamin K_1 deficiency. As a result, Gla-residues are inadequately formed and the Gla-proteins are insufficiently active.

241. True regarding vitamin B_3 are all EXCEPT:
a. Tryptophan is a precursor
b. Milk is a rich source
c. Pellagra results due to deficiency
d. Not excreted in urine

Niacin is found in variety of foods, including liver, chicken, beef, fish, cereal, peanuts, and legumes, and is also synthesized from tryptophan, an essential amino acid found in most forms of protein.

242. Vitamin D is NOT found in high quantities in:
a. Fish fat
b. Egg
c. Halibut liver oil
d. Milk

Vitamin D is found in few dietary sources. Sunlight exposure is the primary source of vitamin D for majority of people, other than supplements. Fish liver oils, such as cod liver oil, 4.5 g (1 teaspoon) provides 450 IU (100 IU/g) are good source of vitamin D.

243. Embryonic hemoglobin is designated as:
a. Alpha2, epsilon2
b. Alpha2, delta2
c. Alpha2, gamma2
d. Alpha2, beta2

Hemoglobin Gower 2 (also referred to as $\alpha_2\varepsilon_2$ or **HbE Gower-2**) is a form of hemoglobin existing at low levels during embryonic and fetal life. It is composed of two alpha chains and two epsilon chains, and is somewhat unstable, though not as much as hemoglobin Gower 1.

244. Amount of hemoglobin catabolized (per 24 hours) in a normal adult:
a. 13.3 gm
b. 12 gm
c. 10 gm
d. 6 gm

Most of the heme degraded in humans comes from hemoglobin. Approximately 6–8 grams of hemoglobin is degraded daily which is equivalent to approximately 300 milligrams of heme per day. Heme is not recycled so it must be degraded and excreted. The iron, however, is conserved.

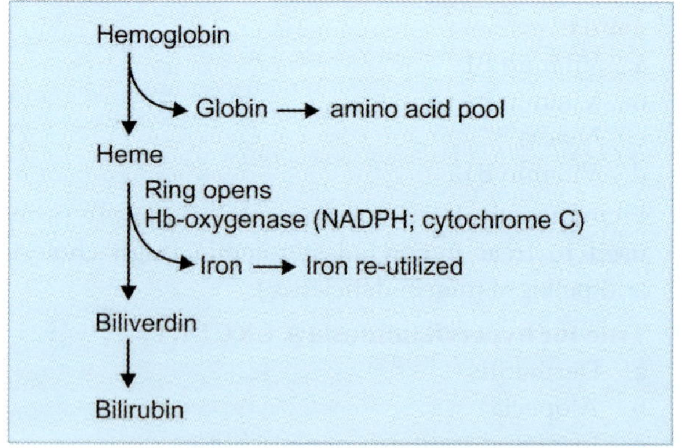

Catabolic pathway of hemoglobin.

245. True for Fetal hemoglobin:
a. Alpha2, beta2
b. Alpha2, delta2
c. Alpha2, theta2
d. Alpha2, gamma2

Fetal hemoglobin, or **foetal hemoglobin** (also **hemoglobin F, HbF**, or $\alpha_2\gamma_2$) is the main oxygen transport protein in the human fetus during the last seven months of development in the uterus and persists in the newborn until roughly 6 months old.

Ans. 237. **d.** 500 microgram 238. **c.** Folic acid 239. **b.** Antioxidant 240. **d.** Vitamin K
241. **b.** Milk is a rich... 242. **d.** Milk 243. **a.** Alpha2, epsilon2 244. **d.** 6 gm
245. **d.** Alpha2, gamma2

246. Which of the following is the correct about breakdown of hemoglobin:

a. Hb – heme – bilirubin – urobilinogen
b. Heme – Hb – biliverdin – bilirubin – urobilinogen
c. Hb – heme – biliverdin – bilirubin – urobilinogen
d. Hb – heme – bilirubin – urobilinogen - biliverdin

The hemoglobin molecule is broken up, and the iron gets recycled. This process also produces one molecule of carbon monoxide for every molecule of heme degraded. When the porphyrin ring is broken up, the fragments are normally secreted as a yellow pigment called bilirubin, which is secreted into the intestines as bile. Intestines metabolise bilirubin into urobilinogen. Urobilinogen leaves the body in faeces, in a pigment called stercobilin. Globulin is metabolised into amino acids that are then released into circulation.

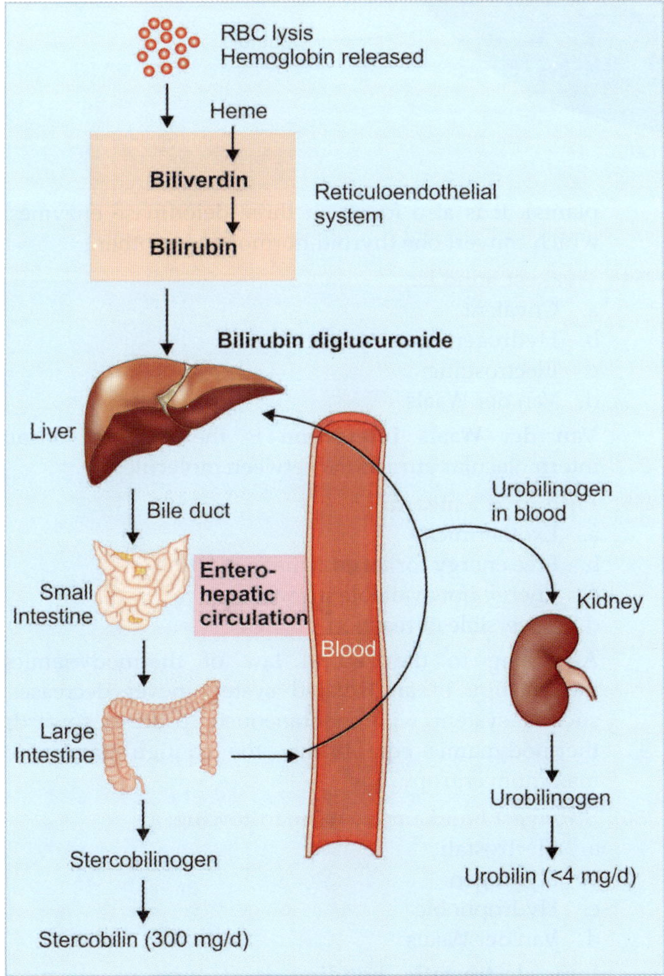

Production and excretion of bilirubin.

247. Which of the following is NOT a part of hemoglobin molecule?

a. Pyrrole rings
b. Vinyl groups
c. Histidine
d. Ferric ions

The iron ion may be either in the Fe^{2+} or in the Fe^{3+} state, but ferrihemoglobin (methemoglobin) (Fe^{3+}) cannot bind oxygen. In binding, oxygen temporarily and reversibly oxidizes (Fe^{2+}) to (Fe^{3+}) while oxygen temporarily turns into superoxide, thus iron must exist in the +2 oxidation state to bind oxygen.

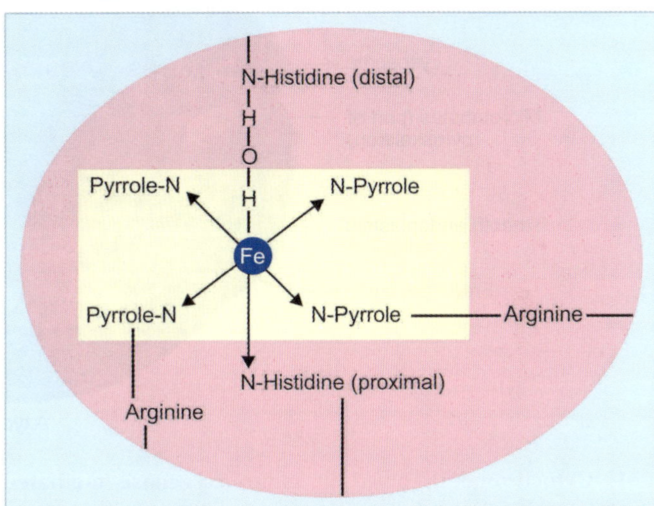

Linkage of heme with globin. Pink circle represents the globin chain. Blue rectangle represents the protoporphyrin ring.

248. Egg yields about .... Kcal of energy:

a. 70
b. 80
c. 90
d. 100

One large (53 g) Grade A egg contains 6 g of protein, 6 g of fats, all vitamins except C and only **70 Kcalories**.

249. Acrodermatitis enteropathica is due to deficiency of:

a. Iron
b. Zinc
c. Calcium
d. Magnesium

Acrodermatitis enteropathica is anautosomal recessive metabolic disorder affecting the uptake of zinc, characterized by periorificial (around the natural orifices) and acral (in the limbs) dermatitis, alopecia (loss of hair), and diarrhea.

250. Secretory proteins are synthesized in:

a. Cytoplasm
b. Endoplasmic reticulum
c. First I cytoplasm, then in ER
d. First in ER, then in cytoplasm

A **secretory protein** is any protein, whether it be endocrine or exocrine, which is secreted by a cell. Secretory proteins include many hormones, enzymes, toxins, and antimicrobial peptides. Secretory proteins are synthesized in the endoplasmic reticulum.

Ans. **246. c.** Hb – heme... **247. d.** Ferric ions **248. a.** 70 **249. b.** Zinc **250. b.** Endoplasmic reticulum

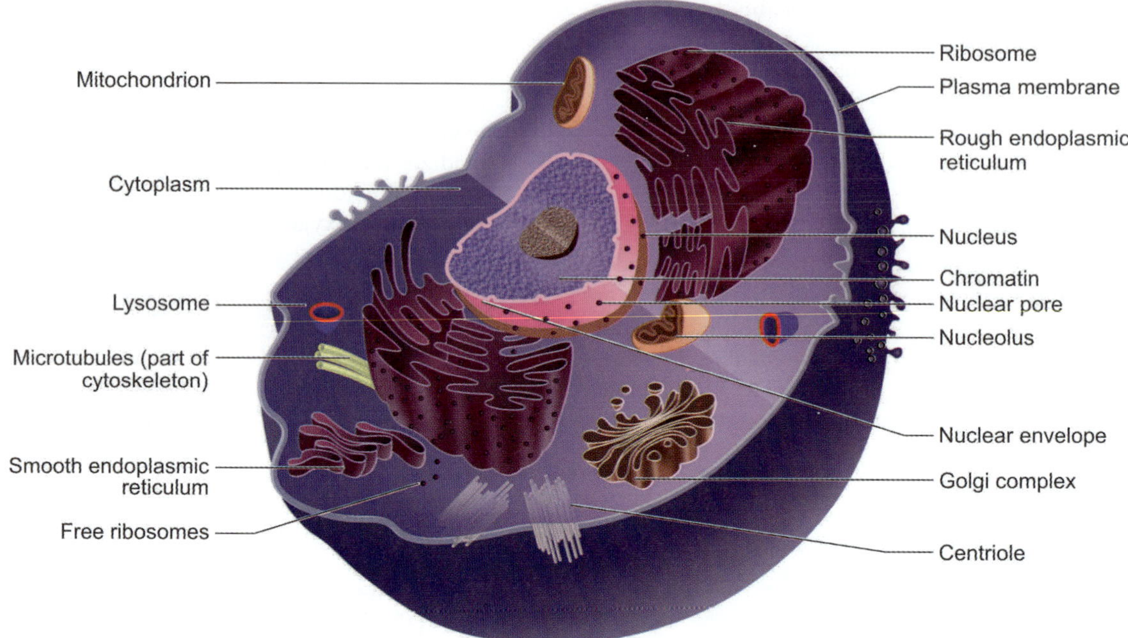

A typical cell.

251. Cytochrome involved in mono-oxygenase mediated detoxification of drugs:

a. Cyt-P-480
b. Cyt-P-450
c. Cyt-P-400
d. Cyt-P-300

Cytochromes P450/CYPs are the major enzymes involved in drug metabolism, accounting for about 75% of the total metabolism. Most drugs undergo deactivation by CYPs, either directly or by facilitated excretion from the body. Also, many substances are bioactivated by CYPs to form their active compounds.

252. Conversion of prothrombin to thrombin requires:

a. Factor X only
b. Factor V only
c. Factors VII, X, V and calcium
d. Factors XI, VI and calcium

Prothrombin is **converted** to **thrombin** by the action of the enzyme factor Xa in a reaction that **requires** calcium ions and is greatly accelerated by factor Va.

253. Element that is known to influence body's ability to handle oxidative stress:

a. Calcium
b. Iron
c. Potassium
d. Selenium

Selenium is an ingredient in many multi-vitamins and other dietary supplements, including infant formula. It is a component of the antioxidant enzymes glutathione peroxidase and thioredoxin reductase (which indirectly reduce certain oxidized molecules in animals and some plants). It is also found in three deiodinase enzymes, which convert one thyroid hormone to another.

254. Weakest bond is:

a. Covalent
b. Hydrogen
c. Electrostatic
d. Van der Waals

Van der Waals interaction is the **weakest** of all intermolecular attractions between molecules.

255. Entropy is a measure of:

a. Exothermicity
b. Free energy for an enzymatic reaction
c. Energy not available for work
d. Reversible of reaction

According to the second law of thermodynamics the entropy of an isolated system never decreases; such a system will spontaneously proceed towards thermodynamic equilibrium, the configuration with maximum entropy.

256. Strongest bond amongst the following:

a. Electrostatic
b. Hydrogen
c. Hydrophobic
d. Van der Waals

Ionic/electrostatic bonding is a type of chemical bond that involves the electrostatic attraction between oppositely charged ions. These ions represent atoms that have lost one or more electrons (known as cations) and atoms that have gained one or more electrons (known as anions).

Ans. **251. b.** Cyt-P-450 **252. c.** Factors VII... **253. d.** Selenium **254. d.** Van der Waals **255. c.** Energy not... **256. a.** Electrostatic

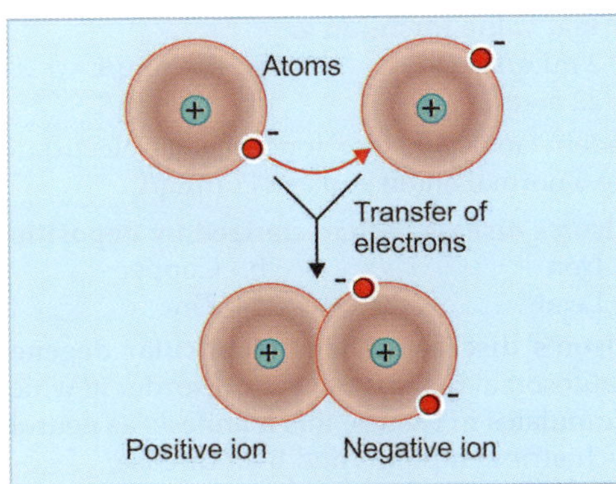

Ionic bond.

257. Major lipid of mitochondrial membrane:

a. Cardiolipin b. Plasmalogen
c. Inositol d. Lecithin

Cardiolipin ("1,3-bis(sn-3'-phosphatidyl)-sn-glycerol") is an important component of the inner mitochondrial membrane, where it constitutes about 20% of the total lipid composition. As well, it can be found is in the membranes of most bacteria.

Metabolic functions of subcellular organelles	
Nucleus	DNA replication, transcription
Endoplasmic reticulum	Biosynthesis of proteins, glycoproteins, lipoproteins, drug metabolism, ethanol oxidation, synthesis of cholesterol (partial)
Golgi body	Maturation of synthesized proteins
Lysosome	Degradation of proteins, carbohydrates, lipids and nucleotides
Mitochondria	Electron transport chain, ATP generation, TCA cycle, beta oxidation of fatty acids, ketone body production, urea synthesis (part), heme synthesis (part), gluconeogenesis (part), pyrimidine synthesis (part)
Cytosol	Protein synthesis, glycolysis, glycogen metabolism, HMP shunt pathway, transaminations, fatty acid synthesis, cholesterol synthesis, heme synthesis (part), urea synthesis (part), pyrimidine synthesis (part), purine synthesis

258. True for ubiquitin:

a. Protein synthesis
b. Seen in prokaryotes
c. Protein destruction
d. Purine metabolism products

The addition of ubiquitin to a substrate protein is called **ubiquitination orubiquitylation**. Ubiquitination can affect proteins in many ways: it can signal for their degradation via the proteasome, alter their cellular location, affect their activity, and promote or prevent protein interactions.

259. Important marker for myocardial infarction:

a. Myoglobin b. CK-MB
c. Troponins d. All of the baove

Markers of myocardial infarction			
Marker	*Onset*	*Peak*	*Duration*
CK-MB	3–6 hours	18–24 hours	36–72 hours
Troponins	4–10 hours	18–24 hours	8–14 days
Myoglobin	1–4 hours	6–7 hours	24 hours

260. Glutathione peroxidase contains which of the following:

a. Selenium b. Zinc
c. Manganese d. Chromium

Mammalian glutathione peroxidase (GPx1, GPx2, GPx3, and GPx4) have been shown to be selenium-containing enzymes, whereas GPx6 is a selenoprotein in humans with cysteine-containing homologues in rodents.

261. Anticoagulant added for estimation of prothrombin time:

a. EDTA b. Sodium citrate
c. Oxalate d. Heparin

In 1914, the Belgian doctor Albert Hustin and the Argentine physician and researcher Luis Agote successfully used sodium citrate as an anticoagulant in blood transfusions. It continues to be used today in blood collection tubes and for the preservation of blood in blood banks. The citrate ion chelates calcium ions in the blood by forming calcium citrate complexes, disrupting the blood clotting mechanism.

262. Glowing of fireflies is due to:

a. Phosphocreatinine
b. GTP
c. NADH
d. ATP

Light production in fireflies is due to a type of chemical reaction called bioluminescence. This process occurs in specialized light-emitting organs, usually on a firefly's lower abdomen. The enzyme luciferase acts on the luciferin, in the presence of magnesium ions, ATP, and oxygen to produce light.

263. FALSE statement:

a. High calcium in diet – Reduced absorption of iron
b. Selenium deficiency – Cardiomyopathy
c. Zinc deficiency – Pulmonary fibrosis
d. Vitamin A deficiency does not occur for a year after stopping its intake

Inhalation of environmental and occupational pollutants, such as metals in asbestosis, silicosis and exposure to certain gases. Coal miners, ship workers and sand blasters among others are at higher risk for developing pulmonary fibrosis.

264. Function of Sertoli cells:

a. Aid in spermiogenesis
b. Seminal fluid secretion
c. Testosterone secretion
d. All of the above

Ans. 257. **a.** Cardiolipin 258. **c.** Protein destruction 259. **d.** All of the above 260. **a.** Selenium
261. **b.** Sodium... 262. **d.** ATP 263. **c.** Zinc... 264. **a.** Aid...

Because its main function is to nourish the developing sperm cells through the stages of spermatogenesis, the Sertoli cell has also been called the "mother" or "nurse" cell. Sertoli cells also act as phagocytes, consuming the residual cytoplasm during spermatogenesis.

265. In monoclonal antibody production, monoclonal cells are differentiated from:

a. Myeloma cell lines
b. Sensitized T cells
c. Sensitized B cells
d. All of the above

Monoclonal antibodies (mAb or moAb) are monospecific antibodies that are made by identical immune cells that are all clones of a unique parent cell, in contrast to polyclonal antibodies which are made from several different immune cells.

266. Hypogonadism, reduced immunity and alopecia may be a deficiency manifestation of:

a. Iron b. Copper
c. Zinc d. Magnesium

Zinc deficiency may manifest as acne, eczema, xerosis (dry, scaling skin), seborrheic dermatitis, or alopecia (thin and sparse hair). There may also be impaired wound healing. Zinc is required to produce testosterone. Thus, zinc deficiency can lead to reduced circulating testosterone, hypogonadism, and delayed puberty.

Impaired immune function in people with zinc deficiency can lead to the development of respiratory, gastrointestinal, or other infections, e.g., pneumonia.

267. Major ECF cation is:

a. Potassium b. Sodium
c. Magnesium d. Calcium

Sodium is the major cation in ECF whereas potassium in ICF.

Electrolyte concentration of body fluid compartments

Solutes	Plasma mEq / L	Interstitial fluid (mEq/L)	Intracellular fluid (mEq/L)
Cations:			
Sodium	140	146	12
Potassium	4	5	160
Calcium	5	3	–
Magnesium	1.5	1	34
Anions:			
Chloride	105	117	2
Bicarbonate	24	27	10
Sulfate	1	1	–
Phosphate	2	2	140
Protein	15	7	54
Other anions	13	1	–

Note - mEq/L = mmol/L × valency

268. Normal value for anion gap:

a. 2 mEq/L b. 10 mEq/L
c. 22 meq/L d. 32 mEq/L

Modern analyzers use ion-selective electro-des which give a normal anion gap as <11 mEq/L.

269. Wilson's disease is characterized by deposition of:

a. Iron b. Copper
c. Lead d. Zinc

Wilson's disease or **hepatolenticular degeneration** is an autosomal recessive genetic disorder in which copper accumulates in tissues; this manifests as neurological or psychiatric symptoms and liver disease.

270. Calcium is more in:

a. Goat milk b. Buffalo milk
c. Human milk d. Cow milk

Buffalo milk contains more calcium, a better calcium to phosphorous ratio and less sodium and potassium which makes it a better nutritional supplement for infants.

Composition of milk

Constituent	Human	Cow	Buffalo	Goat
Water (%)	87.5	87.2	83.6	87.5
Total solids (%)	12.5	12.8	16.4	12.5
Proteins (g/dL)	1.1	3.3	4.3	3.7
Lipids (g/dL)	3.8	3.8	6.0	3.5
Carbohydrate (g/dL)	7.5	4.4	5.3	4.7
Calcium (mg/dL)	34	150	160	170

271. In an acute attack of MI, CPK-MB returns to normal by:

a. 2 days b. 4 days
c. 6 days d. 8 days

CK-MB first appears 4–6 hours after symptom onset, peaks at 24 hours, and returns to normal in 48–72 hours. Its value in the early and late (>72 h) diagnosis of acute MI is limited. However, its release kinetics can assist in diagnosing reinfarction if levels rise after initially declining following acute MI.

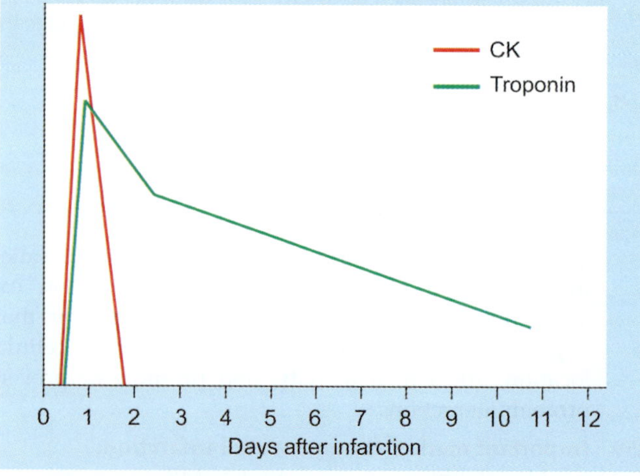

Time course of elevation of CK-MB and cardiac troponins in blood of myocardial infarction patients.

Ans. 265. a. Myeloma... 266. c. Zinc 267. b. Sodium 268. b. 10 mEq/L
269. b. Copper 270. b. Buffalo milk 271. a. 2 days

272. Metabolic acidosis is due to:

a. Raised bicarbonate b. Raised carbon dioxide
c. Decreased bicarbonate d. Decreased carbon dioxide

Metabolic acidosis is a condition that occurs when the body produces excessive quantities of acid or when the kidneys are not removing enough acid from the body. If unchecked, metabolic acidosis leads to acidemia, i.e., blood pH is low (less than 7.35) due to increased production of hydrogen ions by the body or the inability of the body to form bicarbonate (HCO_3^-) in the kidney.

Types of acid-base disturbances

Disturbance	pH	Primary change	Ratio	Secondary change
Metabolic acidosis	Decreased	Deficit of bicarbonate	<20	Decrease in $PaCO_2$
Metabolic alkalosis	Increased	Excess of bicarbonate	>20	Increase in $PaCO_2$
Respiratory acidosis	Decreased	Excess of carbonic acid	<20	Increase in bicarbonate
Respiratory alkalosis	Increased	Deficit of carbonic acid	>20	Decrease in bicarbonate

273. Normal blood pH:

a. 6.95–7.05
b. 7.15–7.25
c. 7.35–7.45
d. 7.65–7.75

Blood pH is regulated to stay within the narrow range of 7.35 to 7.45, making it slightly basic. Blood that has a pH below 7.35 is too acidic, whereas blood pH above 7.45 is too basic.

274. Rate of diffusion in simple diffusion depends on:

a. Energy supply
b. Carrier protein
c. Concentration of the diffusing substance
d. All of the above

Molecular diffusion, often simply called **diffusion**, is the thermal motion of all (liquid or gas) particles at temperatures above absolute zero. The rate of this movement is a function of temperature, viscosity of the fluid and the size (mass) of the particles. Diffusion explains the net flux of molecules from a region of higher concentration to one of lower concentration.

Types of transport mechanisms

	Carrier	*Against gradient*	*Energy required*	*Examples*
Simple diffusion	No	No	Nil	Water
Facilitated diffusion	Yes	No	Nil	Glucose to RBCs
Primary active	Yes	Yes	Directly	Sodium pump
Secondary active	Yes	Yes	Indirect	Glucose to intestine
Ion channels	Yes	No	No	Sodium channel

275. Troponin is a marker for which of the following conditions:

a. Complete heart block
b. Pericardial effusion
c. Myoglobinuria
d. Myocardial infarction

Troponin is a complex of three regulatory proteins (troponin C, troponin I, and troponin T) that is integral to muscle contraction in skeletal muscle and cardiac muscle, but not smooth muscle. An increased level of the cardiac protein isoform of troponin circulating in the blood has been shown to be a biomarker of heart disorders, the most important of which is myocardial infarction.

Markers for cardiac diseases

Serial testing of the following cardiac enzymes is usually done to guide the prognosis (Box 23.1). No single marker can successfully identify or exclude acute MI within the first 6 hour.

i. Creatine kinase (CK-MB)
ii. Cardiac troponin I (CTI) and Cardiac troponin T (CTT). These are not true enzymes.
iii. Brain natriuretic peptide (BNP). It is a reliable marker of ventricular function.
iv. Lactate dehydrogenase (LDH) and aspartate amino transferase (AST) were previously used as markers of myocardial function, but no more used in clinical practice.

276. Serum marker to return to normal level, last in myocardial infarction is:

a. Lactate dehydrogenase
b. Creatine phosphokinase
c. Aspartate transmainase
d. Myoglobin

LDH can also be used as a marker of myocardial infarction. Following a myocardial infarction, levels of LDH peak at 3–4 days and remain elevated for up to 10 days. In this way, elevated levels of LDH (where the level of LDH1 is higher than that of LDH2, i.e. the LDH Flip, as normally, in serum, LDH2 is higher than LDH1) can be useful for determining whether a patient has had a myocardial infarction if they come to doctors several days after an episode of chest pain.

Ans. **272. c.** Decreased... **273. c.** 7.35–7.45 **274. c.** Concentration... **275. d.** Myocardial infarction **276. d.** Myoglobin

Characteristic features of LDH iso-enzymes					
No. of iso-enzyme	*Subunit make up of iso-enzyme*	*Electrophoretic mobility at pH 8.6*	*Activity at 60°C for 30 minutes*	*Tissue from which iso-enzyme has originated*	*Percentage in human serum (Mean)*
LDH-1	H4	Fastest	Not destroyed	Heart muscle	30%
LDH-2	H3M1	Faster	Not destroyed	RBC	35%
LDH-3	H2M2	Fast	Partially destroyed	Brain	20%
LDH-4	H1M3	Slow	Destroyed	Liver	10%
LDH-5	M4	Slowest	Destroyed	Skeletal muscle	5%

277. Body Mass Index is expressed as:

a. Gram/metre^2
b. Gram/centimetre^2
c. Kilogram/metre^2
d. Kilogram/ centimetre^2

The **body mass index (BMI)** or **Quetelet index** is a value derived from the mass (weight) and height of an individual. The BMI is defined as the body mass divided by the square of the body height, and is universally expressed in units of kg/m^2, resulting from mass in kilograms and height in metres.

278. Regarding isoelectric pH, true is:

a. All amino acids exists as zwitter ions
b. Net positive and negative charge on molecule are equal
c. Enzyme activity maximum
d. None of the above

The **isoelectric point (pI, pH(I), IEP)**, is the pH at which a particular molecule carries no net electrical charge. The net charge on the molecule is affected by pH of its surrounding environment and can become more positively or negatively charged due to the gain or loss, respectively, of protons (H^+).

279. The conversion of optically pure isomer (enantiomer) into mixture of equal amounts of both dextro and levo forms is called as:

a. Polymerization
b. Stereo-isomerization
c. Racemization
d. Fractionation

Racemization refers to the conversion of an enantiomerically pure mixture (one where only one enantiomer is present) into a mixture where more than one of the enantiomers are present. If the racemization results in a mixture where the enantiomers are present in equal quantities, the resulting sample is described as racemic or a racemate.

Ans. 277. **c.** Kilogram/metre^2 278. **b.** Net positive... 279. **c.** Racemization

ANSWERS WITH REFERENCES

ENZYMES

1. **Ans. (c) Normal Km, low Vmax**
   Ref: Vasudevan's Biochemistry, 7/e p61

2. **Ans. (c) Mg2+**
   Ref: Vasudevan's Biochemistry 7/e p51

3. **Ans. (c) Holoenzyme**
   Ref: Vasudevan's Biochemistry 7/e p49

4. **Ans. (a) Competitive**
   Ref: Vasudevan's Biochemistry 7/e p62

5. **Ans. (c) The substrate concentration at half maximum velocity**
   Ref: Vasudevan's Biochemistry 7/e p57

6. **Ans. (c) Mitochondrial enzyme**
   Ref: Vasudevan's Biochemistry 7/e p203

7. **Ans. (b) Phosphotriose isomerase**
   Ref: Vasudevan's Biochemistry 7/e p49

8. **Ans. (d) Protein**
   Ref: Vasudevan's Biochemistry 7/e p48

9. **Ans. (a) SGOT**
   Ref: Vasudevan's Biochemistry 7/e p305

10. **Ans. (b) Pepsin**
    Ref: Vasudevan's Biochemistry 7/e p197

11. **Ans. (c) Both**
    Ref: Vasudevan's Biochemistry 7/e p262

12. **Ans. (d) Oxidase**
    Ref: Vasudevan's Biochemistry 7/e p434

13. **Ans. (d) Lipoprotein lipase**
    Ref: Internet resources

14. **Ans. (c) Competitive inhibitor of alcohol dehydrogenase**
    Ref: Internet resources

15. **Ans. (d) Chronic granulomatous disease**
    Ref: Vasudevan's Biochemistry 7/e p434

16. **Ans. (d) Ribozyme**
    Ref: Vasudevan's Biochemistry 7/e p592

17. **Ans. (c) Molybdenum**
    Ref: Vasudevan's Biochemistry 7/e p525

18. **Ans. (d) Phenylethanolamine-N-methyltrasferase**
    Ref: Vasudevan's Biochemistry 7/e p235

19. **Ans. (d) Forms of same enzyme that catalyzes same reaction**
    Ref: Vasudevan's Biochemistry 7/e p66

20. **Ans. (a) V_{max} unchanged**
    Ref: Vasudevan's Biochemistry 7/e p60 (Figure 60)

21. **Ans. (b) Prothrombin**
    Ref: Internet resources

22. **Ans. (c) Molybdenum**
    Ref: Internet resources

23. **Ans. (a) Xanthine oxidase**
    Ref: Vasudevan's Biochemistry 7/e p523

24. **Ans. (b) Glutathione peroxidase**
    Ref: Vasudevan's Biochemistry 7/e p523

25. **Ans. (c) Succinylcholine**
    Ref: Internet resources

26. **Ans. (b) Proteolytic enzyme in gastric juice of infants**
    Ref: Vasudevan's Biochemistry 7/e p197

27. **Ans. (b) Forms of the same enzymes that catalyze same reaction**
    Ref: Vasudevan's Biochemistry 7/e p66

28. **Ans. (a) Phenylethanolamine-N-methyltransferase**
    Ref: Vasudevan's Biochemistry 7/e p235

29. **Ans. (a) Vitamin B1**
    Ref: Vasudevan's Biochemistry 7/e p130

AMINO ACIDS AND PROTEIN METABOLISM

30. **Ans. (d) Covalent peptide bonds**
    Ref: Vasudevan's Biochemistry, 7/e p35

31. **Ans. (d) Kynurenine**
    Ref: Vasudevan's Biochemistry, 7/e p239

32. **Ans. (a) Primary structure**
    Ref: Vasudevan's Biochemistry, 7/e p42

33. **Ans. (c) Cation**
    Ref: Vasudevan's Biochemistry, 7/e p41

34. **Ans. (c) Homogentisate oxidase**
    Ref: Vasudevan's Biochemistry, 7/e p238

35. **Ans. (c) Tyrosine hydroxylase**
    Ref: Vasudevan's Biochemistry, 7/e p234

36. **Ans. (c) Tyrosinemia**
Ref: Vasudevan's Biochemistry 7/e p239

37. **Ans. (d) Isoleucine**
Ref: Vasudevan's Biochemistry 7/e p27

38. **Ans. (b) Decarboxylation**
Ref: Vasudevan's Biochemistry 7/e p29

39. **Ans. (a) Phenylalanine**
Ref: Vasudevan's Biochemistry 7/e p231

40. **Ans. (a) Synthesis of spermine**
Ref: Vasudevan's Biochemistry 7/e p211

41. **Ans. (c) Glutamine**
Ref: Vasudevan's Biochemistry 7/e p202

42. **Ans. (c) Tyrosine**
Ref: Vasudevan's Biochemistry 7/e p238

43. **Ans. (d) Histidine**
Ref: Vasudevan's Biochemistry 7/e p225

44. **Ans. (a) Tryptophan**
Ref: Vasudevan's Biochemistry 7/e p241

45. **Ans. (d) Melatonin**
Ref: Vasudevan's Biochemistry 7/e p233

46. **Ans. (a) Non-polar side chain**
Ref: Vasudevan's Biochemistry 7/e p25

47. **Ans. (c) Tripeptide**
Ref: Vasudevan's Biochemistry 7/e p218

48. **Ans. (c) Net protein utilization**
Ref: Vasudevan's Biochemistry 7/e p534

49. **Ans. (d) Light chains**
Ref: Vasudevan's Biochemistry 7/e p372

50. **Ans. (d) Proline**
Ref: Vasudevan's Biochemistry 7/e p37

51. **Ans. (d) Iron**
Ref: Vasudevan's Biochemistry 7/e p294

52. **Ans. (c) 70**
Ref: Internet resources

53. **Ans. (b) Ferritin**
Ref: Vasudevan's Biochemistry 7/e p724

54. **Ans. (c) Homocysteine**
Ref: Vasudevan's Biochemistry 7/e p221

CARBOHYDRATE METABOLISM

55. **Ans. (c) Enolase**
Ref: Vasudevan's Biochemistry, 7/e p117

56. **Ans. (c) Gluconeogenesis**
Ref: Vasudevan's Biochemistry, 7/e p118

57. **Ans. (c) NADPH**
Ref: Vasudevan's Biochemistry, 7/e p132

58. **Ans. (b) ATP**
Ref: Vasudevan's Biochemistry, 7/e p256

59. **Ans. (b) HMP pathway**
Ref: Vasudevan's Biochemistry 7/e p130

60. **Ans. (b) Glucose-1-phosphate**
Ref: Vasudevan's Biochemistry 7/e p124

61. **Ans. (b) Lactate**
Ref: Vasudevan's Biochemistry 7/e p112

62. **Ans. (b) G-6-phosphatase**
Ref: Vasudevan's Biochemistry 7/e p118

63. **Ans. (c) Thiokinase**
Ref: Vasudevan's Biochemistry 7/e p251

64. **Ans. (d) All of the above**
Ref: Vasudevan's Biochemistry 7/e p115

65. **Ans. (c) Glucose-6-phosphate dehydrogenase**
Ref: Internet resources

66. **Ans. (c) Sodium fluoride**
Ref: Vasudevan's Biochemistry 7/e p111

67. **Ans. (d) Glycolysis**
Ref: Vasudevan's Biochemistry 7/e p108

68. **Ans. (c) Glycosaminoglycans**
Ref: Vasudevan's Biochemistry 7/e p143

69. **Ans. (d) G-6-PD deficients**
Ref: Vasudevan's Biochemistry 7/e p307

70. **Ans. (c) Alpha ketoglutarate dehydrogenase**
Ref: Vasudevan's Biochemistry 7/e p481

71. **Ans. (c) Acetoacetate**
Ref: Vasudevan's Biochemistry 7/e p117

72. **Ans. (d) Vasopressin**
Ref: Vasudevan's Biochemistry 7/e p313

73. **Ans. (d) Cholesterol synthesis**
Ref: Vasudevan's Biochemistry 7/e p165

74. **Ans. (b) Enzyme of TCA cycle**
Ref: Vasudevan's Biochemistry 7/e p248

75. **Ans. (c) Mucopolysacchridosis**
Ref: Vasudevan's Biochemistry 7/e p80

76. **Ans. (a) Ribose**
Ref: Vasudevan's Biochemistry 7/e p70

77. **Ans. (d) Glucose 1,6,diphosphate synthase**
Ref: Vasudevan's Biochemistry 7/e p113

78. **Ans. (a) Branching enzyme**
Ref: Vasudevan's Biochemistry 7/e p129

79. **Ans. (c) Amylo-1, 6-glucosidase**
Ref: Vasudevan's Biochemistry 7/e p124

80. **Ans. (b) Magnesium**
Ref: Vasudevan's Biochemistry 7/e p512

81. **Ans. (b) Conversion to glycogen**
Ref: Vasudevan's Biochemistry 7/e p109

82. **Ans. (c) Glyceraldehyde**
Ref: Vasudevan's Biochemistry 7/e p70

83. **Ans. (c) Both**
Ref: Internet resources

84. **Ans. (c) Alpha ketoglutarate dehydrogenase**
Ref: Vasudevan's Biochemistry 7/e p253

85. **Ans. (a) Galactose-1-phosphate uridyl transferase/ GALT**
Ref: Vasudevan's Biochemistry 7/e p139

86. **Ans. (b) Pyruvate**
Ref: Vasudevan's Biochemistry 7/e p253

87. **Ans. (b) Fructose-2,6-biphosphate**
Ref: Vasudevan's Biochemistry 7/e p114

88. **Ans. (c) NADPH**
Ref: Vasudevan's Biochemistry 7/e p131

89. **Ans. (a) GLUT4**
Ref: Vasudevan's Biochemistry 7/e p106

90. **Ans. (a) Pro-insulin**
Ref: Vasudevan's Biochemistry 7/e p318

91. **Ans. (d) RBC**
Ref: Vasudevan's Biochemistry 7/e p107

92. **Ans. (a) GLUT4**
Ref: Vasudevan's Biochemistry 7/e p106

93. **Ans. (b) Tyrosine kinase activity**
Ref: Vasudevan's Biochemistry 7/e p653

94. **Ans. (b) Cardiac muscle**
Ref: Vasudevan's Biochemistry 7/e p106

95. **Ans. (d) Norpinephrine**
Ref: Vasudevan's Biochemistry 7/e p313

96. **Ans. (c) 40–50 units**
Ref: Vasudevan's Biochemistry 7/e p318

97. **Ans. (c) Promote gluconeogenesis**
Ref: Vasudevan's Biochemistry 7/e p323

98. **Ans. (d) GLUT-4**
Ref: Internet resources

99. **Ans. (c) Glucose-6-phosphatase**
Ref: Vasudevan's Biochemistry 7/e p125

100. **Ans. (d) Glucuronic acid pathway**
Ref: Vasudevan's Biochemistry 7/e p134

101. **Ans. (c) 6**
Ref: Vasudevan's Biochemistry 7/e p205

102. **Ans. (c) Beta (1→4) glycosidic**
Ref: Vasudevan's Biochemistry 7/e p77

103. **Ans. (a) Phosphoglycerate kinase/PGK**
Ref: Vasudevan's Biochemistry 7/e p113

104. **Ans. (a) Fructokinase**
Ref: Vasudevan's Biochemistry 7/e p138

105. **Ans. (a) Enolase**
Ref: Vasudevan's Biochemistry 7/e p111

106. **Ans. (d) Hexokinase**
Ref: Vasudevan's Biochemistry 7/e p109

107. **Ans. (a) RBC**
Ref: Vasudevan's Biochemistry 7/e p106

LIPIDS METABOLISM

108. **Ans. (d) Sphingomyelinase**
Ref: Satyanarayana's Biochemistry, 3/e p307

109. **Ans. (b) LDL receptors**
Ref: Vasudevan's Biochemistry, 7/e p343

110. **Ans. (d) Alpha linolenic acid**
Ref: Vasudevan's Biochemistry, 7/e p84

111. **Ans. (c) Hexosaminidase-A**
Ref: Vasudevan's Biochemistry, 7/e p194

112. **Ans. (d) Reduced NADP$^+$**
Ref: Vasudevan's Biochemistry 7/e p481

113. **Ans. (b) Linoleic acid**
Ref: Vasudevan's Biochemistry 7/e p186

114. **Ans. (a) LT6**
Ref: Vasudevan's Biochemistry 7/e p189

115. **Ans. (d) Niemann Pick's disease**
Ref: Vasudevan's Biochemistry 7/e p193

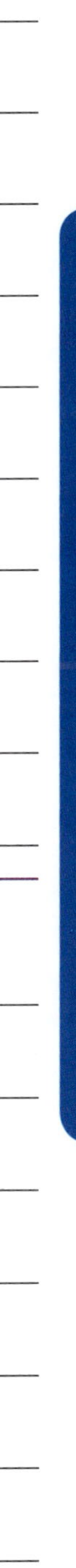

116. **Ans. (b)** Coconut oil
Ref: Vasudevan's Biochemistry 7/e p86

117. **Ans. (c)** Beta hydroxy butyrate
Ref: Vasudevan's Biochemistry 7/e p100

118. **Ans. (d)** Acetoacetate
Ref: Vasudevan's Biochemistry 7/e p164

119. **Ans. (c)** Cholesterol
Ref: Vasudevan's Biochemistry 7/e p169

120. **Ans. (b)** Ketosis
Ref: Internet resources

121. **Ans. (c)** Fatty acid
Ref: Vasudevan's Biochemistry 7/e p101

122. **Ans. (c)** HMG CoA reductase
Ref: Vasudevan's Biochemistry 7/e p172

123. **Ans. (b)** LDL
Ref: Vasudevan's Biochemistry 7/e p175

124. **Ans. (b)** Apolipoprotein A
Ref: Vasudevan's Biochemistry 7/e p179

125. **Ans. (d)** Glucose
Ref: Vasudevan's Biochemistry 7/e p157, 170

126. **Ans. (c)** Propionyl CoA
Ref: Vasudevan's Biochemistry 7/e p154

127. **Ans. (a)** Linoleic acid
Ref: Vasudevan's Biochemistry 7/e p86

128. **Ans. (d)** Hormone sensitive lipase/HSL
Ref: Vasudevan's Biochemistry 7/e p148

129. **Ans. (d)** HDL
Ref: Vasudevan's Biochemistry 7/e p178

130. **Ans. (b)** Thromboxane A2 and prostacyclin (PGI-2)
Ref: Vasudevan's Biochemistry 7/e p190

131. **Ans. (a)** Histamine
Ref: Vasudevan's Biochemistry 7/e p243

132. **Ans. (a)** ApoE
Ref: Vasudevan's Biochemistry 7/e p175

133. **Ans. (d)** ApoA1
Ref: Vasudevan's Biochemistry 7/e p180

134. **Ans. (c)** Hypercholesterolemia
Ref: Vasudevan's Biochemistry 7/e p101

135. **Ans. (d)** Apo-B
Ref: Vasudevan's Biochemistry 7/e p175

136. **Ans. (c)** VLDL
Ref: Vasudevan's Biochemistry/7th/180

137. **Ans. (c)** Propionyl CoA
Ref: Vasudevan's Biochemistry 7/e p156

138. **Ans. (a)** Arachidonic acid metabolites
Ref: Vasudevan's Biochemistry 7/e p191

139. **Ans. (a)** Liver
Ref: Vasudevan's Biochemistry 7/e p164

140. **Ans. (d)** Pentose phosphate pathway
Ref: Vasudevan's Biochemistry 7/e p158

141. **Ans. (d)** Binding to bile acids
Ref: Internet resources

142. **Ans. (b)** Albumin
Ref: Vasudevan's Biochemistry 7/e p151

143. **Ans. (c)** Acetoacetate
Ref: Vasudevan's Biochemistry 7/e p165

144. **Ans. (d)** Triglycerides
Ref: Vasudevan's Biochemistry 7/e p162

145. **Ans. (a)** Arachidonic acid
Ref: Vasudevan's Biochemistry 7/e p189

146. **Ans. (c)** Acetyl CoA
Ref: Vasudevan's Biochemistry 7/e p156

147. **Ans. (b)** Carnitine
Ref: Vasudevan's Biochemistry 7/e p152

148. **Ans. (c)** Bile pigment
Ref: Vasudevan's Biochemistry 7/e p173

149. **Ans. (c)** Taurocholic acid
Ref: Vasudevan's Biochemistry 7/e p276

150. **Ans. (c)** Both
Ref: Vasudevan's Biochemistry 7/e p155

151. **Ans. (c)** Triglyceride and cholesterol
Ref: Vasudevan's Biochemistry 7/e p176

152. **Ans. (d)** Reduced gluconeogenesis
Ref: Vasudevan's Biochemistry 7/e p102

153. **Ans. (b)** Triglyceride
Ref: Vasudevan's Biochemistry 7/e p99

154. **Ans. (b)** $\omega 6$ series
Ref: Vasudevan's Biochemistry 7/e p86

155. **Ans. (b)** Increased fat degradation
Ref: Vasudevan's Biochemistry 7/e p165

NUCLEOTIDE METABOLISM

156. **Ans. (c) Carbamoyl phosphate synthase II**
Ref: Vasudevan's Biochemistry, 7/e p570

157. **Ans. (c) Cytoplasm**
Ref: Vasudevan's Biochemistry, 7/e p569

158. **Ans. (a) Total deficiency of HGPRTase**
Ref: Vasudevan's Biochemistry 7/e p569

159. **Ans. (c) Nucleobase + sugar + phosphate**
Ref: Vasudevan's Biochemistry 7/e p561

160. **Ans. (c) Purine**
Ref: Vasudevan's Biochemistry 7/e p566

161. **Ans. (b) Gout**
Ref: Vasudevan's Biochemistry 7/e p566

162. **Ans. (c) Xanthine oxidase**
Ref: Vasudevan's Biochemistry 7/e p567

163. **Ans. (b) Histidine**
Ref: Vasudevan's Biochemistry 7/e p564

MISCELLANEOUS

164. **Ans. (b) Post-replication repair**
Ref: Vasudevan's Biochemistry, 7/e p583

165. **Ans. (b) Magnesium**
Ref: Vasudevan's Biochemistry, 7/e p639

166. **Ans. (d) Hydrogen bond is between a purine and a pyrimidine only**
Ref: Vasudevan's Biochemistry, 7/e p577

167. **Ans. (b) mRNA**
Ref: Vasudevan's Biochemistry, 7/e p597

168. **Ans. (c) Vitamin K3**
Ref: Vasudevan's Biochemistry, 7/e p474

169. **Ans. (d) Conversion of proline to hydroxyl-proline**
Ref: Vasudevan's Biochemistry, 7/e p498

170. **Ans. (c) Metaphase**
Ref: Vasudevan's Biochemistry 7/e p583

171. **Ans. (b) They play a key role in post-transcription conversion of pre-mRNA to mature mRNA**
Ref: Vasudevan's Biochemistry 7/e p592

172. **Ans. (a) Intron**
Ref: Vasudevan's Biochemistry 7/e p591

173. **Ans. (a) Right handed, anti-parallel**
Ref: Vasudevan's Biochemistry 7/e p576

174. **Ans. (b) Overalapping of codons**
Ref: Vasudevan's Biochemistry 7/e p598

175. **Ans. (b) Uracil**
Ref: Vasudevan's Biochemistry 7/e p575

176. **Ans. (a) Hydrophobic effect**
Ref: Vasudevan's Biochemistry 7/e p576

177. **Ans. (b) Chromosome is seen in interphase**
Ref: Internet resources

178. **Ans. (d) Northern blotting**
Ref: Vasudevan's Biochemistry 7/e p634

179. **Ans. (c) Adenosine**
Ref: Vasudevan's Biochemistry 7/e p575

180. **Ans. (c) Reverse transcriptase**
Ref: Vasudevan's Biochemistry 7/e p593

181. **Ans. (d) Intron**
Ref: Vasudevan's Biochemistry 7/e p592

182. **Ans. (c) RFLP**
Ref: Vasudevan's Biochemistry 7/e p637

183. **Ans. (b) t-RNA**
Ref: Internet resources

184. **Ans. (d) More than one codon for a single amino acid**
Ref: Vasudevan's Biochemistry 7/e p598

185. **Ans. (b) RNA dependent DNA polymerase**
Ref: Vasudevan's Biochemistry 7/e p585

186. **Ans. (d) Protein**
Ref: Vasudevan's Biochemistry 7/e p634

187. **Ans. (c) Promoter site**
Ref: Vasudevan's Biochemistry 7/e p589

188. **Ans. (c) Translation**
Ref: Vasudevan's Biochemistry 7/e p600

189. **Ans. (d) Hydrogen bond**
Ref: Vasudevan's Biochemistry 7/e p576

190. **Ans. (b) Sequence of DNA**
Ref: Internet resources

191. **Ans. (c) G-C**
Ref: Vasudevan's Biochemistry 7/e p575

192. **Ans. (c) Nuclear**
Ref: Vasudevan's Biochemistry 7/e p575

193. **Ans. (b) 35%**
Ref: Vasudevan's Biochemistry 7/e p575

194. **Ans. (a) Hybridization**
Ref: Vasudevan's Biochemistry 7/e p636

195. **Ans. (d) RFLP**
Ref: Vasudevan's Biochemistry 7/e p637

196. **Ans. (c) S phase**
Ref: Vasudevan's Biochemistry 7/e p615

197. **Ans. (b) Helicase**
Ref: Vasudevan's Biochemistry 7/e p581

198. **Ans. (b) Taq polymerase**
Ref: Vasudevan's Biochemistry 7/e p638

199. **Ans. (d) Dideoxynucleotide method**
Ref: Internet resources

200. **Ans. (c) Promoter region**
Ref: Vasudevan's Biochemistry 7/e p590

201. **Ans. (d) Chaperones**
Ref: Vasudevan's Biochemistry 7/e p604

202. **Ans. (d) Protein folding**
Ref: Vasudevan's Biochemistry 7/e p604

203. **Ans. (c) Mediators of post-transitional assembly of protein complexes**
Ref: Vasudevan's Biochemistry 7/e p604

204. **Ans. (b) DNA double helix**
Ref: Vasudevan's Biochemistry 7/e p576

205. **Ans. (d) U**
Ref: Vasudevan's Biochemistry 7/e p603

206. **Ans. (d) ADH**
Ref: Vasudevan's Biochemistry 7/e p659

207. **Ans. (d) Zinc**
Ref: Vasudevan's Biochemistry 7/e p522

208. **Ans. (b) Gonadotropins**
Ref: Vasudevan's Biochemistry 7/e p650

209. **Ans. (d) Decreased testosterone**
Ref: Vasudevan's Biochemistry 7/e p666

210. **Ans. (a) GH**
Ref: Vasudevan's Biochemistry 7/e p145

211. **Ans. (c) Aldosterone**
Ref: Vasudevan's Biochemistry 7/e p669

212. **Ans. (d) Albumin**
Ref: Vasudevan's Biochemistry 7/e p714

213. **Ans. (c) Thyroxine**
Ref: Vasudevan's Biochemistry 7/e p669

214. **Ans. (a) G protein**
Ref: Vasudevan's Biochemistry 7/e p651

215. **Ans. (c) Aromatase**
Ref: Vasudevan's Biochemistry 7/e p666

216. **Ans. (b) Coenzyme A**
Ref: Vasudevan's Biochemistry 7/e p484

217. **Ans. (d) Histidine**
Ref: Vasudevan's Biochemistry 7/e p490

218. **Ans. (d) 1,25 dihydrocholecalciferol**
Ref: Vasudevan's Biochemistry 7/e p470

219. **Ans. (a) Vitamin B1**
Ref: Vasudevan's Biochemistry 7/e p476

220. **Ans. (b) Vitamin B12**
Ref: Vasudevan's Biochemistry 7/e p494

221. **Ans. (d) Carboxylation**
Ref: Vasudevan's Biochemistry 7/e p475

222. **Ans. (b) Proximal convoluted tubules**
Ref: Vasudevan's Biochemistry 7/e p470

223. **Ans. (d) Acetic acid**
Ref: Vasudevan's Biochemistry 7/e p484

224. **Ans. (a) Biotin**
Ref: Vasudevan's Biochemistry 7/e p486

225. **Ans. (b) Vitamin D**
Ref: Vasudevan's Biochemistry 7/e p469

226. **Ans. (c) Folic acid**
Ref: Vasudevan's Biochemistry 7/e p489

227. **Ans. (a) Lysosome**
Ref: Vasudevan's Biochemistry 7/e p469

228. **Ans. (d) Sunflower seeds**
Ref: Vasudevan's Biochemistry 7/e p464

229. **Ans. (c) Biotin**
Ref: Vasudevan's Biochemistry/ 7th/485

230. **Ans. (d) Vitamin K**
Ref: Vasudevan's Biochemistry 7/e p475

231. **Ans. (b) Pyridoxine**
Ref: Vasudevan's Biochemistry 7/e p483

232. **Ans. (c) Folic acid**
Ref: Vasudevan's Biochemistry 7/e p488

233. **Ans. (b) Niacin**
Ref: Vasudevan's Biochemistry 7/e p481

234. **Ans. (c)** Niacin
Ref: Vasudevan's Biochemistry 7/e p482

235. **Ans. (c)** Increased synthesis of peroxidases
Ref: Vasudevan's Biochemistry 7/e p469

236. **Ans. (c)** Ileum
Ref: Vasudevan's Biochemistry 7/e p492

237. **Ans. (d)** 500 microgram
Ref: Vasudevan's Biochemistry 7/e p490

238. **Ans. (c)** Folic acid
Ref: Vasudevan's Biochemistry 7/e p490

239. **Ans. (b)** Antioxidant
Ref: Vasudevan's Biochemistry 7/e p473

240. **Ans. (d)** Vitamin K
Ref: Vasudevan's Biochemistry 7/e p475

241. **Ans. (b)** Milk is a rich source
Ref: Vasudevan's Biochemistry 7/e p482

242. **Ans. (d)** Milk
Ref: Vasudevan's Biochemistry 7/e p473

243. **Ans. (a)** Alpha2, epsilon2
Ref: Internet resources

244. **Ans. (d)** 6 gm
Ref: Vasudevan's Biochemistry 7/e p277

245. **Ans. (d)** Alpha2, gamma2
Ref: Vasudevan's Biochemistry 7/e p288

246. **Ans. (c)** Hb–heme–biliverdin–bilirubin–urobilinogen
Ref: Vasudevan's Biochemistry/ 7th/278

247. **Ans. (d)** Ferric ions
Ref: Vasudevan's Biochemistry 7/e p284

248. **Ans. (a)** 70
Ref: Internet resources

249. **Ans. (b)** Zinc
Ref: Vasudevan's Biochemistry 7/e p522

250. **Ans. (b)** Endoplasmic reticulum
Ref: Vasudevan's Biochemistry 7/e p11

251. **Ans. (b)** Cyt-P-450
Ref: Vasudevan's Biochemistry 7/e p545

252. **Ans. (c)** Factors VII, X, V and calcium
Ref: Internet resources

253. **Ans. (d)** Selenium
Ref: Vasudevan's Biochemistry 7/e p523

254. **Ans. (d)** Vander Waals
Ref: Vasudevan's Biochemistry 7/e p6

255. **Ans. (c)** Energy not available for work
Ref: Internet resources

256. **Ans. (a)** Electrostatic
Ref: Vasudevan's Biochemistry 7/e p5

257. **Ans. (a)** Cardiolipin
Ref: Vasudevan's Biochemistry 7/e p14

258. **Ans. (c)** Protein destruction
Ref: Internet resources

259. **Ans. (d)** All of the baove
Ref: Vasudevan's Biochemistry 7/e p302

260. **Ans. (a)** Selenium
Ref: Vasudevan's Biochemistry 7/e p523

261. **Ans. (b)** Sodium citrate
Ref: Vasudevan's Biochemistry 7/e p442

262. **Ans. (d)** ATP
Ref: Internet resources

263. **Ans. (c)** Zinc deficiency – Pulmonary fibrosis
Ref: Vasudevan's Biochemistry 7/e p522

264. **Ans. (a)** Aid in spermiogenesis
Ref: Internet resources

265. **Ans. (a)** Myeloma cell lines
Ref: Vasudevan's Biochemistry 7/e p690

266. **Ans. (c)** Zinc
Ref: Vasudevan's Biochemistry/ 7th/522

267. **Ans. (b)** Sodium
Ref: Vasudevan's Biochemistry 7/e p408

268. **Ans. (b)** 10 mEq/l
Ref: Internet resources

269. **Ans. (b)** Copper
Ref: Vasudevan's Biochemistry 7/e p521

270. **Ans. (b)** Buffalo milk
Ref: Vasudevan's Biochemistry 7/e p420

271. **Ans. (a)** 2 days
Ref: Vasudevan's Biochemistry 7/e p302

272. **Ans. (c)** Decreased bicarbonate
Ref: Vasudevan's Biochemistry 7/e p398

273. **Ans. (c)** 7.35–7.45
Ref: Internet resources

274. **Ans. (c) Concentration of the diffusing substance**
Ref: Vasudevan's Biochemistry 7/e p21

275. **Ans. (d) Myocardial infarction**
Ref: Vasudevan's Biochemistry 7/e p302

276. **Ans. (d) Myoglobin**
Ref: Vasudevan's Biochemistry 7/e p304

277. **Ans. (c) Kilogram/metre^2**
Ref: Vasudevan's Biochemistry 7/e p536

278. **Ans. (b) Net positive and negative charge on molecule are equal**
Ref: Vasudevan's Biochemistry 7/e p41

279. **Ans. (c) Racemization**
Ref: Internet resources

PRACTICE QUESTIONS

ENZYME

1. **Most important marker of MI:**
   a. Troponin I b. LDH
   c. Myoglobin d. CK-MB

AMINO ACIDS & PROTEINS

2. **A child presented to the clinic with complaints of mental retardation. Phenyllactate, phenylketone & phenylacetate was detected in urine. Which test should be done:**
   a. Marsh test b. Rothera's test
   c. Guthrie test d. Gerhardt's test
3. **Most specific test for HIV detects:**
   a. DNA b. RNA
   c. Proteins d. Nucleic acids
4. **Collagen type II is predominantly found in:**
   a. Skin b. Lung
   c. Cartilage d. Vascular tissues
5. **Proteins which are synthesized in rough endoplasmic reticulum will NOT go to:**
   a. Mitochondria b. Cytosol
   c. Golgi body d. Lysosome

CARBOHYDRATE METABOLISM

6. **Andersen disease is because of deficiency of:**
   a. Debranching enzyme b. Muscle phorphorylase
   c. Branching enzyme d. Liver phosphorylase
7. **Which of the following pathway is cytoplasm to mitochondria substrate shuttle:**
   a. Glycerophosphate shuttle
   b. Malate shuttle
   c. HMP shunt
   d. Cytochrome oxidase pathway
8. **Von Gierke's disease is due to deficiency of:**
   a. G6PD b. GPUT
   c. Glycogen synthase d. Glucose-6-phosphatase

LIPIDS

9. **Ketone body formation occurs in:**
   a. Overfed state b. Hyperinsulinemia
   c. Starvation d. All of the above
10. **Which of the following lipoprotein transports cholesterol to peripheral tissue:**
   a. VLDL b. IDL
   c. LDL d. HDL
11. **Activator of LCAT:**
   a. Apo A-I b. Apo A-II
   c. Apo B-100 d. Apo B-48

NUCLEIC ACID METABOLISM

12. **Xeroderma pigmentosum is due to defect in:**
   a. Defective ATM gene
   b. Defect in hMSH genes
   c. Defective DNA transcriptase
   d. Nucleotide excision repair mechanism
13. **Which of the following is NOT involved in raising uric acid levels in body:**
   a. Xanthine oxidase inhibitors
   b. Phospho-Ribosyl-Pyrophosphate synthetase
   c. Glucose-6-phosphatase
   d. Hypoxanthine-Guanine-Phospho-Ribosyl Transferase
14. **Substance common to both purine & pyrimidine:**
   a. Alanine b. Glutamine
   c. Guanine d. Uracil

MISCELLANEOUS

15. **Reduced stringency between the third base of the codon and the complimentary nucleotide in the anticodon is called:**
   a. Non-overlapping b. Non-punctuated
   c. Degenerate d. Wobbling
16. **Insulin acts via:**
   a. Phosphatidyl inositol b. cGMP
   c. Tyrosine kinase d. cAMP
17. **FAD/ FMN consist of:**
   a. B1 b. B2
   c. B6 d. B12
18. **3′ to 5′ exonuclease activity:**
   a. Proof reading
   b. Repair of damaged DNA
   c. DNA synthesis
   d. DNA polymerase

Ans. 1. a. Troponin I 2. c. Guthrie test 3. c. Proteins 4. c. Cartilage 5. a. Mitochondria 6. c. Branching enzyme 7. b. Malate shuttle 8. d. Glucose-6-phosphatase 9. c. Starvation 10. c. LDL 11. a. Apo A-I 12. d. Nucleotide excision... 13. a. Xanthine oxidase... 14. b. Glutamine 15. d. Wobbling 16. c. Tyrosine kinase 17. b. B2 18. d. DNA polymerase

19. Which of the following is DNA enzyme is responsible for aging:
a. Telo-isomerase
b. Topo-isomerase
c. Telomerase
d. DNA polymerase

20. Which of the following is DNA enzyme is responsible for aging:
a. Substitution of amino acids
b. Changed mRNA base at 3rd nucleotide of codon
c. Stop codon
d. Deletion of 2 bases

21. Frame shift mutation is due to:
a. Phylloquinone b. Menaquinone
c. Menadione d. Cobalamin

22. RBC transketolase activity is reduced in deficiency of which vitamin:
a. B1 b. B2
c. B6 d. B9

23. Presence of urinary Xanthurenic indicates deficiency of:
a. B1 b. B2
c. B3 d. B6

24. Number of ATPs given by $FADH_2$ in electron transport chain:
a. 1 b. 1.5
c. 2 d. 2.5

25. Which of the following is responsible for RNA silencing:
a. tRNA b. mRNA
c. rRNA d. SiRNA

26. Which of the following is associated with DNA repair defect:
a. Xeroderma pigmentosum
b. Li-Fraumani syndrome
c. Retinoblastoma
d. Neuroblastoma

27. Zinc deficiency causes:
a. Iron deficiency anemia
b. Acrodermatitis enteropathica
c. Megaloblastic anemia
d. Enteritis

28. Keshan disease is due to deficiency of:
a. Zinc b. Iron
c. Magnesium d. Selenium

29. True regarding organization of DNA:
a. Single stranded
b. Winds around histones
c. Contains uracil
d. Right handed single helix

30. One amino acid has more than one codon. This is:
a. Triplet b. Unambiguous
c. Non-overlapping d. Degenerate

31. Gene therapy was firstly employed for which condition:
a. Cystic fibrosis b. SCID
c. Retroviral infections d. DMD

32. Uracil is ABSENT in:
a. DNA b. RNA
c. Both d. None

33. Which enzyme is important in synthesis of mRNA:
a. Amino-acyl tRNA synthetase
b. Helicase
c. Topi-isomerase
d. RNA polymerase

34. Transcription process is terminated by:
a. Rh factor b. Rho factor
c. TATA box gene d. RNA polymerase

35. Okazaki fragments are formed during:
a. Transcription b. Translation
c. Transformation d. Replication

36. Mitochondrial DNA is:
a. Open, circular b. Closed, circular
c. Open, straight d. Closed, straight

Ans. **19.** c. Telomerase **20.** d. Deletion of 2 bases **21.** c. Menadione **22.** a. B1
23. d. B6 **24.** b. 1.5 **25.** d. SiRNA **26.** a. Xeroderma...
27. b. Acrodermatitis... **28.** d. Selenium **29.** b. Winds around histones **30.** d. Degenerate
31. b. SCID **32.** a. DNA **33.** d. RNA polymerase **34.** b. Rho factor
35. d. Replication **36.** b. Closed, circular

IMAGE-BASED QUESTIONS

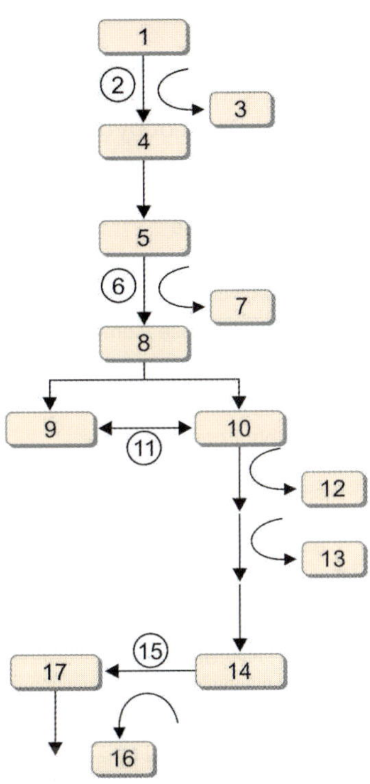

1. **Label 1 is:**
   a. Fructose b. Glucose
   c. Sucrose d. Mannose

   Glucose is phosphorylated to glucose-6-phosphate.

2. **Label 2 is:**
   a. Phosphofructokinase b. Pyruvate kinase
   c. Hexokinase
   d. Phosphoglycerate kinase

   The enzyme is hexokinase (HK), which splits the ATP into ADP, and the Pi is added on to the glucose.

3. **Label 3 is:**
   a. ATP b. NADH
   c. NAD d. ADP

   Hexokinase (HK) splits the ATP into ADP, and the Pi is added on to the glucose.

4. **Label 4 is:**
   a. 2,3-biphosphoglycerate
   b. Glucose 6-phosphate
   c. Pyruvate
   d. Phosphoenol pyruvate

   Glucose is phosphorylated to glucose-6-phosphate

5. **Label 5 is:**
   a. Fructose 6-phosphate b. Glucose 6-phosphate
   c. Pyruvate d. Phosphoenol pyruvate

   Glucose-6-phosphatase is ismoerized to fructose-6-phosphate by phosphohexose isomerise. This is readily reversible.

6. **Label 6 is:**
   a. Hexokinase b. Phosphofructokinase
   c. Pyruvate kinase d. Enolase

   Fructose-6-phosphate is further phosphorylated to fructose-1,6-biphosphate. The enzyme is phosphofructokinase.

7. **Label 7 is:**
   a. ATP b. NADH
   c. ADP d. NAD^+

   PFK is the rate limiting enzyme of glycolysis. The enzyme catalyzes the second phosphorylation step of glycolysis using a second molecule of ATP.

8. **Label 8 is:**
   a. Fructose 1,6-biphosphate
   b. Phosphoenol pyruvate
   c. Pyruvate
   d. Lactate

   Fructose-6-phosphate is further phosphorylated to fructose-1,6-biphosphate. The enzyme is phosphofructokinase.

9. **Label 9 is:**
   a. Phosphofructose
   b. 2,3-BPG
   c. Dihydroxyacetone phosphate
   d. Phosphoenol pyruvate

   The 6 carbon fructose-1,6-biphosphate is cleaved into two 3 carbon units; one glyceraldehydes-3-phosphate and another molecule of dihydoxy acetone phosphate (DHAP).

10. **Label 10 is:**
    a. Phosphofructose
    b. Glyceraldehyde 3-phosphate
    c. 2,3-BPG
    d. Dihydroxyacetone phosphate

    The 6 carbon fructose-1,6-biphosphate is cleaved into two 3 carbon units; one glyceraldehydes-3-phosphate (GAP) and another molecule of dihydoxy acetone phosphate (DHAP).

11. **Label 11 is:**
    a. Hexokinase
    b. Phosphofructokinase
    c. Pyruvate kinase
    d. Triose phosphate isomerase

    DHAP is isomerized to GAP by the enzyme triose phosphate isomerise.

12. Label 12 is:

a. NADH
b. NAD^+
c. ATP
d. ADP

GAP is dehydrogenated and simultaneously phosphorylated to 1,3-biphosphoglycerate (1,3-BPG) with the help of NAD^+. During this reaction, NAD^+ is reduced to NADH.

13. Label 13 is:

a. NADH
b. NAD^+
c. ADP
d. ATP

The energy of 1,3-BPG is trapped to synthesize one ATP molecule with the help of biphosphoglycerate kinase.

14. Label 14 is:

a. Phosphofructose
b. Glyceraldehyde 3-phosphate
c. 2,3-BPG
d. Phosphoenol pyruvte

2-phosphoglycerate is converted to phosphoenol pyruvate (PEP) by the enzyme enolase.

15. Label 15 is:

a. Hexokinase
b. Phosphofructokinase
c. Pyruvate kinase
d. Triose phosphate isomerase

PEP is dephosphorylated to pyruvate, by pyruvate kinase.

16. Label 16 is:

a. NADH
b. NAD^+
c. ADP
d. ATP

One molecule of ATP is generated during this reaction. This is again an example of substrate level phosphorylation.

17. Label 17 is:

a. Phosphofructose
b. Glyceraldehyde 3-phosphate
c. 2,3-BPG
d. Pyruvate

First PEP is made into a transient intermediary of enol private; which is spontaneously isomerized into keto pyruvate, the stable form of pyruvate

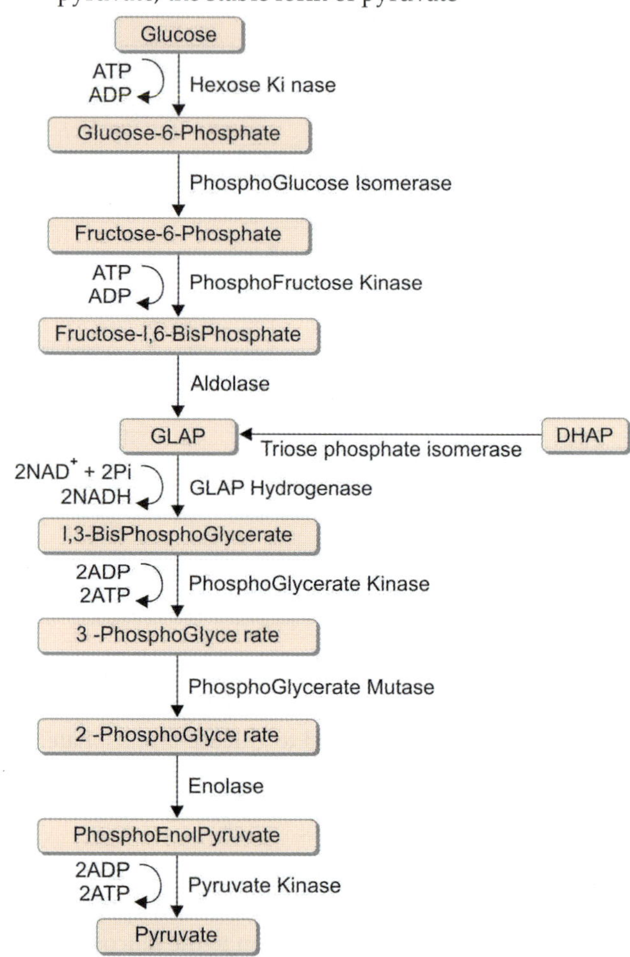

Simplified Glycolysis diagram. Molecule names contain extra capitals to illustrate components.

MCQ POINTS

S. No.	Question statement	Answer
1.	Cofactor for phosphofructokinase	***Magnesium***
2.	Melanin is synthesized from	***Tyrosine***
3.	Successor of phenylalanine	***Tyrosine***
4.	Sulkowitch test is done for	***Urinary calcium***
5.	Reverse folding of protein is carried out by	***Chaperones***
6.	Cysteine is formed from	***Methionine***
7.	RBC Transketolase is associated with	***Thiamine/B1***
8.	Alpha2, beta2 is which hemoglobin	***HbF***
9.	Type 2 hypercholesterolemia is due to	***LDL receptor defect***
10.	Agent added to blood for estimating blood glucose (added to prevent glycolysis)	***Sodium fluoride***
11.	Fluoride inhibits which enzyme	***Enolase***
12.	Rate limiting enzyme in heme synthesis	***ALA synthase***
13.	In TCA cycle, substrate level phosphorylation occurs in reaction catalyzed by enzyme	***Succinyl-CoA-thiokinase***
14.	In sickle cell anemia, translocation on codon 6 is due to substitution of	***Glutamate by valine***
15.	Muscle cannot make use of glycogen as they lack	***Glucose-6-phosphatase***
16.	Protein synthesis occurs in which cellular organelle	***Ribosome***
17.	Number of ATP produced in HMP shunt	***Zero***
18.	Cyanide inhibits which enzyme	***Cytochrome oxidase (complex IV)***
19.	In diabetes, cataract occurs because of the accumulation of	***Sorbitol***
20.	Most essential fatty acid is	***Linoleic acid***
21.	Feature of mitochondrial DNA	***Closed, circular***
22.	Vitamins synthesized by intestinal bacteria	***Vitamins K and B_{12}***
23.	Which organs cannot ketone bodies	***Liver***
24.	Important feature of ketosis in diabetes	***Ketosis with glycosuria***
25.	Function of intrinsic factor	***Absorption of vitamin B_{12} (extrinsic factor)***
26.	Glycogen storage disease due to muscle phosphorylase deficiency is known as	***McArdle's disease***
27.	Another name of glucose	***Dextrose***
28.	Which substance is required for protein destruction	***Ubiquitin***
29.	Deficiency of sphingomyelinase causes	***Niemann-Pick disease***
30.	Uncoupler of electron transport chain	***Dinitrophenol***
31.	Vitamin required for hydroxylation of proline	***Vitamin C***
32.	Cofactor for carbonic anhydrase	***Zinc***
33.	Essential fructosuria is due to deficiency of	***Fructokinase***
34.	Procedure which separates proteins by their mass	***SDS page***
35.	Source of nitrogen in urea cycle	***Ammonia and aspartate***
36.	Limiting amino acids in wheat	***Lysine, threonine***
37.	Amino acid which becomes essential in phenylketonuria	***Tyrosine***
38.	Enzyme used in PCR	***Taq polymerase***

S. No.	Question statement	Answer
39.	Number of ATPs generated in Krebs cycle	***10 ATPS***
40.	Vitamin derived from tryptophan	***Niacin***
41.	Finding on cartilages in a patient with alkaptonuria	***Ochronosis***
42.	Cycle occurring both in cytosol as well as mitochondria	***Urea cycle***
43.	Deficiency of branching enzyme leads to	***Andersen disease***
44.	End product of aerobic glycolysis	***Pyruvate***
45.	Most potent anti-oxidant is vitamin	***Vitamin E***
46.	Location of electron transport chain	***Inner mitochondrial membrane***
47.	End product of pyrimidine metabolism	***Beta alanine***
48.	Hexosaminidase A deficiency leads to	***Tay-Sachs disease***
49.	Nitrogen base + sugar + phosphate group =	***Nucleotide***
50.	Rate limiting step in fatty acid synthesis	***Acetyl-CoA-carboxylase***
51.	Western blotting is done for	***Protein***
52.	Final product of purine metabolism in humans	***Uric acid***
53.	Building block for fatty acid biosynthesis	***Acetyl CoA + NADPH***
54.	Deficiency of aldolase B causes	***Hereditary fructose intolerance***
55.	Good cholesterol is	***HDL***
56.	Biosynthesis of fatty acids occurs in which part of the cell	***Cytoplasm***
57.	Ammonia is detoxified in brain to	***Glutamine***
58.	Thyroxine is synthesized from	***Tyrosine***
59.	Beta oxidation of fatty acids takes place in which part of the cell	***Mitochondria***
60.	Source of nitrogen in urea cycle	***Ammonia and aspartate***
61.	Hormone which inhibits ketogenesis	***Insulin***
62.	Substrate for energy production in brain in well fed state	***Glucose***
63.	Mousy odour of urine is present in	***Phenylketonuria***
64.	Most direct precursor of taurine is	***Cysteic acid (from cysteine)***
65.	Fluoroacetate inhibits which enzyme	***Aconitase***
66.	Ochronosis is because of accumulation of	***Benzoquinone acetate***
67.	End product of protein metabolism is	***Urea***
68.	Cori's disease is due to deficiency of which enzyme	***Debranching enzyme***
69.	End product of anaerobic glycolysis	***Lactate***
70.	Alternative pathway to glycolysis and TCA cycle for the oxidation of glucose is	***Glucuronic acid pathway***
71.	NADPH generated from HMP Shunt is used for biosynthesis of	***Fatty acid and steroid synthesis***
72.	Base present in RNA, but absent in DNA	***Uracil***
73.	Enzyme deficient in essential pentosuria	***Xylitol dehydrogenase***
74.	Cori cycle occurs in	***Skeletal muscle, blood and liver***
75.	Methylmalonic aciduria is seen in deficiency of	***Vitamin B_{12}***

CHAPTER

4

PATHOLOGY

KEY POINTS

Stains and Tissue Stained

- Alcian blue stains: Acid mucin, mast cells
- Masson Fontana stains: Melanin
- Masson's trichrome stains: Collagen

Giant Cells and Associated Diseases

- Langhans: Tuberculosis, Sarcoidosis
- Aschoff: Rheumatic heart disease
- Touton: Xanthomas
- Warthin-Finkeldey: Measles

Intracellular Accumulations and Stains Used

- Fat: Sudan 4, Oil red O
- Glycogen: PAS, Best carmine
- Iron: Prussian blue
- Amyloid: Congo red, crystal violet, methyl green, Thioflavin, toluidine blue DMAB nitrite.

Pathological Calcification

- Dystrophic calcification: Deposition occurs in non viable or dying tissue despite normal serum calcium levels
- Metastatic calcification: Deposition occurs in normal tissues due to hypercalcemia.

Amyloid Proteins

- AL: Primary amyloidosis
- AA: Secondary amyloidosis
- Beta-2-microglobulin: Hemodialysis-associated amyloidosis
- Beta-2 amyloid protein: Alzheimer's disease
- Transthyretin: Hereditary amyloidosis, senile amyloidosis

Exudative Effusion

- Protein: More than 3 gm percent; mostly fibrinogen
- Specific gravity: < 1.018
- pH: >7.3
- LDH: Increased
- Effusion LDH/serum LDH: <0.6
- Effusion protein/serum protein: <0.5

Transudative Effusion

- Protein: <3 gm percent; mostly albumin
- Specific gravity: <1.015
- pH: >7.3
- LDH: Decreased
- Effusion LDH/serum LDH: <0.6
- Effusion protein/serum protein: <0.5

Virchow's Triad

- Endothelial injury
- Abnormal blood flow
- Hypercoagulability

Skin Markers (of Internal Malignancy)

- Acanthosis nigricans
- Lentigines
- Café-au-lait
- Nevi
- Pemphigoid
- Dermatophytosis
- Erythema gyratum repens

Carcinoma and Their Genetic Associations

- RET protooncogene: Medullary carcinoma thyroid, papillary carcinoma
- Rb gene (13q14): Retinoblastoma
- BRCA1: Ca breast (females), Ca ovary
- APC gene: Familial adenomatous polyposis coli
- Chromosome 3: Renal cell carcinoma
- 11p13: Wilm's tumor
- Xp2l: Duchenne muscular dystrophy
- APP gene: Alzheimer's disease

Cytochemical Features of Malignancy

- CML: Decreased leucocyte alkaline phosphatase
- Accelerated and blastic phase of CML: Increased leucocyte alkaline phosphatase
- Lymphoblasts of ALL: Negative for sudan black B, myeloperoxidase, ASD

Chloroacetate Esterase

- Myelobeasts of AML: Positive for Sudan black B, myeloperoxidase, ASD-chloroacetate esterase
- Hairy cell leukemia: Tartrate-resistant acid phosphatase

Psammoma Bodies are Associated with

- Papillary carcinoma thyroid
- Serous cystadenocarcinoma ovary
- Meningioma

Histopathological Characteristics

- H-X bodies, Birbeck granules: Langerhans cell histiocytosis
- Flexner-Wintersteiner rosettes, Homer-Wright rosette, Fleurette: Retinoblastoma
- Neurofibrillary tangles, senile/neuritic plaques, amyloid angiopathy: Alzheimer's disease
- Lewy bodies: Parkinson's disease
- Henderson-Peterson bodies: Molluscum contagiosum
- Russell bodies: Multiple myeloma
- Halberstaedter-Prowazek bodies: Chlamydia trachomatis
- Dohle bodies: Severe inflammatory disease or sepsis

Acute Rheumatic Fever

- Affects all the three layers of heart
- The stenotic mitral value appears like button-hole or fish mouth
- MacCallum's patch – Rough portion of endocardium of left atrium
- Characteristic distribution of erythema marginatum in rheumatic heart disease is bathing suit distribution
- Bread and butter pericarditis

Must Know Facts

- Tree barking of aortic intima – Syphilitic aortitis
- Most common site of coronary atherosclerosis – left anterior descending branch
- Vegetations of NBTE are sterile, nondestructive, small, singly or multiple along the lines of closure of the leaflets or cusps

Blood Transfusion

- Stored at 4 degrees centigrade
- Those who have received HBIG- should not donate for 6 months
- Those who have received Rabies vaccine- should not donate for 1 year

Reid Index

- Thickness of mucous gland layer/Thickness of wall between the epithelium and cartilage
- Normal ratio = 0.14 to 0.36
- Increased in chronic bronchitis.

Crohn's Disease

- Bowel region: Ileum, colon
- Distribution: Skip lesion
- Stricture: Yes
- Wall appearance: Thick
- Inflammation: Transmural
- Pseudopolyps: Moderate
- Ulcers: Deep, knife like
- Lymphoid reaction, fibrosis, serositis: Marked
- Granulomas: Yes (35%)
- Fistulae/Sinuses: Yes
- Perianal fistula: Yes (in colonic disease)
- Fat/vitamin malabsorption: Yes
- Malignant potential: With colonic involvement
- Recurrence after surgery: Common
- Toxic megacolon: No

Centrilobular Necrosis is associated with

- Chronic venous congestion
- Hemorrhagic shock
- Carbon tetrachloride
- Halothane
- Acetaminophen
- Rifampicin

Amyloidosis of the Spleen

- Sago spleen: Deposit mostly limited to splenic follicles
- Lardaceous spleen: Amyloid spares the follicle and involves the walls of the splenic sinuses and connective tissue framework of the red pulp.

Mallory Bodies are associated with

- Alcoholic liver disease
- Primary biliary cirrhosis
- Wilson's disease
- Chronic cholestatic syndromes
- Hepatocellular carcinoma

Hepatitis Markers

- HbsAg: Acute or chronic HBV infection
- Anti- HBs: Immunity against HBV
- IgM Anti-HBc-high titre: Acute HBV infection
- IgM Anti-HBc-low titre/absent: Chronic HBV infection

- IgG Anti-HBc: Past exposure to HBV
- HBV DNA: Continued infectious state
- HBeAg: Continued infectious state, acute or chronic HBV infection
- Anti-HBe: Convlescence

Urinary Casts

- Hyaline casts: Normal
- RBC casts: Glomerular injury
- WBC casts: Interstitial nephritis/pyelonephritis
- Broad granular casts: Chronic renal failure
- Pigmented muddy brown granular casts: Tubular necrosis

Electron Microscopic Features of Glomerulonephritis

- Type I MPGN: Subendothelial and mesangial deposition of IgG and C3
- Type II MPGN: Dense deposit disease, deposits within basement membrane, deposition of C3
- PSGN: Immunofluorescence microscopy shows diffuse granular depositiuon of IgG and C3, giving rise to starry sky appearance

Must Know Facts

- Hyaline arteriosclerosis is seen in benign nephrosclerosis
- Fibrinoid necrosis and hyperplastic arteriosclerosis is seen in malignant hypertension.

Peripheral Smear Features

- Basophilic stippling: Iron deficiency anemia, lead poisoning, thalassemia, sideroblastic anemia
- Heinz bodies: Glucose- 6-phosphate deficiency, Thalassemia
- Acanthocytes: Abetalipoproteinemia
- Spiculated RBC: Pyruvate kinase deficiency
- Burr cells: HUS, uremia

Pentad of Thrombocytopenic Purpura (TTP)

- Thrombocytopenia
- Fever
- Microangiopathic hemolytic anemia
- Transient neurological deficits
- Renal failure

Myelofibrosis

- Marked splenomegaly (tear drop cells)
- Peripheral blood shows leukoerythrocytic anemia
- In bone marrow dysplastic megakaryocytes are characteristically seen
- Characteristic dry tap

Must Know Facts

- Most sensitive and specific test for diagnosis of iron deficiency is –Serum ferritin level.
- Thrombocytopenia indicates platelet count below 1 lac/cu mm
- Wiskott-Aldrich syndrome shows – small platelets
- Crumbling brick wall appearance seen in Hailey- Hailey disease
- Mycosis fungoides is a: T-cell lymphoproliferative disorder
- von Willebrand's factor can be assayed by: Ristocetin aggregation test

Histopathological Pentad of Alzheimer's Disease

- Neuritic plaques
- Neurofibrillary tangles
- Granulovacuolar degeneration
- Amyloid angiopathy
- Gliosis

Neurotransmitters Depletion and Neurological Diseases

- Alzheimer's: Decreased acetylcholine
- Parkinson's disease: Dopamine < acetylcholine
- Schizophrenia: Dopamine> Acetylcholine
- Huntington's disease: Loss of GABA-ergic and Cholinergic neurons

Familial Syndromes associated with Phaeochromocytoma and Extra-Adrenal Paraganglioma

- Multiple endocrine neoplasia (MEN) type-2A: Phaeochromocytoma, Medullary carcinoma of thyroid, Parathyroid hyperplasia
- MEN type-2B: Phaeochromocytoma, Medullary carcinoma of thyroid, Marfanoid habitus
- Neurofibromatosis (NF) type-I: Phaeochromocytoma, Neurofibromatosis, Café-au-lait spots, Optic nerve glioma
- Von-Hippel Lindau: Phaeochromocytoma, paraganglioma, renal cell carcinoma, haemangioblastoma, Pancreatic endocrine neoplasm

Down's Syndrome

- Muscle hypotonia
- Oblique eye fissures with epicanthic skin folds on the inner corner of the eyes

- Flat nasal bridge
- Excessive space between large toe and second toe
- Single palmar fold (Simian crease)
- Protruding tongue
- Short neck
- White spots on the iris known as Brushfield spots
- Single flexion furrow of the fifth finger
- Higher number of ulnar loop dermatoglyphics

Autosomal Dominant Disorders

- Huntington disease
- Familial hypercholesterolemia
- Familial adenomatous polyposis
- Von Hippel-Lindau syndrome
- MEN type 1 and 2
- Retinoblastoma
- Spherocytosis
- Antithrombin III and factor V Leiden
- von Willebrand's disease
- Polycystic kidney disease
- Achondroplasia
- Marfan syndrome
- Amyloidosis

Autosomal Recessive Disorders

- Cystic fibrosis
- Galactosemia
- Alpha-1 antitrypsin deficiency
- Ataxia telangiectasia
- Alkaptonuria
- Phenylketonuria
- Alpha and beta thalassemia
- Sickle cell disease
- Hereditary spherocytosis
- Wilson's disease
- Hemochromatosis
- Gaucher's disease
- Niemann-Pick disease
- Tay-Sachs disease
- MPS I-VII
- Glycogen storage disorders I-VIII
- Congenital adrenal hyperplasia

X-Linked Dominant Disorders

- Vitamin D resistant rickets
- Orofacial digital syndrome
- Incontinentia pigmenti

Mitochondrial Disorders

- Kearns-Sayre syndrome
- MELAS
- Leber's hereditary optic neuropathy
- Myoclonic epilepsy

Traits inherited along Y Chromosome

- Male infertility
- Gonadoblastoma

Chromosomal Breakage Disorders

- Fanconi's syndrome
- Bloom's syndrome
- Ataxia – telangiectasia

Mutations

- Silent mutation: Codon containing the changed base codes for the same amino acid
- Missense mutation: Codon containing the changed base codes for a different amino acid, this mistaken codon may be acceptable, partially acceptable or unacceptable to functioning of that protein molecule
- Nonsense mutation: Codon containing the changed base becomes the termination codon

Prion Diseases

- Kuru
- Creutzfeldt-Jakob disease
- Fatal familial insomnia
- Mad cow disease

Must Know Facts

- Regular trisomy 21 is found in 94 percent cases of Down's syndrome
- Fragile X syndrome is the second most common cause of mental retardation after Down's syndrome in males
- Achondroplasia: Most common disproportionate dwarfism; Trident hand (index and ring finger are divergent)
- Ataxia telangiectasia: Autosomal recessive; Basic defect in abnormal sensitivity to X-ray and certain radiomimetic chemicals which leads to chromosome and chromatid breakage
- G6 PD deficiency is X-linked recessive transmission
- Marfan's syndrome is associated with mutation in fibrillin protein
- Hamartomas: Excessive and focal overgrowth of cells and tissues native to the organ in which it occurs
- Choristoma/heterotopia: Microscopically normal cells or tissues that are present in abnormal locations.

MCQs WITH SHORT EXPLANATIONS

GENERAL PATHOLOGY

1. Feature of malignant neoplasm:

a. Extremely scanty mitoses
b. Increased nuclear to cytoplasm ratio
c. Normal configuration of cell
d. All of the above

Anaplasia

- Lack of differentiation, or anaplasia, is considered a hallmark of malignancy.
- Anaplastic cells display marked pleomorphism.
- The nuclei are characteristically extremely hyperchromatic (darkly stained) and large.
- The nuclear-cytoplasmic ratio may approach 1:1 instead of the normal 1:4 or 1:6.
- Giant cells that are considerably larger than their neighbors may be formed and possess either one enormous nucleus or several nuclei (syncytia).
- Anaplastic nuclei are variable and bizarre in size and shape.
- The chromatin is coarse and clumped, and nucleoli may be of astounding size.
- More important, mitoses are often numerous and distinctly atypical; anarchic multiple spindles may be seen and sometimes appear as tripolar or quadripolar forms.
- Also, anaplastic cells usually fail to develop recognizable patterns of orientation to one another (i.e. they lose normal polarity).
- They may grow in sheets, with total loss of communal structures, such as gland formation or stratified squamous architecture.
- Anaplasia is the most extreme disturbance in cell growth encountered in the spectrum of cellular proliferations.

Contrasting features of benign and malignant tumours.

		Feature	*Benign*	*Malignant*
i.	CLINICAL AND GROSS FEATURES			
	1.	Boundaries	Encapsulated or well-circumscribed	Poorly-circumscribed and irregular
	2.	Surrounding tissue	Often compressed	Usually invaded
	3.	Size	Usually small	Often larger
	4.	Secondary changes	Occur less often	Occur more often
II.	MICROSCOPIC FEATURES			
	1.	Pattern	Usually resembles the tissue of origin closely	Often poor resemblance to tissue of origin
	2.	Basal polarity	Retained	Often lost
	3.	Pleomorphism	Usually not present	Often present
	4.	Nucleo-cytoplasmic ratio	Normal	Increased
	5.	Anisonucleosis	Absent	Generally present
	6.	Hyperchromatism	Absent	Often present
	7.	Mitoses	May be present but are always typical mitoses	Mitotic figures increased and are generally atypical and abnormal
	8.	Tumour giant cells	May be present but without nuclear atypia	Present with nuclear atypia
	9.	Chromosomal abnormalities	Infrequent	Invariably present
	10.	Function	Usually well maintained	May be retained, lost or become abnormal
III.	GROWTH RATE		Usually slow	Usually rapid
IV.	LOCAL INVASION		Often compresses the surrounding tissues without invading or infiltrating them	Usually infiltrates and invades the adjacent tissues

Ans. 1. **b.** Increased nuclear to cytoplasm ratio

Feature		Benign	Malignant
V.	METASTASIS	Absent	Frequently present
VI.	PROGNOSIS	Local complications	Death by local and metastatic complications

2. Ischemia in kidney leads to:

a. Fat necrosis
b. Liquefactive necrosis
c. Caseous necrosis
d. Coagulative necrosis

Coagulative necrosis

- Accidental cell death typically caused by ischemia or infarction.
- Characterized by the 'ghostly' appearance of cells under light microscopy in the affected area of tissue.
- In coagulative necrosis the architecture of dead tissue is preserved for at least a couple of days.
- Injury denatures structural proteins as well as lysosomal enzymes thus blocking the proteolysis of the damaged cells.
- The lack of lysosomal enzymes allows it to maintain a "coagulated" morphology for some time.

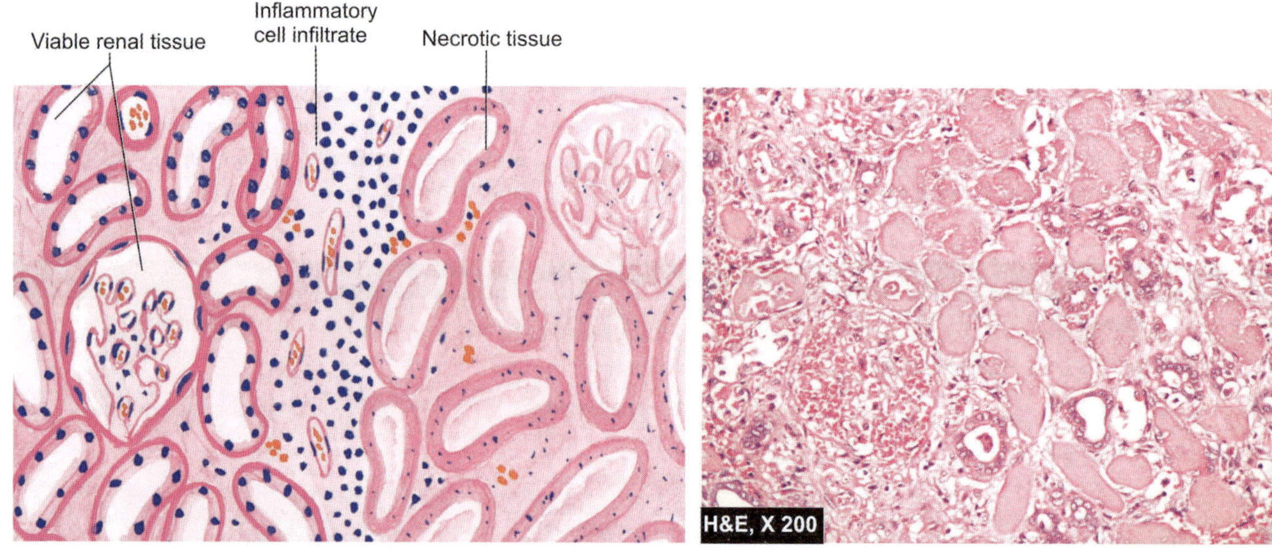

Coagulative necrosis in infarct kidney. The affected area on right shows cells with intensely eosinophilic cytoplasm of tubular cells but the outlines of tubules are still maintained. The nuclei show granular debris. The interface between viable and non-viable area shows non-specific chronic inflammation and proliferating vessels.

3. Tissue thromboplastin activates:

a. Factor IV
b. Factor VI
c. Factor VII
d. All of the above

Tissue Factor/thromboplastin/factor III is the cell surface receptor for the serine protease factor VIIa.

The best known function of tissue factor is its role in blood coagulation. The complex of TF with factor VIIa activates factor IX and catalyzes the conversion of the inactive protease factor X into the active protease factor Xa.

4. Invasive carcinoma differs from carcinoma in situ by:

a. Abnormal nuclear morphology
b. Pleomorphism
c. Basement membrane involvement
d. Mitoses

Few terms

Dysplasia is the earliest form of pre-cancerous lesion recognizable in a biopsy. Dysplasia can be low grade or high grade. High grade dysplasia may also be referred to as carcinoma *in situ*.

Invasive carcinoma, usually simply called cancer, has the potential to invade and spread to surrounding tissues and structures, and may eventually be lethal.

5. All of the following responses are seen in acute inflammation EXCEPT:

a. Vasodilatation
b. Neutrophil migration
c. Granuloma formation
d. Increased vascular permeability

In terms of the underlying cause, the difference between granulomas and other types of inflammation is that granulomas form in response to antigens that are

Ans. 2. **d.** Coagulative... 3. **c.** Factor VII 4. **c.** Basement membrane... 5. **c.** Granuloma formation

resistant to "first-responder" inflammatory cells such as neutrophils and eosinophils. Granulomatous inflammation is a distinctive pattern of chronic inflammatory reactions.

Major differences between acute and chronic inflammation.

Feature	Acute inflammation	Chronic inflammation
1. *Onset and Duration*	❑ Within short time ❑ Lasts for short duration	❑ After delay ❑ Lasts longer
2. *Cardinal Signs*	Invariably present	Generally imperceptible
3. *Pathogenesis*	❑ Vascular events: hemodynamic changes, incresed vascular permeability ❑ Cellular events: exudation of leucocytes, Phagocytosis ❑ Role of chemical mediators and regulators	❑ Following acute inflammation ❑ Recurrent attacks of acute inflammation ❑ Chronic inflammation from beginning
4. *Main Inflammatory Cells*	❑ Neutrophils ❑ Eosinophils ❑ Lymphomononuclear cells (late) ❑ Pus cells	❑ Lymphocytes ❑ Plasma cells ❑ Monocytes/macrophages (epithelioid cells in granulomas) ❑ Giant cells (foreign body, Langhans')
5. *Plasma Exudation*	Present	May or may not be present
6. *Systemic Effects*	❑ Fever: high grade ❑ Leucocytosis (neutrophilic, eosinophilic) ❑ Lymphadenitis-lymphangiitis ❑ Septic shock (in severe acute infection)	❑ Fever: mild ❑ Leucocytosis (lymphocytic, monocytic) ❑ Lymphadenitis-lymphangiitis ❑ Raised ESR ❑ Anaemia ❑ Amyloidosis (in long-term cases)
7. *Main morphology*	❑ Abscesses (suppuration) ❑ Ulcers ❑ Through blood (Bacteraemia, septicaemia, pyaemia)	❑ Chronic non-specific inflammation (infectious, others) ❑ Granulomatous inflammation (tuberculosis, leprosy, sarcoidosis, syphilis, actinomycosis, Crohn's disease etc)
8. *Fate*	❑ Resolution ❑ Healing (regeneration, fibrosis) ❑ Chronicity	❑ Resolution ❑ Healing (regeneration, fibrosis) ❑ Dystrophic calcification
9. *Common Examples*	Pyogenic abscess, cellulitis, bacterial pneumonia, pyaemia	Granulation tissue, granulomatous inflammation (tuberculosis, leprosy etc), chronic osteomyelitis

6. Epithelioid granuloma consists mainly of which type of cells:

a. B cells
b. T cells
c. Monocytes
d. Macrophages

Macrophages (also known as histiocytes) are the cells that define a granuloma. They often, but not invariably, fuse to form multinucleated giant cells (Langhans giant cell). The macrophages in granulomas are often referred to as "epithelioid".

(See Diagram next page)

7. Apoptosis is:

a. Regeneration of cells after injury
b. Reperfusion injury of the cells
c. Programmed internal cell death
d. Uncontrolled multiplication of cells

Apoptosis is the process of programmed cell death that may occur in multicellular organisms. Biochemical events lead to characteristic cell changes (morphology) and death. These changes include blebbing, cell shrinkage, nuclear fragmentation, chromatin condensation, chromosomal DNA fragmentation, and global mRNA decay.

Ans. **6. d.** Macrophages **7. c.** Programmed internal cell death

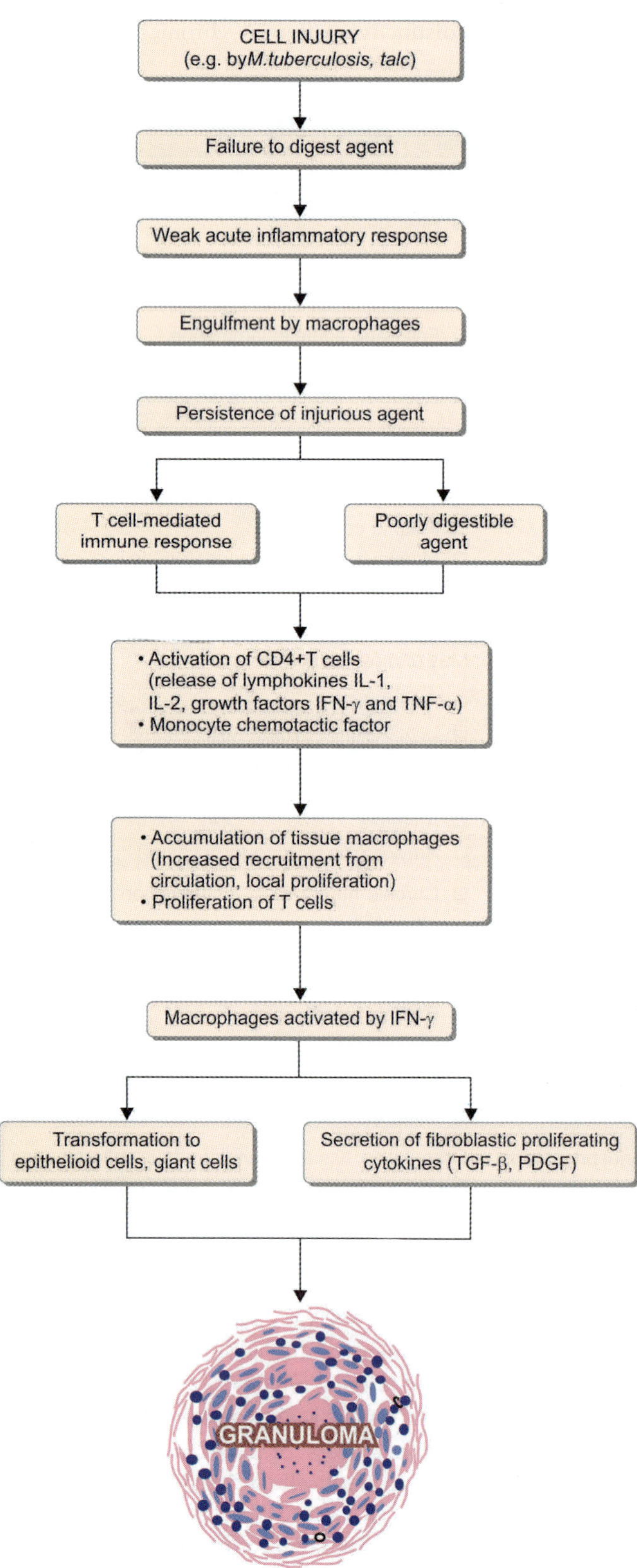

Mechanism of evolution of a granuloma (IL = interleukin; IFN = interferon; TNF = tumour necrosis factor).

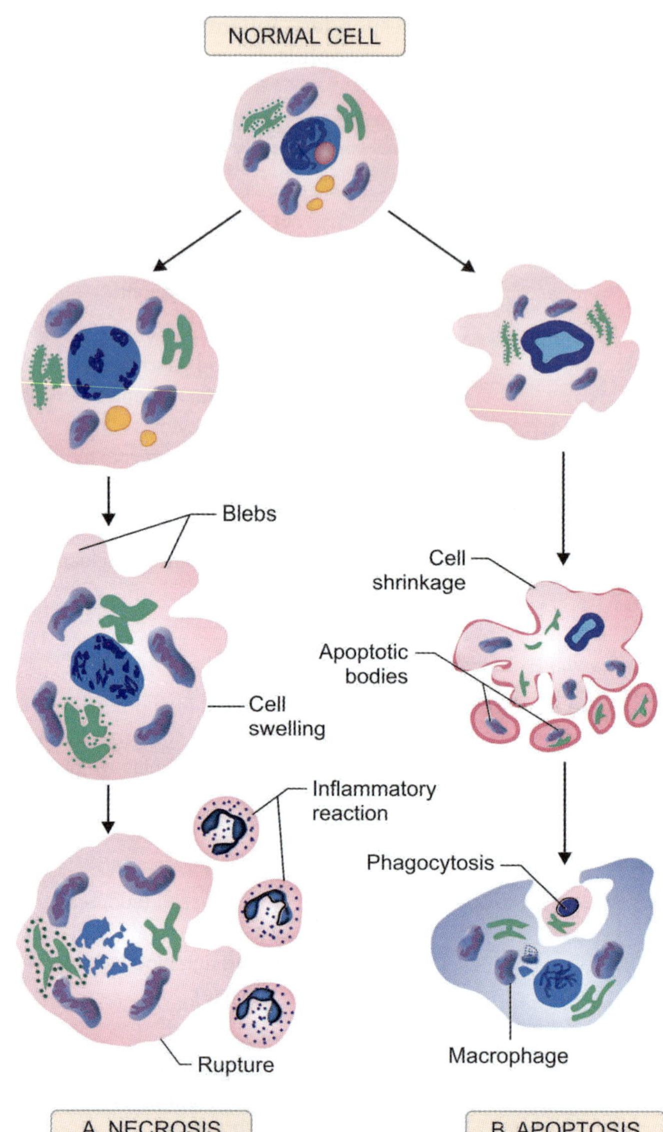

Necrosis and apoptosis. A, Cell necrosis is identified by homogeneous, eosinophilic cytoplasm and nuclear changes of pyknosis, karyolysis, and karyorrhexis. B, Apoptosis consists of condensation of nuclear chromatin and fragmentation of the cell into membrane-bound apoptotic bodies which are engulfed by macrophages.

8. Red infarct is seen in:

a. Kidney
b. Hear
c. Limbs
d. Small intestine

Hemorrhagic infarcts are infarcts commonly caused by occlusion of veins, with red blood cells entering the area of the infarct, or an artery occlusion of an organ with collaterals or dual circulation. This is commonly seen in brain, lungs, liver and the GI tract, areas referred to as having "loose tissue," or dual circulation.

Ans. 8. **d.** Small intestine

	Location	Gross appearance	Outcome
Infarcts of most commonly affected organs.			
1.	*Myocardial infarction*	Pale	Frequently lethal
2.	*Pulmonary infarction*	Hemorrhagic	Less commonly fatal
3.	*Cerebral infarction*	Hemorrhagic or pale	Fatal if massive
4.	*Intestinal infarction*	Hemorrhagic	Frequently lethal
5.	*Renal infarction*	Pale	Not lethal unless massive and bilateral
6.	*Infarct spleen*	Pale	Not lethal
7.	*Infarct liver*	Pale	Not lethal
8.	*Infarcts lower extremity*	Pale	Not lethal

9. Edema results when the plasma proteins fall below:

a. 0.5% b. 5%

c. 15% d. 50%

Albumin comprises 75-80% of normal plasma colloid oncotic pressure and 50% of protein content. When plasma proteins, especially albumin, no longer sustain sufficient colloid osmotic pressure to counterbalance hydrostatic pressure, edema develops.

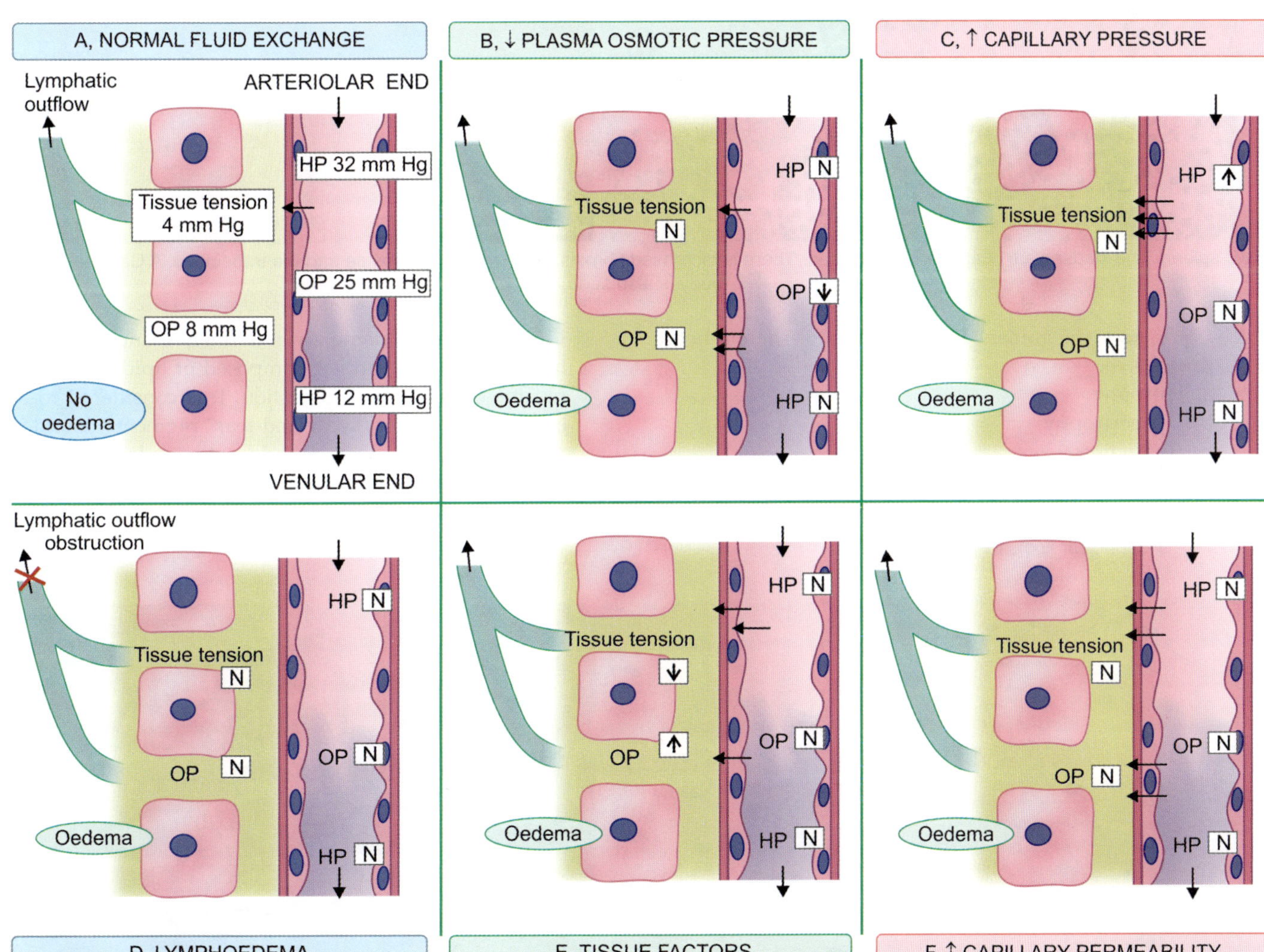

Diagrammatic representation of pathogenesis of oedema (OP = oncotic pressure; HP = hydrostatic pressure). A, Normal pressure gradients and fluid exchanges between plasma, interstitial space and lymphatics. B, Mechanism of oedema by decreased plasma oncotic pressure and hypoproteinemia. C, Mechanism of oedema by increased hydrostatic pressure in the capillary. D, Mechanism of lymphoedema. E, Mechanism by tissue factors (increased oncotic pressure of interstitial fluid and lowered tissue tension). F, Mechanism of oedema by increased capillary permeability.

Ans. **9. d.** 50%

10. Gamna Gandy bodies contain hemosiderin and:

a. Potassium
b. Magnesium
c. Calcium
d. Sodium

Gandy–Gamna nodules or **Gandy-Gamna bodies,** sometimes known as **Gamna-Gandy bodies** or **Gamna-Gandy nodules,** are small yellow-brown, brown, or rust-colored foci found in the spleen in patients with splenomegaly due to portal hypertension and sickle cell disease. They consist of fibrous tissue with hemosiderin and calcium deposits, and probably form due to scarring at sites of small perivascular hemorrhages.

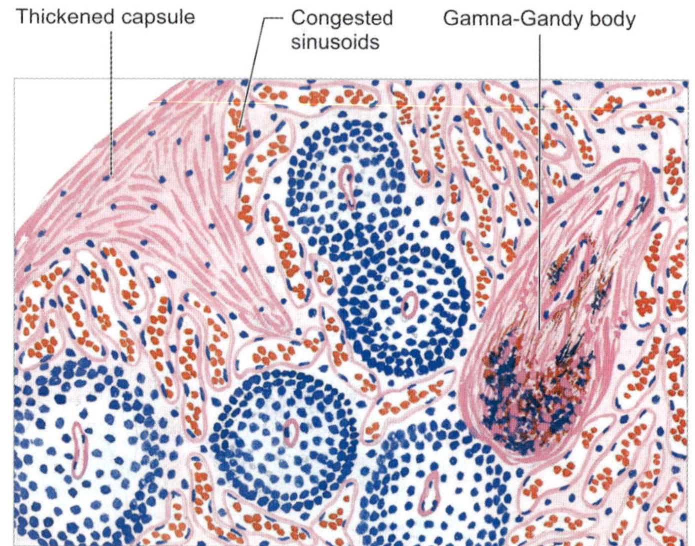

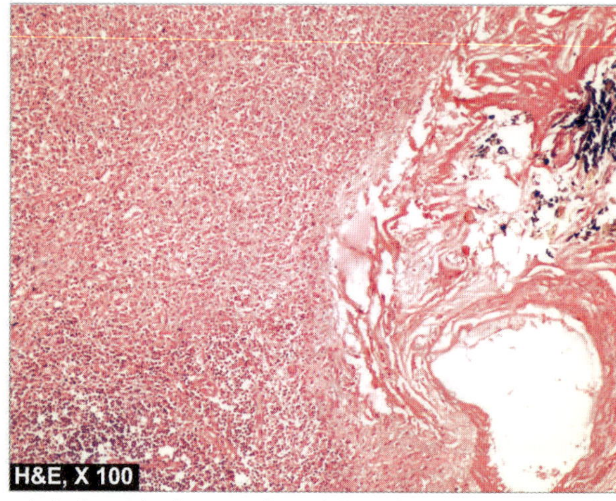

CVC spleen. The sinuses are dilated and congested. There is increased fibrosis in the red pulp, capsule and the trabeculae. A Gamna-Gandy body is also seen.

11. Lipofuscin, the golden yellow pigment is seen in heart muscles in:

a. Atrophy
b. Hypertrophy
c. Infarction
d. Hyperplasia

Lipofuscin is the name given to finely granular yellow-brown pigment granules composed of lipid-containing residues of lysosomal digestion. It is considered to be one of the aging or "wear-and-tear" pigments, found in the liver, kidney, heart muscle, retina, adrenals, nerve cells, and ganglion cells.

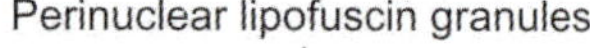

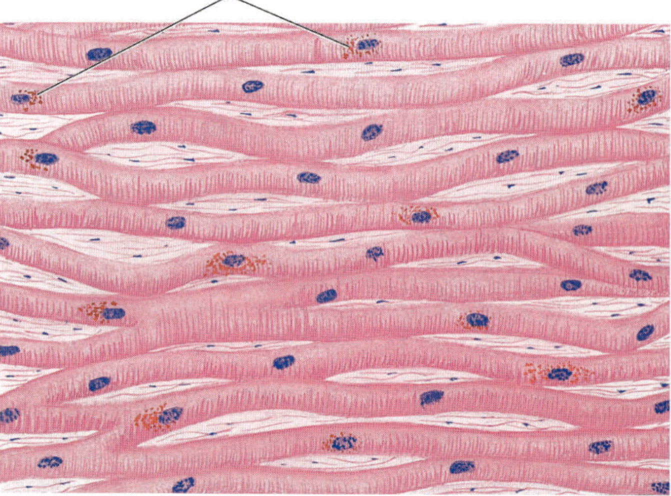

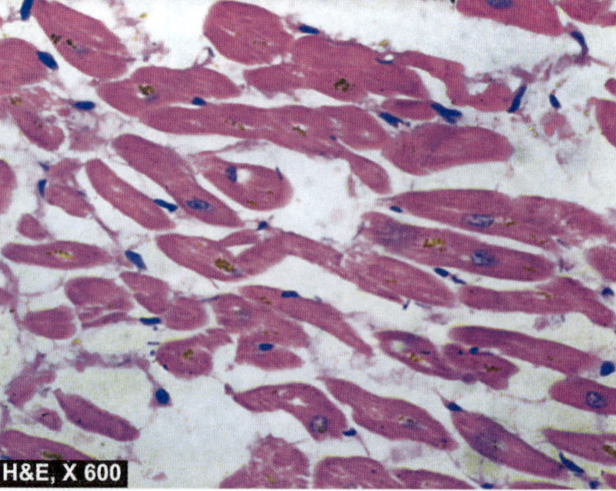

Brown atrophy of the heart. The lipofuscin pigment granules are seen in the cytoplasm of the myocardial fibres, especially around the nuclei.

Ans. **10. c.** Calcium **11. a.** Atrophy

12. **Heart failure cells are:**
   a. Lipofuscin granules in cardiac cells
   b. Pigmented hepatocytes
   c. Pigmented alveolar macrophages
   d. Pigmented cells in pancreas

Heart failure cells are siderophages (hemosiderin-containing macrophages) generated in the alveoli of patients with left heart failure or chronic pulmonary edema, when the high pulmonary blood pressure causes red cells to pass through the vascular wall. Siderophages are not specific of heart failure.

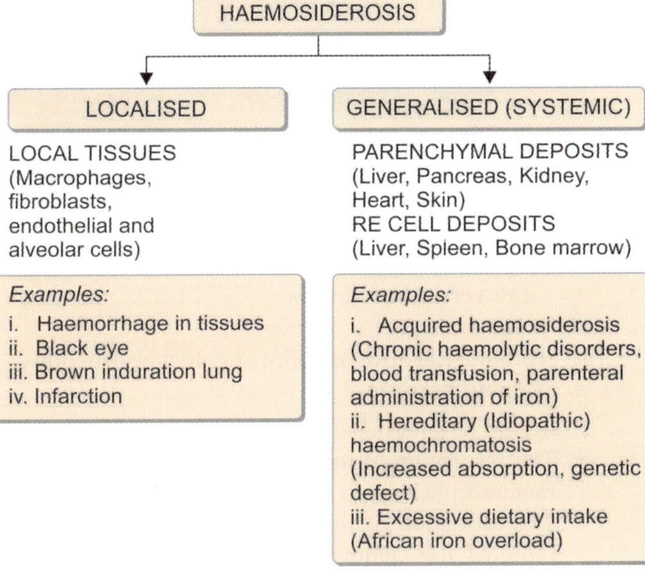

Effects of hemosiderosis.

13. **White infarcts are seen in all EXCEPT:**
   a. Heart
   b. Spleen
   c. Kidney
   d. Liver

Anemic infarcts (also called **white infarcts** or **pale infarcts**) are white or pale infarcts caused by arterial occlusions, and are usually seen in the heart, kidney and spleen. These are referred to as "white" because of the lack of hemorrhaging and limited red blood cells accumulation, (compare to Hemorrhagic infarct). The tissues most likely to be affected are solid organs which limit the amount of hemorrhage that can seep into the area of ischemic necrosis from adjoining capillary beds. The organs typically include single blood supply (no dual arterial blood supply or anastomoses). The infarct generally results grossly in a wedge shaped area of necrosis with the apex closest to the occlusion and the base at the periphery of the organ. The margins will become better defined with time with a narrow rim of congestion attributable to inflammation at the edge of the lesion.

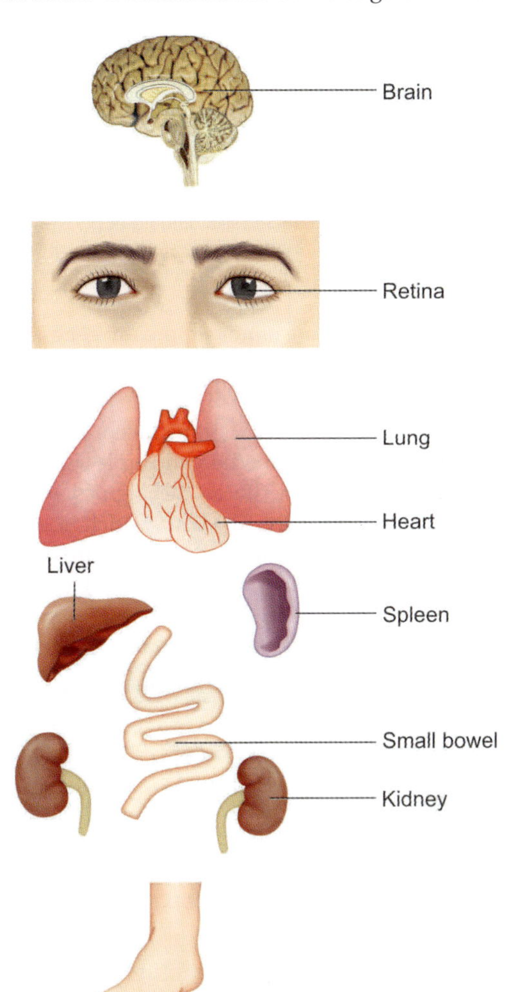

Common locations of systemic infarcts following arterial embolism.

14. **Metastatic calcification does NOT occur in:**
   a. Fundal glands of intestine
   b. Renal tubules
   c. Lungs alveoli
   d. Blood vessels

Metastatic calcification can occur widely throughout the body but principally affects the interstitial tissues of the vasculature, kidneys, lungs, and gastric mucosa. For the latter three, acid secretions or rapid changes in pH levels contribute to the formation of salts.

Differences between dystrophic and metastatic calcification.

	Feature	*Dystrophic calcification*	*Metastatic calcification*
1.	*Definition*	Deposits of calcium salts in dead and degenerated tissues	Deposits of calcium salts in normal tissues

Contd...

Ans. 12. **c.** Pigmented alveolar macrophages 13. **d.** Liver 14. **a.** Fundal glands of intestine

Contd...

	Feature	*Dystrophic calcification*	*Metastatic calcification*
2.	*Calcium metabolism*	Normal	Deranged
3.	*Serum calcium level*	Normal	Hypercalcaemia
4.	*Reversibility*	Generally irreversible	Reversible upon correction of metabolic disorder
5.	*Causes*	Necrosis (caseous, liquefactive, fat), infarcts, thrombi, hematomas, dead parasites, old scars, atheromas, Mönckeberg's sclerosis, certain tumours, cysts, calcinosis cutis	Hyperparathyroidism (due to adenoma, hyperplasia, CRF), bony destructive lesions (e.g. myeloma, metastatic carcinoma), prolonged immobilisation, hypervitaminosis D, milk-alkali syndrome, hypercalcaemia of infancy
6.	*Pathogenesis*	Increased binding of phosphates with necrotic and degenerative tissue, which in turn binds to calcium forming calcium phosphate precipitates	Increased precipitates of calcium phosphate due to hypercalcaemia at certain sites e.g. in lungs, stomach, blood vessels and cornea

15. All of the following are tumor suppressor genes EXCEPT:

a. NF1 b. pRb
c. SMAD1 d. p53

SMAD proteins are signal transducers and transcriptional modulators that mediate multiple signaling pathways. This protein mediates the signals of the bone morphogenetic proteins (BMPs), which are involved in a range of biological activities including cell growth, apoptosis, morphogenesis, development and immune responses.

Important tumour-suppressor anti-oncogenes and associated human tumours.

	Gene	*Location*	*Associated Human Tumours*
1.	*RB*	Nucleus (13q)	Retinoblastoma, osteosarcoma
2.	*p53 (TP53)*	Nucleus (17p)	Most human cancers, common in Ca lung, head and neck, colon, breast
3.	*TGF-β and its receptor*	Extracellular	Ca pancreas, colon, stomach
4.	*APC and β-catenin proteins*	Nucleus, cytosol	Ca colon
5.	*Others*		
	i) BRCA 1 and 2	Nucleus (*BRCA1* 17q21, *BRCA2* 13q12-13)	Ca breast, ovary
	ii) VHL	Nucleus (3p)	Renal cell carcinoma
	iii) WT 1 and 2	Nucleus (11p)	Wilms' tumour
	iv) NF 1 and 2	Plasma membrane	Neurofibromatosis type 1 and 2

16. Following are the examples of apoptosis EXCEPT:

a. Graft versus host disease
b. Menstrual cycle
c. Pathological atrophy following duct obstruction
d. Tumour necrosis

Examples of apoptosis:

- The resorption of the tadpole tail at the time of its metamorphosis into a frog occurs by apoptosis.
- The formation of the fingers and toes of the fetus requires the removal, by apoptosis, of the tissue between them.
- The sloughing off of the inner lining of the uterus (the endometrium) at the start of menstruation occurs by apoptosis.
- The formation of the proper connections (synapses) between neurons in the brain requires that surplus cells be eliminated by apoptosis.
- The elimination of T cells that might otherwise mount an autoimmune attack on the body occurs by apoptosis.
- During the pupal stage of insects that undergo complete metamorphosis, most of the cells of the larva die by apoptosis thus providing the nutrients for the development of the structures of the adult.

Contrasting features of apoptosis and necrosis.

	Feature	*Apoptosis*	*Necrosis*
1.	*Definition*	Programmed and coordinated cell death	Cell death along with degradation of tissue by hydrolytic enzymes
2.	*Causative agents*	Physiologic and pathologic processes	Hypoxia, toxins

Contd...

Ans. **15. c.** SMAD1 **16. d.** Tumour necrosis

Contd...

	Feature	*Apoptosis*	*Necrosis*
3.	*Morphology*	i. No inflammatory reaction ii. Death of single cells iii. Cell shrinkage iv. Cytoplasmic blebs on membrane v. Apoptotic bodies vi. Chromatin condensation vii. Phagocytosis of apoptotic bodies by macrophages	i. Inflammatory reaction always present ii. Death of many adjacent cells iii. Cell swelling initially iv. Membrane disruption v. Damaged organelles vi. Nuclear disruption vii. Phagocytosis of cell debris by macrophages
4.	*Molecular changes*	i. Lysosomes and other organelles intact ii. Initiation of apoptosis by loss of signals of normal cell survival and by action of agents injurious to the cell iii. Triggered by intrinsic (mitochondrial) pathway (pro- and anti-apoptotic members of Bcl-2 family), extrinsic (cell death receptor initiated) pathway (TNF-R1, Fas, Fas-L) and finally by activated caspases	i. Lysosomal breakdown with liberation of hydrolytic enzymes ii. Initiated by various etiologies (ischemia hypoxia, chemicals, physical agents, microbes etc). iii. Cell death by ATP depletion, membrane damage, free radical injury

17. Red infarct is seen in:

a. Spleen
b. Kidney
c. Heart
d. Lung

Red infarct is commonly seen in brain, lungs, liver and the GI tract.

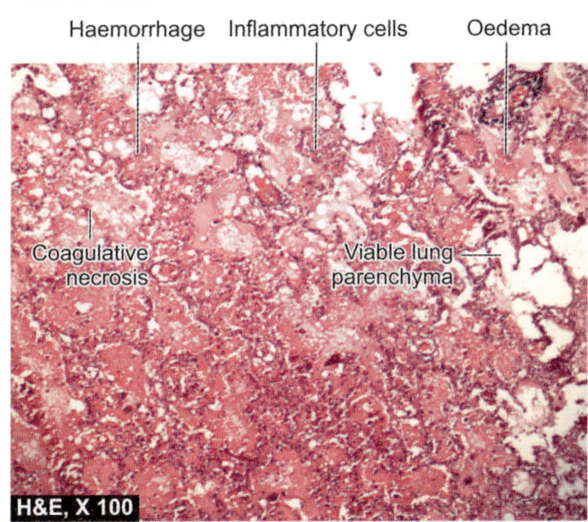

Hemorrhagic infarct lung. Infarcted area shows ghost alveoli filled with blood.

18. If calcium levels are normal, which type of calcification is seen:

a. Metastatic
b. Dystrophic
c. Dysplastic
d. Metaplastic

Dystrophic calcification (**DC**) is the calcification occurring in degenerated or necrotic tissue, as in hyalinized scars, degenerated foci in leiomyomas, and caseous nodules. This occurs as a reaction to tissue damage, including as a consequence of medical device implantation. Dystrophic calcification can occur even if the amount of calcium in the blood is not elevated. (A systemic mineral imbalance would elevate calcium levels in the blood and all tissues and cause metastatic calcification).

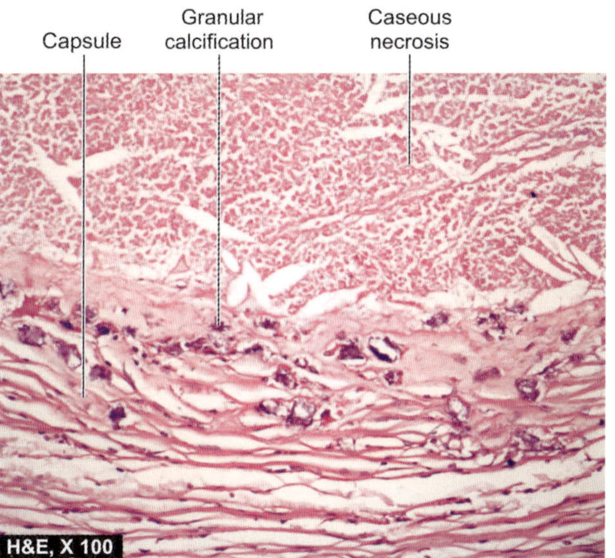

Dystrophic calcification in caseous necrosis in tuberculous lymph node. In H and E, the deposits are basophilic granular while the periphery shows healed granulomas.

19. Metastatic calcification is seen in:

a. Cysts
b. Atheroma
c. Normal tissues
d. Infarcts

Metastatic calcification is deposition of calcium salts in otherwise normal tissue, because of elevated serum levels of calcium, which can occur because of deranged metabolism as well as increased absorption or decreased excretion of calcium and related minerals, as seen in hyperparathyroidism.

Ans. **17. d.** Lung **18. b.** Dystrophic **19. c.** Normal tissues

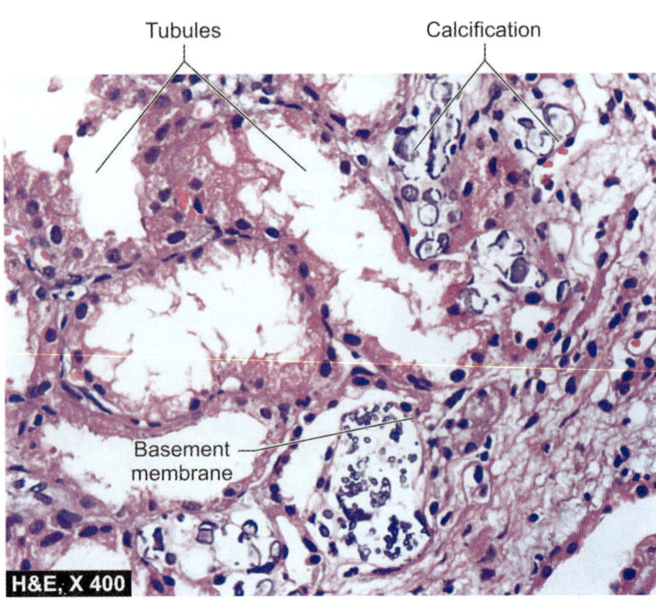

Metastatic calcification in tubular basement membrane in nephrocalcinosis due to hypercalcaemia.

20. Myositis ossificans is differentiated from other reactive fibroblastic proliferations by the presence of:

a. Dysplastic bone
b. Dystrophic bone
c. Metaplastic bone
d. Hypertrophic bone

Myositis ossificans is essentially metaplasia of the intramuscular connective tissue resulting in extraosseous bone formation (without inflammation).

21. Cloudy swelling occurs in all EXCEPT:

a. Lungs
b. Adrenals
c. Liver
d. Kidney

Cloudy swelling

1. Hydropic change or vacuolar degeneration.
2. Appears whenever cells are incapable of maintaining ionic and fluid homeostasis.
3. The first manifestation of almost all forms of sell injury.
4. Reversible injury.

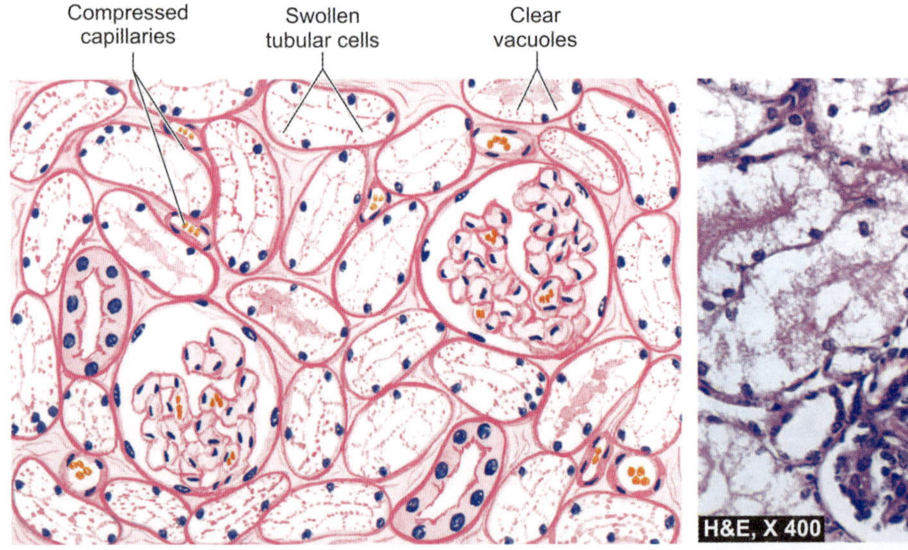

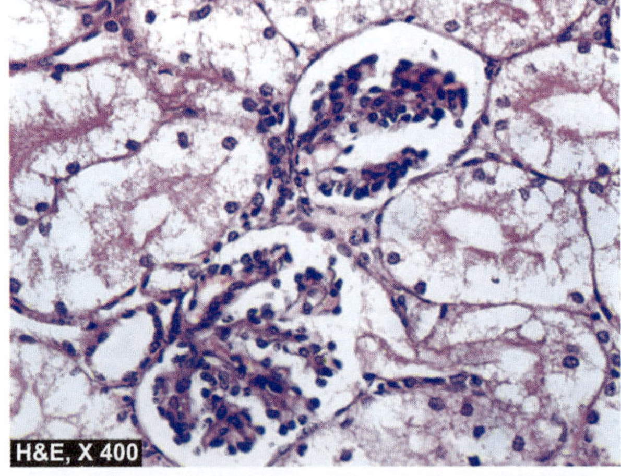

Hydropic change kidney. The tubular epithelial cells are distended with cytoplasmic vacuoles while the interstitial vasculature is compressed. The nuclei of affected tubules are pale.

22. Psammoma bodies shows which type of calcification:

a. Secondary
b. Dystrophic
c. Metastatic
d. All of the above

Psammoma bodies are associated with the papillary (nipple-like) histomorphology and are thought to arise from (1) the infarction and calcification of papillae tips and (2) calcification of intralymphatic tumor thrombi.

23. First change seen in acute inflammation is:

a. Increased permeability
b. Vasodilation
c. Neutrophil migration
d. Vasoconstriction

In acute inflammation, firstly there is transient vasoconstriction of arterioles followed by persistent progressive vasodilatation.

24. Hypercalcemia is seen in all EXCEPT:

a. Multiple myeloma
b. Primary hyperparathyroidism
c. Sarcoidosis
d. Tumour lysis syndrome

Tumour lysis syndrome is a group of metabolic complications that can occur after treatment of cancer,

Ans. 20. c. Metaplastic bone 21. a. Lungs 22. b. Dystrophic 23. d. Vasoconstriction 24. d. Tumour lysis syndrome

usually lymphomas and leukemias, and sometimes even without treatment. These complications are caused by the breakdown products of dying cells and include a high blood potassium, high blood phosphorus, high blood uric acid and high urine uric acid, low blood calcium, and consequent acute uric acid nephropathy and acute kidney failure.

25. Apoptosis is inhibited by:

a. c-Myc b. Ras
c. p53 d. BCL-2

BCL-2 (**B-cell lymphoma 2**), encoded in humans by the *BCL2* gene, is the founding member of the Bcl-2 family of regulator proteins that regulate cell death (apoptosis), by either inducing (pro-apoptotic) or inhibiting (anti-apoptotic) apoptosis. Bcl-2 is specifically considered an important anti-apoptotic protein and is thus classified as an oncogene.

26. The complex process of leukocyte movements through the blood vessels are all EXCEPT:

a. Rolling b. Adhesion
c. Migration d. Phagocytosis

Phagocytosis is a major mechanism used to remove pathogens and cell debris. For example, when a macrophage ingests a pathogenic microorganism, the pathogen becomes trapped in a phagosome which then fuses with a lysosome to form a phagolysosome. Within the phagolysosome, enzymes and toxic peroxides digest the pathogen. Bacteria, dead tissue cells, and small mineral particles are all examples of objects that may be phagocytized.

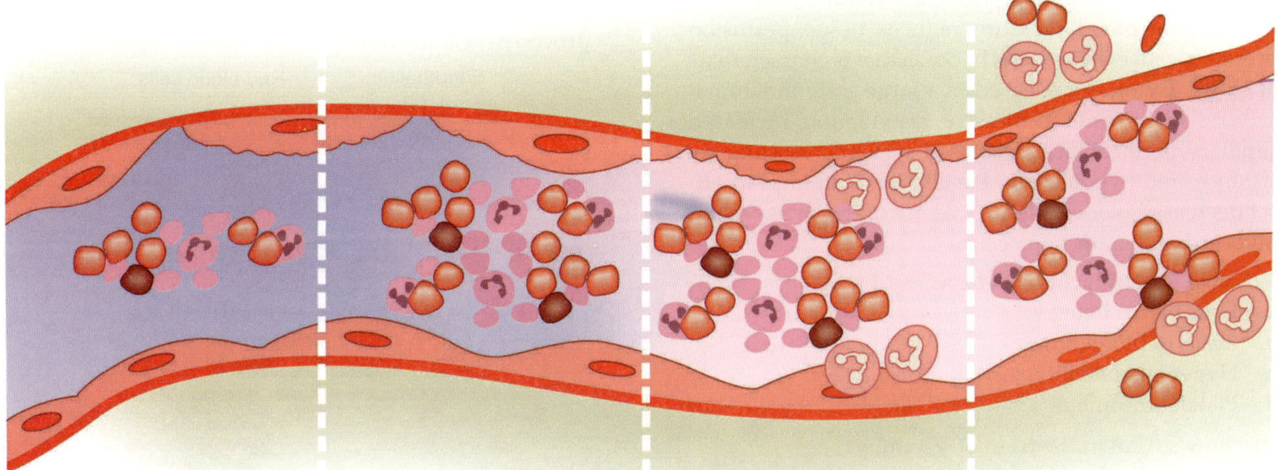

Sequence of changes in the exudation of leucocytes. A, Normal axial flow of blood with central column of cells and peripheral zone of cell-free plasma. B, Margination and pavementing of neutrophils with narrow plasmatic zone. C, Adhesion of neutrophils to endothelial cells with pseudopods in the intercellular junctions. D, Emigration of neutrophils and diapedesis with damaged basement membrane.

27. Primary causes of non-inflammatory edema include all EXCEPT:

a. Increase in intravascular hydrostatic pressure
b. Increased vascular permeability
c. Diminished plasma colloid oncotic pressure
d. Lymphatic obstruction

Differences between Transudate and Exudate.

Feature	Transudate	Exudate
1. *Definition*	Filtrate of blood plasma without changes in endothelial permeability	Oedema of inflamed tissue associated with increased vascular permeability
2. *Character*	Non-inflammatory oedema	Inflammatory oedema
3. *Protein content*	Low (less than 1 gm/dl); mainly albumin, low fibrinogen; hence no tendency to coagulate	High (2.5-3.5 gm/dl), readily coagulates due to high content of fibrinogen and other coagulation factors
4. *Glucose content*	Same as in plasma	Low (less than 60 mg/dl)

Cond...

Ans. **25. d.** BCL-2 **26. d.** Phagocytosis **27. b.** Increased vascular permeability

Cond...

Feature	*Transudate*	*Exudate*
5. *Specific gravity*	Low (less than 1.015)	High (more than 1.018)
6. *pH*	> 7.3	< 7.3
7. *LDH*	Low	High
8. *Effusion LDH/ Serum LDH ratio*	< 0.6	> 0.6
9. *Cells*	Few cells, mainly mesothelial cells and cellular debris	Many cells, inflammatory as well as parenchymal
10. *Examples*	Oedema in congestive cardiac failure	Purulent exudate such as pus

28. Following pathogenetic mechanisms operate in septic shock EXCEPT:

a. Increased peripheral vascular resistance
b. Metabolic abnormality
c. Direct toxic endothelial injury
d. Activation of the complement

Septic shock can be defined as sepsis-induced hypotension that persists despite treatment with intravenous fluids. Low blood pressure reduces tissue perfusion pressure, causing the tissue hypoxia that is characteristic of shock. Cytokines released in a large scale inflammatory response result in massive vasodilation, increased capillary permeability, decreased systemic vascular resistance, and hypotension. Finally, in an attempt to offset decreased blood pressure, ventricular dilatation and myocardial dysfunction occur.

29. Virchow's triad includes all EXCEPT:

a. Endothelial injury
b. Stasis of blood flow
c. Hypercoagulability
d. Platelet thrombus

Virchow's triad or the triad of Virchow

It describes the three broad categories of factors that are thought to contribute to thrombosis.

- Hypercoagulability
- Hemodynamic changes (stasis, turbulence)
- Endothelial injury/dysfunction

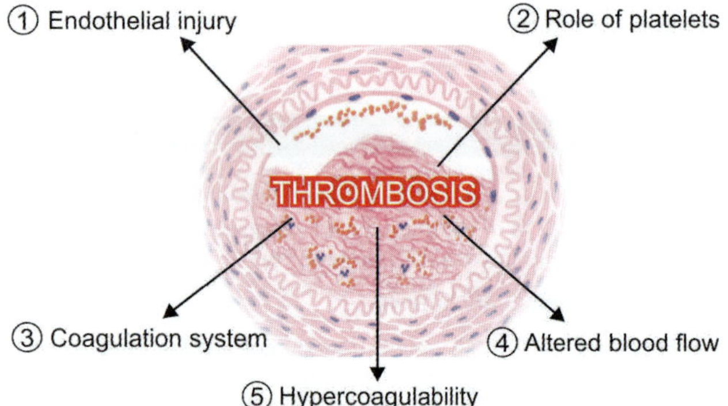

Major factors in pathophysiology of thrombus formation.

30. All of the following occur in hemostasis EXCEPT:

a. Vasospasm of blood vessel
b. Platelet plug formation
c. Dissolution of clot by plasmin
d. Formation of fibrin clot

Hemostasis has three major steps: 1) vasoconstriction, 2) temporary blockage of a break by a platelet plug, and 3) blood coagulation, or formation of a fibrin clot. These processes seal the hole until tissues are repaired.

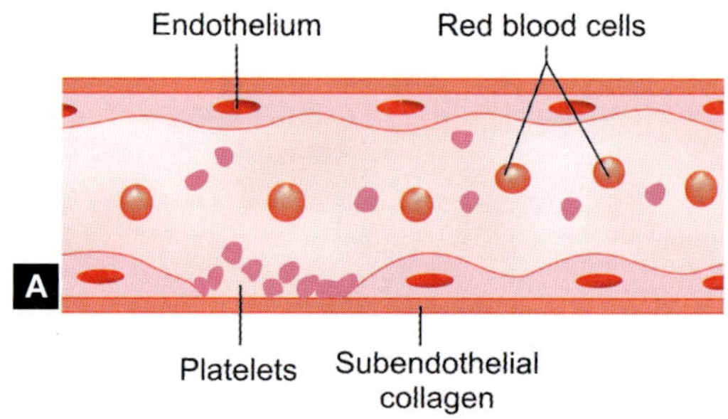

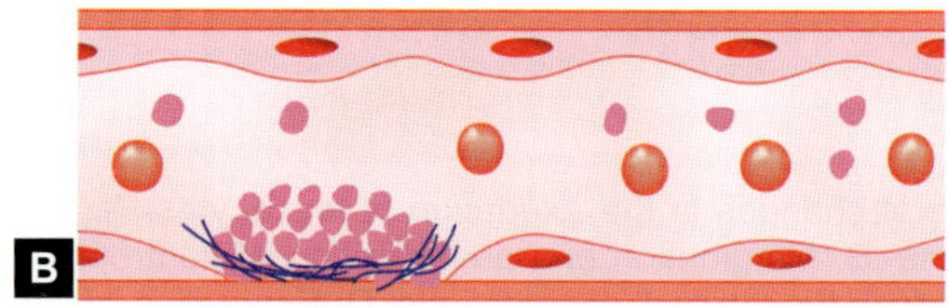

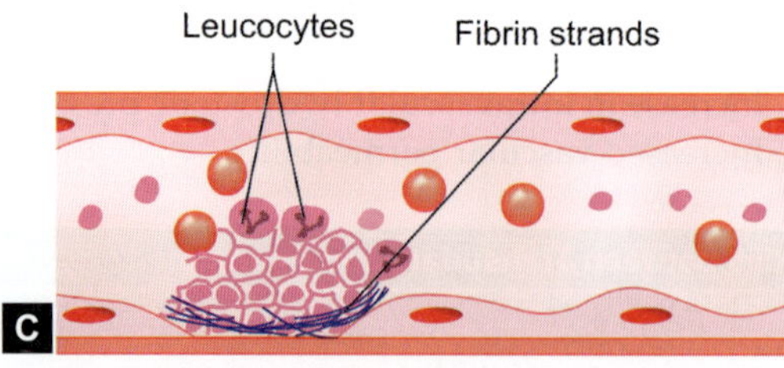

Role of endothelial injury and platelet activation in thrombosis. A, Endothelial injury exposes subendothelial matrix to circulating blood. B, This triggers three platelet steps involving platelet activation: adhesion, release and aggregation. Platelet release is associated with release of granules (alpha granules and dense bodies). C, Concurrent activation of coagulation cascade generates fibrin strands and thrombin forming a tight meshwork called thrombus.

Ans. 28. **a.** Increased per... 29. **d.** Platelet thrombus 30. **c.** Dissolution of clot by plasmin

31. Periodic acid Schiff stain shows black positivity in:

a. Megakaryoblasts b. Monoblasts
c. Lymphoblasts d. Myeloblasts

The periodic acid Schiff stain demonstrates glycogen and related mucopolysaccharides. Myeloid or monocytic blasts are typically weakly positive or negative. A granular (may be fine, coarse, or block) PAS pattern with a negative background is characteristic of lymphoblastic leukemia. PAS staining is positive in the erythroid population in erythroblastic leukemias.

Morphologic characteristics of the blast cells in Romanowsky stains

	Feature	Myeloblast	Lymphoblast
1.	Size	10-18 μm	10-18 μm
2.	Nucleus	Round or oval	Round or oval
3.	Nuclear chromatin	Fine meshwork	Slightly clumped
4.	Nuclear membrane	Very fine	Fairly dense
5.	Nucleoli	2-5	1-2
6.	Cytoplasm	Scanty, blue, agranular, Auer rods may be seen	Scanty, clear blue, agranular

32. Micro-albuminuria is defined as:

a. Protein levels of 10-50 mg/L
b. Protein levels of 51-300 mg/L
c. Protein levels of 301-600 mg/L
d. Protein levels of 601-900 mg/L

Microalbuminuria can be diagnosed from a 24-hour urine collection (between 30–300 mg/24 hours) or, more commonly, from elevated concentrations in a spot sample (30 to 300 mg/L). Both must be measured on at least two of three measurements over a two- to three-month period.

33. Organelle playing an important role in apoptosis:

a. Nucleus b. Mitochondria
c. Golgi complex d. Endoplasmic reticulum

After the cell has been initiated into self destruct mode, cell death signaling mechanisms get activated from intrinsic (mitochondrial) and extrinsic (cell death receptor activated) pathways.

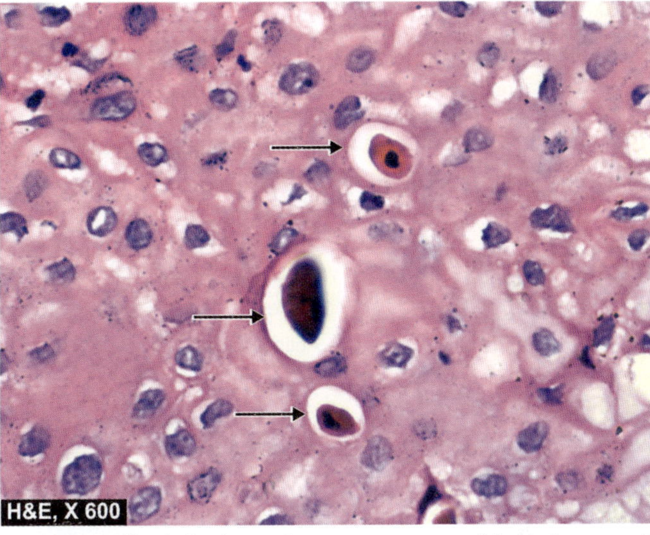

Apoptotic bodies in the layer of squamous mucosa (shown by arrows). The dead cell seen in singles, is shrunken, the nucleus has clumped chromatin, while the cytoplasms in intensely eosinophilic. There is no inflammation, unlike necrosis.

34. All of the following are macrophage EXCEPT:

a. Monocyte b. Kupffer cells
c. Microglia d. RBC

Red blood cells (**RBCs**), also called **erythrocytes**, are the most common type of blood cell and the vertebrate organism's principal means of delivering oxygen (O_2) to the body tissues—via blood flow through the circulatory system.

35. Granuloma is seen in all EXCEPT:

a. TB b. Syphilis
c. Mycoplasma d. Leprosy

Granulomas are seen in a wide variety of diseases, both infectious and non-infectious. Infections that are characterized by granulomas include tuberculosis, leprosy, histoplasmosis, cryptococcosis, coccidioidomycosis, blastomycosis and cat scratch disease. Examples of non-infectious granulomatous diseases are sarcoidosis, Crohn's disease, berylliosis, granulomatosis with polyangiitis, Churg-Strauss syndrome, pulmonary rheumatoid nodules and aspiration of food and other particulate material into the lung.

Principal granulomatous conditions.

		Conditions	Etiologic agent	Special characteristics
i.	BACTERIAL			
	1.	Tuberculosis*	Mycobacterium tuberculosis	Tuberculous granulomas with central caseation necrosis; acid-fast bacilli.
	2.	Leprosy*	Mycobacterium leprae	Foamy histiocytes with acid-fast bacilli (lepromatous); epithelioid cell granulomas (tuberculoid).
	3.	Syphilis*	Treponema pallidum	Gummas composed of histiocytes; plasma cell infiltration; central necrosis.

Contd...

Ans. 31. c. Lymphoblasts 32. b. Protein levels... 33. b. Mitochondria 34. d. RBC 35. c. Mycoplasma

Contd...

	Conditions	Etiologic agent	Special characteristics
4.	Granuloma inguinale (Donovanosis)	C. donovani (Donovan body)	Anal and genital lesions; macrophages and neutrophils show Donovan bodies.
5.	Brucellosis (Mediterranean fever)	Brucella abortus	Dairy infection to humans; enlarged reticuloendothelial organs (lymph nodes, spleen, bone marrow); non-specific granulomas.
6.	Cat scratch disease	Coccobacillus	Lymphadenitis; reticuloendothelial hyperplasia; granulomas with central necrosis and neutrophils.
7.	Tularaemia (Rabbit fever)	Francisella (Pasteurella) tularensis	Necrosis and suppuration (acute); tubercles hard or with minute central necrosis (chronic).
8.	Glanders	Actinobacillus mallei	Infection from horses and mules; subcutaneous lesions and lymphadenitis; infective granulomas.
II.	FUNGAL		
1.	Actinomycosis* (bacterial)	Actinomycetes israelii	Cervicofacial, abdominal and thoracic lesions; granulomas and abscesses with draining sinuses; sulphur granules.
2.	Blastomycosis	Blastomyces dermatitidis	Cutaneous, systemic and lung lesions; suppuration; ulceration and granulomas.
3.	Cryptococcosis	Cryptococcus neoformans	Meninges, lungs and systemic distribution; organism yeast-like with clear capsule.
4.	Coccidioidomycosis	Coccldioides immitis	Meninges, lungs and systemic distribution; granulomas and abscesses; organism cyst containing endospores.
III.	PARASITIC		
	Schistosomiasis (Bilharziasis)	*Schistosoma mansoni, hematobium, japonicum*	Eggs and granulomas in gut, liver, lung; schistosome pigment; eosinophils in blood and tissue.
IV.	MISCELLANEOUS		
1.	Sarcoidosis*	Unknown	Non-caseating granulomas (hard tubercles); asteroid and Schaumann bodies in giant cells.
2.	Crohn's disease (Regional enteritis)	Unknown ? Bacteria, ?? Viruses	Transmural chronic inflammatory infiltrates; non-caseating sarcoid-like granulomas.
3.	Silicosis	Silica dust	Lung lesions, fibrocollagenous nodules.
4.	Berylliosis	Metallic beryllium	Sarcoid-like granulomas in lungs; fibrosis; inclusions in giant cells (asteroids, Schaumann bodies, crystals).
5.	Foreign body granulomas	Talc, suture, oils, wood splinter etc.	Non-caseating granulomas with foreign body giant cells; demonstration of foreign body.

*Diseases discussed in this chapter.

36. All of the following are true for lactoferrin EXCEPT:

a. It is present in secondary granules of neutrophil
b. It is present in exocrine secretion of body
c. It has great affinity for iron
d. It transports iron for erythropoiesis

The main role of transferrin is to deliver iron from absorption centers in the duodenum and white blood cell macrophages to all tissues. Transferrin plays a key role in areas where erythropoiesis and active cell division occur.

37. All of the following vascular changes are observed in acute inflammation EXCEPT:

a. Vasodilation
b. Stasis of blood
c. Increased vascular permeability
d. Decreased hydrostatic pressure

Acute inflammation is characterized by marked vascular changes, including vasodilation, increased permeability and decreased blood flow, which are induced by the actions of various inflammatory mediators. Vasodilation occurs first at the arteriole level, progressing to the capillary level, and brings about a net increase in the amount of blood present, causing the redness and heat of inflammation. Increased permeability of the vessels results in the movement of plasma into the tissues, with resultant *stasis* due to the increase in the concentration of the cells within blood—a condition characterized by enlarged vessels packed with cells.

Ans. **36. d.** It transports iron... **37. d.** Decreased hydrostatic pressure

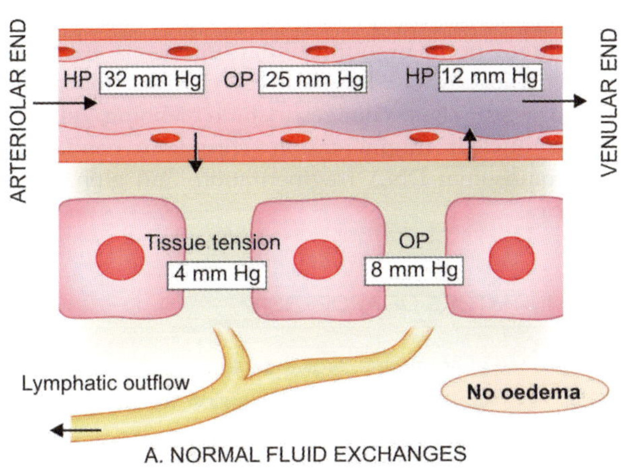

A. NORMAL FLUID EXCHANGES

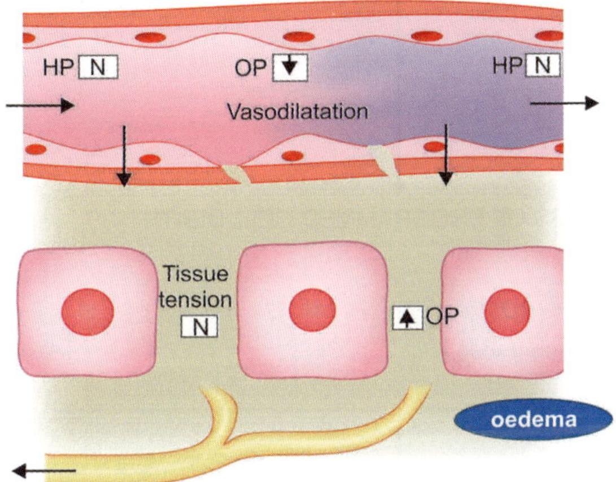

B. IN ACUTE INFLAMMATION

Fluid interchange between blood and extracellular fluid (ECF). (HP = hydrostatic pressure, OP = osmotic pressure).

38. Dystrophic calcification occurs in all EXCEPT:

a. Rheumatic heart disease b. TB Lymph node
c. Normal kidney d. Aneurysm

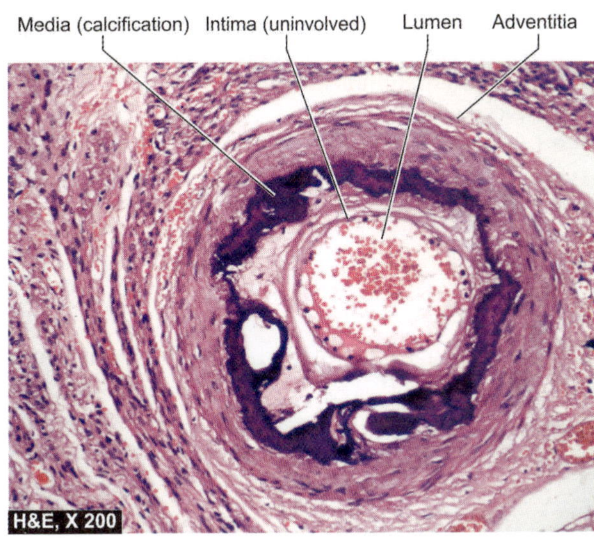

Dystrophic calcification in degenerated tunica media of muscular artery of uterine myometrium in Mönckeberg's arteriosclerosis.

Metastatic calcification is deposition of calcium salts in otherwise normal tissue, because of elevated serum levels of calcium, which can occur because of deranged metabolism as well as increased absorption or decreased excretion of calcium and related minerals, as seen in hyperparathyroidism.

39. Coagulative necrosis is seen in all EXCEPT:

a. Myocardial infarction b. Burns
c. TB d. Hypoxic injury to brain

For unclear reasons, hypoxic death of cells within the central nervous system can result in liquefactive necrosis. This is a process in which lysosomes turn tissues into pus as a result of lysosomal release of digestive enzymes. Loss of tissue architecture means that the tissue can be liquefied. This process is not associated with bacterial action or infection.

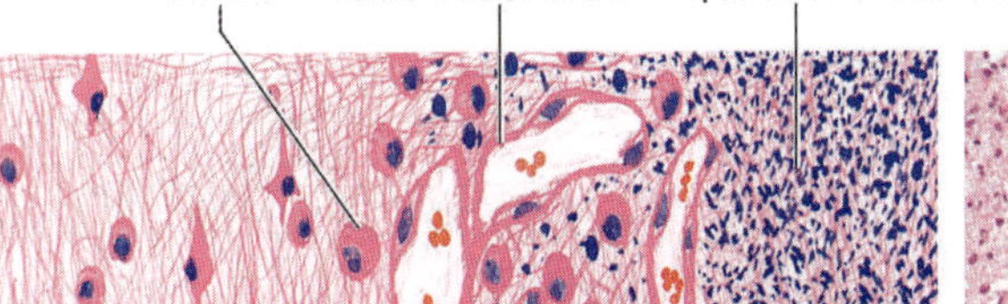
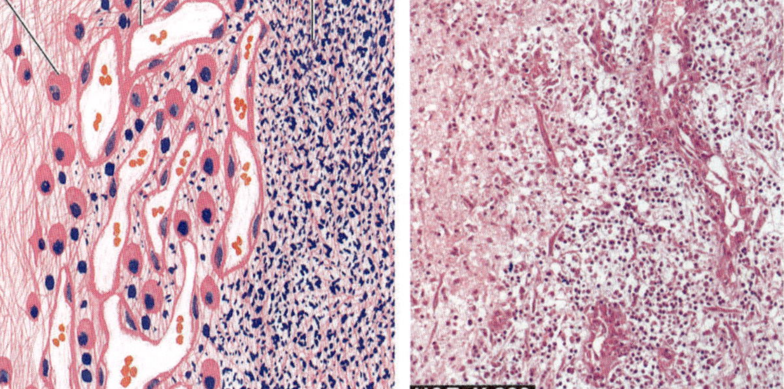

Liquefactive necrosis brain. The necrosed area on right side of the field shows a cystic space containing cell debris, while the surrounding zone shows granulation tissue and gliosis.

Ans. **38. c.** Normal kidney **39. d.** Hypoxic injury to brain

40. The process of programmed gene directed cell death characterized by cell shrinkage, nuclear condensation and fragmentation is known as:

a. Necrosis
b. Chromatolysis
c. Pyknosis
d. Apoptosis

Apoptosis is the process of programmed cell death that may occur in multicellular organisms. Biochemical events lead to characteristic cell changes (morphology) and death. These changes include blebbing, cell shrinkage, nuclear fragmentation, chromatin condensation, chromosomal DNA fragmentation, and global mRNA decay.

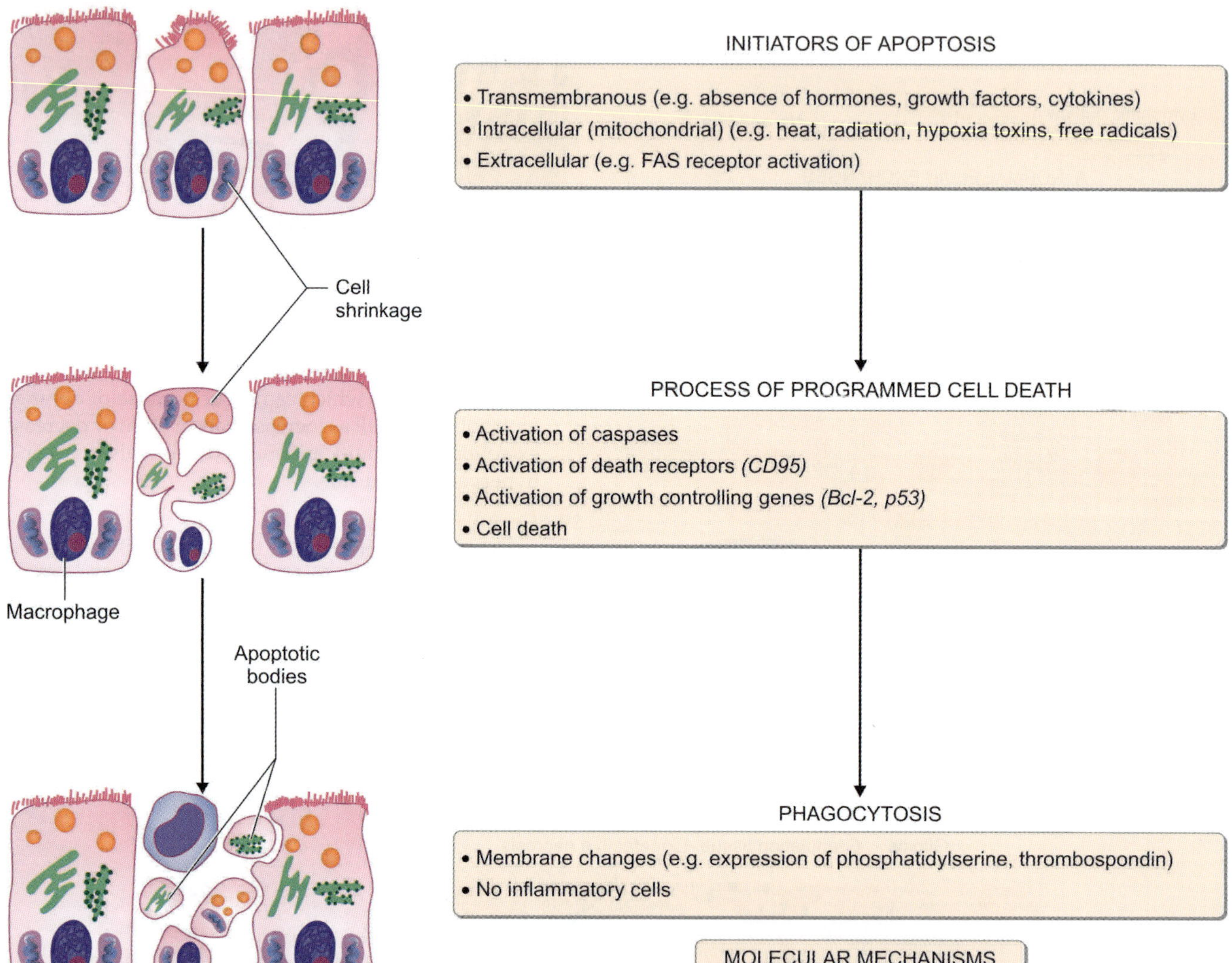

Molecular mechanism of apoptosis contrasted with sequence of morphologic changes.

41. True for reversible cell injury:

a. Formation of small amorphous densities in the mitochondrial matrix
b. Dilation of the ER
c. Formation of blebs in the plasma membrane
d. All of the above

The ultrastructural changes of reversible cell injury include:

- Blebbing
- Blunting
- Distortion of microvilli
- Loosening of intercellular attachments
- Mitochondrial changes
- Dilation of the endoplasmic reticulum

Ans. **40. d.** Apoptosis **41. d.** All of the above

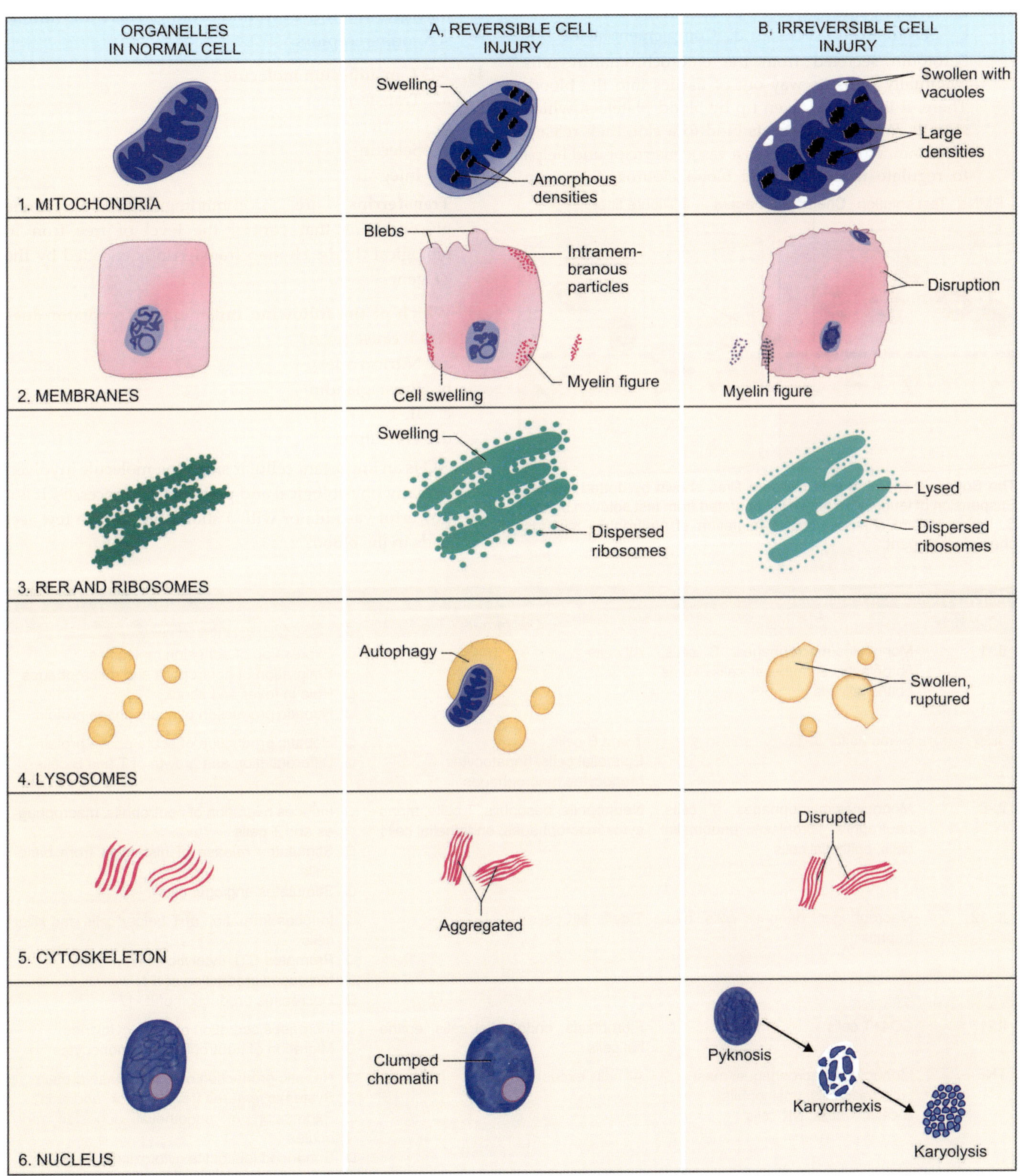

Ultrastructural changes during cell injury due to hypoxia-ischemia.

42. Chemotaxis is promoted by all EXCEPT:

a. Lymphokine
b. Kallikrein
c. Serotonin
d. Complement factor 5

Serotonin secreted from the enterochromaffin cells eventually finds its way out of tissues into the blood. There, it is actively taken up by blood platelets, which store it. When the platelets bind to a clot, they release serotonin, where it serves as a vasoconstrictor and helps to regulate hemostasis and blood clotting. Serotonin also is a growth factor for some types of cells, which may give it a role in wound healing. There are various serotonin receptors.

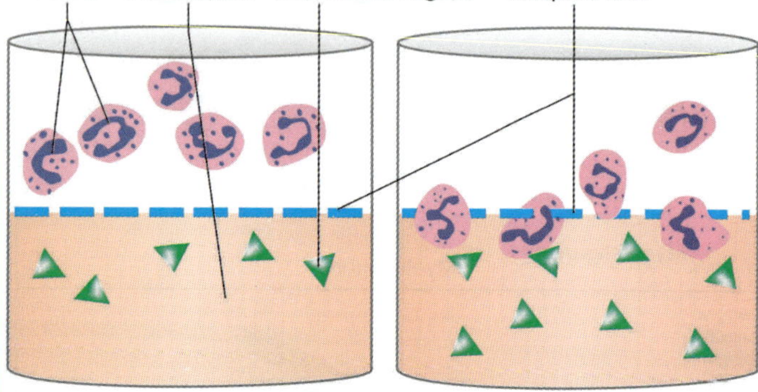

The Boyden's chamber with millipore filter, shown by dotted line. A, Suspension of leucocytes above is separated from test solution below. B, Lower half of chamber shows migration of neutrophils towards chemotactic agent.

43. NOT an adhesion molecule:

a. Transferrin
b. Interferon
c. Selectin
d. Integrin

Transferrins are iron-binding blood plasma glycoproteins that control the level of free iron in biological fluids. Human transferrin is encoded by the *TF* gene.

44. Which of the following inflammatory mediator does NOT cause fever?

a. Nitric oxide
b. Prostaglandin
c. IL-1
d. TNF-alpha

NO is an important cellular signaling molecule involved in many physiological and pathological processes. It is a powerful vasodilator with a short half-life of a few seconds in the blood.

Major cytokines in Inflammation

Cytokine	*Cell source*	*Cell target*	*Main actions*
IL-1	Monocytes/macrophages, B cells, fibroblasts, endothelial cells, some epithelial cells	All cells	❑ Expression of adhesion molecules ❑ Emigration of neutrophils and macrophages ❑ Role in fever and shock ❑ Hepatic production of acute phase protein
IL-6	Same as for IL-1	T and B cells, Epithelial cells, hepatocytes, Monocytes/macrophages	❑ Hepatic production of acute phase protein ❑ Differentiation and growth of T and B cells
IL-8	Monocytes/macrophages, T cells, neutrophils, fibroblasts, endothelial cells, epithelial cells	Neutrophils, basophils, T cells, monocytes/macrophages, endothelial cells	❑ Induces migration of neutrophils, macrophages and T cells ❑ Stimulates release of histamine from basophils ❑ Stimulates angiogenesis
IL-12	Macrophages, dendritic cells, neutrophils	T cells, NK cells	❑ Induces formation of T helper cells and killer cells ❑ Promotes CTL cytolytic activity ❑ Increases production of IFN-γ ❑ Decreases production of IL-17
IL-17	CD4+T cells	Fibroblasts, endothelial cells, epithelial cells	❑ Increases secretion of other cytokines ❑ Migration of neutrophils and monocytes
TNF-α	Monocytes/macrophages, mast cells/basophils, eosinophils, B cells, T cells, NK cells	All cells except RBCs	❑ Hepatic production of acute phase protein ❑ Systemic features (fever, shock, anorexia) ❑ Expression of endothelial adhesion molecules ❑ Enhanced leucocyte cytotoxicity ❑ Induction of pro-inflammatory cytokines

Contd...

Ans. **42. c.** Serotonin **43. a.** Transferrin **44. a.** Nitric oxide

Contd...

Cytokine	*Cell source*	*Cell target*	*Main actions*
IFN- γ	T cells, NK cells	All cells	❑ Activation of macrophages and NK cells ❑ Stimulates secretion of Igs by B cells ❑ Differentiation of T helper cells
MCP-1	Fibroblasts, smooth muscle cells, blood mononuclear cells	Monocytes/macrophages, NK cells, T cells	❑ Chemoattractant for monocytes, T cells and NK cells ❑ Stimulates release of histamine from basophils
Eotaxin	Alveolar cells, myocardium	Eosinophils, basophils	❑ Chemoattractant for eosinophils and Basophils ❑ Induces allergic pulmonary disease
PF-4	Platelets, megakaryocytes	Fibroblasts, endothelial cells	❑ Chemoattractant for fibroblasts ❑ Inhibitory to hematopoietic precursors and endothelial cell proliferation

IL= interleukin; TNF = tumour necrosis factor; IFN = interferon; MCP = monocyte chemotactic protein; PF = platelet factor.

45. In shock all happens EXCEPT:

a. Constrcition of capacitance vessels
b. Dilatation of arterioles
c. Decrease in cardiac output
d. Heart rate decreases

The baroreceptors in the arteries detect the resulting hypotension, and cause the release of epinephrine and norepinephrine. Norepinephrine causes predominately vasoconstriction with a mild increase in heart rate, whereas epinephrine predominately causes an increase in heart rate with a small effect on the vascular tone; the combined effect results in an increase in blood pressure.

STAGE	*PATHOGENESIS*	*EFFECTS*
COMPENSATED (INITIAL) SHOCK	i) Widespread vasoconstriction ii) Fluid conservation by kidney iii) Stimulation of adrenal medulla	• Tachycardia • Cool clammy skin
PROGRESSIVE DECOMPENSATED SHOCK	i) Pulmonary hypoperfusion ii) Tissue ischaemia	• ↓ Cardiac output • Mental confusion • ↓ Urinary output • Tachypnoea
IRREVERSIBLE DECOMPENSATED SHOCK	i) Progressive vasodilatation ii) ↑ Vascular permeability iii) Myocardial depressant factor (MDF) iv) Pulmonary hypoperfusion v) Anoxic damage vi) Hypercoagulability	• Brain: Hypoxic encephalopathy • Heart: Focal myocardial necrosis • Lungs: ARDS • Kidney: ATN • Adrenals: Necrosis • GI: Haemorrhagic gastroenteropathy • Liver: Necrosis • Blood : DIC

Mechanisms and effects of three stages of shock.

46. True about apoptosis are all EXCEPT:

a. Inflammation is present
b. Chromosomal breakage
c. Clumping of chromatin
d. Cell shrinkage

Apoptosis is a highly regulated and controlled process that confers advantages during an organism's lifecycle. For example, the separation of fingers and toes in a developing human embryo occurs because cells between the digits undergo apoptosis. Characteristically, unlike necrosis, there is no acute inflammatory reaction around apoptosis.

47. Von Brun's nest is seen in:

a. Normal urothelium
b. Transitional cell carcinoma
c. Squamous cell carcinoma
d. Adenocarcinoma

Cystitis glandularis arises from and merges with **Von Brunn's nests**, which are groups of urothelial cells (cells of urinary tract) within the lamina propria and submucosa, formed from budding from the surface mucosa. They are considered normal.

Ans. 45. **d.** Heart rate decreases 46. **a.** Inflammation is present
47. **a.** Normal urothelium

48. N-Myc amplification is associated with which tumour:

a. Burkitt lymphoma
b. Squamous cell carcinoma lung
c. Astrocytoma
d. Neuroblastoma

Amplification and overexpression of N-Myc can lead to tumorigenesis. Excess N-Myc is associated with a variety of tumors, most notably neuroblastomas where patients with amplification of the N-Myc gene tend to have poor outcomes.

Important Oncogenes, their Mechanism of Activation and Associated Human Tumours

Type	Proto-oncogene	Mechanism	Associated Human Tumours
1. Growth factors			
i. *PDGF-β*	*SIS*	Overexpression	Gliomas, sarcoma
ii. *TGF-α*	*RAS*	Overexpression	Carcinomas, astrocytoma
iii. *FGF*	*HST-1* INT-2	Overexpression Amplification	Bowel cancers Breast cancer
iv. *c-MET*	HGF	Overexpression	Follicular carcinoma thyroid
2. Receptors for growth factors			
i. *EGF* receptors	*ERB B1(HER 1)* ERB B2 (*HER 2/neu*)	Overexpression Amplification	Squamous cell carcinoma lung, glioblastoma Ca breast, ovary, stomach, lungs
ii. *c-KIT* receptor (Steel factor)	c-KIT	Point mutation	GIST
iii. RET receptor	RET	Point mutation	MEN type 2A and type 2B, medullary ca thyroid
iv. FMS-like tyrosine kinase receptor	FLT-3 gene	Point mutation	Acute myeloid leukaemia
3. Cytoplasmic signal transduction proteins			
GTP-bound	*RAS*	Point mutation	Common in 1/3rd human tumours, Ca lung, colon, pancreas
Non-GF receptor tyrosine kinase	*ABL-BCR*	Translocation	CML, acute leukaemias
4. Nuclear transcription factors			
C-MYC	MYC	Translocation	Burkitt's lymphoma
N-MYC	*MYC*	Amplification	Neuroblastoma, small cell Ca lung
L-MYC	*MYC*	Amplification	Small cell Ca lung
5. Cell cycle regulatory proteins			
Cyclins	*Cyclin D* *Cyclin E*	Translocation Overexpression	Ca breast, liver, mantle cell lymphoma Ca breast
CDKs	*CDK4*	Amplification	Glioblastoma, melanoma, sarcomas

49. The cell most sensitive to ischemia is:

a. Myocardial fibres
b. Glial cells of brain
c. Renal tubular epithelium
d. Cortical neuron

Neurons are more susceptible than glial cells to ischemia, hypoxia or hypoglycemia; and the phylogenetically newer regions of the brain, including the cortex and cerebellum, are affected to a greater extent than the brainstem.

50. The percentage of pulmonary emboli, that proceed to pulmonary infarction, is approximately:

a. 0-5%
b. 5-15%
c. 20-30%
d. 30-40%

Only 10% to **15%** of all **pulmonary emboli** result in pulmonary **infarction**.

Ans. **48. d.** Neuroblastoma **49. d.** Cortical neuron **50. b.** 5-15%

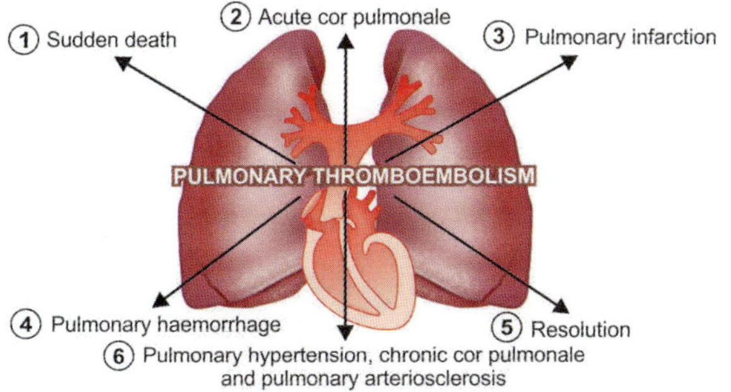

Major consequences of pulmonary embolism.

51. **Myofibroblast is seen in:**
   a. Normal connective tissue
   b. Muscle septa
   c. Wound margin
   d. Bronchus

Myofibroblasts can contract by using smooth muscle type actin-myosin complex, rich in a form of actin called alpha-smooth muscle actin. These cells are then capable of speeding wound repair by contracting the edges of the wound.

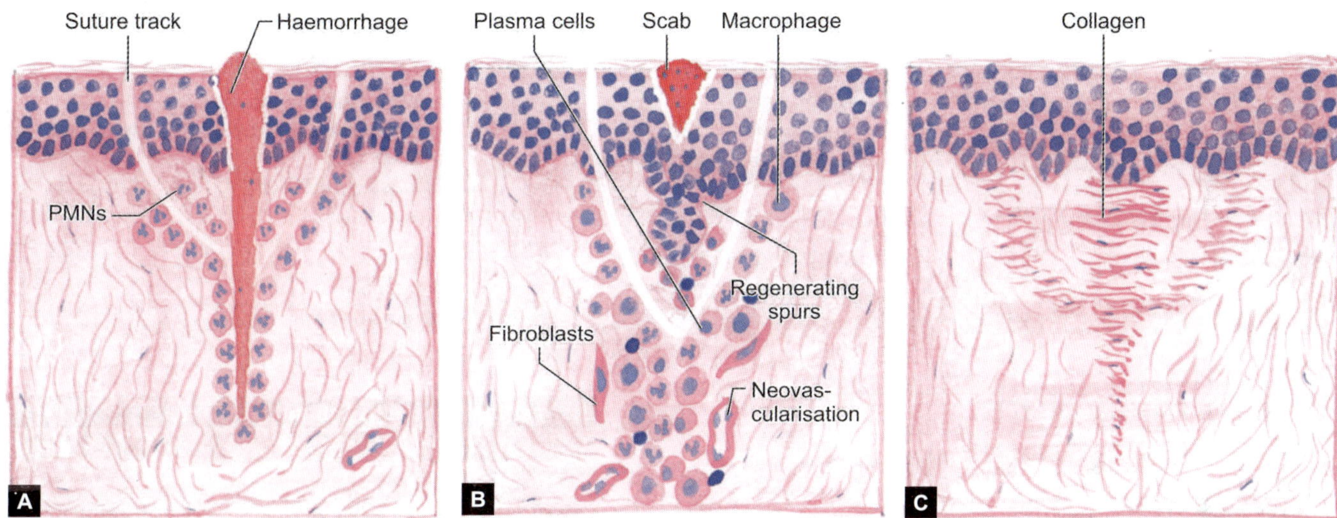

Primary union of skin wounds. A, The incised wound as well as suture track on either side are filled with blood clot and there is inflammatory response from the margins. B, Spurs of epidermal cells migrate along the incised margin on either side as well as around the suture track. Formation of granulation tissue also begins from below. C, Removal of suture at around 7th day results in scar tissue at the sites of incision and suture track.

52. **Articular cartilage is made up of:**
   a. Type I collagen
   b. Type II collagen
   c. Type III collagen
   d. Type IV collagen

Collagen, type II, alpha 1 (primary osteoarthritis, spondyloepiphyseal dysplasia, congenital), also known as **COL2A1**, is a human gene that provides instructions for the production of the pro-alpha1(II) chain of type II collagen. This gene encodes the alpha-1 chain of type II collagen, a fibrillar collagen found in cartilage and the vitreous humor of the eye.

53. **Macrophages are seen in:**
   a. Early inflammation
   b. Chronic inflammation
   c. Wound repair
   d. Healing

In general, acute inflammation is mediated by granulocytes, whereas chronic inflammation is mediated by mononuclear cells such as monocytes and lymphocytes.

Morphology and functions of inflammatory cells.

Morphology	*Features*	*Mediators*
A, Polymorph	i. Initial phagocytosis of bacteria and foreign body ii. Acute inflammatory cell	i. Primary granules (MPO, lysozyme, cationic proteins, acid hydrolases, elastase) ii. Secondary granules (lysozyme, alk. phosph, collagenase, lactoferrin) iii. Tertiary granules (gelatinase, cathepsin) iv. Reactive oxygen metabolites

Contd...

Ans. **51. c.** Wound margin **52. b.** Type II collagen **53. b.** Chronic inflammation

Contd...

Morphology	*Features*	*Mediators*
B, Monocyte/Macrophage	i. Bacterial phagocytosis ii. Chronic inflammatory cell iii. Regulates lymphocyte response	i. Acid and neutral hydrolases (lysosomal) Cationic protein ii. Phospholipase iii. Prostaglandins, leukotrienes iv. IL-1 v.
C, Lymphocyte	i. Humoral and cell-mediated immune responses ii. Chronic inflammatory cell iii. Regulates macrophage response	i. B cells: antibody production ii. T cells: delayed hypersensitivity, cytotoxicity
D, Plasma Cell	i. Derived from B cells ii. Chronic inflammatory cell	i. Antibody synthesis ii. Antibody secretion
E, Eosinophil	i. Allergic states ii. Parasitic infestations iii. Chronic inflammatory cell	i. Reactive oxygen metabolites ii. Lysosomal (major basic protein, cationic protein, eosinophil peroxidase, neurotoxin) iii. PGE_2 synthesis
F, Basophil/Mast Cell	i. Receptor for IgE molecules ii. Electron-dense granules	i. Histamine ii. Leukotrienes iii. Platelet activating factor

CLINICAL PATHOLOGY

54. Decreased ESR is found in:

a. TB
b. Multiple myeloma
c. Polycythemia
d. Rheumatoid arthritis

Raised ESR

- Pregnancy
- Inflammation
- Anemia or
- Rheumatoid arthritis

ESR is decreased in

- Polycythemia
- Sickle cell anemia
- Hereditary spherocytosis and
- Congestive heart failure

55. Leukocytosis is seen in all EXCEPT:

a. Brucellosis
b. Acute MI
c. Megaloblastic anemia
d. Diphtheria

In megaloblastic anemia, neutrophil granulocytes may show multisegmented nuclei ("senile neutrophil"). This is thought to be due to decreased production and a compensatory prolonged lifespan for circulating neutrophils, which increase numbers of nuclear segments with age.

Normal white blood cell counts in health.

	Absolute Count
TLC	
Adults	4,000–11,000/µl
Infants (Full term, at birth)	10,000–25,000/µl
Infants (1 year)	6,000–16,000/µl
Children (4–7 years)	5,000–15,000/µl
Children (8–12 years)	4,500–13,500/µl
DLC in Adults	
Polymorphs (neutrophils) 40–75%	2,000–7,500/µl
Lymphocytes 20–50%	1,500–4,000/µl
Monocytes 2–10%	200–800/µl
Eosinophils 1–6%	40–400/µl
Basophils <l%	10–100/µl

56. Biomarker to rise earliest in myocardial infarction is:

a. Troponin-I
b. Creatine kinase-MB
c. Myoglobin
d. Troponin-T

Myoglobin is a sensitive marker for muscle injury, making it a potential marker for heart attack in patients with chest pain. However, elevated myoglobin has low specificity for acute myocardial infarction (AMI) and thus CK-MB, cTnT, ECG, and clinical signs should be taken into account to make the diagnosis. Levels of **myoglobin** start to **rise** within 2-3 hours of a **heart attack.**

Ans. **54. c.** Polycythemia **55. c.** Megaloblastic anemia **56. c.** Myoglobin

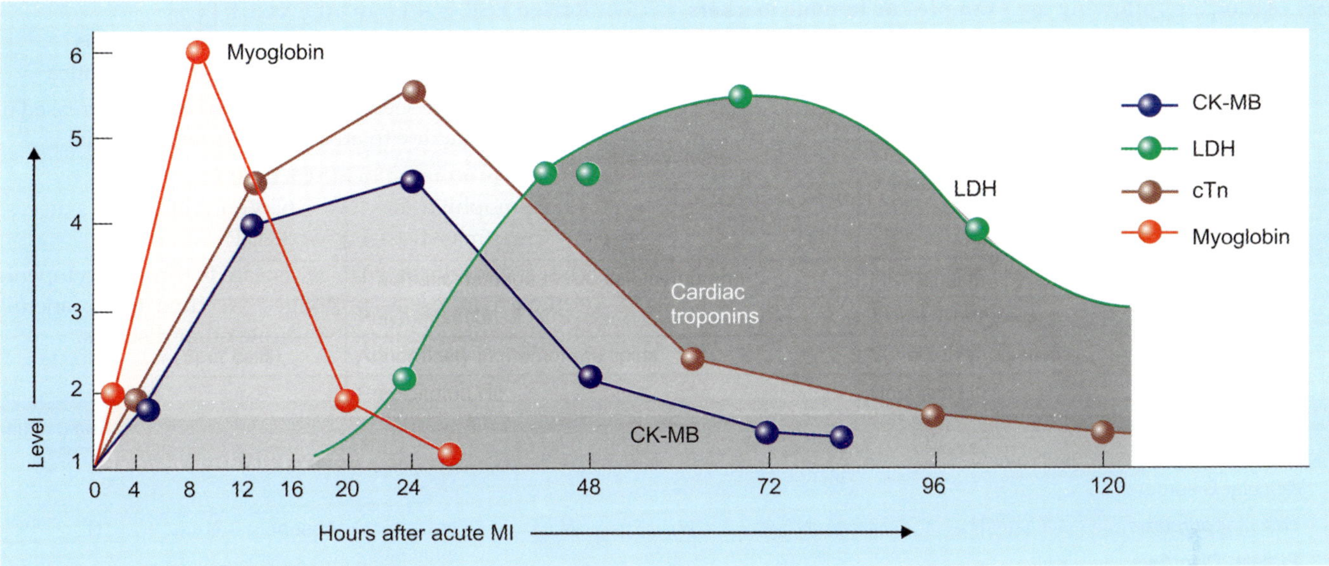

Time course of serum cardiac markers for the diagnosis of acute MI.

57. CEA is elevated in all of the following EXCEPT:

a. Alcoholic cirrhosis b. Ca colon
c. Ulcerative colitis
d. Emphysema

CEA measurement is mainly used as a tumor marker to monitor colorectal carcinoma treatment, to identify recurrences after surgical resection, for staging or to localize cancer spread through measurement of biological fluids. CEA levels may also be raised in gastric carcinoma, pancreatic carcinoma, lung carcinoma, breast carcinoma, and medullary thyroid carcinoma, as well as some non-neoplastic conditions like ulcerative colitis, pancreatitis, cirrhosis, Crohn's disease, hypothyroidism as well as in smokers.

Important tumour markers.

Marker	*Cancer*
1. Oncofoetal antigens	
i. *Alpha-foetoprotein (AFP)*	Hepatocellular carcinoma, non-seminomatous germ cell tumours of testis
ii. *Carcinoembryonic antigen (CEA)*	Cancer of bowel, pancreas, breast
2. Enzymes	
i. *Prostate acid phosphatase (PAP)*	Prostatic carcinoma
ii. *Neuron-specific enolase (NSE)*	Neuroblastoma, oat cell carcinoma lung
iii. *Lactic dehydrogenase (LDH)*	Lymphoma, Ewing's sarcoma
3. Hormones	
i. *Human chorionic gonadotropin (hCG)*	Trophoblastic tumours, non-seminomatous germ cell tumours of testis
ii. *Calcitonin*	Medullary carcinoma thyroid
iii. *Catecholamines and vanillylmandelic acid (VMA)*	Neuroblastoma, pheochromocytoma
iv. *Ectopic hormone production*	Paraneoplastic syndromes
4. Cancer associated proteins	
i. *CA-125*	Ovary
ii. *CA 15-3*	Breast
iii. *CA 19-9*	Colon, pancreas, breast
iv. *CD30*	Hodgkin's disease, anaplastic large cell lymphoma (ALCL)
v. *CD25*	Hairy cell leukaemia (HCL), adult T cell leukaemia lymphoma (ATLL)
vi. *Monoclonal immunoglobulins*	Multiple myeloma, other gammopathies
vii. *Prostate specific antigen (PSA)*	Prostate carcinoma

Ans. **57. d.** Emphysema

58. All of the following are examples of tumour markers EXCEPT:

a. Alpha fetoprotein
b. Prostatic alkaline phosphatase
c. Calcitonin
d. Metabolites of catecholamines

Prostatic acid phosphatase (PAP), also **prostatic specific acid phosphatase** (PSAP), is an enzyme produced by the prostate. It may be found in increased amounts in men who have prostate cancer or other diseases. The highest levels of acid phosphatase are found in metastasized prostate cancer.

59. Raised ESR is seen in all EXCEPT:

a. Polycythemia rubra
b. Giant cell arteritis
c. Multiple myeloma
d. Myositis rheumatica

The erythrocyte sedimentation rate (ESR) is decreased in polycythemia due to an increase in zeta potential.

60. aPTT is prolonged in all EXCEPT:

a. Hemophilia
b. Von Willebrand's disease
c. Christmas disease
d. ITP

The hallmark of ITP is isolated thrombocytopenia (which manifest as prolonged bleeding time); anemia and/or neutropenia may indicate other diseases.

Major laboratory findings in common hemostatic disorders.

Disorder	*Platelet Count*	*BT*	*PT*	*APTT*	*TT*	*FDP's*	*F-VIII*	*F-IX*
I. Vascular Disorders								
Vascular purpuras	N	N	N	N	N	Absent	N	N
II. Platelet Disorders								
1. *ITP*	↓	↑	N	N	N	Absent	N	N
2. *Heparin*	↓	↑	N	↑	↑	Absent	N	N
3. *TTP*	↓	↑	N	N	N	Absent	N	N
III. Coagulation Disorders								
1. *Hemophilia A*	N	↑	N	↑	↑	Absent	↓	N
2. *Hemophilia B*	N	↑	N	↑	↑	Absent	N	↓
3. *von Willebrand's*	N	↑	N	↑	↑	Absent	↓	N
4. *Vit. K deficiency*	N	↑	↑	↑	↑	Absent	N	N
5. *Liver disease*	N	↑	↑	↑	N	Absent	N	N
IV. DIC	↓	↑	↑	↑	↑	Present	↓	↓

61. ASO titres are used in the diagnosis of:

a. Osteo-arthritis
b. Ankylosing spondylitis
c. Acute rheumatic fever
d. Acute rheumatoid arthritis

When the body is infected with streptococci, it produces antibodies against the various antigens that the streptococci produce. ASO is one such antibody. A raised or rising levels can indicate past or present infection. Historically it was one of the first bacterial markers used for diagnosis and follow up of rheumatic fever or scarlet fever.

62. Increase in leukocyte/neutrophilic alkaline phosphatase is a feature of:

a. Malaria
b. Eosinophilia
c. Leukemoid reaction
d. CML

Serum leukocyte alkaline phosphatase is normal or elevated in leukemoid reaction, but is depressed in chronic myelogenous leukemia.

63. Marker for carcinoma colon is:

a. AFP
b. CA-125
c. CEA
d. HCG

CEA are glycosylphosphatidylinositol (GPI) cell surface anchored glycoproteins whose specialized sialofucosylated glycoforms serve as functional colon carcinoma L-selectin and E-selectin ligands, which may be critical to the metastatic dissemination of colon carcinoma cells.

64. AFP (alpha feta protein) is raised in:

a. Renal carcinoma
b. Pancreatic carcinoma
c. Prostatic carcinoma
d. Hepatic carcinoma

AFP is a marker that is useful in HCC, if it is markedly elevated. At levels less >20 sensitivity is 41-65% and specificity is 80-94%. However, at levels >200 sensitivity is 31, specificity is 99%.

65. CA-125 is marker for:

a. Breast cancer
b. Ovarian cancer
c. Pancreatic cancer
d. Colon cancer

CA-125 is the most frequently used biomarker for ovarian cancer detection.

Ans. **58. b.** Prostatic alka... **59. a.** Polycythemia rubra **60. d.** ITP **61. c.** Acute rheumatic... **62. c.** Leukemoid react... **63. c.** CEA **64. d.** Hepatic... **65. b.** Ovarian cancer

66. **Tumor marker related to both colon carcinoma and pancreatitis:**
a. CA-125 b. CA-19-9
c. CD-15-3 d. All of the above

CA 19-9 can be elevated in many types of gastrointestinal cancer, such as colorectal cancer, esophageal cancer and hepatocellular carcinoma. Apart from cancer, elevated levels may also occur in pancreatitis, cirrhosis, and diseases of the bile ducts. It can be elevated in people with obstruction of the bile ducts.

67. **Alpha fetoprotein is raised in all EXCEPT:**
a. Teratocarcinoma
b. Down syndrome
c. Embryonal cell carcinoma
d. Hepatocellular carcinoma

In Down syndrome, AFP and uE3 levels are low whereas HCG levels are high.

68. **CA 19-9 is a marker for which of the following:**
a. Pancreatic carcinoma b. Breast carcinoma
c. Ovarian carcinoma d. Lung carcinoma

CA19-9 (carbohydrate antigen 19.9) is a tumor marker that is frequently elevated in pancreatic cancer. However, it lacks sensitivity and specificity, not least because 5% of people lack the Lewis (a) antigen and cannot produce CA19-9. It has a sensitivity of 80% and specificity of 73% in for detecting pancreatic adenocarcinoma, and is used for following known cases rather than diagnosis.

69. **Leucopenia is NOT seen in:**
a. Viral infection
b. Acute pyogenic bacterial infection
c. Malnutrition
d. Enteric fever

Acute pyogenic bacterial infections causes neutrophilic leuocytosis.

70. **Low LAP score may be seen in the following EXCEPT:**
a. CML
b. Paroxysmal nocturnal hemoglobinuria
c. Autoimmune hemolytic anemia
d. Polycythemia vera

Higher levels of leucocytic alkaline phosphatase are seen in polycythemia vera (PV), essential thrombocytosis (ET), primary myelofibrosis (PM), and the leukemoid reaction.

71. **A patient Shweta presented with raised serum alkaline phosphate and raised parathormone level along with low calcium and low phosphate level is likely to have:**
a. Primary hyperparathyroidism
b. Paget's disease
c. Osteoporosis
d. Vitamin D deficiency

Typical biochemical findings in osteomalacia
- Low serum and urinary calcium
- Low serum phosphate, ***except*** in cases of renal osteodystrophy
- Elevated serum alkaline phosphatase (due to an increase in compensatory osteoblast activity)
- Elevated parathyroid hormone (due to low calcium)

72. **Alkaline phosphatase is increased beyond 30 KA units in:**
a. Obstructive jaundice b. Thyrotoxicosis
c. Polycythemia vera d. Erythroblastosis fetalis

Diagnosis of obstructive jaundice is based on elevated Alkaline phosphatase (twice the normal value more, 30 K.A. units), SGPT and total serum bilirubin.

Liver function tests

Tests	*Significance*
I. Tests for Manufacture and Excretion of Bile	
1. *Bilirubin:*	
i. Serum bilirubin (0.3-1.3 mg/dl)	Increased in hepatocellular, obstructive and hemolytic disease, Gilbert's disease
ii. In faeces	Absent in biliary obstruction
iii. In urine	Conjugated bilirubinuria in patients of hepatitis
2. *Urobilinogen:*	Increased in hepatocellular and hemolytic diseases, absent in biliary obstruction
3. *Bile acid (Bile salts):*	Increased in serum and detectable in urine in cholestasis
II. Serum Enzyme Assays	
1. *Alkaline phosphatase* (33-96 U/L)	Increased in hepatobiliary disease (highest in biliary obstruction), bone diseases, pregnancy
2. *γ-Glutamyl transpeptidase (γ-GT)* (9-58 IU/L)	Rise parallels alkaline phosphatase but is specific for hepatobiliary diseases
3. *Transaminases:*	

Contd...

Ans. 66. **b.** CA-19-9 67. **b.** Down... 68. **a.** Pancreatic... 69. **b.** Acute...
70. **d.** Polycythemia... 71. **d.** Vitamin... 72. **a.** Obstructive...

Contd...

Tests	*Significance*
i. SGOT (AST) (12-38 U/L)	Increased in tissue injury to liver as well as to other tissues like in myocardial infarction
ii. SGPT (ALT) (7-41 U/L)	Increase is fairly specific for liver cell injury
4. *Other enzymes:*	
i. 5'-Nucleotidase	Rise parallels alkaline phosphatase but more specific for diseases of hepatic origin
ii. Lactate dehydrogenase (115-221 U/L)	Increased in tumours involving the liver
iii. Cholinesterase	Decreased in hepatocellular disease, malnutrition
III. Tests for Metabolic Functions	
1. *Amino acid and protein metabolism:*	
i. Serum proteins (total = 6.7-8.6 g/dl; A/G ratio = 1.5-3:1)	Hypoalbuminaemia in hepatocellular diseases; hyperglobulinaemia in cirrhosis and chronic active hepatitis
ii. Immunoglobulins	Nonspecific alterations in IgA, IgG and IgM
iii. Clotting factors	Prothrombin time and partial thromboplastin time prolonged in patients with hepatocellular disease
iv. Plasma ammonia (19-60 μg/dl)	Increased in acute fulminant hepatitis, cirrhosis, hepatic encephalopathy
v. Aminoaciduria	In fulminant hepatitis
2. *Lipid and lipoprotein metabolism:*	
Blood lipids (total serum cholesterol <200 mg/dl; triglycerides < 150 mg/dl; and lipoprotein fractions)	Increased in cholestasis, decreased in acute and chronic diffuse liver disease and in malnutrition
3. *Carbohydrate metabolism:*	
Blood glucose and GTT	Decreased in hepatic necrosis
IV. Immunologic Tests	
1. *Nonspecific immunologic reactions:*	
i. Smooth muscle antibody	In hepatic necrosis
ii. Mitochondrial antibody	In primary biliary cirrhosis
iii. Antinuclear antibody and LE cell test	In chronic active hepatitis
2. *Antibodies to specific etiologic agents:*	
i. Antibodies to hepatitis B (HBsAg, HBc, HBeAg)	In hepatitis B
ii. Amoeba antibodies	Amoebic liver abscess
V. Ancillary Diagnostic Tests	
1. *Ultrasound examination*	Cholestasis of various etiologies; SOLs, US-guided-FNAC/ liver biopsy
2. *FNAC and/or percutaneous liver biopsy*	Unknown cause of hepatocellular disease, hepatomegaly and splenomegaly; long-standing hepatitis; PUO and SOLs of the liver

73. Medullary carcinoma of thyroid is associated with increase in:

a. Calcitonin
b. Thyroglobulin
c. T3
d. T4

Medullary thyroid cancer (MTC) is a form of thyroid carcinoma which originates from the parafollicular cells (C cells), which produce the hormone calcitonin. Medullary tumors are the third most common of all thyroid cancers. They make up about 3% of all thyroid cancer cases.

Ans. 73 a. Calcitonin

Contrasting features of main histologic types of thyroid carcinoma.

	Feature	*Papillary carcinoma*	*Follicular carcinoma*	*Medullary carcinoma*	*Anaplastic carcinoma*
1.	*Frequency*	75-80%	10-20%	5%	5%
2.	*Age*	All ages	Middle to old age	Middle to old age; familial too	Old age
3.	*Female/male ratio*	3:1	2.5:1	1:1	1.5:1
4.	*Relation to radiation*	Maximum	Present	None	Present
5.	*Genetic alterations*	*RET* gene over-expression, *NTRK* gene rearrangement	*RAS* mutation, *PAX-PPAR γ1* fusion	*RET* point mutation	*p53* loss, β-catenin mutation
6.	*Cell of origin*	Follicular	Follicular	Parafollicular	Follicular
7.	*Gross*	Small, multifocal	Moderate size, nodular	Moderate size	Invasive growth
8.	*Pathognomonic* microscopy	Nuclear features, papillary pattern	Vascular and capsular invasion	Solid nests, amyloid stroma	Undifferentiated, spindle-shaped, giant cells
9.	*Regional metastases*	Common	Rare	Common	Common
10.	*Distant metastases*	Rare	Common	Rare	Common
11.	*10-year survival*	80-95%	50-70%	60-70%	5-10% (median survival about 2 months)

74. Which is NOT a tumour marker?

a. HCG b. HPL
c. CEA d. AFP

Human placental lactogen (**hPL**), also called **human chorionic somatomammotropin** (**HCS**), is a polypeptide placental hormone. Its structure and function is similar to that of human growth hormone. It modifies the metabolic state of the mother during pregnancy to facilitate the energy supply of the fetus. hPL has anti-insulin properties. hPL is a hormone secreted by the syncytiotrophoblast during pregnancy. Like human growth hormone, hPL is encoded by genes on chromosome 17q22-24.

75. All of the following conditions cause thrombocytopenia EXCEPT:

a. Giant hemangioma
b. Infectious mononucleosis
c. HIV infection
d. Iron deficiency anemia

Very commonly, the platelet count is slightly above the high limit of normal in iron deficiency anemia (this is mild thrombocytosis). This effect was classically postulated to be due to high erythropoietin levels in the body as a result of anemia, cross-reacting to activate thrombopoietin receptors in the precursor cells that make platelets; however, this process has not been corroborated. Such slightly increased platelet counts present no danger, but remain valuable as an indicator even if their origin is not yet known.

Causes of thrombocytopenia.
I. Impaired Platelet Production
1. *Generalised bone marrow failure e.g.*
Aplastic anaemia, leukaemia, myelofibrosis, megaloblastic anaemia, marrow infiltrations (carcinomas, lymphomas, multiple myeloma, storage diseases).
2. *Selective suppression of platelet production e.g.*
Drugs (quinine, quinidine, sulfonamides, PAS, rifampicin, anticancer drugs, thiazide diuretics), (heparin, diclofenac, acyclovir), alcohol intake.
II. Accelerated Platelet Destruction
1. *Immunologic thrombocytopenias e.g.*
ITP (acute and chronic), neonatal and post-transfusion (isoimmune), drug-induced, secondary immune thrombocytopenia (post-infection, SLE, AIDS, CLL, lymphoma).
2. *Increased consumption e.g.*
DIC, TTP, giant hemangiomas, microangiopathic hemolytic anaemia.
III. Splenic Sequestration
Splenomegaly
IV. Dilutional Loss
Massive transfusion of old stored blood to bleeding patients

Ans. **74. b.** HPL **75. d.** Iron deficiency anemia

76. A patient presented with fever, night sweats and weight loss. Clinical examination revealed painless lymphadenopathy. Microscopy shows Reed Sternberg cells. Most likely condition is:

a. HIV
b. Chronic lymphocytic leukemia
c. Hodgkin's lymphoma
d. Secondary TB

Contrasting features of Hodgkin's disease and non-Hodgkin's lymphoma.

Feature	Hodgkin's	Non-Hodgkin's
1. *Cell derivation*	B-cell mostly	90% B 10% T
2. *Nodal involvement*	Localised, may spread to contiguous nodes	Disseminated nodal spread
3. *Extranodal spread*	Uncommon	Common
4. *Bone marrow involvement*	Uncommon	Common
5. *Constitutional symptoms*	Common	Uncommon
6. *Chromosomal defects*	Aneuploidy	Translocations, deletions
7. *Spill-over*	Never	May spread to blood
8. *Prognosis*	Better (75-85% cure)	Bad (30-40% cure)

Features of Hodgkin's lymphoma:

- **Lymph nodes:** The most common symptom of Hodgkin's is the painless enlargement of one or more lymph nodes, or lymphadenopathy. The nodes may also feel rubbery and swollen when examined. The nodes of the neck and shoulders (cervical and supraclavicular) are most frequently involved (80–90% of the time, on average). The lymph nodes of the chest are often affected, and these may be noticed on a chest radiograph.
- Itchy skin
- Night sweats
- Unexplained weight loss
- **Splenomegaly:** Enlargement of the spleen occurs in about 30% of people with Hodgkin's lymphoma. The enlargement, however, is seldom massive and the size of the spleen may fluctuate during the course of treatment.
- **Hepatomegaly:** Enlargement of the liver, due to liver involvement, is present in about 5% of cases.

ABDOMINAL PATHOLOGY

77. Councilman bodies is a histological feature of:

a. Hemochromatosis
b. Acute viral hepatitis
c. Chronic viral hepatitis
d. Hepatocellular carcinoma

Councilman body, also known as **Councilman hyaline body**,

- It represents a hepatocyte that is undergoing apoptosis.
- It is an eosinophilic globule often surrounded by normal parenchyma found in the liver of individuals suffering from
  - Acute viral hepatitis,
  - Yellow fever, or other
  - Viral syndrome.

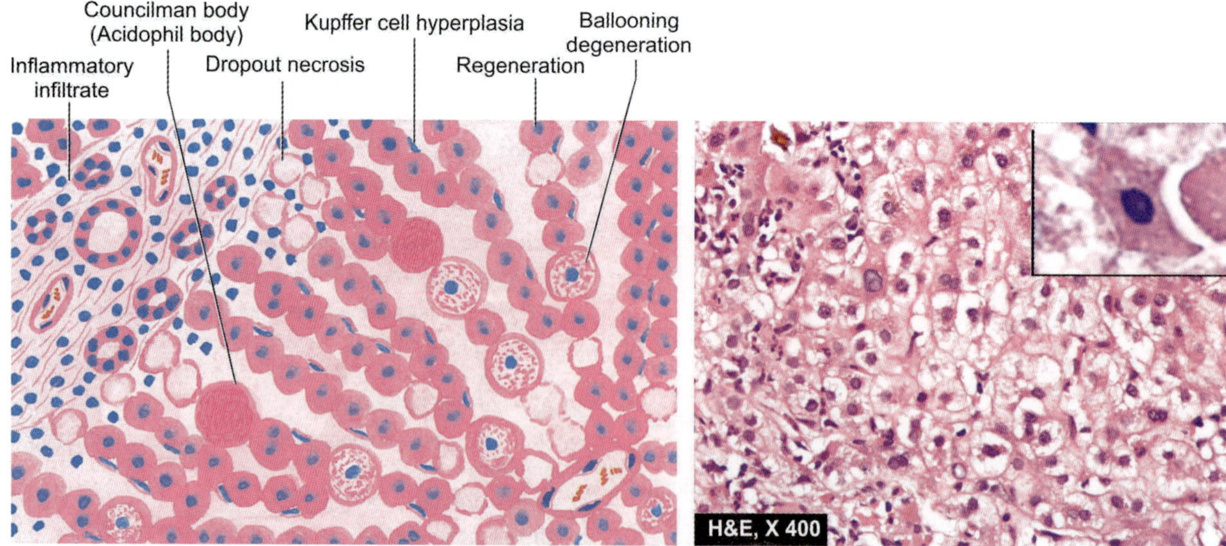

Acute viral hepatitis. The predominant histologic changes are: variable degree of necrosis of hepatocytes, most marked in zone 3 (centrilobular); and mononuclear cellular infiltrate in the lobule. Mild degree of liver cell necrosis is seen as ballooning degeneration while acidophilic Councilman bodies (inbox) are indicative of more severe liver cell injury.

Ans. **76. c.** Hodgkin's lym... **77. b.** Acute viral hepatitis

78. **Which of the following is a hallmark of chronic active hepatitis?**

a. Necrosis
b. Fibrosis
c. Councilman bodies
d. Ballooning degeneration

Chronic hepatitis with piecemeal (periportal) necrosis (or interface hepatitis) with or without fibrosis (formerly chronic active hepatitis)

- It is any case of hepatitis occurring for more than 6 months with portal based inflammation, fibrosis, disruption of the terminal plate, and piecemeal necrosis.
- This term has now been replaced by the diagnosis of 'chronic hepatitis'.

Chronic hepatitis without piecemeal necrosis (formerly called chronic persistent hepatitis)

- It has no significant periportal necrosis or regeneration with a fairly dense mononuclear portal infiltrate.
- Councilman bodies are frequently seen within the lobule.
- Instead it includes persistent parenchymal focal hepatocyte necrosis (apoptosis) with mononuclear sinusoidal infiltrates.

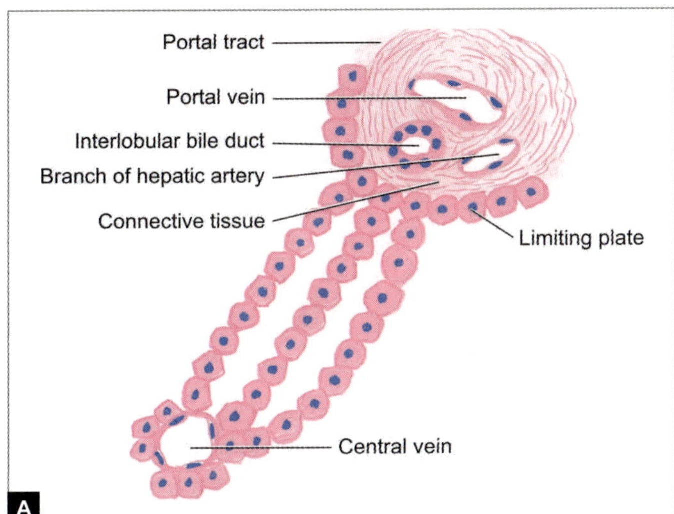

NORMAL HEPATIC LOBULE

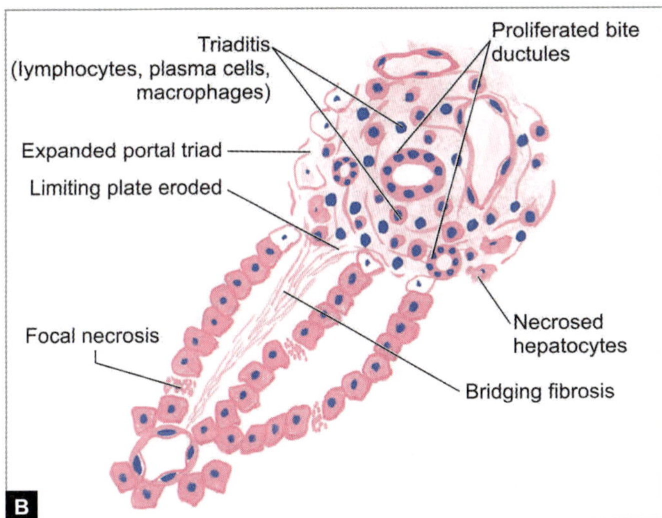

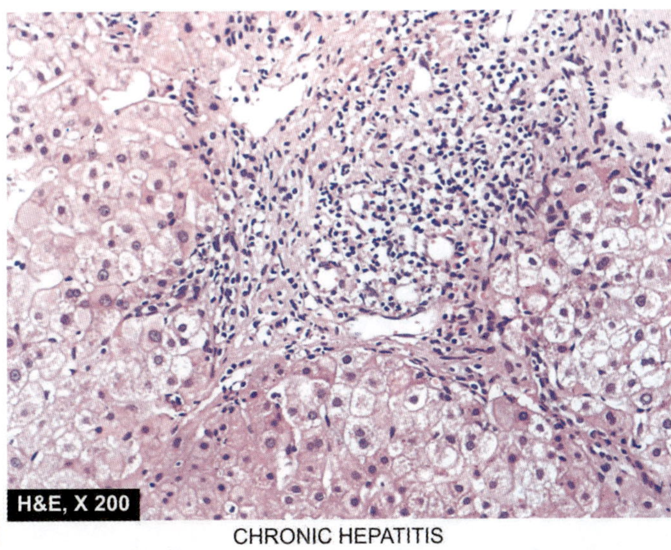

CHRONIC HEPATITIS

Chronic hepatitis. Diagrammatic representation of pathologic changes in chronic hepatitis (B) contrasted with normal morphology (A). Photomicrograph on right (C) shows stellate-shaped portal triad, with extension of fibrous spurs into lobules. The portal tract is expanded due to increased lymphomononuclear inflammatory cells which are seen to breach the limiting plate (i.e. hepatocytes at the interface of portal tract and lobule are destroyed).

Ans. 78. **a.** Necrosis

79. MC benign tumour of liver:
a. Nodular focal hyperplasia
b. Adenoma
c. Hemangioma
d. Hematoma

A **cavernous liver hemangioma** or **hepatic hemangioma** is a benign tumour of the liver composed of hepatic endothelial cells. It is the most common liver tumour, and is usually asymptomatic and diagnosed incidentally on radiological imaging.

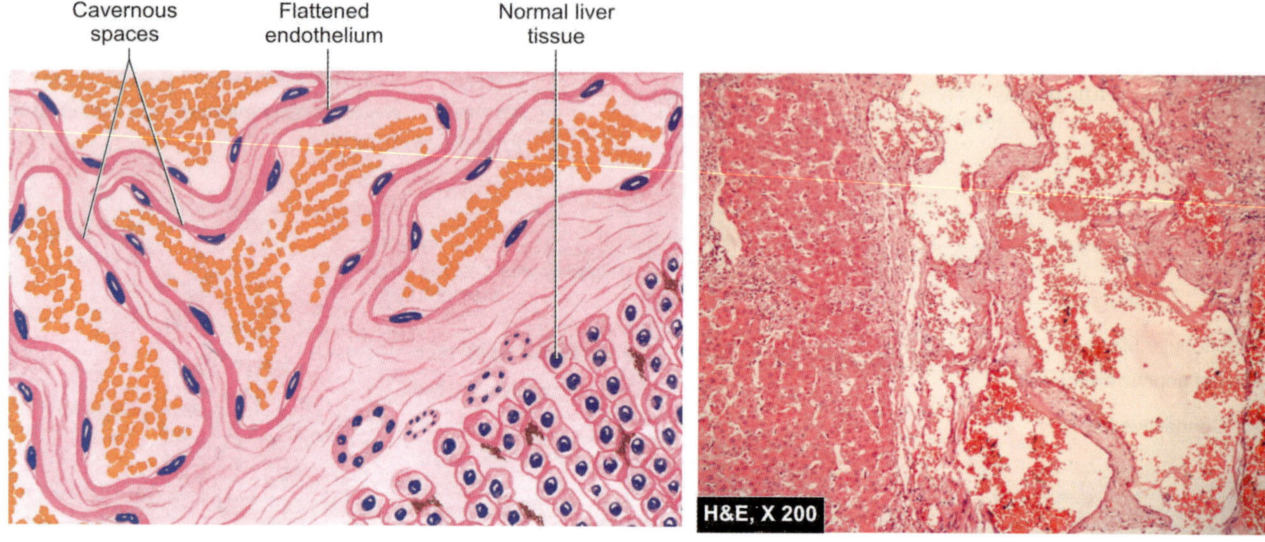

Cavernous hemangioma of the liver.

80. All are correctly matched EXCEPT:
a. Hepatitis B – ground glass hepatocytes
b. Reye's syndrome – ground glass hepatocytes
c. Alcohol and Wilson disease – Mallory hyaline
d. Acute hepatitis – councilman bodies

Liver biopsy in Reyes syndrome reveals diffuse, small lipid deposits in the hepatocytes (microvesicular steatosis) without significant necrosis or inflammation.

81. Call-Exner bodies are seen in:
a. Theca cell tumour
b. Yolk sac tumour
c. Granulosa cell tumour
d. Fibroma of ovary

Call–Exner bodies are small eosinophilic fluid-filled spaces between granulosa cells. The granulosa cells are usually arranged haphazardly around the space.
They are usually associated with Granulosa cell tumors.

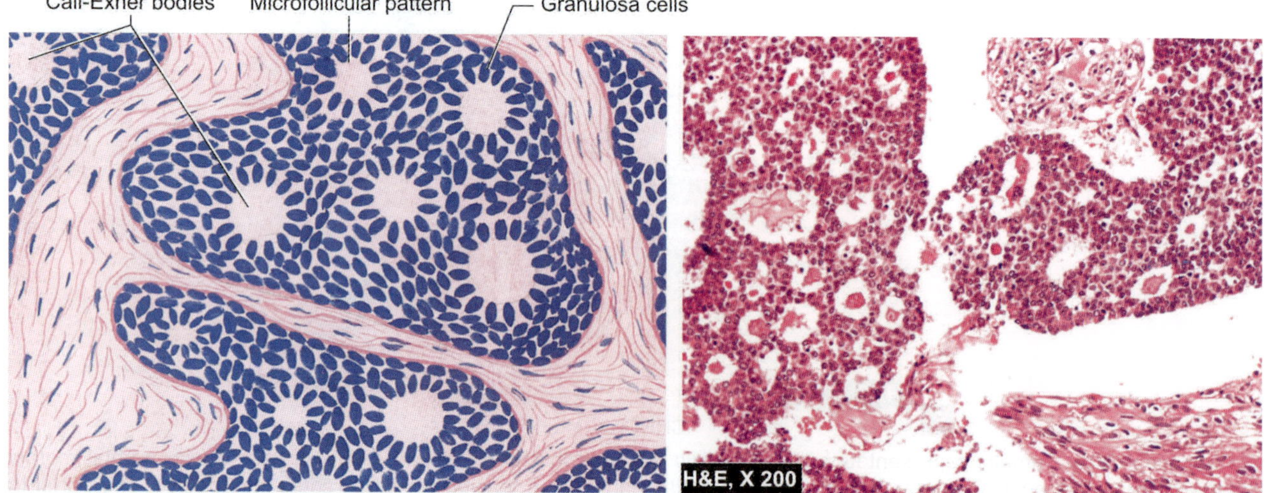

Granulosa cell tumour showing uniform granulosa cells and numerous rosette-like Call-Exner bodies containing central amorphous pink material surrounded by granulosa cells.

Ans. **79. c.** Hemangioma **80. b.** Reye's... **81. c.** Granulosa cell tumour

82. Mallory hyaline is present in all EXCEPT:
a. Alcoholic cirrhosis
b. Indian childhood cirrhosis
c. Primary biliary cirrhosis
d. Secondary biliary cirrhosis

Histology of secondary biliary cirrhosis
- Fibrosis divides liver into jigsaw-like pattern
- Septa contain large and small bile ducts with inspissated pigment
- Extensive proliferation of bile ductules and edema, particularly at interface of septa and parenchyma
- May have bile lakes, extensive feathery degeneration.

Contrasting features of major forms of biliary cirrhosis.

Feature	Primary biliary cirrhosis	Secondary biliary cirrhosis	Primary sclerosing cholangitis
1. *Etiology*	Possibly autoimmune; association with other autoimmune diseases	Extrahepatic biliary obstruction; biliary atresia	Possibly autoimmune; association with inflammatory bowel disease
2. *Age and sex*	Middle-aged women Male: Female = 1:9	Any age and either sex	Middle age Male: Female = 2:1
3. *Laboratory tests*	↑ Alkaline phosphatase ↑ Conjugated bilirubin Autoantibodies present	↑ Alkaline phosphatase ↑ Conjugated bilirubin	↑ Alkaline phosphatase ↑ Conjugated bilirubin Hypergammaglobulinaemia
4. *Pathologic changes*	Chronic destructive; cholangitis of intrahepatic bile ducts	Bile stasis in bile ducts, and sterile or pyogenic cholangitis	Fibrosing cholangitis with periductal fibrosis

83. Hepatocellular carcinoma – all are true EXCEPT:
a. Fibrolamellar variety has better prognosis
b. Uncommon in Asians
c. Associated with aflatoxin
d. Serum markers of hepatitis B and C are inc-reased frequently

The risk factors of HCC (which are most important) varies widely from country to country. In countries where Hepatitis B is endemic, such as China, Hepatitis B will be the predominant cause of Hepatocellular Carcinoma. Whereas in countries, such as the United States, where Hepatitis B is rare because of high vaccination rates, the major cause of HCC is Cirrhosis (often due to alcohol abuse).

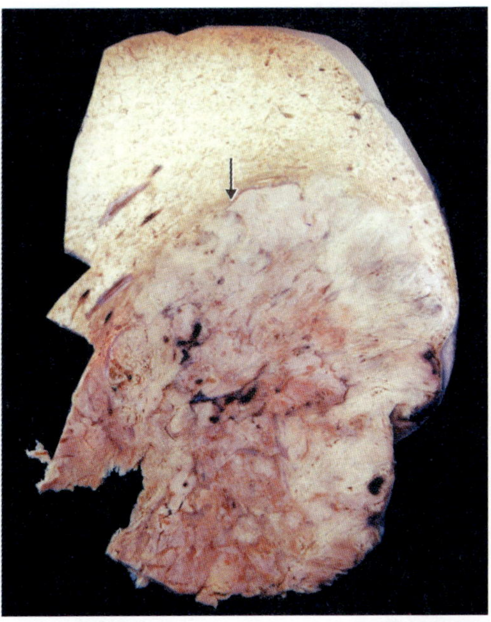

Hepatocellular carcinoma. Sectioned surface shows a single, large mass (arrow) with irregular borders and having central areas of necrosis, while rest of the hepatic parenchyma in the upper part of the picture shows many nodules of variable sizes owing to co-existent macronodular cirrhosis.

Ans. 82. **d.** Secondary bili... 83. **b.** Uncommon in Asians

84. Hydatid cyst is commonly found in:
a. Lungs
b. Liver
c. Kidney
d. Brain

In the human manifestation of the disease, *E. granulosus*, *E. multilocularis*, *E. oligarthrus* and *E. vogeli* are localized in the liver (in 75% of cases), the lungs (in 5–15% of cases) and other organs in the body such as the spleen, brain, heart, and kidneys (in 10–20% of cases).

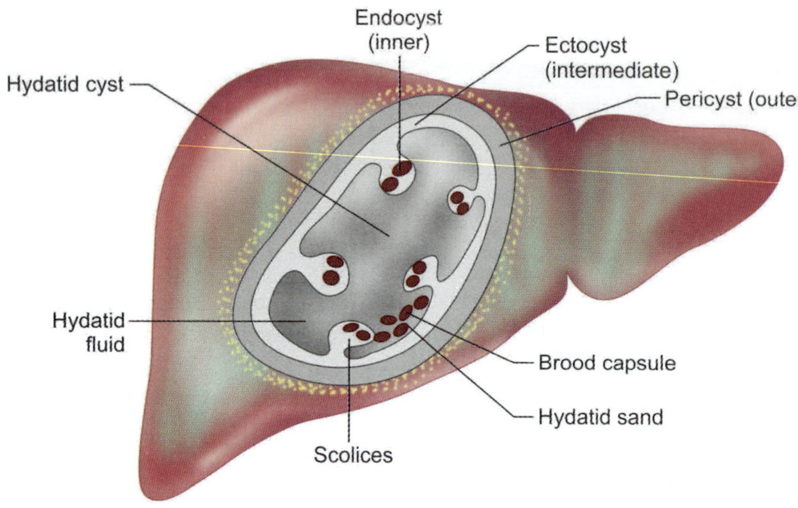

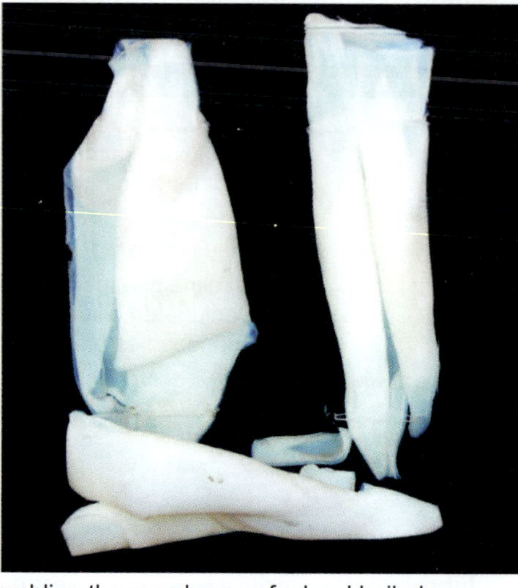

Hydatid cyst in the liver. The cyst wall is composed of whitish membrane resembling the membrane of a hard boiled egg.

85. Most common site of abscess formation due to amoeba is:
a. Lungs
b. Liver
c. Kidney
d. Brain

E. histolytica, as its name suggests (*histo–lytic* = tissue destroying), is pathogenic; infection can be asymptomatic or can lead to amoebic dysentery or amoebic liver abscess.

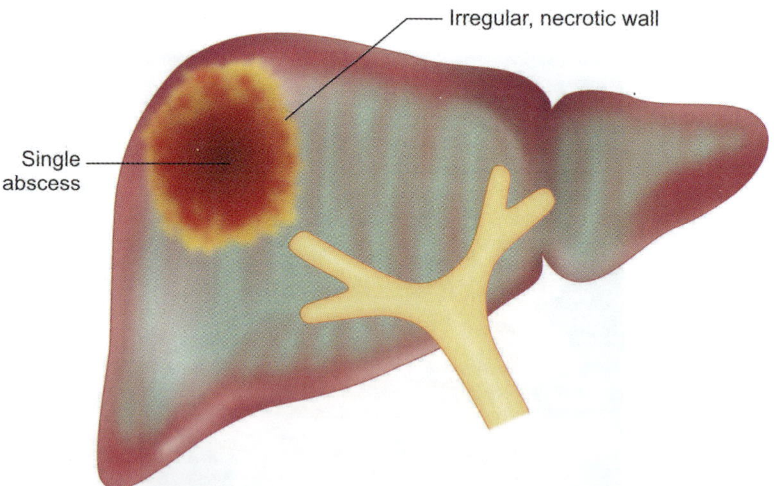

Amoebic liver abscess is commonly solitary and its wall is irregular and necrotic.

86. All of the following are features of non-alcoholic steatohepatitis EXCEPT:
a. Hepatocyte ballooning
b. Steatosis
c. Histological features are different from alcoholic steatohepatitis
d. Mallory bodies

It is difficult to distinguish alcoholic fatty liver disease (FLD) from nonalcoholic FLD, and both show microvesicular and macrovesicular fatty changes at different stages.

Ans. **84. b.** Liver **85. b.** Liver **86. c.** Histological features...

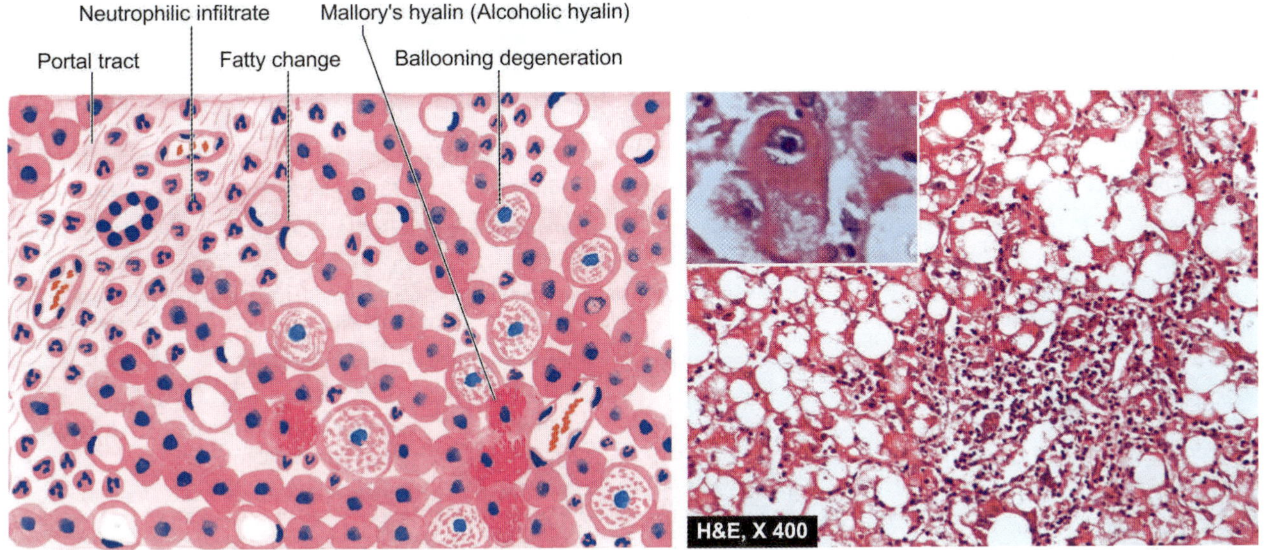

Alcoholic hepatitis. Liver cells show ballooning degeneration and necrosis with some containing Mallory's hyalin (Inbox). Fatty change and clusters of neutrophils are also present.

87. **Serum marker indicating active viral replication in Hepatitis B is:**
    a. HBsAg
    b. HBeAg
    c. HBcAg
    d. Anti-HBs

HBeAg (extracellular antigen) is a hepatitis B viral protein. It is an indicator of active viral replication; this means the person infected with Hepatitis B can likely transmit the virus on to another person (i.e. the person is infectious).

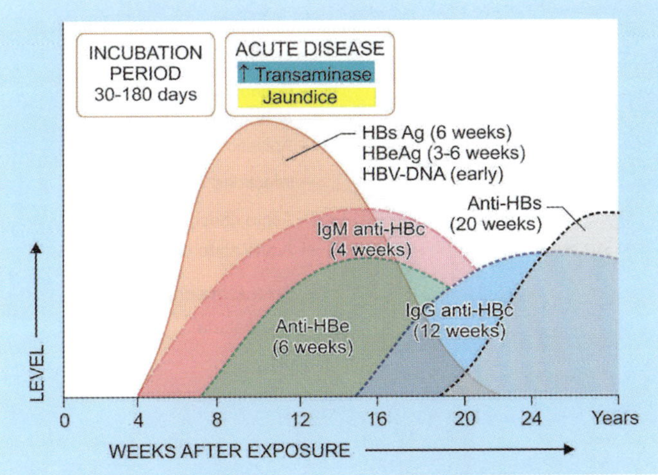

Sequence of serologic and viral markers in acute hepatitis B.

88. **Which of the following is also known as Australia antigen?**
    a. HBsAg
    b. HBeAg
    c. HBcAg
    d. HBV DNA

HBsAg (also known as the **Australia antigen**) is the surface antigen of the hepatitis B virus (HBV). It indicates current hepatitis B infection.

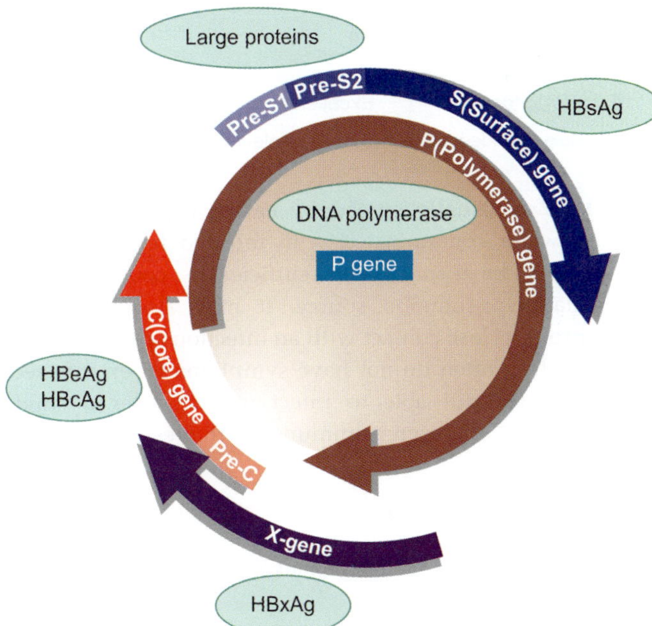

Genomic structure of hepatitis B virus (Dane particle).

89. **Hepatitis which spreads by fecal-oral route is:**
    a. Hepatitis A
    b. Hepatitis B
    c. Hepatitis C
    d. Hepatitis D

Ans. 87. **b.** HBeAg 88. **a.** HBsAg 89. **a.** Hepatitis A

Features of various types of hepatitis viruses.

	Feature	Hepatitis A	Hepatitis B	Hepatitis C	Hepatitis D	Hepatitis E
1.	*Agent*	HAV	HBV	HCV	HDV	HEV
2.	*Year identified*	1973	1965	1989	1977	1980
3.	*Viral particle*	27 nm	42 nm	30-60 nm	35-37 nm	32-34 nm
4.	*Genome*	RNA, ss, linear	DNA, ss/ds	RNA, ss, linear circular	RNA, ss, circular	RNA, ss, linear
5.	*Morphology*	Icosahedral non-enveloped	Double-shelled, enveloped	Enveloped	Enveloped, replication defective	Icosahedral, non-enveloped
6.	*Spread*	Faeco-oral	Parenteral, close contact	Parenteral, close contact	Parenteral, close contact	Water-borne
7.	*Incubation period*	15-45 days	30-180 days	20-90 days	30-50 days (In superinfection)	15-60 days
8.	*Antigen(s)*	HAV	HBsAg HBcAg HBeAg HBxAg	HCV RNA C 100-3 C 33c NS5	HBsAg HDV	HEV
9.	*Antibodies*	anti-HAV	anti-HBs anti-HBc anti-HBe	anti-HCV	anti-HBs anti-HDV	anti-HEV
10.	*Severity*	Mild	Occasionally severe	Moderate	Occasionally severe	Mild
11.	*Chronic hepatitis*	None	Occasional	Common	Common	None
12.	*Carrier state*	None	<1%	<1%	1-10%	Unknown
13.	*Hepatocellular carcinoma*	No	+	+	±	None
14.	*Prognosis*	Excellent	Worse with age	Moderate	Acute good; chronic poor	Good

(ss = single-stranded; ss/ds = partially single-stranded partially double-stranded)

HAV is usually spread by eating or drinking food or water contaminated with infected feces. Shellfish which have not been sufficiently cooked are a relatively common source. It may also be spread through close contact with an infectious person. While children often do not have symptoms when infected, they are still able to infect others. After a single infection, a person is immune for the rest of his or her life.

90. Massive splenomegaly is NOT seen in:

a. Malaria
b. Chronic myelogenous leukemia
c. Syphilis
d. Sickle cell anemia

Because of its narrow vessels and function in clearing defective red blood cells, the spleen is frequently affected. It is usually infarcted (autosplenectomy) before the end of childhood in individuals suffering from sickle-cell anemia. This spleen damage increases the risk of infection from encapsulated organisms.

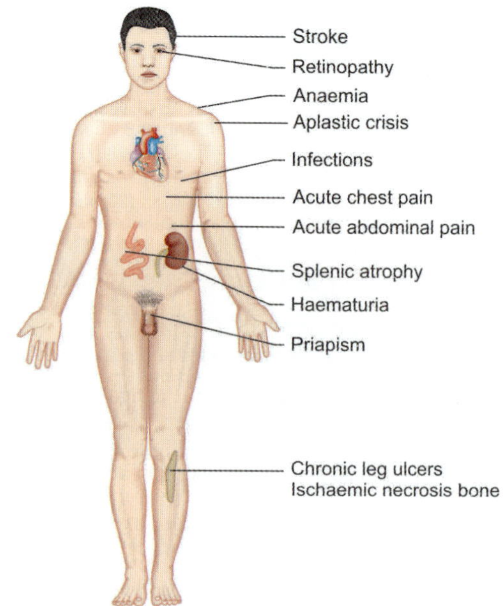

Major clinical manifestations of sickle cell disease.

Ans. **90. d.** Sickle cell anemia

91. True regarding infectivity period of hepatitis A:

a. 1-2 weeks before and 2 weeks after the onset of jaundice
b. 1-2 weeks before and 1 week after the onset of jaundice
c. 2-3 weeks before and 2 weeks after the onset of jaundice
d. 2-3 weeks before and 1 week after the onset of jaundice

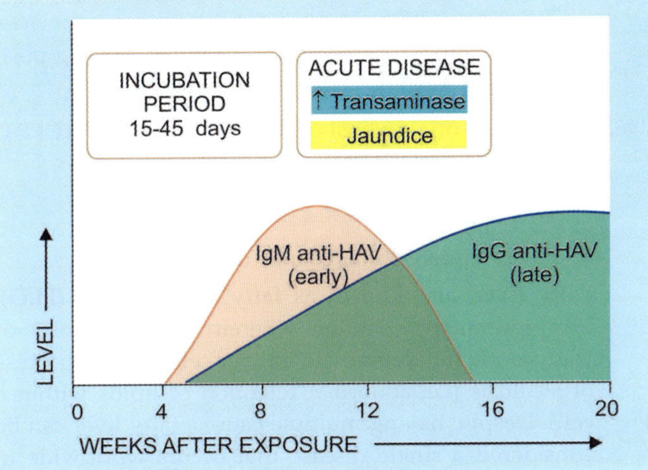

Sequence of appearance of antibodies to HAV.

HAV is excreted in large quantities about 11 days prior to appearance of symptoms or anti-HAV IgM antibodies in the blood. The incubation period is 15–50 days and mortality is less than 0.5%.

92. Presence of HBeAg in serum of a patient of hepatitis-B indicates:

a. Acute, non-infectious stage
b. Acute, infectious stage
c. Chronic, non-infectious stage
d. Chronic, infectious stage

HBeAg is a viral protein that is secreted by hepatitis B infected cells. It is associated with chronic hepatitis B infections and is used as a marker of active viral disease and a patient's degree of infectiousness.

93. Associated with primary hepatic malignancy:

a. Cadmium
b. Vinyl chloride
c. Chromium compounds
d. Asbestos

According to ICAR, Vinyl Chloride is Group 1 human carcinogen posing elevated risks of rare Angiosarcoma, brain and lung tumors and malignant hematopoeitic, lymphatic tumors. Decreased male libido, spontaneous abortion and birth defects are major reproductive defects.

Important chemical carcinogens.

Carcinogen	Tumour
I. DIRECT-ACTING CARCINOGENS	
i. *Alkylating agents* a. Anti-cancer drugs (e.g. cyclophosphamide, chlorambucil, busulfan, melphalan, nitrosourea etc) b. β-propiolactone c. Epoxides ii. *Acylating agents* a. Acetyl imidazole b. Dimethyl carbamyl chloride	❑ Lymphomas ❑ AML ❑ Bladder cancer
II. INDIRECT-ACTING CARCINOGENS (PROCARCINOGENS)	
i. *Polycyclic, aromatic hydrocarbons (in tobacco, smoke, fossil fuel, soot, tar, minerals oil, smoked animal foods, industrial and atmospheric pollutants)* a. Anthracenes (benza-, dibenza-, dimethyl benza-) b. Benzapyrene c. Methylcholanthrene	❑ Lung cancer ❑ Skin cancer ❑ Cancer of upper aerodigestive tract
ii. *Aromatic amines and azo-dyes* a. β-naphthylamine b. Benzidine c. Azo-dyes (e.g. butter yellow, scarlet red etc)	❑ Bladder cancer ❑ Hepatocellular carcinoma
iii. *Naturally-occurring products* a. Aflatoxin BI b. Actinomycin D c. Mitomycin C d. Safrole e. Betel nuts	❑ Hepatocellular carcinoma

Contd...

Ans. **91. d.** 2-3 weeks before... **92. d.** Chronic, infectious... **93. b.** Vinyl chloride

Contd...

Carcinogen	*Tumour*
iv. *Miscellaneous*	
a. Nitrosamines and nitrosamides	❑ Gastric carcinoma
b. Vinyl chloride monomer	❑ Angiosarcoma of liver
c. Asbestos	❑ Bronchogenic carcinoma, mesothelioma
d. Arsenical compounds	❑ Cancer, skin, lung
e. Metals (e.g. nickel, lead, cobalt, chromium etc)	❑ Lung cancer
f. Insecticides, fungicides (e.g. aldrin, dieldrin, chlordane etc)	❑ Cancer in experimental animals
g. Saccharin and cyclomates	

94. Early diagnosis of acute hepatitis B infection is done by:
a. Presence of HBeAg in serum
b. Presence of IgM anti-HBc in serum
c. Presence of HBsAg in serum
d. Presence of IgG anti-HBc in serum

During this 'window' in which the host remains infected but is successfully clearing the virus, IgM antibodies specific to the hepatitis B core antigen (*anti-HBc IgM*) may be the only serological evidence of disease. Therefore, most hepatitis B diagnostic panels contain HBsAg and total anti-HBc (both IgM and IgG).

95. A young man presents with HBsAg positive, HBeAg negative and normal levels of AST and ALT. He is asymptomatic. What is the next line of management:
a. Wait and watch
b. Lamivudine
c. Immunoglobulin
d. Liver transplant

Non-infectious carriers (HBeAg negative, HBsAg positive) of HBV need no active treatment.

96. In post-necrotic cirrhosis of liver, all are seen EXCEPT:
a. Loss of normal architecture
b. Degeneration of hepatocytes
c. Fatty infiltration
d. Loss of intercellular connective tissue matrix

Fatty liver, also known as **fatty liver disease** (**FLD**), is a reversible condition wherein large vacuoles of triglyceride fat accumulate in liver cells via the process of steatosis (i.e. abnormal retention of lipids within a cell). Despite having multiple causes, fatty liver can be considered a single disease that occurs worldwide in those with excessive alcohol intake and the obese (with or without effects of insulin resistance). The condition is also associated with other diseases that influence fat metabolism.

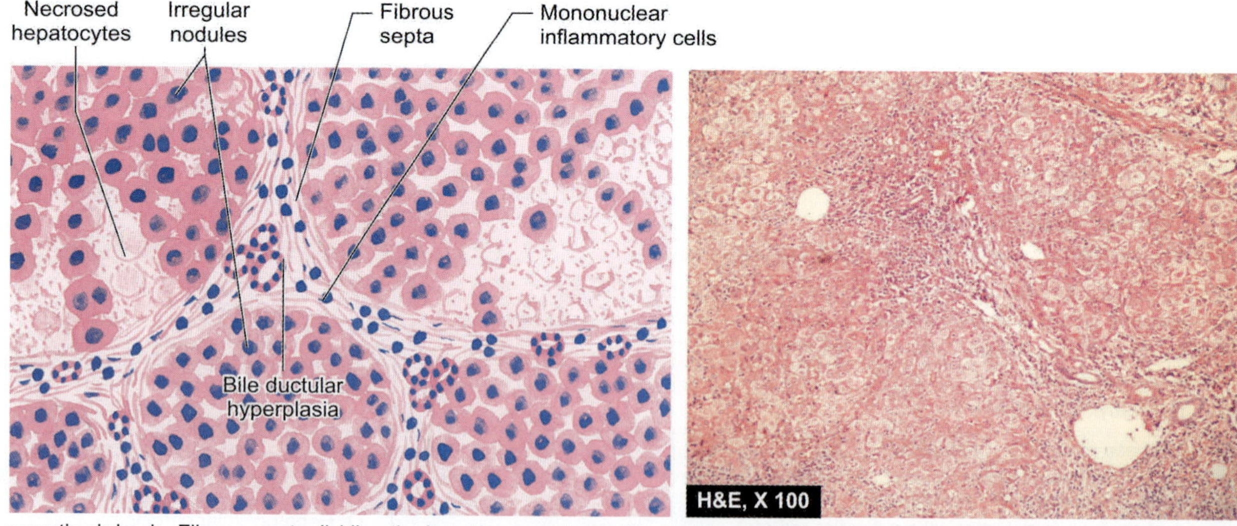

Post-necrotic cirrhosis. Fibrous septa dividing the hepatic parenchyma into nodules are thick and contain prominent mononuclear inflammatory cell infiltrate and bile ductular hyperplasia. A few intact hepatic lobules remain.

97. In India, splenectomy is most commonly performed for:
a. Hydatid cyst
b. Carcinoma thyroid
c. Trauma
d. Portal hypertension

Splenectomy has been considered the treatment of choice for patients with bleeding from sinistral portal hypertension (SPH) and varices, but is controversial for asymptomatic patients.

Ans. **94. b.** Presence of IgM... **95. a.** Wait and watch **96. c.** Fatty infiltration **97. d.** Portal hypertension

NERVOUS SYSTEM PATHOLOGY

98. Berry aneurysm can lead to:

a. Subdural hemorrhage
b. Subarachnoid hemorrhage
c. Brain parenchymal hemorrhage
d. All of the above

Subarachnoid hemorrhage

- If an aneurysm ruptures, blood leaks into the space around the brain, it is called a subarachnoid hemorrhage.

The circle of Willis showing principal sites of berry (saccular) aneurysms. The serial numbers indicate the frequency of involvement.

- The risk of a subarachnoid hemorrhage is greater with a saccular aneurysm than a fusiform aneurysm
- Onset is usually sudden with no prodrome, classically presenting as a "thunderclap headache" worse than previous headaches.
- Symptoms of a subarachnoid hemorrhage differ depending on the site and size of the aneurysm.

Symptoms of a ruptured aneurysm can include:
- A sudden severe headache that can last from several hours to days
- Nausea and vomiting
- Drowsiness, confusion and/or loss of consciousness
- Visual abnormalities
- Meningism

99. All of the following are true regarding Guillain-Barre syndrome EXCEPT:

a. Peripheral nervous system is affected
b. Histologically there is inflammation of peripheral nerve
c. Descending paralysis
d. Elevated CSF proteins

Guillain-Barré syndrome (GBS) can be described as a collection of clinical syndromes that manifests as an acute inflammatory polyradiculoneuropathy with resultant weakness and diminished reflexes.

Although the classic description of GBS is that of a demyelinating neuropathy with ascending weakness, many clinical variants have been well documented in the medical literature.

100. Negri bodies are characteristic of:

a. Tetanus b. Rabies
c. Polio d. AIDS

Negri bodies are eosinophilic, sharply outlined, pathognomonic inclusion bodies (2–10 μm in diameter) found in the cytoplasm of certain nerve cells containing the virus of rabies, especially in Ammon's horn of the hippocampus.

101. Damage to nervous tissue is repaired by:

a. Microglia b. Axons
c. Fibroblasts d. Neuroglia

Glial cells, sometimes called **neuroglia** or simply **glia**, are non-neuronal cells that maintain homeostasis, form myelin, and provide support and protection for neurons in the central nervous system and peripheral nervous system.

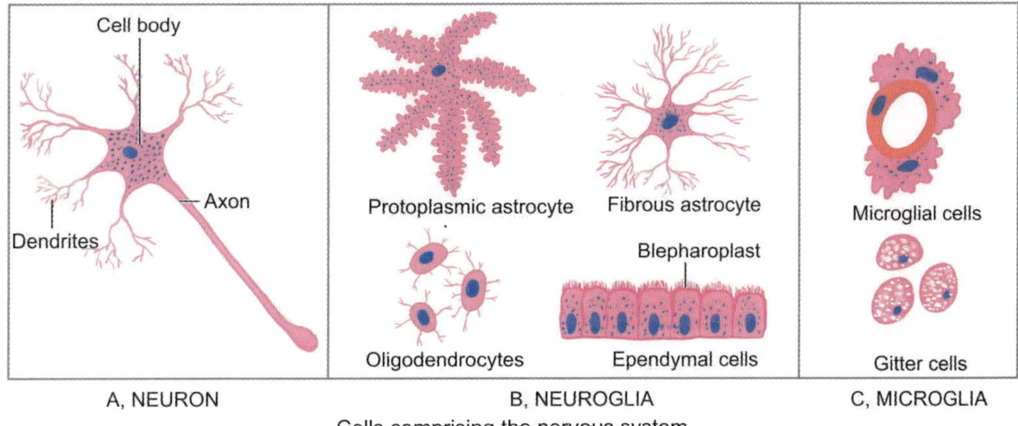

Cells comprising the nervous system.

Ans. 98. **b.** Subarachnoid... 99. **c.** Descending paralysis 100. **b.** Rabies 101. **d.** Neuroglia

102. All are true about pyogenic meningitis EXCEPT:

a. Increased CSF protein
b. Purulent CSF
c. Markedly decreased CSF glucose
d. Lymphocytic pleocytosis

Lymphocytic pleocytosis is an abnormal increase in the amount of lymphocytes in the cerebrospinal fluid (CSF). It is usually considered to be a sign of TB infection (not pyogenic bacterial) or inflammation within the nervous system, and is encountered in a number of neurological diseases, such as pseudomigraine, Susac's syndrome, and encephalitis.

CSF Findings in Health and Various Types of Meningitis

	Feature	*Normal*	*Acute Pyogenic (Bacterial) Meningitis*	*Acute Lymphocytic (Viral) Meningitis*	*Chronic (Tuberculous) Meningitis*
1.	*Naked eye appearance*	Clear and colourless	Cloudy or frankly purulent	Clear or slightly turbid	Clear or slightly turbid, forms fibrin coagulum on standing
2.	*CSF pressure*	60-150 mm water	Elevated (above 180 mm water)	Elevated (above 250 mm water)	Elevated (above 300 mm water)
3.	*Cells*	0-4 lymphocytes/μl	10-10,000 neutrophils/μl	10-100 lymphocytes/μl	100-1000 lymphocytes/μl
4.	*Proteins*	15-45 mg/dl	Markedly raised	Mildly raised	Raised
5.	*Glucose*	50-80 mg/dl	Markedly reduced	Normal	Reduced
6.	*Bacterlology*	Sterilc	Causative organisms present	Sterile	Tubercle bacilli present

103. Rosette shaped arrangement of cells is a feature of:

a. Lymphoma
b. Neurofibroma
c. Ependymoma
d. Thecoma ovary

In ependymoma, more frequently present are perivascular pseudorosettes in which tumor cells are arranged around vessels with an intervening zone consisting of thin ependymal processes directed toward the wall of the vessel.

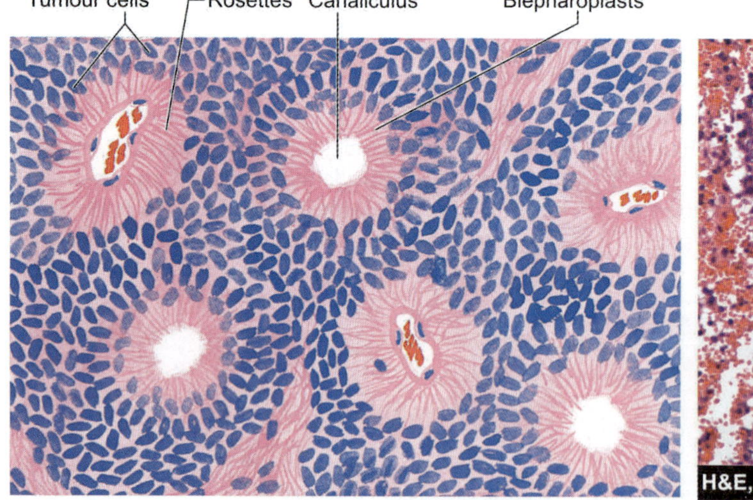

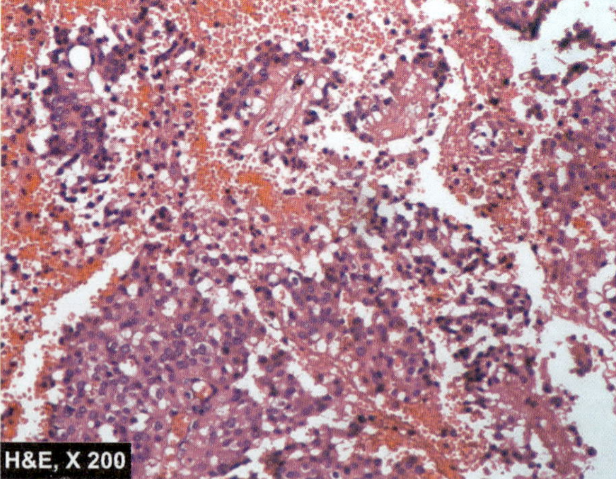

Ependymoma showing uniform ependymal tumour cells forming rosettes and canaliculi.

104. Commonest type of intracranial tumours:

a. Secondaries
b. Meningioma
c. Medulloblastoma
d. Astrocytoma

Secondary tumors of the brain are very common in the terminal phases of patients with an incurable metastasized cancer; the most common types of cancers that bring about secondary tumors of the brain are lung cancer, breast cancer, malignant melanoma, kidney cancer, and colon cancer (in decreasing order of frequency).

Ans. **102. d.** Lymphocytic... **103. c.** Ependymoma **104. a.** Secondaries

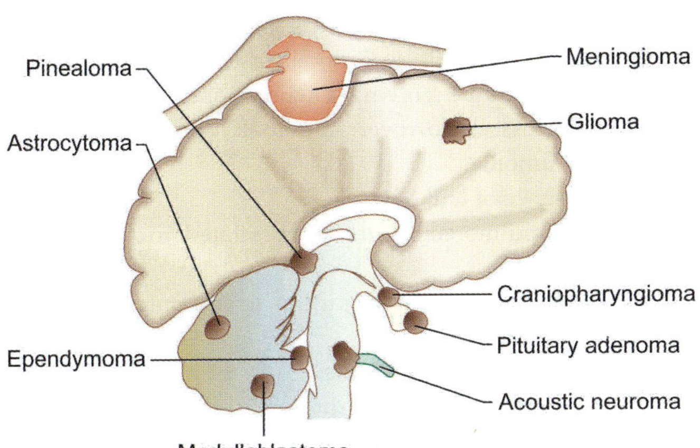

The anatomic distribution of common intracranial tumours.

105. True for carotid body tumour:

a. Sympathetic paraganglioma
b. Parasympathetic paraganglioma
c. Arises from carotid artery
d. None of the above

Paragangliomas originate from paraganglia in chromaffin-negative glomus cells derived from the embryonic neural crest, functioning as part of the sympathetic nervous system (a branch of the autonomic nervous system). These cells normally act as special chemoreceptors located along blood vessels, particularly in the carotid bodies (at the bifurcation of the common carotid artery in the neck) and in aortic bodies (near the aortic arch).

106. Which of the following cancer metastasize to brain LEASTLY:

a. Hypernephroma
b. Breast carcinoma
c. Choriocarcinoma
d. Prostatic carcinoma

Most prostate cancers are slow growing; however, some grow relatively quickly. The cancer cells may spread from the prostate to other parts of the body, particularly the bones (osteoblastic osseous metastases) and lymph nodes.

107. Parkinson triad contains all EXCEPT:

a. Rigidity
b. Resting tremors
c. Bradykinesia
d. Preserved postural reflexes

Postural instability is one of the axial symptoms of Parkinsonism Disease and it is due to the loss of **postural reflexes**.

108. In myasthenia gravis, antibodies are present against:

a. Muscarinic receptor proteins
b. Nicotinic receptor proteins
c. Protein actin
d. Protein myosin

In the most common cases of myasthenia gravis, muscle weakness is caused by circulating antibodies that block acetylcholine receptors at the postsynaptic neuromuscular junction, inhibiting the excitatory effects of the neurotransmitter acetylcholine on nicotinic receptors at neuromuscular junctions.

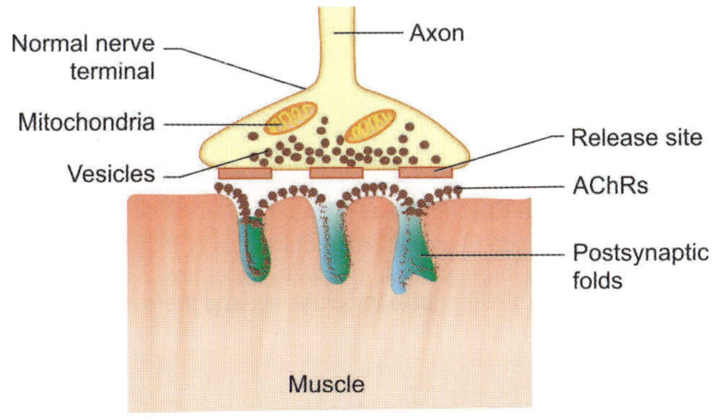

A, NORMAL NEUROMUSCULAR JUNCTION

Nerve terminal
AChRs reduced
Widened synaptic space
Flattened and simplified postsynaptic folds

B, JUNCTION IN MYASTHENIA GRAVIS

Neuromuscular junction in normal transmission (A) and in myasthenia gravis (B). The junction in MG shows reduced number of AChRs, flattened and simplified postsynaptic folds, a widened synaptic space but a normal nerve terminal.

109. Pathognonmic finding of rabies is:

a. Obliterative endarteritis
b. Microglial nodules
c. Neuronophagia
d. Negri bodies

Negri bodies are eosinophilic, sharply outlined, pathognomonic inclusion bodies (2–10 μm in diameter) found in the cytoplasm of certain nerve cells containing the virus of rabies, especially in Ammon's horn of the hippocampus. They are also often found in the cerebellar cortex of postmortem brain samples of rabies victims.

Ans. **105. b.** Parasympath... **106. d.** Prostatic carcinoma **107. d.** Preserved postural... **108. b.** Nicotinic receptor... **109. d.** Negri bodies

RESPIRATORY SYSTEM PATHOLOGY

110. Infective foci of TB spread to other organs by:

a. Direct
b. Lymphatic
c. Hematogenous
d. None of the above

TB

- The primary site of infection in the lungs, known as the "Ghon focus", is generally located in either the upper part of the lower lobe, or the lower part of the upper lobe
- Tuberculosis of the lungs may also occur via infection from the blood stream.
- This is known as a Simon focus and is typically found in the top of the lung.
- This hematogenous transmission can also spread infection to more distant sites, such as peripheral lymph nodes, the kidneys, the brain, and the bones.
- All parts of the body can be affected by the disease, though for unknown reasons it rarely affects the heart, skeletal muscles, pancreas, or thyroid.

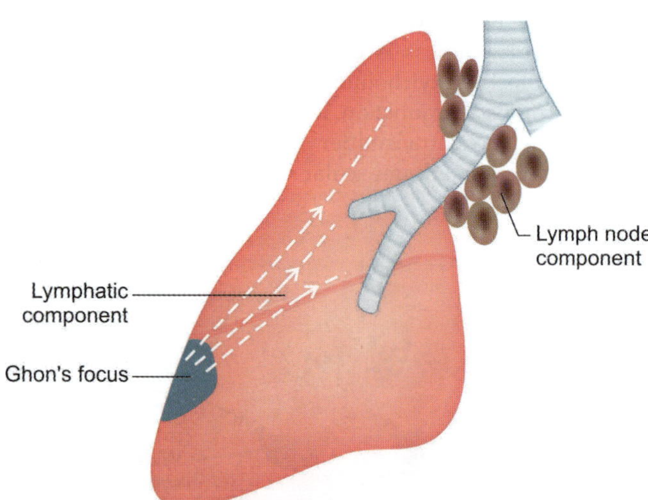

The primary complex is composed of 3 components: Ghon's focus, draining lymphatics, and hilar lymph nodes

111. All of the following are features of viral pneumonia EXCEPT:

a. Presence of interstitial inflammation
b. Predominance of alveolar exudates
c. Bronchiolitis
d. Multinucleate giant cells in the bronchiolar walls

- Usually the atypical causes also involve atypical symptoms:
- No response to common antibiotics such as sulfonamide and beta-lactams like penicillin.
- No signs and symptoms of lobar consolidation, meaning that the infection is restricted to small areas, rather than involving a whole lobe. As the disease progresses, however, the look can tend to lobar pneumonia.
- Absence of leukocytosis.
- Extrapulmonary symptoms, related to the causing organism.
- Moderate amount of sputum, or no sputum at all (i.e. non-productive).
- Lack of alveolar exudate.
- Despite general symptoms and problems with the upper respiratory tract (such as high fever, headache, a dry irritating cough followed later by a productive cough with radiographs showing consolidation), there are in general few physical signs. The patient looks better than the symptoms suggest.

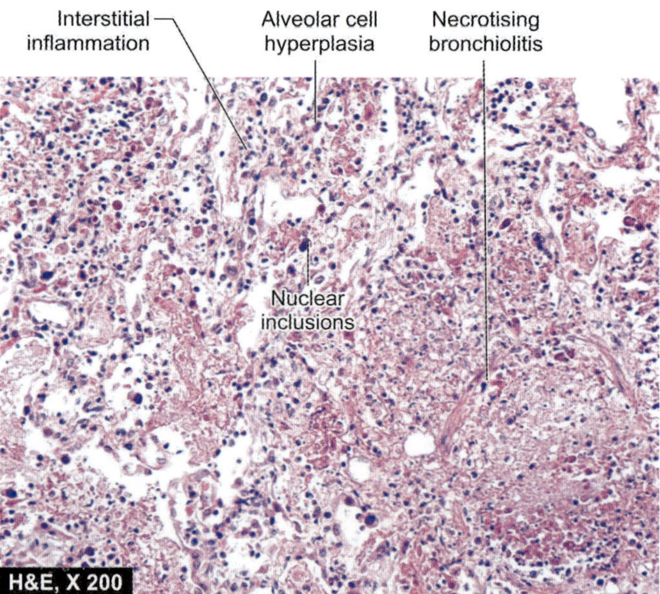

Microscopic appearance of interstitial pneumonitis (viral pneumonia). There is necrotising bronchiolitis, reactive hyperplasia of alveolar epithelial cells, some having nuclear inclusions, and there is interstitial inflammation.

112. Earliest feature of TB:

a. Granuloma
b. Giant cells (Langerhans)
c. Lymphocytosis
d. Caseation

Tuberculosis is classified as one of the granulomatous inflammatory diseases. Macrophages, T lymphocytes, B lymphocytes, and fibroblasts aggregate to form granulomas, with lymphocytes surrounding the infected macrophages.

Ans. 110. c. Hematogenous **111. b.** Predominance... **112. c.** Lymphocytosis

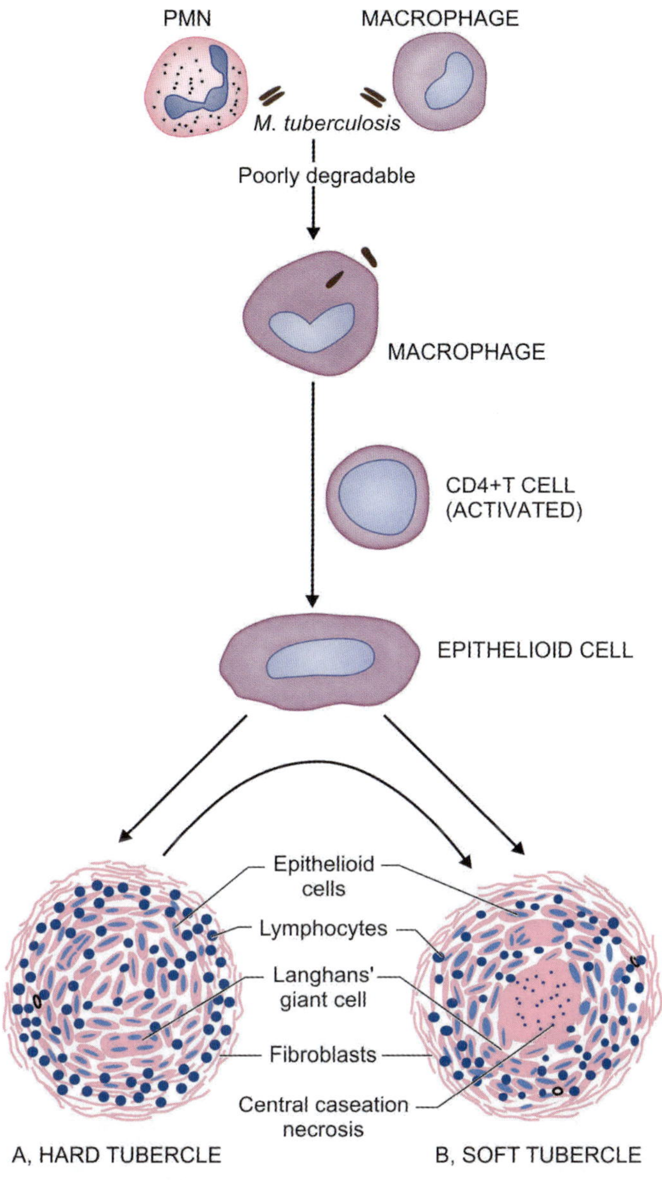

Schematic evolution of tubercle. In fully formed granuloma, the centre is composed of granular caseation necrosis, surrounded by epithelioid cells and Langhans' giant cells and peripheral rim of lymphocytes bounded by fibroblasts.

113. True for Reid's index:

a. Increased in bronchial asthma
b. Increased in chronic bronchitis
c. Decreased in bronchial asthma
d. Decreased in chronic bronchitis

The **Reid Index** is a mathematical relationship that exists in a human bronchus section observed under the microscope. It is defined as ratio between the thickness of the submucosal mucus secreting glands and the thickness between the epithelium and cartilage that covers the bronchi.

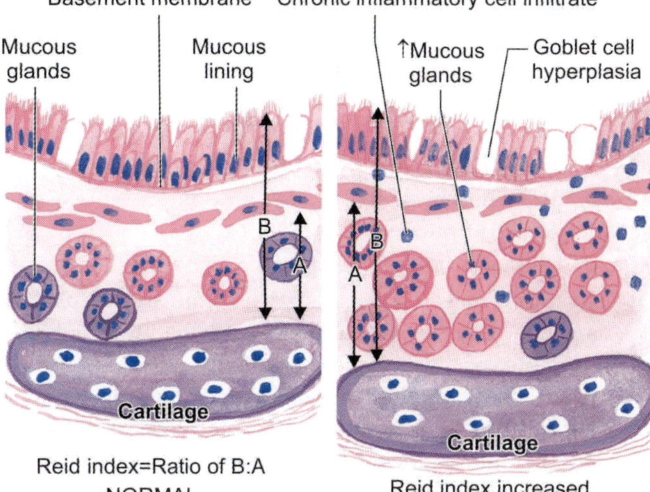

Diagrammatic representation of increased Reid's index in chronic bronchitis.

114. Reactivation of pulmonary tuberculosis always occurs at:

a. Lower part of upper lobe
b. Upper part of lower lobe
c. Lower part of lower lobe
d. Apex of the upper lobe

Post-primary tuberculosis, also known as **reactivation tuberculosis** or **secondary tuberculosis** usually occurs during the first and second years time following the initial infection later. Reactivation frequently in the setting of a decreased immune status and usually involves the lung apex.

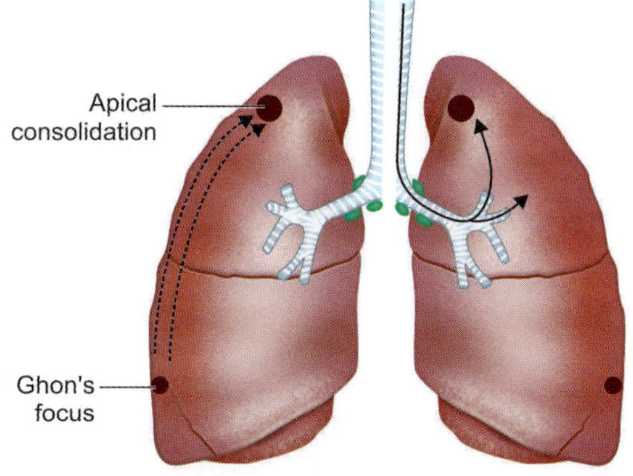

Progressive secondary tuberculosis. A, Endogenous infection from reactivation of dormant primary complex. B, Exogenous infection from fresh dose of tubercle bacilli.

115. Cavernous breathing is seen in:

a. Pleural effusion
b. Consolidation
c. Carcinoma lung
d. Cavity lung

Ans. 113. b. Increased in... **114. d.** Apex of the upper lobe **115. d.** Cavity lung

Abnormal breath sounds marked by a peculiar prolonged hollow resonance, usually due to an underlying **cavity** in the lung. Called also **cavernous respiration**.

116. Clinical manifestation of cystic fibrosis includes all EXCEPT:

a. Cor pulmonale
b. Bronchiectasis
c. Malabsorption
d. Hypertension

Cystic fibrosis (CF), also known as **mucoviscidosis**, is a genetic disorder that affects mostly the lungs but also the pancreas, liver, kidneys, and intestine. Long-term issues include difficulty breathing and coughing up mucus as a result of frequent lung infections. Other signs and symptoms include sinus infections, poor growth, fatty stool, clubbing of the finger and toes, and infertility in males among others.

117. Alpha1 antitrypsin deficiency occurs in:

a. Emphysema
b. Bronchiectasis
c. Empyema
d. Bronchogenic carcinoma

In absence of A1AT, neutrophil elastase is free to break down elastin, which contributes to the elasticity of the lungs, resulting in respiratory complications such as emphysema, or COPD (chronic obstructive pulmonary disease) in adults and cirrhosis in adults or children.

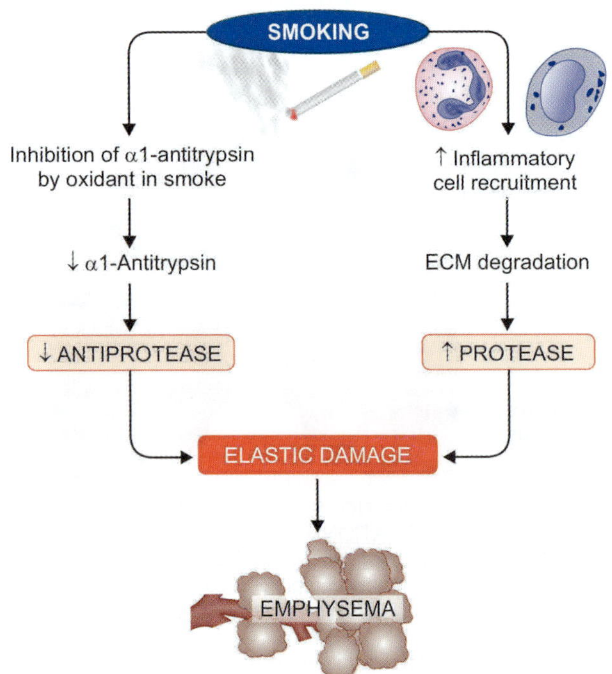

Pathogenesis of alveolar wall destruction in emphysema by protease-antiprotease mechanism.

CARDIOVASCULAR SYSTEM PATHOLOGY

118. Which is NOT seen in acute rheumatic fever?

a. Aschoff bodies
b. Pericarditis
c. Myocarditis
d. Mitral valve stenosis

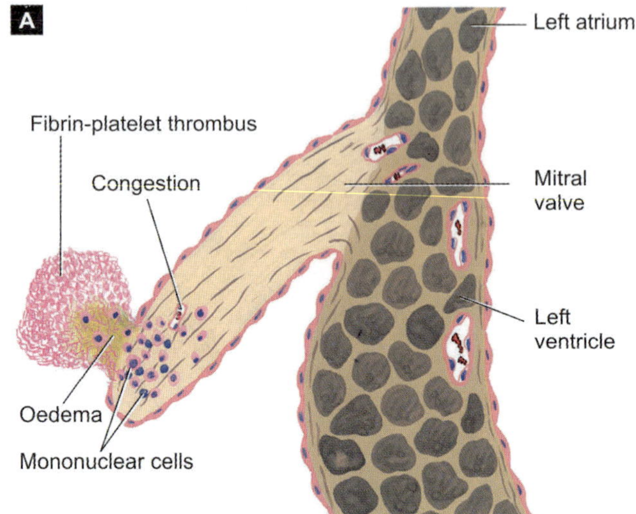

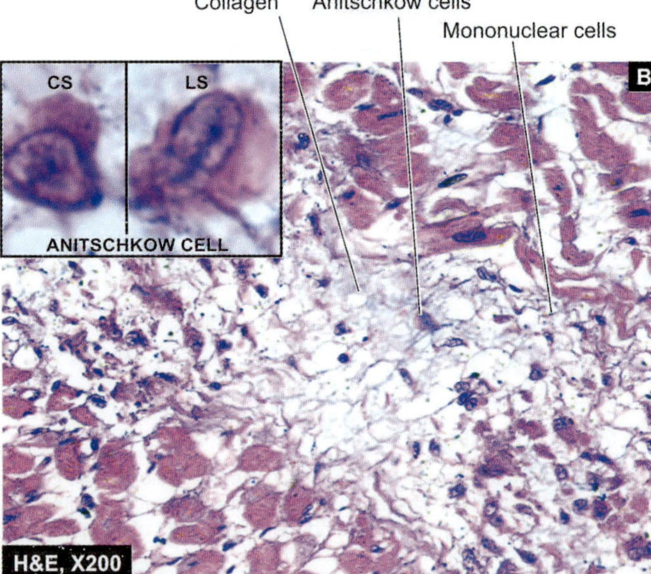

Rheumatic heart disease. A, Microscopic structure of the rheumatic valvulitis and a vegetation on the cusp of mitral valve in sagittal section. B, Section of the myocardium shows a healed Aschoff nodule in the interstitium having collagen, sparse cellularity, a multinucleate giant cell and Anitschkow cells. Inbox shows an Anitschkow cell in cross section (CS) and in longitudinal section (LS).

Acute rheumatic fever

- Characteristic Aschoff bodies, composed of swollen eosinophilic collagen surrounded by lymphocytes and macrophages can be seen on light microscopy.
- The larger macrophages may become Anitschkow cells or Aschoff giant cells.

Ans. **116. d.** Hypertension **117. a.** Emphysema **118. d.** Mitral valve stenosis

- In acute rheumatic fever, these lesions can be found in any layer of the heart and is hence called pancarditis.

Chronic rheumatic heart disease (RHD)

- It is characterized by repeated inflammation with fibrinous repair.
- The cardinal anatomic changes of the valve include leaflet thickening, commissural fusion, and shortening and thickening of the tendinous cords.
- It is caused by an autoimmune reaction to Group A β-hemolytic streptococci (GAS) that results in valvular damage.
- Fibrosis and scarring of valve leaflets, commissures and cusps leads to abnormalities that can result in valve stenosis or regurgitation

119. NOT a granulomatous condition:

a. Takayasu arteritis b. Polyarteritis nodosa
c. Wegener's granulomatosis
d. Giant cell arteritis

Polyarteritis nodosa, also known as **panarteritis nodosa**, **periarteritis nodosa**, Kussmaul **disease** or **Kussmaul-Maier disease**

- It is a vasculitis of medium and small-sized arteries, which become swollen and damaged from attack by rogue immune cells.
- Infantile polyarteritis nodosa is restricted to infants.
- In polyarteritis nodosa, small aneurysms are strung like the beads of a rosary, therefore making "rosary sign" an important diagnostic feature of the vasculitis.

120. Hypertrophic cardiomyopathy presents as impaired:

a. Diastolic filling
b. Ventricular contractions
c. Ventricular ejection
d. None

HOCM/ HCM

- About 25% of individuals with HCM demonstrate an obstruction to the inflow of blood to the left ventricle during rest.
- In as much as 70% of patients however obstruction can be provoked under certain conditions.
- This is known as dynamic outflow obstruction, because the degree of obstruction is variable and is dependent on the loading conditions (ventricular filling and arterial blood pressure) and the contractility state of the left ventricle.

Classification of primary cardiomyopathies.	
1.	IDIOPATHIC DILATED (OR CONGESTIVE) CARDIOMYOPATHY
2.	IDIOPATHIC HYPERTROPHIC CARDIOMYOPATHY
	i) Obstructive type
	ii) Non-obstructive type
3.	IDIOPATHIC RESTRICTIVE (OR OBLITERATIVE OR INFILTRATIVE) CARDIOMYOPATHY
	i) Cardiac amyloidosis
	ii) Endocardial fibroelastosis
	iii) Endomyocardial fibrosis
	iv) Löeffler's endocarditis (fibroplastic parietal endocarditis with peripheral blood eosinophilia)
	v) Other forms

121. Extracellular hyaline change is seen in:

a. Hyaline arteriosclerosis
b. Chronic glomerulonephritis
c. Leiomyoma
d. Alcoholic hyaline

Hyaline arteriosclerosis, also referred to as arterial hyalinosis and arteriolar hyalinosis, refers to lesions that are caused by the deposition of homogenous pink hyaline.

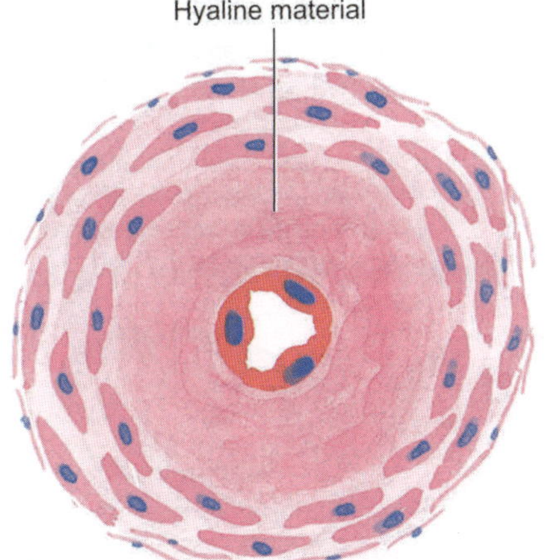

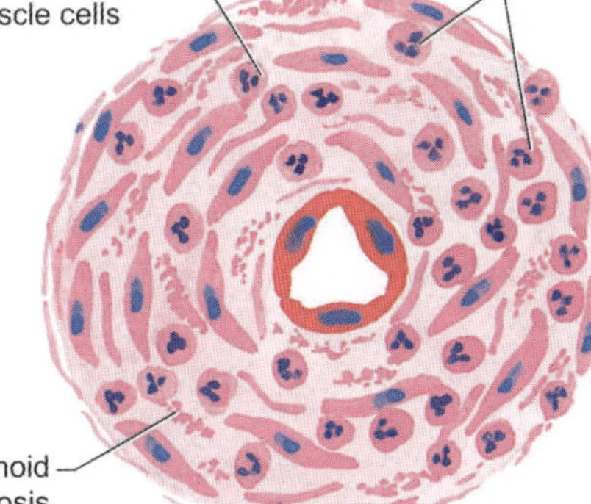

A, HYALINE ARTERIOLOSCLEROSIS B, HYPERPLASTIC ARTERIOLOSCLEROSIS C, NECROTISING ARTERIOLITIS

Diagrammatic representation of three forms of arteriolosclerosis, commonly seen in hypertension.

Ans. 119. b. Polyarteritis.... **120. a.** Diastolic filling **121. a.** Hyaline arteriosc...

122. Ascending aorta is commonly involved in:

a. Mycotic aneurysm
b. Syphilitic aneurysm
c. Atherosclerotic aneurysm
d. All of the above

Syphilitic aortitis takes place during the stage of tertiary syphilis between 5 to 30 years after initiation of primary syphilis. This is normally due to infection of aorta secondary to endarteritis obliterans of vasa vasorum. The responsible organism is a spirochete Treponema pallidum and the ascending aorta is most commonly involved.

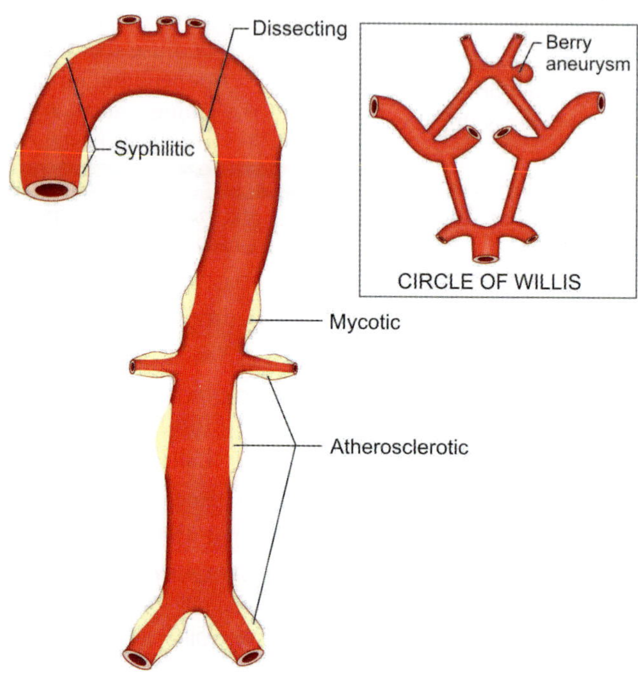

Sites of major forms of aneurysms.

123. All of the following are true regarding marantic endocarditis EXCEPT:

a. Vegetation may embolize
b. Vegetations along the line of closure of leaflets
c. Affects damaged valves
d. May be associated with hypercoagulable states

Nonbacterial thrombotic endocarditis (NBTE) or **marantic endocarditis** is a noninfectious process **affecting normal** or degenerative cardiac **valves** that is due to fibrin thrombi deposits in patients with hypercoagulable states associated with adenocarcinoma of lung, colon, or pancreas that produce mucin.

Distinguishing features of vegetations in major forms of endocarditis.

Feature	Rheumatic	Libman-sacks	Non-bacterial thrombotic	Bacterial (infective)
1. Valves commonly affected	Mitral alone; mitral and aortic combined	Mitral, tricuspid	Mainly mitral; less often aortic and tricuspid	Mitral; aortic; combined mitral and aortic
2. Location on valve cusps or leaflets	Occur along the line of closure, atrial surface of atrioventricular valves and ventricular surface of semilunar valves	Occur on both surfaces of valve leaflets or cusps, in the valve pockets	Occur along the line of closure	SABE more often on diseased valves: ABE on previously normal valves; location same as in RHD
3. Macroscopy	Small, multiple, warty, grey brown, translucent, firmly attached, generally produce permanent valvular deformity	Medium-sized, multiple, generally do not produce significant valvular deformity	Small but larger than those of rheumatic, single or multiple, brownish, firm, but more friable than those of rheumatic	Often large, grey-tawny to greenish, irregular, single or multiple, typically friable

Ans. 122. **b.** Syphilitic ane... 123. **c.** Affects dama...

Feature	Rheumatic	Libman-sacks	Non-bacterial thrombotic	Bacterial (infective)
4. Microscopy	Composed of fibrin with superimposed platelet thrombi and no bacteria, Adjacent and underlying endocardium shows oedema, proliferation of capillaries, mononuclear inflammatory infiltrate and occasional Aschoff bodies.	Composed of fibrinoid material with superimposed fibrin and platelet thrombi and no bacteria. The underlying endocardium shows fibrinoid necrosis, proliferation of capillaries and acute and chronic inflammatory infiltrate including the haematoxylin bodies of Gross.	Composed of degenerated valvular tissue, fibrinplatelets thrombi and no bacteria. The underlying valve shows swelling of collagen, fibrinoid change, proliferation of capillaries but no significant inflammatory cell infiltrate.	Composed of outer eosinophilic zone of fibrin and platelets, covering colonies of bacteria and deeper zone of non-specific acute and chronic inflammatory cells. The underlying endocardium may show abscesses in ABE and inflammatory granulation tissue in the SABE.

124. NOT a component of Jones criteria for diagnosing acute rheumatic fever:

a. Pancarditis
b. Migratory polyarthritis
c. Erythema nodosum
d. Sydenham chorea

One of the major criteria of Rheumatic fever (Jones criteria) is erythema marginatum: A long-lasting reddish rash that begins on the trunk or arms as macules, which spread outward and clear in the middle to form rings, which continue to spread and coalesce with other rings, ultimately taking on a snake-like appearance. This rash typically spares the face and is made worse with heat.

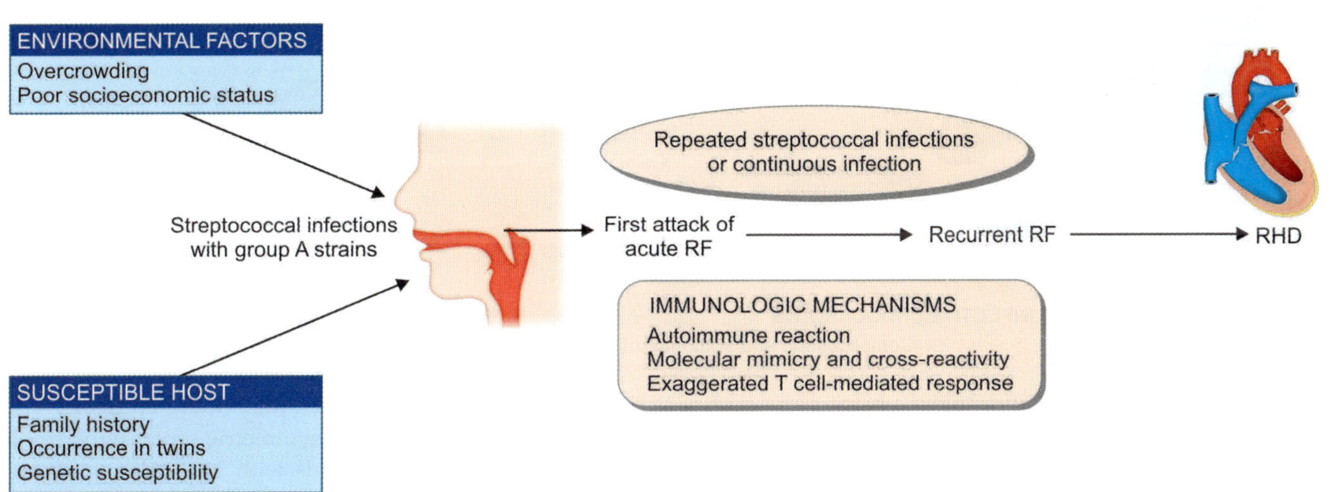

Pathogenesis of RHD, schematic evolution.

125. All of the following are true regarding Wegener's granulomatosis EXCEPT:

a. Affects large size blood vessels
b. May affect lungs and kidneys
c. Necrotizing granuloma may be seen on microscopy
d. PR3-ANCAs are present in upto 95% of cases

Granulomatosis with polyangiitis (**GPA**), also known as **Wegener's granulomatosis** (**WG**), is a systemic disorder that involves both granulomatosis and polyangiitis. It is a form of vasculitis (inflammation of blood vessels) that affects small- and medium-size vessels in many organs.

126. All of the following are features of atrial myxoma EXCEPT:

a. Clubbing b. Hypertension
c. Murmur d. Fever

The symptoms and signs of left atrial myxomas often mimic mitral stenosis. General symptoms may also be present, such as:

- Cough
- Fever
- Cachexia - Involuntary weight loss
- General discomfort (malaise)
- Joint pain
- Blue discoloration of the skin, especially the fingers (Raynaud's phenomenon)
- Fingers that change color upon pressure or with cold or stress
- Clubbing - Curvature of nails accompanied with soft tissue enlargement of the fingers
- Swelling - any part of the body
- Presystolic heart murmur

Ans. 124. c. Erythema nodo... **125. a.** Affects large size... **126. b.** Hypertension

127. Infective endocarditis can cause all EXCEPT:

a. Bulky friable vegetations
b. Myocardial abscess
c. Septal perforation
d. Left atrial thrombus

The most common complication of infective endocarditis on the left side of the heart is ring abscess, which can lead to a number of complications, such as ventricular septal defect, pericarditis, complete heart block, or a high-degree bundle-branch block.

Patients with infection on the right side of the heart present primarily with pulmonary complications, that is, septic emboli to the lung. Vegetations on the tricuspid valve should be removed primarily to prevent pulmonary emboli, which is usually the killer in patients with right-sided infective endocarditis.

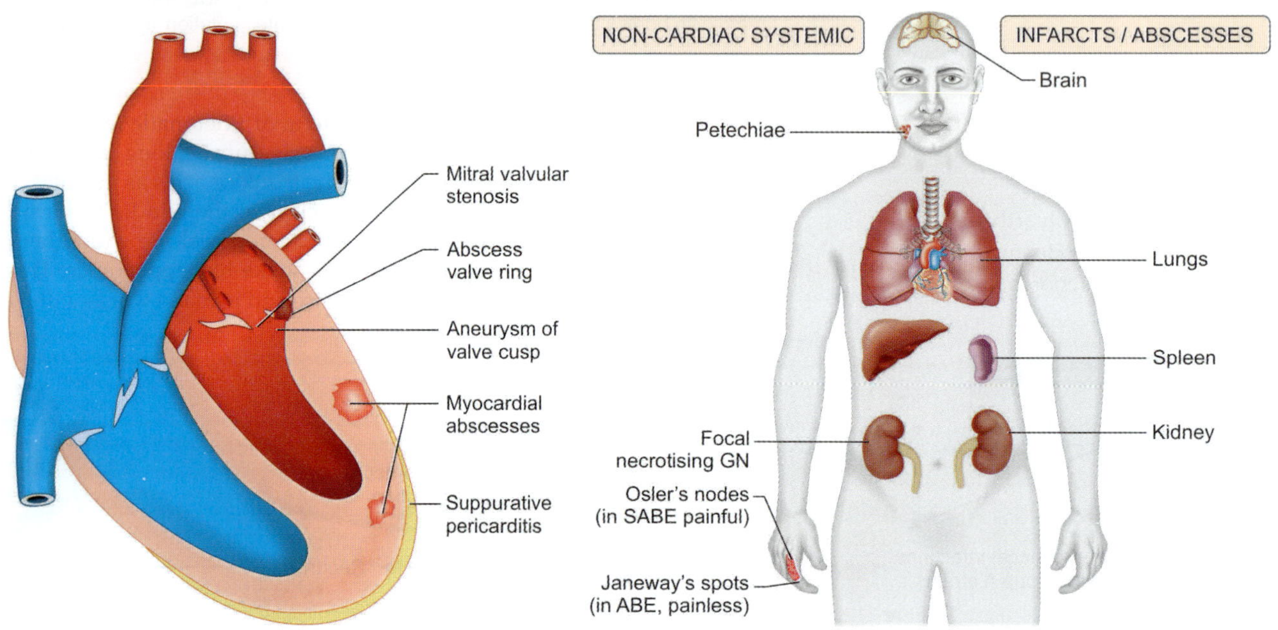

Complications and sequelae of infective endocarditis.

128. All are true of hypertrophic obstructive cardiomyopathy EXCEPT:

a. Asymmetrical septal hypertrophy
b. Dilatation of the atria
c. Dilatation of ventricles
d. Outflow obstruction

Individuals with HCM have some degree of left ventricular hypertrophy. Usually this is an asymmetric hypertrophy, involving the inter-ventricular septum, and is known as asymmetric septal hypertrophy. About 25% of individuals with HCM demonstrate an obstruction to the outflow of blood from the left ventricle during rest. Myocardial hypertrophy and extracellular fibrosis predispose to increased left ventricular stiffness.

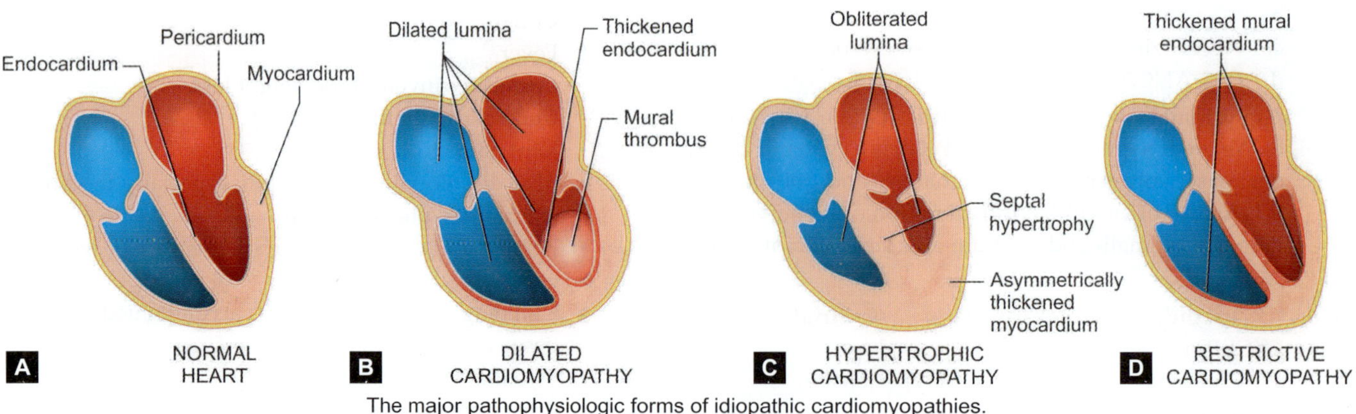

The major pathophysiologic forms of idiopathic cardiomyopathies.

Ans. **127. d.** Left atrial thrombus **128. c.** Dilatation of ventricles

129. **Which of the following is NOT a major criteria for diagnosing rheumatic fever?**
a. Carditis b. Subcutaneous nodules
c. Increased ASLO d. Arthritis

According to revised Jones criteria, the diagnosis of rheumatic fever can be made when two of the major criteria, or one major criterion plus two minor criteria, are present along with evidence of streptococcal infection: elevated or rising antistreptolysin O titre or DNAase.

130. **All are used in the treatment of myocardial infarction EXCEPT:**
a. Antiplatelets b. Thrombolytics
c. Antithrombotics
d. Plasminogen activator inhibitors

Plasminogen Activator Inhibitor-1 is a serine protease inhibitor (serpin) that functions as the principal inhibitor of tissue plasminogen activator (tPA) and urokinase (uPA), the activators of plasminogen and hence fibrinolysis (the physiological breakdown of blood clots).

131. **Right coronary artery supplies all EXCEPT:**
a. Apex of heart
b. Posterior part of interventricular septum
c. Interatrial septum
d. SA node

Apex of heart is supplied by left coronary artery.

132. **Rheumatic fever is commonly associated with affection of:**
a. Tricuspid valve b. Mitral valve
c. Aortic valve d. Pulmonary valve

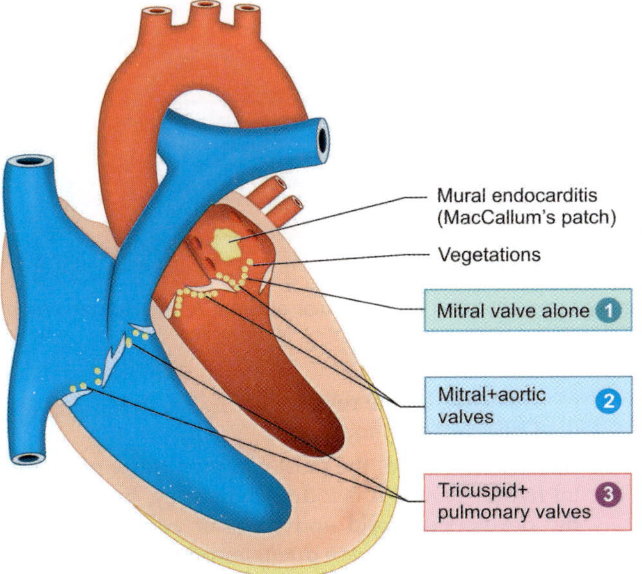

Schematic representation of the anatomic regions of involvement and location of vegetations in rheumatic endocarditis (both valvular and mural). Serial numbers 1, 2 and 3 are denoted for the frequency of valvular involvement.

Rheumatic heart disease chronically manifests as congestive heart failure form valvular involvement. Most commonly the mitral valve is affected resulting in mitral stenosis or mitral regurgitation. Less commonly the aortic valve can be involved and tricuspid valve involvement is rare, but reported.

133. **MC primary tumour of heart:**
a. Lipoma b. Myxoma
c. Fibroma d. Rhabdomyosarcoma

A **myxoma** is a myxoid tumor of primitive connective tissue. It is the most common primary tumor of the heart in adults, but can also occur in other locations.

134. **Which is NOT true of hypersensitivity vasculitis?**
a. May be due to deposition of immune complexes or delayed hypersensitivity
b. Affects small, medium sized and larger arteries commonly
c. Immunologic response to an antigen
d. None of the above

Cutaneous small-vessel vasculitis (also known as "Cutaneous leukocytoclastic angiitis," "Cutaneous leukocytoclastic vasculitis," "Cutaneous necrotizing venulitis," and "Hypersensitivity angiitis") is inflammation of small blood vessels (usually post-capillary venules in the dermis), characterized by palpable purpura. It is the most common vasculitis seen in clinical practice.

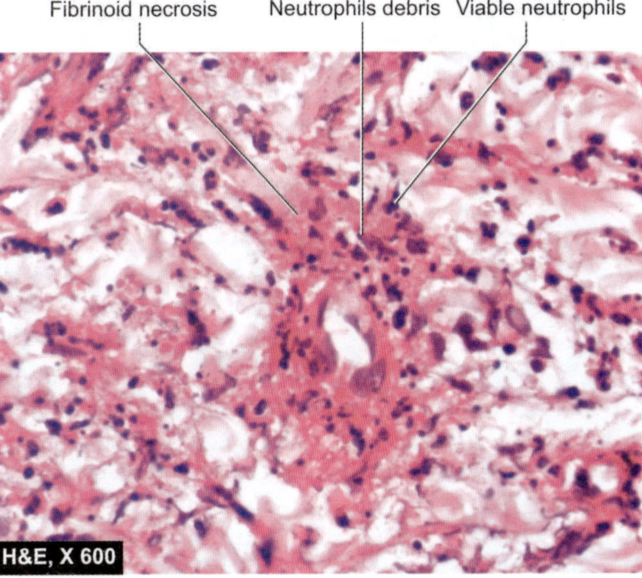

Leucocytoclastic vasculitis. The vessel wall shows fibrinoid necrosis surrounded by viable as well as fragmented neutrophils.

135. **For the management of intra-operative myocardial ischemia, all of the following are advised EXCEPT:**
a. Heparin
b. Intravenous nitroglycerine
c. Calcium channel blocker
d. Atropine

Ans. 129. **c.** Increased ASLO 130. **d.** Plasminogen... 131. **a.** Apex of heart 132. **b.** Mitral valve
133. **b.** Myxoma 134. **b.** Affects small... 135. **a.** Heparin

Heparin is not given for fear of bleeding during operative procedure.

136. Aneurysms in polyarteritis nodosa usually spares:

a. Spleen b. Liver
c. Kidney d. Periphery

Polyarteritis nodosa, also known as **panarteritis nodosa, periarteritis nodosa, Kussmaul disease, Kussmaul-Maier disease** or **PAN**, is a systemic vasculitis of small- or medium-sized muscular arteries, typically involving renal and visceral vessels but sparing the pulmonary circulation.

137. Wegener's granulomatosis involve all EXCEPT:

a. Lung b. Liver
c. Kidney d. Heart

Granulomatosis with polyangiitis (**GPA**), formerly referred to as **Wegener's granulomatosis** (**WG**), is a systemic disorder that involves both granulomatosis and polyangiitis. It is a form of vasculitis (inflammation of blood vessels) that affects small- and medium-size vessels in many organs. Damage to the lungs and kidneys can be fatal. It requires long-term immunosuppression.

138. Most common tumour of heart is:

a. Myxoma
b. Secondaries
c. Papillary fibroelastoma
d. Rhabdomyomas

MC tumour of heart is metastasis whereas MC primary tumour is myxoma (left atrial)

ENDOCRINE SYSTEM PATHOLOGY

139. All of the following statements are true about neuroblastoma EXCEPT:

a. MC abdominal tumour in infants
b. Radiography shows calcification
c. Spontaneous regression though rare
d. Urine contains 5-HIAA

About 90% of neuroblastomas, regardless of location, produce catecholamines (similar to catecholamines associated with phaeochromocytoma), which are important diagnostic feature (i.e. elevated blood levels of catecholamines and elevated urine levels of catecholamine metabolites such as vanillylmandelic acid/ VMA) & homovanillic acid/ HVA

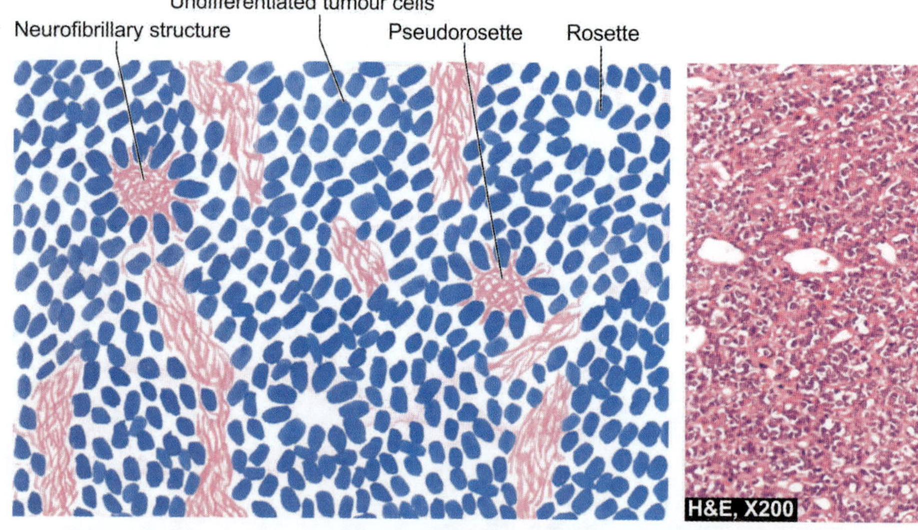

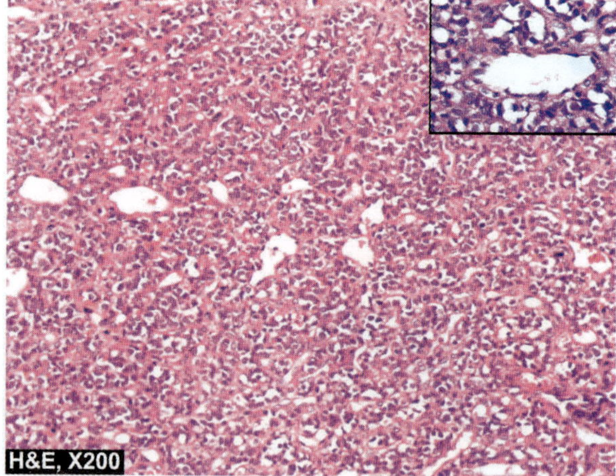

Neuroblastoma, It shows small, round to oval cells forming irregular sheets separated by fibrovascular stroma. A few Homer-Wright's pseudorosettes are also present. *Inset* shows a close-up view of pseudorosette.

140. Hutchinson's secondaries in skull are due to:

a. Adrenals b. Liver
c. Breast d. Lungs

Hutchinson's type is left sided adrenal neuro-blastoma with **secondaries** in orbit and **skull. Pepper type is right sided.**

141. The commonest cause of congenital hypo-thyroidism:

a. Thyroid dysgenesis
b. Pendred syndrome
c. Defective iodine release
d. Deficiency of de-iodinase

Around the world, the most common cause of congenital hypothyroidism is iodine deficiency, but in most of the developed world and areas of adequate environmental iodine, cases are due to a combination of known and unknown causes. Most commonly there is a defect of development of the thyroid gland itself, resulting in an absent (athyreosis) or underdeveloped (hypoplastic) gland.

Ans. 136. **d.** Periphery 137. **b.** Liver 138. **b.** Secondaries 139. **d.** Urine contains 5-HIAA
140. **a.** Adrenals 141. **a.** Thyroid dysgenesis

142. Hurthle cell is a feature of:

a. Acute thyroiditis
b. Thyroid carcinoma
c. Granulomatous thyroiditis
d. Hashimoto's thyroiditis

A **Hürthle cell** is a cell in the thyroid that is often associated with Hashimoto's thyroiditis as well as follicular thyroid cancer.

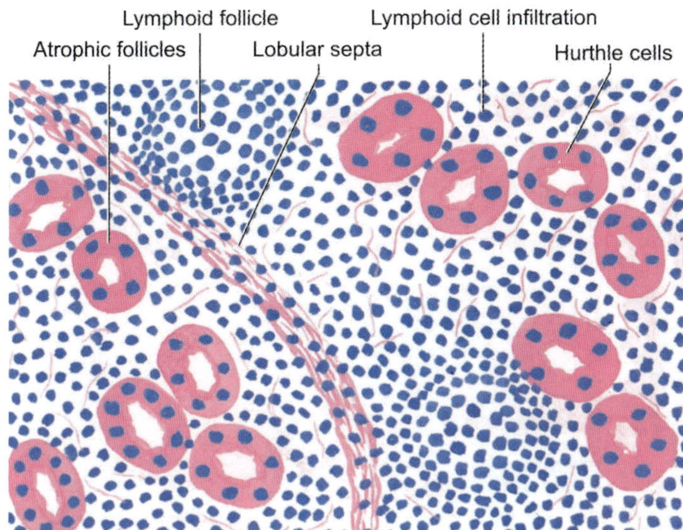

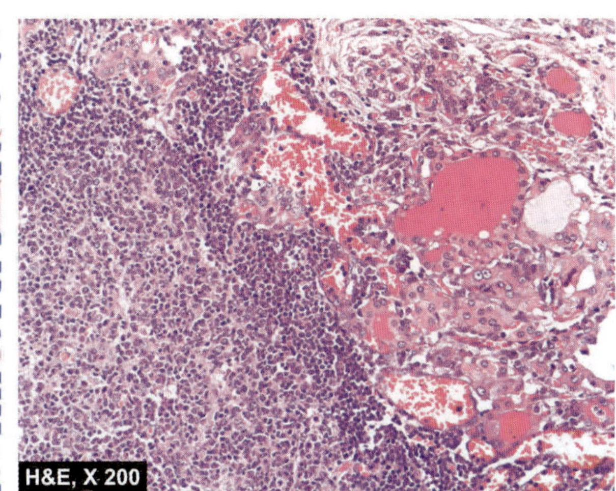

Hashimoto's thyroiditis. Histologic features include: Lymphoid cell infiltration with formation of lymphoid follicles having germinal centres; small, atrophic and colloid-deficient follicles; presence of Hurthle cells which have granular oxyphil cytoplasm and large irregular nuclei; and slight fibrous thickening of lobular septa.

143. All are associated with pheochromocytoma EXCEPT:

a. MEN IIa
b. MEN IIb
c. Von Hippel Lindau syndrome
d. Weber syndrome

Weber's syndrome (superior alternating hemiplegia) is a form of stroke characterized by the presence of an ipsilateral oculomotor nerve palsy and contralateral hemiparesis or hemiplegia.

144. 'Orphan annie eye nuclei' is seen in which carcinoma of thyroid:

a. Follicular b. Anaplastic
c. Medullary d. Papillary

Characteristic Orphan Annie eye nuclear inclusions (nuclei with uniform staining, which appear empty) and psammoma bodies on light microscopy. The former is useful in identifying the follicular variant of papillary thyroid carcinomas.

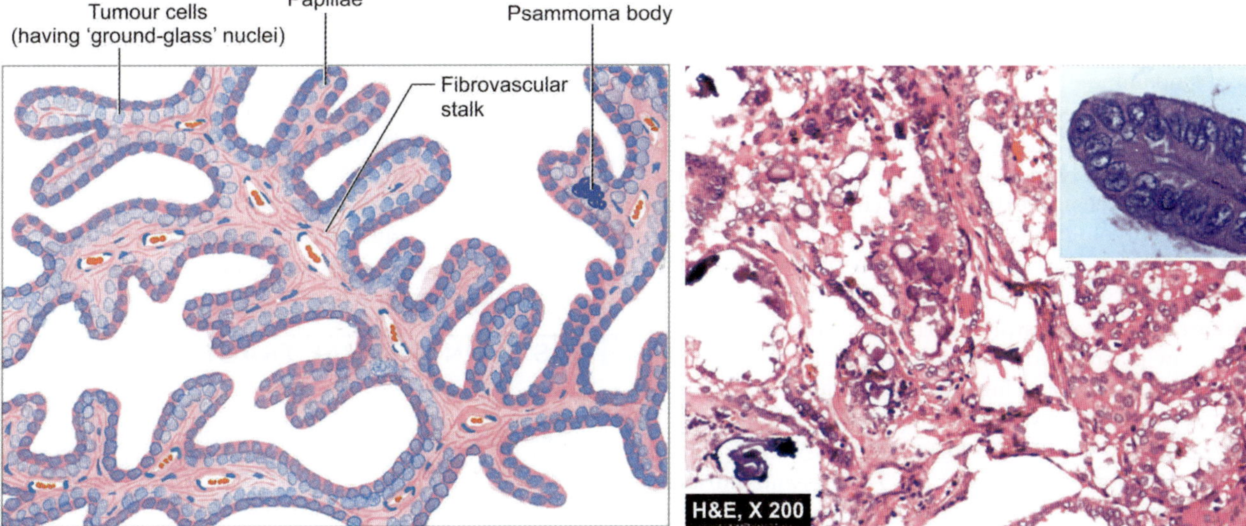

Papillary carcinoma thyroid. Microscopy shows branching papillae having fibrovascular stalk covered by a single layer of cuboidal cells having ground-glass nuclei (inbox). Colloid-filled follicles and solid sheets of tumour cells are also present.

Ans. 142. d. Hashimoto's... **143. d.** Weber syndrome **144. d.** Papillary

145. Commonest cause of solitary thyroid adenoma:

a. Adenomatous goitre b. Papillary carcinoma
c. Follicular carcinoma d. Follicular adenoma

Almost all thyroid adenomas are follicular adenomas. Follicular adenomas can be described as "cold", "warm" or "hot" depending on their level of function.

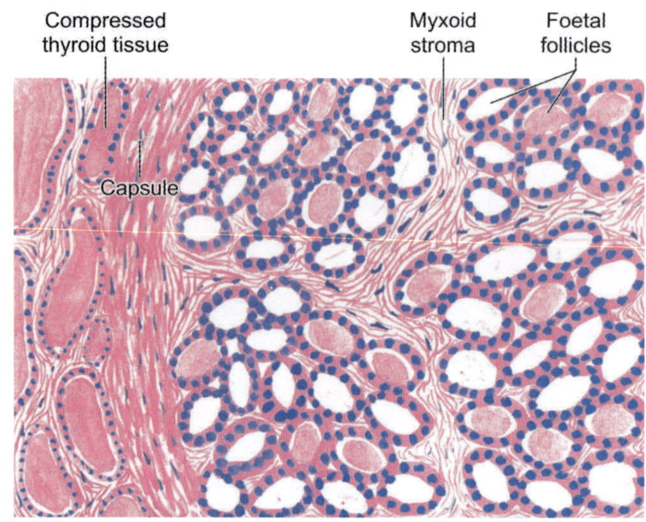

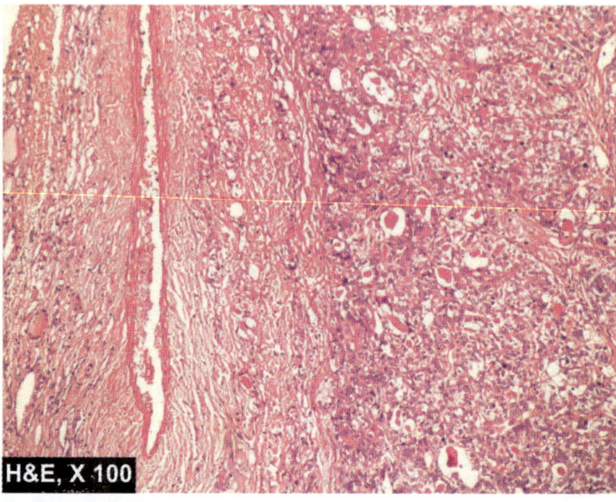

Follicular adenoma, foetal (microfollicular) type. The tumour is well encapsulated with compression of surrounding thyroid parenchyma. The tumour consists of small follicles lined by cuboidal epithelium and contain little or no colloid and separated by abundant loose stroma.

146. Which is NOT a feature of hypothyroidism:

a. Myxedema
b. Carpal tunnel syndrome
c. Menorrhagia
d. Increased appetite

Voracious appetite is a feature of hyperthyroidism.

147. Hypothyroidism is caused by all EXCEPT:

a. PAS b. Lithium
c. Phenytoin d. Amiodarone

Side effects of phenytoin include fetal hydantoin syndrome, gum hyperplasia, megaloblastic anemia, pseudolymphoma etc.

148. Pheochromocytoma predominantly secretes:

a. Epinephrine b. Nor-epinephrine
c. Dopamine d. Dobutamine

A **pheochromocytoma** (*phaios* "dark", *chroma* "color", *kytos* "cell",*-oma* "tumor") is a neuroendocrine tumor of the medulla of the adrenal glands (originating in the chromaffin cells), or extra-adrenal chromaffin tissue that failed to involute after birth, that secretes high amounts of catecholamines, mostly norepinephrine, plus epinephrine to a lesser extent.

149. Central diabetes insipidus is characterized by:

a. Low plasma and low urine osmolality
b. High plasma and high urine osmolality
c. Low plasma and high urine osmolality
d. High plasma and low urine osmolality

A urinary specific gravity of 1.005 or less and a urinary osmolality of less than 200 mOsm/kg are the hallmark of DI. Random plasma osmolality generally is greater than 287 mOsm/kg.

150. Which of the following is the earliest manifestation of Cushing's syndrome:

a. Loss of diurnal variation
b. Increased ACTH
c. Decreased plasma cortisol
d. Increased urinary metabolites of cortisol

Cushing's syndrome refers to excess cortisol of any etiology (as syndrome means a group of symptoms). One of the causes of Cushing's syndrome is a cortisol-secreting adenoma in the cortex of the adrenal gland (primary hypercortisolism/hypercorticism). The adenoma causes cortisol levels in the blood to be very high, and negative feedback on the pituitary from the high cortisol levels causes ACTH levels to be very low.

151. Syndrome of inappropriate ADH secretion is commonly associated with:

a. Breast carcinoma b. Ovarian carcinoma
c. Lung carcinoma
d. Hepatocellular carcinoma

SIADH was originally described in people with small-cell carcinoma of the lung, but it can be caused by a number of underlying medical conditions.

GASTROINTESTINAL TRACT PATHOLOGY

152. Ulcerative colitis is associated with:

a. AMA b. ANA
c. c-ANCA d. p-ANCA

p-ANCA is associated with several medical conditions:

- It is fairly specific, but not sensitive for ulcerative colitis, so is not useful as a sole diagnostic test.

Ans. **145. d.** Follicular aden... **146. d.** Increased... **147. c.** Phenytoin **148. b.** Nor-epinephrine
149. d. High... **150. a.** Loss of diurnal... **151. c.** Lung carcinoma **152. d.** p-ANCA

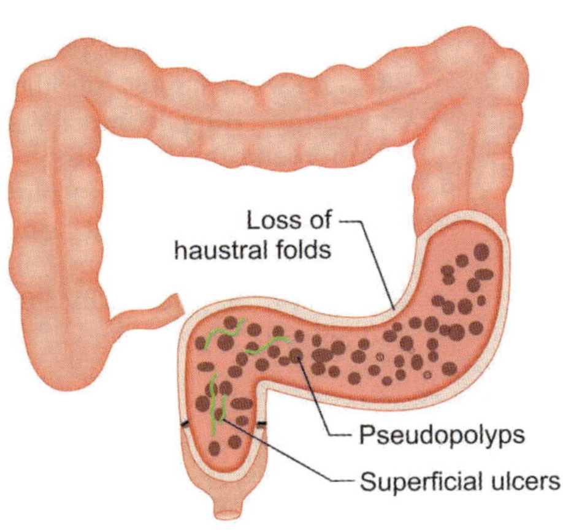

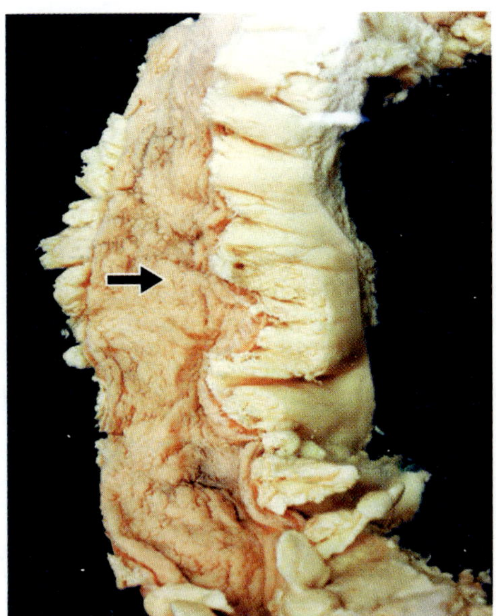

Ulcerative colitis. Continuous involvement of the rectum and colon without any uninvolved skip areas. The ulcers are superficial with intervening inflammatory pseudopolyps. The lumen is narrow and the haustral folds are lost giving 'garden-hose appearance'.

- When measured together with Anti-saccharomyces cerevisiae antibodies (ASCA), p-ANCA has been estimated to have a specificity of 97% and a sensitivity of 48% in differentiating patients with ulcerative colitis from normal controls.
- About 50% of cases of Churg Strauss syndrome
- A majority of primary sclerosing cholangitis
- Sometimes polyarteritis nodosa (only in the variant microscopic polyangiitis, usually negative in typical polyarteritis nodosa)
- Microscopic polyangitis
- Focal necrotising and crescentic glomerulonephritis
- Rheumatoid arthritis

153. Condition associated with Type A gastritis:

a. Autoimmunity
b. Drugs
c. Crohns disease
d. Beta haemolytic streptococci

Type A Gastritis

- Those with the type A/autoimmune version of atrophic gastritis are statistically more likely to develop gastric Ca, Hashimoto's thyroiditis, and achlorhydria
- Type A gastritis primarily affects the body/fundus of the stomach, and
- Is more common with pernicious anemia.

Type B gastritis

- Most common overall
- Primarily affects the antrum, and
- Is more common with H. pylori infection.

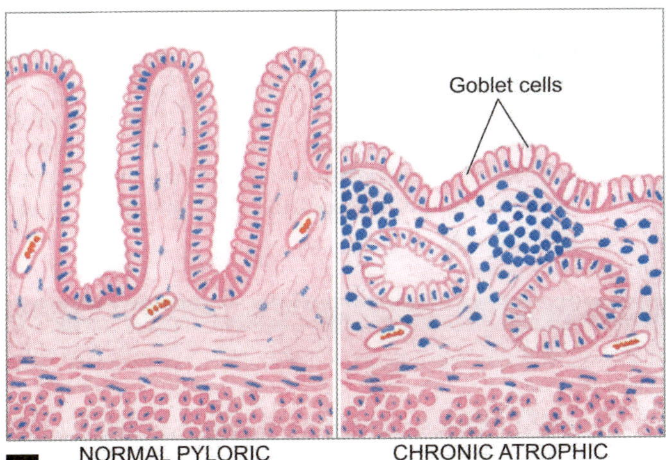

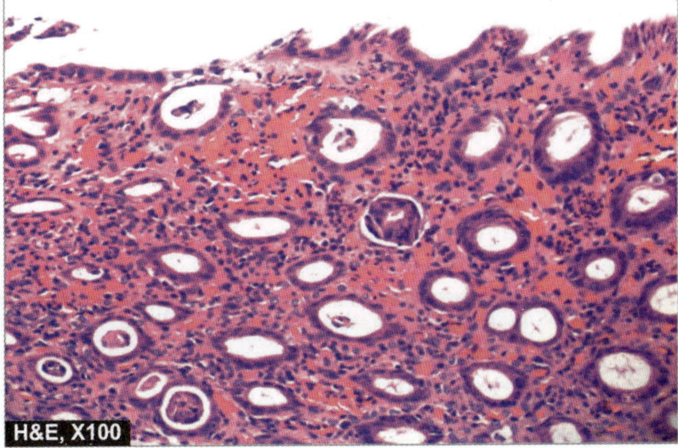

A, Chronic atrophic gastritis (right) contrasted with normal pyloric mucosa (left). There is marked gastric atrophy with disappearance of gastric glands and appearance of goblet cells (intestinal metaplasia). B, Photomicrograph showing chronic atrophic gastritis with intestinal metaplasia.

Ans. 153. a. Autoimmunity

154. Condition associated with Toxic megacolon:

a. Crohns disease
b. Ulcerative colitis
c. Typhoid
d. TB

Toxic megacolon (megacolon toxicum)

- It is an acute form of colonic distension.
- It is characterized by a very dilated colon (megacolon), accompanied by abdominal distension (bloating), and sometimes fever, abdominal pain, or shock.
- Toxic megacolon is usually a complication of:
  - Inflammatory bowel disease, such as ulcerative colitis and, more rarely, Crohn's disease, and
  - Of some infections of the colon, including Clostridium difficile infections, which have led to pseudomembranous colitis.
  - Other forms of megacolon exist and can be congenital (present since birth, such as Hirschprung's disease).
  - Also, it can be caused by Entamoeba histolytica and Shigella.

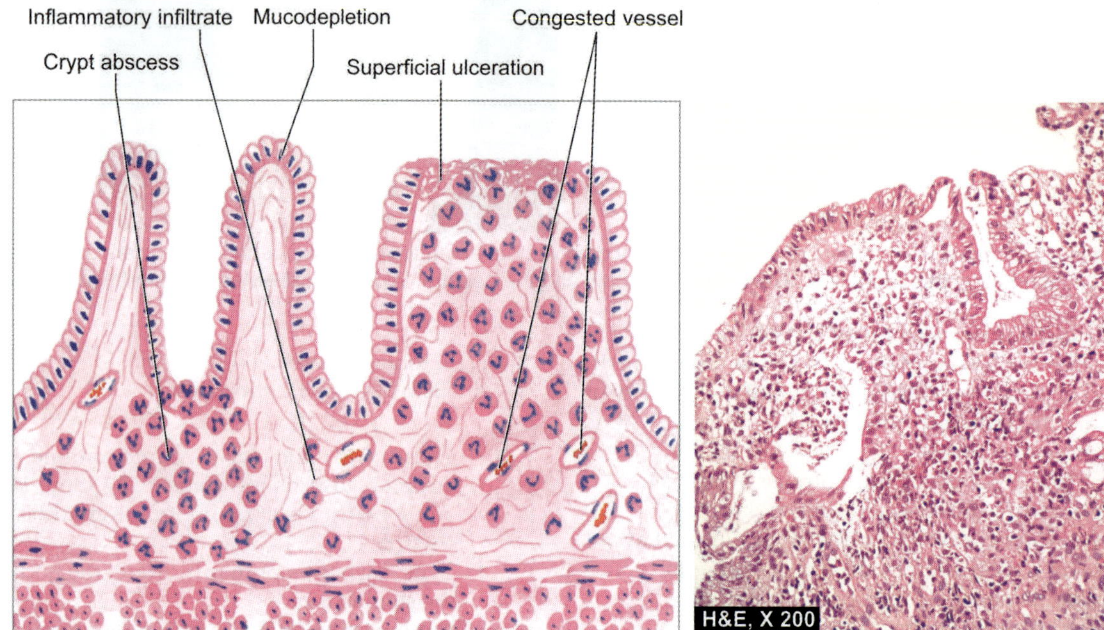

Ulcerative colitis in active phase. The microscopic features seen are superficial ulcerations, with mucosal infiltration by inflammatory cells and a 'crypt abscess'.

155. Features of Crohn's disease are all EXCEPT:

a. Absence of granuloma
b. Skip lesion
c. Transmural involvement
d. Crypt abscess

Under a microscope, biopsies of the colon affected by Crohn's disease may show mucosal inflammation, characterized by focal infiltration of neutrophils, a type of inflammatory cell, into the epithelium. This typically occurs in the area overlying lymphoid aggregates. These neutrophils, along with mononuclear cells, may infiltrate the crypts, leading to inflammation (cryptitis) or abscess (crypt abscess). Granulomas, aggregates of macrophage derivatives known as giant cells, are found in 50% of cases and are most specific for Crohn's disease. The granulomas of Crohn's disease do not show "caseation", a cheese-like appearance on microscopic examination characteristic of granulomas associated with infections, such as tuberculosis.

Distinguishing features of Crohn's disease and ulcerative colitis

Feature	*Crohn's disease*	*Ulcerative colitis*
a. MACROSCOPIC FEATURES		
1. Distribution	Segmental with skip areas	Continuous without skip areas
2. Location	Commonly terminal ileum and/or ascending colon	Commonly rectum, sigmoid colon and extending upwards

Contd...

Ans. 154. b. Ulcerative colitis **155. a.** Absence of granuloma

Contd...

Feature	*Crohn's disease*	*Ulcerative colitis*
3. Extent	Usually involves the entire thickness of the affected segment of bowel wall	Usually superficial, confined to mucosal layers
4. Ulcers	Serpiginous ulcers, may develop into deep fissures	Superficial mucosal ulcers without fissures
5. Pseudopolyps	Rarely seen	Commonly present
6. Fibrosis	Common	Rare
7. Shortening	Due to fibrosis	Due to contraction of muscularis
B. MICROSCOPIC FEATURES		
1. Depth of inflammation	Typically transmural	Mucosal and submucosal
2. Type of inflammation	Non-caseating granulomas and infiltrate of mononuclear cells (lymphocytes, plasma cells and macrophages)	Crypt abscess and non-specific acute and chronic inflammatory cells (lymphocytes, plasma cells, neutrophils, eosinophils, mast cells)
3. Mucosa	Patchy ulceration	Hemorrhagic mucosa with ulceration
4. Submucosa	Widened due to oedema and lymphoid aggregates	Normal or reduced in width
5. Muscularis	Infiltrated by inflammatory cells	Usually spared ***except*** in cases of toxic megacolon
6. Fibrosis	Present	Usually absent
C. IMMUNOLOGIC FEATURES		
1. Lymphocyte type	CD4+ TH1	CD4+ TH2
2. Cytokines	INF-γ, TNF, IL-12	TGF-β, IL-4, IL-5, IL-13
3. ANCA-P antibodies	Positive in a few	Positive in most
D. COMPLICATIONS		
1. Fistula formation	Internal and external fistulae in 10% cases	Extremely rare
2. Malignant changes	Rare	May occur infrequently in disease of more than 10 years' duration
3. Type of malignancy	Lymphoma more often than carcinoma	Carcinoma more often than lymphoma
4. Fibrous strictures	Common	Never

156. Conditions associated with increased risk of squamous cell carcinoma of the esophagus include all EXCEPT:

a. Barrett's esophagus
b. Achalasia cardia
c. Smoking
d. Tylosis

Barrett's esophagus, sometimes called **Barrett syndrome, Barrett esophagus**, or **columnar epithelium lined lower esophagus** (**CELLO**), refers to an abnormal change (metaplasia) in the cells of the lower portion of the esophagus. It is characterized by the replacement of the normal stratified squamous epithelium lining of the esophagus by simple columnar epithelium with goblet cells (which are usually found lower in the gastrointestinal tract). The medical significance of Barrett's esophagus is its strong association (about 0.5% per patient-year) with esophageal adenocarcinoma, a very often deadly cancer, because of which it is considered to be a premalignant condition.

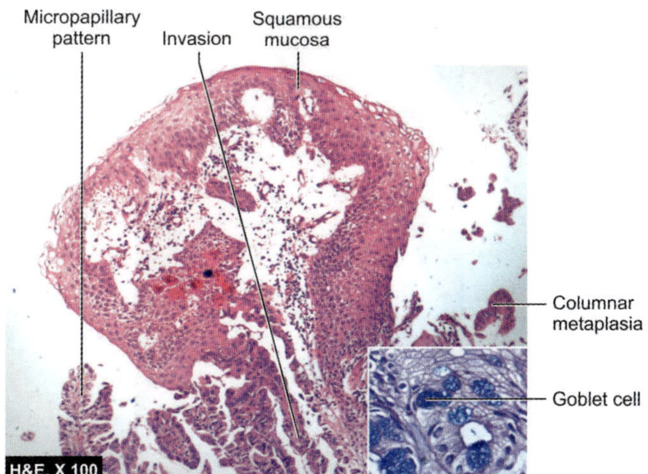

Barrett's esophagus. The central part of the image shows squamous mucosa bounded on either side by metaplastic columnar mucosa showing anaplastic change and micropapillary pattern of adenocarcinoma. Inbox shows goblet cells in the metaplastic columnar epithelium strained positive for alcian blue.

Ans. 156. a. Barrett's esophagus

157. All are seen in ulcerative colitis EXCEPT:

a. Pseudopolyps
b. Skip lesions
c. Rectum involvement
d. Malabsorption

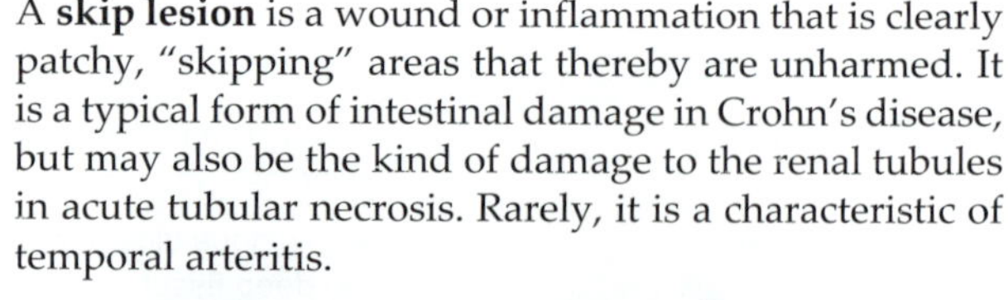

A **skip lesion** is a wound or inflammation that is clearly patchy, "skipping" areas that thereby are unharmed. It is a typical form of intestinal damage in Crohn's disease, but may also be the kind of damage to the renal tubules in acute tubular necrosis. Rarely, it is a characteristic of temporal arteritis.

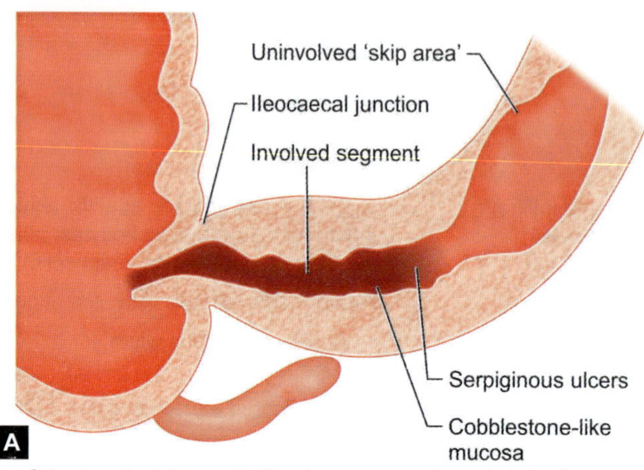

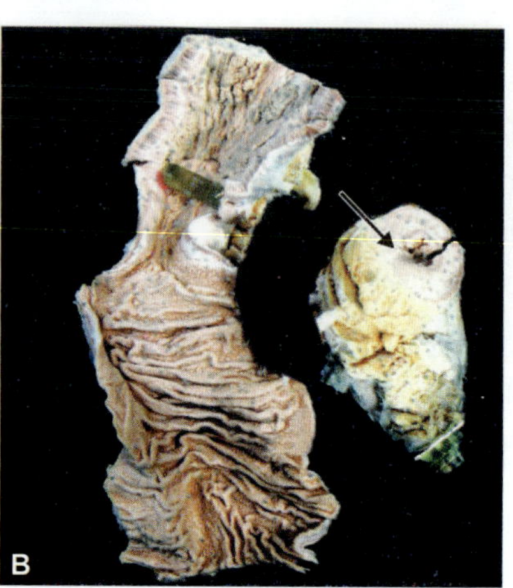

Crohn's disease of the terminal ileum. A, The lesions are characteristically segmental with intervening uninvolved 'skip areas'. The bowel wall is thickened and the lumen narrowed, giving hose-pipe appearance. Serpiginous ulcers, some deep fissures and swollen intervening surviving mucosa giving 'cobblestone appearance', are present. B, The specimen of small intestine is shown in longitudinal section along with a segment in cross-section. External surface shows increased mesenteric fat, thickened wall and narrow lumen. Luminal surface of longitudinal cut section shows segment of thickened wall with narrow lumen which is better appreciated in cross-section (arrow) while intervening areas of the bowel are uninvolved or skipped.

158. All have high malignant potential EXCEPT:

a. Hyperplastic polyp
b. Pseudoneuroma
c. Villous adenoma
d. Tubular adenoma

Most hyperplastic polyps are found in the distal colon and rectum. They have no malignant potential, which means that they are no more likely than normal tissue to eventually become a cancer.

159. MC site for amoebiasis:

a. Liver
b. Caecum
c. Transverse colon
d. Sigmoid colon

Intestinal amebiasis may involve any part of the bowel. It usually involves caecum and ascending colon followed by sigmoid colon, rectum, and appendix.

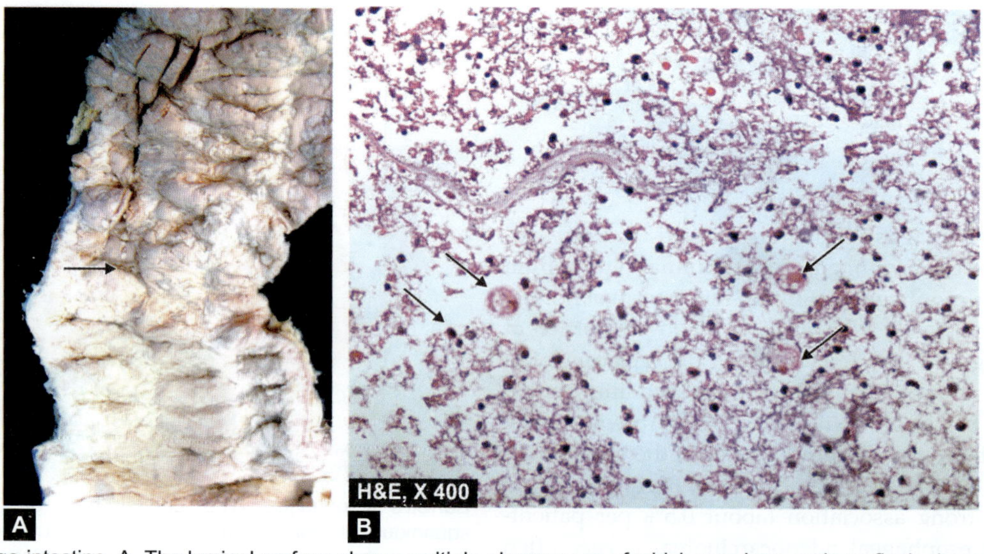

Amoebic ulcers large intestine. A, The luminal surface shows multiple ulcers some of which are deep and are flask-shaped with narrow neck and broad base (arrow) containing necrotic tissue and undermined margins. B, Trophozoites of Entamoeba histolytica are seen at the margin of ulcer (arrow).

Ans. **157. b.** Skip lesions **158. a.** Hyperplastic polyp **159. b.** Caecum

160. All are complications of typhoid ulcer EXCEPT:

a. Perforation b. Stricture
c. Hemorhage d. Sepsis

Stricture is a common complication of tuberculous intestinal ulcers as they lied circumferentially. Typhoid ulcers lie longitudinally.

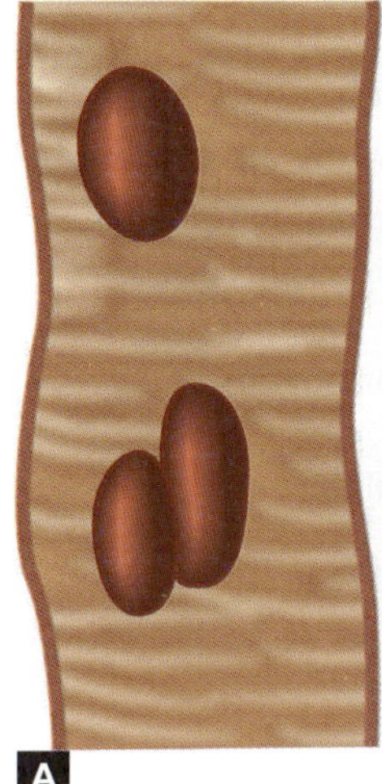

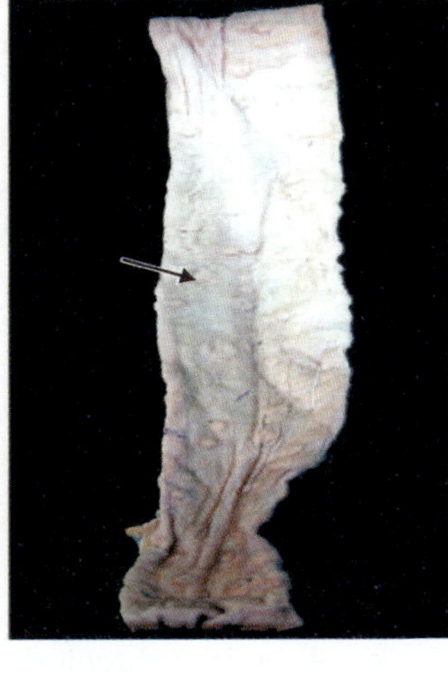

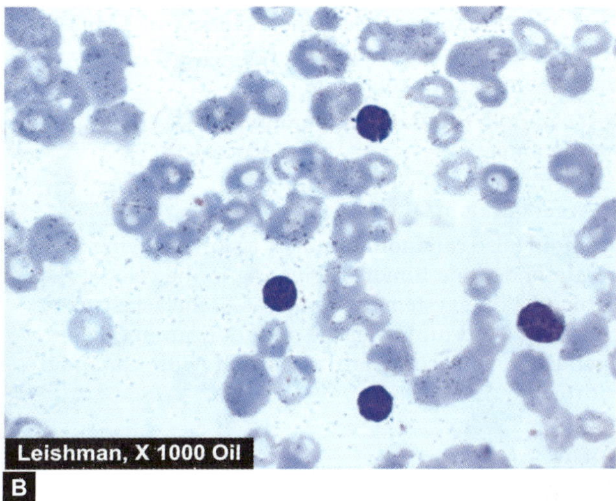

A, Typhoid ulcers in the small intestine appear characteristically oval with their long axis parallel to the long axis of the bowel. B, Blood picture in typhoid fever showing neutropenia and relative lymphocytosis.

161. MC site of diverticulosis:

a. Sigmoid colon b. Descending colon
c. Transverse colon d. Ascending colon

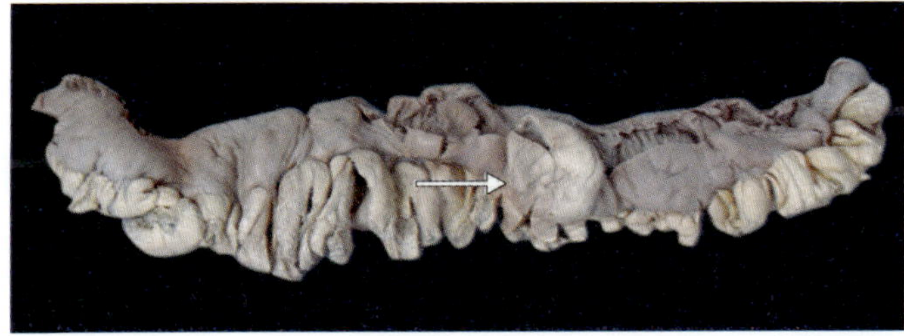

Diverticulosis coli. The outpouchings on the mesentery communicate with lumen of colon.

Diverticulosis, also known as "**diverticular disease**", is the condition of having diverticula in the colon, which are outpocketings of the colonic mucosa and submucosa through weaknesses of muscle layers in the colon wall. These are more common in the sigmoid colon, which is a common place for increased pressure.

162. All of the following are pathological features associated with Crohn's disease EXCEPT:

a. Skip lesions
b. Non caseating granulomas
c. Cobblestone appearance
d. Toxic megacolon

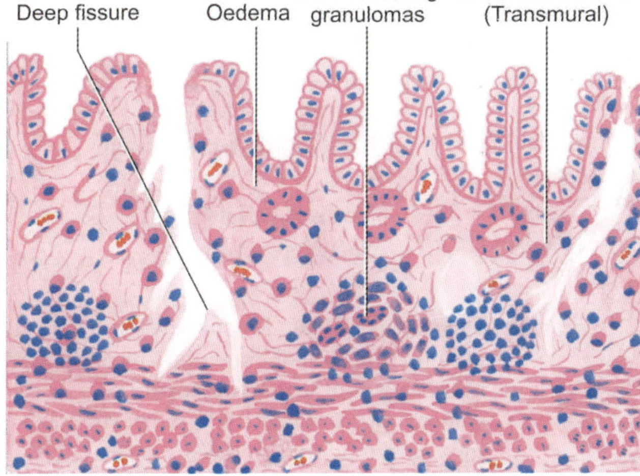

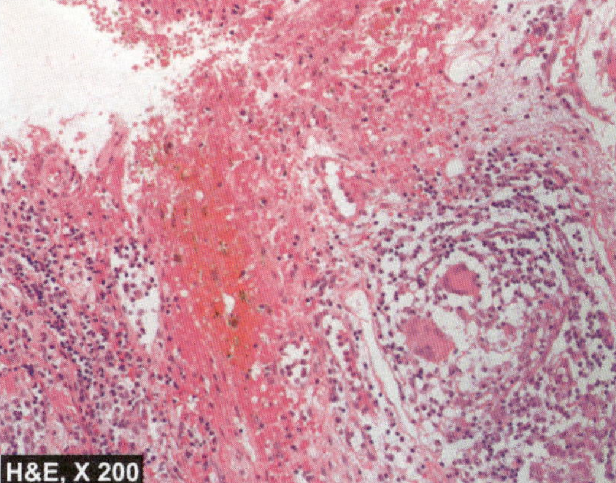

Crohn's disease of the ileum. The histological features present are: transmural chronic inflammatory cell infiltration, deep fissures into the bowel wall, submucosal widening due to oedema, some prominent lymphoid follicles and a few non-caseating epithelioid cell granulomas in the bowel wall.

Ans. **160. b.** Stricture **161. a.** Sigmoid colon **162. d.** Toxic megacolon

Toxic Megacolon (toxic colitis) was first thought to be a complication only of ulcerative colitis. In fact, TM (TC) may complicate any number of colitides, including inflammatory, ischemic, infectious, radiation, and pseudomembranous. Indeed, the incidence of TM (TC) is expected to increase due to the rising prevalence of pseudomembranous colitis.

163. Most common tumour of appendix is:

a. Adenoma b. Mucocoele
c. Pseudomyxoma peritonei
d. Argentaffinoma

Carcinoid (also **carcinoid tumor**) is a slow-growing type of neuroendocrine tumor originating in the cells of the neuroendocrine system. In some cases, metastasis may occur. Carcinoid tumors of the midgut (jejunum, ileum, appendix, and cecum) are associated with carcinoid syndrome.

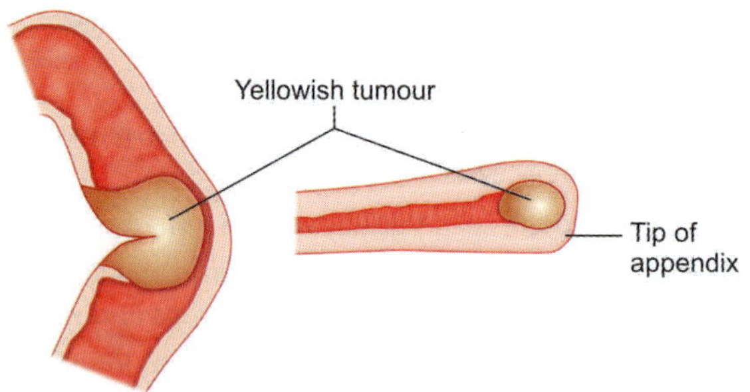

Carcinoid tumour. Gross appearance at common locations in longitudinal section.

HEMATOPOIETIC SYSTEM PATHOLOGY

164. Common subtype of ALL:

a. T cell b. B cell
c. Pre B cell d. Pre T cell

Precursor B-cell lymphoblastic leukemia

- It is a form of lymphoid leukemia in which too many B-cells lymphoblasts (immature WBCs) are found in the blood and bone marow.
- It is the most common type of acute lymphoblastic leukemia (ALL).
- It is sometimes additionally classified as a lymphoma, as designated leukemia/ lymphoma.
- It consists of the following subtypes
  - t(9;22)—BCR/ AB
  - t(v;11q23)—MLL rearrangement
  - t(1;19)—E2A/PBX1
  - t(12;21)—ETV/ CBFalpha
  - t (17;19)—E2A-HLF

165. Low iron & low TIBC is suggestive of:

a. Sideroblastic anemia
b. Iron deficiency anemia
c. Anemia of chronic diseases
d. Aplastic anemia

Anemia

- In anemia of chronic disease without iron deficiency, ferritin levels should be normal or high, reflecting the fact that iron is stored within cells, and ferritin is being produced as an acute phase reactant but the cells are not releasing their iron. In IDA ferritin should be low.
- TIBC should be high in genuine iron deficiency, reflecting efforts by the body to produce more transferrin and bind up as much iron as possible; TIBC should be low or normal in anemia of chronic disease.

Laboratory diagnosis of hypochromic anaemias.

	Test	*Iron deficiency*	*Chronic disorders*	*Thalassaemia minor*	*Sideroblastic anaemia*
1.	*MCV, MCH, MCHC*	Reduced	Low normal-to- reduced	Very low	Very low (except MCV raised in aquired type)
2.	*Serum iron*	Reduced	Reduced	Normal	Raised
3.	*TIBC*	Raised	Low-to-normal	Normal	Normal
4.	*Serum ferritin*	Reduced	Raised	Normal	Raised (complete saturation)
5.	*Marrow-iron stores*	Absent	Present	High	High
6.	*Iron in normoblasts*	Absent	Absent	Present	Ring sideroblasts
7.	*Hb electrophoresis*	Normal	Normal	Abnormal	Normal

166. Splenectomy would be most useful in:

a. Goodpasture syndrome b. TB
c. Sickle cell anemia d. Idiopathic ITP

Idiopathic thrombocytopenic purpura (ITP), often called **primary immune thrombocytopenia** and also known as **primary immune thrombocytopenic purpura** and **autoimmune thrombocytopenic purpura**

- Defined as isolated low platelet count (thrombocytopenia) with normal bone marrow and the absence of other causes of thrombocytopenia.
- Causes a characteristic purpuric rash and an increased tendency to bleed.
- The acute form often follows an infection and has a spontaneous resolution within 2 months.

Ans. 163. d. Argentaffinoma **164. c.** Pre B cell **165. c.** Anemia of chronic... **166. d.** Idiopathic ITP

- Chronic idiopathic thrombocytopenic purpura persists longer than 6 months with a specific cause being unknown.
- ITP is an autoimmune condition with antibodies detectable against several platelet surface antigens.
- ITP is diagnosed by a low platelet count in a complete blood count
- However, since the diagnosis depends on the exclusion of other causes of a low platelet count, additional investigations (such as a bone marrow biopsy) may be necessary in some cases.

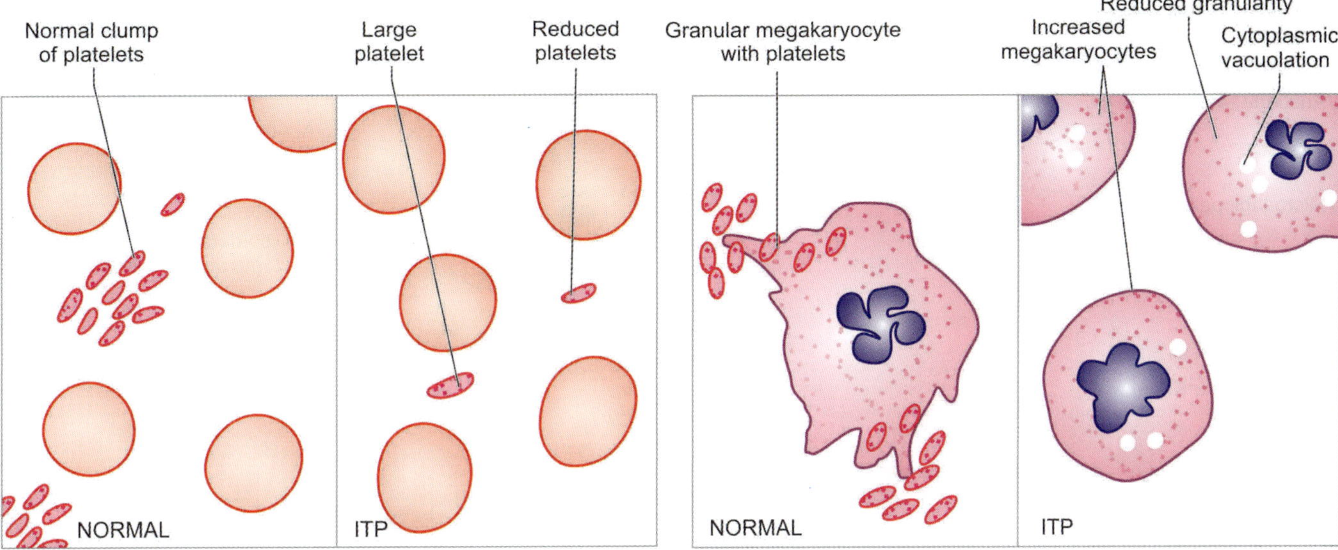

A, BLOOD FILM

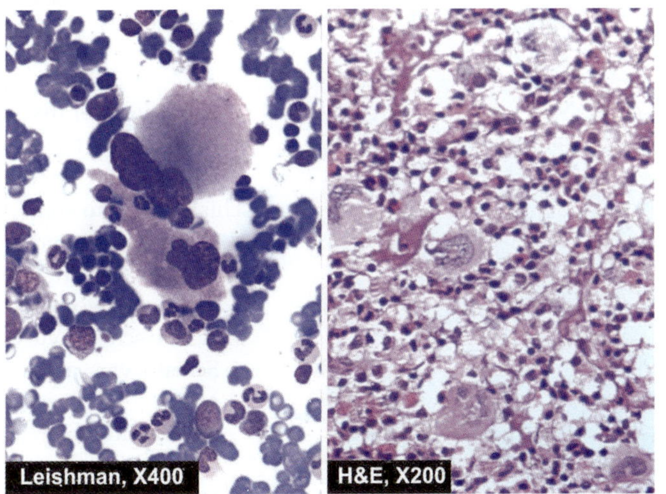

B, BONE MARROW ASPIRATE C, BONE MARROW TREPHINE

Laboratory findings of ITP contrasted with those found in a normal individual. A, Peripheral blood in ITP shows presence of reduced number of platelets which are often large. B, C, Bone marrow aspirate and trephine in ITP show characteristically increased number of megakaryocytes with single non-lobulated nuclei and reduced cytoplasmic granularity.

167. G-6-PD helps in maintaining the integrity of RBC by:
a. Component of electron transport chain
b. Maintain flexibility of cell membrane
c. Controlling reduction stress of RBC
d. Controlling oxidation stress of RBC

Glucose-6-phosphate dehydrogenase (G6PD or G6PDH)

- This enzyme is in the pentose phosphate pathway, a metabolic pathway that supplies reducing energy to cells (such as erythrocytes) by maintaining the level

Ans. **167. d.** Controlling oxidation stress of RBC

of the co-enzyme nicotinamide adenine dinucleotide phosphate (NADPH).

- The NADPH in turn maintains the level of glutathione in these cells that helps protect the red blood cells against oxidative damage.
- Notable in humans when there is a genetic deficiency of G6PD which predisposes to non-immune haemolytic anemia.

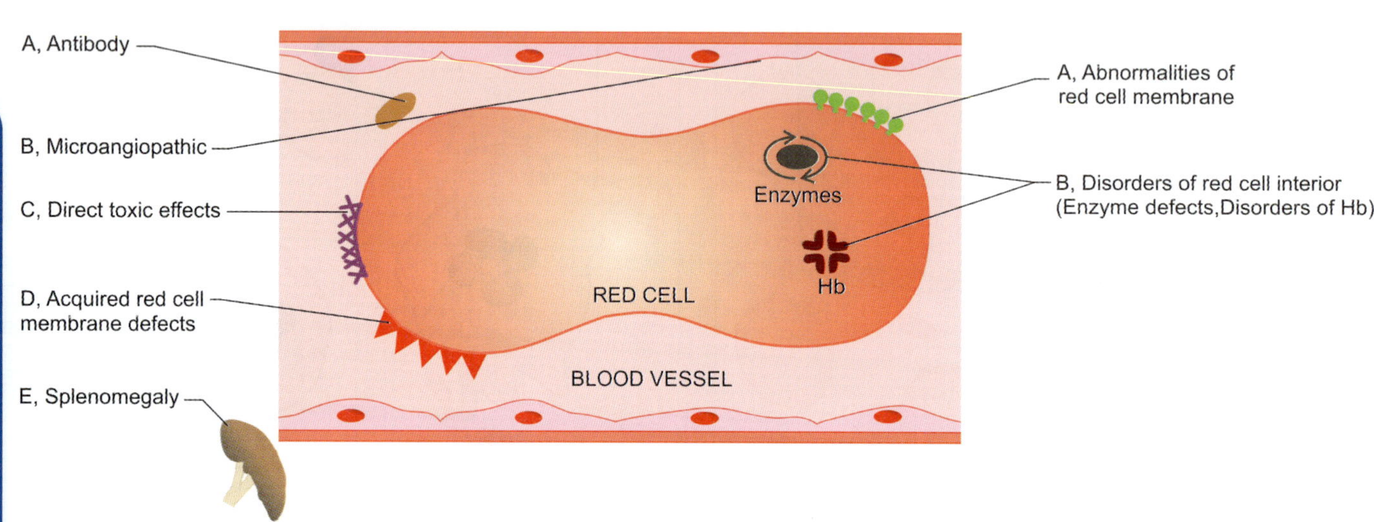

Diagrammatic representation of classification of haemolytic anaemias based on principal mechanisms of haemolysis

168. Which of the following does NOT predispose to Disseminated intravascular coagulation?

a. Retained dead fetus
b. Amniotic fluid embolism
c. Placenta praevia
d. Burns

Risk-factors for DVT

- Cancer,
- Trauma and
- Antiphospholipid syndrome.
- **Older age:** The frequency of occurrence increases dramatically from childhood to old age; in adulthood, about 1 in 1000 adults develops DVT annually.
- Surgery,
- Immobilization (as with bed rest, orthopaedic casts, and sitting on long flights),
- Combined oral contraceptives,
- Pregnancy,
- Postnatal period, and
- Genetic factors such as a non-O blood type.

169. Schistocytes are seen in:

a. Hemolytic uremic syndrome
b. Malaria
c. Chronic liver disease
d. Iron deficiency anemia

A **schistocyte** or **schizocyte** (schistos for "divided" or schistein for "to split", and kytos for "hollow" or "cell")

- It is a fragmented part of a red blood cell.
- Schistocytes are typically irregularly shaped, jagged, and have two pointed ends.
- A true schistocyte does not have central pallor.
- Schistocytes are sometimes referred to as "helmet cells".
- Several microangiopathic diseases, including disseminated intravascular coagulation and thrombotic microangiopathies, generate fibrin strands that sever red blood cells as they try to move past a thrombus, creating schistocytes.
- Schistocytes are often seen in patients with haemolytic anemia.
- They are frequently a consequence of mechanical artificial heart valves and haemolytic uremic syndrome, among other causes.
- Excessive schistocytes present in blood can be a sign of microangiopathic hemolytic anemia (MAHA) where the most common cause is aortic stenosis.

Ans. 168. c. Placenta praevia **169. a.** Hemolytic uremic syndrome

Red cell morphologic features in various types of haemolytic anaemias.		
Feature	*Etiology*	*Type of haemolytic anaemia*
1. Spherocytes	Loss of spectrin from membrane	Hereditary spherocytosis AIHA
2. Target cells (Leptocytes)	Increased ratio of surface area: volume	Thalassaemias Liver disease HbS disease HbC disease
3. Schistocytes	Traumatic damage to red cell membrane	Microangiopathy
4. Sickle cells	Polymerisation of HbS	Sickle syndromes
5. Acanthocytes (Spur cells)	Abnormality in membrane lipids	Severe liver disease
6. Heinz bodies	Precipitated Hb	Unstable Hb

170. DIC is seen with all EXCEPT:

a. Accidental hemorrhage
b. Black water fever
c. Amniotic fluid embolism
d. Anticoagulants

Disseminated intravascular coagulation (**DIC**), also known as **disseminated intravascular coagulopathy** or less commonly as **consumptive coagulopathy**, is a pathological process characterized by the widespread activation of the clotting cascade that results in the formation of blood clots in the small blood vessels throughout the body.

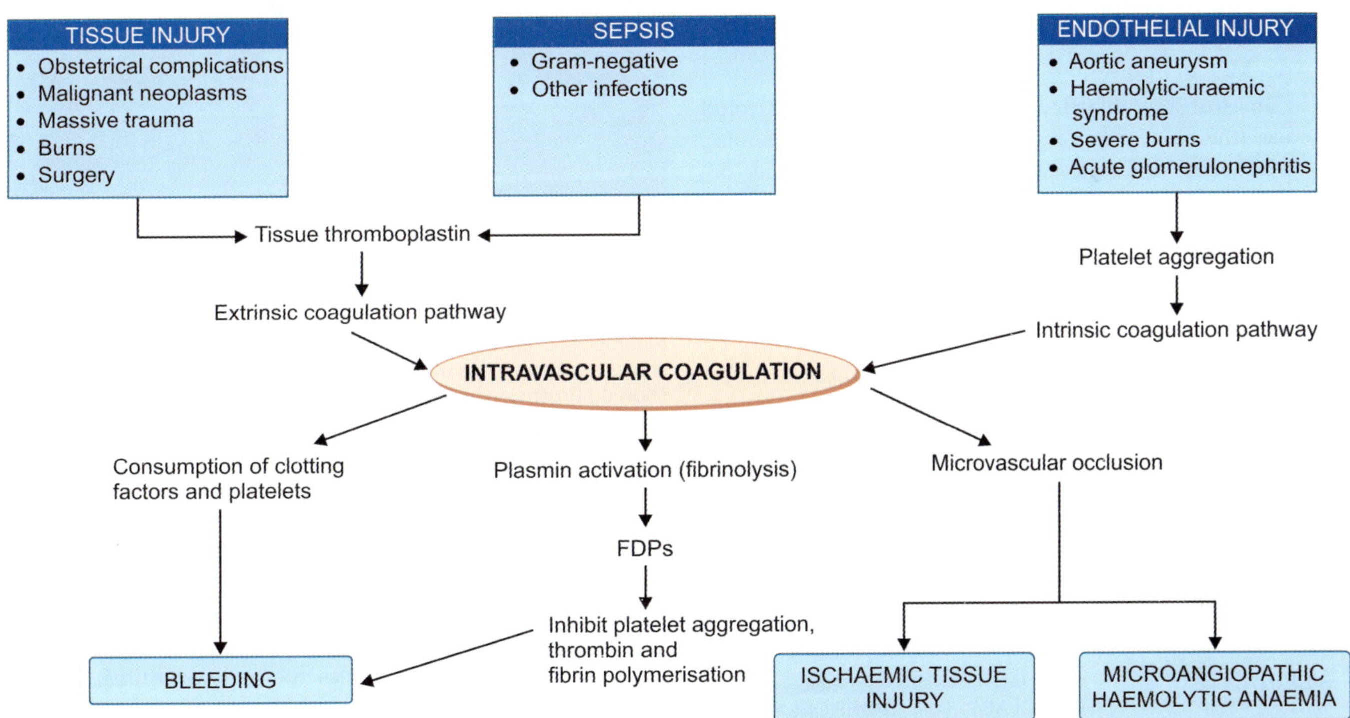

Pathophysiology of disseminated intravascular coagulation.

171. True for DIC are all EXCEPT:

a. Release of tissue factor
b. Decreased fibrinogen products
c. Fibrin deposition in microcirculation
d. Platelet aggregation

In DIC, the processes of coagulation and fibrinolysis are dysregulated, and the result is widespread clotting with resultant bleeding. Excess circulating thrombin assists in the conversion of plasminogen to plasmin, resulting in fibrinolysis. The breakdown of clots results in an excess of Fibrin Degradation Products, which have powerful anticoagulant properties, contributing to hemorrhage.

Ans. 170. d. Anticoagulants **171. b.** Decreased fibrinogen products

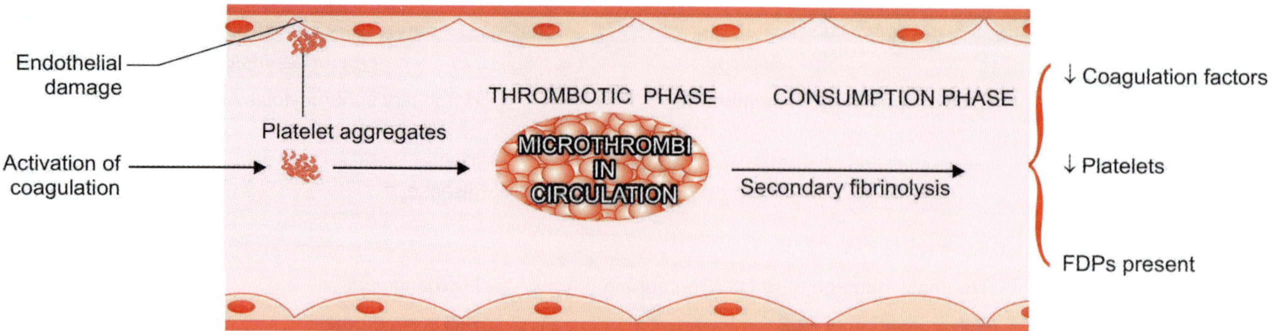

The pathogenesis of disseminated intravascular coagulation.

172. Echinocytes are:

a. Platelets b. Monocytes
c. WBC d. RBC

Echinocytosis is a reversible condition of red blood cells that is often merely an artifact produced by EDTA, which is used as an anticoagulant in sampled blood.

173. Sideroblastic anemia is seen in:

a. Lead poisoning
b. Arsenic poisoning
c. Copper poisoning
d. Mercury poisoning

Causes of sideroblastic anemia include excessive alcohol use (the most common cause of sideroblastic anemia), pyridoxine deficiency, lead poisoning, and copper deficiency. Excess zinc can indirectly cause sideroblastic anemia by decreasing absorption and increasing excretion of copper. Antimicrobials that may lead to sideroblastic anemia include isoniazid, chloramphenicol, cycloserine, and linezolid.

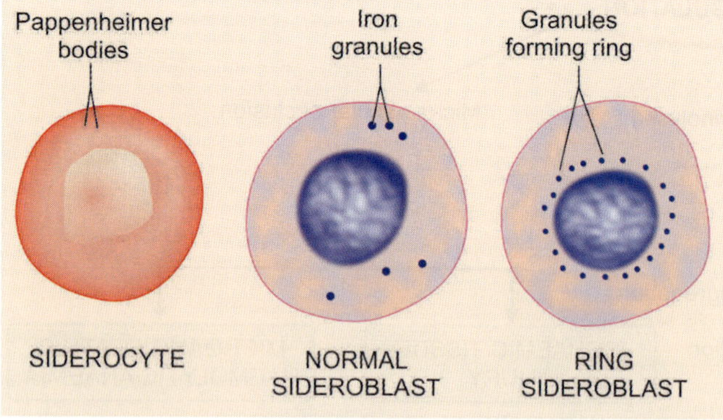

A siderocyte containing Pappenheimer bodies, a normal sideroblast and a ring sideroblast.

174. Lead causes all of the following EXCEPT:

a. Uroporphyrinuria b. Sideroblastic anemia
c. Basophilic stippling d. Macrocytic anemia

Blood film examination in lead poisoning may reveal basophilic stippling of red blood cells (dots in red blood cells visible through a microscope), as well as the changes normally associated with iron-deficiency anemia (microcytosis and hypochromasia).

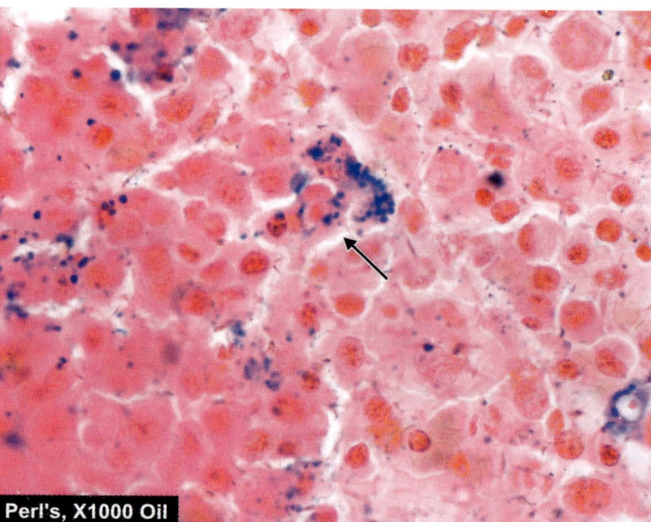

Sideroblastic anemia. Bone marrow aspirate smear in Perls' stain shows marked excess of reticular iron and a ringed sideroblast (arrow) showing Prushsian blue granules in the cytoplasm.

175. Mycosis fungoides is:

a. Cutaneous lymphoma
b. Exfoliative erythroderma
c. Leukemia
d. Fungal infection of skin

Mycosis fungoides, also known as **Alibert-Bazin syndrome** or **granuloma fungoides**, is the most common form of cutaneous T-cell lymphoma. It generally affects the skin, but may progress internally over time.

176. Earliest feature of correction of iron deficiency of anemia:

a. Increase in serum iron level immediately
b. Raised RBCC count
c. Raised serum ferritin
d. Reticulocytosis

The therapeutic goal of oral iron therapy is to induce reticulocytosis within days and raise serum hemoglobin by 1–2 g/dl every 2 weeks, ultimately restoring iron stores in approximately 3–4 months.

Ans. 172. **d.** RBC 173. **a.** Lead poisoning 174. **d.** Macrocytic... 175. **a.** Cutaneous lymphoma 176. **d.** Reticulocytosis

	LABORATORY FINDINGS	NORMAL	IRON-DEFICIENCY ANAEMIA
BLOOD	RED CELL MORPHOLOGY	Normal red cell	Microcytic hypochromic red cell
	RED CELL INDICES	MCV, MCH, MCHC all normal	MCV ↓, MCH ↓, MCHC ↓
BONE MARROW	MARROW ERYTHROPOIESIS	Normoblastic	Micronormoblastic
	MARROW IRON STORES	Normal	Deficient

Laboratory findings in iron deficiency anemia.

177. Blood can be stored at 4°C for:

a. 7 days
b. 14 days
c. 21 days
d. 28 days

Shelf-life of **blood stored** in CPD at 2-**4** °C was **21 days**.

178. CML is characterized by all of the following EXCEPT:

a. Leukocytosis
b. Thrombocytosis
c. Increased leucocyte alkaline phosphatase
d. Increased serum vitamin B12

Serum leukocyte alkaline phosphatase is normal or elevated in leukemoid reaction, but is depressed in chronic myelogenous leukemia.

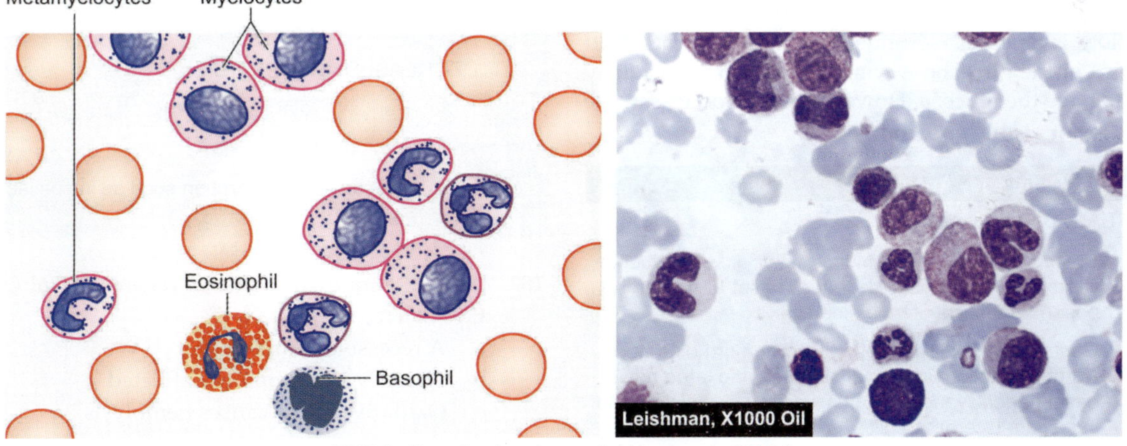

PBF findings in chronic myeloid leukemia (CML).

179. Which one of the following is NOT a feature of polycythemia vera:

a. Elevated RBC mass
b. Normal arterial oxygen tension
c. Splenomegaly
d. Elevated plasma erythropoietin levels

Because polycythemia vera results from an essential increase in erythrocyte production, patients have a low erythropoietin (EPO) level.

180. Auer rods are a feature of:

a. CLL
b. CML
c. AML
d. ALL

Auer rods are clumps of azurophilic granular material that form elongated needles seen in the cytoplasm of leukemic blasts. They can be seen in the leukemic blasts of acute myeloid leukemia with maturation

Ans. 177. **c.** 21 days 178. **c.** Increased leucocyte... 179. **d.** Elevated plasma... 180. **c.** AML and acute promyelocytic leukemia (known as acute myeloid leukemia M2 and M3, in the FAB classification, respectively) and in high grade myelodysplastic syndromes and myeloproliferative syndromes.

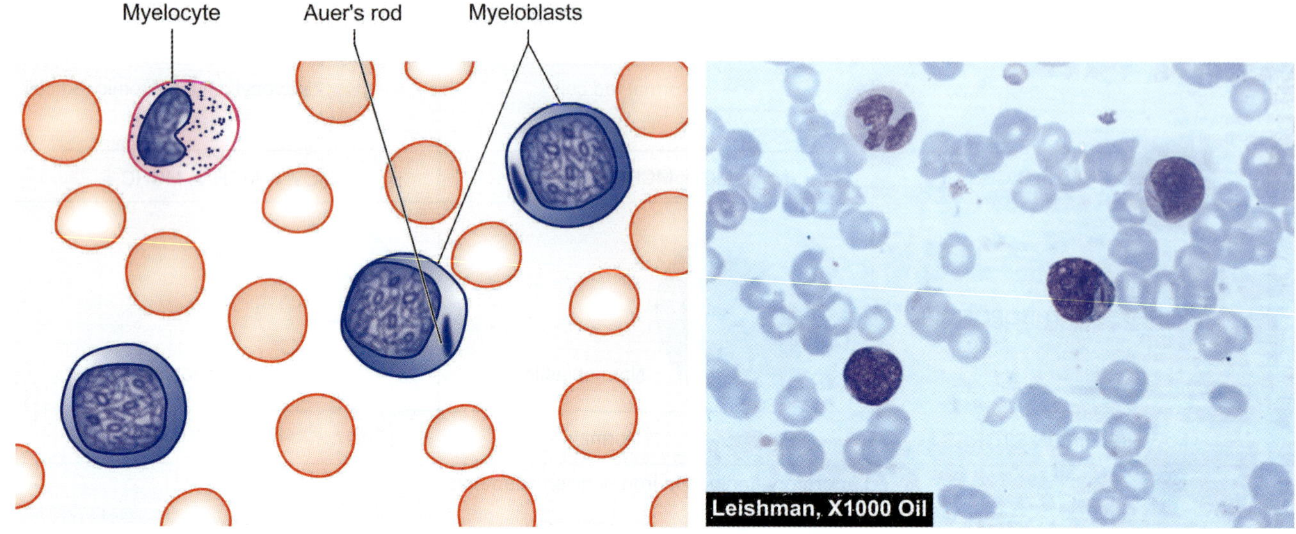

PBF findings in a case of acute myeloblastic leukaemia (AML).

181. In humans, anemia is caused by:

a. Tapeworm
b. Strongyloides
c. Hookworm
d. Roundworm

Hookworm infections include ancylostomiasis and necatoriasis. The most significant risk of hookworm infection is anemia, secondary to loss of iron (and protein) in the gut. The worms suck blood voraciously and damage the mucosa. However, the blood loss in the stools is not visibly apparent.

Etiology of Iron Deficiency Anemia
I. INCREASED BLOOD LOSS
1. *Uterine* e.g. excessive menstruation in reproductive years, repeated miscarriages, at onset of menarche, post-menopausal uterine bleeding
2. *Gastrointestinal* e.g. peptic ulcer, hemorrhoids hookworm infestation, cancer of stomach and large bowel, oesophageal varices, hiatus hernia, chronic aspirin ingestion, ulcerative colitis, diverticulosis
3. *Renal tract* e.g. hematuria, hemoglobinuria
4. *Nose* e.g. repeated epistaxis
5. *Lungs* e.g. hemoptysis
II. INCREASED REQUIREMENTS
1. Spurts of growth in infancy, childhood and adolescence
2. Prematurity
3. Pregnancy and lactation
III. INADEQUATE DIETARY INTAKE
1. Poor economic status
2. Anorexia e.g. in pregnancy
3. Elderly individuals due to poor dentition, apathy and financial constraints
IV. DECREASED ABSORPTION
1. Partial or total gastrectomy
2. Achlorhydria
3. Intestinal malabsorption such as in coeliac disease

182. All of the following are true regarding G6PD deficiency EXCEPT:

a. A recessive X-linked trait
b. Females are commonly affected
c. Oxidative stress causes hemolysis
d. Protective against plasmodium falciparum malaria

Most individuals with G6PD deficiency are asymptomatic.

Symptomatic patients are almost exclusively male, due to the X-linked pattern of inheritance, but female carriers can be clinically affected due to unfavorable lyonization, where random inactivation of an X-chromosome in certain cells creates a population of G6PD-deficient red blood cells coexisting with normal red cells.

Ans. **181. c.** Hookworm **182. b.** Females are commonly affected

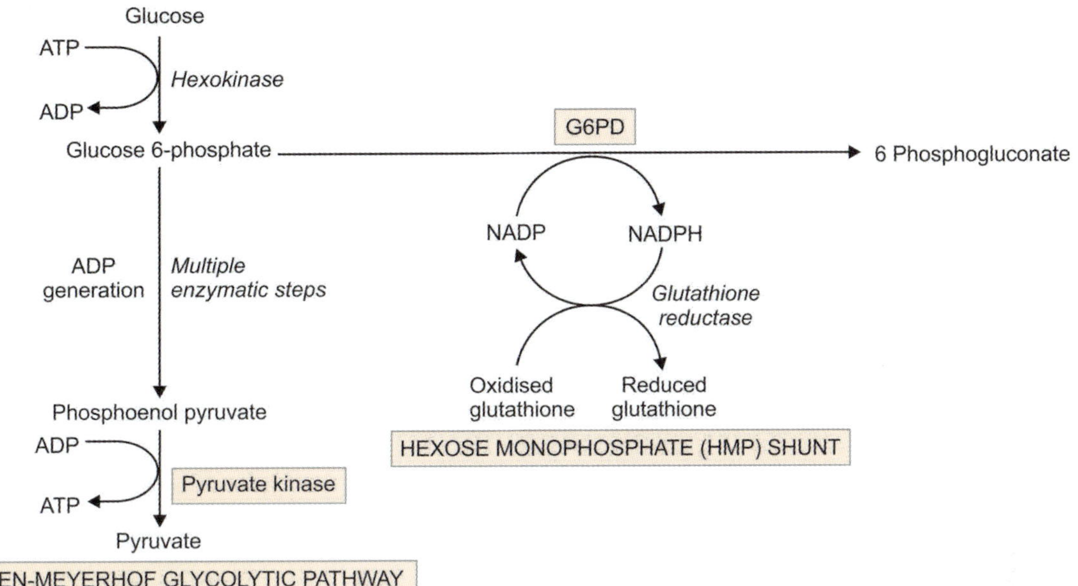

Abbreviated pathways of anaerobic glycolysis (Embden-Meyerhof) and hexose monophosphate (HMP) shunt in the metabolism of erythrocyte. The two red cell enzyme defects, glucose-6 phosphate dehydrogenase (G6PD) and pyruvate kinase, are shown in bold.

183. Bone infarcts are seen in:

a. Hereditary spherocytosis
b. Sickle cell anemia
c. Thalassemia
d. Iron deficiency anemia

The vaso-occlusive crisis is caused by sickle-shaped red blood cells that obstruct capillaries and restrict blood flow to an organ resulting in ischemia, pain, necrosis, and often organ damage.

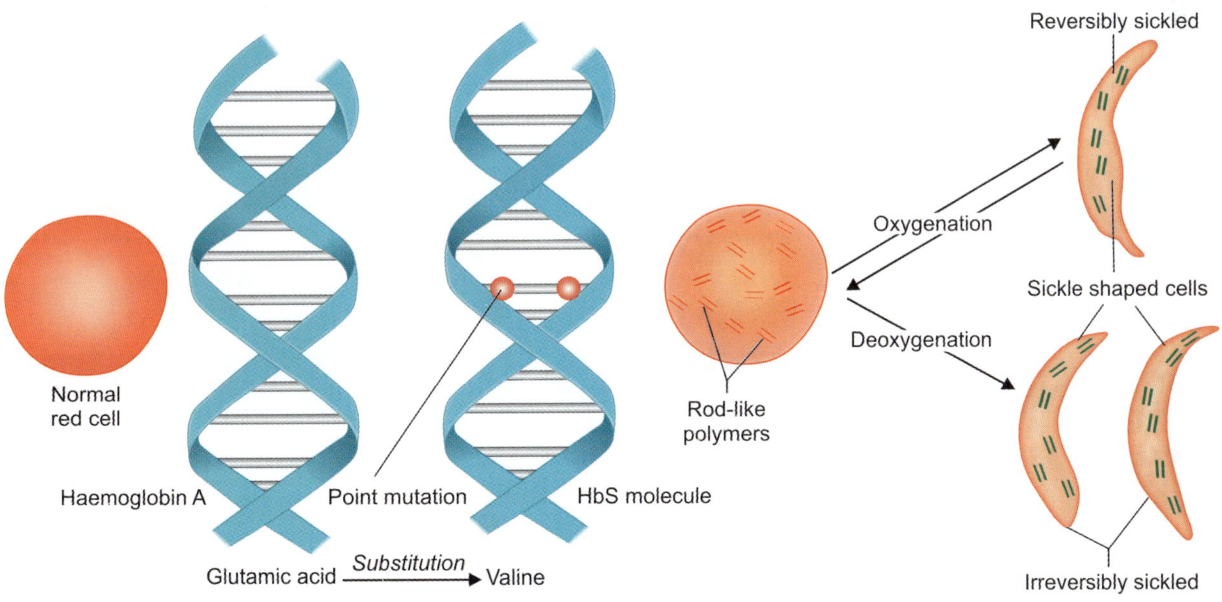

Pathogenesis of sickle cell anemia. A Basic molecular defect, B Mechanism of polymerisation and consequent sickling of red cells containing HbS. C, Mechanism of sickling on oxygenation-deoxygenation.

Ans. 183. b. Sickle cell anemia

184. A patient with Von-Willebrand disease will show:

a. Normal PT and increased PTT
b. Normal PT and normal PTT
c. Decreased PT and increased PTT
d. Increased PT and increased PTT

Patients with von-Willebrand disease will typically display a normal prothrombin time and a variable prolongation of partial thromboplastin time.

Screening tests for hemostasis (coagulation tests)

Laboratory test	Factor/function measured	Associated disorders
1. *Bleeding time*	Platelet function, vascular integrity	i. Qualitative disorders of platelets ii. von-Willebrand's disease iii. Quantitative disorders of platelets iv. Acquired vascular disorders
2. *Platelet count*	Quantification of platelets	i. Thrombocytopenia ii. Thrombocytosis
3. *Prothrombin time*	Evaluation of extrinsic and common pathway (deficiency of factors I, II, V, VII, X)	i. Oral anticoagulant therapy ii. DIC iii. Liver disease
4. *Partial thromboplastin time*	Evaluation of intrinsic and common pathway (deficiency of factors I, II, V, VIII, IX, X, XI, XII)	i. Parenteral heparin therapy ii. DIC iii. Liver disease
5. Thrombin time	Evaluation of common pathway	i. Afibrinogenaemia ii. DIC iii. Parenteral heparin therapy

185. Cabot's ring (RBC) is a feature of:

a. Post splenectomy
b. Thalassemia
c. Hemochromatosis
d. Acquired hemolytic anemia

Cabot rings are thin, red-violet staining, threadlike strands in the shape of a loop that are found on rare occasions in red blood cells (erythrocytes). They are believed to be microtubules that are remnants from a mitotic spindle, and their presence indicates an abnormality in the production of red blood cells.

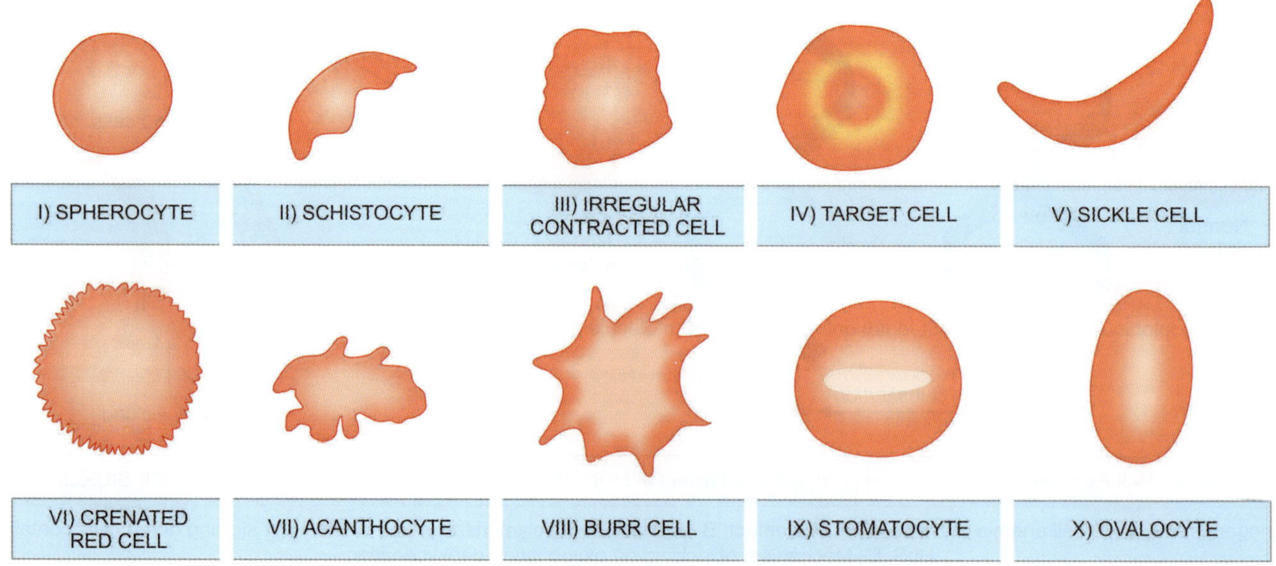

Some of the common morphologic abnormalities of red cells

Ans. 184. b. Normal PT and normal PTT **185. a.** Post splenectomy

186. MC extranodal site of lymphoma in AIDS patient is:

a. Mediastinum
b. GIT
c. Retroperitoneum
d. CNS

People with AIDS have an increased risk of developing various viral-induced cancers, including Kaposi's sarcoma, Burkitt's lymphoma, primary central nervous system lymphoma, and cervical cancer.

187. True for iron deficiency anemia:

a. Macrocytic hypochromic anemia
b. Marrow is normoblastic
c. Decreased TIBC
d. Increased ferritin

Purely IDA anemia usually give rise to a microcytic hypochromic anemia with a normoblastic bone marrow, while that due to iron plus folic acid or vitamin B12 give rise to a megaloblastic hypochromic anemia with or without megaloblastic bone marrow.

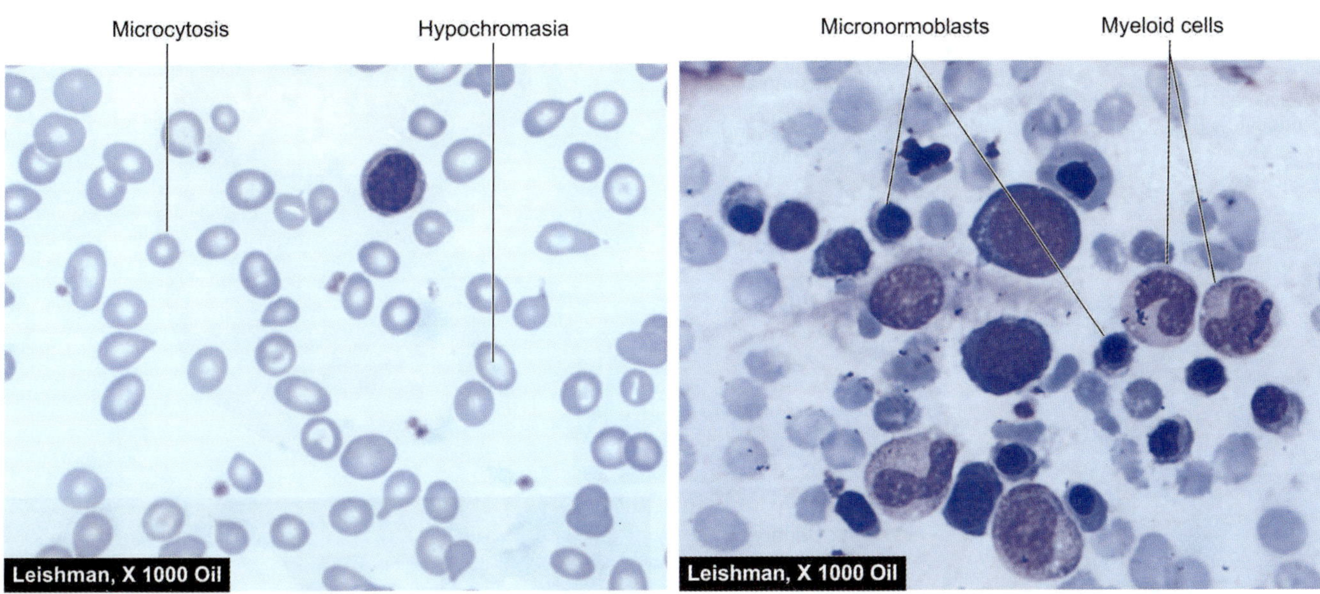

A, PERIPHERAL BLOOD SMEAR B, BONE MARROW ASPIRATE SMEAR

Iron deficiency anaemia. A, PBF showing microcytic hypochromic anaemia. There is moderate microcytosis and hypochromia. B, Examination of bone marrow aspirate showing micronormoblastic erythropoiesis.

188. Auer rods are formed in:

a. Myeloperoxidases
b. Primary granules
c. Secondary granules
d. None of the above

Auer rods are clumps of azurophilic granular material that form elongated needles seen in the cytoplasm of leukemic blasts. They can be seen in the leukemic blasts of acute myeloid leukemia with maturation and acute promyelocytic leukemia (known as acute myeloid leukemia M2 and M3, in the FAB classification, respectively) and in high grade myelodysplastic syndromes and myeloproliferative syndromes. They are composed of fused lysosomes/primary neutrophilic granules and contain peroxidase, lysosomal enzymes, and large crystalline inclusions.

EXCRETORY SYSTEM PATHOLOGY

189. Urinary RBC casts are seen in:

a. Lipoid nephrosis
b. Thrombosis of renal vein
c. Schistosomiasis of urinary bladder
d. Rapidly progressive glomerulonephritis

Rapidly progressive glomerulonephritis (RPGN)

- It is a syndrome of the kidney that is characterized by a rapid loss of renal function, (usually a 50% decline in the glomerular filtration rate (GFR) within 3 months) with glomerular crescent formation seen in at least 50% or 75% of glomeruli seen on kidney biopsies.
- If left untreated, it rapidly progresses into acute renal failure and death within months.

Ans. 186. **d.** CNS 187. **b.** Marrow is norm... 188. **b.** Primary granules 189. **d.** Rapidly progressive...

- Regardless of the underlying cause, RPGN involves severe injury to the kidneys' glomeruli, with many of the glomeruli containing characteristic glomerular screscents (crescent-shaped scars).
- Because of this microscopic feature, RPGN is also called crescentic glomerulonephritis

A schematic illustration of the structure of a nephron (in longitudinal section) and associated blood supply.

190. Cause of Renal osteodystrophy in chronic renal failure patient:

a. Primary hypoparathyroidism
b. Secondary hypoparathyroidism
c. Primary hyperparathyroidism
d. Secondary hyperparathyroidism

Renal osteodystrophy

- It is thought to be the result of hyperparathyroidism secondary to hyperphosphatemua combined with hypocalcemia, both of which are due to decreased excretion of phosphate by the damaged kidney.
- Low activated vitamin D_3 levels are a result of the damaged kidneys' inability to convert vitamin D_3 into its active form, calcitriol, and result in further hypocalcemia.

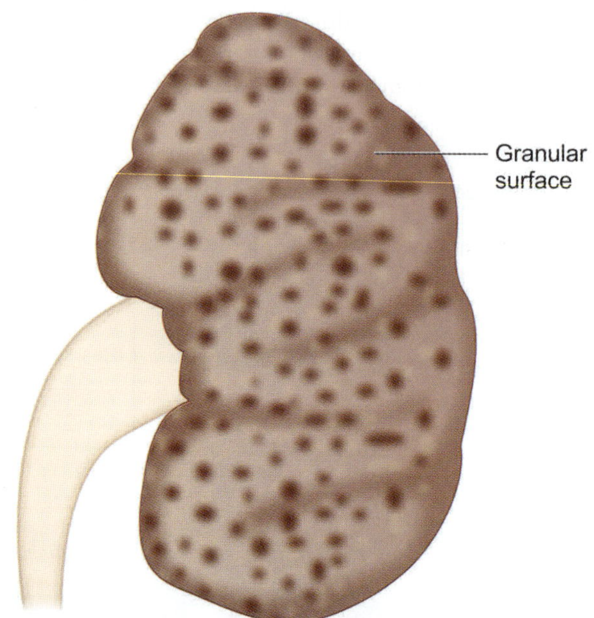

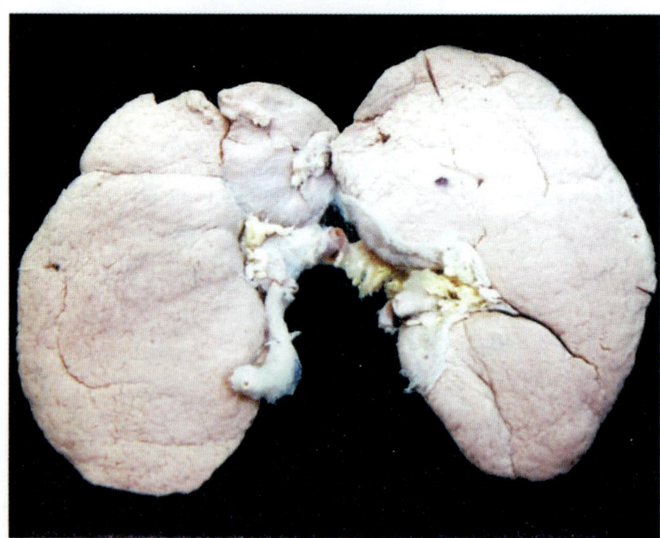

End-stage kidney, gross appearance of short contract kidney in chronic glomerulonephritis. The kidney is small and contracted. The capsule is adherent to the cortex and has diffusely granular cortical surface.

191. Periglomerular fibrosis is considered typical of:

a. Malignant hypertension
b. Arterio-nephrosclerosis
c. Chronic GN
d. Chronic pyelonephritis

Ans. **190. d.** Secondary hyp... **191. d.** Chronic pyelonephritis

Histologically, the kidney in chronic pyelonephritis has irregular areas of interstitial fibrosis with chronic inflammatory cell infiltration. Tubules are atrophic or may be dilated and contain proteinaceous material. Glomeruli show periglomerular fibrosis and many demonstrate complete hyalinization.

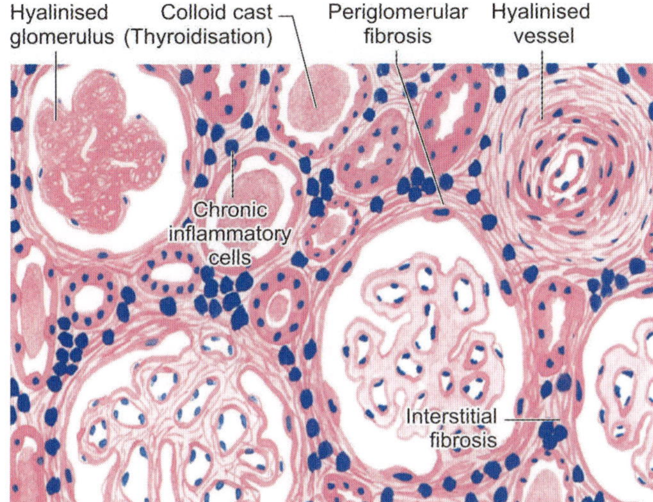

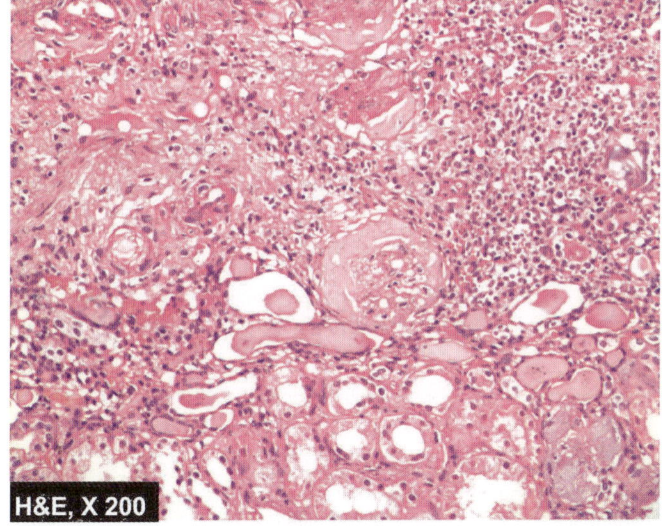

Chronic pyelonephritis. The scarred area shows atrophy of some tubules and dilatation of others which contain colloid casts (thyroidisation). The tubules are surrounded by abundant fibrous tissue and chronic interstitial inflammatory reaction. The blood vessels included are thick-walled and the glomeruli show periglomerular fibrosis.

192. Which does NOT occur in malignant hypertension?

a. Petechial hemorrhages on cortical surfaces
b. Fibrinoid necrosis of arterioles
c. Intimal concentric thickening
d. Hyaline arteriosclerosis

Hyaline arteriolosclerosis is a major morphologic characteristic of benign nephrosclerosis, in which the arteriolar narrowing causes diffuse impairment of renal blood supply, with loss of nephrons.

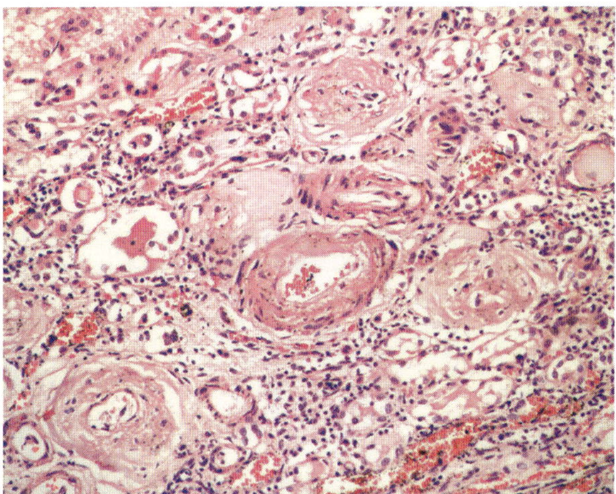

A, BENIGN NEPHROSCLEROSIS

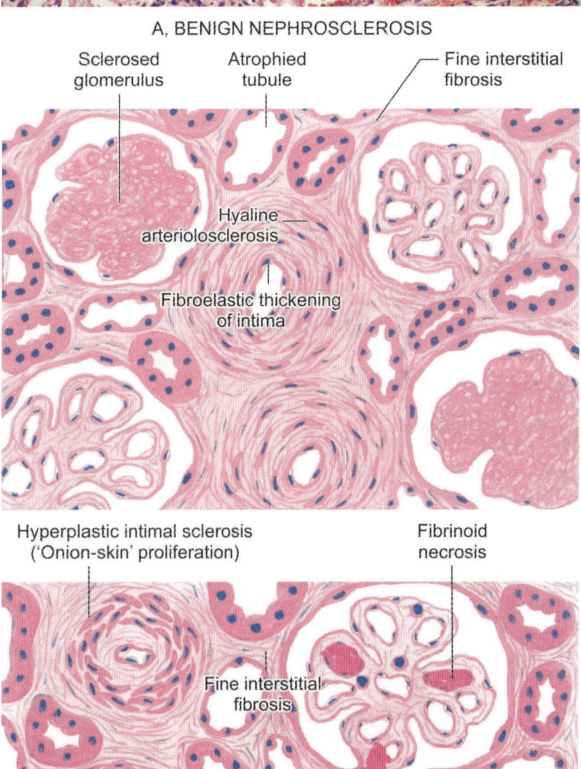

B. Malignant NF

Microscopic changes in kidney in hypertension. A, Benign nephrosclerosis. The vascular changes are hyaline arteriolosclerosis and intimal thickening of small blood vessels in the glomerular tuft. The parenchymal changes include sclerosed glomeruli, tubular atrophy and fine interstitial fibrosis. B, Malignant nephrosclerosis. The vascular changes are necrotising arteriolitis and hyperplastic intimal sclerosis or onion-skin proliferation. The parenchymal changes are tubular loss, fine interstitial fibrosis and foci of infarction necrosis.

Ans. 192. **d.** Hyaline arteriosclerosis

193. Crescent forming GN is:
- a. MPGN
- b. MGN
- c. RPGN
- d. All of the above

Rapidly progressive glomerulonephritis (**RPGN**) is a syndrome of the kidney that is characterized by a rapid loss of renal function, (usually a 50% decline in the glomerular filtration rate (GFR) within 3 months) with glomerular **crescent formation** seen in at least 50% or 75% of glomeruli seen on kidney biopsies.

Comparative features of major forms of primary glomerulonephritis.

Type	Clinical Features	Pathogenesis	Pathology		
			LM	EM	IFM
1. *Acute GN*	Acute nephrotic syndrome	Immune complex disease (local or circulating)	Diffuse proliferation, leucocytic infiltration	Subepithelial deposits ('humps')	Irregular IgG, C3
2. *RPGN*	Acute renal failure	i. Type I: anti-GBM type ii. Type II: immune complex type iii. Type III: pauci-immune RPGN	Proliferation, crescents	i. Linear deposits along GBM ii. Subepithelial deposits iii. No deposits	i. Linear IgG, C3 ii. Granular IgG, C3 iii. Negative
3. *Minimal change disease*	Nephrotic syndrome (highly selective proteinuria)	Reduction of normal negative charge on GBM ?Cell-mediated mechanism	Normal glomeruli, lipid vacuolation in tubules	Loss of foot processes, no deposits	Negative
4. *Membranous GN*	Nephrotic syndrome	Immune complex disease (local)	Diffuse thickening of capillary wall	Subepithelial deposits ('spikes')	Granular IgG, C3
5. *Membrano-proliferative GN*	Nephrotic syndrome	Type I: immune complex disease Type II: dense deposit disease (alternate pathway activation) Type III: rare, with systemic diseases and drugs	Lobular proliferation of mesangial cells, increased mesangial matrix, double contour of GBM	Type I: Subendothelial deposits Type II: Dense intramembranous deposits Type III: Subendothelial and subepithelial deposits	Type I: IgG, C3 Type II: C3 properdin Type III: C3, IgG, IgM
6. *Focal GN*	Variable, hematuria common	Variable, possibly immune complex disease	Focal and segmental proliferation	Mesangial deposits	IgA ± IgG, C3 and fibrin
7. *Focal segmental glomerulo-sclerosis*	Nephrotic syndrome	i) Idiopathic ii) With superimposed primary glomerular disease iii) Secondary type	Focal and segmental sclerosis and hyalinosis	Loss of foot processes, electron dense deposits in regions of sclerosis and hyalinosis	IgM, C3
8. *IgA nephropathy*	Recurrent hematuria, mild proteinuria	Unknown, possibly alternate pathway disease	Variable, commonly focal proliferative GN	Mesangial electron-dense deposits	IgA ± IgG, C3, properdin
9. *Chronic GN*	Chronic renal failure	Variable	Hyalinised glomeruli	Variable	Variable

(GN = glomerulonephritis; LM = light microscopy; EM = electron microscopy; IFM = immunofluorescence microscopy)

194. Hyaline arteriosclerosis is seen in which of the following conditions:
- a. Tuberculosis
- b. Hypertension
- c. Syphilis
- d. Leprosy

Hyaline arteriosclerosis is associated with aging, hypertension, diabetes mellitus and may be seen in response to certain drugs (calcineurin inhibitors).

Ans. 193. c. RPGN **194. b.** Hypertension

Volume I Non-Clinical Subjects

It is often seen in the context of kidney pathology. In hypertension only the afferent arteriole is affected, while in diabetes mellitus, both the afferent and efferent arteriole are affected.

195. Bilateral contracted granular kidneys are seen in all of the following EXCEPT:

a. Chronic pyelonephritis
b. Chronic glomerulonephritis
c. Benign nephrosclerosis
d. Early diabetic nephropathy

In the early stages of diabetic nephropathy, kidney size may be enlarged from hyperfiltration. With progressive kidney disease from diabetes, the kidneys diminish in size from glomerulosclerosis.

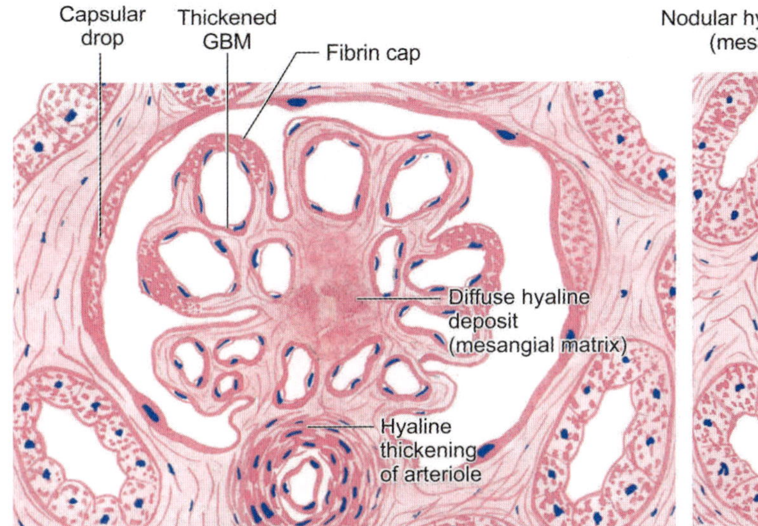

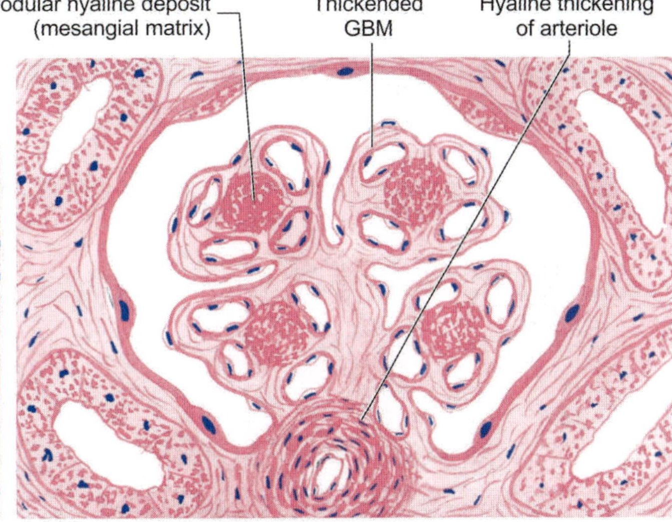

Diabetic glomerulosclerosis. A, Diffuse lesions. The characteristic features are diffuse involvement of the glomeruli showing thickening of the GBM and diffuse increase in the mesangial matrix with mild proliferation of mesangial cells and exudative lesions (fibrin caps and capsular drops). B, Nodular lesion (Kimmelstiel-Wilson Lesion). There are one or more hyaline nodules within the lobules of glomeruli, surrounded peripherally by glomerular capillaries with thickened walls.

196. All cause nephrotic syndrome EXCEPT:

a. Minimal lesion glomerulonephritis
b. Membranous glomerulonephritis
c. Post streptococcal glomerulonephritis
d. Focal glomerulosclerosis

Acute proliferative glomerulonephritis is a disorder of the glomeruli (glomerulonephritis), or small blood vessels in the kidneys. It is a common complication of bacterial infections, typically skin infection by *Streptococcus* bacteria types 12, 4 and 1 (impetigo) but also after streptococcal pharyngitis, for which it is also known as postinfectious or poststreptococcal glomerulonephritis.

Causes of nephrotic syndrome
I. PRIMARY GLOMERULONEPHRITIS
1. Minimal change disease *(most common in children)*
2. Membranous GN *(most common in adults)*
3. Membranoproliferative GN
4. Focal segmental glomerulosclerosis
5. Focal and diffuse proliferative GN
6. IgA nephropathy
II. SYSTEMIC DISEASES
1. Diabetes mellitus
2. Amyloidosis
3. SLE
III. SYSTEMIC INFECTIONS
1. Viral infections (HBV, HCV, HIV)
2. Bacterial infections (bacterial endocarditis, syphilis, leprosy)
3. Protozoa and parasites (*P. falciparum* malaria, filariasis)
IV. HYPERSENSITIVITY REACTIONS
1. Drugs (heavy metal compounds like gold and mercury, other drugs like penicillamine, trimethadione and tolbutamide, heroin addiction)
2. Bee stings, snake bite, poison ivy
V. MALIGNANCY
1. Carcinomas

Ans. 195. None > D **196. c.** Post streptococcal glomerulonephritis

Causes of nephrotic syndrome	
	2. Myeloma
	3. Hodgkin's disease
VI.	PREGNANCY
	Toxaemia of pregnancy
VII.	CIRCULATORY DISTURBANCES
	1. Renal vein thrombosis
	2. Constrictive pericarditis
VIII.	HEREDITARY DISEASES
	1. Alport's disease

Contd...

Contd...

Causes of nephrotic syndrome
2. Fabry's disease
3. Nail-patella syndrome

197. All are true regarding minimal change disease EXCEPT:
a. Selective proteinuria
b. IgG deposition in mesangium
c. Common in age group 2-9 years
d. Respond to steroids

The pathology of minimal change disease is unclear and is currently considered idiopathic. The pathology does not appear to involve complement, immunoglobulins, or immune complex deposition (Nil deposit disease).

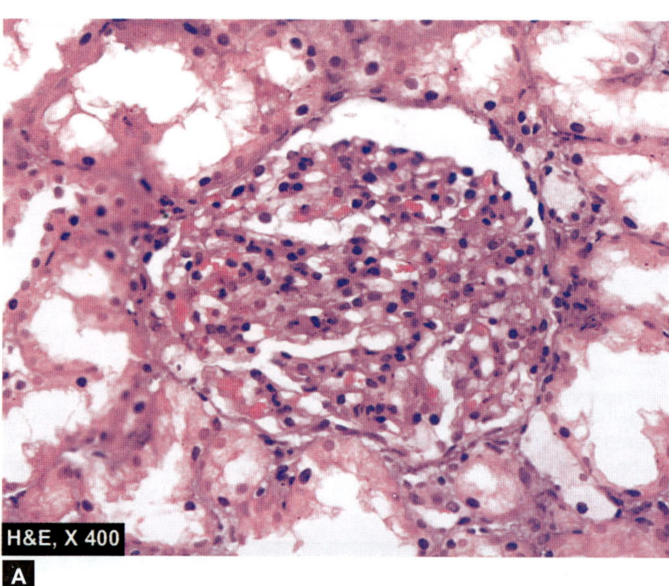

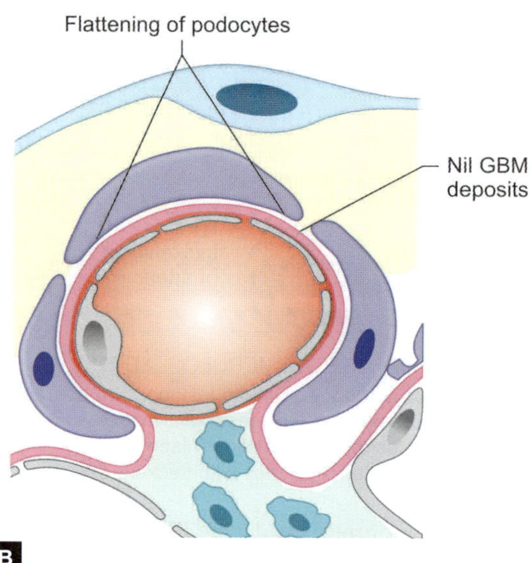

Minimal change disease. A, Light microscopy shows a normal glomerulus while tubules show cytoplasmic vacuolation and proteinaceous material. B, Diagrammatic representation of ultrastructure of a portion of glomerular lobule showing diffuse fusion or flattening of foot processes of visceral epithelial cells (podocytes). The GBM is normal and there are no deposits.

198. Nephrotic syndrome is characterized by all of the following EXCEPT:
a. Hypoalbuminemia
b. Hypolipidemia
c. Lipiduria
d. Proteinuria more than 3.5 gm per 1.73 sq. m. per day

There is hyperlipidemia which results in lipiduria.

Contrasting features of acute nephritic and nephrotic syndromes

Feature	*Acute nephritic syndrome*	*Nephrotic syndrome*
1. *Proteinuria*	Mild (< 3 gm per 24 hrs)	Heavy (> 3 gm per 24 hrs)
2. *Hypoalbuminaemia*	Uncommon	Present
3. *Oedema*	Mild, in loose tissues	Marked, generalised peripheral
4. *Mechanism of oedema*	Na^+ and water retention	↓ plasma osmotic pressure, Na^+ and water retention
5. *Hematuria*	Present, microscopic	Absent
6. *Hypertension*	Present	Present in advanced disease
7. *Hyperlipidaemia*	Absent	Present

Contd...

Ans. **197. b.** IgG deposition... **198. b.** Hypolipidemia

Contd...

Feature	Acute nephritic syndrome	Nephrotic syndrome
8. *Lipiduria*	Absent	Present
9. *Oliguria*	Present	Present in advanced disease
10. *Hypercoagulability*	Absent	Present

199. Michaelis-Gutmann bodies are found in:

a. Xanthelsma
b. Nail patella syndrome
c. Xanthogranulomatous pyelonephritis
d. Malakoplakia

Malakoplakia or **Malacoplakia** is a rare inflammatory condition which makes its presence known as a papule, plaque or ulceration that usually affects the genitourinary tract. Microscopically it is characterized by the presence of foamyhistiocytes with basophilic inclusions called Michelis–Gutmann bodies.

200. Organism causing pyelonephritis in renal allografts:

a. Rotavirus b. HB
c. Herpes virus d. Polyomavirus

Diseases caused by human polyomavirus infections are most common among persons who become immunosuppressed by AIDS, old age or after transplantation and include Merkel cell carcinoma, PML and BK nephropathy.

201. Glomerulosclerosis is a feature of:

a. Diabetes mellitus
b. Hypertension
c. Acute glomerular injury
d. Nephrotic syndrome

Nodular deposits
Compressed capillaries
Increased mesangial matrix
H&E, X 200

Diabetic nephropathy—nodular (Kimmelstiel-Wilson or KW) lesions.

Both children and adults can develop glomerulosclerosis and it can result from different types of kidney conditions. One frequently encountered type of glomerulosclerosis is caused by diabetes. Drug use or infections may cause focal segmental glomerulosclerosis (FSGS), a very chronic kidney condition. FSGS may also occur in patients with AIDS but most are of unknown cause.

202. Salt losing nephropathy:

a. Interstitial nephritis b. Amyloidosis
c. Lupus nephritis d. Post-streptococcal GN

Granulomatous TINU (tubulointerstitial nephritis with uveitis) has also been associated with a salt wasting nephropathy.

203. In Chronic Renal Failure, all are seen EXCEPT:

a. Hyperphosphatemia b. Hyponatremia
c. Hyperkalemia d. Metabolic acidosis

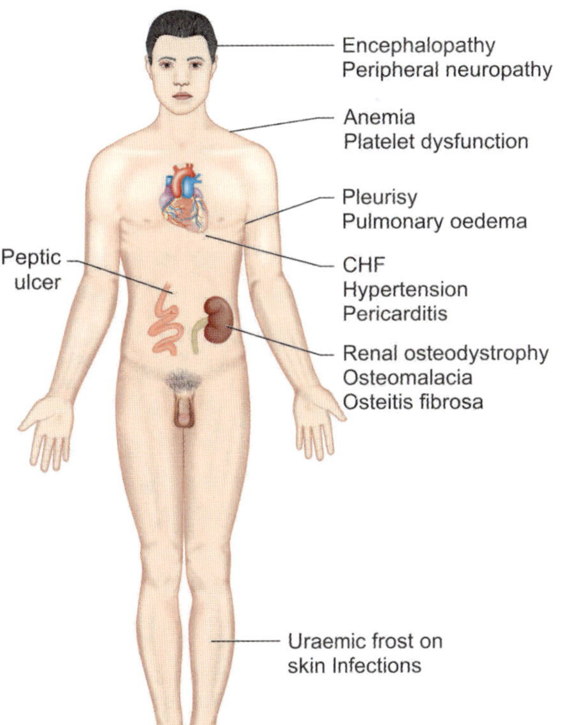

Clinical manifestations in chronic kidney disease.

Hyperphosphatemia, due to reduced phosphate excretion, follows the decrease in glomerular filtration.

Ans. 199. **d.** Malakoplakia 200. **d.** Polyoma virus 201. **a.** Diabetes mellitus 202. **a.** Interstitial nephritis
203. **b.** Hyponatremia

Hyperphosphatemia is associated with increased cardiovascular risk, being a direct stimulus to vascular calcification.

Metabolic acidosis (due to accumulation of sulfates, phosphates, uric acid etc.) may cause altered enzyme activity by excess acid acting on enzymes; and also increased excitability of cardiac and neuronal membranes by the promotion of hyperkalemia due to excess acid (acidemia).

204. All are true for nephrotic syndrome EXCEPT:

a. Edema b. Massive proteinuria
c. Hyperlipidemia d. Hypertension

Hypertension is a feature of nephritic syndrome.

Relationship of physiologic role of glomerular components with consequences in glomerular injury.

Component	Physiologic function	Consequence of injury	Related glomerular disease
1. *Endothelial cells*	i. Maintain glomerular perfusion	Vasoconstriction	Acute renal failure
	ii. Prevent leucocyte adhesion	Leucocyte infiltration	Focal/diffuse proliferative GN
	iii. Prevent platelet aggregation	Intravascular microthrombi	Thrombotic microangiopathies
2. *Mesangial cells*	Control glomerular filtration	Proliferation and increased matrix	Membranoproliferative GN
3. *Visceral epithelial cells*	Prevent plasma protein filtration	Proteinuria	Minimal change disease, FSGS
4. *GBM*	Prevents plasma protein filtration	Proteinuria	Membranous GN, ? MPGN
5. *Parietal epithelial cells*	Maintain Bowman's space	Crescent formation	RPGN

205. Condition which can present both as nephritic syndrome and nephrotic syndrome, is:

a. Minimal change disease
b. Acute proliferative glomerulonephritis
c. Rapidly progressive glomerulonephritis
d. Membranoproliferative glomerulonephritis

Membranoproliferative glomerulonephritis primarily affects children and young adults, with patients presenting with nephrotic or nephritic syndrome or with asymptomatic renal disease. This type of glomerulonephritis often progresses slowly to end-stage renal disease, and it tends to recur after renal transplantation, especially type II.

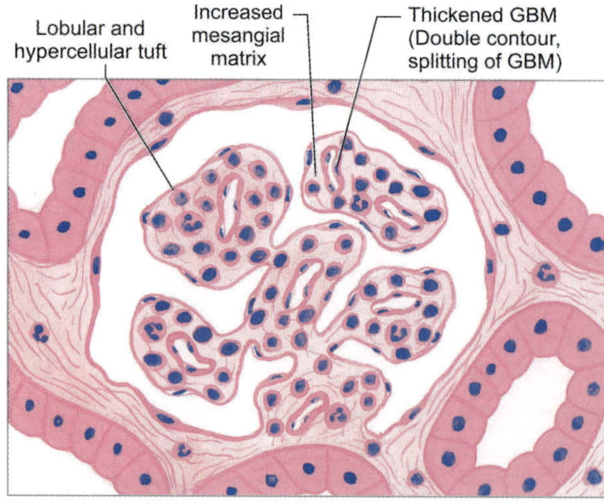

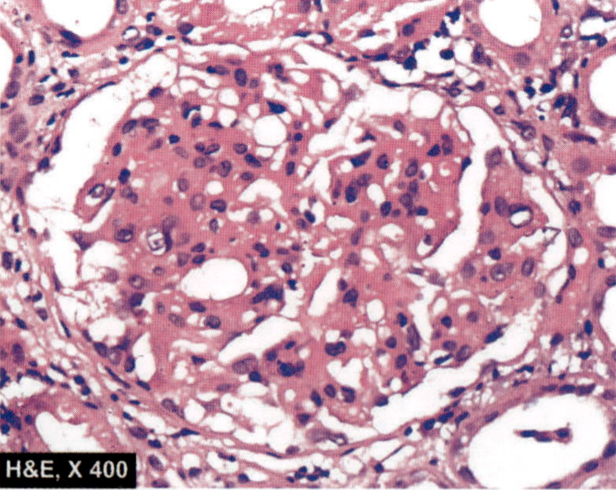

Membranoproliferative GN, light microscopic appearance. The glomerular tufts show lobulation and mesangial hypercellularity. There is increase in the mesangial matrix between the capillaries. There is widespread thickening of the GBM.

206. Papillary necrosis is seen in all EXCEPT:

a. Sickle cell anemia
b. Analgesic nephropathy
c. Diabetes mellitus
d. Chronic alcoholism

In terms of cause, most any condition that involves ischemia can lead to renal papillary necrosis. A mnemonic for the causes of renal papillary necrosis is POSTCARDS: pyelonephritis, obstruction of the urogenital tract, sickle cell disease, tuberculosis, cirrhosis of the liver, analgesia/

Ans. 204. d. Hypertension 205. d. Membranop... 206. d. Chronic alcoholism alcohol abuse, renal vein thrombosis, diabetes mellitus, and systemic vasculitis.

207. Condition which presents as nephritic syndrome with features of loss of foot processes on electron microscopy and poor response to corticosteroid therapy is:

a. Postinfectious glomerulonephritis
b. Membranoproliferative glomerulonephritis type I
c. Minimal change disease
d. Focal segmental glomerulonephritis

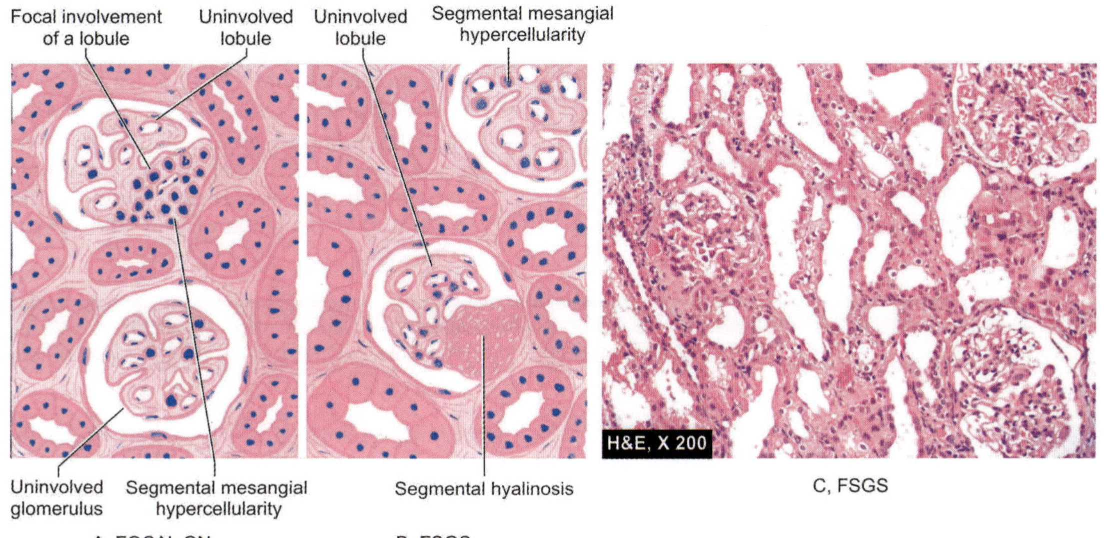

(A) Focal GN. The characteristic feature is the cellular proliferation in some glomeruli and in one or two lobules of the affected glomeruli i.e. focal and segmental proliferative change. (B and C) Focal segmental glomerulosclerosis. The features are focal and segmental involvement of the glomeruli by sclerosis and hyalinosis and mesangial hypercellularity.

The most common clinical presenting feature of FSGS (>70% of patients) is nephrotic syndrome, characterized by generalized edema, massive proteinuria, hypoalbuminemia, and hyperlipidemia. However, the natural history of FSGS is variable and can range from edema that is difficult to manage, to proteinuria that is refractory to corticosteroids and other immunosuppressive agents, to worsening hypertension and a progressive loss of renal function.

GENETICS

208. All of the following are autosomal dominant disorders EXCEPT:

a. Tuberous sclerosis
b. Polyposis coli
c. Cystic fibrosis
d. Myotonic dystrophy

Cystic Fibrosis is inherited in an autosomal recessive manner. It is caused by the presence of mutations in both copies of the gene for the cystic fibrosis transmembrane conductance regulator (CFTR) protein.

Important examples of Mendelian disorders (single gene defects)
I. AUTOSOMAL RECESSIVE INHERITANCE
1. β-thalassaemia
2. Sickle cell anaemia

Contd...

Contd...

Important examples of Mendelian disorders (single gene defects)
3. Hemochromatosis
4. Cystic fibrosis of pancreas
5. Albinism
6. Wilson's disease
7. Xeroderma pigmentosum
8. Inborn errors of metabolism (Lysosomal storage diseases, glycogenosis, alkaptonuria, phenylketonuria)
II. AUTOSOMAL CODOMINANT INHERITANCE
1. ABO blood group antigens
2. α 1-antitrypsin deficiency
3. HLA antigens
III. AUTOSOMAL DOMINANT INHERITANCE
1. Familial polyposis coli
2. Adult polycystic kidney
3. Hereditary spherocytosis
4. Neurofibromatosis (von Recklinghausen's disease)
5. Marfan's syndrome
6. von Willebrand's disease
7. Hereditary hemorrhagic telangiectasia
8. Acute intermittent porphyria

Contd...

Ans. **207.** **d.** Focal segmental... **208.** **c.** Cystic fibrosis

Contd...

Important examples of Mendelian disorders (single gene defects)
9. Familial hypercholesterolaemia
10. Osteogenesis imperfecta
IV. SEX-(X-) LINKED RECESSIVE INHERITANCE
1. Hemophilia A
2. G6PD deficiency
3. Diabetes insipidus
4. Chronic granulomatous disease
5. Colour blindness
6. Bruton's agammaglobulinaemia
7. Muscular dystrophies
V. SEX-(X-) LINKED DOMINANT INHERITANCE
1. Hypophosphataemic rickets
2. Incontinentia pigmenti

Contd...

Contd...

209. Which is NOT a X-linked recessive:

a. Beta thalassemia
b. G6PD deficiency
c. Hemophilia A
d. Colour blindness

Thalassaemia is a form of inherited autosomal recessive blood disorder characterized by abnormal formation of hemoglobin. The abnormal hemoglobin formed results in improper oxygen transport and destruction of red blood cells.

Classification of thalasaemias.

Type	*Hb*	*Hb-electrophoresis*	*Genotype*	*Clinical syndrome*
α-THALASSEMIAS				
1. Hydrops foetalis	3-10 gm/dl	Hb Barts (g_4) (100%)	Deletion of four α-genes	Fatal *in utero* or in early infancy
2. Hb-H disease	2-12 gm/dl	HbF (10%), HbH (2-4%)	Deletion of three α-genes	Hemolytic anemia
3. α-*Thalasaemia trait*	10-14 gm/dl	Almost normal	Deletion of two α-genes	Microcytic hypochromic blood picture but no anaemia
β-THALASSAEMIAS				
1. β-*Thalasaemia major*	< 5 gm/dl	HbA (0-50%), HbF(50-98%)	$\beta^{thal}/\beta^{thal}$	Severe congenital hemolytic anaemia, requires blood transfusions
2. β-*Thalasaemia intermedia*	5-10 gm/dl	Variable	Multiple mechanisms	Severe anaemia, but regular blood transfusions not required
3. β-*Thalasaemia minor*	10-12 gm/dl	HbA_2 (4-9%), HbF (1-5%)	β^{A}/β^{thal}	Usually asymptomatic

210. Which of the following are autosomal recessive disorders EXCEPT:

a. Hereditary spherocytosis
b. Hemochromatosis
c. Wilsons disease
d. Cystic fibrosis

Hereditary spherocytosis (also known as **Minkowski–Chauffard syndrome**) is an autosomal dominant abnormality of erythrocytes. The disorder is caused by mutations in genes relating to membrane proteins that allow for the erythrocytes to change shape. The abnormal erythrocytes are sphere-shaped (spherocytosis) rather than the normal biconcave disk shaped.

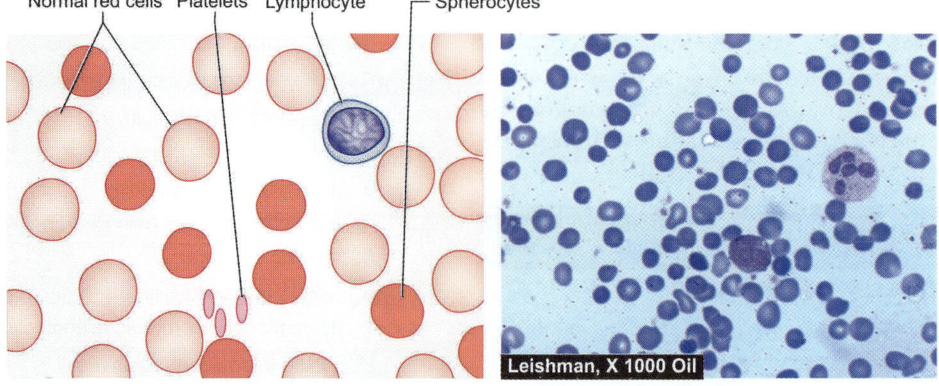

Peripheral blood film findings in hereditary spherocytosis.

Ans. 209. a. Beta thalassemia **210. a.** Hereditary spherocytosis

211. The following are X-linked disorders EXCEPT:

a. Cystic fibrosis
b. Hemophilia A
c. Duchenne muscular dystrophy
d. Hemophilia B

CF is inherited in an autosomal recessive manner. It is caused by the presence of mutations in both copies of the gene for the cystic fibrosis transmembrane conductance regulator (CFTR) protein.

212. Males are more commonly affected than females in:

a. Autosomal dominant
b. Autosomal recessive
c. X-linked dominant
d. X-linked recessive

X-linked inheritance means that the gene causing the trait or the disorder is located on the X chromosome. Females have two X chromosomes, while males have one X and one Y chromosome. Carrier females who have only one copy of the mutation do not usually express the phenotype, although differences in X chromosome inactivation can lead to varying degrees of clinical expression in carrier females since some cells will express one X allele and some will express the other.

213. True for palindromic sequence are all EXCEPT:

a. Short stretches of DNA
b. Recognised by specific restriction endonuclease
c. Code for bacterial resistance
d. Complementary strands

A **palindromic sequence** is a nucleic acid sequence on double-stranded DNA or RNA wherein reading 5′ (five-prime) to 3′ (three prime) forward on one strand matches the sequence reading backward 5′ to 3′ on the complementary strand with which it forms a double helix. This definition of palindrome thus depends on complementary strands being palindromic of each other.

IMMUNITY AND AMYLOIDOSIS

214. Lardaceous spleen is a feature of:

a. Thalassemia
b. Amyloidosis
c. Sickle cell anemia
d. Malaria

Amyloidosis of the spleen is seen in two forms - the sago spleen in which amyloid deposits are limited to the follicles, and the lardaceous spleen in which amyloid is deposited in the walls of the splenic sinusoids and spares the follicles.

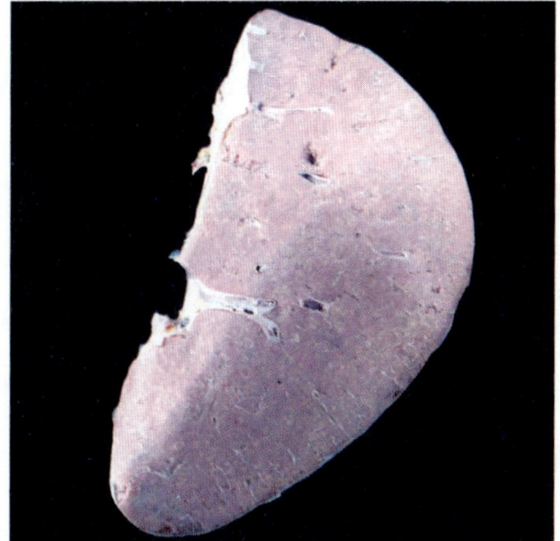

Lardaceous amyloidosis of the spleen. The sectioned surface shows presence of pale waxy translucency in a map-like pattern.

215. Immunoglobulin is produced by:

a. T cell
b. B cell
c. Both
d. None

Antibodies/Ig are secreted by cells of the adaptive immune system (B cells), and more specifically, differentiated B cells called plasma cells.

Differences between T and B lymphocytes.

Feature	T Cells	B Cells
1. *Origin*	Bone marrow → Thymus	Bone marrow → Bursa (in fowl); mucosa-associated lymphoid tissue (MALT)
2. *Lifespan*	Small T cells: months to years T cell blasts: several days	Small B cells: less than 1 month B cell blasts : several days
3. *Location* i. Lymph nodes ii. Spleen iii. Peyer's patches	 Perifollicular (paracortical) Periarteriolar Perifollicular	 Germinal centres, medullary cords Germinal centres, red pulp Central follicles
4. *Presence in circulation*	75-80%	10-15%
5. *Surface markers* i. Ag receptors ii. Surface Ig iii. Fc receptor iv. Complement receptor v. CD markers	 Present Absent Absent Absent T_H cells CD4, 3, 7, 2 T_S cells CD8, 3, 7, 2	 Absent Present Present Present CD19, 20, 21, 23

Contd...

Ans. **211. a.** Cystic... **212. d.** X-linked... **213. c.** Code... **214. b.** Amyloidosis **215. b.** B cell

Contd...

Feature	T Cells	B Cells
6. *Functions*	i. CMI via cytotoxic T cells positive for CD3 and CD4 ii. Delayed hypersensitivity via CD4+ T cells iii. Immunoregulation of other T cells, B cells and stem cells via T helper (CD4+) or T suppressor (CD8+) cells	i. Role in humoral immunity by synthesis of specific antibodies (Igs) ii. Precursors of plasma cells

216. All of the following are immune complexes disease/ type III HS reactions EXCEPT:

a. Serum sickness b. Farmers lung

c. SLE d. Pernicious anemia

Antireceptor antibodies: IgG antibody is directed against receptors in target cells, resulting in complement-mediated destruction of the receptors. Diseases (type II hypersensitivity reaction) caused by this mechanism include:

- Myasthenia gravis: acetylcholine receptor antibody.
- Graves disease (thyrotoxicosis): anti-TSH receptor antibody.
- Pernicious anemia: anti-parietal cell antibody.

Comparative features of 4 types of hypersensitivity reactions

Feature	Type I (Anaphylactic, atopic)	Type II (Antibody-mediated, cytotoxic)	Type III (Immune-complex, Arthus reaction)	Type IV (Delayed, T cell-mediated)
1. *Definition*	Rapidly developing immune response in a previously sensitised person	Reaction of humoral antibodies that attack cell surface antigens and cause cell lysis	Results from deposition of antigen-antibody complexes on tissues	Cell-mediated slow and prolonged response
2. *Peak action time*	15-30 minutes	15-30 minutes	Within 6 hours	After 24 hours
3. *Mediated by*	IgE antibodies	IgG or IgM antibodies	IgG, IgM antibodies	Cell-mediated
4. *Etiology*	Genetic basis, pollutants, viral infections	HLA-linked, exposure to foreign tissues/cells	Persistence of low grade infection, environmental antigens, autoimmune process	CD8+ T cells, cutaneous antigens
5. *Examples*	i. Systemic anaphylaxis (administration of antisera and drugs, stings) ii. Local anaphylaxis (hay fever, bronchial asthma, food allergy, cutaneous, angioedema)	i. Cytotoxic antibodies to blood cells (autoimmune hemolytic anaemia, transfusion reactions, erythroblastosis foetalis, ITP, leucopenia, drug-induced) ii. Cytotoxic antibodies to tissue components (Graves' disease, myasthenia gravis, male sterility, type I DM, hyperacute reaction against organ transplant)	i. Immune complex glomerulonephritis ii. Goodpasture's syndrome, iii. Collagen diseases (SLE, rheumatoid arthritis) iv. PAN v. Drug-induced vasculitis	i. Reaction against mycrobacterial antigen (tuberculin reaction, tuberculosis, tuberculoid leprosy) ii. Reaction against virus-infected cells iii. Reaction against tumour cells

217. Secondary amyloidosis complicates:

a. Chronic osteomyelitis

b. Irritable bowel syndrome

c. Chronic glomerulonephritis

d. Pneumonia

Complications of chronic osteomyelitis include pathological fractures, secondary amyloidosis or squamous cell carcinoma of sinus tract.

Contrasting features of primary and secondary amyloidosis.

Feature	Primary amyloid	Secondary amyloid
1. *Biochemical composition*	AL (Light chain proteins); lambda chains more common than kappa; sequence homology of chains	AA (Amyloid associated proteins); derived from larger precursor protein SAA; no sequence homology of polypeptide chain
2. *Associated diseases*	Plasma cell dyscrasias e.g. multiple myeloma, B cell lymphomas, others	Chronic inflammation e.g. infections (TB, leprosy, osteomyelitis, bronchiectasis), autoimmune diseases (rheumatoid arthritis, IBD), cancers (RCC, Hodgkin's disease), FMF

Contd...

Ans. 216. d. Pernicious... **217. a.** Chronic osteomyelitis

Contd...

Feature	*Primary amyloid*	*Secondary amyloid*
3. *Pathogenesis*	Stimulus → Monoclonal B cell proliferation → Excess of Igs and light chains → Partial degradation → Insoluble AL fibril	Stimulus → Chronic inflammation → Activation of macrophages → Cytokines (IL1,6) → Partial degradation → AEF → Insoluble AA fibril
4. *Incidence*	Most common in US and other developed countries	Most common worldwide, particularly in developing countries
5. *Age*	>40 years	Any age including children
6. *Course and prognosis*	Rapidly progressive, dismal	Better, treat the underlying cause
7. *Organ distribution*	Kidney, heart, bowel, nerves	Kidney, liver, spleen, adrenals
8. *Stains to distinguish*	Congophilia persists after permanganate treatment of section; specific immunostains anti-λ, anti-κ	Congophilia disappears after permanganate treatment of section; specific immunostain anti-AA

218. Congo red staining for amyloid under polarized light shows:

a. Silver birefringence b. Golden birefringence
c. Blue birefringence d. Green birefringence

Diagnosis of amyloidosis requires tissue biopsy. Biopsy is assessed for evidence of characteristic amyloid deposits. The tissue is treated with various stains. The most useful stain in the diagnosis of amyloid is Congo red, which, combined with polarized light, makes the amyloid proteins appear apple-green on microscopy. Also, thioflavin T stain may be used.

Atrophied white pulp
Pink acellular material
Expanded red pulp
A H&E, X 200
B Congo red, X 200
C

Amyloidosis spleen. A, The pink acellular amyloid material is seen in the red pulp causing atrophy of while pulp. B, Congo red staining shows Congophilia as seen by red-pink colour. C, When viewed under polarising microscopy the corresponding area shows apple-green birefringence.

219. Stain used to diagnose amyloidosis:

a. Methylene blue b. Acid fast stain
c. Rose Bengal d. Congo red

Congo red also shows a fluorescent activity when bound to amyloid fibrils, which tends to be used as a sensitive diagnosis tool for amyloidosis, instead of the traditional histological birefringence test.

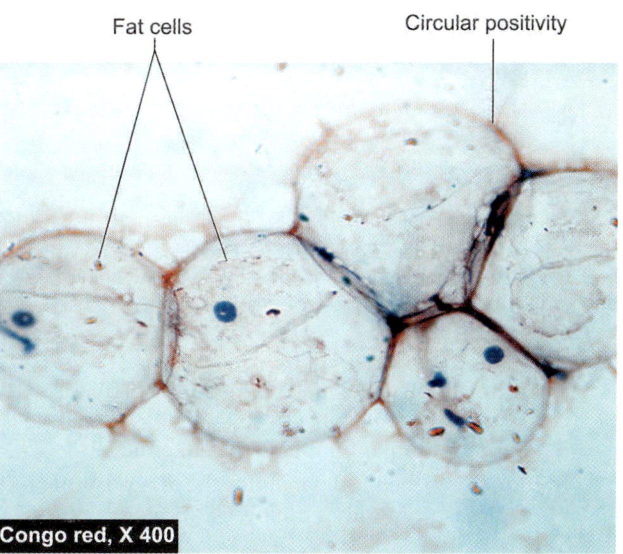

Abdominal fat aspirate smear stained with Congo red.

220. CD-10 is seen in:

a. CML b. HCL
c. CLL d. ALL

Neprilysin/**membrane metallo-endopeptidase** (MME), **neutral endopeptidase** (NEP), **cluster of differentiation 10** (CD10), and **common acute lymphoblastic leukemia antigen** (CALLA) is expressed in a wide variety of tissues and is particularly abundant in kidney. It is also a common acute lymphocytic leukemia antigen that

Ans. 218. d. Green birefring... **219. d.** Congo red **220. d.** ALL is an important cell surface marker in the diagnosis of human acute lymphocytic leukemia (ALL). This protein is present on leukemic cells of pre-B phenotype, which represent 85% of cases of ALL.

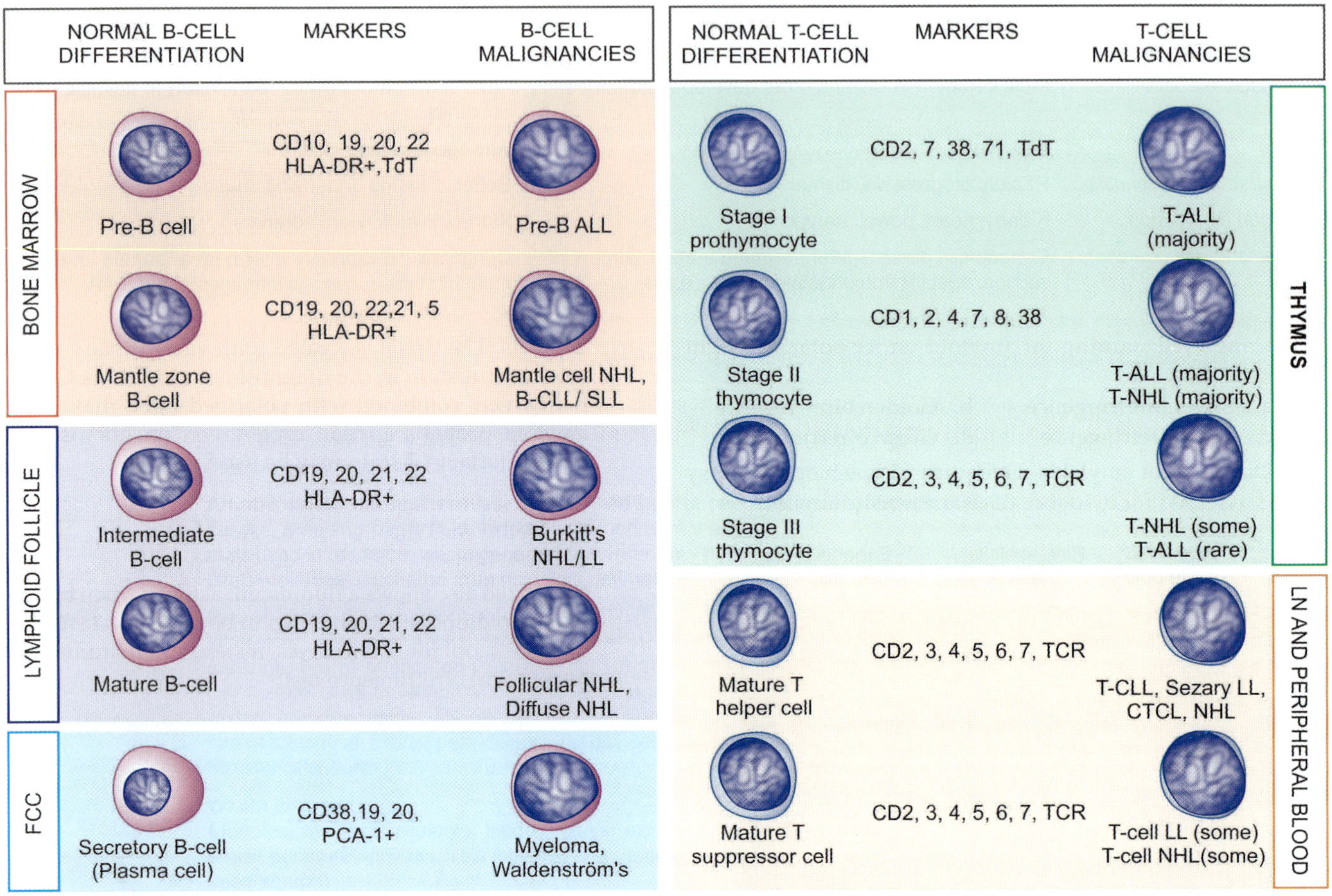

	NORMAL B-CELL DIFFERENTIATION	MARKERS	B-CELL MALIGNANCIES
BONE MARROW	Pre-B cell	CD10, 19, 20, 22 HLA-DR+,TdT	Pre-B ALL
BONE MARROW	Mantle zone B-cell	CD19, 20, 22,21, 5 HLA-DR+	Mantle cell NHL, B-CLL/ SLL
LYMPHOID FOLLICLE	Intermediate B-cell	CD19, 20, 21, 22 HLA-DR+	Burkitt's NHL/LL
LYMPHOID FOLLICLE	Mature B-cell	CD19, 20, 21, 22 HLA-DR+	Follicular NHL, Diffuse NHL
FCC	Secretory B-cell (Plasma cell)	CD38,19, 20, PCA-1+	Myeloma, Waldenström's

NORMAL T-CELL DIFFERENTIATION	MARKERS	T-CELL MALIGNANCIES	
Stage I prothymocyte	CD2, 7, 38, 71, TdT	T-ALL (majority)	THYMUS
Stage II thymocyte	CD1, 2, 4, 7, 8, 38	T-ALL (majority) T-NHL (majority)	THYMUS
Stage III thymocyte	CD2, 3, 4, 5, 6, 7, TCR	T-NHL (some) T-ALL (rare)	THYMUS
Mature T helper cell	CD2, 3, 4, 5, 6, 7, TCR	T-CLL, Sezary LL, CTCL, NHL	LN AND PERIPHERAL BLOOD
Mature T suppressor cell	CD2, 3, 4, 5, 6, 7, TCR	T-cell LL (some) T-cell NHL(some)	LN AND PERIPHERAL BLOOD

(PCA = Plasma cell antigen; TCR = T cell receptor; FCC = Follicular centre B cells; LN = Lymph node; LL = Lymphoid leukaemia)

Schematic representation of WHO-REAL classification of lymphoid neoplasms. Various immunophenotypes of B and T-cell malignancies are correlated with normal immunophenotypic differentiation/maturation stages of B and T-cells in the bone marrow, lymphoid tissue, peripheral blood and thymus.

221. CD-15 helps in assessment of:

a. Adult T-cell leukemia b. Hodgkin's disease

c. Mycosis fungoides

d. Larger granular lymphocytic leukemia

Immunohistochemical panels for the diagnosis of Hodgkin's disease typically employ CD15 along with CD30 and CD45; the latter does not stain Reed-Sternberg cells, but does stain almost all other lymphoid cells. CD15 is also present in about 50% of adenocarcinoma cells and can be used to distinguish such conditions from mesothelioma, which is typically negative.

Modified WHO classification of Hodgkin's Disease				
Histologic subtype	*Incidence*	*Main pathology*	*RS cells*	*Prognosis*
I. CLASSIC HD				
Lymphocyte-predominance	5%	Proliferating lymphocytes, a few histiocytes	Few, classic and polyploid type, CD15–, CD30–, CD20+	Excellent
Nodular sclerosis	70%	Lymphoid nodules, collagen bands	Frequent, lacunar type, CD15+, CD30+	Very good
Mixed cellularity	22%	Mixed infiltrate	Numerous, classic type, CD15+, CD30+	Good

Contd...

Ans. 221. a. Adult T-cell leukemia

Contd...

Histologic subtype	*Incidence*	*Main pathology*	*RS cells*	*Prognosis*
Lymphocyte-depletion (Diffuse fibrotic and reticular variants)	1%	Scanty lymphocytes, atypical histiocytes, fibrosis	Numerous, pleomorphic type, CD15+, CD30+	Poor
II. NODULAR LYMPHOCYTE-PREDOMINANT HD				
	2%	Proliferation of small lymphocytes, nodular pattern of growth	Sparse number of RS cells, CD45+, EMA+, CD15-, CD30-	Chronic relapsing, may transform into large B cell NHL

222. HMB-45 is a marker of:

a. Sarcoma
b. Melanoma
c. Carcinoma
d. All of the above

HMB-45 is a monoclonal antibody that reacts against an antigen present in melanocytic tumors such as melanomas, and stands for **human melanoma black 45**. It is used in anatomic pathology as a marker for such tumors. The specific antigen recognized by HMB-45 is now known as Pmel 17.

Common panel of immunohistochemical stains for tumours of uncertain origin

Tumour	*Immunostain*
1. *Epithelial tumours (Carcinomas)*	i. Pankeratin (fractions: high and low molecular weight keratins, HMW-K, LMW-K) ii. Epithelial membrane antigen (EMA) iii. Carcinoembryonic antigen (CEA) iv. Neuron-specific enolase (NSE)
2. *Mesenchymal tumours (Sarcomas)*	i. Vimentin (general mesenchymal) ii. Desmin (for general myogenic) iii. Muscle specific actin (for general myogenic) iv. Myoglobin (for skeletal myogenic) v. α-1-anti-chymotrypsin (for malignant fibrous histiocytoma) vi. Factor VIII (for vascular tumours) vii. CD34 (endothelial marker)
3. *Special groups*	
a. Melanoma	i. HMB-45 (most specific) ii. Vimentin iii. S-100
b. Lymphoma	i. Leucocyte common antigen (LCA/CD45) ii. Pan-B (Immunoglobulins, CD20) iii. Pan-T (CD3) iv. CD15, CD30 (RS cell marker for Hodgkin's)
c. Neural and neuro- endocrine tumours	i. Neurofilaments (NF) ii. NSE iii. GFAP (for glial tumours) iv. Chromogranin (for neuroendocrine)

223. Anti-U1 RNP antibody is associated with:

a. Dermatomyositis b. MCTD
c. SLE d. Scleroderma

Antibodies towards snRNP70 are associated with mixed connective tissue disease.

224. Confirmatory test for diagnosing amyloidosis:

a. Whole body CT scan b. Rectal biopsy
c. Tongue biopsy
d. Diagnostic peritoneal lavage

Diagnosis of amyloidosis requires tissue biopsy. Biopsy is assessed for evidence of characteristic amyloid deposits. Tissue can come from any involved organ. But in systemic disease first line site of biopsy is subcutaneous abdominal fat, known as a fat pad biopsy, because it's simple to acquire and less invasive than biopsy of the rectum, salivary gland or internal organs. An abdominal fat biopsy is not completely sensitive and so, sometimes, biopsy of an involved organ (such as the kidney) is required to achieve a diagnosis. For example, in AL amyloidosis only 85% of people will have a positive fat-pad biopsy using Congo red stain. By comparison, rectal biopsy has sensitivity of 74-94%

225. Stain NOT used for lipid:

a. Oil red O b. Congo red
c. Sudan III d. Sudan black

Congo red is used to stain microscopic preparations, especially as a cytoplasm and erythrocyte stain. Apple-green birefringence of Congo red stained preparates under polarized light is indicative for the presence of amyloid fibrils. Additionally, Congo red is used in microbiological epidemiology to rapidly identify the presence of virulent serotype 2a *Shigella flexneri*, where the dye binds the bacterium's unique lipopolysaccharide structure.

Staining characteristics of amyloid.

Stain	*Appearance*
1. *H and E*	Pink, hyaline, homogeneous
2. *Methyl violet/Crystal violet*	Metachromasia: rose-pink
3. *Congo red*	Light microscopy: pink-red Polarising light: red-green birefringence
4. *Thioflavin-T/Thioflavin-S*	Ultraviolet light: fluorescence
5. *Immunohistochemistry (antibody against fibril protein)*	Immunoreactivity: Positive

Ans. 222. **b.** Melanoma 223. **b.** MCTD 224. **b.** Rectal biopsy 225. **b.** Congo red

226. CD-99 is a marker of:

a. Ewing sarcoma
b. Chronic lymphocytic leukemia
c. Mantle cell lymphoma
d. All of the above

Antibodies to CD99 are used in diagnostic immunohistochemistry to distinguish Ewing's sarcoma from other tumours of similar histological appearance, as well as for the identification of thymic tumours, and of spindle cell tumours, such as synovial sarcoma, hemangiopericytoma, and meningioma.

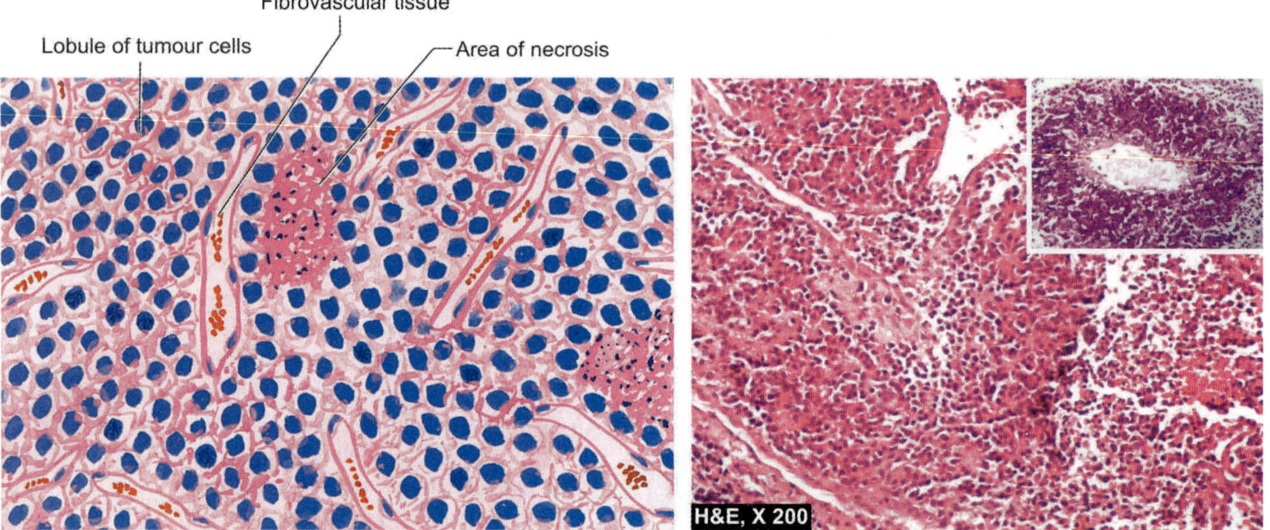

Ewing's sarcoma. Characteristic microscopic features are irregular lobules of uniform small tumour cells with indistinct cytoplasmic outlines which are separated by fibrous tissue septa having rich vascularity. Areas of necrosis and inflammatory infiltrate are also included. Inbox in the right photomicrograph shows PAS positive tumour cells in perivascular location.

227. The HLA class III region genes are important elements in:

a. Transplant rejection phenomenon
b. Governing susceptibility to autoimmune disease
c. Immune surveillance
d. Antigen presentation and elimination

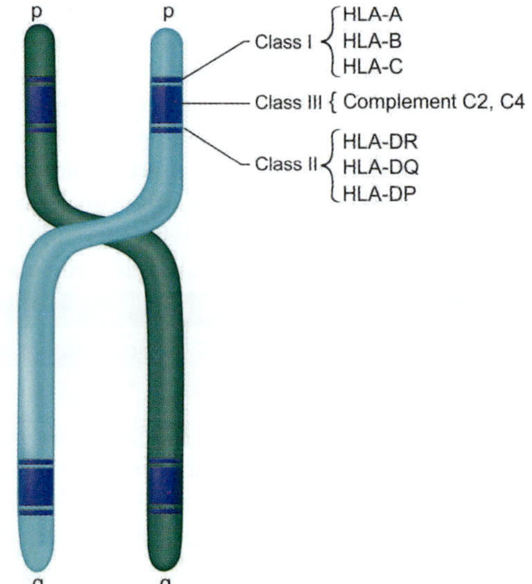

HLA system and loci on short arm of chromosome 6.

MHC Class III region has the highest gene density but some of the genes are not involved in the immune system.

Since class III genes encode several components of the complement system (i.e. C2, C4a, C4b, Bf), they are responsible for the levels of components of compliment system.

In addition to components of the complement system MHC III genes code inflammatory cytokines, tumor necrosis factor a and 0 (TNF a and P), two heat shock proteins (HSP) etc. They are not membrane proteins and have no role in Ag presentation. MHC Class III molecules are not structurally related to class I and class II molecules but are important in immune response.

228. Which of the following marker is specific for GastroIntestinal Stromal Tumor (GIST):

a. CD117
b. CD34
c. CD23
d. S-100

Antibodies to CD117 are widely used in immunohistochemistry to help distinguish particular types of tumour in histological tissue sections. It is used primarily in the diagnosis of GISTs, which are positive for CD117, but negative for markers such as desmin and S-100, which are positive in smooth muscle and neural tumors, which have a similar appearance. In GISTs, CD117 staining is typically cytoplasmic, with stronger accentuation along the cell membranes.

Ans. **226. a.** Ewing sarcoma **227. b.** Governing suscep... **228. a.** CD117

229. Which of the following best denotes classical complement pathway activation in immune-inflammatory conditions:

a. C2, C3 and C4 decreased
b. C2 and C4 is normal; C3 is decreased
c. C3 normal; C2 and C4 decreased
d. C1 and C3 normal; C2 is increased

The classical pathway is triggered by activation of the C1-complex. The C1-complex is composed of 1 molecule of C1q, 2 molecules of C1r and 2 molecules of C1s, or *C1qr²s²*. This occurs when C1q binds to IgM or IgG complexed with antigens. A single pentameric IgM can initiate the pathway, while several, ideally six, IgGs are needed. This also occurs when C1q binds directly to the surface of the pathogen. Such binding leads to conformational changes in the C1q molecule, which leads to the activation of two C1r molecules. C1r is a serine protease. They then cleave C1s (another serine protease). The C1r²s² component now splits C4 and then C2, producing C4a, C4b, C2a, and C2b. C4b and C2a bind to form the classical pathway C3-convertase (C4b2a complex), which promotes cleavage of C3 into C3a and C3b; C3b later joins with C4b2a (the C3 convertase) to make C5 convertase (C4b2a3b complex).

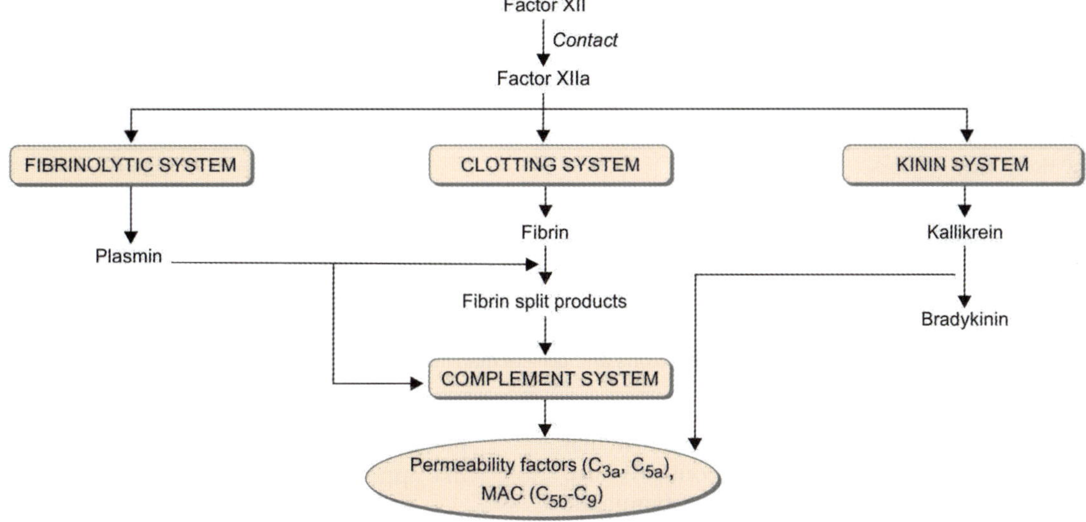

Inter-relationship among clotting, fibrinolytic, kinin and complement systems.

230. Which tumor is NOT seen in AIDS:

a. Kaposi sarcoma
b. GI adenocarcinoma
c. Non Hodgkin's lymphoma
d. Astrocytoma

Astrocytomas are a type of cancer of the brain. They originate in a particular kind of glial cells, star-shaped brain cells in the cerebrum called astrocytes. This type of tumor does not usually spread outside the brain and spinal cord and it does not usually affect other organs. Astrocytomas are the most common glioma and can occur in most parts of the brain and occasionally in the spinal cord. *(See Diagram on next page)*

231. HLA-B27 is associated with all EXCEPT:

a. Ankylosing spondylitis
b. Behcet's syndrome
c. Psoriasis
d. Reiter's syndrome

Behçet's disease is considered more prevalent in the areas surrounding the old silk trading routes in the Middle East and in Central Asia. Thus, it is sometimes known as *Silk Road Disease*. However, this disease is not restricted to people from these regions. A large number of serological studies show a linkage between the disease and HLA-B51.

232. HLA is located on:

a. Short arm of chr-6
b. Long arm of chr-6
c. Short arm of chr-3
d. Long arm of chr-3

The **human leukocyte antigen (HLA)** system is the locus of genes that encode for proteins on the surface of cells that are responsible for regulation of the immune system in humans.

This group of genes resides on chromosome 6 (***exception***: the gene for β2-microglobulin which is located on chromosome 15), and encodes cell-surface antigen-presenting proteins and has many other functions.

233. Multifocal tumor of vascular origin in a patient of AIDS is:

a. Kaposi sarcoma
b. Astrocytoma
c. Gastric carcinoma
d. Primary CNS lymphoma

Ans. **229. a.** C2, C3 and C4... **230. d.** Astrocytoma **231. b.** Behcet's syndrome **232. a.** Short arm of chr-6 **233. a.** Kaposi sarcoma

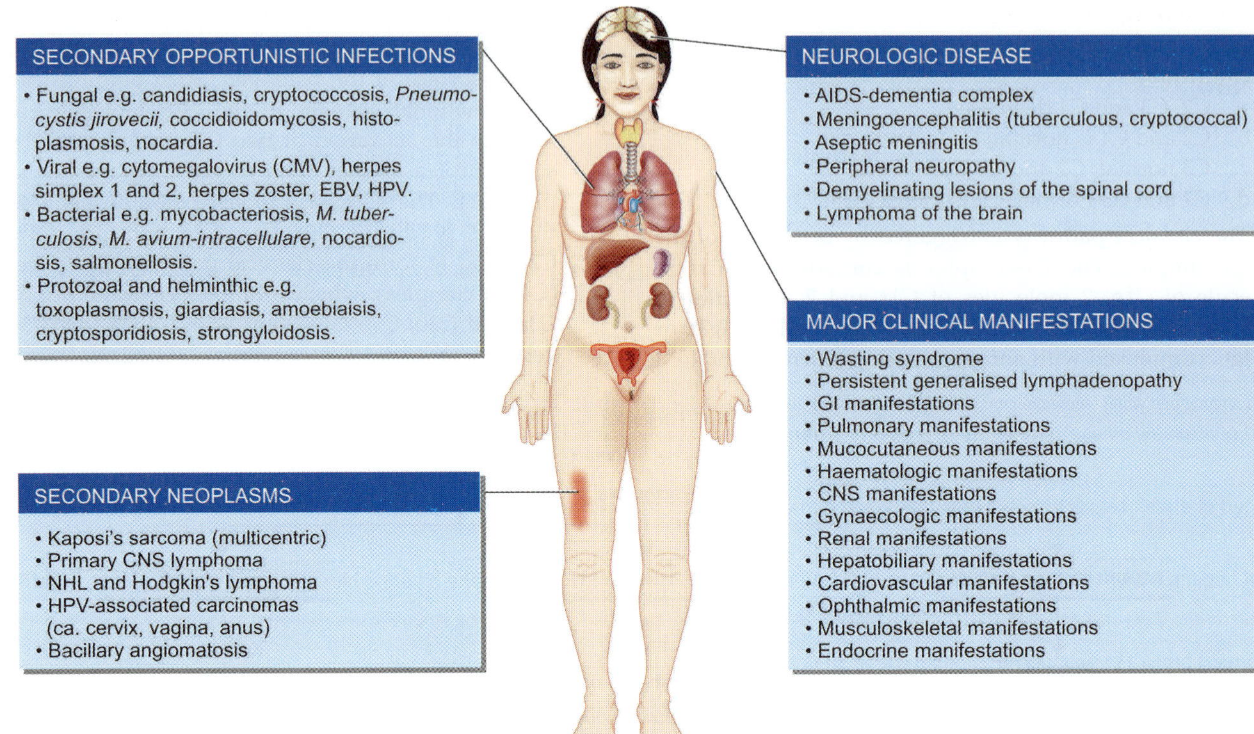

Major pathological lesions and clinical manifestations of HIV/AIDS.

Despite its name, in general it is not considered a true sarcoma, which is a tumor arising from mesenchymal tissue. The histogenesis of KS remains cont-roversial. According to some, KS arises as a cancer of lymphatic endothelium and forms vascular channels that fill with blood cells, giving the tumor its characteristic bruise-like appearance.

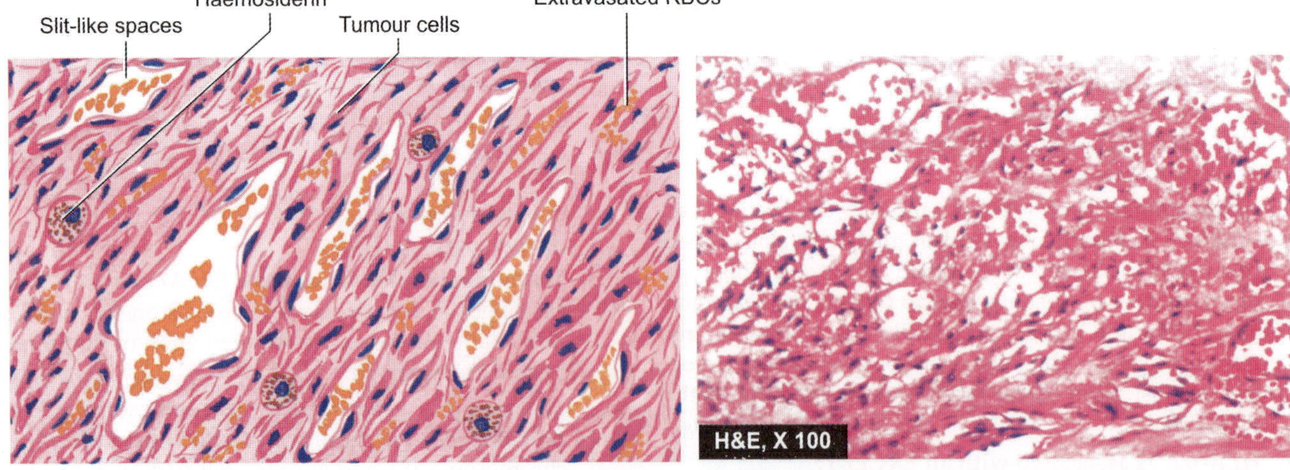

Kaposi's sarcoma in late nodular stage. There are slit-like blood-filled vascular spaces with extravasated RBCs. Between them are present bands of plump spindle-shaped tumour cells.

234. Which of the following combinations of cytogenetic abnormality and associated leukemia/lymphoma is INCORRECT:

a. t(8; 14): Burkitt's lymphoma
b. t(15; 17): AML-M3
c. t(9; 22): CML
d. t(9; 20): ALL

12;21 is the most common translocation in ALL and portends a good prognosis. 14;11 is the most common in children under 12 months and portends a poor prognosis.

Ans. 234. d. t(9; 20): ALL

FAB classification of ALL				
A. MORPHOLOGIC CRITERIA				
Fab Class		Percent Cases	Morphology	Cytochemistry
L1:	Childhood-ALL (B-ALL, and T-ALL)	More common in children	Homogeneous small lymphoblasts; scanty cytoplasm, regular round nuclei, inconspicuous nucleoli	PAS ± Acid phosphatase ±
L2:	Adult-ALL (mostly T-ALL)	More frequent in adults	Heterogeneous lymphoblasts; variable amount of cytoplasm, irregular or cleft nuclei, large nucleoli	PAS ± Acid phosphatase ±
L3:	Burkitt type-ALL (B-ALL)	Uncommon	Large homogeneous lymphoblasts; round nuclei, prominent nucleoli, cytoplasmic vacuolation	PAS – Acid phosphatase –
B. CYTOGENETIC AND IMMUNOLOGIC CRITERIA				
Subtype	Incidence	Markers	Fab Subtype	Cytogenetic Abnormalities
Pre-B ALL	75%	CD10+ (90%), TdT+	L1, L2	t(9;22) i.e. Philadelphia+ALL
B cell ALL	5%	CD10+ (50%), TdT-	L3	t(8;14) (Burkitt's leukaemia)
T cell ALL	20%	CD10+ (30%), TdT+	L1, L2	14q11

(TdT = terminal deoxynucleotidyl transferase)

235. Amyloidosis is associated with all of the following EXCEPT:

a. Multiple myeloma
b. Renal failure
c. Alzheimer's disease
d. Acute inflammatory conditions

Most classification systems included primary (i.e., idiopathic) amyloidosis, in which no associated clinical condition was identified, and secondary amyloidosis (i.e., secondary to chronic inflammatory conditions). Some classification systems included myeloma-associated, familial, and localized amyloidosis.

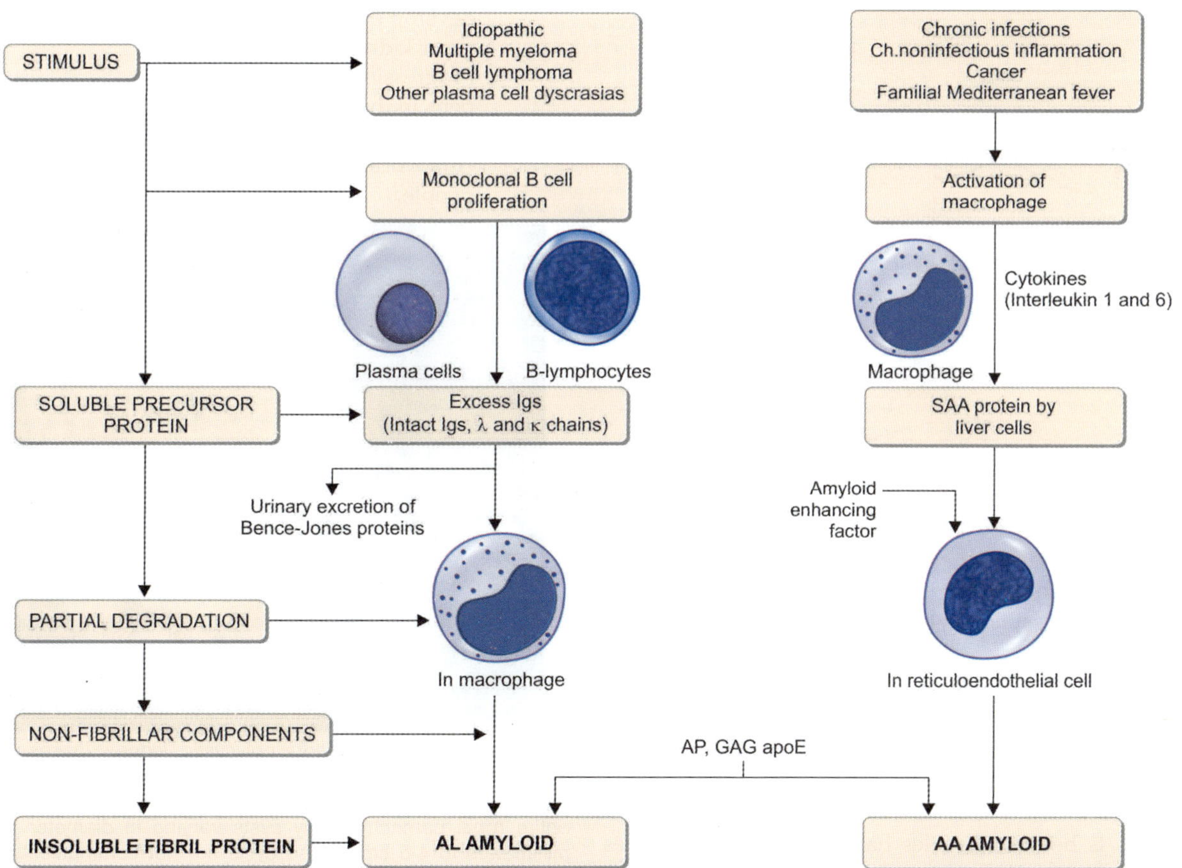

Pathogenesis of two main forms of amyloid deposition (AL = Amyloid light chain; AA = Amyloid-associated protein; GAG = Glycosaminoglycan; AP = Amyloid P component). The sequence on left shows general schematic representation common to both major forms of amyloidogenesis.

Ans. **235. d.** Acute inflammatory conditions

MISCELLANEOUS

236. Which of the following is a X-linked dominant disorder?

a. Achondroplasia
b. Red green color blindness
c. Familial hypercholesterolemia
d. Vitamin D resistant rickets

X-linked hypophosphatemia (XLH), also called **X-linked dominant hypophosphatemic rickets**, **X-linked vitamin d-resistant rickets**

- It is an X-linked dominant form of rickets (or osteomalacia) that differs from most cases of rickets in that ingestion of vitamin D is relatively ineffective.
- It can cause bone deformity including short stature and genu varum (bow leggedness).
- It is associated with a mutation in the PHEX gene sequence (Xp.22) and subsequent inactivity of the PHEX protein.
- The prevalence of the disease is 1:20000

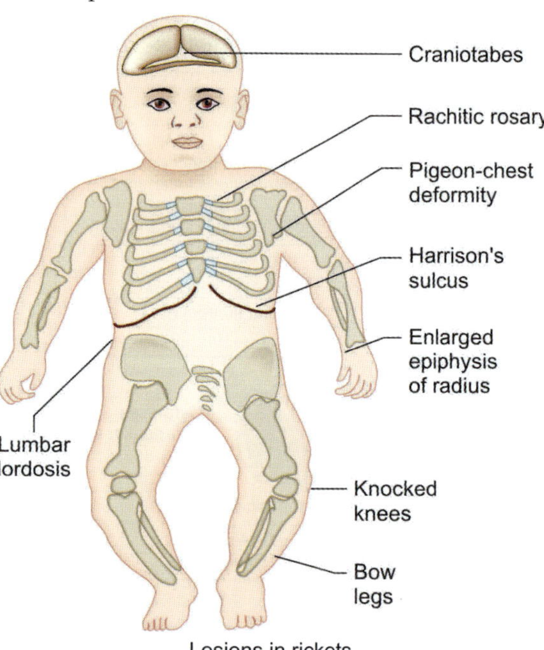

Lesions in rickets.

237. X-linked recessive inheritance is for:

a. Neurofibromatosis
b. Hereditary spherocytosis
c. Hemophilia
d. Cystic fibrosis

Hemophilia

- Like most recessive sex-linked, X chromosome disorders, haemophilia is more likely to occur in males than females.
- This is because females have two X chromosomes while males have only one, so the defective gene is guaranteed to manifest in any male who carries it.
- Because females have two X chromosomes and haemophilia is rare, the chance of a female having two defective copies of the gene is very remote, so females are almost exclusively asymptomatic carriers of the disorder.
- Female carriers can inherit the defective gene from either their mother or father, or it may be a new mutation.
- Although it is not impossible for a female to have haemophilia, it is unusual: a female with haemophilia A or B would have to be the daughter of both a male haemophiliac and a female carrier, while the non-sex-linked haemophilia C due to coagulant factor XI deficiency, which can affect either sex

238. Adult Polycystic kidney disease is inherited as:

a. Autosomal dominant
b. Autosomal recessive
c. X linked dominant
d. X linked recessive

Autosomal dominant polycystic kidney disease ("ADPKD", "autosomal dominant PKD" or "Adult-onset PKD")

- It is an inherited systemic disorder that predominantly affects the kidneys, but may affect other organs including the liver, pancreas, brain, and arterial blood vessels.
- Approximately 50% of people with this disease will develop end stage kidney disease and require dialysis or kidney transplantation.
- Progression to end stage kidney disease usually happens in the 4th to 6th decades of life.
- Autosomal dominant polycystic kidney disease occurs worldwide and affects about 1 in 400 to 1 in 1000 people.

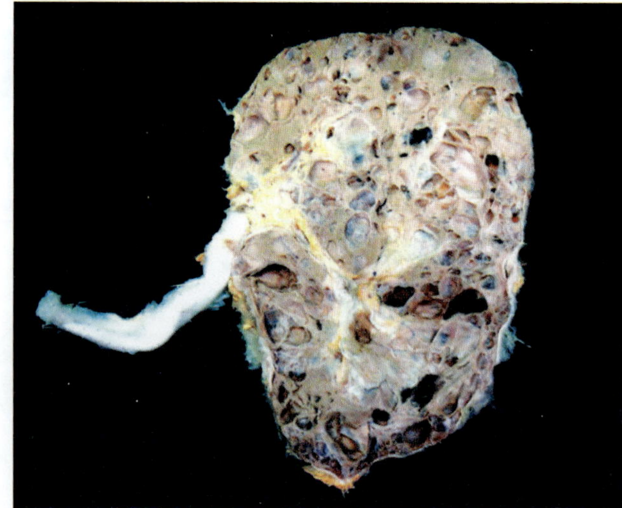

Adult (autosomal dominant) polycystic kidney disease (ADPKD). The kidney is enlarged and heavy. Sectioned surface shows loss of demarcation between cortex and medulla and replacement of the entire renal parenchyma by cysts varying in diameter from a few millimeters to 4-5 cm. These cysts are not communicating with the pelvi-calyceal system. The renal pelvis and calyces are distorted due to cystic change.

Ans. **236. d.** Vitamin D resis... **237. c.** Hemophilia **238. a.** Autosomal dominant

239. All are examples of round cell tumour EXCEPT:
- a. Neuroblastoma
- b. Ewing's sarcoma
- c. Non-Hodgkin's lymphoma
- d. Osteosarcoma

Osteosarcoma is an aggressive malignant neoplasm that arises from primitive transformed cells of mesenchymal origin (and thus a sarcoma) and that exhibits osteoblastic differentiation and produces malignant osteoid.

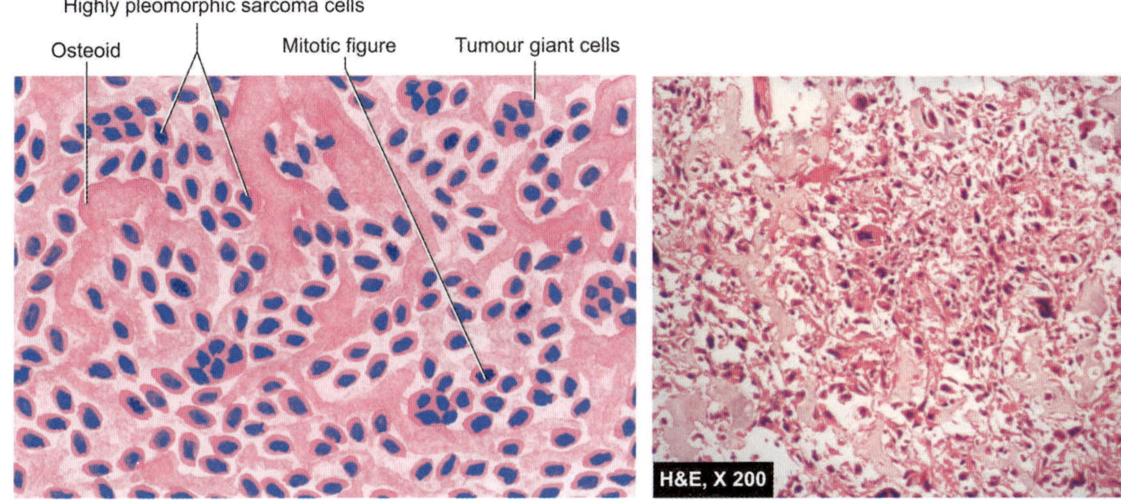

Osteosarcoma. Hallmarks of microscopic picture of the usual osteosarcoma are the sarcoma cells characterised by variation in size and shape of tumour cells, bizarre mitosis and multinucleate tumour giant cells, and osteogenesis i.e. production of osteoid matrix and bone directly by the tumour cells.

240. Bone tumour arising from metaphysis:
- a. Osteogenic sarcoma
- b. Ewing sarcoma
- c. Osteoclastoma
- d. Osteoid osteoma

An **osteosarcoma** is a cancerous tumor in a bone. Specifically, it is an aggressive malignant neoplasm that arises from primitive transformed cells of mesenchymal origin (and thus a sarcoma) and that exhibits osteoblastic differentiation and produces malignant osteoid.

BENIGN
MALIGNANT
DIAPHYSIS
METAPHYSIS
EPIPHYSIS
METAPHYSIS
DIAPHYSIS
Osteoid osteoma
Nonossifying fibroma
Osteoblastoma
Osteochondroma
Chondroblastoma
Giant cell tumour
Chondromyxoid fibroma
Enchondroma
Adamantinoma
Ewing's sarcoma
Lymphoma
Osteosarcoma
Chondrosarcoma
FEMUR
KNEE JOINT
TIBIA

Anatomic locations of common primary bone and cartilage tumours.

241. Charcot's joint includes all of the following EXCEPT:
- a. Syringomyelia
- b. Leprosy
- c. Diabetes
- d. Arthrogryposis multiplex congenita

Arthrogryposis multiplex congenita (AMC), or simply **arthrogryposis**, describes congenital joint contractures in two or more areas of the body.

242. 'Biphasic pattern' on histology is seen in which tumor:
- a. Rhabdomyosarcoma
- b. Synovial cell sarcoma
- c. Osteosarcoma
- d. Neurofibroma

Two cell types can be seen microscopically in synovial sarcoma. One fibrous type, known as a spindle or sarcomatous cell, is relatively small and uniform, and found in sheets. The other is epithelial in appearance. Classical synovial sarcoma has a biphasic appearance with both types present.

Ans. **239. d.** Osteosarcoma **240. a.** Osteogenic sarcoma **241. d.** Arthrogryposis... **242. b.** Synovial cell sarcoma

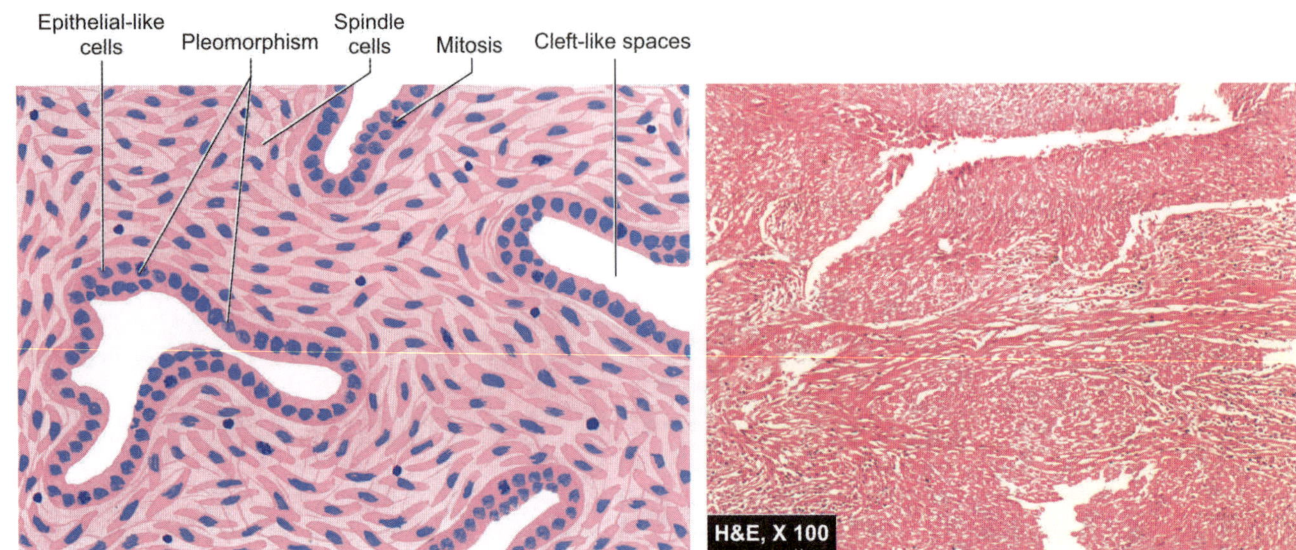

Classic synovial sarcoma, showing characteristic biphasic cellular pattern. The tumour is composed of epithelial-like cells lining cleft-like spaces and gland-like structures, and spindle cell areas forming fibrosarcoma-like growth pattern.

243. Lactic acidosis is seen in all EXCEPT:

a. Respiratory failure
b. Circulatory failure
c. Phenformin therapy
d. Acute renal failure

Lactic acidosis is a physiological condition characterized by low pH in body tissues and blood (acidosis) accompanied by the buildup of lactate, especially L-lactate, and is considered a distinct form of metabolic acidosis. Lactic acidosis is characterized by lactate levels >5 mmol/L and serum pH <7.35.

244. Human papilloma virus-8 infection is associated with:

a. Anogenital warts
b. Kaposi sarcoma
c. Cervical carcinoma in situ
d. Flat warts

Verruca plana, also known as a "flat wart", is a reddish-brown or flesh-colored, slightly raised, flat-surfaced, well-demarcated papule of 2 to 5 mm in diameter. Upon close inspection, these lesions have a surface that is "finely verrucous". Warts are caused by a viral infection, specifically by one of the many types of human papillomavirus (HPV).

Correlation of HPV types with disease

	Disease	Common type	Malignant potential
1.	Common wart (verruca vulgaris)	1, 2	41
2.	Palmoplantar wart	1, 2	—
3.	Flat wart (verruca plana)	3, 10	41
4.	Anogenital warts (condyloma acuminatum)	6, 11	30, 45
5.	Bowen's disease	16	31
6.	Bowenoid papulosis	16	39, 45
7.	Laryngeal papilloma	6, 11	—
8.	Conjunctival papilloma	6, 11, 16	16
9.	Epidermodysplasia verruciformis	2, 3, 9, 10	5, 8
10.	Cervical carcinoma	16, 18	16, 18, 31, 33

Ans. **243. a.** Respiratory... **244. d.** Flat warts

ANSWERS WITH REFERENCES

GENERAL PATHOLOGY

1. **Ans. (b) Increased nuclear to cytoplasm ratio**
Ref: Harsh Mohan's Pathology, 7/e p186

2. **Ans. (d) Coagulative necrosis**
Ref: Harsh Mohan's Pathology, 7/e p27

3. **Ans. (c) Factor VII**
Ref: Internet resources

4. **Ans. (c) Basement membrane involvement**
Ref: Harshmohan's Pathology 7/e p200

5. **Ans. (c) Granuloma formation**
Ref: Harshmohan's Pathology 7/e p137

6. **Ans. (d) Macrophages**
Ref: Harshmohan's Pathology 7/e p136

7. **Ans. (c) Programmed internal cell death**
Ref: Harshmohan's Pathology 7/e p30

8. **Ans. (d) Small intestine**
Ref: Harshmohan's Pathology 7/e p112

9. **Ans. (d) 50%**
Ref: Harshmohan's Pathology 7/e p82

10. **Ans. (c) Calcium**
Ref: Harshmohan's Pathology 7/e p94

11. **Ans. (a) Atrophy**
Ref: Harshmohan's Pathology 7/e p25

12. **Ans. (c) Pigmented alveolar macrophages**
Ref: Harshmohan's Pathology 7/e p24

13. **Ans. (d) Liver**
Ref: Harshmohan's Pathology 7/e p111

14. **Ans. (a) Fundal glands of intestine**
Ref: Harshmohan's Pathology 7/e p37

15. **Ans. (c) SMAD1**
Ref: Harshmohan's Pathology 7/e p205

16. **Ans. (d) Tumour necrosis**
Ref: Harshmohan's Pathology 7/e p31

17. **Ans. (d) Lung**
Ref: Harshmohan's Pathology 7/e p113

18. **Ans. (b) Dystrophic**
Ref: Harshmohan's Pathology 7/e p35

19. **Ans. (c) Normal tissues**
Ref: Harshmohan's Pathology 7/e p36

20. **Ans. (c) Metaplastic bone**
Ref: Harshmohan's Pathology 7/e p854

21. **Ans. (a) Lungs**
Ref: Harshmohan's Pathology 7/e p17

22. **Ans. (b) Dystrophic**
Ref: Harshmohan's Pathology 7/e p35

23. **Ans. (d) Vasoconstriction**
Ref: Harshmohan's Pathology 7/e p117

24. **Ans. (d) Tumour lysis syndrome**
Ref: Internet resources

25. **Ans. (d) BCL-2**
Ref: Harshmohan's Pathology 7/e p208

26. **Ans. (d) Phagocytosis**
Ref: Harshmohan's Pathology 7/e p119

27. **Ans. (b) Increased vascular permeability**
Ref: Harshmohan's Pathology 7/e p81

28. **Ans. (a) Increased peripheral vascular resistance**
Ref: Harshmohan's Pathology 7/e p97

29. **Ans. (d) Platelet thrombus**
Ref: Harshmohan's Pathology 7/e p100

30. **Ans. (c) Dissolution of clot by plasmin**
Ref: Harshmohan's Pathology 7/e p100

31. **Ans. (c) Lymphoblasts**
Ref: Harshmohan's Pathology 7/e p326

32. **Ans. (b) Protein levels of 51-300 mg/L**
Ref: Harshmohan's Pathology 7/e p677

33. **Ans. (b) Mitochondria**
Ref: Harshmohan's Pathology 7/e p30

34. **Ans. (d) RBC**
Ref: Harshmohan's Pathology 7/e p130

35. **Ans. (c) Mycoplasma**
Ref: Harshmohan's Pathology 7/e p138

36. **Ans. (d) It transports iron for erythropoiesis**
Ref: Harshmohan's Pathology 7/e p272

37. **Ans. (d) Decreased hydrostatic pressure**
Ref: Harshmohan's Pathology 7/e p118

38. **Ans. (c)** Normal kidney
Ref: Harshmohan's Pathology 7/e p35

39. **Ans. (d)** Hypoxic injury to brain
Ref: Harshmohan's Pathology 7/e p28

40. **Ans. (d)** Apoptosis
Ref: Harshmohan's Pathology 7/e p32

41. **Ans. (d)** All of the above
Ref: Harshmohan's Pathology 7/e p12

42. **Ans. (c)** Serotonin
Ref: Harshmohan's Pathology 7/e p120

43. **Ans. (a)** Transferrin
Ref: Harshmohan's Pathology 7/e p120

44. **Ans. (a)** Nitric oxide
Ref: Harshmohan's Pathology 7/e p125

45. **Ans. (d)** Heart rate decreases
Ref: Harshmohan's Pathology 7/e p97

46. **Ans. (a)** Inflammation is present
Ref: Harshmohan's Pathology 7/e p29

47. **Ans. (a)** Normal urothelium
Ref: Internet resources

48. **Ans. (d)** Neuroblastoma
Ref: Harshmohan's Pathology 7/e p203

49. **Ans. (d)** Cortical neuron
Ref: Internet resources

50. **Ans. (b)** 5-15%
Ref: Harshmohan's Pathology 7/e p107

51. **Ans. (c)** Wound margin
Ref: Harshmohan's Pathology 7/e p158

52. **Ans. (b)** Type II collagen
Ref: Internet resources

53. **Ans. (b)** Chronic inflammation
Ref: Harshmohan's Pathology 7/e p129

CLINICAL PATHOLOGY

54. **Ans. (c)** Polycythemia
Ref: Internet resources

55. **Ans. (c)** Megaloblastic anemia
Ref: Harshmohan's Pathology 7/e p326

56. **Ans. (c)** Myoglobin
Ref: Harshmohan's Pathology 7/e p415

57. **Ans. (d)** Emphysema
Ref: Harshmohan's Pathology 7/e p229

58. **Ans. (b)** Prostatic alkaline phosphatase
Ref: Harshmohan's Pathology 7/e p229

59. **Ans. (a)** Polycythemia rubra
Ref: Internet resources

60. **Ans. (d)** ITP
Ref: Harshmohan's Pathology 7/e p317

61. **Ans. (c)** Acute rheumatic fever
Ref: Harshmohan's Pathology 7/e p423

62. **Ans. (c)** Leukemoid reaction
Ref: Harshmohan's Pathology 7/e p332

63. **Ans. (c)** CEA
Ref: Harshmohan's Pathology 7/e p229

64. **Ans. (d)** Hepatic carcinoma
Ref: Harshmohan's Pathology 7/e p229

65. **Ans. (b)** Ovarian cancer
Ref: Harshmohan's Pathology 7/e p229

66. **Ans. (b)** CA-19-9
Ref: Harshmohan's Pathology 7/e p229

67. **Ans. (b)** Down syndrome
Ref: Harshmohan's Pathology 7/e p229

68. **Ans. (a)** Pancreatic carcinoma
Ref: Harshmohan's Pathology 7/e p229

69. **Ans. (b)** Acute pyogenic bacterial infection
Ref: Harshmohan's Pathology 7/e p327

70. **Ans. (d)** Polycythemia vera
Ref: Harshmohan's Pathology 7/e p339

71. **Ans. (d)** Vitamin D deficiency
Ref: Harshmohan's Pathology 7/e p245

72. **Ans. (a)** Obstructive jaundice
Ref: Harshmohan's Pathology 7/e p579

73. **Ans. (a)** Calcitonin
Ref: Harshmohan's Pathology 7/e p802

74. **Ans. (b)** HPL
Ref: Harshmohan's Pathology 7/e p229

75. **Ans. (d)** Iron deficiency anemia
Ref: Harshmohan's Pathology 7/e p310

76. **Ans. (c)** Hodgkin's lymphoma
Ref: Harshmohan's Pathology 7/e p353

ABDOMINAL PATHOLOGY

77. **Ans. (b)** Acute viral hepatitis
Ref: Harsh Mohan's Pathology, 7/e p596

78. **Ans. (a) Necrosis**
Ref: Harsh Mohan's Pathology, 7/e p597

79. **Ans. (c) Hemangioma**
Ref: Harshmohan's Pathology 7/e p619

80. **Ans. (b) Reye's syndrome – ground glass hepatocytes**
Ref: Harshmohan's Pathology 7/e p587

81. **Ans. (c) Granulosa cell tumour**
Ref: Harshmohan's Pathology 7/e p739

82. **Ans. (d) Secondary biliary cirrhosis**
Ref: Harshmohan's Pathology 7/e p612

83. **Ans. (b) Uncommon in Asians**
Ref: Harshmohan's Pathology 7/e p620

84. **Ans. (b) Liver**
Ref: Harshmohan's Pathology 7/e p602

85. **Ans. (b) Liver**
Ref: Harshmohan's Pathology 7/e p600

86. **Ans. (c) Histological features are different from alcoholic steatohepatitis**
Ref: Harshmohan's Pathology 7/e p607

87. **Ans. (b) HBeAg**
Ref: Harshmohan's Pathology 7/e p592

88. **Ans. (a) HBsAg**
Ref: Harshmohan's Pathology 7/e p592

89. **Ans. (a) Hepatitis A**
Ref: Harshmohan's Pathology 7/e p591

90. **Ans. (d) Sickle cell anemia**
Ref: Harshmohan's Pathology 7/e p295

91. **Ans. (d) 2-3 weeks before and 1 week after the onset of jaundice**
Ref: Harshmohan's Pathology 7/e p590

92. **Ans. (d) Chronic, infectious stage**
Ref: Harshmohan's Pathology 7/e p592

93. **Ans. (b) Vinyl chloride**
Ref: Harshmohan's Pathology 7/e p212

94. **Ans. (b) Presence of IgM anti-HBc in serum**
Ref: Harshmohan's Pathology 7/e p592

95. **Ans. (a) Wait and watch**
Ref: Harshmohan's Pathology 7/e p595

96. **Ans. (c) Fatty infiltration**
Ref: Harshmohan's Pathology 7/e p610

97. **Ans. (d) Portal hypertension**
Ref: Internet resources

NERVOUS SYSTEM PATHOLOGY

98. **Ans. (b) Subarachnoid hemorrhage**
Ref: Harsh Mohan's Pathology, 7/e p874

99. **Ans. (c) Descending paralysis**
Ref: Harshmohan's Pathology 7/e p885

100. **Ans. (b) Rabies**
Ref: Harshmohan's Pathology 7/e p178

101. **Ans. (d) Neuroglia**
Ref: Harshmohan's Pathology 7/e p863

102. **Ans. (d) Lymphocytic pleocytosis**
Ref: Harshmohan's Pathology 7/e p868

103. **Ans. (c) Ependymoma**
Ref: Harshmohan's Pathology 7/e p881

104. **Ans. (a) Secondaries**
Ref: Harshmohan's Pathology 7/e p879

105. **Ans. (b) Parasympathetic paraganglioma**
Ref: Harshmohan's Pathology 7/e p503

106. **Ans. (d) Prostatic carcinoma**
Ref: Harshmohan's Pathology 7/e p708

107. **Ans. (d) Preserved postural reflexes**
Ref: Harshmohan's Pathology 7/e p877

108. **Ans. (b) Nicotinic receptor proteins**
Ref: Harshmohan's Pathology 7/e p849

109. **Ans. (d) Negri bodies**
Ref: Harshmohan's Pathology 7/e p178

RESPIRATORY SYSTEM PATHOLOGY

110. **Ans. (c) Hematogenous**
Ref: Harsh Mohan's Pathology, 7/e p142

111. **Ans. (b) Predominance of alveolar exudates**
Ref: Harshmohan's Pathology 7/e p454

112. **Ans. (c) Lymphocytosis**
Ref: Harshmohan's Pathology 7/e p141

113. **Ans. (b) Increased in chronic bronchitis**
Ref: Harshmohan's Pathology 7/e p459

114. **Ans. (d) Apex of the upper lobe**
Ref: Harshmohan's Pathology 7/e p144

115. **Ans. (d) Cavity lung**
Ref: Internet resources

116. **Ans. (d) Hypertension**
Ref: Harshmohan's Pathology 7/e p631

117. **Ans. (a) Emphysema**
Ref: Harshmohan's Pathology 7/e p460

CARDIOVASCULAR SYSTEM PATHOLOGY

118. **Ans. (d) Mitral valve stenosis**
Ref: Harsh Mohan's Pathology, 7/e p422

119. **Ans. (b) Polyarteritis nodosa**
Ref: Robbin's Pathology, 7/e p349

120. **Ans. (a) Diastolic filling**
Ref: Harsh Mohan's Pathology, 7/e p434

121. **Ans. (a) Hyaline arteriosclerosis**
Ref: Harshmohan's Pathology 7/e p372

122. **Ans. (b) Syphilitic aneurysm**
Ref: Harshmohan's Pathology 7/e p387

123. **Ans. (c) Affects damaged valves**
Ref: Harshmohan's Pathology 7/e p426

124. **Ans. (c) Erythema nodosum**
Ref: Harshmohan's Pathology 7/e p419

125. **Ans. (a) Affects large size blood vessels**
Ref: Harshmohan's Pathology 7/e p383

126. **Ans. (b) Hypertension**
Ref: Internet resources

127. **Ans. (d) Left atrial thrombus**
Ref: Harshmohan's Pathology 7/e p428

128. **Ans. (c) Dilatation of ventricles**
Ref: Harshmohan's Pathology 7/e p435

129. **Ans. (c) Increased ASLO**
Ref: Harshmohan's Pathology 7/e p423

130. **Ans. (d) Plasminogen activator inhibitors**
Ref: Internet resources

131. **Ans. (a) Apex of heart**
Ref: Internet resources

132. **Ans. (b) Mitral valve**
Ref: Harshmohan's Pathology 7/e p421

133. **Ans. (b) Myxoma**
Ref: Harshmohan's Pathology 7/e p439

134. **Ans. (b) Affects small, medium-sized and larger arteries commonly**
Ref: Harshmohan's Pathology 7/e p383

135. **Ans. (a) Heparin**
Ref: Internet resources

136. **Ans. (d) Periphery**
Ref: Harshmohan's Pathology 7/e p383

137. **Ans. (b) Liver**
Ref: Harshmohan's Pathology 7/e p384

138. **Ans. (b) Secondaries**
Ref: Harshmohan's Pathology 7/e p439

ENDOCRINE SYSTEM PATHOLOGY

139. **Ans. (d) Urine contains 5-HIAA**
Ref: Harsh Mohan's Pathology, 7/e p792

140. **Ans. (a) Adrenals**
Ref: Internet resources

141. **Ans. (a) Thyroid dysgenesis**
Ref: Harshmohan's Pathology 7/e p794

142. **Ans. (d) Hashimoto's thyroiditis**
Ref: Harshmohan's Pathology 7/e p796

143. **Ans. (d) Weber syndrome**
Ref: Harshmohan's Pathology 7/e p819

144. **Ans. (d) Papillary**
Ref: Harshmohan's Pathology 7/e p803

145. **Ans. (d) Follicular adenoma**
Ref: Harshmohan's Pathology 7/e p801

146. **Ans. (d) Increased appetite**
Ref: Harshmohan's Pathology 7/e p793

147. **Ans. (c) Phenytoin**
Ref: Internet resources

148. **Ans. (b) Nor-epinephrine**
Ref: Harshmohan's Pathology 7/e p790

149. **Ans. (d) High plasma and low urine osmolality**
Ref: Harshmohan's Pathology 7/e p786

150. **Ans. (a) Loss of diurnal variation**
Ref: Internet resources

151. **Ans. (c) Lung carcinoma**
Ref: Harshmohan's Pathology 7/e p785

GASTROINTESTINAL TRACT PATHOLOGY

152. **Ans. (d) p-ANCA**
Ref: Harsh Mohan's Pathology, 7/e p551

153. **Ans. (a) Autoimmunity**
Ref: Harsh Mohan's Pathology, 7/e p532

154. **Ans. (b) Ulcerative colitis**
Ref: Harsh Mohan's Pathology, 7/e p551

155. Ans. (a) Absence of granuloma
Ref: Harshmohan's Pathology 7/e p552

156. Ans. (a) Barrett's esophagus
Ref: Harshmohan's Pathology 7/e p523

157. Ans. (b) Skip lesions
Ref: Harshmohan's Pathology 7/e p549

158. Ans. (a) Hyperplastic polyp
Ref: Harshmohan's Pathology 7/e p566

159. Ans. (b) Caecum
Ref: Harshmohan's Pathology 7/e p556

160. Ans. (b) Stricture
Ref: Harshmohan's Pathology 7/e p555

161. Ans. (a) Sigmoid colon
Ref: Harshmohan's Pathology 7/e p564

162. Ans. (d) Toxic megacolon
Ref: Harshmohan's Pathology 7/e p550

163. Ans. (d) Argentaffinoma
Ref: Harshmohan's Pathology 7/e p560

HEMATOPOIETIC SYSTEM PATHOLOGY

164. Ans. (c) Pre-B cell
Ref: Robbin's Pathology, 7/e p423

165. Ans. (c) Anemia of chronic diseases
Ref: Harsh Mohan's Pathology, 7/e p278

166. Ans. (d) Idiopathic ITP
Ref: Harsh Mohan's Pathology, 7/e p312

167. Ans. (d) Controlling oxidation stress of RBC
Ref: Harsh Mohan's Pathology, 7/e p286

168. Ans. (c) Placenta praevia
Ref: Robbin's Pathology, 7/ed p445

169. Ans. (a) Hemolytic uremic syndrome
Ref: Harsh Mohan's Pathology, 7/e p288

170. Ans. (d) Anticoagulants
Ref: Harshmohan's Pathology 7/e p316

171. Ans. (b) Decreased fibrinogen products
Ref: Harshmohan's Pathology 7/e p316

172. Ans. (d) RBC
Ref: Internet resources

173. Ans. (a) Lead poisoning
Ref: Harshmohan's Pathology 7/e p277

174. Ans. (d) Macrocytic anemia
Ref: Harshmohan's Pathology 7/e p278

175. Ans. (a) Cutaneous lymphoma
Ref: Harshmohan's Pathology 7/e p359

176. Ans. (d) Reticulocytosis
Ref: Harshmohan's Pathology 7/e p276

177. Ans. (c) 21 days
Ref: Internet resources

178. Ans. (c) Increased leucocyte alkaline phosphatase
Ref: Harshmohan's Pathology 7/e p338

179. Ans. (d) Elevated plasma erythropoietin levels
Ref: Harshmohan's Pathology 7/e p339

180. Ans. (c) AML
Ref: Harshmohan's Pathology 7/e p342

181. Ans. (c) Hookworm
Ref: Harshmohan's Pathology 7/e p274

182. Ans. (b) Females are commonly affected
Ref: Harshmohan's Pathology 7/e p293

183. Ans. (b) Sickle cell anemia
Ref: Harshmohan's Pathology 7/e p295

184. Ans. (b) Normal PT and normal PTT
Ref: Harshmohan's Pathology 7/e p307

185. Ans. (a) Post splenectomy
Ref: Harshmohan's Pathology 7/e p270

186. Ans. (d) CNS
Ref: Harshmohan's Pathology 7/e p882

187. Ans. (b) Marrow is normoblastic
Ref: Harshmohan's Pathology 7/e p276

188. Ans. (b) Primary granules
Ref: Harshmohan's Pathology 7/e p324

EXCRETORY SYSTEM PATHOLOGY

189. Ans. (d) Rapidly progressive glomerulonephritis
Ref: Harsh Mohan's Pathology, 7/e p637

190. Ans. (d) Secondary hyperparathyroidism
Ref: Harsh Mohan's Pathology, 7/e p662

191. Ans. (d) Chronic pyelonephritis
Ref: Harshmohan's Pathology 7/e p671

192. Ans. (d) Hyaline arteriosclerosis
Ref: Harshmohan's Pathology 7/e p679

193. Ans. (c) RPGN
Ref: Harshmohan's Pathology 7/e p663

194. Ans. (b) Hypertension
Ref: Harshmohan's Pathology 7/e p678

195. **Ans.** None > d
Ref: Harshmohan's Pathology 7/e p664

196. **Ans. (c)** Post streptococcal glomerulonephritis
Ref: Harshmohan's Pathology 7/e p648

197. **Ans. (b)** IgG deposition in mesangium
Ref: Harshmohan's Pathology 7/e p657

198. **Ans. (b)** Hypolipidemia
Ref: Harshmohan's Pathology 7/e p649

199. **Ans. (d)** Malakoplakia
Ref: Harshmohan's Pathology 7/e p686

200. **Ans. (d)** Polyomavirus
Ref: Harshmohan's Pathology 7/e p219

201. **Ans. (a)** Diabetes mellitus
Ref: Harshmohan's Pathology 7/e p665

202. **Ans. (a)** Interstitial nephritis
Ref: Internet resources

203. **Ans. (b)** Hyponatremia
Ref: Harshmohan's Pathology 7/e p642

204. **Ans. (d)** Hypertension
Ref: Harshmohan's Pathology 7/e p649

205. **Ans. (d)** Membranoproliferative glomerulonephritis
Ref: Harshmohan's Pathology 7/e p659

206. **Ans. (d)** Chronic alcoholism
Ref: Harshmohan's Pathology 7/e p669

207. **Ans. (d)** Focal segmental glomerulonephritis
Ref: Harshmohan's Pathology 7/e p660

GENETICS

208. **Ans. (c)** Cystic fibrosis
Ref: Harshmohan's Pathology 7/e p255

209. **Ans. (a)** Beta thalassemia
Ref: Harshmohan's Pathology 7/e p297

210. **Ans. (a)** Hereditary spherocytosis
Ref: Harshmohan's Pathology 7/e p292

211. **Ans. (a)** Cystic fibrosis
Ref: Harshmohan's Pathology 7/e p255

212. **Ans. (d)** X-linked recessive
Ref: Harshmohan's Pathology 7/e p255

213. **Ans. (c)** Code for bacterial resistance
Ref: Internet resources

IMMUNITY AND AMYLOIDOSIS

214. **Ans. (b)** Amyloidosis
Ref: Harshmohan's Pathology 7/e p75

215. **Ans. (b)** B cell
Ref: Harshmohan's Pathology 7/e p47

216. **Ans. (d)** Pernicious anemia
Ref: Harshmohan's Pathology 7/e p58

217. **Ans. (a)** Chronic osteomyelitis
Ref: Harshmohan's Pathology 7/e p71

218. **Ans. (d)** Green birefringence
Ref: Harshmohan's Pathology 7/e p76

219. **Ans. (d)** Congo red
Ref: Harshmohan's Pathology 7/e p73

220. **Ans. (d)** ALL
Ref: Harshmohan's Pathology 7/e p347

221. **Ans. (a)** Adult T-cell leukemia
Ref: Harshmohan's Pathology 7/e p349

222. **Ans. (b)** Melanoma
Ref: Harshmohan's Pathology 7/e p228

223. **Ans. (b)** MCTD
Ref: Internet resources

224. **Ans. (b)** Rectal biopsy
Ref: Harshmohan's Pathology 7/e p73

225. **Ans. (b)** Congo red
Ref: Harshmohan's Pathology 7/e p73

226. **Ans. (a)** Ewing sarcoma
Ref: Harshmohan's Pathology 7/e p840

227. **Ans. (b)** Governing susceptibility to autoimmune disease
Ref: Harshmohan's Pathology 7/e p49

228. **Ans. (a)** CD117
Ref: Internet resources

229. **Ans. (a)** C2, C3 and C4 decreased
Ref: Harshmohan's Pathology 7/e p127

230. **Ans. (d)** Astrocytoma
Ref: Harshmohan's Pathology 7/e p56

231. **Ans. (b)** Behcet's syndrome
Ref: Internet resources

232. **Ans. (a)** Short arm of chr-6
Ref: Harshmohan's Pathology 7/e p49

233. **Ans. (a) Kaposi sarcoma**
Ref: Harshmohan's Pathology 7/e p396

234. **Ans. (d) t(9; 20): ALL**
Ref: Harshmohan's Pathology 7/e p346

235. **Ans. (d) Acute inflammatory conditions**
Ref: Harshmohan's Pathology 7/e p69

MISCELLANEOUS

236. **Ans. (d) Vitamin D resistant rickets**
Ref: Harsh Mohan's Pathology, 7/e p244

237. **Ans. (c) Hemophilia**
Ref: Robbin's Pathology, 7/e p450

238. **Ans. (a) Autosomal dominant**
Ref: Harsh Mohan's Pathology, 7/e p645

239. **Ans. (d) Osteosarcoma**
Ref: Harshmohan's Pathology 7/e p834

240. **Ans. (a) Osteogenic sarcoma**
Ref: Harshmohan's Pathology 7/e p833

241. **Ans. (d) Arthrogryposis multiplex congenita**
Ref: Internet resources

242. **Ans. (b) Synovial cell sarcoma**
Ref: Harshmohan's Pathology 7/e p861

243. **Ans. (a) Respiratory failure**
Ref: Internet resources

244. **Ans. (d) Flat warts**
Ref: Harshmohan's Pathology 7/e p763

PRACTICE QUESTIONS

GENERAL PATHOLOGY

1. Caspases are important in:
- a. Necrosis
- b. Cell regeneration
- c. Nerve regeneration
- d. Apoptosis

2. Malignant tumours differ from benign tumours in the fact that they:
- a. Are poorly cirumscribed
- b. Retain polarity
- c. Are slow growing
- d. Are small in size

3. Which of the following is FALSE statement for reversible cell injury:
- a. Reduced generation of ATPs
- b. Membranous bleb formation
- c. Nuclear chromatin condensation
- d. Detachment of ribosomes from the granular endoplasmic reticulum

4. Which of the following is the earliest feature of reversible cell injury:
- a. Amorphous densities
- b. Ribosomal detachment
- c. Hydropic swelling
- d. Bleb formation

5. Which of the following is NOT a site for fat necrosis:
- a. Pancreas
- b. Liver
- c. Breast
- d. Peritoneum

6. All of the following may show cell swelling EXCEPT:
- a. Infection
- b. Malignancy
- c. Pathologic calcification
- d. Hypoxia

7. All of the following are sure sign of malignancy EXCEPT:
- a. Chromosomal diploidy
- b. Pleomorphism
- c. Anisonucleosis
- d. Tumour giant cells

8. All are causes of dystrophic calcification EXCEPT:
- a. Necrosis
- b. Milk alkali syndrome
- c. Dead parasites
- d. Calcinosis cutis

9. Lardaceous spleen is due to deposition of:
- a. Lipofuscin
- b. Hemosiderin
- c. Amyloid in red pulp
- d. Amyloid in white pulp

10. Which of the following is NOT associated with deep venous thrombosis:
- a. Epithelial injury
- b. Platelets
- c. Hypercoagulability
- d. Altered blood flow

11. Dystrophic calcification is seen in:
- a. Hyperparathyroidism
- b. Multiple myeloma
- c. Atheromatous plaque
- d. Prolonged immobilization

12. Uterus size increase by:
- a. Hypertrophy
- b. Hyperplasia
- c. Both
- d. None

13. Proto-oncogene for gastro-intestinal stromal tumour/ GIST:
- a. C-myc
- b. N-myc
- c. L-myc
- d. c-KIT

14. Hallmark of acute inflammation:
- a. Vasoconstriction
- b. Macrophages
- c. Exudate
- d. Increased vascular permeability

15. Leukotrienes are produced due to:
- a. Cyclo-oxygenase pathway
- b. Lipo-oxygenase pathway
- c. Both
- d. None

16. All of the following inflammatory mediators cause pain EXCEPT:
- a. Histamine
- b. Serotonin
- c. Nitric oxide
- d. Vasoactive intestinal polypeptide

CLINICAL PATHOLOGY

17. Tumour marker for trophoblastic tumours:
- a. AFP
- b. CEA
- c. CA-125
- d. Beta-HCG

18. Diagnosis of a case who had >10% myeloma cells in marrow with lytic lesions of skull & presence of M-protein in serum:
- a. Smoldering myeloma
- b. Multiple myeloma
- c. Monoclonal gammopathy of unknown significance
- d. Non-secretory myeloma

Ans.
1. **d.** Apoptosis 2. **a.** Are poorly cirum... 3. **c.** Nuclear chromatin... 4. **c.** Hydropic swelling
5. **b.** Liver 6. **c.** Pathologic calcification 7. **a.** Chromosomal... 8. **b.** Milk alkali syndrome
9. **c.** Amyloid in red... 10. **a.** Epithelial injury 11. **c.** Atheromatous plaque 12. **c.** Both
13. **d.** c-KIT 14. **d.** Increased vascular... 15. **b.** Lipo-oxygenase... 16. **c.** Nitric oxide
17. **d.** Beta-HCG 18. **b.** Multiple myeloma

Volume I Non-Clinical Subjects

19. **Which of the following diseases with oral ulceration, may show absence of auto-antibodies:**
    a. Behcet disease b. SLE
    c. Pemphigus d. Celiac disease

20. **Normal value of HDL cholesterol should be more than:**
    a. 50 mg/dl b. 100 mg/dl
    c. 150 mg/dl d. 200 mg/dl

21. **A young lady presented with cauliflower like growth around vulva. It may be caused by:**
    a. HIV b. HPV
    c. HTLV d. HBV

ABDOMINAL PATHOLOGY

22. **Which of the following term is associated with mucinous tumour of ovary:**
    a. Psammoma bodies
    b. Pseudomyxoma peritoneii
    c. Coffee bean nuclei
    d. Rokitansky's protuberance

23. **Angiosarcoma of liver are associated with exposure of:**
    a. Asbestos b. Nickel
    c. Vinyl chloride d. Beta-naphthylamine

24. **What is deposited in haemochromatosis:**
    a. Amyloid b. Hemosiderin
    c. Zinc d. Lipofuchsin

25. **Psamomma bodies is a histological feature of which of the following:**
    a. Seminoma
    b. Serous cystadenocarcinoma
    c. Mucinous cystadenoma
    d. Dysgerminoma

26. **Pseudomyxoma peritoneii is seen in which condition:**
    a. Dysgerminoma b. Brenners tumour
    c. Theca cell tumour d. Mucinous cystadenoma

27. **Reinke's crystals are seen in:**
    a. Leydig cell tumour b. Arrhenoblastoma
    c. Seminoma d. Granulosa cell tumour

CNS

28. **MC cause of cerebral ischemia:**
    a. Diabetes
    b. Thromboembolism
    c. Vasospastic conditions
    d. Compression from outside

29. **MC cause of stroke in elderly:**
    a. Spasm b. Haemorrhage
    c. Embolism d. Aneurysm

30. **Another term for glioma retinae:**
    a. Retinoblastoma b. Meningioma
    c. Optic nerve glioma d. Giant cell astrocytoma

CVS

31. **Which is seen in early stages of hypertension:**
    a. Eccentric hypertrophy of left ventricle
    b. Concentric hypertrophy of left ventricle
    c. Eccentric hypertrophy of left ventricle
    d. Concentric hypertrophy of left ventricle

32. **MC organism causing acute infective/bacterial endocarditis/ABE:**
    a. Staphylococcus aureus
    b. Streptococcus viridans
    c. Streptococcus faecium
    d. Staphylococcus epidermidis

33. **Which of the following is a cause of left sided heart failure:**
    a. Pulmonary hypertension
    b. Left atrial myxoma
    c. Left to right shunts
    d. Restrictive pericarditis

34. **Libman Sack endocarditis occur in:**
    a. Rheumatic fever
    b. SLE
    c. Rheumatoid arthritis
    d. Osteoarthritis

35. **Trure regarding Wegener's granumolatosis:**
    a. Mainly affects heart
    b. Granuloma is seen
    c. p-ANCA positive
    d. Caused by Ebstein Barr virus

36. **MC organism causing endocarditis in prosthetic valves:**
    a. Staphylococcus aureus
    b. Streptococcus viridans
    c. Streptococcus faecium
    d. Staphylococcus epidermidis

37. **Regarding Buergers disease, FALSE statement is:**
    a. Ischemia of nerves
    b. Deep vein thrombosis
    c. Segmental inflammation
    d. Superficial thrombophlebitis

Ans.				
	19. a. Behcet disease	**20. a.** 50 mg/dl	**21. b.** HPV	**22. b.** Pseudomyxoma...
	23. c. Vinyl chloride	**24. b.** Hemosiderin	**25. b.** Serous cystadeno...	**26. d.** Mucinous cysta...
	27. a. Leydig cell tumour	**28. b.** Thromboem...	**29. c.** Embolism	**30. a.** Retinoblastoma
	31. b. Concentric...	**32. a.** Staphylococcus...	**33. d.** Restrictive...	**34. b.** SLE
	35. b. Granuloma is...	**36. b.** Streptococcus viridans	**37. b.** Deep vein...	

Practice Questions

ENDOCRINO

38. **MC cause of primary hyperparathyroidism:**
    a. Carcinoma of parathyroid
    b. Parathyroid hyperplasia
    c. Parathyroid gland hyperplasia
    d. MEN-II

39. **Which of the following is NOT a component of MEN-IIB:**
    a. Phaeochromocytoma
    b. Hyperparathyroidism
    c. Mucosal neuroma
    d. Marfanoid habitus

40. **Pseudo-rosette is seen in:**
    a. Retinitis pigmentosa
    b. Osteogenesis imperfecta
    c. Neuroblastoma
    d. Ameloblastoma

41. **Which of the following condition does NOT present with hyerparathyrdoism:**
    a. MEN-I
    b. MEN-IIA
    c. MEN-IIB
    d. Parathyroid hyperplasia

42. **Which of the following is NOT a feature of primary hyperparathyroidis:**
    a. Raised PTH
    b. Hypercalciuria
    c. Hypercalcemia
    d. Renal osteodystrophy

GIT

43. **Which of the following entity is NOT associated with carcinoma of tongue:**
    a. Alcohol
    b. Smoking
    c. Chewing of tobacco
    d. Aphthous ulcers

44. **Whipple disease is caused by:**
    a. Campylobacter jejunii
    b. H. pylori
    c. E. coli
    d. Trophermyma whippelii

HAEMATO

45. **Which is NOT true for sickle cell anemia:**
    a. Single point mutation
    b. Protection against falciparum malaria
    c. Organ infarctions
    d. Severe anaemia

46. **Which of the following condition presents with IgA, C3 and fibrin deposition in vessel wall:**
    a. Haemolytic uraemic syndrome
    b. Ehler-Danlos syndrome
    c. Wegener's granulomatosis
    d. Henoch Schonlein purpura

47. **What is needed for RBC synthesis:**
    a. Iro
    b. Folate
    c. Ascorbic acid
    d. Cyanocobalamin

48. **Low serum ferritin, elliptocytosis & poikilocytosis is seen in which type of anemia:**
    a. Megaloblastic anemia
    b. Iron deficiency anemia
    c. Sickle cell anemia
    d. Thalassemia

RENAL

49. **HIV associated nephropathy:**
    a. Post-streptococcal GN
    b. Minimal change disease
    c. Focal segmental GN
    d. Rapidly progressive GN

50. **All of the followings statements are true regarding polycystic kidney disease EXCEPT:**
    a. Adult polycystic kidney disease is inherited autosomal dominantly
    b. Involvement of chromosome 4 & 16
    c. Cysts in liver & pancreas
    d. Fully curable

51. **In Alport syndrome, which collagen is at fault:**
    a. Collagen I
    b. Collagen II
    c. Collagen III
    d. Collagen IV

52. **Selective proteinuria is seen in:**
    a. Post streptococcal GN
    b. SLE
    c. Rapidly progressive GN
    d. Minimum change disease

53. **A 8 year old child presented with highly selective proteinuria. Most likely diagnosis:**
    a. Post streptococcal GN
    b. Rapidly progressive GN
    c. Minimal change disease
    d. Chronic GN

54. **Which of the following glomerulonephritis shows proliferation of mesangial cells:**
    a. Rapidly progressive GN
    b. Post-streptococcal GN
    c. Membrano-proliferative GN
    d. Minimal change disease

Ans. 38. **c.** Parathyroid gland... 39. **b.** Hyperparath... 40. **c.** Neuroblastoma 41. **c.** MEN-IIB
42. **d.** Renal osteody... 43. **d.** Aphthous ulcers 44. **d.** Trophermyma whip... 45. **d.** Severe anaemia
46. **d.** Henoch Schon... 47. **a.** Iron 48. **b.** Iron deficiency anemia 49. **c.** Focal segmental...
50. **d.** Fully curable 51. **d.** Collagen IV 52. **d.** Minimum change... 53. **c.** Minimal change...
54. **c.** Minimal change...

55. Anti-GBM antibodies are seen in:
a. Caplan syndrome
b. Minimal change disease
c. Lipoid nephrosis
d. Goodpasture's syndrome

RESPI

56. Centri-acinar emphysema is more common in:
a. Alcoholics
b. Obese
c. Smokers
d. Diabetics

57. Haemoptysis seen in:
a. Mitral stenosis
b. Small cell carcinoma lungs
c. TB
d. All of the above

58. Increased susceptibility to TB may be seen in:
a. Asthma
b. Bronchitis
c. Silicosis
d. Bronchiectasis

MISCELLANEOUS

59. Which of the following is the main cause of childhood otitis media:
a. Streptococcus viridans
b. H. influenzae
c. Streptococcus pneumoniae
d. Staphylococcus aureus

60. Total number of chromosomes in Patau's syndrome:
a. 45
b. 46
c. 47
d. 48

61. Angelman's syndrome is:
a. Deletion of chromosome 14
b. Addition to chromosome 15
c. Deletion of chromosome 15
d. Addition to chromosome 14

62. Complement C1 is associated with which of the following:
a. Magnesium
b. Manganese
c. Phosphate
d. Calcium

63. Action of gp120 antigen exposed on the surface of HIV envelope:
a. Fusion
b. Attachment
c. Resistance
d. Entery of virus

64. Which of the following mediates primary immune response:
a. B cell
b. T cell
c. Both
d. None

65. Which of the following is NOT an anti-cancer gene preventing development of breast carcinoma:
a. BRCA1
b. p53
c. p16
d. PTEN

66. HLA involved in graft rejection:
a. MHC-I
b. MHC-II
c. MHC-III
d. MHC-IV

67. Which of the following is an effect of manganese deficiency:
a. Parkinsonism like disorder
b. Impairment of skeletal growth
c. Imapirment of glucose tolerance
d. Anemia

68. Which of the following interleukin is associated with growth of natural killer cells:
a. IL-2
b. IL-7
c. IL-8
d. IL-13

69. All of the following are antigen presenting cells EXCEPT:
a. Bipolar cells
b. Dendritic cells
c. Follicular dendritic cells
d. Tissue macrophages

70. Barr body is present in:
a. Klinefelters syndrome
b. Turner syndrome
c. Both
d. None

71. Use of Nitro-blue tetrazolium test:
a. For chronic glomerulonephritis
b. For chronic granulomatous diseases
c. For acute granulomatous diseases
d. For severe combined immunodeficiency

Ans. **55. d.** Goodpasture's... **56. c.** Smokers **57.** d. All of the above **58. c.** Silicosis
59. c. Streptococcus... **60. c.** 47 **61. c.** Deletion of... **62. d.** Calcium
63. b. Attachment **64. a.** B cell **65. c.** p16 **66. a.** MHC-I
67. b. Impairment... **68. a.** IL-2 **69. a.** Bipolar cells **70. a.** Klinefelters syndrome
71. b. For chronic granulomatous diseases

IMAGE-BASED QUESTIONS

1. Likely pathology in a case presenting with the following peripheral blood smear:

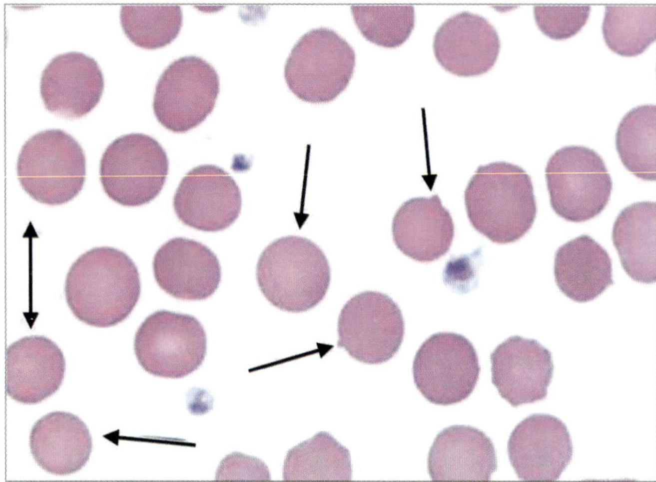

a. Replacement of glutamate by valine
b. Replacement of valine by glutamate
c. Defect in ankyrin
d. Deficiency of G-6PD enzyme

Arrow shows spherocytes, which are indicative of hereditary spherocytosis characterized by defect in spectrin (almost all cases) and defect in ankyrin (in about half of the cases).

2. This presentation is related to which of the following entity:

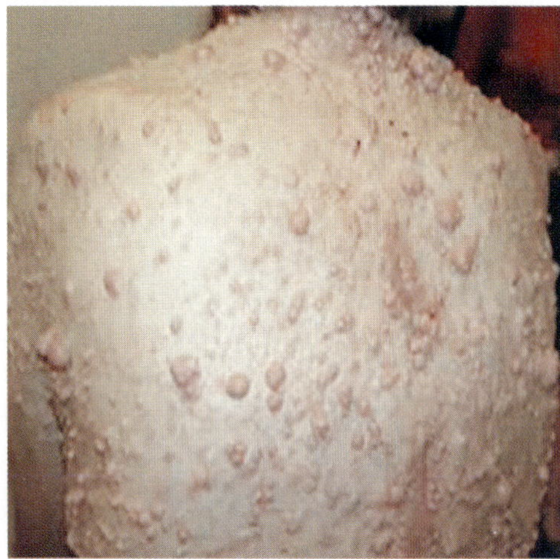

a. Von Willebrand disease
b. Von Recklinghausen disease
c. Von-Hippel Lindau disease
d. Lichen planus

The image shows multiple neurofibromas, associated with Von Recklinghausen's disease

3. Following image is of angiosarcoma of liver. Which of the following is associated with it:

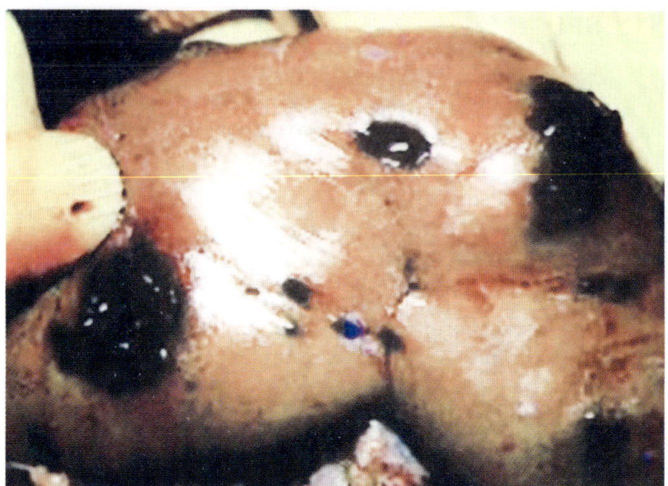

a. HBV
b. HCV
c. Carbon tetrachloride
d. Vinyl chloride

Exposure to Polyvinyl chloride is associated with development of angiosarcoma

4. This kind of kidney is associated with:

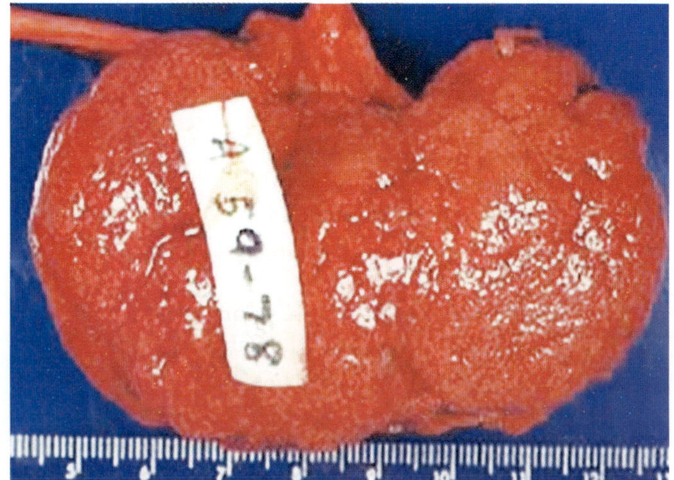

a. Benign hypertension
b. Diabetes mellitus
c. Post-streptococcal glomerulonephritis
d. Renal cell carcinoma

This image is of Flea bitten kidney, suggestive of PSGN (also seen in malignant hypertension), RPGN, hemolytic uremic syndrome, thrombotic thrombocytopenic purpura and Henoch Schonlein purpura).

5. **Electron microscopic view suggests the diagnosis of:**

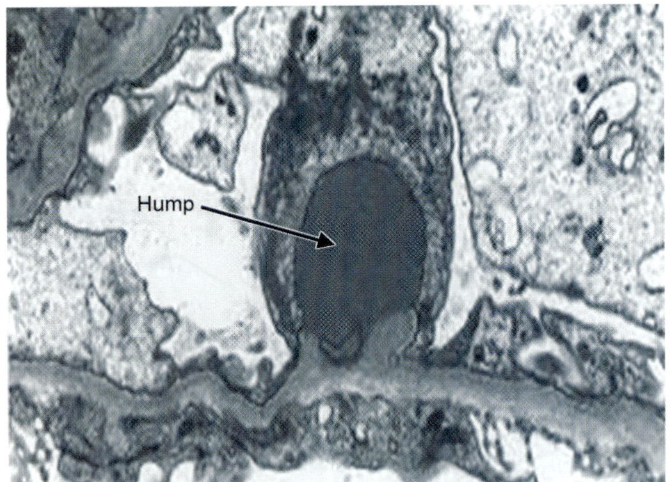

a. MGN
b. PSGN
c. Minimal change disease
d. MPGN

Electron microscopy of Post-streptococcal glomerulonephritis shows electron dense irregular deposits (Hump) on the epithelial side of glomerular basement membrane

6. **Electron microscopic view suggests the diagnosis of:**

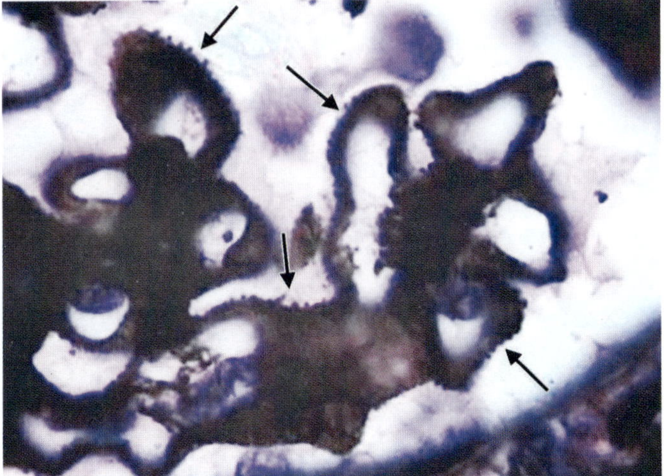

a. MGN
b. RPGN
c. Minimal change disease
d. MPGN

Electron microscopy of membranous glomerulonephritis shows electron dense deposits in subepithelial location. Basement membrane material protrudes between deposits as spikes (arrows)

7. **Light microscopic view of glomeruli suggests the diagnosis of:**

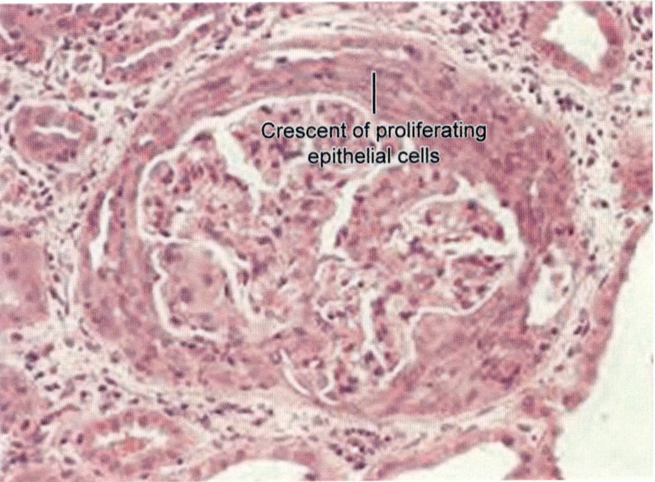

a. MGN
b. RPGN
c. Minimal change disease
d. MPGN

Formation of crescent on the inside of Bowman's capsule suggest the diagnosis of crescentic/rapidly progressive GN

8. **Light microscopic view suggests the diagnosis of:**

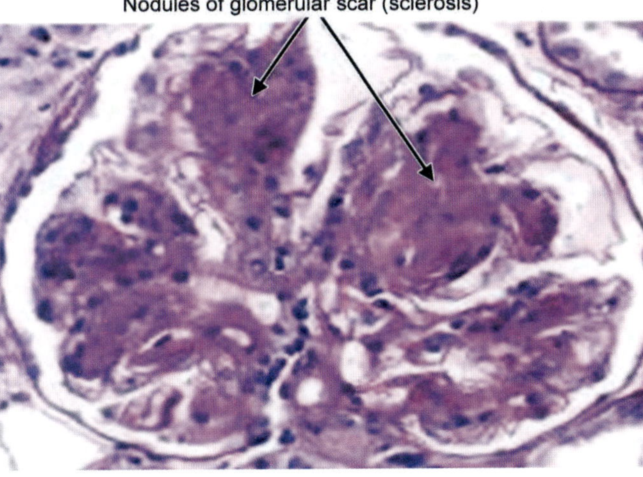

a. Diabetes mellitus type II
b. Diabetes mellitus type I
c. Post-streptococcal glomerulonephritis
d. Renal cell carcinoma

Nodular lesions of diabetic glomerulosclerosis are also called as Kimmelstiel Wilson (KW) lesions or intercapillary glomerulosclerosis. These lesions are specific for type I diabetes (juvenile onset diabetes) or islet cell antibody positive DM.

9. Histology suggests which thyroid carcinoma:

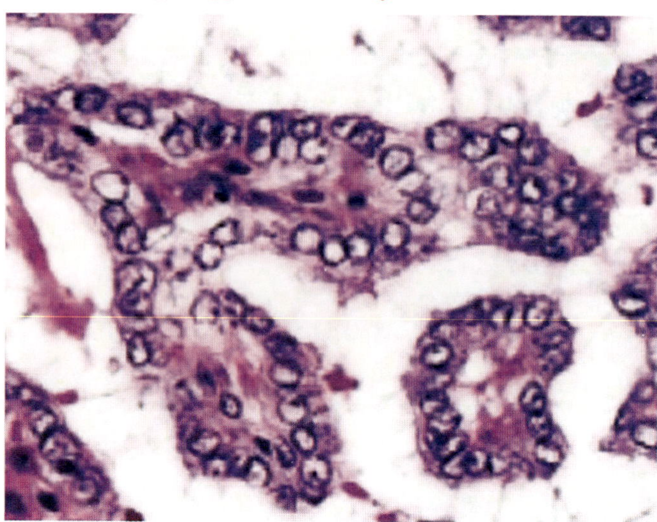

a. Medullary
b. Follicular
c. Anaplastic
d. Papillary

Orphan annie eye appearance of nucleus is a feature of papillary carcinoma of thyroid

10. Peripheral blood smear is suggestive of:

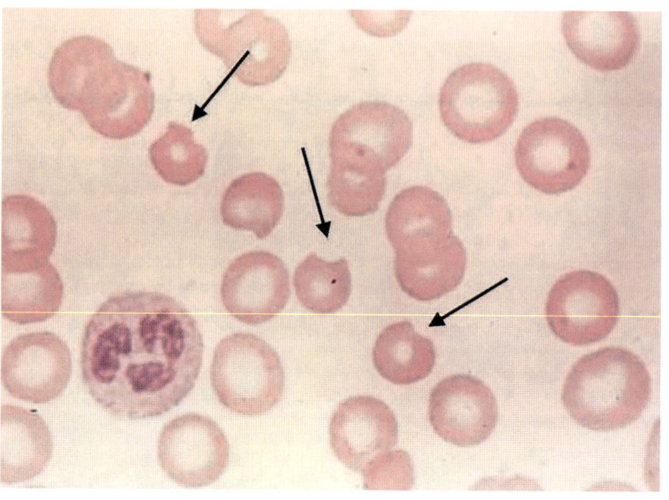

a. Thalassemia
b. Iron deficiency anemia
c. G-6-PD deficiency
d. Sickle cell anemia

Bite cells (arrows) are suggestive of G-6-PD deficiency

MCQ POINTS

S. No	Question statement	Answer
1.	Hypertrophy is defined as	***Increase in size of cell***
2.	Irreversible cell injury is demonstrated by	***Amorphous densities in mitochondria***
3.	Programmed cell death is known as	***Apoptosis***
4.	Most important source of histamine	***Mast cell***
5.	Following injury to a blood vessel, immediate hemostasis is achieved by:	***Vasoconstriction***
6.	Cell mediated immune response is which type of hypersensitivity	***Type IV***
7.	Neurofibromatosis is inherited as	***Autosomal dominant***
8.	Duchenne muscular dystrophy is inherited as:	***X-linked recessive***
9.	Edwards syndrome is known as trisomy....	***18***
10.	Best tumour marker for lung carcinoma	***Carcinoembryonic antigen***
11.	Tumour marker for squamous cell carcinoma	***Cytokeratin***
12.	Poorly differentiated carcinoma expresses which tumour marker	***Cytokeratin***
13.	Virus associated with Kaposi sarcoma	***HHV-8***
14.	Heart failure cells are seen in which organ	***Lungs***
15.	MC site of coronary atherosclerosis	***Left anterior descending***
16.	Location of vegetations in Libman Sack endocarditis	***Undersurface of valves***
17.	Which worm causes myocarditis	***Trichinella***
18.	HbA2 is written as	***Alpha2, delta2***
19.	Primary defect which leads to sickle cell anemia	***Replacement of glutamic acid by valine at beta 6***
20.	Earliest sign of iron deficiency anemia	***Decreased serum ferritin***
21.	Hodgkin's disease subtype with best prognosis	***Lymphocytic predominant (prognosis is directly proportional to lymphocye status)***
22.	Lacunar cells are seen in which subtype of Hodgkin's disease	***Nodular sclerosis***
23.	Starry sky appearance is seen in	***Burkitt's lymphoma***
24.	MC type of carcinoma lung	***Adenocarcinoma***
25.	Marker of small cell carcinoma of lung	***Chromogranin***
26.	Tamm Horsfalll protein is produced in which part of kidney	***Loop of Henle***
27.	Cause of edema in nephritic syndrome	***Salt and water retention***
28.	Common pathological changes seen in kidney in benign hypertension is	***Hyaline arteriosclerosis***
29.	Cause of flea bitten kidney	***Malignant hypertension***
30.	Renal papillary necrosis is associated with	***Diabetes mellitus, analgesic nephropathy***
31.	MC site of carcinoma of esophagus	***Lower ⅓rd***
32.	MC site of GIST is	***Stomach***
33.	Osteomas, adenomatous polyps of intestine and peri-ampullary carcinoma are seen in which syndrome	***Gardeners syndrome***
34.	Klatskin tumour is another term for	***Cholangiocarcinoma***
35.	Schiller Duval bodies are seen in:	***Endodermal sinus/yolk sac tumour***
36.	MC malignant bone tumour	***Secondaries***
37.	Macrophage in the brain is	***Microglia***
38.	MC site of metastasis of medulloblastoma	***Bone***
39.	Mode of inheritance of Wilson disease	***Autosomal recessive***

S. No	Question statement	Answer
40.	HLA complex in human is located on chromosome number	***6***
41.	HLA associated with Rheumatoid arthritis	***DR4***
42.	CD marker for angiosarcoma	***31***
43.	Localized Langerhans cells histiocytosis affecting head and neck is	***Eosinophilic granuloma***
44.	Burkitt's lymphoma is positive for	***CD19***
45.	An anti-apoptotic gene is	***Bcl-2***
46.	Michelis Gutmann bodies are seen in	***Malakoplakia***
47.	In xeroderma pigmentosum, defect lies in	***DNA repair/nucleotid excision repair defect***
48.	A patient having cystic medial necrosis with necrotizing arteritis is suffering from	***Giant cell arteritis***
49.	Tram track appearance of glomeruli is found in which condition	***MembranoProliferative GN***
50.	Duchenne's muscular dystrophy is inherited as	***XLR***
51.	Range of microalbuminuria	***30-300 mg/day***
52.	Most sensitive test for DIC is	***Raised FDP***
53.	Female with mantle radiation will suffer from which thyroid malignancy	***Papillary***
54.	HMB 45 is used as a marker of	***Malignant melanoma***
55.	Ascending aorta is involved in which aneurysm commonly	***Syphilis***
56.	Caterpillar cells are seen in which heart condition	***Rheumatic fever***
57.	Albumino-cytological (CSF examination) dissociation is seen in	***Guillain Barre syndrome***
58.	MC primary tumour of heart	***Myxoma***
59.	Myxoma of heart commonly arises from which chamber	***Left atrium***
60.	Reactivated TB is MC located near	***Apex of lung***
61.	MC heart tumour	***Secondaries***
62.	Type of calcification seen in normal tissues with raised serum calcium levels	***Metastatic calfication***
63.	Brown induration of lung is seen in	***Chronic venous congestion of lungs***
64.	Protein which transport iron	***Transferrin***
65.	Type of necrosis in infarction	***Coagulative/ischemic***
66.	Arthus reaction is type ..... hypersensitivity reaction	***III***
67.	Creola bodies are seen in	***Asthma***
68.	Lardaceous spleen in seen in	***Amyloidosis***
69.	Only immunoglobulin that crosses placenta	***IgG***
70.	Complement component which helps in chemotaxis	***C5a***
71.	Beta2 microglobulin protein is seen in amyloidosis due to	***Hemodialysis***
72.	Small protein which degrades many intracellular proteins	***Ubiquitin***
73.	Ovarian counterpart of testicular seminoma	***Dysgerminoma***
74.	MC involved artery in peripheral aneurysm	***Popliteal artery***
75.	Parasite which can cause carcinoma of bladder	***Schistosoma***
76.	Transverse ulcers in GIT are seen in which infection	***TB***
77.	MC CNS neoplasm	***Secondaries***
78.	Marker for squamous cell carcinoma	***Cytokeratin***
79.	MC cause of nephrotic syndrome in adults	***Membranous GN***
80.	Psammoma bodies are seen in .... carcinoma of thyroid	***Papillary***
81.	Multisegmented neutrophils are seen in	***Megaloblastic anemia***
82.	Feature of intestinal ulcers in amoebiasis	***Flask shaped ulcer***

S. No	Question statement	Answer
83.	MC bilateral tumour of breast	***Lobular***
84.	Commonest histological finding in benign hypertension	***Hyaline arteriosclerosis***
85.	Micro Munro abscesses is seen in	***Psoriasis***
86.	Congo red staining for amyloid under normal light shows	***Pink***
87.	Serum marker indicating active viral replication in HBV infection	***HbeAg, HBV DNA***
88.	Which cells are important source of histamine	***Mast cell***
89.	Rheumatic fever MC affects .... valve	***Mitral***
90.	Heart failure cells are pigmented alveolar macrophages. The pigment is	***Hemosiderin***
91.	Biomarker which rises lastly in MI	***LDH***
92.	Flask shaped ulcer are seen in	***Amoebiasis***
93.	MC site of affection in syphilitic aortitis	***Ascending aorta***
94.	Pulmonary artery is NOT involved in which type of vasculitis	***Churg strauss syndrome***
95.	Loss of intercellular connections between cells is known as	***Acantholysis***
96.	Decreased osmotic fragility is characteristic of	***Thalassemia***
97.	Hemochromatosis is a defect in metabolism of	***Iron***
98.	Duchenne muscular dystrophy is a ...... protein defect	***Sarcolemmal***
99.	MC site of GIST is	***Stomach***
100.	Call Exner bodies are seen in	***Granulosa cell tumour***
101.	MC type of lung Ca in young age group	***Adenocarcinoma***
102.	Takayasu arteritis does NOT affect which arteries	***Coronary artery***
103.	Werner syndrome is MEN type ...	***Type I***
104.	Bilateral hilar lymphadenopathy is a feature of	***Sarcoidosis***
105.	Antibodies associated with primary biliary cirrhosis	***anti-mitochondrial***
106.	Wilson disease is due to accumulation of	***Copper***
107.	Auto-splenectomy is seen in	***Sickel cell anemia***
108.	Orphan annie eyed nuclei appearance is characteristic of which thyroid tumour	***Papillary***
109.	Organ MC involved in hydatid disease	***Liver***
110.	Schilling test is done for	***Vitamin B_{12} malabsorption***
111.	Congo red staining for amyloid under normal light shows	***Pink***
112.	Serum marker indicating active immunity in HBV infection	***Anti-HBs***
113.	Negri bodies are seen in which part of CNS	***Hippocampus***
114.	MC cause of endocarditis in native but previously damaged valve	***Streptococcus viridans***
115.	Heart failure cells are seen in	***Left ventrcular failure***
116.	Biomarker which is specific for MI	***Troponin T and I***
117.	Piecemeal necrosis on liver histology suggest which condition	***Chronic hepatitis***
118.	Anti-endomysial antibodies are seen in	***Coeliac sprue***
119.	MC type of glomerulonephritis in HIV	***Focal Segmental GN***
120.	In AML, Auer rods are numerous in	***M3***
121.	Increased osmotic fragility is characteristic of	***Hereditary spherocytosis***
122.	Christmas disease is due to deficiency of	***Factor IX***
123.	Adult polycystic kidney is inherited as	***Autosomal dominant***
124.	Community acquired pneumonia is MC caused by	***Streptococcus pneumoniae***
125.	Pneumoconiosis, as a result of prolonged cotton dust inhalation	***Byssinosis***

S. No	Question statement	Answer
126.	MC type of lung Ca in non-smokers	***Adenocarcinoma***
127.	Loss of foot process on electron microscopy of kidney tissue suggests	***Minimal change disease/lipoid nephrosis***
128.	MC feature of sarcoidosis on chest X-ray	***Bilateral hilar lymphadenopathy***
129.	SLE is type ….. hypersensitivity reaction	***III***
130.	HIV affects ….. cells	***CD4***
131.	Bronze diabetes is associated with	***Hemochromatosis***
132.	Enlarged kidney is seen in	***Diabetes mellitus, polycystic kidney, amyloidosis***
133.	MC type of stomach malignancy	***Leiomyoma***
134.	Effect of paracetamol toxicity on kidney	***Renal papillary necrosis***
135.	Nodular glomerulosclerosis is classically associated with	***Diabetes mellitus***

CHAPTER

5

MICROBIOLOGY

KEY POINTS

Bacteria

- Sterols absent
- They are prokaryotes; nucleus and cytoplasm not well-developed
- Divide by binary fission
- Do not show true branching EXCEPT actinomycetes.

Immunodeficiencies

- **Humoral immunodeficiencies:**
  - Common variable immunodeficiency: Late onset hypogammaglobulinemia, infection with Giardia.
- **Cellular immunodeficiencies**
  - DiGeorge syndrome: Thymus hypoplasia, Fallot's tetralogy.
- Combined immunodeficiencies:
  - Ataxia telangiectasia
  - Wiskott-Aldrich syndrome: X-linked thrombocytopenia, decreased cell mediated immunity.
- **Subacute chronic immunodeficiency:** Adenosine deaminase deficiency.
- **Phagocytosis defects:**
  - Chediak-Higashi syndrome: Decreased pigments, photophobia, nystagmus
  - Lazy leucocyte syndrome: Peripheral neutropenia, decreased phagocytosis.

Genetics

- **Conjugation:** Transfer of genetic elements after actual physical contact between a male donor bacterium and female recipient
- **Transposons:** Jumping genes consisting of inverted repeat sequences, responsible for transferable drug resistance
- **Transformation:** Transfer of genetic information through the agency of free DNA
- **Transduction:** Transfer of a portion of DNA from one bacterium to another through the agency of a bacteriophage.

Some Important Terms

- **Quellung reaction:** When a suspension of a capsulated bacterium is mixed with its specific anticapsular serum, and examined under microscope, capsule becomes very prominent and appears swollen
- Chemical present in gram-positive bacterial wall but absent in gram-negative bacteria is: Teichoic acid.

Mechanism of Action of Toxins

- **ADP ribosylation of G-protein:** Pertussis toxin
- **Activation of cyclic amp:** LT (ETEC), cholera toxin
- **Activation of cGMP:** Heat stable E. coli toxin
- **Irreversible protein synthesis inhibition:** Shiga toxin (shigella dysenteriae-1), EHEC, diphtheria toxin, exotoxin A (Pseudomonas aeruginosa).

Staphylococcus

- Spherical cocci, grape like clusters, gram-positive
- Nonmotile, nonsporing, aerobes and facultative anaerobes
- Produce golden yellow pigment on nutrient agar slope-oil paint appearance
- Ferment sugar, producing acid but no gas
- On blood agar-beta hemolysis
- Macconkey's agar-pink colonies
- Mannitol is fermented anaerobically by S aureus but NOT by other species
- Catalase positive S aureus gives prompt phosphatase
- S epidermidis is the most common cause of infection of central nervous system shunts.

Streptococcus Pyogenes

- Nonmotile, nonsporing, gram-positive
- Aerobes and facultative anaerobes
- Spherical, arranged in chains
- Catalase negative

- Do not ferment inulin
- Ferment sugar producing acid but no gas
- Does not grow on simple media, requires blood or serum, sugars
- Virulent forms give matt/granular colonies, while avirulent give glossy colonies
- Blood agar—Circular, small colonies with area of hemolysis around them.

Pneumococcus

- Aerobes and facultative anaerobes
- Small, Lanceolate, Diplococci
- Capsulated, Gram-positive
- Blood agar—Under aerobic conditions, small, dome shaped, shiny colonies with greenish discoloration (alpha hemolysis), with central umbonation, giving carom coin or draughtsman appearance
- Under anaerobic conditions—they show beta hemolysis
- Catalase and oxidase negative, sensitive to optochin
- Ferment inulin, bile soluble.

Gonococcus

- Kidney shaped, Aerobic and facultatively anaerobic
- N. gonorrhea ferments glucose, but not maltose
- N. meningitides ferments both.

Neisseria Meningitides

- Gram-negative, aerobic, nonsporing, nonmotile
- Strict aerobes
- Oxidase positive
- Weak hemolysis on based agar
- Exacting growth requirements
- Solid media—round, bluish grey smooth, glistening, butyrous.

Corynebacterium diphtheriae/Klebs-Loeffler bacillus

- Slender rod, clubbing at end, pleomorphic, nonsporing, nonmotile, noncapsulated, gram-positive
- Bacilli are arranged in Chinese letter or cuneiform pattern
- Tellurite blood agar is the selective medium (Grey/black).

Bacillus Anthracis

- Aerobic and facultatively anaerobic
- Sporing
- Large capsulated bacilli (polypeptide capsule)
- Arranged in long chains, giving bamboo stick appearance
- Gelatin swab culture—Inverted fir tree appearance
- String of pearls reaction—When grown solid media containing penicillin, cells become large, spherical and in chains
- Grows on ordinary media
- Agar—Round, grayish colonies with frosted glass appearance which under low power resembles locks of matted hair, called medusa head appearance
- McFadyen's reaction—When blood films containing anthrax bacilli are stained with polychrome-Methylene blue, and examined under microscope, capsule is detected as amorphous purplish material around the bacilli.

E. Coli

- Gram-negative, straight rod, motile by peritrichous flagella
- Aerobe and facultatively anaerobe
- Hemolytic on blood agar
- MacConkey's medium-bright pink colonies, due to lactose fermentation.

Proteus Mirabilis

- Gram-negative, noncapsulated, pleomorphic, motile rod
- Cultures give a fishy or seminal odour
- Swarming growth
- Lactose fermenters
- Produces urease, rapidly hydrolyses urea to ammonia and carbon dioxide
- MacConkey's medium—Colorless colonies
- Weil-Felix reaction-Heterophilic agglutination due to the sharing of carbohydrates hapten by proteus and rickettsiae.

Shigella

- Gram-negative, rods, nonmotile, nonsporing, noncapsulated
- Aerobes and facultative anaerobes
- Grow on ordinary media
- Deoxycholate citrate agar/DCA—Selective medium
- MacConkey's—Colorless colonies, EXCEPT Shigella sonnei which is late lactose fermenter.

Salmonella

- Gram-negative, motile with peritrichous flagella
- Aerobic and facultatively anaerobic
- Ferment sugars producing acid and gas, EXCEPT salmonella typhi which is anaerogenic
- MacConkey's agar and Deoxycholate citrate—colonies are colorless due to absence of lactose fermentation

- Wilson and Blair medium—jet black colonies, due to H_2S production
- Selenite F broth and tetrathionate broth are enrichment media.

Vibrio Cholera

- Comma shaped, actively motile by polar flagella, characteristic vibratory/darting motility, like a swarm of gnats
- Venkatraman—Ramakrishnan medium and Cary Blair medium-Holding of transport medium
- Alkaline peptone water and Monsur's taurocholate tellurite peptone water are transport and enrichment medium
- TCBS is the preferred plating medium (yellowish green).

Pseudomonas Aeruginosa

- Aerobic, nonsporing, gram-negative, motile by polar flagella
- Grows on simple media—colonies give musty or earthy smell
- **Produces pigments:** Pyocyanin-bluish green; Fluorescein/pyoverdine-greenish yellow; Pyorubin-red, Pyomelanin –brown
- MacConkey's and DCA—Colorless colonies.

Yersinia Pestis

- Reservoir of plague
- Gives safety pin appearance (Bipolar staining) [Similar safety pin appearance in Burkholderia pseudomallei]
- Ghee broth culture—Stalactite growth.

Haemophilus Influenzae/Pfeiffer Bacillus

- Gram-negative, capsulated
- Fastidious growth requirements, require accessory growth factors, named X and V.

Haemophilus Ducreyi

- Shows bipolar staining
- Bacilli are arranged in whorls or parallel chains, giving school of fish or rail road track appearance.

Bordetella Pertussis/Bordet Gengou Bacillus

- Gram-negative, strict aerobes, produce toxins
- Capsulated
- **Bordet-Gengou glycerin-potato-blood agar:** Selective medium
- Dome shaped, smooth, opaque, grayish-white colonies, bisected pearls or mercury drops appearance
- In culture films, thumb print appearance
- Colonies are surrounded by a hazy zone of hemolysis; confluent growth gives aluminum paint appearance.

Brucella

- Gram-negative, strict aerobic
- Catalase, oxidase and urease positive
- Antigenic cross reactions between Brucella and Vibrio cholera
- Brucellosis is also known as Mediterranean fever, Malta fever, undulant fever
- Transmitted through unpasteurised milk.

Mycobacterium Tuberculosis

- Acid fast (due to presence of mycolic acid)
- Generation time is 14-15 hours
- Lowenstein Jensen medium is the most widely used solid medium.

Mantoux Test

- 0.5 ml of PPD is injected intradermally, on the flexor aspect of forearm
- Result is read after 72 hours
- Positive tuberculin test indicates hypersensitivity to tuberculin protein due to infection with tubercle bacillus or BCG immunization
- Induration > 10 mm is positive
- 5 mm or less is negative.

Mycobacterium Leprae

- Gram-positive and acid fast
- Bacteriological index—Number of bacilli in tissues
- Morphological index—Live bacilli appear solid and uniformly stained, whereas dead bacilli appear fragmented (The percentage of uniformly stained bacilli is called morphological index)
- They agglomerate, as globi (giving a cigar bundle appearance)
- They are not cultivable (Can be grown in footpads of mice kept at 200 and in nine banded armadillo.

Treponema Pallidum

- Thin, spiral
- It can be stained with silver impregnation method
- It can be seen in low microscope by negative staining with India ink
- Morphology and motility can be seen under dark ground or phase contrast microscope.

Leptospira

- Generation time is 12-16 hours
- Actively motile
- Coiled appearance seen under dark ground microscopy
- Their ends are hooked, resembling umbrella handles.

Mycoplasma

- Gram-negative
- Aerobic and facultatively anaerobic
- Require cholesterol for growth
- Devoid of cell wall, pleomorphic
- Show true branching
- Biphasic colonies, with a fried egg appearance
- Hemolytic.

Rickettsiae

- They are obligate intracellular parasites transmitted by arthropod vectors.

Chlamydiae

- Called energy parasites
- They are obligate intracellular parasites
- **Occur in two forms:**
  Reticulate body/initial body: Intracellular, growing and replicative form
  Elementary body: Extracellular, infective form.

Inclusion Bodies

- **Molluscum bodies:** Molluscum contagiosum
- **Torres bodies/Councilman bodies:** Yellow fever
- **Warthin-Finkeldey cells:** Measles
- **Negri bodies:** Rabies
- **Guarnieri bodies:** Vaccinia
- **Bollinger bodies:** Fowl pox
- **Cowdry A inclusion bodies (Lipschutz):** Herpes, yellow fever
- **Cowdry B inclusion bodies:** Adenovirus, polio virus.

Infectious Mononucleosis

- Kissing disease is another name for infectious mononucleosis, as kissing is the predominant mode of transport
- Paul-Bunnell test is used for diagnosing infectious mononucleosis.

Yeast Like Fungi

- Partly yeast, partly hyphae
- Candida.

Yeast

- Unicellular fungi
- Cryptococcus.

Moulds/filamentous Fungi

- True mycelia
- Dermatophytes.

Dimorphic

- **Yeast at 37 degrees and Mould at 22 degrees:** Paracoccidioides, histoplasma
- **Filaments and yeasts at different temperature:** Coccidioides, blastomyces.

MCQs WITH SHORT EXPLANATIONS

GENERAL MICROBIOLOGY

1. What is the percentage of sulfuric acid used in AFB staining for mycobacterium leprae?

a. 5%
b. 10%
c. 15%
d. 20%

Modifications in AFB

- 5% sulfuric acid is used for destaining Mycobacterium leprae instead of the 20% used for Mycobacterium tuberculosis.
- 1% sulfuric acid for actinomycetes, nocardia.
- 0.5–1% sulfuric acid for oocysts of isospora, cyclospora.
- 0.25–0.5% sulfuric acid for bacterial endospores.

2. In which phase of bacterial growth curve, bacterium produces exotoxin?

a. Lag phase
b. Log phase
c. Stationary phase
d. Phase of decline

The stationary phase

- It is often due to a growth-limiting factor such as the depletion of an essential nutrient, and/or the formation of an inhibitory product such as an organic acid.
- Stationary phase results from a situation in which growth rate and death rate are equal.
- The number of new cells created is limited by the growth factor and as a result the rate of cell growth matches the rate of cell death.
- The result is a "smooth," horizontal linear part of the curve during the stationary phase.

3. Father of Microbiology:

a. Elie Metchnikoff
b. Robert Koch
c. Joseph Lister
d. Louis Pasteur

Louis Pasteur is regarded as one of the three main founders of bacteriology, together with Ferdinand Cohn and Robert Koch, and is popularly known as the "father of microbiology".

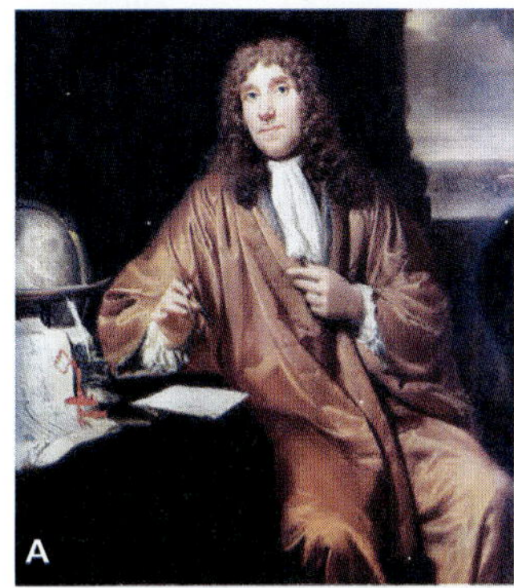

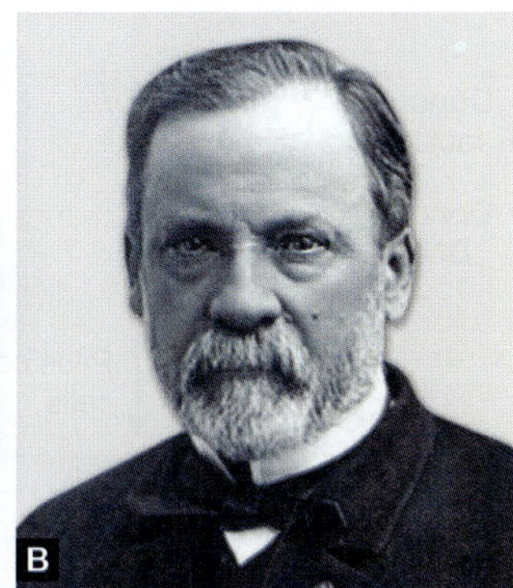

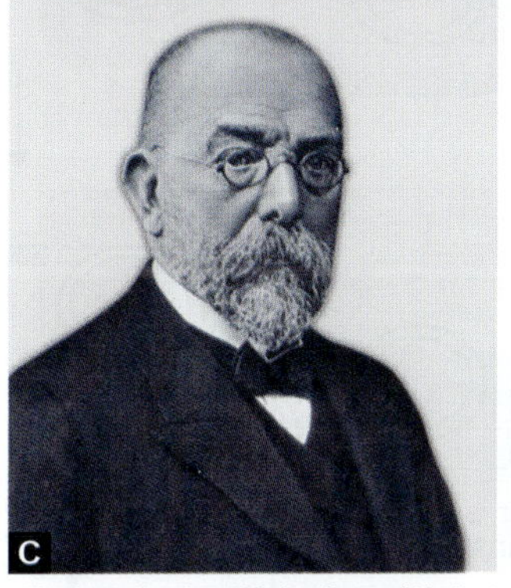

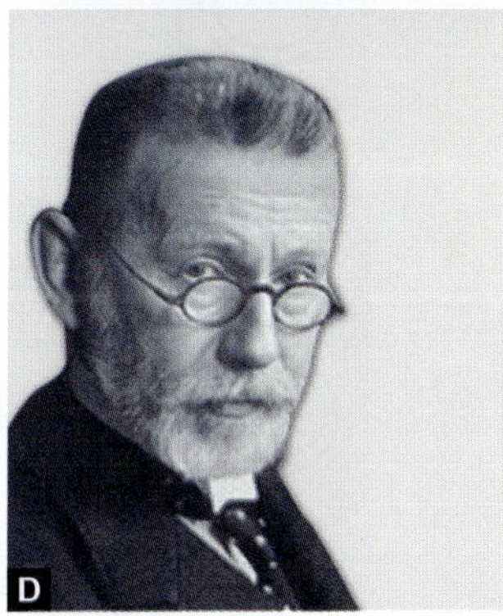

Eminent microbiologists. (A) Antonie van Leeuwenhoek; (B) Louis Pasteur; (C) Robert Koch; (D) Paul Ehrlich.

4. Best medium to grow anaerobic bacteria exclusively is:

a. Blood agar
b. Robertson's cooked meat medium
c. Thioglycollate medium
d. Sabouraud Dextrose agar

RCMM is used to grow anaerobic bacteria, for example, Clostridium species.

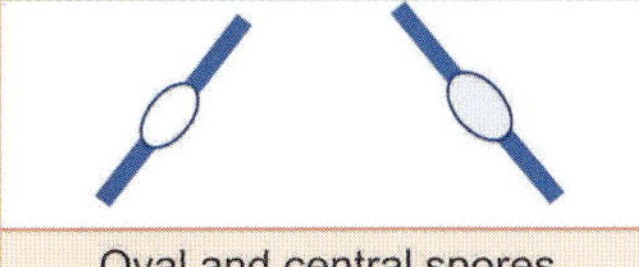
Oval and central spores (e.g. *Clostridium bifermentans*)

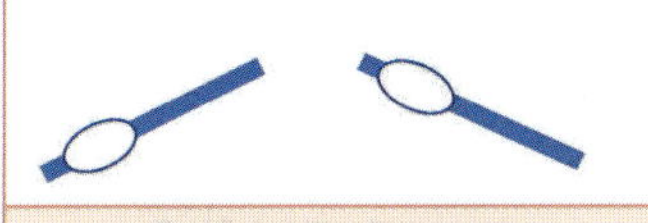
Subterminal spores (e.g. *Clostridium perfringens*)

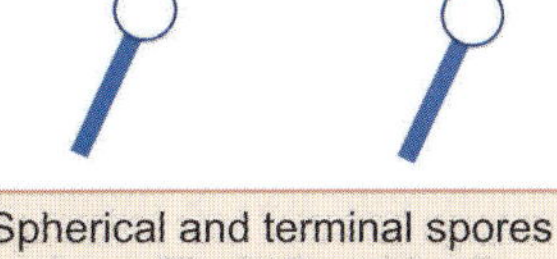
Spherical and terminal spores (e.g. *Clostridium tetani*)

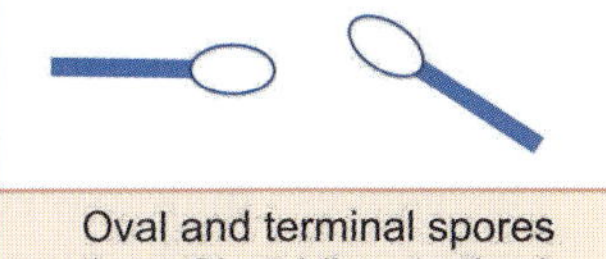
Oval and terminal spores (e.g. *Clostridium tertium*)

Types of spores of various clostridia species.

Ans. 1. **a.** 5% 2. **c.** Stationary phase 3. **d.** Louis Pasteur 4. **b.** Robertson's cooked...

5. Multiple drug resistance is transmitted by:
- a. Conjugation
- b. Mutation
- c. Transduction
- d. Transformation

Bacterial conjugation is the transfer of genetic material between bacterial cells by direct cell-to-cell contact or by a bridge-like connection between two cells. Discovered in 1946 by Joshua Lederberg and Edward Tatum, conjugation is a mechanism of horizontal gene transfer as are transformation and transduction although these two other mechanisms do not involve cell-to-cell contact.

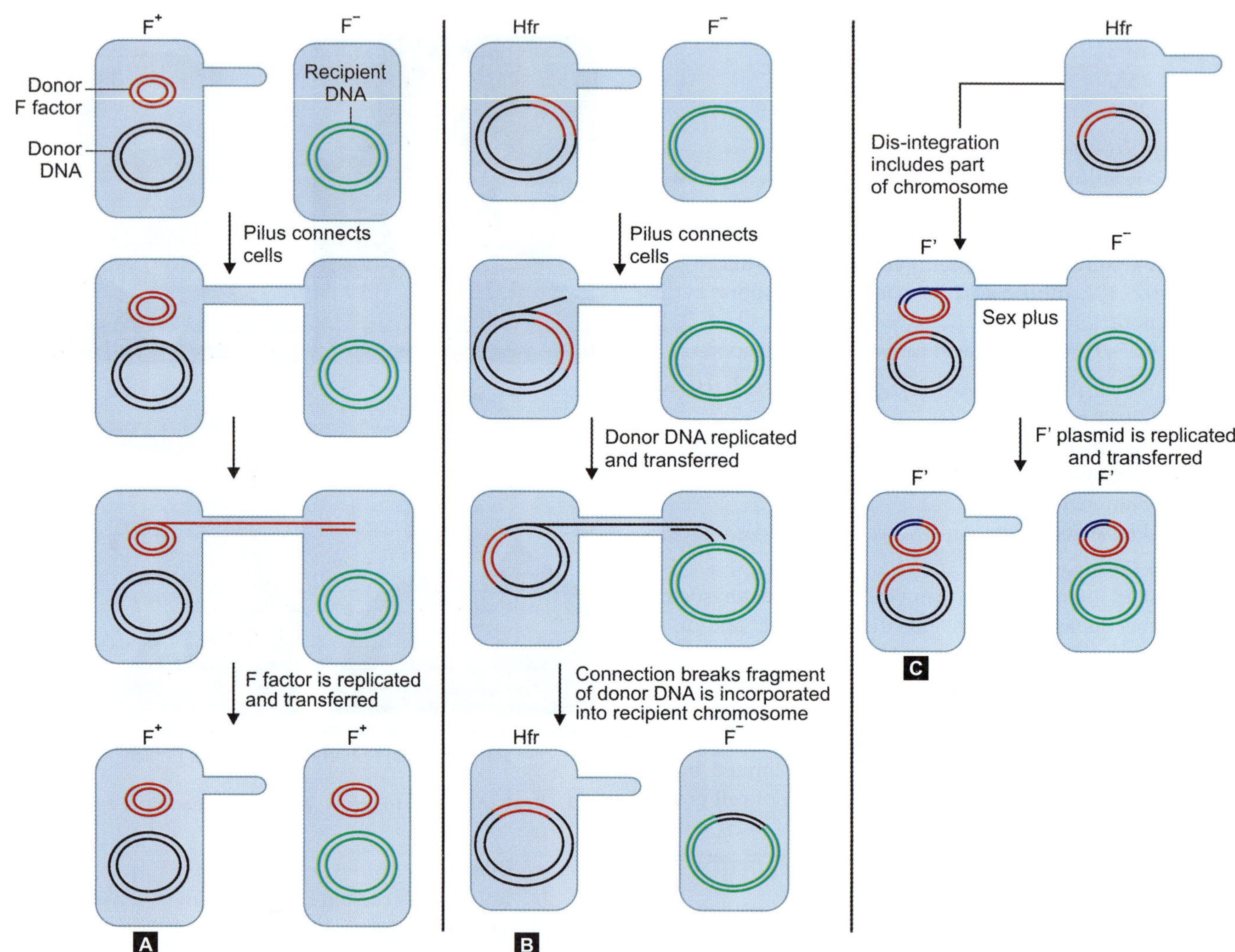

Bacterial conjugation. (A) F+ × F− mating; (B) Hfr × F− mating; (C) F′ × F− mating.

6. Efficacy of pasteurization is determined by:
- a. Nitric acid
- b. Phosphatase
- c. Turbidity test
- d. Paper chromatography

As a result of the unsuitability of microbiological techniques, milk pasteurization efficacy is typically monitored by checking for the presence of alkaline phosphatase, which is denatured by pasteurization. B. tuberculosis, the bacterium that requires the highest temperature to be killed of all milk pathogens is killed at ranges of temperature and time similar to those that denature alkaline phosphatase. For this reason, presence of alkaline phosphatase is an ideal indicator of pasteurization efficacy.

7. The mechanism of genetic transfer where a phage serves as a vehicle is:
- a. Transformation
- b. Translation
- c. Conjugation
- d. None of the above

Ans. 5. **a.** Conjugation 6. **b.** Phosphatase 7. **d.** None of the above

Transduction is the process by which DNA is transferred from one bacterium to another by a virus. It also refers to the process whereby foreign DNA is introduced into another cell via a viral vector. Transduction does not require physical contact between the cell donating the DNA and the cell receiving the DNA (which occurs in conjugation), and it is DNase resistant (transformation is susceptible to DNase).

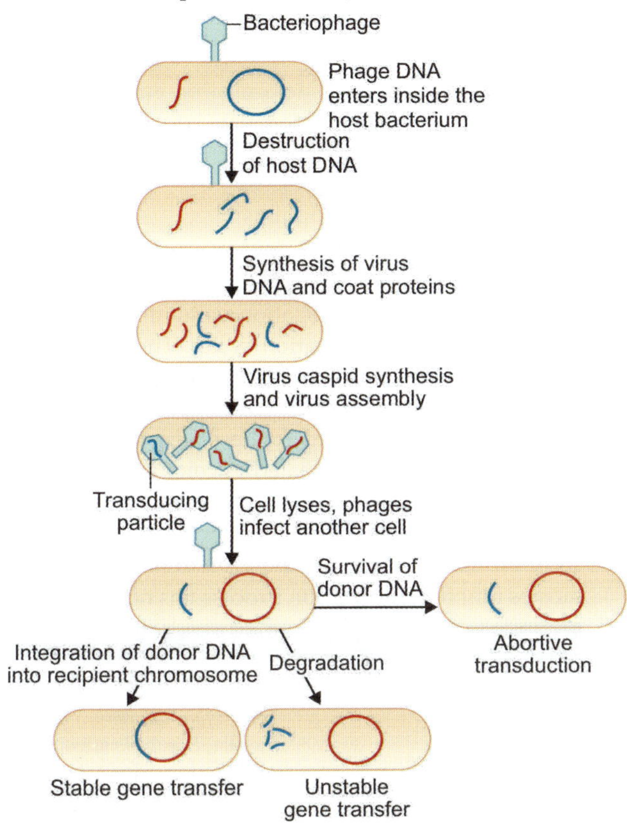

Generalized transduction.

8. **Jumping gene:**
   a. Transposons
   b. Episome
   c. Cosmid
   d. Plasmid

A **transposable element** (**TE** or **transposon**) is a DNA sequence that can change its position within the genome, sometimes creating or reversing mutations and altering the cell's genome size. Transposition often results in duplication of the TE. Barbara Mc Clintock's discovery of these **jumping genes** earned her a Nobel prize in 1983.

9. **Which of the following is an enrichment media?**
   a. Alkaline peptone water
   b. Monsour's taurocholate Tellurite peptone water
   c. Selenite F broth
   d. All of the above

An **enrichment culture** is a medium with specific and known qualities that favors the growth of a particular microorganism. The enrichment culture's environment will support the growth of a selected microorganism, while inhibiting the growth of others. Lourens Baas Becking succinctly summarized enrichment cultures' abilities when he said "everything is everywhere; the environment selects."

10. **Blood agar is an example of:**
    a. Enrichment media
    b. Enriched media
    c. Selective media
    d. Transport media

Enriched media contain the nutrients required to support the growth of a wide variety of organisms, including some of the more fastidious ones. They are commonly used to harvest as many different types of microbes as are present in the specimen.

11. **Horizontal transmission of 'R' factor is by:**
    a. Transduction
    b. Transformation
    c. Conjugation
    d. Fusion

Bacterial conjugation is often regarded as the bacterial equivalent of sexual reproduction or mating since it involves the exchange of genetic material. During conjugation the *donor* cell provides a conjugative or mobilizable genetic element that is most often a plasmid or transposon. Most conjugative plasmids have systems ensuring that the *recipient* cell does not already contain a similar element.

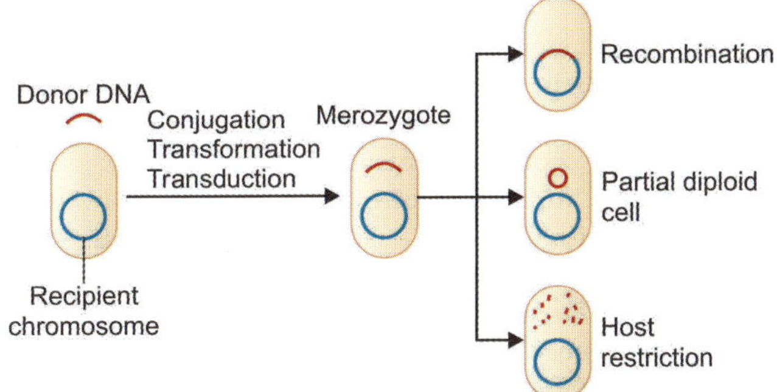

Fate of the donor DNA following horizontal transfer.

12. **Louis Pasteur is NOT associated with:**
    a. Introduction of complex media
    b. Discovery of Rabies vaccine
    c. Discovery of M. tuberculosis
    d. Disproved spontaneous generation theory

Robert Heinrich Herman Koch (German: 11 December 1843 – 27 May 1910) was a celebrated German physician and pioneering microbiologist. As the founder of modern bacteriology, he is known for his role in identifying

Ans. 8. **a.** Transposons 9. **d.** All of the above 10. **b.** Enriched media 11. **c.** Conjugation 12. **c.** Discovery of M. tuberculosis

the specific causative agents of tuberculosis, cholera, and anthrax and for giving experimental support for the concept of infectious disease.

13. Vibrio cholera was discovered by:

a. Koch
b. Metchnikoff
c. John snow
d. Virchow

In India, Koch was indeed able to determine the causative agent of cholera, isolating *Vibrio cholerae*. The bacterium had originally been isolated in 1854 by Italian anatomist Filippo Pacini, but its exact nature and his results were not widely known.

14. Tellurite stimulates growth of:

a. E. coli
b. Cl. Tetani
c. C. diphtheriae
d. Salmonella

An enrichment medium, such as Löffler's medium, is used to preferentially grow *C. diphtheriae*. After that, a differential plate known as tellurite agar, allows all *Corynebacteria* (including *C. diphtheriae*) to reduce tellurite to metallic tellurium. The tellurite reduction is colorimetrically indicated by brown colonies for most *Corynebacteria* species or by a black halo around the *C. diphtheriae* colonies.

15. Pike's medium is employed for transport of:

a. Vibrio
b. Shigella
c. Streptococci
d. Staphylococci

Transport media

- Cary Blair medium and Venkatraman Ramakrishnan (VR) medium are used to transport feces from suspected cholera patients.
- Sach's buffered glycerol saline is used to transport feces from patients suspected to be suffering from bacillary dysentery.
- Pike's medium is used to transport streptococci from throat specimens.

Transport media used for common bacteria.

Transport media	*Organism*
Streptococcus	Pike's medium
Neisseria	❑ Amies medium and Stuart's medium
Vibrio cholerae	❑ VR (Venkatraman-Ramakrishnan) medium ❑ Autoclaved sea water ❑ Cary Blair medium
Shigella, Salmonella	❑ Buffered glycerol saline ❑ Cary Blair medium

STERILIZATION

16. Proctoscope is sterilized by:

a. Soap solution
b. Formalin
c. Glutaraldehyde
d. Autoclave

A glutaraldehyde solution of 0.1% to 1.0% concentration may be used for system disinfection and as a preservative for long term storage. It is a sterilant, killing endospores in addition to many microorganisms and viruses.

17. Biological indicator for determining efficacy of autoclaving is:

a. Pseudomonas aeruginosa
b. Clostridium Perfringens
c. Bacillus stearothermophilus
d. Salmonella typhi

Bacillus stearothermophilus is commonly used as a challenge organism for sterilization validation studies and periodic check of sterilization cycles. The biological indicator contains spores of the organism on filter paper inside a vial. After sterilizing, the cap is closed, an ampoule of growth medium inside of the vial is crushed and the whole vial is incubated. A color and/or turbidity change indicates the results of the sterilization process; no change indicates that the sterilization conditions were achieved, otherwise the growth of the spores indicates that the sterilization process has not been met.

Biological indicators of sterilization.

Methods	*Indicator*
Hot air oven	*Clostridium tetani* non toxigenic strain, *B.subtilis* subsp. *niger*
Autoclave	*Bacillus stearothermophilus*
Filtration	*Brevundimonas diminuta* or *Serratia*
Ionizing radiation	*Bacillus pumilus*
Ethylene oxide	*Bacillus globigi*
Plasma sterilization	*Bacillus stearothermophilus* or *Bacillus subtilis* subsp. *niger*

18. Autoclaving is done at what temperature for 15 minutes:

a. 118 degree C
b. 121 degree C
c. 126 degree C
d. 134 degree C

An **autoclave** is a pressure chamber used to sterilize equipment and supplies by subjecting them to high pressure saturated steam at 121°C (249°F) for around 15–20 minutes depending on the size of the load and the contents. It was invented by Charles Chamberland in 1879.

Ans. **13. a.** Koch **14. c.** C. diphtheriae **15. c.** Streptococci **16. c.** Glutaraldehyde **17. c.** Bacillus... **18. b.** 121 degree C

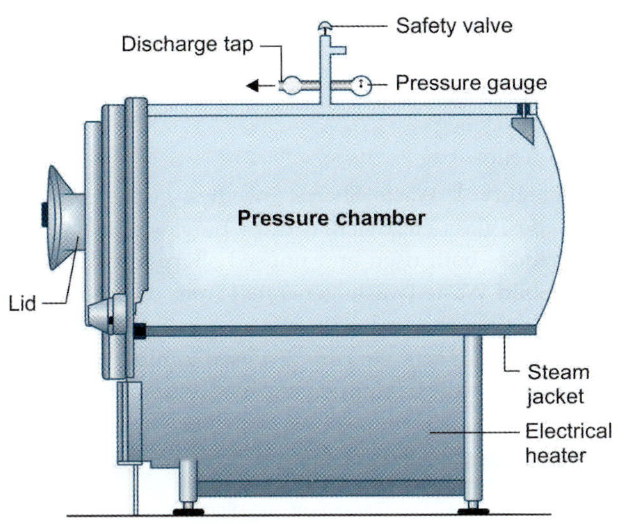

Schematic diagram of horizontal autoclave.

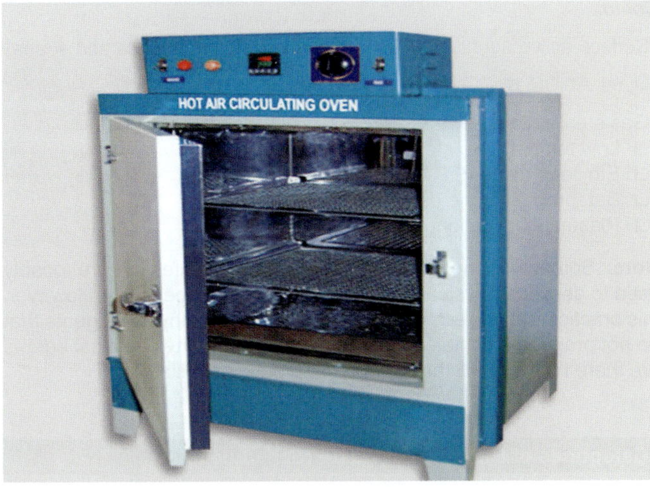

Hot air oven.

19. Incineration is done for:
a. Liquid waste
b. Anatomy waste
c. Sharp waste
d. All of the above

Incineration has particularly strong benefits for the treatment of certain waste types in niche areas such as clinical wastes and certain hazardous wastes where pathogens and toxins can be destroyed by high temperatures. Examples include chemical multi-product plants with diverse toxic or very toxic wastewater streams, which cannot be routed to a conventional wastewater treatment plant.

20. Operation theatres are sterilized by:
a. Ethylene oxide gas
b. Formaldehyde fumigation
c. Washing with soap water
d. Carbolic acid spraying

An aqueous solution of formaldehyde can be useful as a disinfectant as it kills most bacteria and fungi (including their spores). Formaldehyde solutions are applied topically in medicine to dry the skin, such as in the treatment of warts. It is also used for fumigation of closed areas, like operation theatres.

21. Best way to sterilize all-glass syringes:
a. Boiling
b. Autoclave
c. Hot air oven
d. Formaldehyde

Hot air oven are widely used to sterilize articles that can withstand high temperatures and not get burnt, like glassware and powders. Linen gets burnt and surgical sharps lose their sharpness.

22. Cold sterilization is done by:
a. Steam
b. Ionizing radiation
c. Infra red
d. UV

Cold sterilization is a process in which sterilization is carry out at low temperature with the help of chemicals, radiations, membranes and all other means excluding high temperature. Ionizing radiation such as X-rays, gamma rays and cosmic rays, cause no appreciable increase in temperature in this method, it is referred as cold sterilization.

Classification of sterilization/disinfection methods	
Physical methods	
Drying	
Heat	
❑ Dry heat: ❑ Flaming ❑ Incineration ❑ Hot air oven	❑ Moist heat: ❑ Temperature below 100°C, e.g. pasteurization, water bath and inspissation ❑ Temperature at 100°C, e.g. boiling, steaming and tyndallization ❑ Temperature above 100°C, e.g. autoclave
Filtration: Depth filters and membrane filters	
Radiation ❑ Ionizing radiation: γ rays, X-rays and cosmic rays ❑ Nonionizing radiation: Ultraviolet (UV) and infrared rays	
Ultrasonic vibration	
Chemical methods	
Alcohols: Ethyl alcohol, isopropyl alcohol	
Aldehydes: Formaldehyde, glutaraldehyde, Ortho-phthalaldehyde	
Phenolic compounds: Cresol, lysol, chlorhexidine, chloroxylenol, hexachlorophene	
Halogens: Chlorine, iodine, iodophors	
Oxidizing agents: Hydrogen peroxide, peracetic acid	
Salts: Mercuric chloride, copper salts	

Contd...

Ans. 19. **b.** Anatomy waste 20. **b.** Formaldehyde... 21. **c.** Hot air oven 22. **b.** Ionizing radiation

Contd...

Surface active agents: Quaternary ammonium compounds and soaps
Dyes: Aniline dyes and acridine dyes
Gas sterilization: ❑ Low temperature steam formaldehyde ❑ Ethylene oxide (ETO) ❑ Betapropiolactone (BPL) ❑ Plasma sterilization

Note: Sometimes the words sterilization and disinfection are loosely used to describe physical and chemical agents respectively. However, this practice is incorrect, because there are some physical agents that do not produce complete sterilization; similarly many chemical agents are there that may kill the spores and produce sterilization.

23. Sharp instrument should be disposed in:

a. Blue bag
b. Red bag
c. Black beg
d. Yellow bag

Category 4: Waste Sharps (needles, syringes, scalpels blades, glass, etc. that may cause puncture and cuts. This includes both used and unused sharps) and Category 7: Solid Waste (waste generated from disposable items other than the waste sharps such as tubing, catheters, intravenous sets, etc.) are disposed in Blue/White translucent (Plastic bag/puncture proof container).

Categories of Bio-Medical Waste (Schedule I).

Categories	*Waste category*	*Treatment and disposal*
category No 1	**Human anatomical waste** (human tissues, organs and body parts)	Incineration*/deep burial**
Category No 2	**Animal waste** (animal tissues, organs, body parts carcasses, bleeding parts, fluid, blood and experimental animals used in research, waste generated by veterinary hospitals/ colleges, discharge from hospitals, animal houses)	Incineration*/deep burial**
Category No 3	**Microbiology and biotechnology waste** (wastes from laboratory cultures, stocks or specimens of micro-organisms, live or attenuated vaccines, human and animal cell culture used in research and infectious agents from research and industrial laboratories, wastes from production of biological, toxins, petri dishes and devices used for transfer of cultures)	Local autoclaving/microwaving/incineration*
Category No 4	**Waste sharps** (needles, syringes, scalpels, blades, glass, etc that may cause puncture and cuts. This includes both used and unused sharps)	Disinfection (chemical treatment*/autoclaving/microwaving) and mutilation/shredding
Category No 5	**Discarded medicines and cytotoxic drugs** (wastes comprising of outdated contaminated and discarded medicines)	Incineration/destruction/disposal in secured landfills
Category No 6	**Solid waste** (items contaminated with blood and body fluids including cotton, dressings, soiled plaster casts, line beddings, other material contaminated with blood)	Incineration*/autoclaving/microwaving
Category No 7	**Solid waste** (disposable items other than the waste sharps such as tubing, catheters, intravenous sets, etc.)	Disinfection by chemical treatment#/autoclaving/ microwaving and mutilation/ shredding##
Category No 8	**Liquid waste** (waste generated from laboratory and washing, cleaning, house-keeping and disinfecting activities)	Disinfection by chemical treatment# and discharge into drains
Category No 9	**Incineration ash** (ash from incineration of any biomedical waste)	Disposal in municipal landfill
Category No 10	**Chemical waste** (chemicals used in production of biological, chemicals, used in disinfection, as insecticides, etc)	Chemical treatment# and discharge into drains for liquids and secured landfill for solids

*There will be no chemical pretreatment before incineration. Chlorinated plastics shall not be incinerated.

**Deep burial shall be an option available only in towns with population less than five lakhs and in rural areas.

#Chemicals treatment using at least 1% hypochlorite solution or any other equivalent chemical reagent. It must be ensured that chemical treatment ensures disinfection.

##Mutilation/shredding must be such so as to prevent unauthorized reuse.

Ans. **23. a.** Blue bag

24. Effective mode of sterilization is:

a. Hot water
b. Steam under pressure
c. Steam at atmospheric pressure
d. Dry heat

Of all the methods available for sterilization, moist heat in the form of saturated **steam under pressure** is the most widely used and the most dependable. **Steam** sterilization is nontoxic, inexpensive rapidly microbicidal, sporicidal, and rapidly heats and penetrates fabrics.

25. Phenol coefficient indicates:

a. Efficiency of a disinfectant
b. Dilution of a disinfectant
c. Quantity of a disinfectant
d. Purity of a disinfectant

The **Phenol coefficient**, is now largely of historical interest, although the principles upon which it is based are still used. It is a measure of the bactericidal activity of a chemical compound in relation to phenol. When listed numerically, the figure expressing the disinfecting power of a substance by relating it to the disinfecting power of phenol may be a function of the standardized test performed. For example, the Rideal-Walker method, introduced in 1903 gives a Rideal-Walker coefficient and the US Department of Agriculture method gives a US Department of Agriculture coefficient.

Common disinfectants and their spectrum of action.

Germicide and their concentrations	*Level of disinfectant*	*Bacteria and enveloped viruses*	*Fungi*	*Un-enveloped viruses*	*M. tuberculosis*	*Spore*	*Inactivated by organic matter*
Glutaraldehyde (2%)	High/CS	+	+	+	+	+	–
Formaldehyde (3–8%)	High/CS	+	+	+	+	+	–
H_2O_2 (3–25%)	High/CS	+	+	+	+	+	±
Chlorine (100–1000 ppm of free chlorine)	High	+	+	+	+	+/–	+
Isopropyl alcohol (60–95%)	Intermediate	+	+	±	+	–	±
Phenol (0.4–5%)	Intermediate	+	+	±	+	–	–
Iodophore (30–50 ppm of free iodine)	Intermediate	+	+	+	±	–	+
Quaternary ammonium compounds (0.4–1.6%)	Low	+	±	–	–	–	+

CS, chemical sterilant; +, effectively kills; –, unable to kill; ±, variably kills; ppm, parts per million

26. Autoclaving is a method of sterilization. The process involves heating by steam at:

a. 10 lb pressure, 100°C temperature for 10 minutes
b. 15 lb pressure, 120°C temperature for 15 minutes
c. 20 lb pressure, 120°C temperature for 20 minutes
d. 25 lb pressure, 120°C temperature for 25 minutes

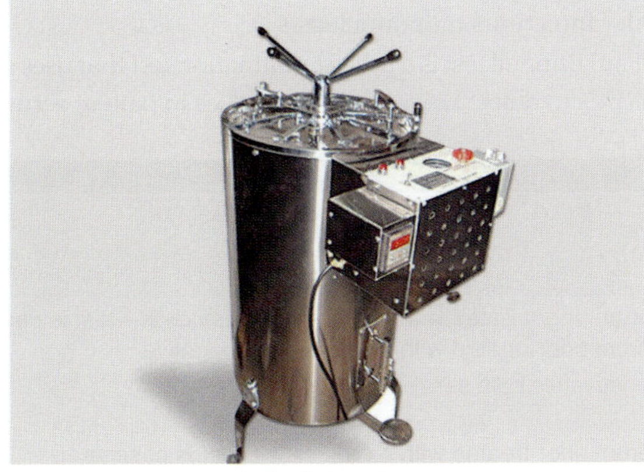

Vertical autoclave.

Some computer-controlled autoclaves use an F_0 (F-nought) value to control the sterilization cycle. F_0 values are set for the number of minutes of sterilization equivalent to 121°C (250°F) at 100 kPa (15 psi) above atmospheric pressure for 15 minutes. Since exact temperature control is difficult, the temperature is monitored, and the sterilization time adjusted accordingly.

27. Endoscopes are sterilized by:

a. Formaldehyde
b. Absolute alcohol
c. Glutaraldehyde
d. Sodium hypochlorite

Glutaraldehyde is one of the most commonly used disinfectants in endoscopy units. It is effective and relatively inexpensive, and does not damage endoscopes, accessories, or automated processing units.

Methods of sterilization/disinfection used in different clinical situations.

Material	*Method of sterilization/ disinfection*
Clinical thermometer	Isopropyl alcohol

Ans. 24. **b.** Steam under... 25. **a.** Efficiency of a... 26. **b.** 15 lb pressure, 120°C... 27. **c.** Glutaraldehyde

Material	Method of sterilization/ disinfection
Paraffin, glass syringe, flask, slide, oil, grease, fat, glycerol	Hot air oven
Operation theater, entryway, ward, lab fumigation , Preservation of anatomical specimen, woolen blanket	Formaldehyde gas > UV > BPL
Cystoscope, bronchoscope	Orthophthaldehyde > glutaraldehyde 2% (cidex)
Heart lung machine, respirator, dental equipments	Ethylene oxide
Vaccine, sera, antibiotic and sugar solution and body fluids	Filtration
Sharp instruments	Cresol
Milk	Pasteurization
Plastic syringe, catgut suture, swab, catheter, bone and tissue grafts, adhesive dressing	Ionizing radiation
Culture media, metal instruments, glassware and all suture materials except catgut	Autoclave
Metallic inoculation wire	Red hot by Bunsen burner
Infective material like soiled dressing, bedding, animal carcasses	Burning (incineration)
Metallic surgical instruments	Autoclave and infra-red radiation
Water	Chlorine as hypochlorite 0.2%
Skin	Tincture iodine, spirit (70% ethanol) and savlon
Contact lenses	H_2O_2 (hydrogen peroxide)

IMMUNITY

28. Site of maturation of T cells:

a. Peyer's patches b. Lymph node
c. Thymus d. Bursa of Fabricius

T cells

- All T cells originate from hematopoietic stem cells in the bone marrow.
- Hematopoietic progenitors (lymphoid progenitor cells) from hematopoietic stem cells populate the thymus and expand by cell division to generate a large population of immature thymocytes.

29. VDRL is:

a. Slide flocculation test b. Tube flocculation test
c. Gel precipitation test
d. Indirect haemagglutination test

The VDRL is a nontreponemal serological screening for syphilis that is also used to assess response to therapy, to detect central nervous system involvement, and as an aid in the diagnosis of congenital syphilis. The basis of the test is that an antibody produced by a patient with syphilis reacts with an extract of ox heart (diphosphatidyl glycerol). It therefore detects anticardiolipin antibodies (IgG, IgM or IgA), visualized through foaming of the test tube fluid, or "flocculation".

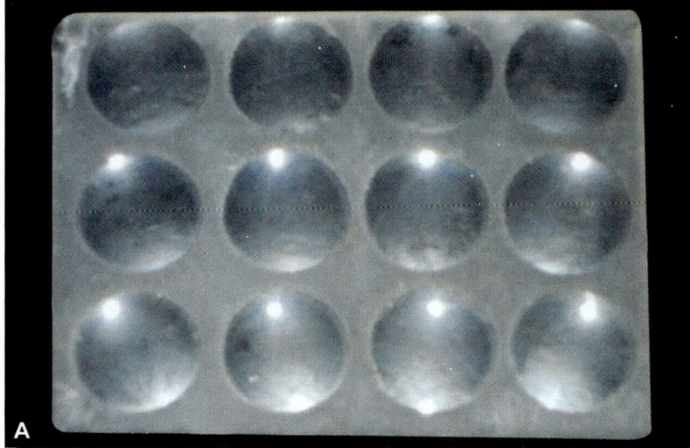

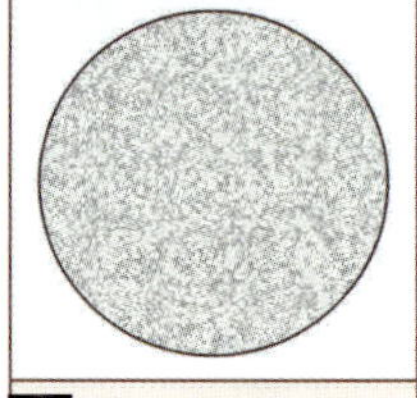

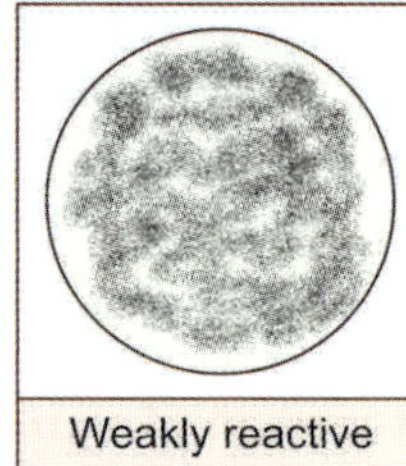

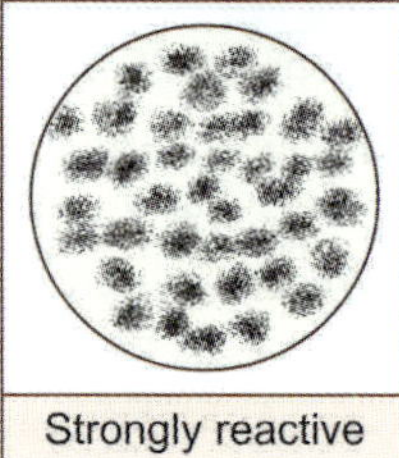

(A) VDRL slide and (B) VDRL test results.

30. Paul Bunnell test is used for:

a. Mycoplasmal pneumonia
b. Enteric fever
c. Typhus fever
d. Infectious mononucleosis

Paul Bunnell test is a tube agglutination test that uses sheep RBCs to detect heterophile antibodies in patient serum.

Paul-Bunnell test and its confirmation by differential absorption test.

Features	Paul-Bunnell test (performed first)	Treated with		Paul-Bunnell test (repeated)
		Guinea pig kidney cells	Ox red cells	
Infectious mononucleosis	Positive	Not absorbed	Absorbed	Serum prior treated with guinea pig kidney cells—test is positive Serum prior treated with ox red cells—Negative
Antibody after serum therapy	Positive	Absorbed	Absorbed	Negative for both sera
Normal serum	Positive	Absorbed	Not absorbed	Serum prior treated with ox red cells—test is positive Serum prior treated with guinea pig kidney cells—test is negative

Ans. 28. **c.** Thymus 29. **a.** Slide flocculation test 30. **d.** Infectious mononucleosis

31. All of the following are functions of CD4 helper T-cells EXCEPT:

a. Immunogenic memory
b. Produce immunoglobulins
c. Activate macrophage
d. Activate cytotoxic cells

An **antibody** (Ab), also known as an **immunoglobulin** (Ig), is a large, Y-shape protein produced by plasma cells (B cells) that is used by the immune system to identify and neutralize pathogens such as bacteria and viruses. The antibody recognizes a unique molecule of the harmful agent, called an antigen, via the variable region.

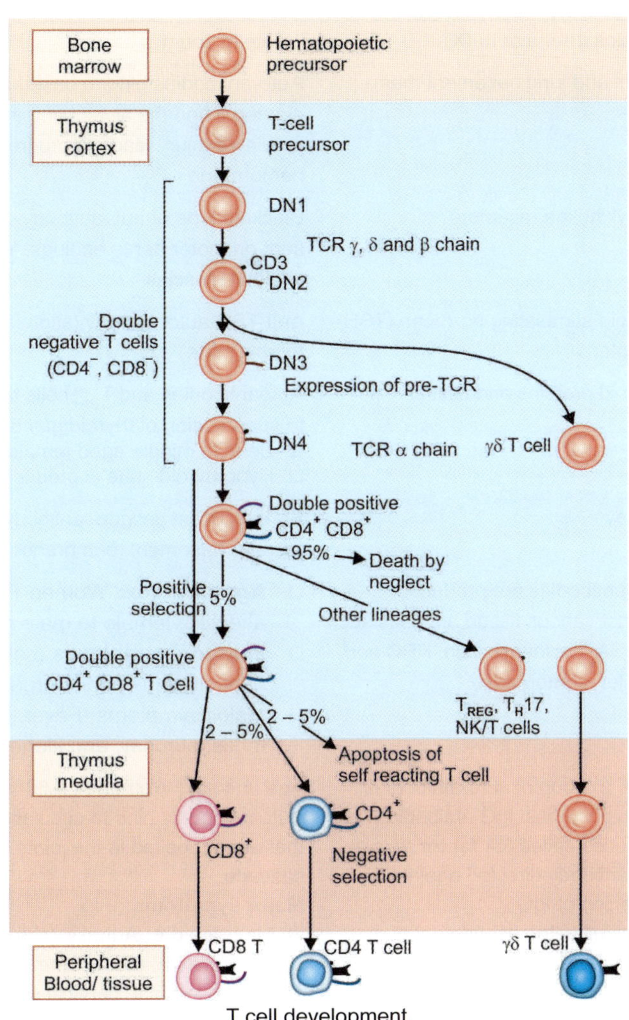

T cell development.

32. Rheumatoid factor is:

a. 19S globulin
b. 8S globulin
c. 17S globulin
d. Albumin

Franklin and co-workers found both **19S rheumatoid factor** and 7S **gamma globulin** as a 22S complex when the sera of rheumatoid arthritis patients were studied by ultracentrifugation.

Autoimmune diseases and immune response produced with their clinical manifestations.		
Single organ or cell type autoimmune diseases		
Disease	*Self-antigen present on*	*Type of immune response and Important features*
Autoimmune anemias		
Autoimmune hemolytic anemia	RBC membrane proteins	Autoantibodies to RBC antigens trigger complement mediated lysis or antibody-mediated opsonization of the RBCs
Drug-induced hemolytic anemia	Drugs alter the red cell membrane antigens	Drugs such as penicillin or methyldopa interact with RBCs so that the cells become antigenic

Contd...

Ans. **31. b.** Produce immu... **32. a.** 19S globulin

Contd...

Single organ or cell type autoimmune diseases		
Disease	*Self-antigen present on*	*Type of immune response and important features*
Pernicious anemia	Intrinsic factor (a membrane-bound protein on gastric parietal cells)	Autoantibodies to intrinsic factor block the uptake of vitamin B 12; leads to megaloblastic anemia
Idiopathic thrombocytopenic purpura	Platelet membrane proteins (glyco-proteins IIb-IIIa or Ib-IX)	Auto-antibodies against platelet membrane antigens leads to ↓platelet count
Goodpasture syndrome	Renal and lung basement membranes	Auto-antibodies bind to basement-membrane antigens on kidney glomeruli and the alveoli of the lungs followed by complement mediated injury leads to progressive kidney damage and pulmonary hemorrhage
Myasthenia gravis	Acetylcholine receptors	Blocking type of autoantibody directed against ACh receptors present on motor nerve endings, leads to progressive weakening of the skeletal muscles
Graves' disease	Thyroid-stimulating hormone (TSH) receptor	Anti-TSH-autoantibody (stimulates thyroid follicles, leads to hyper-thyroid state)
Hashimoto's thyroiditis	Thyroid proteins and cells	Autoantibodies and T_{DTH} cells targeted against thyroid antigen leads to suppression of thyroid gland. ❑ Seen in middle aged females ❑ Hypothyroid state is produced (↓ production of thyroid hormones)
Post-streptococcal glomerulonephritis	Kidney	Streptococcal antigen–antibody complexes are deposited in glomerular basement membrane
Systemic lupus erythematosus (SLE)	Autoantibodies are produced against various tissue antigens such as DNA, nuclear protein, RBC and platelet membranes.	❑ **Age and sex:** Women (20-40 years of age) are commonly affected; female to male ratio is 10:1. ❑ **Immune complexes** (self Ag-autoAb) are formed; which are deposited in various organs ❑ Major symptoms: Fever, **butterfly rash** over the cheeks, arthritis, pleurisy, and kidney dysfunction
Rheumatoid arthritis	Here, a group of auto-antibodies against the host IgG antibodies are produced called **RA factor**. It is an IgM antibody directed against the Fc region of IgG. Anticitrullinated peptide antibodies (**ACPA**) are also produced	Age and sex: Women (40–60 years of age) affected Autoantibodies bind to circulating IgG, forming IgM-IgG complexes that are deposited in the joints and can activate the complement cascade. **Major symptoms:** ❑ Main feature: Arthritis (chronic inflammation of the joints, begins at synovium; most common joints involved are-small joints of the hands, feet and cervical spine) ❑ Other features: Hematologic, cardiovascular, and respiratory systems are also frequently affected
Sjögren syndrome	Ribonucleoprotein (RNP) antigens SS-A (Ro) and SS-B (La) present on salivary gland, lacrimal gland, liver, kidney, thyroid	Auto-antibodies to the RNP antigens SS-A (Ro) and SS-B (La); leads to immune-mediated destruction of the lacrimal and salivary glands resulting in dry eyes (*keratoconjunctivitis sicca*) and dry mouth (xerostomia)
Systemic autoimmune diseases		
Scleroderma (Systemic sclerosis)	Nuclear antigens such as DNA topoisomerase and centromere present in heart, lungs, GIT, kidney, etc.	Helper T cell (mainly) and auto-antibody mediated. Excessive fibrosis of the skin, throughout the body **Two types** ❑ Diffuse scleroderma: Autoantibodies against DNA topoisomerase I (anti-Scl 70) is elevated ❑ Limited scleroderma: ↑Anticentromere antibody, characterized by CREST syndrome—calcinosis, Raynaud phenomenon, esophageal dysmotility, sclerodactyly, and telangiectasia

Contd...

Systemic autoimmune diseases		
Seronegative spondyloarthropathies	Sacroiliac joints and other vertebrae Several types: ❑ Ankylosing spondylitis ❑ Reiter syndrome ❑ Psoriatic arthritis ❑ Spondylitis with inflammatory Bowel disease ❑ Reactive arthritis	**Common characteristics:** They present as rheumatoid arthritis like features, but differ from it by: ❑ Association with HLA-B27 ❑ Pathologic changes begin in the ligamentous attachments to the bone rather than in the synovium ❑ Involvement of the sacroiliac joints, and/or arthritis in other peripheral joints ❑ Absence of RA (hence the name "seronegative") ❑ Auto-Ab and immune complex mediated
Multiple sclerosis	Brain (white matter)	Self-reactive T cells produce characteristic inflammatory lesions in brain that **destroys the myelin** sheath of nerve fibers; leads to numerous neurologic dysfunctions

33. True regarding IgM:

a. Activates alternate complement
b. Activates classical complement
c. Crosses placenta
d. None of the above

Classical complement pathway is triggered by antigen-bound antibody molecules. (The only antibodies capable of binding are two units of IgG or one IgM, although IgM is more effective at activating complement. IgG4 cannot bind, but the other three IgG types can.) It is the binding of Fc region to the C1 component that initiates this pathway. The classical pathway can also be triggered by binding of C1 to some types of structures on the target microbe. Also, it can be triggered by C-Reactive Protein binding to microbical polysaccharides such as phosphocholine.

Properties of various immunoglobulins.

Property	*IgG*	*IgA*	*IgM*	*IgD*	*IgE*
Usual form	Monomer	Monomer, dimer	Monomer, pentamer	Monomer	Monomer
Valency	2	2 or 4	2 or 10	2	2
Other chains	None	J chain, secretory component	J chain	None	None
Subclasses	G1, G2, G3, G4	A1, A2	None	None	None
Molecular weight (kDa)	150	150–600	900	150	190
Serum level (mg/mL)	9.5–12.5	IgA 1–3.0 IgA 2–0.5	1.5	0.03	0.0003
% of total serum Ig	75–85%	10–15%	5–10%	0.3%	0.019%
Half-life, days	23*	6	5	3	2.5
Daily production (mg/kg)	34	24	3.3	0.4	0.0023
Intravascular distribution (%)	45	42	80	75	50
Sedimentation coefficient	7	7	19	7	8
Complement activation					
Classical	++ (IgG3>1>2)	–	+++	–	–
Alternate	–	+	–	–	–
Binds to Fc receptors of phagocytes	++	–	? **	–	–
Placental transfer	Yes (except IgG2)	–	–	–	–
Mediates coagglutination	Yes (except IgG3)	–	–	–	–
Mucosal transport	–	Yes	–	–	–
Mast cell degranulation	–	–	–	–	Yes
Marker for B cells	–	–	+	+	–
Heat stability	+	+	+	+	–

*Half-life of IgG3 is 8 days; **?- Questionable

Ans. 33. **b.** Activates classical complement

34. Which one of the following is a major component in activation of the complement via alternative pathway:

a. C1 b. C2
c. C3 d. C4

Classical complement pathway is initiated by the spontaneous hydrolysis of C3, which is abundant in the blood plasma. "Tickover" occurs through the spontaneous cleavage of the thioester bond in C3 to form C3(H_2O).

Differences between the three complement pathways.

Features	*Classical pathway*	*Alternative pathway*	*Lectin pathway*
Activator (initiator)	Antigen–antibody complex	Endotoxin IgA, IgD, cobra venom, Nephritic factor	Carbohydrate residue of bacterial cell wall (mannose binding protein) that binds to host lectin antigen.
First complement activated	C1	C3b	C4
C3 convertase	C14b2a	C3bBb	MBL/MASP-C4b2a
C5 convertase (C3 convertase + 3b)	C14b2a3b	C3bBb3b	MBL/MASP-C4b2a3b
Complement levels in the serum	All C1-C9: Low	❑ C1,C4,C2: Normal ❑ Others: Low	❑ C1: Normal ❑ Others: Low
Immunity	Acquired	Innate	Innate

35. Defect seen in DiGeorge syndrome:

a. Humoral immunity
b. Cell mediated immunity
c. Thymic hyperplasia
d. Autoimmune hemolytic anaemia

Characteristic signs and symptoms of DiGeorge syndrome may include birth defects such as congenital heart disease, defects in the palate, most commonly related to neuromuscular problems with closure (velopharyngeal insufficiency), learning disabilities, mild differences in facial features, and recurrent infections. Infections are common in children due to problems with the immune system's T-cell-mediated response that in some patients is due to an absent or hypoplastic thymus.

Classification of primary immunodeficiency diseases.

Humoral immunodeficiency (B cell defects)
❑ Bruton disease (X-linked agammaglobulinemia) ❑ Common variable immunodeficiency ❑ Isolated IgA deficiency ❑ Hyper-IgM syndrome ❑ Transient hypogammaglobulinemia of infancy
Cellular immunodeficiencies (T cell defects)
❑ DiGeorge syndrome (thymic hypoplasia) ❑ Chronic mucocutaneous candidiasis ❑ Purine nucleoside phosphorylase (PNP) deficiency
Combined immunodeficiencies (B and T cell defects)
❑ Severe combined immunodeficiencies – Cytokine receptor mutation – Adenosine deaminase (ADA) deficiency ❑ Wiskott-Aldrich syndrome ❑ Ataxia telangiectasia ❑ Nezelof syndrome
Disorders of phagocytosis
❑ Chronic granulomatous disease ❑ Myeloperoxidase deficiency ❑ Chediak-Higashi syndrome ❑ Leukocyte adhesion deficiency ❑ Lazy leukocyte syndrome ❑ Job's syndrome or Hyper-IgE syndrome ❑ Tuftsin deficiency ❑ Shwachman's disease
Disorders of complement
❑ Complement component deficiencies ❑ Complement regulatory protein deficiencies

36. Which Immunoglobulin is involved in anaphylaxis:

a. IgA
b. IgE
c. IgG
d. IgM

In the immunologic mechanism of anaphylaxis, immunoglobulin E (IgE) binds to the antigen (the foreign material that provokes the allergic reaction). Antigen-bound IgE then activates FcεRI receptors on mast cells and basophils. This leads to the release of inflammatory mediators such as histamine. These mediators subsequently increase the contraction of bronchial smooth muscles, trigger vasodilation, increase the leakage of fluid from blood vessels, and cause heart muscle depression.

Type of heavy chain in each immunoglobulin class.

Immunoglobulin class	*Heavy chain type*
IgG	γ (gamma)
IgA	α (alpha)
IgM	μ (mu)
IgD	δ (delta)
IgE	ε (epsilon)

37. All are type II hypersensitivity reaction EXCEPT:

a. Stevens-Johnson syndrome
b. Drug induced hemolytic anemia
c. Drug induced thrombocytopenia
d. Hemolytic disease of newborn

Stevens-Johnson syndrome is type IV hypersensitivity reaction.

Ans. **34. c.** C3 **35. b.** Cell mediated immu... **36. b.** IgE **37. a.** Stevens-Johnson...

Features of various types of hypersensitivity reactions.				
	Type I	*Type II*	*Type III*	*Type IV*
Immune response altered	Humoral	Humoral	Humoral	Cell mediated
Immediate or delayed	Immediate	Immediate	Immediate	Delayed
Duration between appearance of symptoms and antigen contact	2 to 30 minutes	5–8 hour	2–8 hours	24–72 hours
Antigen	Soluble	Cell surface bound	Soluble	Soluble or bound
Mediator	IgE	IgG	Ag-Ab complex	T_{DTH} cell
Effector mechanism	Mast cell degranulation	ADCC Complement- mediated cytolysis	Complement activation and inflammatory response	Macrophage activation leads to phagocytosis or cell cytotoxicity
Desensitization to the allergen	Easy, but short lasting	Easy, but short lasting	Easy, but short lasting	Difficult, but sustained
Typical manifestations	❑ Anaphylaxis ❑ Asthma ❑ Atopic dermatitis	❑ Transfusion reactions ❑ Rh incompatibility ❑ Hemolytic anemia	❑ Arthus reaction ❑ Serum sickness ❑ Glomerulonephritis ❑ Rheumatoid arthritis	❑ Tuberculin test ❑ Granuloma formation in tuberculosis, leprosy, etc ❑ Contact dermatitis

38. Intravascular hemolysis is mediated by:

a. IgA
b. IgD
c. IgE
d. IgG

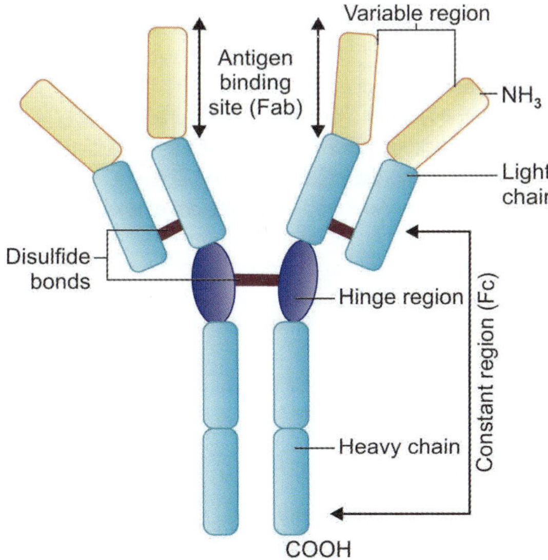

General structure of antibody.

An example of type II hypersensitivity is the ABO blood incompatibility where the red blood cells have different antigens, causing them to be recognized as different; B cell proliferation will take place and antibodies to the foreign blood type are produced. IgG and IgM antibodies bind to these antigens to form complexes that activate the classical pathway of complement activation to eliminate cells presenting foreign antigens. That is, mediators of acute inflammation are generated at the site and membrane attack complexes cause cell lysis and death. The reaction takes hours to a day.

39. Erythroblastosis fetalis is which type of hypersensitivity:

a. Type I
b. Type II
c. Type III
d. Type IV

Type II reactions can affect healthy cells. Examples include Red blood cells in Haemolytic Anaemia, Acetylcholine receptors in Myasthenia Gravis, and TSH receptors in Grave's Disease.

Another example of type II hypersensitivity reaction is Goodpasture's syndrome where the basement membrane (containing collagen type IV) in the lung and kidney is attacked by one's own antibodies.

Another form of type II hypersensitivity is called antibody-dependent cell-mediated cytotoxicity (ADCC). Here, cells exhibiting the foreign antigen are tagged with antibodies (IgG or IgM). These tagged cells are then recognised by natural killer cells (NK) and macrophages (recognised via IgG bound (via the Fc region) to the effector cell surface receptor, CD16 (FcγRIII)), which in turn kill these tagged cells.

Ans. 38. **d.** IgG 39. **b.** Type II

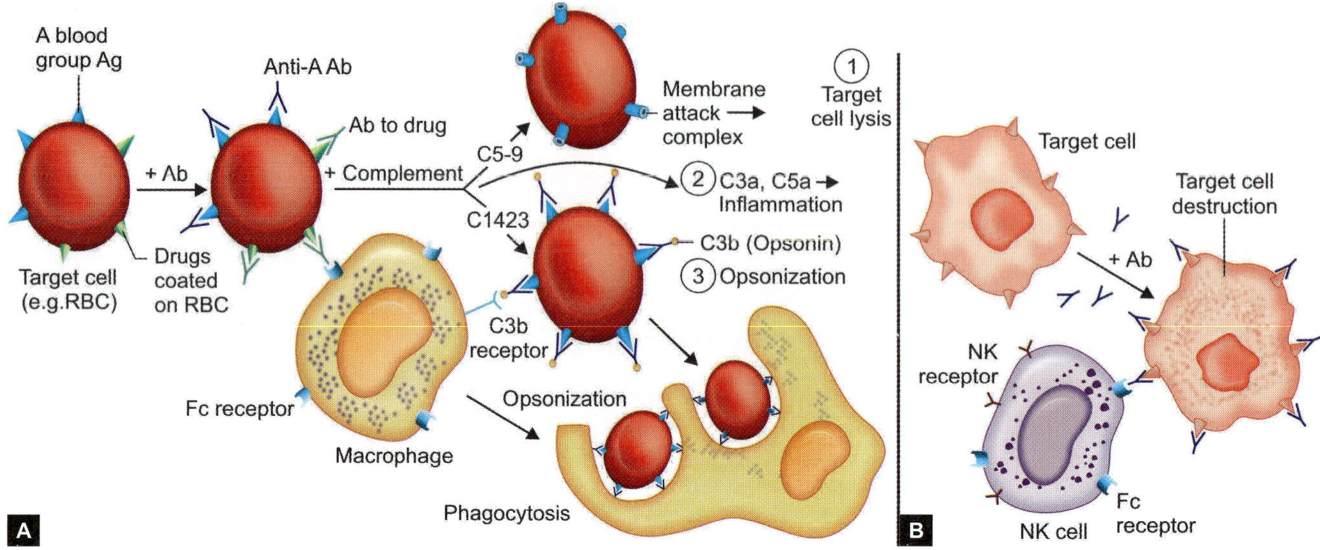

Different mechanisms of antibody mediated type II hypersensitivity reactions. (A) Complement-dependent reactions; (B) Antibody-dependent cellular cytotoxicity (ADCC).

40. Cells associated with humoral immunity are:

a. NK cells b. B cells
c. T cells d. Null cells

Humoral immunity, also called the **antibody-mediated beta cellularis immune system**, is the aspect of immunity that is mediated by macromolecules (as opposed to cell-mediated immunity) found in extracellular fluids such as secreted antibodies, complement proteins and certain antimicrobial peptides. Humoral immunity is so named because it involves substances found in the humours, or body fluids.

The principal function of B cells is to make antibodies against soluble antigens.

Differences between innate and acquired immunity.

Innate immunity	*Acquired / Adaptive immunity*
Resistance to infection that an individual possesses from birth	Resistance to infection that an individual acquires during his lifetime
Immune response occurs in minutes	Immune response occurs in days
Prior exposure to the antigen is not required	Develops following the antigenic exposure
Diversity is limited, acts through a restricted set of reactions	More varied and specialized responses
Immunological memory responses are absent	Immunological memory responses are present
Microbial antigen: Innate immunity develops against antigens that are shared by many microbes (called microbes-associated molecular patterns)	Microbial antigen: Acquired immunity develops against antigens that are specific for each microbes.
Host cell receptors of innate immunity (called pattern recognition receptors) are non-specific, e.g. Toll-like receptor	Host cell receptors are specific, e.g. T cell receptors and B cell immunoglobulin receptors
Components of innate immunity ❑ Anatomical barriers such as skin and mucosa ❑ Physiological barriers (e.g. body temperature) ❑ Phagocytes (neutrophils, macrophages and monocytes) ❑ Natural killer (NK) cells ❑ Other classes of lymphocytes— – γδ T cells, NK-T cells – B-1 cells and marginal-zone B cells ❑ Mast cells and dendritic cells ❑ Complement pathways—alternate and mannose binding pathways ❑ Fever and inflammatory responses ❑ Normal resident flora ❑ Cytokines: TNF-α, interleukins (IL-1, IL-6, IL-8, IL-12, IL-16, IL-18), IFN-α, β and TGF- β ❑ Acute phase reactant proteins (APRs)	**Components of acquired immunity** T cell B cell Classical complement pathway Antigen presenting cells Cytokines (IL-2, IL-4, IL-5, IFN-γ) **Types of acquired immunity** It can be classified in two ways: ❑ Active and passive immunity ❑ Artificial and natural immunity

TNF: tumor necrosis factor; TGF-β: transforming growth factor; β; IFN: interferon

Ans. **40. b.** B cells

41. Which of the following is type III hypersensitivity reaction:

a. Prausnitz-kustner reaction
b. Contact dermatitis
c. Arthus reaction
d. Rh incompatibility

Vasculitis, glomerulonephritis and arthritis are commonly associated conditions as a result of type III hypersensitivity responses.

As observed under methods of histopathology, acute necrotizing vasculitis within the affected tissues is observed concomitant to neutrophilic infiltration, along with notable eosinophilic deposition (fibrinoid necrosis). Often, immunofluorescence microscopy can be used to visualize the immune complexes. Skin response to a hypersensitivity of this type is referred to as an Arthus reaction, and is characterized by local erythema and some induration. Platelet aggregation, especially in microvasculature, can cause localized clot formation, leading to blotchy hemorrhages. This typifies the response to injection of foreign antigen sufficient to lead to the condition of serum sickness.

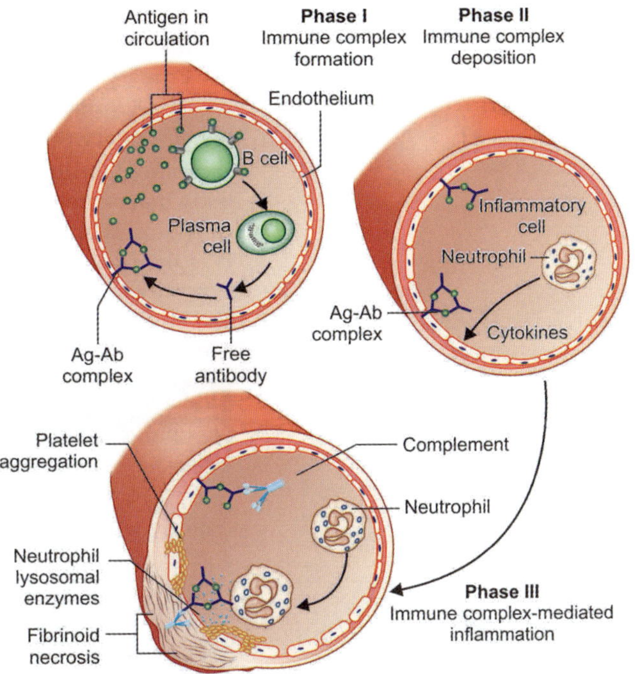

Mechanism of systemic type III hypersensitivity reaction.

42. True about Chediak-Higashi syndrome:

a. Neutrophilia
b. Impaired bacteriolysis
c. Autosomal dominant
d. Associated with polycythemia

Chédiak-Higashi syndrome is a rare autosomal recessive disorder that arises from a mutation of a lysosomal trafficking regulator protein, which leads to a decrease in phagocytosis. The decrease in phagocytosis results in recurrent pyogenic infections, partial albinism and peripheral neuropathy.

43. Widal test is:

a. Agglutination
b. Flocculation
c. Both
d. None of the above

Widal Test is an agglutination test which detects the presence of serum agglutinins (H and O) in patients serum with typhoid and paratyphoid fever.

Types of antigen–antibody reactions.
Conventional techniques
❑ Precipitation reaction
❑ Agglutination reaction
❑ Complement fixation test
❑ Neutralization test
Newer techniques
❑ Enzyme linked immunosorbent assay (ELISA)
❑ Immunofluorescence assay (IFA)
❑ Radioimmunoassay (RIA)
❑ Chemiluminescence-linked immunoassay (CLIA)
❑ Immunohistochemistry
❑ Rapid tests – Lateral flow assay (Immunochromatographic test) – Flow through assay
❑ Western blot
❑ Immunoassays using electron microscope

Ans. **41. c.** Arthus reaction **42. b.** Impaired bacteriolysis **43. a.** Agglutination

44. Wheal-and-flare reaction is:

a. Type I hypersensitivity b. Type II hypersensitivity
c. Type III hypersensitivity d. Type IV hypersensitivity

Type I hypersensitivity reaction: If the antigen is injected beneath the skin—for example, by the sting of an insect or in the course of some medical procedure—the local reaction may be extensive. Called a wheal-and-flare reaction, it includes swelling, produced by the release of serum into the tissues (wheal), and redness of the skin, resulting from the dilation of blood vessels (flare).

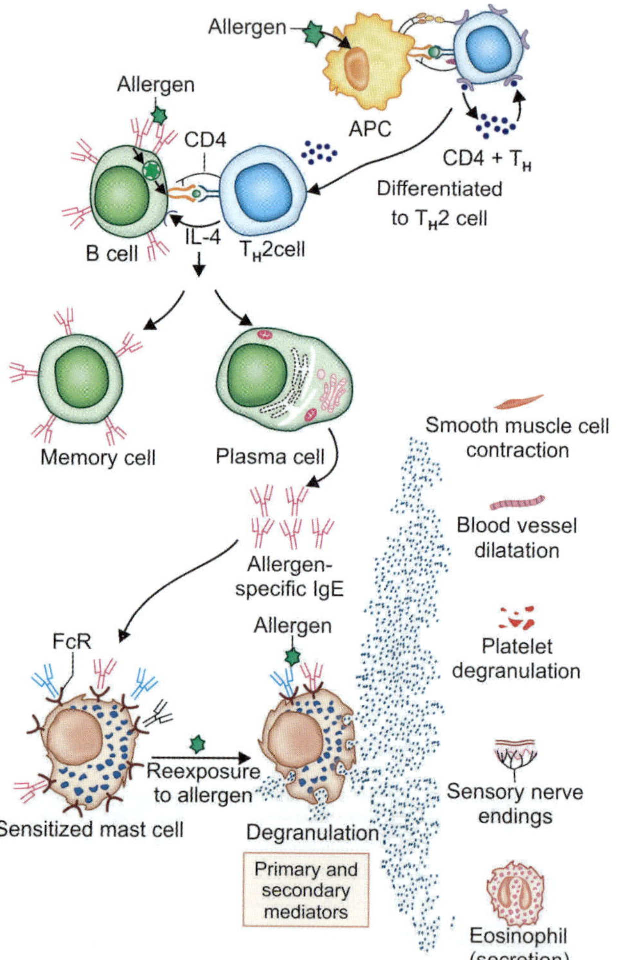

Mechanism of type I hypersensitivity reaction.

45. Which immunoglobulin is present in the breast milk:

a. Ig A
b. Ig E
c. Ig D
d. Ig M

IgA has two subclasses (IgA1 and IgA2) and can exist in a dimeric form called *secretory IgA* (**sIgA**). In its secretory form, IgA is the main immunoglobulin found in mucous secretions, including tears, saliva, sweat, colostrum and secretions from the genitourinary tract, gastrointestinal tract, prostate and respiratory epithelium. It is also found in small amounts in blood.

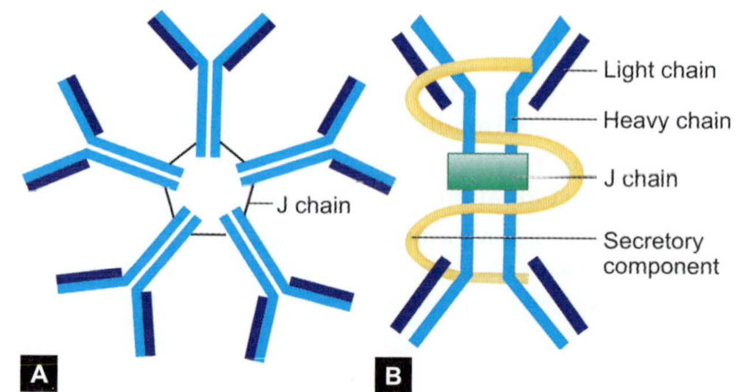

(A) Pentameric IgM; (B) Dimeric IgA.

46. True about IgM is:

a. Mediates Prausnitz-kustner reaction
b. Primary response
c. Transported across placenta
d. Secondary response

Immunoglobulin M, or **IgM** for short, is a basic antibody that is produced by B cells. IgM is by far the physically largest antibody in the human circulatory system. It is the first antibody to appear in response to initial exposure to an antigen. The spleen, where plasmablasts responsible for antibody production reside, is the major site of specific IgM production.

Differences between primary and secondary immune response.	
Primary immune response	*Secondary immune response*
Immune response against primary antigenic challenge	Immune response against subsequent antigenic challenge
Slow, sluggish (appear late) and short lived	Prompt, powerful and prolonged (long lasting)
❑ Lag period is longer (4–7 days)	Lag period is absent or short (1–3 days)
❑ No negative phase	Negative phase may occur
❑ Antibody produced in low titer and is of IgM type. ❑ Antibodies are more specific but less avid	Antibody produced in high titer and is of IgG type Antibodies are less specific but more avid
Antibody producing cells—Naive B cells	Antibody producing cells—Memory B cells
Both T dependent and T independent antigens are processed	Only T dependent antigens are processed

47. True regarding agglutination reaction are all EXCEPT:

a. It is less sensitive than precipitation reaction for detecting antibodies
b. Works on the same principle as that of precipitation reaction
c. It is the method used for cross matching and blood grouping
d. Agglutination occurs optimally when antigens and antibody react in equivalent proportions

Ans. **44. a.** Type I hypersen... **45. a.** Ig A **46. b.** Primary response **47. a.** It is less sensitive...

Agglutination is commonly used as a method of identifying specific bacterial antigens, and in turn, the identity of such bacteria. Because the clumping reaction occurs quickly and is easy to produce, agglutination is an important technique in diagnosis.

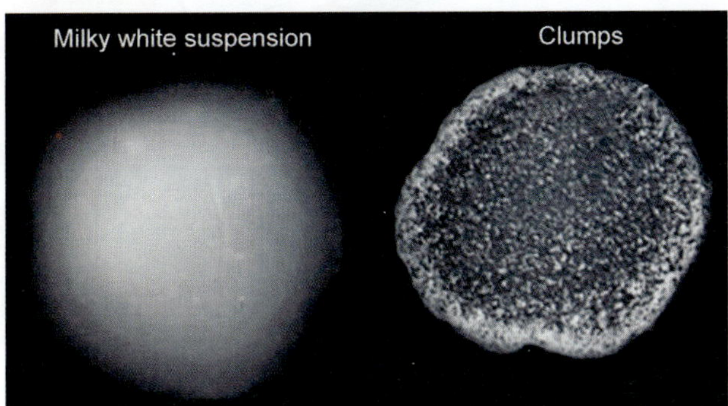

Slide agglutination test.

48. Type-IV hypersensitivity reaction:

a. Anaphylaxis
b. Casoni's test
c. PK reaction
d. Mantoux test

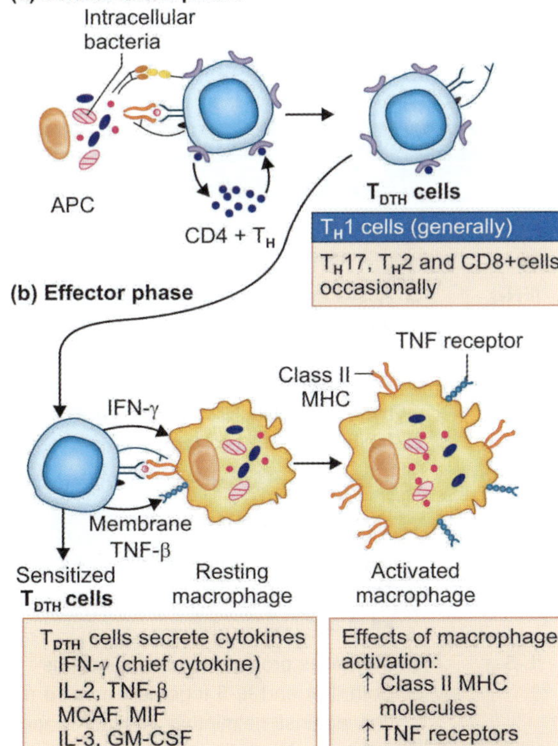

Mechanism of delayed type hypersensitivity. (A) Sensitization phase; (B) Effector phase.
APCs: Antigen presenting cells; MHC: Major histocompatibility complex; TNF: Tumor necrosis factor; IFN: Interferons; DTH: Delayed type hypersensitivity; MCAF: Monocyte chemotactic and activating factor; MIF: Migration inhibitory factor.

A classic example of delayed **type IV hypersensitivity** is the **Mantoux tuberculin** test in which skin induration indicates exposure to tuberculosis.

49. Complement Fixation test is:

a. Widal
b. Coombs test
c. Wassermann reaction
d. VDRL

The **Wassermann test** or **Wassermann reaction** (**WR**) is an antibody test for syphilis, named after the bacteriologist August Paul von Wassermann, based on complement-fixation.

50. Weil-Felix is:

a. Immunoassay test
b. Complement fixation test
c. Agglutination test
d. Precipitin test

The **Weil–Felix test** is an agglutination test for the diagnosis of rickettsial infections. It was first described in 1916. By virtue of its long history and of its simplicity, it has been one of the most widely employed tests for rickettsia on a global scale, despite being superseded in many settings by more sensitive and specific diagnostic tests.

51. NitroBlue Tetrazolium test is employed for:

a. B-cell
b. T-cell
c. Complement
d. Phagocytes

The nitroblue-tetrazolium (NBT) test is the original and most widely known test for chronic granulomatous disease. It is negative in CGD, meaning that it does not turn blue. The higher the blue score, the better the cell is at producing reactive oxygen species. This test depends upon the direct reduction of NBT to the insoluble blue compound formazan by NADPH oxidase; NADPH is oxidized in the same reaction. This test is simple to perform and gives rapid results, but only tells whether or not there is a problem with the PHOX enzymes, not how much they are affected.

52. E-rosetting is a means of identifying:

a. T-cells
b. B-cells
c. NK cells
d. Null cells

Erythrocyte rosetting or **E-rosetting** is a phenomenon seen through a microscope where red blood cells *(erythrocytes)* are arranged around a central cell to form a cluster that looks like a flower. The red blood

Ans. **48. d.** Mantoux test **49. c.** Wassermann reaction **50. c.** Agglutination test **51. d.** Phagocytes **52. a.** T-cells

cells surrounding the cell form the *petal,* while the central cell forms the *stigma* of the flower shape. This formation occurs due to an immunological reaction between an epitope on the central cells surface and a receptor or antibody on a red blood cell. The presence of E-rosetting can be used as a test for T cells although more modern tests such as immunohistochemistry are available. May be caused by *Plasmodium* in malaria.

53. Which is NOT true about secondary immunoglobulin response is:

a. Predominance of IgG
b. Takes 5 days to appear
c. Depends on immunologic memory
d. May be repeated in physiological limits

2° Immune Response

1. If a second dose of the same antigen is given days or even years later, an accelerated 2° or anamnestic immune response (IR) occurs. This lag phase is usually very short (e.g. 3 or 4 days) due to the presence of memory cells.
2. The amount of antibody produced rises to a high level.
3. Antibody level tends to remain high for longer.
4. The main type of antibody produced is IgG (although small amounts of IgM are sometimes produced).

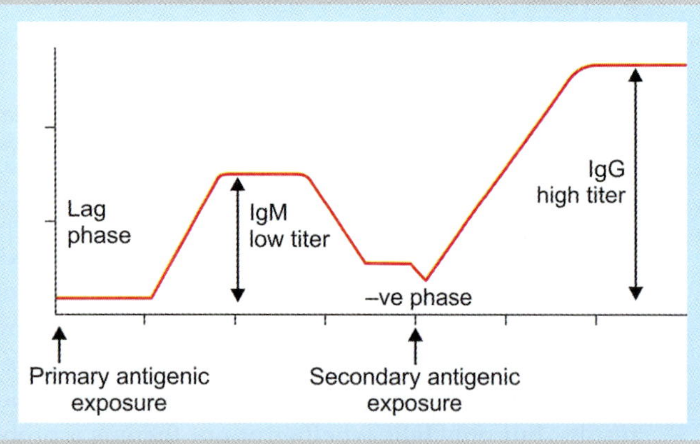

Primary and secondary immune responses.

54. Process of coating of pathogen for efficient phagocytosis is known as:

a. Agglutination
b. Transduction
c. Conjugation
d. Opsonization

An **opsonin** (*opsōneîn*, to prepare for eating) is any molecule that enhances phagocytosis by marking an antigen for an immune response (i.e., causes the phagocyte to "relish" the marked cell).

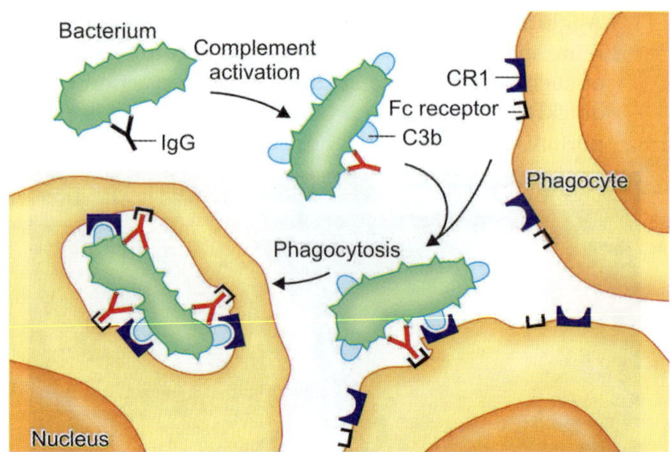

Complement-mediated opsonization.

55. IL-5 is released in which hypersensitivity reaction?

a. Type I
b. Type II
c. Type III
d. Type IV

Interleukin-5 has long been associated with the cause of several allergic diseases including allergic rhinitis and asthma, wherein a large increase in the number of circulating, airway tissue, and induced sputum eosinophils have been observed.

Role of cytokines secreted by T_H1 and T_H2 cells	
T_H1 cytokines and their functions	
IL-2	❑ Promotes activation of T_H and T_C cells ❑ Activates NK cells to become LAK cells
IFN-γ	❑ Activates the resting macrophages into activated macrophage ❑ Activates B cells to produce IgG ❑ Promotes inflammation of delayed type of hypersensitivity (along with TNF-β) ❑ Inhibits T_H2 cell proliferation
TNF-β	❑ Enhances phagocytic activity of macrophage
T_H2 cytokines and their functions	
IL-4	❑ Inhibits T_H1 cell differentiation ❑ Stimulates B cells to produce IgE and also IgG4 and IgG1
IL-5	❑ Enhances proliferation of eosinophils ❑ Both IL-4 and IL-5 together provide protection against helminthic infections and also mediate allergic reaction
IL-6	❑ Promotes B cell proliferation and antibody production
IL-10	❑ Inhibits T_H1 cell differentiation

LAK cell: Lymphokine-activated killer cells; IFN: Interferons; IgG: Immunoglobulin G; TNF: Tumor necrosis factor; NK: Natural killer.

Ans. **53. b.** Takes 5 days to appear **54. d.** Opsonization
55. a. Type I

56. Which of the following immunoglobulin mediates primary immune response?

a. IgA b. IgM
c. IgG d. IgD

IgM antibodies appear early in the course of an infection and usually reappear, to a lesser extent, after further exposure. IgM antibodies do not pass across the human placenta (only isotype IgG).

These two biological properties of IgM make it useful in the diagnosis of infectious diseases. Demonstrating IgM antibodies in a patient's serum indicates recent infection, or in a neonate's serum indicates intrauterine infection (e.g. congenital rubella).

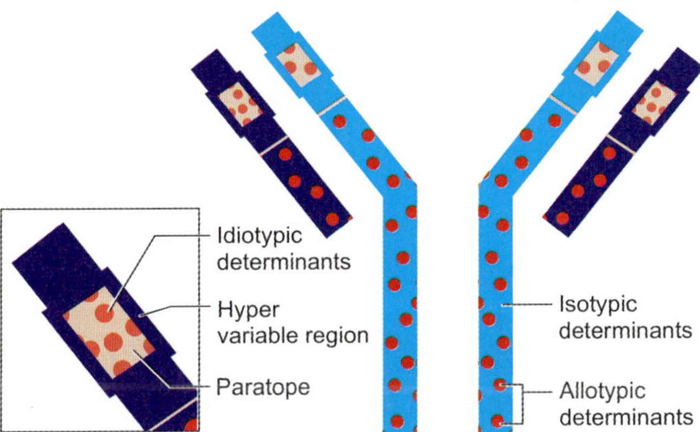

Antigenic determinants of immunoglobulins.

57. Which of the following immunoglobulin crosses placenta?

a. IgA
b. IgM
c. IgG
d. IgD

IgG antibodies are generated following class switching and maturation of the antibody response and thus participate predominantly in the secondary immune response. IgG is secreted as a monomer that is small in size allowing it to easily perfuse tissues. It is the only isotype that has receptors to facilitate passage through the human placenta, thereby providing protection to the fetus *in utero*.

58. Serum sickness is which type of hypersensitivity reaction:

a. Type I
b. Type II
c. Type III
d. Type IV

Serum sickness in humans is a reaction to proteins in antiserum derived from a non-human animal source, occurring 4–10 days after exposure. It is a type of hypersensitivity, specifically immune complex hypersensitivity (type III).

Diseases associated with generalized type III hypersensitivity reactions.
Connective tissue disorders: Due to autoantibodies forming immunocomplexes with self-antigens
❑ SLE (systemic lupus erythematosus): Anti-DNA Ab
❑ Rheumatoid arthritis: Ab against human immunoglobulin
❑ PAN (polyarteritis nodosa)
Parasitic diseases: Resulting from immunocomplex deposition
❑ Nephrotic syndrome in *Plasmodium malariae*
❑ Katayama fever in schistosomiasis
❑ African trypanosomiasis
❑ **Bacterial diseases:** Resulting from immunocomplex deposition
❑ *Streptococcus pyogenes*: Post-streptococcal glomerulonephritis
❑ *Mycobacterium leprae* (Lepra reaction type 2)
Viral diseases: With immunocomplex deposition
❑ Hepatitis B (arthritis)
❑ Hepatitis C (arthritis)
❑ Infectious mononucleosis (Epstein-Barr virus)
❑ Dengue (arthritis)
Others
❑ Hyperacute graft rejection
❑ Subacute bacterial endocarditis
❑ Serum sickness

59. The valency of IgM:

a. 1 b. 3
c. 4 d. 5

IgM forms polymers where multiple immunoglobulins are covalently linked together with disulfide bonds, mostly as a pentamer but also as a hexamer. IgM has a molecular mass of approximately 970 kDa (in its pentamer form). Because each monomer has two antigen binding sites, a pentameric IgM has 10 binding sites. Typically, however, IgM cannot bind 10 antigens at the same time because the large size of most antigens hinders binding to nearby sites.

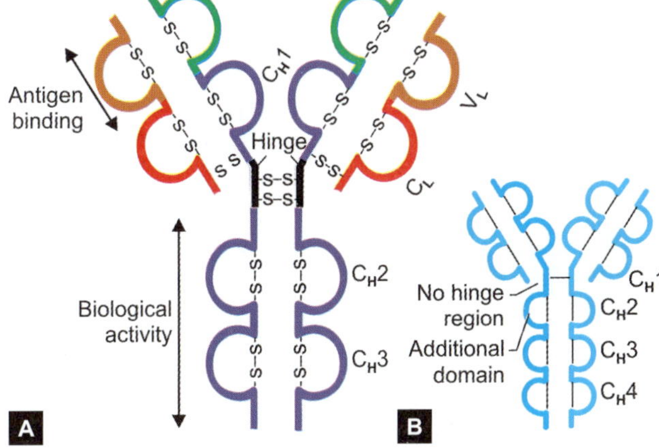

Immunoglobulin domains. (A) Ig with γ, δ and α heavy chains; (B) Ig with μ and ε heavy chains.

Ans. 56. b. IgM 57. c. IgG 58. c. Type III 59. d. 5

60. Components of innate immunity that are active against viral cell include:

a. NK cells
b. Cytotoxic T cells
c. B cells
d. Memory B cells

Natural killer cells or **NK cells** are a type of cytotoxic lymphocyte critical to the innate immune system. The role NK cells play is analogous to that of cytotoxic T cells in the vertebrate adaptive immune response. NK cells provide rapid responses to viral-infected cells, acting at around 3 days after infection, and respond to tumor formation.

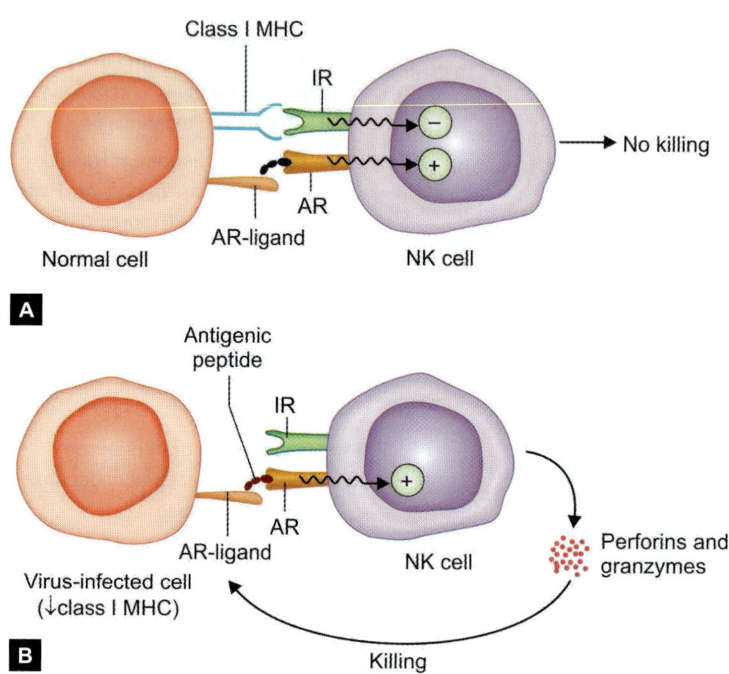

NK cell-mediated cytotoxicity. (A) In normal cell; (B) In virus infected cell. AR: Activation receptor; IR: Inhibition receptor.

61. Type IV hypersensitivity reaction is:

a. Serum sickness
b. Anaphylaxis
c. Arthus reaction
d. Granuloma

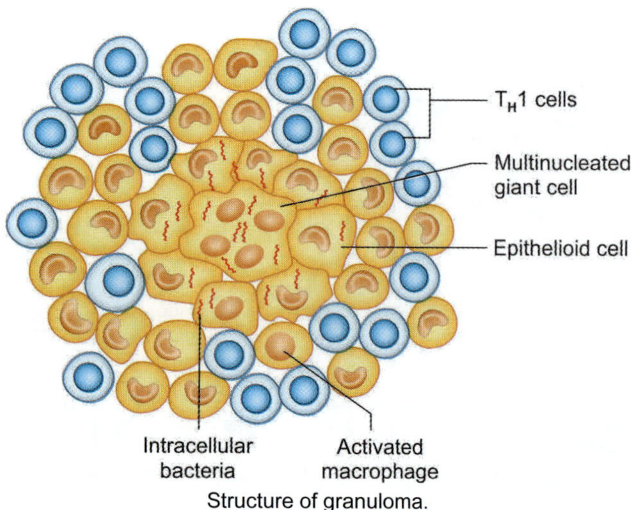

Structure of granuloma.

Type IV hypersensitivity is involved in the pathogenesis of many autoimmune and infectious diseases (tuberculosis, leprosy, blastomycosis, histoplasmosis, toxoplasmosis, leishmaniasis, etc.) and granulomas due to infections and foreign antigens.

62. Which of the following complement component is the common link in the classical and alternate pathway of the complement system:

a. C1
b. C2
c. C3
d. C4

The proteins and glycoproteins that constitute the complement system are synthesized by hepatocytes. But significant amounts are also produced by tissue macrophages, blood monocytes, and epithelial cells of the genitourinal tract and gastrointestinal tract. The three pathways of activation all generate homologous variants of the protease C3-convertase.

Ans. **60. a.** NK cells **61. d.** Granuloma **62. c.** C3

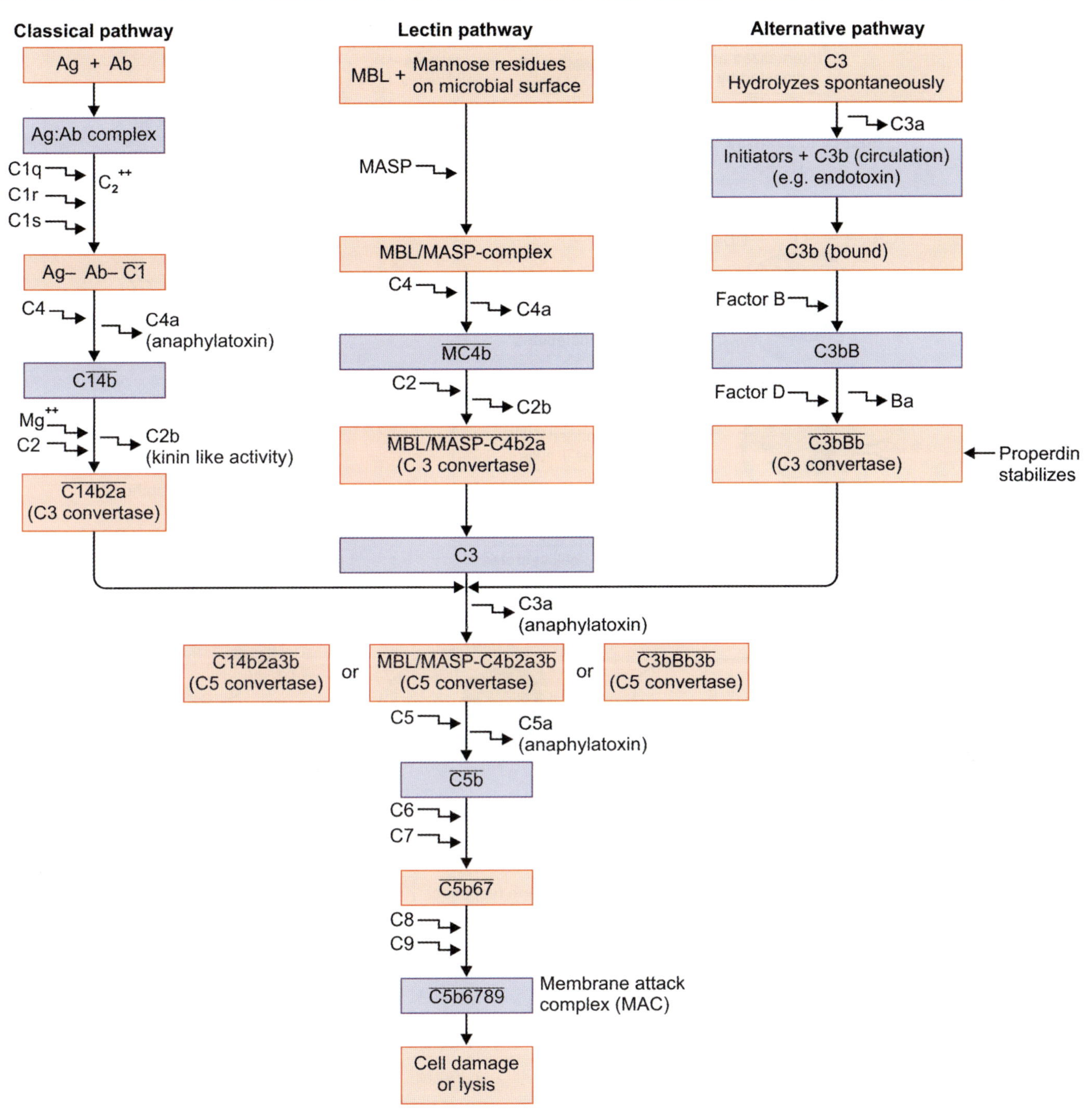

The complement pathways. MBL: Mannose binding lectins; MASP: MBL-associated serine protease.

63. Killer cells and helper cells are part of:

a. B cells b. T cells
c. Monocytes d. Macrophages

Natural killer T cells (NKT cells – not to be confused with natural killer cells of the innate immune system) bridge the adaptive immune system with the innate immune system. Unlike conventional T cells that recognize peptide antigens presented by major histocompatibility complex (MHC) molecules, NKT cells recognize glycolipid antigen presented by a molecule called CD1d. T helper cells (T_H cells) assist other white blood cells in immunologic processes, including maturation of B cells into plasma cells and memory B cells, and activation of cytotoxic T cells and macrophages. These cells are also known as **CD4⁺ T cells** because they express the CD4 glycoprotein on their surfaces.

Ans. **63. b.** T cells

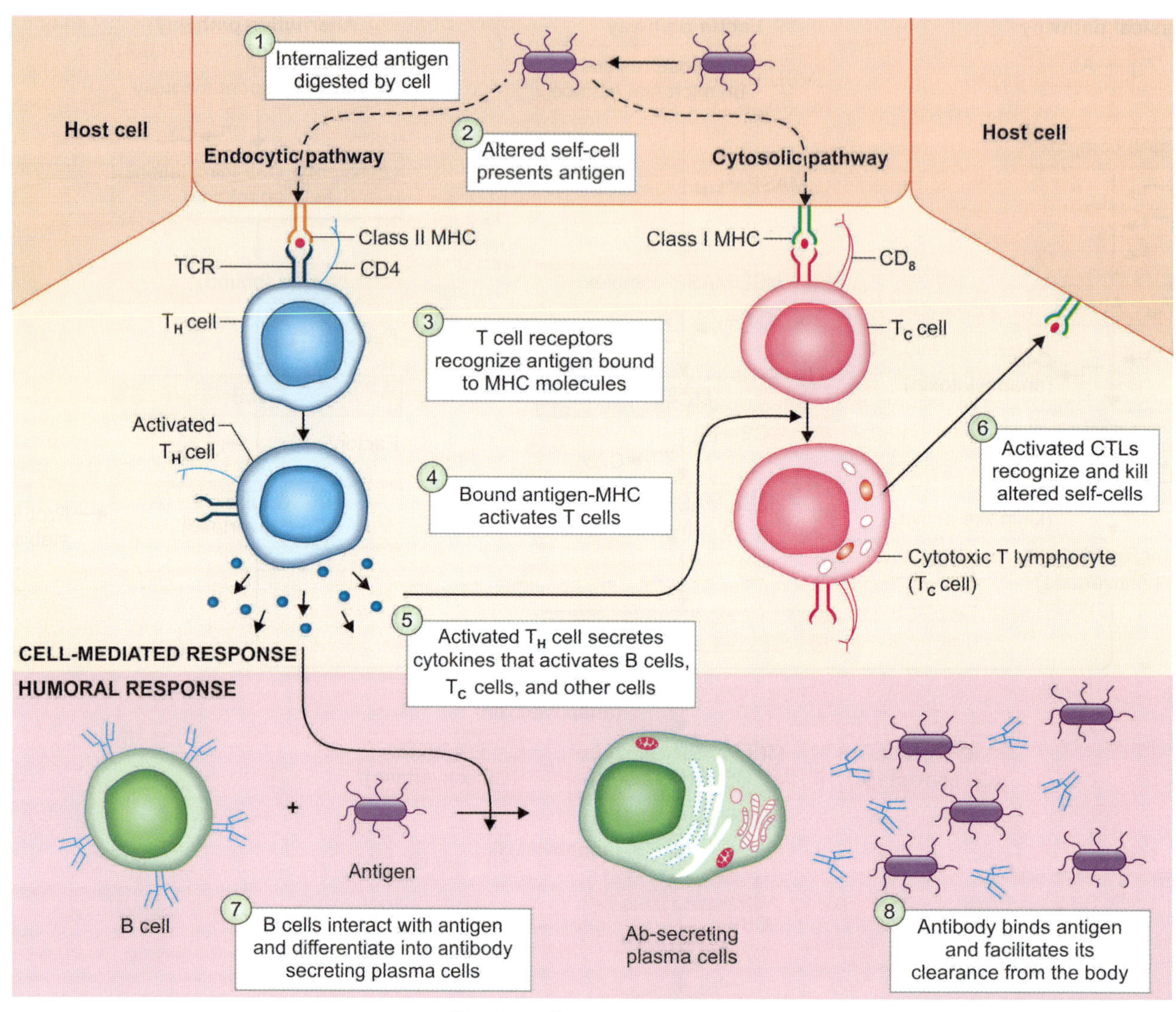

Overview of immune response.

64. Which is true about Widal reaction:

a. Antibody to H antigen appears first and persists
b. Antibody to O antigen appears first and persists
c. Antibodies to H and O antigen appears simultaneously and persists
d. None of the above

The Widal test is positive if TO antigen titer is more than 1:160 in an active infection, or if TH antigen titer is more than 1:160 in past infection or in immunized persons. A single Widal test is of little clinical relevance.

Interpretation of Widal test.

Widal test result	*Suggestive of*
Rise of TO and TH antibody	Enteric fever due to *S.* Typhi
Rise of TO and AH antibody	Enteric fever due to *S.* Paratyphi A
Rise of TO and BH antibody	Enteric fever due to *S.* Paratyphi B
Rise of only TO antibody	Recent infection: Due to any serotype-*S.* Typhi or *S.* Paratyphi A or B
Rise of only TH antibody	? Convalescent stage/ Anamnestic response
Rise of all TH, AH, BH antibodies	Post TAB vaccination

65. Wiskott Aldrich syndrome, NOT true is:

a. Raised IgE
b. Raised IgM
c. Thrombocytopenia
d. CD4 and CD8 defect

Wiskott-Aldrich syndrome (WAS) is a rare X-linked recessive disease characterized by eczema, thrombocy-

Ans. **64. a.** Antibody to H... **65. b.** Raised IgM

topenia (low platelet count), immune deficiency, and bloody diarrhea (secondary to the thrombocytopenia). Immunoglobulin M (IgM) levels are reduced, IgA and IgE are elevated, and IgG levels can be normal, reduced, or elevated.

66. Rheumatoid factor is:
a. IgM antibody against Fc fragment of IgG
b. IgG antibody against Fc fragment of IgG
c. IgM antibody against Fc fragment of IgM
d. IgE antibody against Fc fragment of IgM

Rheumatoid factor (RF) is the autoantibody (antibody directed against an organism's own tissues) that was first found in rheumatoid arthritis. It is defined as an antibody against the Fc portion of IgG (an antibody against an antibody). RF and IgG join to form immune complexes that contribute to the disease process.

67. HLA typing is useful in:
a. Blood grouping
b. Assessing prognosis of disease
c. Cancer therapy
d. Cases of paternal dispute

Typing is also used along with blood typing and DNA tests to determine the parentage (that is, for paternity testing). The HLA antigens of the mother, child, and alleged father can be compared. When an HLA antigen of the child cannot be attributed to the mother or the alleged father, then the latter is excluded as the father of the child.

68. T-cell mature in:
a. Peyer's patch b. Lymph node
c. Thymus d. Bursa of fabricius

They are called T cells because they mature in the thymus (although some also mature in the tonsils)

Differences between T cell and B cell.

Property	T cell	B cell
Origin	Bone marrow	Bone marrow
Maturation	Thymus	Bone marrow
Peripheral blood	70–80% of total lymphocytes	10–15% of total lymphocytes
Antigen recognition receptors	T cell receptors complexed with CD3	B cell receptor-surface IgM or IgD complexed with Igα/Igβ
CD markers	CD 3, 4, 8	CD19, 21, 24
Thymus specific Ag	Present	Absent
Microvilli on the surface	Absent	Present

69. Function of IgA:
a. Acts as a mucosa barrier for infection
b. Circulating antibody
c. Kills virus infected cells
d. Activates macrophages

Immunoglobulin A (**IgA**, also referred to as **sIgA**) is an antibody that plays a critical role in mucosal immunity. More IgA is produced in mucosal linings than all other types of antibody combined; between three and five grams are secreted into the intestinal lumen each day. This accumulates up to 15% of the total immunoglobulin produced in the entire body.

70. The immunoglobulin which passes through placenta and gives immunity to newborns:
a. IgM b. IgA
c. IgG d. IgE

IgG is the only subtype which can cross placenta.

71. An example of heterophile agglutination reaction:
a. Weil Felix
b. Paul Bunnell test
c. Cold agglutinin test
d. All of the above

Heterophile agglutination test
- Typhus fever (Weil Felix reaction)
- Infectious mononucleosis (Paul Bunnell test)
- Mycoplasma pneumonia (Cold agglutination test).

72. Which one of the following is a precipitation reaction:
a. Widal test
b. Weil Felix reaction
c. Wassermann reaction
d. VDRL

Ring test and flocculation test (VDRL) are **examples** of **precipitation** in solution.

73. NOT an immune complex hypersensitivity reaction:
a. Goodpasture syndrome
b. SLE
c. Arthus reaction
d. Post-streptococcal glomerulonephritis

Example of type II hypersensitivity reaction is Goodpasture's syndrome where the basement membrane (containing collagen type IV) in the lung and kidney is attacked by one's own antibodies.

74. Cytokines are released by:
a. Monocyte
b. Macrophage
c. T lymphocyte
d. All of the above

Cytokines include Chemokines, interferons, interleukins, lymphokines, tumour necrosis factor but generally not hormones or growth factors (despite some terminologic overlap). Cytokines are produced by a broad range of cells, including immune cells like macrophages, B lymphocytes, T lymphocytes and mast cells, as well as endothelial cells, fibroblasts, and various stromal cells; a given cytokine may be produced by more than one type of cell.

Ans. 66. **a.** IgM antibody... 67. **d.** Cases of... 68. **c.** Thymus 69. **a.** Acts as a mucosa... 70. **c.** IgG 71. **d.** All of the above 72. **d.** VDRL 73. **a.** Goodpasture synd... 74. **d.** All of the above

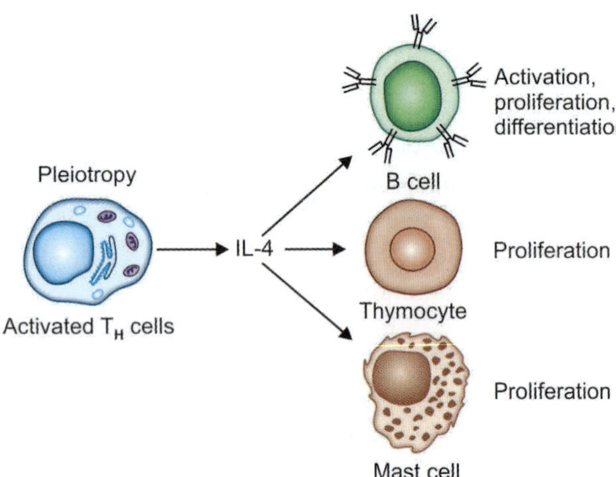

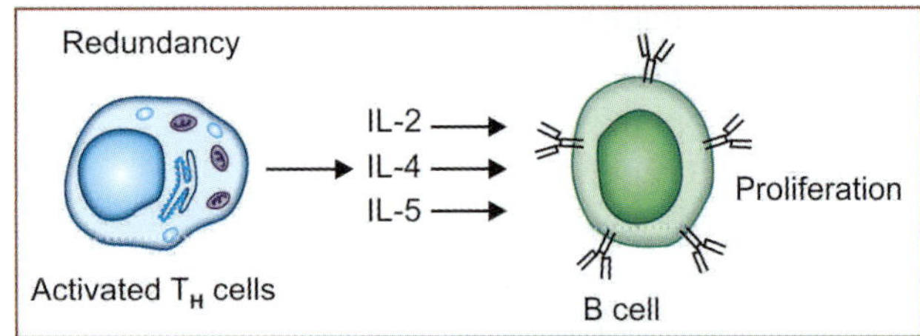

Pleiotropy and redundancy effect of cytokines.

BACTERIOLOGY

75. Which of the following bacterium can be cultured on Cetrimide agar?

a. Staphylococcus
b. Streptococcus
c. Salmonella
d. Pseudomonas

Cetrimide agar

- It is a type of agar used for the selective isolation of the gram-negative bacterium, Pseudomonas aeruginosa.
- As the name suggests, it contains cetrimide, which is the selective agent against alternate microbial flora.
- Cetrimide also enhances the production of Pseudomonas pigments such as pyocyanin and fluorescein, which show a characteristic blue-green and yellow-green color, respectively.

76. Which of the following bacterium can cause hemolytic uremic syndrome:

a. Enterotoxigenic E. coli
b. Enterohemorrhagic E. coli
c. Shigella
d. Salmonella

Hemolytic-uremic syndrome (or **haemolytic-uraemic syndrome**), abbreviated **HUS**,

- It is a disease characterized by hemolytic anemia (anemia caused by destruction of red blood cells), acute kidney failure (uremia), and a low platelet count (thrombocytopenia).
- It predominantly, but not exclusively, affects children.
- Most cases are preceded by an episode of infectious, sometimes bloody, diarrhea acquired as a food-borne illness or from a contaminated water supply and caused by E. coli O157:H7, although Shigella, Campylobacter and a variety of viruses have also been implicated.

77. Clostridium difficile associated diarrhea occurs after consumption of:

a. Trauma
b. Dairy products
c. Fried rice
d. Antibiotic use

Clostridium difficile colitis or pseudomembranous colitis

- It is colitis (inflammation of the large intestine) resulting from infection with Clostridium difficile, a type of spore-forming bacteria.
- It causes an infectious diarrhea called **C. difficile diarrhea**.
- The colitis is thought to occur when this bacteria replaces normal gut flora that has been compromised, usually following antibiotic treatment for an unrelated infection.

78. Which of the following is a Gram-negative cocci?

a. Neisseria gonorrhoeae
b. Bacillus
c. Staphylococci
d. Streptococci

Negative Gram staining

- The outer lipid-based membrane of gram-negative bacteria is removed by an alcohol solution.
- The alcohol also decolorizes the then exposed peptidoglycan layer by dissolving away the previously applied crystal violet.
- A counterstain (safranin or fuchsine) is then added which recolorizes the bacteria red or pink.

79. Which of the following organism requires tryptophan for growth:

a. H. influenzae
b. Vibrio
c. Gonococci
d. Salmonella typhi

Salmonella are non-spore-forming, predominantly motile enterobacteria with cell diameters between approximately 0.7 and 1.5 μm, lengths from 2 to 5 μm, and peritrichous flagella (flagella that are all around the cell body). They are chemo-organotrophs, obtaining their energy from oxidation and reduction reactions using organic sources, and are facultative anaerobes, capable of surviving with or without oxygen.

Ans. 75. **d.** Pseudomonas 76. **b. and c.** Enterohemorr... 77. **d.** Antibiotic use 78. **a.** Neisseria gonorrhoeae 79. **d.** Salmonella typhi

Bacterial vitamins.	
Vitamins	*Bacteria requiring vitamin*
Biotin	*Leuconostoc* species
Cyanocobalamin (B12)	*Lactobacillus* species
Folic acid	*Enterococcus faecalis*
Pantothenic acid	*Morganella morganii*
Pyridoxine (B6)	*Lactobacillus species*
Niacin (nicotinic acid)	*Brucell abortus, Haemophilus influenzae*
Riboflavin (B2)	*Bacillus anthracis*

80. Anton test is used in the diagnosis of:

a. C. diphtheriae b. H. influenzae
c. L. monocytogenes d. S. pneumoniae

The Anton test is used in the identification of *L. monocytogenes;* instillation of a culture into the conjunctival sac of a rabbit or guinea pig causes severe keratoconjunctivitis within 24 hours.

81. Commonest complication of infective endocarditis is:

a. Thromboembolism b. Mycotic aneurysm
c. Fibrinous pericarditis d. Myocardial abscess

Infective endocarditis (IE) has become the most common condition underlying **myocardial abscesses**.

Agents of endocarditis.

Agents of endocarditis

- Streptococci (Viridans streptococci and others)
- Pneumococci
- Enterococci
- *Staphylococcus aureus*
- Coagulase-negative staphylococci
- (e.g. *Staphylococcus epidermidis)*
- Fastidious gram-negative coccobacilli (HACEK group)
- Gram-negative bacilli
- *Candida* species
- Diphtheroids
- Culture-negative endocarditis: Such as *Bartonella, Coxiella*

Most common agent in specific types of endocarditis.

Native valve endocarditis: *Staphylococcus aureus*

Prosthetic valve endocarditis: It occurs following cardiac valve replacement

- Early prosthetic valve endocarditis (occurs within 12 months of valve replacement)—*Staphylococcus epidermidis* is the commonest agent
- Late prosthetic valve endocarditis (occurs after 12 months of valve replacement)— Viridans streptococci is the commonest agent

Endocarditis in IV drug abusers: Young males are the most common victims. The skin is the commonest source of infection.

- Right sided: Most common agent is *Staphylococcus aureus*
- Left sided: Most common agent is *Enterococcus,* followed by *S.aureus*
- Over all: Most common agent is *Staphylococcus aureus*

Most common cause of Subacute endocarditis: Viridians streptococci

82. Which of the following is a lanceolate:

a. Cl. tetani b. Donovania
c. Pneumococci d. Meningococci

S. pneumoniae can be differentiated from *Streptococcus viridans*, some of which are also alpha-hemolytic, using an optochin test, as *S. pneumoniae* is optochin-sensitive. *S. pneumoniae* can also be distinguished based on its sensitivity to lysis by bile, the so-called "bile solubility test". The encapsulated, Gram-positive coccoid bacteria have a distinctive morphology on Gram stain, lancet-shaped diplococci. They have a polysaccharide capsule that acts as a virulence factor for the organism.

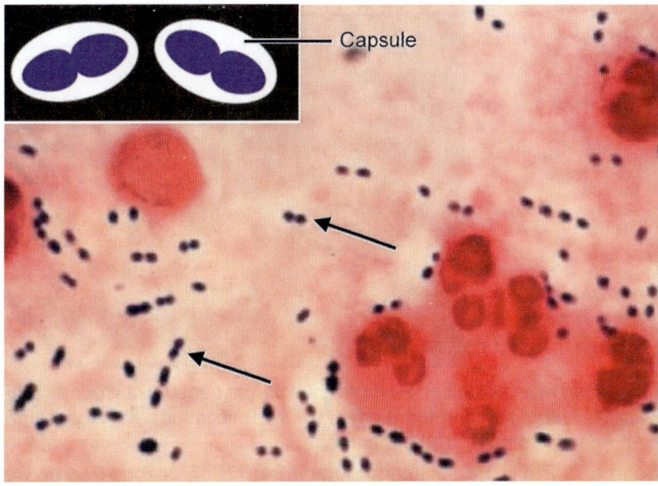

Pneumococci in Gram stained smear of sputum [lanceolate shaped gram-positive cocci in pair surrounded by clear halo (capsule)] (arrows showing).

83. Shock with bullous skin lesion is seen in infection with:

a. E. coli b. Pseudomonas
c. Meningococci d. Candida

P. aeruginosa is an opportunistic human pathogen, most commonly affecting immunocompromised patients, such as those with cystic fibrosis or AIDS. Infection can affect many different parts of the body, but infections typically target the respiratory tract (e.g. patients with Cystic Fibrosis or those on mechanical ventilation), causing bacterial pneumonia. Treatment of such infections can be difficult due to multiple antibiotic resistance. Pseudomonas is the most common organism to infect the burn wounds.

84. McFadyean reaction is seen with:

a. Cl. welchii b. B. anthrax
c. Brucellosis d. H. influenzae

The poly-D-glutamyl capsule of Bacillus anthracis is formed in vivo or in the laboratory when the bacterium is grown on serum plates in a 5% CO_2 atmosphere. The capsular material can be detected by the McFadyean reaction which involves staining with polychrome methylene blue. Blue rods in a background of purple/pink-stained capsular material is a positive test.

Ans. 80. **c.** L. monocytogenes 81. **d.** Myocardial abscess 82. **c.** Pneumococci 83. **b.** Pseudomonas 84. **b.** B. anthrax

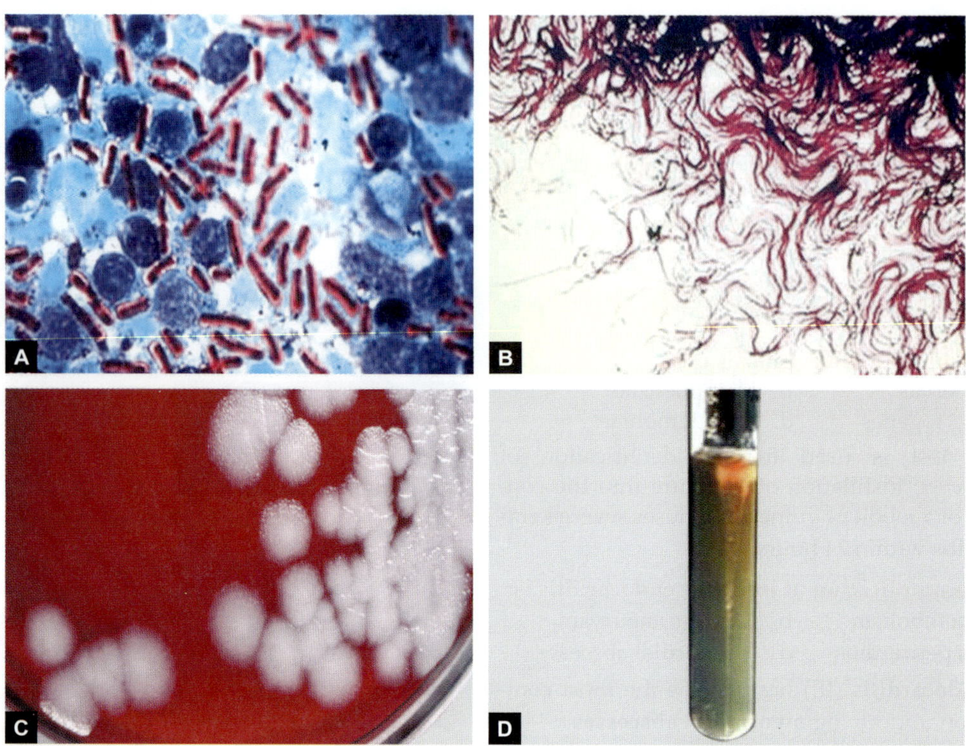

(A) McFadyean's reaction—amorphous purple capsule surrounding blue bacilli (polychrome methylene blue stain); (B) Medusa head colonies of *Bacillus anthracis* on nutrient agar (10× magnification); (C) Non-hemolytic dry wrinkled colonies of *Bacillus anthracis* on blood agar; (D). Gelatin stab agar-inverted fir tree appearance.

Source: C. Public Health Image Library/ID#: 17097/Dr Todd Parker, Centers for Disease Control and Prevention (CDC), Atlanta *(with permission)*.

85. Endemic typhus is transmitted by:

a. Mite b. Rat flea
c. Louse d. None of the above

Murine typhus (also called **endemic typhus**) is a form of typhus transmitted by fleas (Xenopsylla cheopis), usually on rats. (This is in contrast to epidemic typhus, which is usually transmitted by lice.) Murine typhus is an under-recognized entity, as it is often confused with viral illnesses. Most people who are infected do not realize that they have been bitten by fleas.

86. Actinomycetes is a:

a. Gram positive bacteria b. Gram negative bacteria
c. Fungus d. A yeast like form

Actinomycetales are Gram-positive, but several species have complex cell wall structures that make the Gram staining unsuitable (e.g. Mycobacteriaceae).

Differences between *Actinomyces* and *Nocardia*.

Features	*Actinomyces*	*Nocardia*
Acid-fastness	Nonacid-fast	Partially acid-fast
Oxygen requirement	Anaerobe	Obligate aerobe
Sugar	Fermenter	Utilizes sugar oxidatively

Contd...

Contd...

Features	*Actinomyces*	*Nocardia*
Habitat	❑ Found as oral flora ❑ Infections occur endogenously	❑ Usual habitat is soil ❑ Infections occur exogenously
Risk factors	Disease occurs in immunocompetent host also	Usually affects people with low immunity
Clinical forms	Cervicofacial, abdominal and others	Pulmonary, CNS forms, Actinomycetoma
Granules	**Sulfur granules** are hard and not emulsifiable, consist of branching filamentous bacilli and surrounded by clubs **(sun-ray appearance)**	❑ Granules are soft and lobulated and also show sun-ray appearance. ❑ Commonly found in mycetoma, rare in other conditions
Culture	❑ **Spidery molar** teeth colony in solid media ❑ **Fluffy ball** at bottom of the liquid medium	Colonies are creamy, wrinkled and pink. Isolation is done in: ❑ Selective media ❑ Paraffin bait technique ❑ LJ medium
Drug of choice	Penicillin	Sulfonamide or cotrimoxazole

Ans. **85. b.** Rat flea **86. a.** Gram positive bacteria

87. Q fever is caused by:

a. Rickettsia tsutsugamushi
b. R. prowazekii
c. R. quintana
d. C. burnetii

Q fever is a disease caused by infection with *Coxiella burnetii*, a bacterium that affects humans and other animals. This organism is uncommon, but may be found in cattle, sheep, goats and other domestic mammals, including cats and dogs. The infection results from inhalation of a spore-like small cell variant, and from contact with the milk, urine, feces, vaginal mucus, or semen of infected animals.

88. The following is the etiological agent for Rocky Mountain Spotted Fever:

a. Rickettsia rickettsii
b. Rochalimaea Quintana
c. Rickettsia tsutsugmashi
d. Coxialla burnetti

RMSF disease is caused by *Rickettsia rickettsii*, a species of bacterium that is spread to humans by *Dermacentor* ticks. Initial signs and symptoms of the disease include sudden onset of fever, headache, and muscle pain, followed by development of rash.

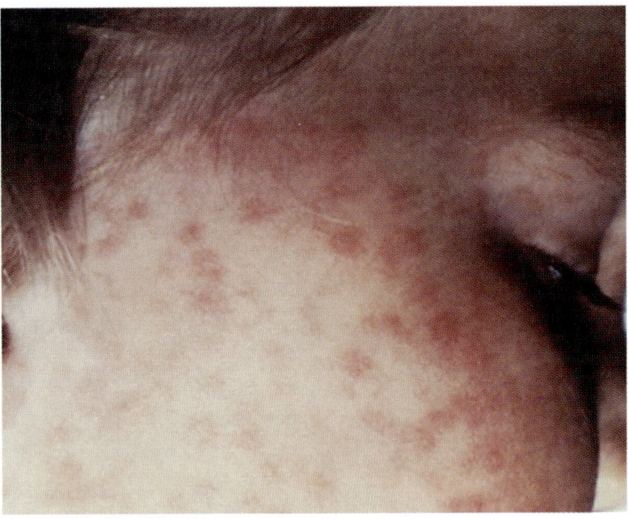

Characteristic rash seen in Rocky mountain spotted fever.
Source: Public Health Image Library, ID#:14489/Centers for Disease Control and Prevention (CDC), Atlanta (with permission).

89. Chlamydia causes all of the following EXCEPT:

a. Trachoma
b. Non-gonococcal urethritis
c. Pneumonia
d. Parotitis

Features of *Chlamydia* infections.

Species	*Character*	*Biovar*	*Serotype*	*Disease*
C. trachomatis	❑ Forms compact inclusions mixed with glycogen matrix ❑ Sensitive to sulfonamide ❑ Natural human pathogen ❑ Leaves the host cell with a scar	TRIC	A, B, Ba, C	Trachoma
			D-K	❑ Genital chlamydiasis ❑ Inclusion conjunctivitis ❑ Infant pneumonia
		LGV	L1, L2, L3	Lymphogranuloma venereum
C. psittaci	❑ Forms diffuse vacuolated inclusions without glycogen matrix ❑ Resistant to sulfonamide ❑ Natural pathogen of birds ❑ Leaves the host cell by lysis	Nil	Many serotypes	❑ Psittacosis (Atypical pneumonia) ❑ Transmission-Inhalational route - pet birds (parrots) and poultry (turkeys and ducks) ❑ No man-to-man transmission
C. pneumoniae TWAR agent	❑ Exclusive human pathogen ❑ Forms inclusions without glycogen matrix ❑ Resistant to sulfonamide	Nil	Only 1 serotype	❑ Community-acquired atypical pneumonia ❑ Associated with– – Atherosclerosis – Asthma

Biovar TRIC: Trachoma Inclusion conjunctivitis; Biovar LGV: Lymphogranuloma venereum; TWAR agent: Taiwan acute respiratory agent.

Acute bacterial parotitis: is most often caused by a bacterial infection of Staphylococcus aureus but may be caused by any commensal bacteria. The most common viral cause of parotitis is mumps. Routine vaccinations have dropped the incidence of mumps to a very low level. Mumps resolves on its own in about ten days.

90. Which of the following is NOT true regarding chlamydiae trachomatis:

a. Elementary body is metabolically active
b. It is biphasic
c. Reticulate body divides by binary fission
d. Inside the cell it evades phagolysosome

Ans. **87. d.** C. burnetii **88. a.** Rickettsia rickettsii **89. d.** Parotitis **90. a.** Elementary body...

Chlamydia may be found in the form of an elementary body and a reticulate body. The elementary body is the nonreplicating infectious particle that is released when infected cells rupture. It is responsible for the bacteria's ability to spread from person to person and is analogous to a spore.

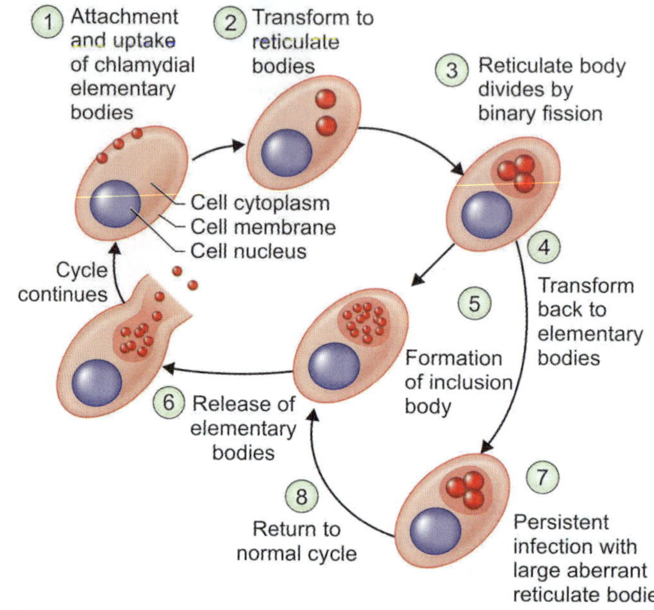

Life cycle of *Chlamydia*. EB: Elementary body; RB: Reticulate body; IFN: Interferons.

91. True for clostridium tetani:

a. Gram negative, non-spore forming
b. Gram positive, non-spore forming
c. Gram negative, spore forming
d. Gram positive, spore forming

Clostridium tetani is a rod-shaped, anaerobic species of pathogenic bacteria, of the genus *Clostridium*. Like other *Clostridium* genus species, it is Gram-positive, and its appearance on a gram stain resembles drumsticks.

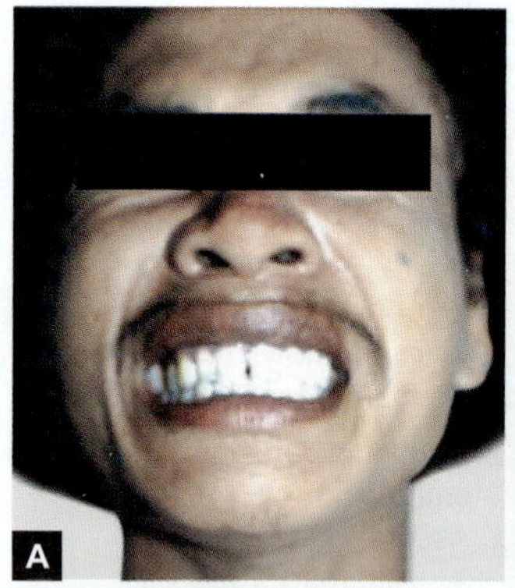

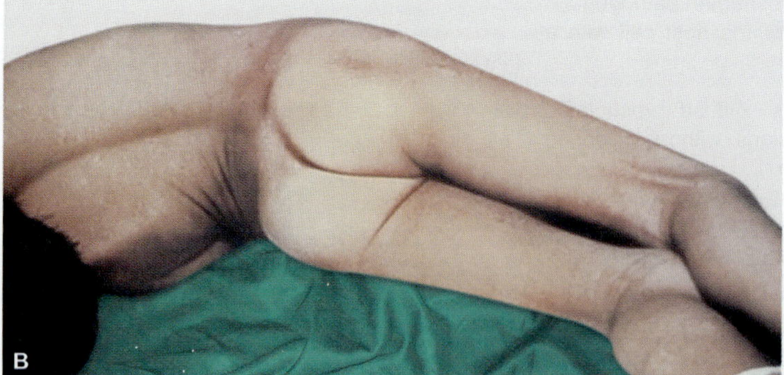

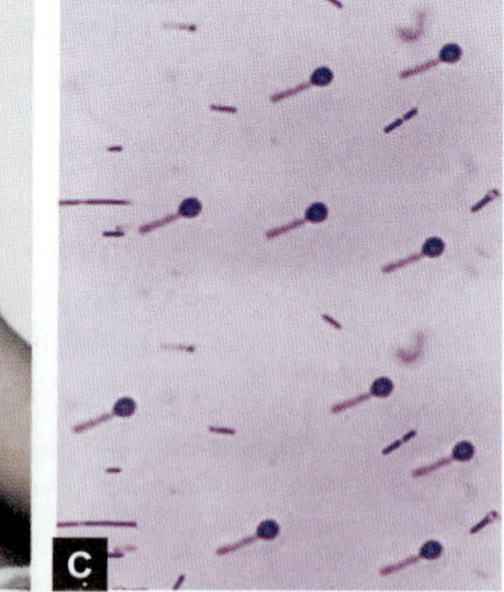

(A) Lockjaw and the facial spasms (risus sardonicus); (B) Patient with opisthotonos seen in tetanus; (C) Gram-stained smear of Clostridium tetani showing round terminal spore bearing gram-positive bacilli.
Source: A. Wikia/Hoidkempuhtust, B. Public Health Image Library, ID# 6373, C. ID# 12056/Dr Holdeman/Centers for Disease Control and Prevention (CDC), Atlanta (with permission)

92. The minimum of treponema that must be present to be detected by dark ground microscopy:

a. 100/mL
b. 1000/mL
c. 10000/mL
d. 100000/mL

Dark field microscopy remains a sensitive, direct, and quick method for diagnosing syphilis in active lesions. However, it requires a special dark field equipped microscope and skilled technicians that are not usually available at most medical facilities today, including many large hospitals in the U.S. Specimens for microscopic

Ans. **91. d.** Gram positive... **92. c.** 10000/mL

examination are best obtained from serous transudate of moist lesions such as such as a primary chancre, condyloma latum (wart like lesions, sometimes extensive), or mucous patches (shallow ulcers on mucous membranes, non-painful unless secondarily infected).

93. Yaws is caused by:

a. T. pertunae
b. T. pallidum
c. T. caraetum
d. Hemophilus

Other pathogenic treponemes (apart from treponema pallidum) for man include *T. pallidum* subspecies pertenue, the causative agent of yaws; *T. carateum*, the causative agent of pinta; and *T. pallidum* subspecies endemicum, the agent associated with non-venereal or endemic syphilis.

Pathogenic spirochetes.

Spirochetes	Disease	Transmission
Treponema		
T. pallidum	Syphilis	Sexual
T. pertenue	Yaws	Direct contact
T. endemicum	Endemic syphilis	
T. carateum	Pinta	
Borrelia		
B. recurrentis	Relapsing fever (epidemic)	Louse borne
B. duttonii, B. hermsii	Relapsing fever (endemic)	Tick borne
B. burgdorferi	Lyme disease	Tick borne
B. vincentii	Vincent's angina	Direct contact
Leptospira		
L. interrogans	Leptospirosis ❑ Milder form ❑ Severe form (Weil's disease)	Contact with rodent urine

94. True about mycoplasma is:

a. Not sensitive to antibiotics
b. Differs from L forms
c. Culture in Sabourad's media
d. MC cause of non-gonococcal urethritis

Several species of Mycoplasma are pathogenic in humans, including *M. pneumoniae*, which is an important cause of atypical pneumonia and other respiratory disorders, and *M. genitalium*, which is believed to be involved in pelvic inflammatory diseases. *Mycoplasma* species are the smallest bacterial cells yet discovered, can survive without oxygen, and are typically about 0.1micrometre in diameter. Mycoplasmas lack cell wall permanently and differ from L-forms in many ways.

Comparison of *Mycoplasma* and L-forms.

Mycoplasma	*L-forms*
Stable, cell wall is absent permanently	**Two types:** **Unstable L-forms:** They usually revert back to normal state once the antibiotic exposure is withdrawn **Stable L-forms:** They are permanently cell wall deficient but resemble parent bacteria both biochemically and antigenically
Absence of precursors of peptidoglycan	Though cell wall deficient, remnants of cell wall components can be demonstrated
Cell membrane contains sterols	Sterols absent
Filterable like viruses	Not filterable
Mycoplasma can cause disease in cell wall deficient form	L-forms do not cause disease but they play an important role in persistence of infection during antibiotic therapy

95. In reference to mycoplasmas, the following are true EXCEPT:

a. They are inhibited by penicillins
b. They can reproduce in cell free media
c. They have an affinity for mammalian cell membranes
d. They can pass through filters of 450 mm pore size

Mycoplasma is a genus of bacteria that lack a cell wall around their cell membrane. Without a cell wall, they are unaffected by many common antibiotics such as penicillin or other beta-lactam antibiotics that target cell wall synthesis.

96. Botulism toxin acts by:

a. Inhibit acetylcholine release
b. Muscle nerve block
c. Increased synthesis of acetylcholine
d. Decreased synthesis of acetylcholine

There are eight serological varieties of the bacterium clostridium botulinum, denoted by the letters A to H. The toxin from all of these acts in the same way and produces similar symptoms: the motor nerve endings are prevented from releasing acetylcholine, causing flaccid paralysis and symptoms of blurred vision, ptosis, nausea, vomiting, diarrhea and/or constipation, cramps, and respiratory difficulty.

97. Elek test is done for:

a. Brucellosis b. Cholera
c. Diphtheria d. Influenza

Elek's test, also known as the immuno diffusion technique, is an in vitro virulence test performed upon *Corynebacterium diphtheriae*. It is used to test for toxigenicity of *C. diphtheriae*.

Ans. 93. **a.** T. pertunae 94. **b.** Differs from L forms 95. **a.** They are inhibited... 96. **a.** Inhibit acetylch... 97. **c.** Diphtheria

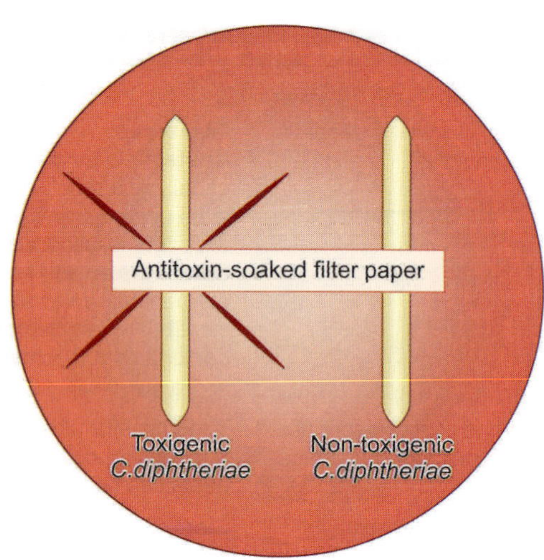

Elek's gel precipitation test.

98. Eaton agent is:

a. Gonococcus
b. Mycoplasma
c. Pseudomonas
d. Corynebacterium

In 1898, Nocard and Roux were the first to isolate a mycoplasma species in culture from bovine, however it wasn't until 1944 when *Mycoplasma pneumoniae*, known then as Eaton agent or Eaton's agent, was isolated and described from a patient with primary atypical pneumonia.

Bacteria named after the discoverers.	
Common name	*Scientific name*
Kleb-Loeffler bacillus	*Corynebacterium diphtheriae*
Preisz Nocard bacillus	*Corynebacterium pseudotuberculosis*
Koch Week bacillus	*Haemophilus aegyptius*
Pfeiffer's bacillus	*Haemophilus influenzae*
Whitmore's bacillus	*Burkholderia pseudomallei*
Battey bacillus	*Mycobacterium intracellulare*
Johne's bacillus	*Mycobacterium paratuberculosis*
Eaton's agent	*Mycoplasma pneumoniae*
Gaffky-Eberth bacillus	*Salmonella* Typhi

99. Lepra cells are:

a. Neutrophils
b. Lymphocytes
c. Histiocytes
d. Plasma cells

Lepra cells are distinctive and large, mononuclear phagocytes (macrophages) with a foam like cytoplasm, and also poorly staining sac like structures resulting from degeneration of such cells, observed characteristically in leprous inflammation reactions; indistinct staining results from numerous, fairly closely packed leprosy bacilli, which are acid fast and resistant to staining by ordinary methods.

Differences between lepromatous leprosy and tuberculoid leprosy.		
Characters	*Lepromatous leprosy (LL)*	*Tuberculoid leprosy (TT)*
Bacillary load	Multibacillary	Paucibacillary
Bacteriological index	4–6+	0–1+
Skin lesions	Many, symmetrical Margin is irregular Lesions appear as: ❑ Multiple nodules (lepromata) ❑ Plaques and xanthoma-like papules Leonine facies and eyebrow alopecia is seen	One or few, asymmetrical Margin is sharp Lesions appear as: Hypopigmented, annular macules with elevated borders Tendency towards central clearing
Nerve lesion	Nerve lesions appear late Hypoesthesia is a late sign	Early anesthetic skin lesion, Enlarged thickened nerves, Nerve abscess seen (common in BT)
Cell-mediated immunity (CMI)	CMI low	CMI normal
Lepromin test	Negative	Positive
Lymphocyte transformation test	Negative	Positive
CD4/CD8 T-cell ratio	1:2	2:1 (normal)
Humoral immunity	Exaggerated	Normal
Autoantibodies	Elevated	Not seen
VDRL test	Biological false positive	VDRL test negative
Antibodies to phenolic glycolipid-1(PGL-1)	Elevated in 95% of cases	Elevated in 60% of cases
Macrophages	Foamy type (lipid-laden)	Epithelioid type
Langhans giant cells	Not seen	Found

VDRL: Venereal disease research laboratory; BT: Borderline tuberculoid leprosy.

Ans. **98. b.** Mycoplasma **99. c.** Histiocytes

100. Fastest microbicidal agent against M-leprae:

a. Clofazimine b. Dapsone
c. Rifampicin d. Minocycline

Leprosy is curable with a treatment known as multidrug therapy (MDT). Treatment for paucibacillary leprosy is with the medications dapsone and rifampicin for six months. Treatment for multibacillary leprosy consists of rifampicin, dapsone, and clofazimine for 12 months.

Clinical classification of leprosy and WHO treatment regimens.

Criteria	*Paucibacillary*	*Multibacillary*
Skin lesions	1–5	6 or more
Nerve involvement	1	2 or more
Microscopy	Smear negative	Smear positive
Leprosy type	TT, BT and Intermediate	BB, BL, LL
Treatment regimen	❑ Dapsone (100 mg) given daily, self administered ❑ Rifampicin (600 mg) given once a month under supervision	❑ Dapsone (100 mg) given daily ❑ Rifampicin (600 mg) given once a month ❑ Clofazimine–300 mg once a month under supervision, followed by 50 mg daily, self administered
Duration of treatment	Up to 6 months	Up to 1 year or till smear negative
Follow up	Annually till 2 years	Annually till 5 years

101. Generation time of lepra bacilli:

a. 12 days
b. 5 minutes
c. 10 hours
d. 24 hours

Mycobacterium leprae has the longest doubling time (14 days) of all known bacteria and has never been cultured in the laboratory without a surrogate host. Despite this it is possible to grow *M. leprae* in nine banded armadillos, and the foot pads of mice.

102. Buruli ulcer is caused by:

a. Mycobacterium ulcerans
b. Mycobacterium marinum
c. Mycobacterium kansasii
d. Mycobacterium fortuitum

Buruli ulcer (also known as the **Bairnsdale ulcer**, **Searls ulcer**, or **Daintree ulcer**) is an infectious disease caused by *Mycobacterium ulcerans*. The early stage of the infection is characterised by a painless nodule or area of swelling. This nodule can turn into an ulcer. The ulcer may be larger inside than at the surface of the skin, and can be surrounded by swelling. As the disease worsens, bone can be infected. Buruli ulcers most commonly affect the arms or legs; fever is uncommon.

Runyon's classification of nontuberculous mycobacteria.

Runyon group	*Property*	*Species*
I. Photochromogens	Produce pigments only in light	*M. marinum, M. asiaticum, M. simiae, M. kansasii, M. genavense*
II. Scotochromogens	Produce pigments both in dark and light	*M. scrofulaceum, M. szulgai, M. gordonae M. celatum, M. flavescens*
III. Non-photochromogens	Do not produce pigments	*M. avium-intracellulare complex (MAC) M. xenopi, M. ulcerans, M. paratuberculosis, M. malmoense*
IV. Rapid growers	Grow within one week	*M. chelonae, M. fortuitum, M. smegmatis, M. abscessus*

103. Pleomorphism is most commonly seen with:

a. Brucella abortus
b. Corynebacterium diphtheria
c. H. influenzae
d. Anaerobic streptococci

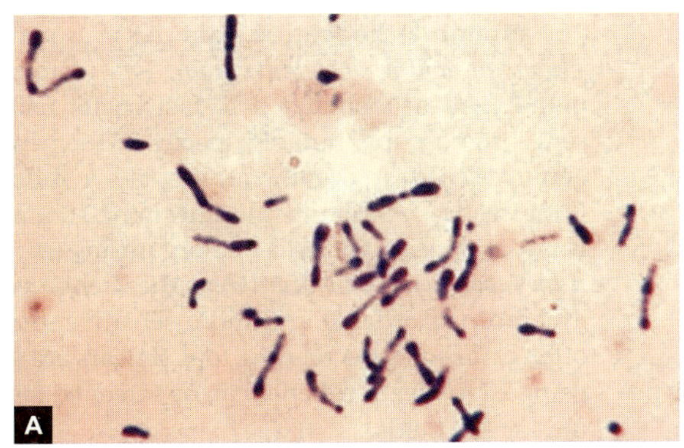
A

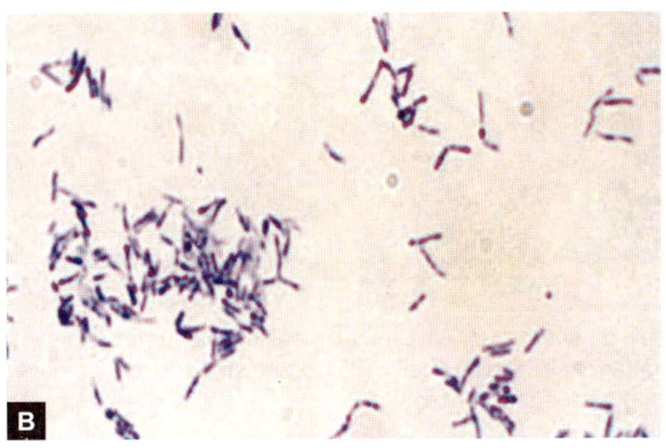
B

Contd...

Ans. 100. c. Rifampicin 101. a. 12 days 102. a. Mycobacterium... 103. b. Corynebacterium...

Contd...

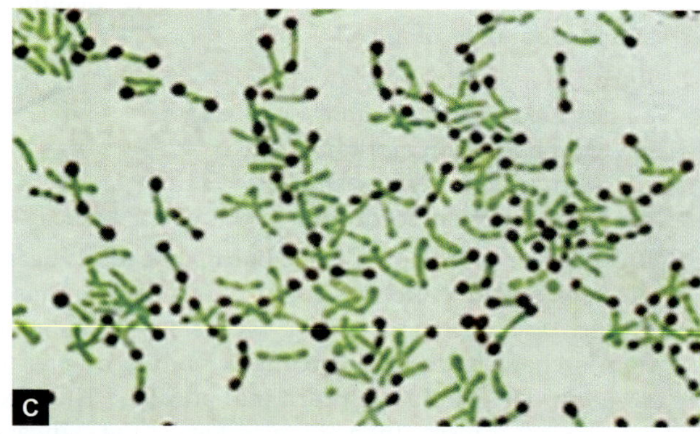

Corynebacterium diphtheriae. (A) Club-shaped bacilli in methylene blue-stained smear; (B) Gram-stained smear shows V- or L-shaped bacilli with cuneiform arrangement; (C) Albert's stain shows dark blue metachromatic granules at the ends of the bacilli.
Source: Public Health Image Library, A. ID# /7323/P.B. Smith, B. ID# /1943, Centers for Disease Control and Prevention (CDC), Atlanta (with permission).

To accurately identify *C. diphtheriae*, a Gram stain is performed to show Gram-positive, highly pleomorphic organisms with no particular arrangement. Special stains like Albert's stain and Ponder's stain are used to demonstrate the metachromatic granules formed in the polar regions. The granules are called as polar granules, Babes Ernst granules, volutin, etc. An enrichment medium, such as Löffler's medium, is used to preferentially grow *C. diphtheriae*. After that, a differential plate known as tellurite agar, allows all *Corynebacteria* (including *C. diphtheriae*) to reduce tellurite to metallic tellurium. The tellurite reduction is colorimetrically indicated by brown colonies for most *Cornyebacterium* species or by a black halo around the *C. diphtheriae* colonies.

104. All are motile EXCEPT:

a. Anthrax b. Clostridia
c. Diphtheria d. Proteus

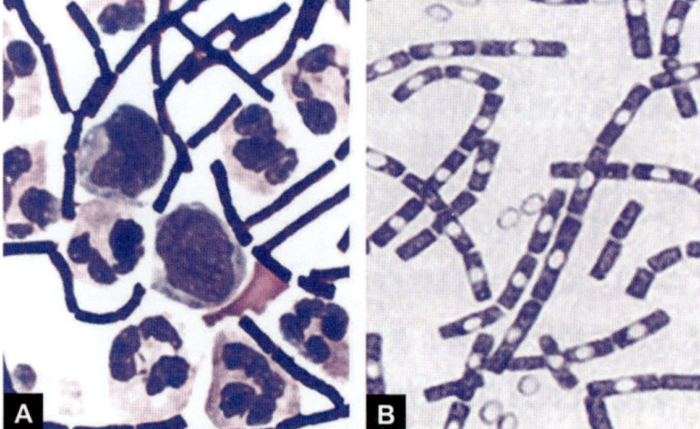

Gram-stain of *B. anthracis:* (A) Direct smear-shows gram-positive, large rectangular bacilli and pus cells; (B) Culture smear-gram-positive bacilli (bamboo stick appearance).
Source: Wikipedia

B. anthracis is a Gram-positive, endospore-forming, rod-shaped bacterium, with a width of 1.0–1.2 μm and a length of 3–5 μm. It can be grown in an ordinary nutrient medium under aerobic or anaerobic conditions. It is one of few bacteria known to synthesize a protein capsule (poly-D-gamma-glutamic acid). Like *Bordetella pertussis,* it forms a calmodulin-dependent adenylate cyclase exotoxin known as (edema factor), along with lethal factor.

105. Babesiosis is most commonly transmitted by:

a. Pigs b. Rats
c. Sand fly d. Ticks

Ticks transmit the human strain of babesiosis, so it often presents with other tick-borne illnesses such as Lyme disease.

Arthropod vectors transmitting human infections.

Vectors	*Human infections transmitted*
Mosquito	Malaria, filariasis, yellow fever, Japanese encephalitis, dengue fever
Sandfly	Kala-azar, oriental sore, sandfly fever, Oroya fever
Hard tick	Tick typhus, Kyasanur forest disease (KFD), babesiosis, tularemia,
Soft tick	Q fever, endemic relapsing fever
Rat flea	Bubonic plague, endemic typhus, *Hymenolepis diminuta*
Trombiculid mite	Scrub typhus, rickettsial pox
Tsetse fly	Sleeping sickness
House fly	Typhoid fever, paratyphoid fever, cholera, gastroenteritis, trachoma
Louse	Epidemic typhus, epidemic relapsing fever, trench fever
Reduvild bug	Chagas disease
Cyclops	Guinea worm disease, fish tape worm

106. Rapid diagnosis of TB is possible by:

a. Auramine rhodamine stain
b. Ziehl-Neelsen stain
c. Giemsa stain
d. Leishman stain

The **auramine-rhodamine stain** (AR), also known as the *Truant auramine-rhodamine stain,* is a histological technique used to visualize acid-fast bacilli using fluorescence microscopy, notably species in the *Mycobacterium* genus. Acid-fast organisms display a reddish-yellow fluorescence. Although the auramine-rhodamine stain is not as specific for acid-fast organisms (i.e. *Mycobacterium tuberculosis* or *Nocardia*) as the Ziehl-Neelsen stain, it is more affordable and more sensitive, therefore it is often utilized as a screening tool. Smears are screened by using 20 × objective, hence can be screened faster (2-minute for 100 fields).

Ans. 104. a. Anthrax **105. d.** Ticks **106. a.** Auramine rhodamine...

107. Mycobacterium TB can be differentiated from other mycobacterium by:
a. Production of niacin
b. Beryl-sulphate test
c. Coagulase test
d. Bile solubility test

Niacin is formed as a metabolic byproduct by all mycobacteria, but some species possess an enzyme that converts free niacin to niacin ribonucleotide. *M. tuberculosis* (and some other species) lack this enzyme, and accumulate niacin as a water-soluble byproduct in the culture medium.

Differences between *M. tuberculosis* and *M. bovis*.

Property	*M. tuberculosis*	*M. bovis*
Acid-fast stain	Curved, long, beaded, less uniformly stained	Straight, short, stout, uniformly stained acid fast bacilli
LJ media	Rough, tough, buff colony	White, smooth, moist colony
Growth	Eugonic	Dysgonic
Glycerol	Helps in growth	No effect on growth
TCH	Resistant to TCH	Sensitive to TCH
Niacin test	Positive	Negative
Nitrate test	Positive	Negative
Rabbit pathogenicity	Not pathogenic	Pathogenic
Oxygen	Obligate aerobe	Microaerophilic
Both are pathogenic to guinea pig and human beings		

TCH: Thiophene caroboxylic acid hydrazide.

108. Selective media for TB bacilli is:
a. NNN medium
b. LJ media
c. Nutrient agar
d. MacConkeys media

The **Löwenstein-Jensen medium**, more commonly known as **LJ medium**, is a growth medium specially used for culture of **Mycobacterium**, notably *Mycobacterium tuberculosis*.

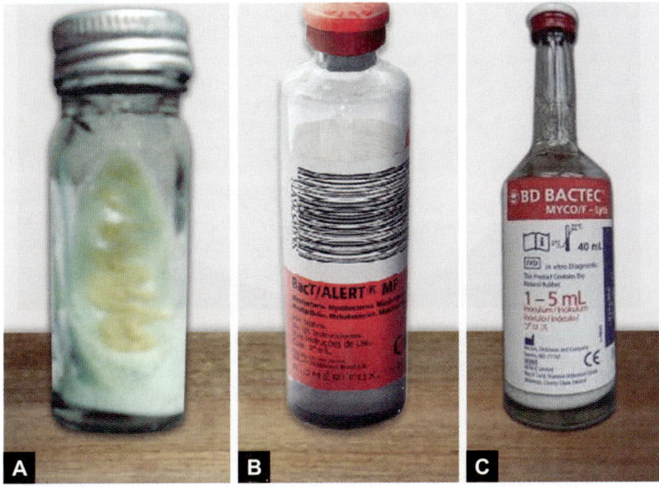

Culture medium for *M. tuberculosis*. (A) Lowenstein-Jensen medium (rough, tough and buff colored colonies); (B) BacT/ALERT bottle; (C) BACTEC bottle.

109. Leprosy spreads by:
a. Skin to skin contact
b. Blood transfusion
c. Breast milk
d. Ingestion

Transmission of leprosy occurs during close contact with those who are infected. Transmission is believed to be by nasal droplets.

110. Leprosy bacilli are cultured on:
a. LJ media
b. Foot pad of mice
c. Agar plate
d. None of the above

While the causative organisms have to date been impossible to culture *in vitro*, it has been possible to grow them in animals such as mice and armadillos.

111. Causative agent of Lyme's disease:
a. Borrelia burgdorferi
b. Borrelia recurrentis
c. Leptospira icterohaemorrhagiae
d. Clostridium difficile

Lyme disease, also known as **Lyme borreliosis**, is an infectious disease caused by bacteria of the *Borrelia* type. The most common sign of infection is an expanding area of redness, known as erythema migrans, that begins at the site of a tick bite about a week after it has occurred. The rash is typically neither itchy nor painful.

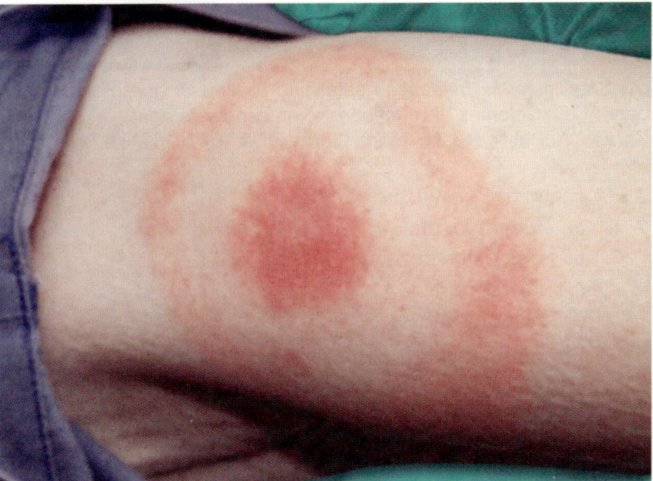

Erythema migrans: Annular bull's eye pattern rash.
Source: Public Health Image Library, Centers for Disease Control and Prevention (CDC), Atlanta, ID# 9874/J. Gathany (with permission).

112. Satellitism on culture is seen in:
a. Proteus
b. Klebsiella
c. Streptococcus
d. Haemophilus

Haemophilus is sometimes cultured using the "Staph streak" technique: both *Staphylococcus* and *Haemophilus* organisms are cultured together on a single blood agar plate. In this case, *Haemophilus* colonies will frequently grow in small "satellite" colonies around the larger *Staphylococcus* colonies because the metabolism of *Staphylococcus* produces the necessary blood factor byproducts required for *Haemophilus* growth.

Ans. 107. **a.** Production... 108. **b.** LJ media 109. **a.** Skin to skin contact 110. **b.** Foot pad of mice
111. **a.** Borrelia... 112. **d.** Haemophilus

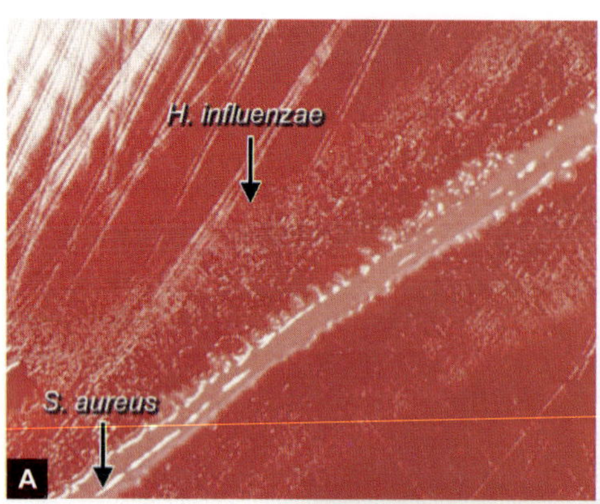

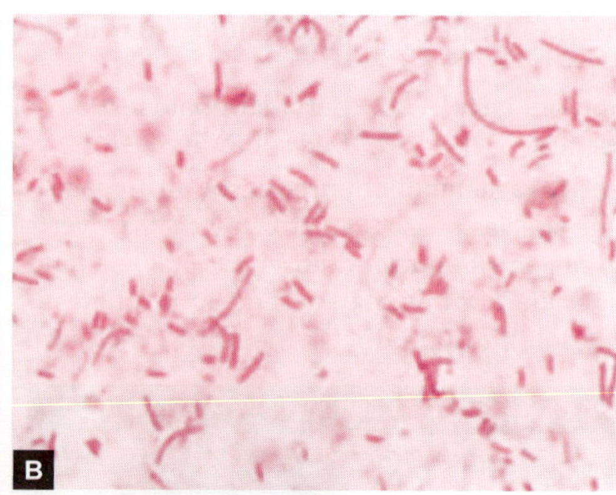

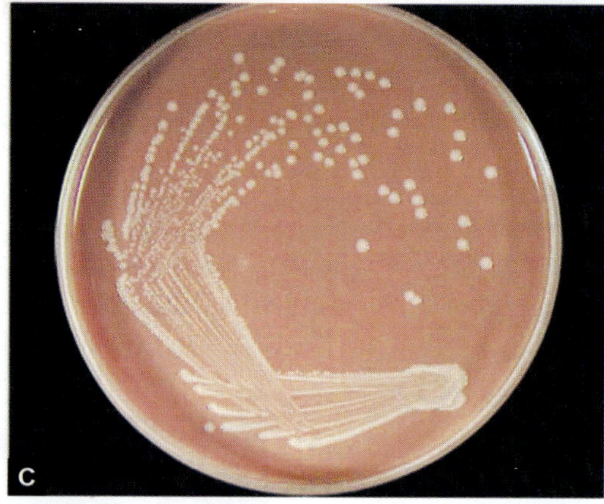

(A) Satellitism: *H. influenzae* satelliting around *S. aureus* streak line; (B) *H. influenzae* in Gram-stained smear (pleomorphic gram-negative bacilli); (C) Colonies of *H. influenzae* on chocolate agar.
Source: A. Public Health Image Library, ID# 1047/Dr. Mike Miller/Centers for Disease Control and Prevention (CDC), Atlanta (with permission).

113. Stalactite growth is a feature of:

a. Mycoplasma
b. Corynebacterium
c. Pasteurella
d. Haemophilus

Stalactite growth pattern is seen for the **growth** of **Yersinia pestis** in ghee broth culture.

114. True regarding typhoid are all EXCEPT:

a. Urinary carriers are more dangerous
b. Vi antibody is used for detecting carrier
c. Vi antibody is seen in normal population
d. Urine carrier is associated with anomalies

The Vi antibody usually disappears early in convalescence, but if persists, indicates the development of the carrier state.

115. Vibrio cholera was discovered by:

a. Koch b. Mekintoff
c. John snow d. Virchow

V. cholerae was first isolated as the cause of cholera by Italian anatomist Filippo Pacini in 1854, but his discovery was not widely known until Robert Koch, working independently 30 years later, publicized the knowledge and the means of fighting the disease.

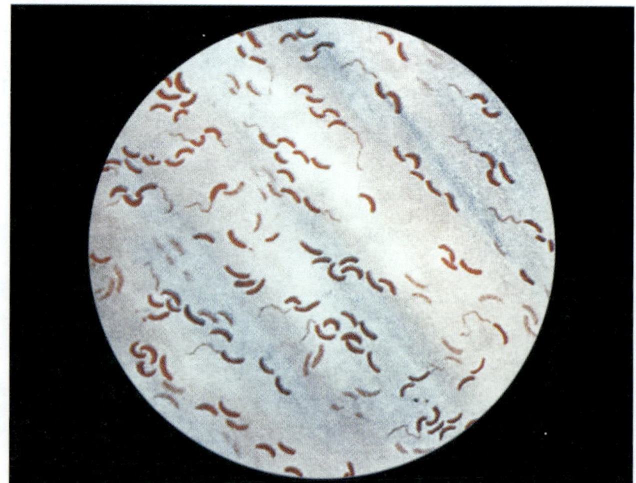

Vibrio cholerae (Gram-stain): Curved comma-shaped gram-negative rods (fish in stream appearance).
Source: Public Health Image Library, ID#:5324/Centers for Disease Control and Prevention (CDC) (with permission).

116. All of the following vibrio species are halophilic EXCEPT:

a. V. cholerae b. V. parahaemolyticus
c. V. alginolyticus d. V. fluvialis

Ans. 113. c. Pasteurella **114. c.** Vi antibody is seen... **115. a.** Koch **116. a.** V. cholerae

The genus vibrios can be divided into **non-halophilic** vibrios, including V. cholerae and other species that are able to grow in a media without added salt and halophilic species like vibrio parahaemolyticus, vibrio alginolyticus and vibrio vulnificus that require salt for growth.

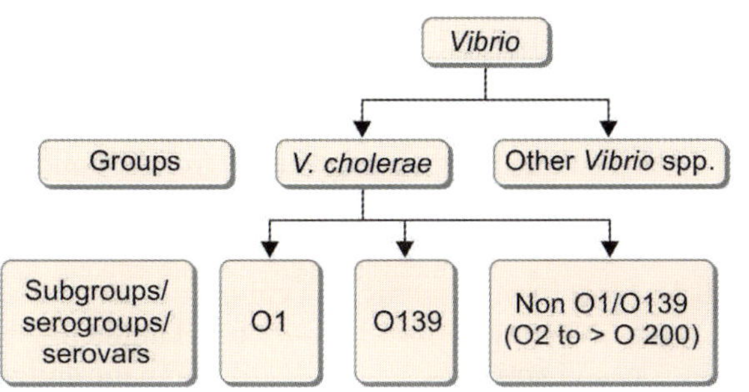

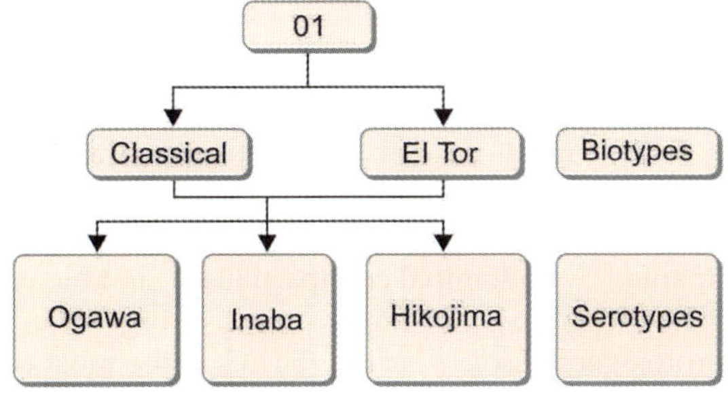

Gardner and Venkatraman classification of V. cholerae.

117. Acid fastness of tubercle bacilli is attributed to:

a. Presence of mycolic acid
b. Integrity of cell wall
c. Both of the above
d. None of the above

The high mycolic acid content of certain Protozoa cell walls, and those of *Mycobacteria*, is responsible for the staining pattern of poor absorption followed by high retention. The most common staining technique used to identify acid-fast genetically engineered bacteria are the Ziehl-Neelsen stain, in which the acid fast mycobacterium are stained bright red and stand out clearly against a blue background. Another method is the Kinyoun method, in which the bacteria are stained bright red and stand out clearly against a green background. Acid-fast Mycobacteria can also be visualized by fluorescence microscopy using specific fluorescent dyes (auramine-rhodamine stain, for example).

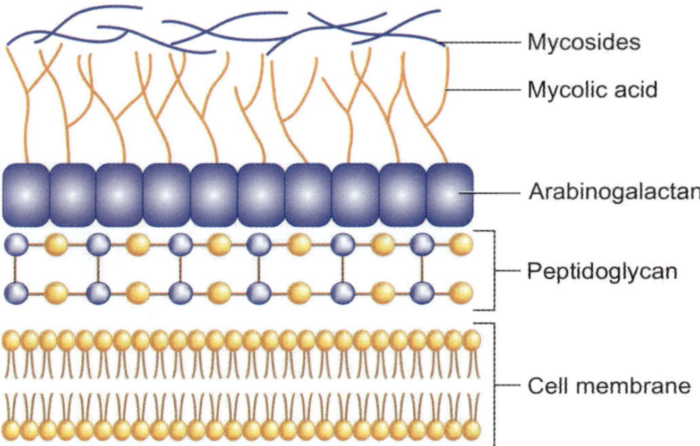

Cell wall of *M. tuberculosis*.

118. The factor which promotes virulence of M. tuberculosis:

a. Wax D
b. Cord factor
c. Muramyl dipeptide
d. Mycolic acid

Cord factor is virulent towards mammalian cells and critical for survival of *M. tuberculosis* in hosts, but not outside of hosts. Cord factor has been observed to influence immune responses, induce the formation of granulomas, and inhibit tumor growth.

119. Tumbling motility is shown by:

a. Listeria
b. Vibrio
c. Proteus mirabilis
d. Proteus vulgaris

Outside the body, *Listeria* has flagellar-driven motility, sometimes described as a "tumbling motility". However, at 37°C, flagella cease to develop and the bacterium instead usurps the host cell's cytoskeleton to move.

Types of motility shown by different bacteria.

Types of motility	*Bacteria*
Tumbling motility	*Listeria*
Gliding motility	*Mycoplasma*
Stately motility	*Clostridium*
Darting motility	*Vibrio cholerae, Campylobacter*
Swarming motility	*Proteus, Clostridium tetani*
Corkscrew, lashing, flexion extension motility	*Spirochete*

120. Organism causing pseudo-membranous colitis:

a. Clostridium botulinum
b. Clostridium tetani
c. Clostridium perfringens
d. Clostridium difficile

***Clostridium difficile* colitis** or **pseudomembranous colitis** is colitis (inflammation of the large intestine) resulting from infection with *Clostridium difficile*, a spore-forming bacterium. It causes an infectious diarrhea called **C. difficile associated diarrhea** (CDAD).

Ans. **117. c.** Both of the above **118. b.** Cord factor **119. a.** Listeria **120. d.** Clostridium difficile

121. MC cause of Traveller's diarrhea:
a. Enterotoxigenic E. coli
b. Enterohemorrhagic E. coli
c. Enteropathogenic E. coli
d. Enteroinvasive E. coli

Traveler's diarrhea (TD), sometimes **tourist diarrhea** or **traveler's dysentery**, is a stomach and intestinal infection, and the most common illness affecting travelers. It is defined as three or more unformed stools passed by a traveler within a 24-hour period. It is commonly accompanied by abdominal cramps, nausea, and bloating. The diagnosis does not imply causative organism, but enterotoxigenic *Escherichia coli* (ETEC) is the most common pathogen.

Agents causing traveler's diarrhea.

Etiologic agent	*Comments*
Bacteria (50–75%)	
Enterotoxigenic *E. coli* (10–45%)	Single most important agent
Enteroaggregative *E. coli* (5–35%)	Emerging enteric pathogen with worldwide distribution
Campylobacter jejuni (5–25%)	More common in Asia
Shigella	Major cause of dysentery
Salmonella	Common agent in India
Others	Including *Aeromonas, Plesiomonas*, and *Vibrio cholerae*
Viruses (<20%)	
Norovirus (<10%)	Associated with cruise ships
Rotavirus (<5%)	Common among children
Parasites (0–10 %)	*Giardia lamblia, Cryptosporidium, Entamoeba histolytica, Cyclospora*

122. Shigellosis is best diagnosed by:
a. Stool examination
b. Stool culture
c. Sigmoidoscopy
d. Enzyme studies

The diagnosis of shigellosis is made by isolating the organism from diarrheal fecal sample cultures. *Shigella* species are negative for motility and are generally not lactose fermenters, but *S. sonnei* can ferment lactose. They typically do not produce gas from carbohydrates (with the exception of certain strains of *S. flexneri*) and tend to be overall biochemically inert. *Shigella* should also be urea hydrolysis negative. When inoculated to a triple sugar iron (TSI) slant, they react as follows: K/A, gas -, and H_2S -. Indole reactions are mixed, positive and negative, with the exception of *S. sonnei*, which is always indole negative. Growth on *Hektoen enteric agar* will produce bluish-green colonies for *Shigella* and bluish-green colonies with black centers for *Salmonella*.

123. Classification of shigella is done on the basis of:
a. Lactose b. Sucrose
c. Mannitol d. Glucose

Shigella dysenteriae (Group A) does not ferment mannitol while the rest three serogroups ferment. Shigella sonnei (group D) is a late lactose fermenter and can be identified by a **positive ONPG test**. It is difficult to differentiate S. flexneri (group B) from S. boydii (group C). Confirmation of their identities can be made by **slide agglutination** using specific antisera.

124. Most immunogenic in Typhoid:
a. O antigen b. H antigen
c. Vi antigen d. Somatic antigen

The **H antigen** is strongly **immunogenic** and induces antibody formation.

Difference between somatic (O) and flagellar (H) antigen.

O antigen	*H antigen*
Somatic antigen It is a part of cell wall lipopolysaccharide (LPS)	**Flagellar antigen** Made up of proteins flagellin It confers motility to the bacteria
Heat stable, Alcohol stable	Heat labile, Alcohol labile
Formaldehyde labile	Formaldehyde stable
In Widal test, O antigen of *S.*Typhi is used	In Widal test, H antigens of *S.*Typhi, *S.*Paratyphi A and B are used
O Ag is less immunogenic	H Ag is more immunogenic
O antibody appears early, disappears early: indicates recent infection	H antibody appears late, disappears late: indicates convalescent stage
When O antigen reacts with O antibody forms compact, granular, chalky clumps ❑ Agglutination takes place slowly ❑ Optimum temperature for agglutination is 55°C	When H antigen reacts with H antibody forms large, loose, fluffy clumps. ❑ Agglutination takes place rapidly. ❑ Optimum temperature for agglutination is 37°C
Serogrouping of salmonellae is based on the O antigen	Serogroups are differentiated into serotypes based on H antigen.
O antigen is also called the Boivin antigen because it can be extracted from the bacterial cell by treatment with trichloracetic acid—this property was first shown by Boivin.	❑ Flagellar antigens exist in two alternative phases—Phase I and II. ❑ Most of them are biphasic except *S.* Typhi which is monophasic.

125. Culture medium in a patient with Legionnaire's disease:
a. Bordet Gengou b. Chocolate agar
c. BCYE medium d. Thayer-Martin medium

Legionella is traditionally detected by culture on buffered charcoal yeast extract (BCYE) agar. *Legionella* requires the presence of cysteine and iron to grow, so does not grow on common blood agar media used for laboratory-based total viable counts or on-site diplslides.

Ans. **121. a.** Enterotoxigenic... **122. b.** Stool culture **123. c.** Mannitol **124. b.** H antigen
125. c. BCYE medium

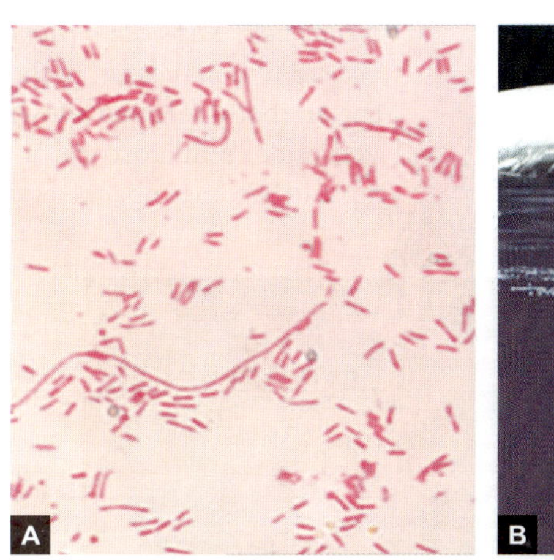
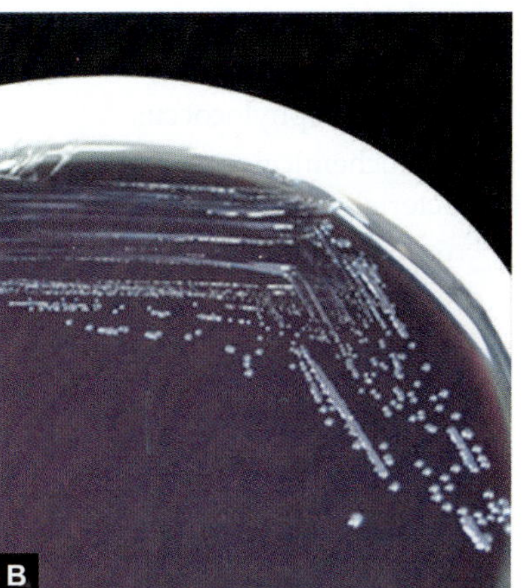

Legionella: (A) Gram-staining; (B) Growth on BCYE agar.
Source: Public Health Image Library, A. ID#: 15328/ Dr. Gilda Jones, B. ID#: 11766/Megan Mathias and J. Todd Parker/Centers for Disease Control and Prevention (CDC), Atlanta (with permission).

126. Bread crumb colony is a feature of:

a. M. leprae
b. Actinomyces israelii
c. Vibrio cholerae
d. Bordetella pertussis

In thioglycollate broth, the Actinomyces israelii grows at the bottom with a large lobulated **'bread-crumb' appearance**.

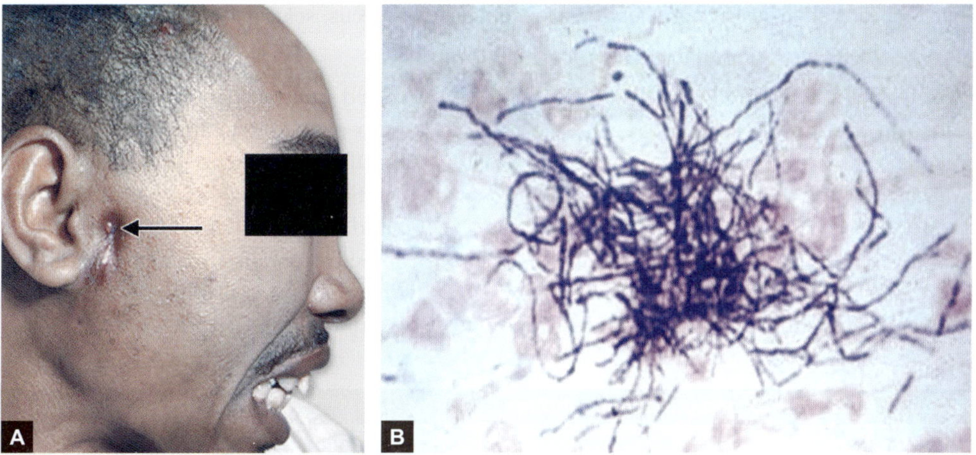
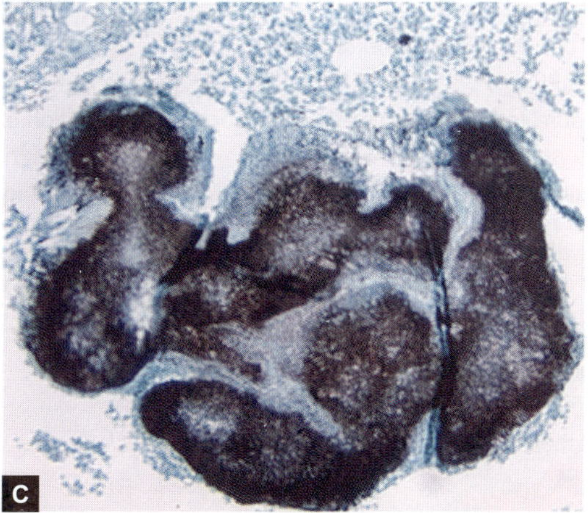

(A) Actinomycosis (painless, slow-growing, hard mass with cutaneous fistula) (arrow showing); *Actinomyces israelii;* (B) Gram-positive filamentous bacilli; (C) Gomori's stained smear showing sun-ray appearance.
Source: A. Public Health Image Library, ID# 2856, C. ID# 10601/Centers for Disease Control and Prevention (CDC), Atlanta (with permission).

Ans. 126. b. Actinomyces...

127. Quellung reaction is seen with:

a. Pneumococcus
b. Gonococcus
c. Streptococcus
d. Staphylococcus

The **Quellung reaction** is a biochemical reaction in which antibodies bind to the bacterial capsule of *Streptococcus pneumoniae, Klebsiella pneumoniae, Neisseria meningitidis, Haemophilus influenzae,* Escherichia coli, and Salmonella. The antibody reaction allows these species to be visualized under a microscope. If the reaction is positive, the capsule becomes opaque and appears to enlarge.

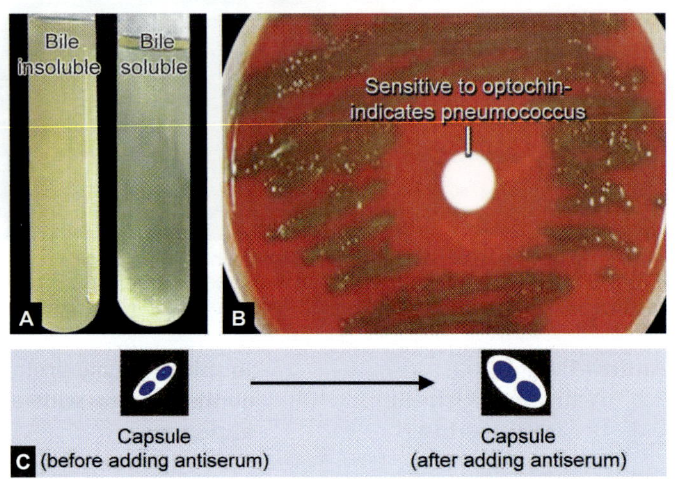

(A) Bile solubility test (left-Viridans streptococci, not soluble in bile; right-pneumococcus, soluble in bile); (B) Optochin sensitivity; (C) Quellung reaction.

128. True about Woolsorter's disease:

a. Pneumonic form of anthrax
b. Pneumonic plague
c. Hydatid disease of lung
d. Caused by psittacosis

Inhalational anthrax is also known as woolsorters or ragpicker's disease. These professions were more susceptible to the disease due to their exposure to infected animal products. Other practices associated with exposure include the slicing up of animal horns for the manufacture of buttons, the handling of hair bristles used for the manufacturing of brushes, and the handling of animal skins. Whether these animal skins came from animals that died of the disease or from animals that had simply lain on ground with spores on it is unknown.

Differences between cutaneous anthrax and pulmonary anthrax.

Features	*Cutaneous anthrax*	*Pulmonary anthrax*
Other name	**Hide porter's disease** (As it commonly occurs in dock workers carrying loads of hides and skins on their bare backs)	**Wool sorter's disease** (As it is seen in workers of wool factory, acquire infection by inhalation of dust from infected wool)
Transmission	Cutaneous exposure to spores (enter through abraded skin)	Inhalation of spores
Characterized by	**Malignant pustule** The lesion begins as a papule that evolves into a painless vesicle followed by the development of a coal-black, necrotic **eschar** surrounded by non-pitting indurated **edema** ❑ The name anthrax, which means coal, comes from the black color of the eschar ❑ However, it is a non-malignant condition.	**Hemorrhagic pneumonia** Bacilli spread by lymphatics or blood, leading to— ❑ Bacteremia ❑ Hemorrhagic mediastinitis ❑ Hemorrhagic meningitis
Occupational exposures	Dock worker, butcher, abattoir and farmer	Workers of wool factory
Occurrence	Most common (95%)	Rare
Prognosis	Self-limiting, rarely becomes fatal if untreated	Fatal
Bioterrorism	Rarely causes bioterrorism	Most common form to cause bioterrorism

Ans. 127. a. Pneumococcus **128. a.** Pneumonic...

129. Botulinum acts at:
- a. Sympathetic system
- b. Parasympathetic system
- c. Amygdala
- d. Motor cortex

The mechanism of action involves toxin-mediated blockade of neuromuscular transmission in cholinergic nerve fibers. This is accomplished by either inhibiting acetylcholine release at the presynaptic clefts of the myoneural junctions or by binding acetylcholine itself.

Bacterial exotoxins and their mechanism of action.

Organisms	*Toxins (Exotoxins)*	*Mechanism*
Staphylococcus aureus	Enterotoxin, Toxic shock syndrome toxin	Act as super antigen; stimulate T cell nonspecifically, to release large amounts of cytokines
Streptococcus pyogenes	Streptococcal pyrogenic exotoxin	
Corynebacterium diphtheriae	Diphtheria toxin (DT)	Inhibits protein synthesis (by inhibiting elongation factor-2)
Bacillus anthracis	Anthrax toxin	↑cAMP in target cell, edema
Clostridium perfringens	α toxin and other major and minor toxins	Lecithinase and phospholipase activity → causes myonecrosis
Clostridium tetani	Tetanus toxin (tetanospasmin)	Decrease in neurotransmitter (GABA and glycine) release from the inhibitory neurons → spastic paralysis
Clostridium botulinum	Botulinum toxin (BT)	Decrease in neurotransmitter (acetyl choline) release from neurons → spastic paralysis
Escherichia coli (diarrheagenic)	Heat labile toxin (LT)	Activation of adenylate cyclase, → cAMP in target cell → secretory diarrhea
	Heat stable toxin (ST)	↑cGMP in target cell → secretory diarrhea
	Verocytotoxin	Inhibit protein synthesis (by inhibiting ribosome)
Shigella dysenteriae type-1	Shiga toxin	
Vibrio cholerae	Cholera toxin (CT)	Activation of adenylate cyclas → cAMP in target cell → secretory diarrhea
Pseudomonas	Exotoxin-A	Inhibit protein synthesis (by inhibiting elongation factor-2)

130. Enteropathogenic E. coli causes:
- a. Causes acute gastroenteritis in infants
- b. Invades intestinal epithelium
- c. Produces cholera like toxin
- d. Non-motile

Flat pink lactose fermenting colonies of *E. coli* on MacConkey agar (arrow showing).

Enteropathogenic E. coli frequently causes infantile diarrhea (outbreaks) and occasionally cause sporadic diarrhea in adults.

131. Species of Pseudomonas, causing infection in intravenous cannulated individuals, most commonly:
- a. P. mallei
- b. P. maltiphila
- c. P. aeruginosa
- d. P. cepacia

Because Pseudomonas aeruginosa thrives on moist surfaces, this bacterium is also found on and in medical equipment, including catheters, causing cross-infections in hospitals and clinics.

132. Staphylococcus aureus virulence is due to:
- a. Pathogenicity correlated with coagulase
- b. Endotoxin
- c. Hemolysis
- d. Pigmented colonies

Coagulase is tightly bound to the surface of the bacterium *S. aureus* and can coat its surface with fibrin upon contact with blood. The fibrin clot may protect the bacterium from phagocytosis and isolate it from other defenses of the host. It has been proposed that fibrin-coated staphylococci resist phagocytosis, making the bacteria more virulent.

Ans. **129. b.** Parasympat... **130. a.** Causes acute... **131. c.** P. aeruginosa **132. a.** Pathogenicity correlated...

Virulence factors of *Staphylococcus aureus.*
Cell wall associated factors
Peptidoglycan Teichoic acid Cell surface adhesins—e.g. clumping factor Protein A
Toxins
Membrane active toxins ❑ Hemolysins—α, β, γ, δ ❑ Leukocidin (or panton valentine toxin)
Epidermolytic toxin (exfoliative toxin) Enterotoxins Toxic shock syndrome toxin
Extracellular enzymes
Coagulase Heat stable thermonuclease Deoxyribonuclease Staphylokinase (fibrinolysin) Others—hyaluronidase, lipase, and protease

133. True regarding streptococcus pneumoniae:

a. Vaccine made from capsular polysaccharide
b. Vaccine is routinely given to Indian children
c. Catalase and oxidase positive
d. Bile insoluble and optochin sensitive

The polysaccharide pneumococcal vaccine most commonly used today consists of purified polysaccharides from 23 serotypes (1, 2, 3, 4, 5, 6b, 7F, 8,9N, 9V, 10A, 11A, 12F, 14, 15B, 17F, 18C, 19F, 19A, 20, 22F, 23F, and 33F). Immunity is induced primarily through stimulation of B-cells which release IgM without the assistance of T cells.

Differences between *Streptococcus pneumoniae* and Viridans streptococci

Features	*S. pneumoniae*	*Viridans streptococci*
Arrangement	Gram-positive cocci in pairs	Gram-positive cocci in long chains
Morphology	Lanceolate or flame shaped	Round/oval
Capsule	Present	Absent
On blood agar	Draughtsman or carom coin colony	Convex shaped colony
Liquid medium	Uniform turbidity	Granular turbidity
Bile solubility	Soluble in bile	Insoluble in bile
Inulin fermentation	Fermenter	Non fermenter
Optochin	Sensitive	Resistant
Mice pathogenicity	Pathogenic	Non-pathogenic

134. Gonococcus ferments:

a. Glucose
b. Maltose
c. Sucrose
d. Fructose

Neisseria is usually isolated on Thayer-Martin agar (or VPN agar)—an agar plate containing antibiotics (vancomycin, colistin, nystatin, and trimethoprim) and nutrients that facilitate the growth of *Neisseria* species while inhibiting the growth of contaminating bacteria and fungi. Further testing to differentiate the species includes testing for oxidase (all clinically relevant *Neisseria* show a positive reaction) and the carbohydrates maltose, sucrose, and glucose test in which *N. gonorrhoeae* will oxidize (that is, utilize) only the glucose.

Differences between *Neisseria meningitidis* and *Neisseria gonorrhoeae.*

N. meningitidis	*N. gonorrhoeae*
Capsulated	Noncapsulated
Lens-shaped/half moon-shaped (diplococci with adjacent sides flattened)	Kidney-shaped (diplococci with adjacent sides concave)
Ferment glucose and maltose	Ferments only glucose
Rarely have plasmids	Usually possess plasmids, coding for drug-resistant genes
Exist in both intra- and extracellular forms	Predominantly exist in intracellular form
Colony—circular	Colony—varies in size with irregular margin
Habitat—nasopharynx	Habitat—genital tract (urethra, cervix), rarely pharynx

135. Gonococcus is:

a. Extracellular gram positive
b. Intracytoplasmic gram positive
c. Intracytoplasmic gram negative
d. Intranuclear gram positive

Neisseria are fastidious Gram-negative cocci that require nutrient supplementation to grow in laboratory cultures. To be specific, they grow on chocolate agar with carbon dioxide. These cocci are facultatively intracellular and typically appear in pairs (diplococci), in the shape of coffee beans.

136. WRONG statement about Corynebacterium diphtheriae:

a. Gram negative
b. Ernest Babes granules
c. Chinese letter pattern
d. Prevented by immunization

Corynebacterium diphtheriae is the gram positive pathogenic bacterium that causes diphtheria. It is also known as the **Klebs-Löffler bacillus**, because it was discovered in 1884 by German bacteriologists Edwin Klebs (1834–1912) and Friedrich Löffler (1852–1915).

Ans. **133. a.** Vaccine made... **134. a.** Glucose **135. c.** Intracytoplasmic... **136. a.** Gram negative

Classification of bacteria depending on their morphology and Gram staining property.	
Bacteria	*Example*
Gram-positive cocci arranged in	
Cluster	Staphylococcus
Chain	*Streptococcus*
Pairs, lanceolate shaped	*Pneumococcus*
Pair or in short chain, spectacle eyed shape	*Enterococcus*
Tetrads	*Micrococcus*
Octate	*Sarcina*
Gram-negative cocci arranged in	
Pairs, lens shaped	Meningococcus
Pairs, kidney shaped	Gonococcus
Gram-positive bacilli arranged in	
Chain (bamboo stick appearance)	*Bacillus anthracis*
Chain	*Streptobacillus*
Chinese letter or cuneiform pattern	*Corynebacterium diphtheriae*
Palisade pattern	Diphtheroids
Branched and filamentous form	*Actinomyces* and *Nocardia*
Gram-negative bacilli arranged in	
Pleomorphic (various shapes)	*Haemophilus, Proteus*
Thumb print appearance	*Bordetella pertussis*
Comma shaped (fish in stream appearance)	*Vibrio cholerae*
Curved	*Campylobacter* (Gull-wing shaped) and *Helicobacter*
Spirally coiled, flexible	*Spirochetes*
Rigid spiral forms	*Spirillum*
Bacteria that lack cell wall	*Mycoplasma*

137. FALSE regarding Campylobacter:

a. C. jejuni may cause GB syndrome
b. Campylobacteriosis is due to C. jejuni
c. Source of infection is poultry
d. Human is the only reservoir

Campylobacter (meaning "curved bacteria") is a genus of Gram-negative, microaerophilic, oxidase-positive, nonfermentative bacteria. *Campylobacter* species are typically spiral-shaped and able to move via unipolar or bipolar flagella. Most *Campylobacter* species are pathogenic and can infect humans and other animals.

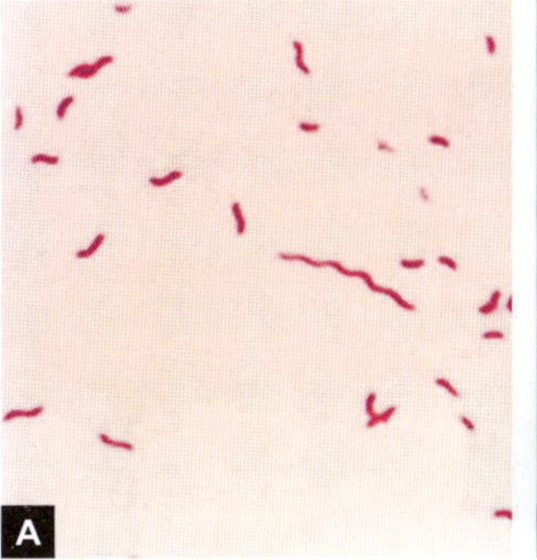

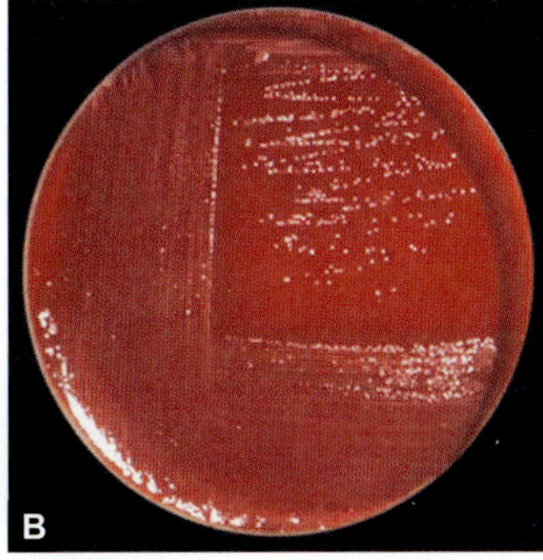

Campylobacter—(A) Gram-negative spiral rods; (B) Growth on Skirrow's media.
Source: Public Health Image Library: A. ID#: 6657; B. D#: 3918/ Centers for Disease Control and Prevention (CDC), Atlanta (with permission).

138. FALSE for N. gonorrhoeae:

a. Some strains may cause disseminated disease
b. Highly sensitive to penicillin
c. Acute urethritis is the MC manifestation in males
d. Exclusive human pathogen

If *N. gonorrhoeae* is resistant to the penicillin family of antibiotics, then ceftriaxone (a third-generation cephalosporin) is often used. Sexual partners should also be notified and treated.

Drug resistance in gonococci.	
PPNG	Penicillinase producing strains of *Neisseria gonorrhoeae*: ❑ Originated from Africa and Asia in 1976; later on, spread worldwide ❑ Plasmids coding for β-lactamases are transferred horizontally by conjugation
CMRNG	Chromosomally mediated resistant *N. gonorrhoeae*: ❑ Show resistance to penicillin and also to tetracycline ❑ It is due to mutations at multiple sites, which decrease the permeability of the cell to antibiotics
TRNG	Tetracycline-resistant *N. gonorrhoeae*; plasmid-borne
QRNG	Quinolone-resistant *N. gonorrhoeae*

139. NOT a constituent of HACEK group of organisms:

a. Eikenella corrodens
b. Cardiobacterium hominis
c. Acinetobacter baumannii
d. Haemophilus aphrophilus

HACEK is an abbreviation of the initials of the genera of this group of bacteria: *Haemophilus, Aggregatibacter* (previously *Actinobacillus*), *Cardiobacterium, Eikenella corrodens, Kingella.* The HACEK organisms are a normal part of the human flora, living in the oralpharyngeal region.

Ans. **137. d.** Human is the... **138. b.** Highly sensitive... **139. c.** Acinetobacter...

140. Malta fever is caused by:

a. Pseudomonas aeruginosa
b. Brucella melitensis
c. Borrelia burgdorferi
d. Treponema pallidum

Brucellosis, **Bang's disease**, **Crimean fever**, **Gibraltar fever**, **Malta fever**, **Maltese fever**, **Mediterranean fever**, **rock fever**, or **undulant fever**, is a highly contagious zoönosis caused by ingestion of unpasteurized milk or undercooked meat from infected animals or close contact with their secretions.

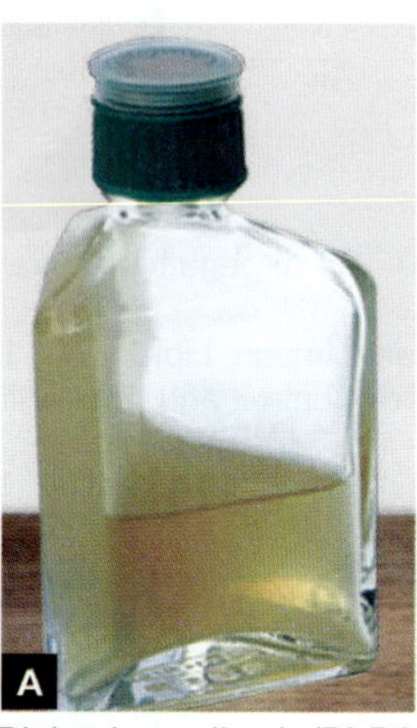

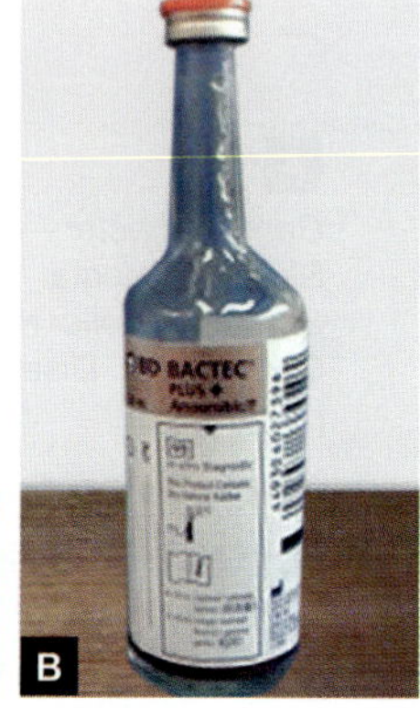

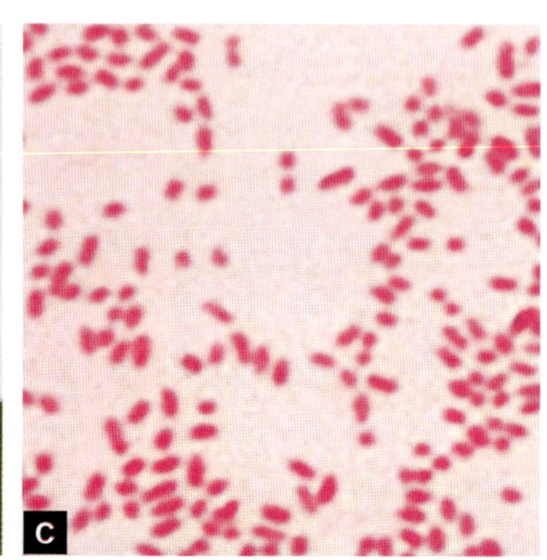

(A) Blood culture bottles (Biphasic medium); (B) BACTEC; (C) Gram-stained smear of Brucella species showing small gram-negative coccobacilli.
Source: C. Public Health Image Library, ID# /15243, Dr. W.A. Clark/Centers for Disease Control and Prevention (CDC), Atlanta (with permission).

141. Neisseria meningitis can be differentiated from Neisseria gonorrhoeae as:

a. It reduces nitrates
b. It ferments maltose
c. It ferments glucose
d. It is oxidase positive

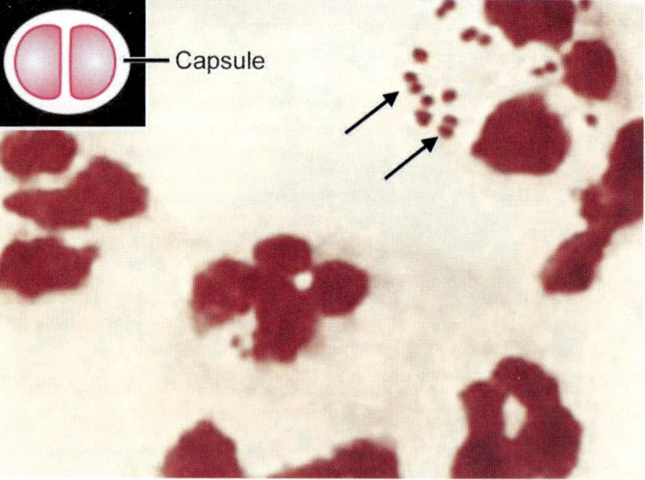

Meningococci in CSF smear (gram-negative diplococci, lens-shaped) (arrows showing).
Source: Centers for Disease Control and Prevention (CDC), Atlanta (with permission).

142. Colour of granules produced by actinomycetes:

a. White
b. Blue
c. Yellow
d. Black

When the vial of pus is rotated, the yellow sulfur granules, characteristic of this organism, can be seen with the naked eye. These granules can also be seen by running sterile water over the gauze used to cover the lesion. The water washes away the purulent material leaving the golden granules on the gauze. This organism, which occurs worldwide, can be seen histologically as "sulfur granules" surrounded by polymorphonuclear cells (PMN) forming the purulent tissue reaction.

143. Cholera toxin:

a. Increases the level of intracellular cyclic GMP
b. Acts through the receptor of opiates
c. Causes continued activation of adenylate cyclase
d. Inhibits the enzyme phosphor-di-esterase

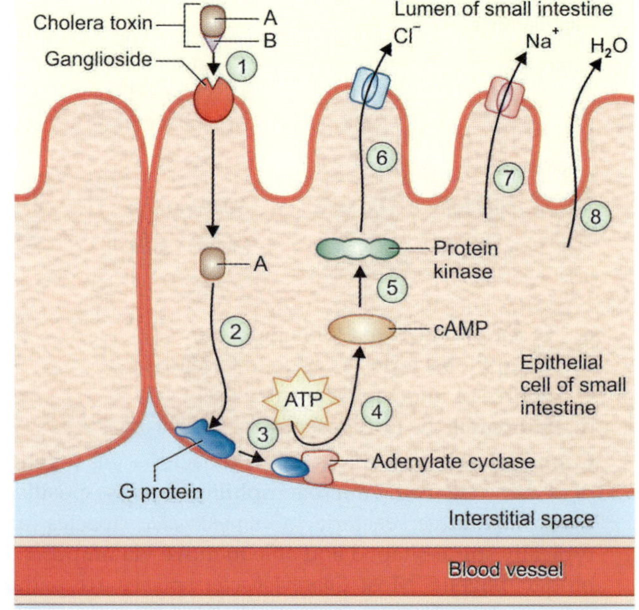

Mechanism of action of cholera toxin.

Ans. **140. b.** Brucella... **141. b.** It ferments maltose **142. c.** Yellow **143. c.** Causes continued...

The cholera toxin is an oligomeric complex made up of six protein subunits: a single copy of the A subunit (part A, enzymatic), and five copies of the B subunit (part B, receptor binding), denoted as AB_5. Subunit B binds while subunit A activates the G protein which activates adenylate cyclase.

144. Dorset's egg medium is used for:

a. Staphylococcus b. Streptococcus
c. Gonococcus d. Mycobacterium

Dorset egg culture medium: A **medium** for cultivating **Mycobacterium** tuberculosis; it consists of the whites and yolks of four fresh **eggs** and a solution of sodium chloride.

145. Which of the following are bounded by membrane containing sterols:

a. Klebsiella b. Staphylococcus
c. Mycobacteria d. Mycoplasma

Mycoplasma species are the smallest free-living organisms. These organisms are unique among prokaryotes in that they lack a cell wall, a feature largely responsible for their biologic properties such as their lack of a reaction to Gram stain and their lack of susceptibility to many commonly prescribed antimicrobial agents, including beta-lactams. Mycoplasmal organisms are usually associated with mucosal surfaces, residing extracellularly in the respiratory and urogenital tracts. They rarely penetrate the submucosa, except in the case of immunosuppression or instrumentation, when they may invade the bloodstream and disseminate to different organs and tissues throughout the body.

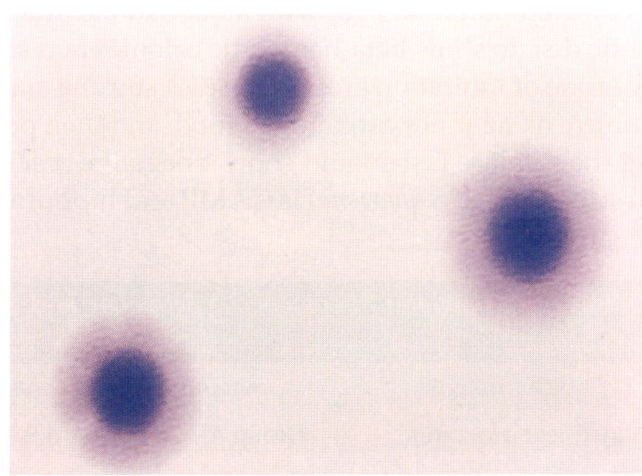

Mycoplasma colonies (typical fried egg appearance).
Source: Public Health Image Library, ID# 11024/Dr. E. Arum; Dr. N. Jacobs/Centers for Disease Control and Prevention (CDC), Atlanta (with permission).

146. Stain employed for mycoplasma is:

a. Acid fast b. Giemsa stain
c. Methylene blue d. Congo red

Mycoplasma is the smallest free living organism. It is polymorphic, coccid or coccobacilli when stained by Giemsa stain or Dienes stain. Mycoplasma is weakly Gram-ve, has no cell wall but possesses triple layered plasma membrane.

147. Number of bacteria in urine sample (per ml) to label it as significant bacteriuria is:

a. 100/mL b. 1,000/mL
c. 10,000/mL d. 100,000/mL

As Per Infectious Disease Society of America guidelines, bacteriuria can be confirmed if a single bacterial species is isolated in a concentration greater than 100,000 colony forming units per millilitre of urine in clean-catch midstream urine specimens (one for men, two consecutive specimens with the same bacterium for women). For urine collected via bladder catheterization in men and women, a single urine specimen with greater than 100,000 colony forming units of a single species per millilitre is considered diagnostic. The threshold is also 100 colony forming units of a single species per millilitre for women displaying UTI symptoms.

Common microorganisms causing UTIs.

Bacterial agents	*Other agents*
Gram-negative Bacilli: ❑ ***Escherichia coli:*** Most common ❑ Klebsiella pneumoniae ❑ Proteus mirabilis ❑ Pseudomonas aeruginosa	**Fungus:** *Candida albicans* **Parasites:** ❑ *Schistosoma hematobium* ❑ *Trichomonas vaginalis*
❑ *Acinetobacter* species ❑ *Enterobacter* species ❑ *Serratia* species	
Gram-positive Cocci: ❑ *Staphylococcus saprophyticus* ❑ *Staphylococcus aureus* ❑ *Staphylococcus epidermidis* ❑ *Enterococcus* species	**Viruses:** ❑ Herpes simplex virus ❑ Adenovirus ❑ JC and BK virus ❑ Cytomegalovirus

UTI: Urinary tract infection; JC: John Cunningham

148. Which of the following is responsible for crepitations in wounds:

a. Staphylococcus b. Mycobacterium
c. Streptococcus d. Clostridium

Gas gangrene (also known as clostridial myonecrosis and myonecrosis) is a bacterial infection that produces gas in tissues in gangrene. This deadly form of gangrene usually is caused by *Clostridium perfringens* bacteria.

Classification of *Clostridium perfringens*

Types	*Major toxin produced*	*Disease*
A	Alpha	Gas gangrene, food poisoning
B	Alpha, beta and epsilon	Lamb dysentery
C	Alpha and beta	Enteritis necroticans in humans
D	Alpha and epsilon	Enterotoxemia and pulpy kidney disease in sheep
E	Alpha and iota	Possible pathogen of sheep and cattle

Ans. 144. **d.** Mycobacterium 145. **d.** Mycoplasma 146. **b.** Giemsa stain 147. **d.** 100,000/mL
148. **d.** Clostridium

149. E. coli causes:

a. Diarrhea
b. Septicemia
c. Urinary tract infection
d. All of the above

Most *E. coli* strains do not cause disease, but virulent strains can cause gastroenteritis, urinary tract infections, and neonatal meningitis.

Sample collection in *E. coli* infections.	
Specimens collected	*Disease*
Pus, exudates and wound swab	Cellulitis or wound infection
Urine	Urinary tract infections (UTI)
Stool	Diarrhea
Cerebrospinal fluid (CSF)	Meningitis
Peritoneal exudate	Peritonitis
Sputum	Pneumonia
Tracheal aspirate	Ventilator-associated pneumonia
Blood	Bacteremia

150. In the small intestine, cholera toxin acts by:

a. ADP ribosylation of the G regulatory protein
b. Inhibition of adenylyl cyclase
c. Activation of GTPase
d. Active absorption of NaCl

When cholera toxin is released from the bacteria in the infected intestine, it binds to the intestinal cells known as enterocytes (epithelial cell in above diagram) through the interaction of the pentameric B subunit of the toxin with the GM1 ganglioside receptor on the intestinal cell, triggering endocytosis of the toxin. Next, the A/B cholera toxin must undergo cleavage of the A1 domain from the A2 domain in order for A1 to become an active enzyme. Once inside the enterocyte, the enzymatic A1 fragment of the toxin A subunit enters the cytosol, where it activates the G protein G_s through an ADP-ribosylation reaction that acts to lock the G protein in its GTP-bound form, thereby continually stimulating adenylate cyclase to produce cAMP. The high cAMP levels activate the cystic fibrosis transmembrane conductance regulator (CFTR), causing a dramatic efflux of ions and water from infected enterocytes, leading to watery diarrhea.

Complications of cholera.	
Loss of body weight by	*Symptoms*
<5%	Increased thirst
At 5–10%	❑ Postural hypotension ❑ Weakness ❑ Tachycardia ❑ Decreased skin turgor
At >10%	Renal failure (due to acute tubular necrosis) and fluid loss result in— ❑ Oliguria ❑ Weak or absent pulses ❑ Sunken eyes ❑ Sunken fontanelles in infants ❑ Wrinkled ("washerwoman") skin ❑ Somnolence and coma

151. Darting motility, which occur in V. cholera, also found in:

a. Shigella
b. Campylobacter jejuni
c. Pneumococcus
d. Bacillus anthrax

Campylobacter: Characteristic rapid **darting motility** by means of long sheathed polar flagellum at one (**polar**) or both (**bipolar**) ends of the cell that may be up to several times the length of the cell; motility slows quickly in wet mount microscopy preparation due to entangling of flagella and aerotoxicity (oxygen sensitivity).

152. Bacitracin sensitivity is used for:

a. Streptococcus viridans
b. Streptococcus pneumoniae
c. Streptococcus agalactiae
d. Streptococcus pyogenes

Streptococcus pyogenes: A Gram stain is performed to show Gram-positive cocci in chains. Then, the organism is cultured on blood agar with an added bacitracin antibiotic disk to show beta-hemolytic colonies and sensitivity (zone of inhibition around the disk) for the antibiotic. Culture on agar not containing blood, and then performing the catalase test should show a negative reaction for all streptococci. *S. pyogenes* is CAMP and hippurate tests negative.

Differences between *Streptococcus pyogenes* and *S. agalactiae.*		
Characters	*S. pyogenes*	*S. agalactiae*
Lancefield grouping	Group A	Group B
Bacitracin sensitivity test	Sensitive	Resistant
PYR test	Positive	Negative
Hippurate hydrolysis test	Negative	Positive
CAMP test	Negative	Positive
β hemolytic colonies	0.5–1 mm, pin point	Mucoid, larger (2 mm)

153. Staph food poisoning includes the following feature:

a. Incubation period of 24 hours
b. Requires immediate antibiotics
c. Common with dairy products
d. Heat labile enterotoxin

Ans. **149. d.** All of the above **150. a.** ADP ribosylation... **151. b.** Campylobacter... **152. d.** Streptococcus... **153. c.** Common with...

Staphylococcus aureus is a common bacterium found in the nose and on the skin of about 25 percent of healthy people and animals. It is a common cause of food poisoning; in fact, it is capable of making seven different toxins that frequently cause food poisoning. It is most commonly transferred to food products such as milk and cheese through contact with contaminated food workers.

Infectious agents of food poisoning.

Incubation period, Organism	*Symptoms*	*Common food sources*
1–6 h		
Staphylococcus aureus	Nausea, vomiting, diarrhea	Ham, poultry, potato or egg salad, mayonnaise, pastries
Bacillus cereus	Nausea, vomiting, diarrhea	Fried rice
Clostridium botulinum	Nausea, vomiting, diarrhea	Canned food
8–16 h		
Clostridium perfringens	Abdominal cramps, diarrhea (vomiting rare)	Beef, poultry, legumes, gravies
B. cereus	Abdominal cramps, diarrhea (vomiting rare)	Meats, vegetables, dried beans, cereals
>16 h		
Vibrio cholerae	Watery diarrhea	Shellfish, water
Enterotoxigenic *E. coli*	Watery diarrhea	Salads, cheese, meat, water
Enterohemorrhagic *E. coli*	Bloody diarrhea	Ground beef, salami, raw milk, raw vegetables, apple juice
Salmonella species	Inflammatory diarrhea	Beef, poultry, eggs, dairy products
Campylobacter jejuni	Inflammatory diarrhea	Poultry, raw milk
Shigella species	Dysentery	Potato or egg salad, lettuce, raw vegetables
Vibrio parahaemolyticus	Dysentery	Mollusks, crustaceans

154. A bacterial disease that has been associated with the 3 'Rs' i.e. rats, ricefields, and rainfall is:
a. Leptospirosis
b. Plague
c. Melioidosis
d. Rodent-bite fever

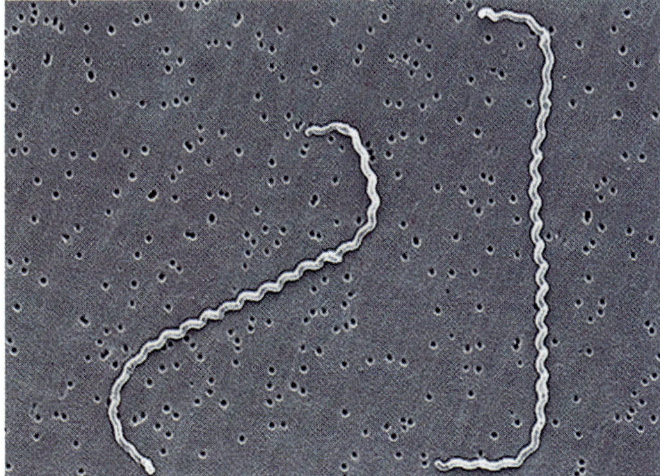

Leptospira interrogans (hooked ends). Dark ground microscopy.
Source: Public Health Image Library, ID# 1220/ NCID/ Rob Weyant/ Centers for Disease Control and Prevention (CDC), Atlanta (with permission).

Up to 13 different genetic types of *Leptospira* may cause disease in humans. It is transmitted by both wild and domestic animals. The most common animals that spread the disease are rodents. It is often transmitted by animal urine or by water or soil containing animal urine coming into contact with breaks in the skin, eyes, mouth, or nose. In the developing world the disease most commonly occurs in farmers and poor people who live in cities.

155. Xanthogranulomatous pyelonephritis is often associated with infection by:
a. Proteus
b. E. coli
c. H. influenzae
d. Klebsiella

Xanthogranulomatous pyelonephritis is an uncommon chronic destructive granulomatous process of renal parenchyma in association with long-term urinary tract obstruction and infection. It affects females more often than males, with a wide range of age, from newborn to elderly. Almost all patients are symptomatic and the most common symptoms are flank or abdominal pain, lower urinary tract symptoms, fever, palpable mass, gross hematuria, and weight loss. The common laboratory findings are leukocytosis and anemia. Urine cultures most often reveal Escherichia coli and Proteus mirabilis.

Ans. 154. a. Leptospirosis **155. a.** Proteus

156. The characteristic feature of Eltor vibrio are all EXCEPT:

a. More of subclinical cases
b. Mortality is less
c. Secondary attack rate is high in family
d. Eltor vibrio is harder and able to survive longer

An El Tor infection is relatively mild, or at least rarely fatal, and patients are asymptomatic for about a week. El Tor is able to survive in the body longer than classical cholera vibrios. This characteristic allows carriers to infect a greater population of people. In fact, *V. cholerae* biotype eltor can be isolated from water sources in the absence of an outbreak of cases. In extreme cases, persons can become long-term carriers; for example, Cholera Dolores, who tested vibrio positive nine years after her primary infection. El Tor is transmitted by the fecal-oral route. This route is the consequence of infected persons defeca.

Differences between classical and El Tor *V. cholerae*.

*Biotypes of **V. cholerae** O1*	*Classical biotype*	*El Tor biotype*
β hemolysis on sheep blood agar	Negative	Positive
Chick erythrocyte agglutination	Negative	Positive
Polymyxin B (50 IU)	Susceptible	Resistant
Group IV phage susceptibility	Susceptible	Resistant
El Tor Phage V susceptibility	Resistant	Susceptible
VP (Voges Proskauer) test	Negative	Positive
CAMP test	Negative	Positive
Cholera toxin gene	CTX-1	CTX-2

CAMP test: Christie Atkins Munch-Petersen test.

157. About Helicobacter pylori, all are true EXCEPT:

a. Is a gram negative bacteria
b. Uncommon in developing Asian countries
c. Urea breath test +ve
d. Associated with duodenal ulcer

More than 50% of the world's population harbor *H. pylori* in their upper gastrointestinal tract. Infection is more prevalent in developing countries, and incidence is decreasing in Western countries. *H. pylori's* helical shape (from which the genus name is derived) is thought to have evolved to penetrate the mucoid lining of the stomach.

158. Ascending UTI caused by all EXCEPT:

a. Salmonella
b. E. coli
c. Chlamydia
d. Klebsiella

E. coli is the cause of 80–85% of community-acquired urinary tract infections, with *Staphylococcus saprophyticus* being the cause in 5–10%. Rarely they may be due to viral or fungal infections. Healthcare-associated urinary tract infections (mostly related to urinary catheterization) involve a much broader range of pathogens including: *E. coli* (27%), *Klebsiella* (11%), *Pseudomonas* (11%), the fungal pathogen *Candida albicans* (9%), and *Enterococcus* (7%) among others. Urinary tract infections due to *Staphylococcus aureus* typically occur secondary to blood-borne infections. *Chlamydia trachomatis* and *Mycoplasma genitalium* can infect the urethra but not the bladder. These infections are usually classified as a urethritis rather than urinary tract infection.

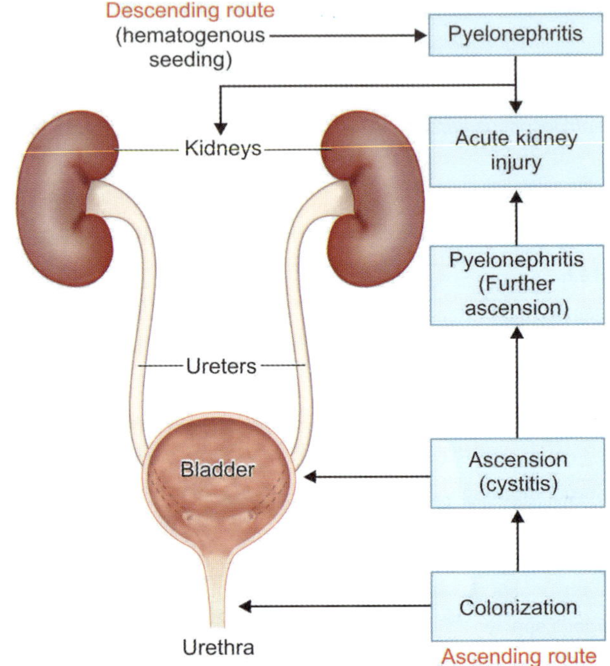

Pathogenesis of urinary tract infection.

159. Gas gangrene is caused by:

a. Clostridium welchii
b. Clostridium tetani
c. Clostridium botulinum
d. Clostridium difficile

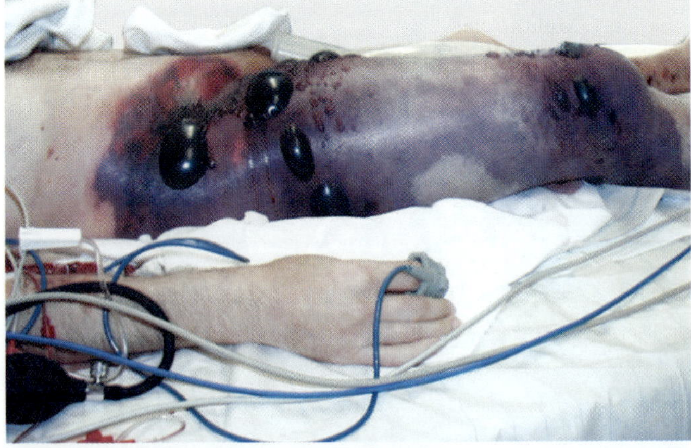

Gas gangrene of the right leg showing swelling and discoloration of the right thigh with bullae, and palpable crepitus.

Source: Wikipedia/Cases/Engelbert Schröpfer, Stephan Rauthe and Thomas Meyer (with permission).

Gas gangrene and clostridial myonecrosis are interchangeable terms used to describe an infection of muscle tissue by toxin-producing clostridia. In 1861, Louis Pasteur identified the first clostridial species, *Clostridium*

Ans. **156. c.** Secondary attack... **157. b.** Uncommon in... **158. a.** Salmonella **159. a.** Clostridium...

butyricum. In 1892 and later, Welch, Nuttall, and other scientists isolated a gram-positive anaerobic bacillus from gangrenous wounds. This organism, originally known as *Bacillus aerogenes capsulatus,* was later renamed *Bacillus perfringens,* and then *Clostridium welchii.* The organism is now named *Clostridium perfringens.*

160. Clostridium botulinum toxin mode of action is by:

a. Presynaptic block
b. Postsynaptic block
c. Competitive inhibition of acetylcholine
d. Destruction of acetylcholine

After entry (either ingested, inhaled, or produced in a wound), botulinum toxin is transported via blood to peripheral cholinergic nerve terminals. The most common nerve terminal sites are neuromuscular junctions, postganglionic parasympathetic nerve endings, and peripheral ganglia. It does NOT affect CNS.

Pathogenic mechanisms of diarrheal agents.

Toxins production		
Enterotoxins Cholera toxin *Vibrio parahaemolyticus* *E. coli* ❑ LT and ST of ETEC ❑ EAST of EAEC ❑ VT of EHEC *Clostridium difficile* (toxin A) *Aeromonas* *Rotavirus (NSP4)* *Campylobacter jejuni*	**Cytotoxins** *Shigella dysenteriae* type 1 Enterohemorrhagic *E.coli* *Clostridium difficile* (toxin B)	**Neurotoxins** *Staphylococcus aureus* enterotoxin *Bacillus cereus* toxin *Clostridium botulinum* toxin
E. coli ❑ Enteropathogenic ❑ Enterohemorrhagic *Cryptosporidium* species *Cyclospora* species Rotavirus Norovirus	*Shigella* species Enteroinvasive *E. coli* *Campylobacter jejuni* *Yersinia enterocolitica* *Plesiomonas shigelloides* *Entamoeba histolytica* *Balantidium coli*	

LT: Heat labile toxin; ST: Heat stable toxin; ETEC: Enterotoxigenic E. coli; EAST: Enteroaggregative *E. coli* heat-stable enterotoxin; EAEC: Enteroaggregative *E. coli*; VT: verocytotoxin; EHEC: Enterohaemorrhagic *E. coli*; NSP4: non-structural protein-4

161. Most common cause of meningitis in adults:

a. Neisseria meningitidis
b. Streptococcus pneumoniae
c. L. monocytogenes
d. H. influenzae

In adults, *Neisseria meningitidis* and *Streptococcus pneumoniae* together cause 80% of bacterial meningitis cases. Risk of infection with *Listeria monocytogenes* is increased in persons over 50 years old. The introduction of pneumococcal vaccine has lowered rates of pneumococcal meningitis in both children and adults.

Causes of pyogenic meningitis.

Age	*Common causes*
Neonates or Infants of 0–2 months	❑ *Escherichia coli* ❑ Group B *Streptococcus* (*S. agalactiae)* ❑ Other gram-negative *bacilli* (like *Klebsiella pneumoniae)* ❑ *Listeria monocytogenes*
2–20 years	❑ *Neisseria meningitidis:* Most common ❑ *Haemophilus influenzae* ❑ *Streptococcus pneumoniae*
> 20 years (adults)	❑ *Streptococcus pneumoniae:* Most common agent ❑ *Haemophilus influenzae** ❑ *Neisseria meningitidis*
Overall	Most common agent is: *Streptococcus pneumoniae*

*Incidence of *H. influenzae* meningitis has been dramatically reduced after the start of Hib vaccination.

162. Enteric fever diagnosis in 2nd week is best made by:

a. Blood
b. Widal test
c. Stool
d. Widal

Typhoid in second week

- During the second week the patient has a toxic appearance with apathy and sustained pyrexia.
- High fever around 40°C (104°F), often swinging.
- Malaise and weakness.
- Relative bradycardia, with dicrotic pulse wave.
- Confusional state, which gave typhoid the name of 'nervous fever'.
- Rose spots on the lower chest and abdomen - seen in around one third of Caucasian patients; difficult to see in darker skin. Rose spots are caused by bacterial emboli. They are crops of macules 2–4 mm in diameter that blanch on pressure.
- Lung base rhonchi.
- Abdominal distension with right lower quadrant tenderness and increased borborygmi.
- Diarrhoea, typically green, with a characteristic foul smell, often compared to pea soup.
- Constipation may also occur.
- Hepatosplenomegaly is common.
- Elevated liver transaminases.
- Positive Widal's test.

Various tests used for diagnosis of enteric fever depending upon duration of illness.

Duration of illness	*Specimen used and test(s) done*
First week	Culture of: ❑ Blood ❑ Bone marrow aspirate ❑ Duodenal aspirate

Contd...

Ans. 160. a. Presynaptic... **161. b.** Streptococcus... **162. b.** Widal test

Contd...

Duration of illness	*Specimen used and test(s) done*
Second week and Third week	Serum: ❑ For antibody detection by Widal test ❑ For antigen detection ❑ Stool and urine culture
Fourth week	Stool and urine culture
Carriers	Stool and urine culture Serum for detection of antibodies to Vi antigen Sewage culture—indirect way

163. A patient was on long term antibiotic therapy for peritonitis. During the course of treatment, he develops mucus diarrhea. Most likely cause of diarrhea is:

a. Peritonitis
b. Antibiotic associated diarrhea
c. Immunocompromised state
d. Altered bowel habits

Antibiotic-associated diarrhea (**AAD**) results from an imbalance in the colonic microbiota caused by antibiotic therapy. Microbiota alteration changes carbohydrate metabolism with decreased short-chain fatty acid absorption and an osmotic diarrhea as a result. Another consequence of antibiotic therapy leading to diarrhea is overgrowth of potentially pathogenic organisms such as *Clostridium difficile*. It is defined as frequent loose and watery stools with no other complications.

VIROLOGY

164. Family of Rabies virus:

a. Filoviridae
b. Bunyaviridae
c. Rhabdoviridae
d. Parvoviridae

The rabies virus has a cylindrical morphology and is the type species of the Lyssavirus genus of the Rhabdoviridae family. These viruses are enveloped and have a single stranded RNA genome with negative-sense.

165. Infection NOT transmitted transplacentally is:

a. Polio
b. CMV
c. Mumps
d. Herpes simplex

Poliovirus is usually spread from person to person through infected feces entering the mouth. It may also be spread by food or water containing human feces and less commonly from infected saliva. Those who are infected may spread the disease for up to six weeks even if no symptoms are present. The disease may be diagnosed by finding the virus in the feces or detecting antibodies against it in the blood.

Transmission and spread of viruses.

Mode of transmission	*Produce local infection at the portal of entry*	*Spread to distant sites from the portal of entry*
Respiratory route (probably the most common route)	**Produce respiratory infection** ❑ Influenza virus ❑ Parainfluenza virus ❑ Respiratory syncytial virus (RSV) ❑ Rhinovirus ❑ Adenovirus ❑ Coronavirus ❑ Herpes simplex virus (HSV)	Measles virus ❑ Mumps virus ❑ Rubella virus ❑ Varicella-zoster virus ❑ Cytomegalovirus (CMV) ❑ Parvovirus ❑ Smallpox virus
Oral route	**Produce gastroenteritis** ❑ Rotavirus ❑ Adenovirus-40,41 ❑ Calicivirus ❑ Astrovirus	❑ Poliovirus ❑ Coxsackie virus ❑ Hepatitis virus – A and E ❑ Cytomegalovirus ❑ Epstein-Barr virus (EBV)
Cutaneous route	**Produce skin lesions** ❑ Herpes simplex virus (HSV) ❑ Human papillomavirus (HPV) ❑ Molluscum contagiosum virus	Herpes simplex virus
Vector bite	–	Arboviruses such as: ❑ Dengue virus (*Aedes*) ❑ Chikungunya virus (*Aedes*) ❑ Japanese encephalitis virus (*Culex*) ❑ Yellow fever virus (*Aedes*) ❑ Kyasanur Forest disease virus (Tick)

Contd...

Ans. 163. b. Antibiotic... **164. c.** Rhabdoviridae **165. a.** Polio

Contd...

Mode of transmission	*Produce local infection at the portal of entry*	*Spread to distant sites from the portal of entry*
Animal bite	–	Rabies virus
Sexual route	**Produce genital lesions** ❑ Herpes simplex virus (HSV) ❑ Human papillomavirus (HPV)	❑ Hepatitis B, C and rarely D viruses ❑ Human immunodeficiency virus (HIV)
Blood transfusion	–	❑ Hepatitis B, C and rarely D viruses ❑ HIV ❑ Parvovirus
Injection	–	❑ Hepatitis B, C and rarely D viruses ❑ HIV
Transplacental route	**Produce congenital manifestations in fetus** ❑ Rubella virus ❑ Cytomegalovirus ❑ Herpes simplex virus ❑ Varicella-zoster virus ❑ Parvovirus	**Transmitted through placenta to fetus, without congenital manifestations** ❑ Measles virus ❑ Mumps virus ❑ Hepatitis B, C and rarely D viruses ❑ HIV
Conjunctival route	❑ Adenovirus ❑ Enterovirus 70 ❑ Coxsackie virus A-24 ❑ Herpes simplex virus	–

166. True for Hepatitis B:

a. Caused by RNA virus
b. HBsAg may be present in saliva
c. Incubation period of 2-4 weeks
d. HBeAg is protective

Salivary HBsAg is probably due to admixture of blood or exudate.

Features of hepatitis viruses.

Properties	*HAV*	*HBV*	*HCV*	*HDV*	*HEV*
Common name	Infectious hepatitis	Serum hepatitis	Non A non B or post-transfusion hepatitis	Delta agent	Non A non B enteric transmitted hepatitis
Family	Enterovirus-72 (Picornaviridae)	Hepadnaviridae	Flaviviridae	Unclassified viroid-like	Unclassified Caliciviridae-like
Genus	Hepatovirus	Orthohepadnavirus	Hepacivirus	Deltavirus	Hepevirus
Virion	27 nm, icosahedral	42 nm, spherical	60 nm, spherical	35 nm, spherical	30–32 nm, icosahedral
Envelope	No	Yes (HBsAg)	Yes	Yes (HBsAg)	No
Genome	ssRNA	dsDNA	ssRNA	ssRNA	ssRNA
Stability	Heat and acid-stable	Acid-sensitive	Ether-sensitive, acid-sensitive	Acid-sensitive	Heat-stable
Onset	Abrupt	Insidious	Insidious	Insidious	Abrupt
Age	❑ Children ❑ Young adults	❑ Young adults ❑ Toddlers and babies	Any age, but more common in adults	Any age (similar to HBV)	Young adults (20–40 years)
Route	Fecal-oral	❑ Blood (MC) ❑ Sexual ❑ Vertical	❑ Blood (MC) ❑ Sexual (±) ❑ Vertical (±)	❑ Blood (MC) ❑ Sexual (++) ❑ Vertical (+)	Fecal-oral
I.P (days)	15–45 (Average 30)	30–180 (Average 60–90)	15–160 (Average 50)	30–180 (Average 60–90)	14–60 (Average 40)
Fulminant disease	Rare (0.1%)	Rare (0.1–1%)	Rare (0.1%)	Frequent (5–20%)	❑ Usually rare (1–2%) ❑ Pregnancy: 20–40%
Carrier	None	Yes (0.1–30%)	Yes (1.5–3.2%)	Variable	None
Chronicity	None	Occasional (1–10%)	Common (85%)	Common	None

Contd...

Ans. 166. b. HBsAg may be present...

Contd...

Properties	*HAV*	*HBV*	*HCV*	*HDV*	*HEV*
Oncogenic	No	Yes (neonate)	Yes	±	No
Prevalence	High	High	Moderate	Low, regional	Regional
Associated other feature	Secondary attack rate 10–20%	HCC, cirrhosis, Autoimmune disorder like AGN, arthritis, PAN	HCC, cirrhosis, Autoimmune disorders like AGN, arthritis, cryoglobulinemia	HCC, cirrhosis, fulminant hepatitis	❑ Secondary attack rate (1–2%) ❑ Rarely seen in western countries
Prognosis	Excellent	Worse with age	Moderate	❑ Acute-good ❑ Chronic- poor	Good
Prophylaxis	❑ Immunoglobulin ❑ Inactivated vaccine	❑ HBIG ❑ Recombinant vaccine	None	HBV vaccine (no vaccine for HBV carriers)	Vaccine (HEV239) (only in China)
Therapy	None	❑ Pegylated interferon ❑ Lamivudine	Pegylated interferon plus ribavirin	Interferon ±	None

MC: Most common; HCC: Hepatocellular carcinoma; HBsAg: Hepatitis B surface antigen; AGN: Acute glomerulonephritis; HBIG: Hepatitis B immunoglobulin; IP: Incubation period; PAN: Polyarteritis nodosa.

167. HIV virus has predilection for affecting:

a. Plasma cells
b. Macrophages
c. CD 8 cells
d. CD4⁺ T-cells

HIV infects vital cells in the human immune system such as helper T cells (specifically CD4⁺ T cells), macrophages, and dendritic cells. HIV infection leads to low levels of CD4⁺ T cells through a number of mechanisms, including pyroptosis of abortively infected T cells, apoptosis of uninfected bystander cells, direct viral killing of infected cells, and killing of infected CD4⁺ T cells by CD8 cytotoxic lymphocytes that recognize infected cells. When CD4⁺ T cell numbers decline below a critical level, cell-mediated immunity is lost, and the body becomes progressively more susceptible to opportunistic infections.

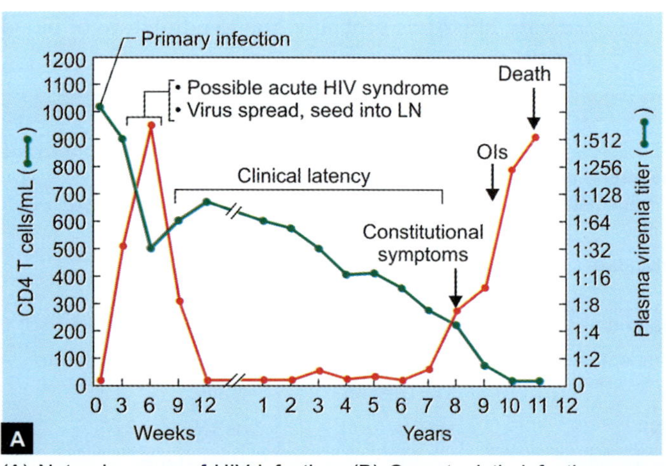

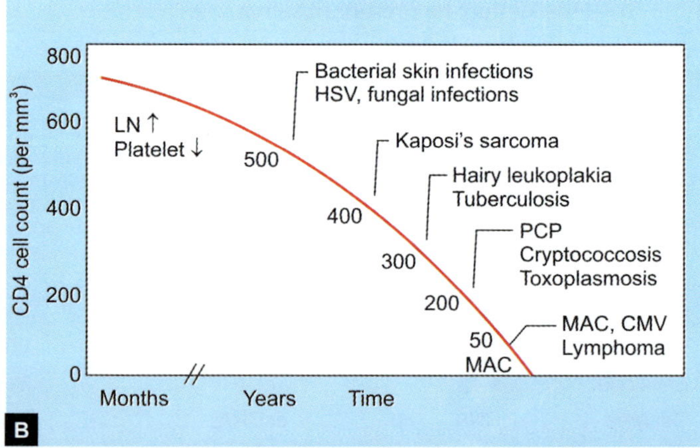

(A) Natural course of HIV infection; (B) Opportunistic infections associated with HIV infection and correlation with CD4 T cell counts. PCP: Pneumocystis *pneumonia*; MAC: *Mycobacterium* avium complex; CMV: Cytomegalovirus.; OIs: Opportunistic infections.

168. Intracytoplasmic inclusion bodies are pathognoonic of:

a. Mumps
b. Measles
c. Adenovirus
d. Rabies

Negri bodies are eosinophilic, sharply outlined, pathognomonic inclusion bodies (2–10 μm in diameter) found in the cytoplasm of certain nerve cells containing the virus of rabies, especially in Ammon's horn of the hippocampus. They are also often found in the cerebellar cortex of postmortem brain samples of rabies victims.

Inclusion bodies.
Intracytoplasmic inclusion bodies
❑ Negri bodies—seen in rabies virus ❑ Paschen body—seen in variola virus ❑ Guarnieri bodies—seen in vaccinia virus ❑ Bollinger bodies—seen in fowlpox virus ❑ Molluscum bodies—seen in molluscum contagiosum virus ❑ Perinuclear cytoplasmic body—seen in reovirus
Intranuclear inclusion bodies

Contd...

Ans. 167. d. CD4⁺ T-cells **168. d.** Rabies

Contd...

Cowdry type A inclusions
❑ Torres body—seen in yellow fever virus ❑ Lipschultz body—seen in herpes simplex virus
Cowdry type B inclusions
❑ Poliovirus ❑ Adenovirus
Intracytoplasmic and intranuclear inclusion bodies
❑ Owl's eye appearance seen in cytomegalovirus ❑ Measles virus

169. Epstein Barr virus is implicated in all of the following EXCEPT:

a. Leukemia
b. Infectious mononucleosis
c. Burkitt's lymphoma
d. Nasopharyngeal carcinoma

Leukemia, is a group of cancers that usually begin in the bone marrow and result in high numbers of abnormal white blood cells. These white blood cells are not fully developed and are called *blasts* or *leukemia cells*.

170. Best laboratory test to diagnose HIV infection:

a. ELISA b. Western blot
c. Complement fixation test
d. RIA

The confirmatory HIV test employs a western blot to detect anti-HIV antibody in a human serum sample. Proteins from known HIV-infected cells are separated and blotted on a membrane. Then, the serum to be tested is applied in the primary antibody incubation step; free antibody is washed away, and a secondary anti-human antibody linked to an enzyme signal is added. The stained bands then indicate the proteins to which the patient's serum contains antibody.

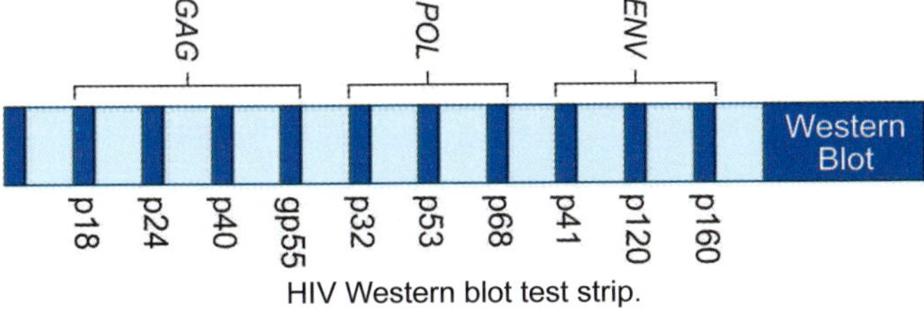

HIV Western blot test strip.

171. HIV can be detected and confirmed by:

a. Mimic PCR b. Real time PCR
c. Reverse transcriptase PCR
d. PCR

Detection of viral RNA is the gold standard method for confirmation of HIV diagnosis. Various formats available are: Reverse transcriptase PCR/ RT-PCR, branched DNA assay, NASBA (nucleic acid sequence based amplification) etc.

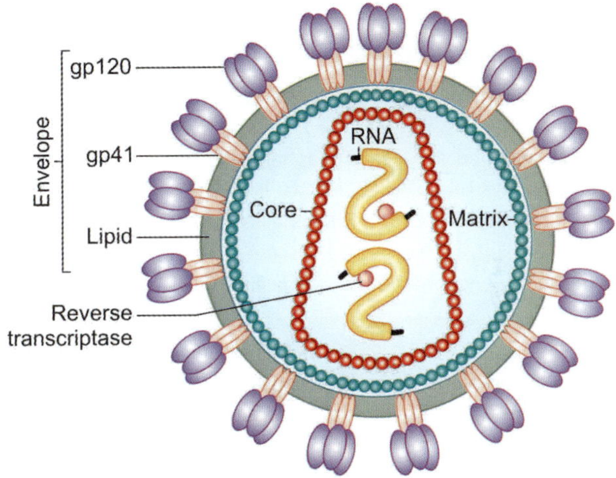

Structure of HIV.

172. NOT a constituent of HIV virus:

a. Endonuclease b. Integrase
c. Reverse transcriptase d. Protease

Endonucleases are enzymes that cleave the phosphodiester bond within a polynucleotide chain. Some, such as Deoxyribonuclease I, cut DNA relatively nonspecifically (without regard to sequence), while many, typically called restriction endonucleases or restriction enzymes, cleave only at very specific nucleotide sequences.

173. Dengue virus belongs to:

a. Bunyaviridae b. Flaviviridae
c. Reoviridae d. Alphaviridae

The **dengue virus** (DENV) is the cause of dengue fever. It is a mosquito-borne single positive-stranded RNA virus of the family *Flaviviridae;* genus *Flavivirus*. Five serotypes of the virus have been found, all of which can cause the full spectrum of disease.

General features of arbovirus.

Virus	*Manifestation*	*Distribution*	*Vector*	*Reservoir*
Family: Togaviridae				
Chikungunya virus	Fever and arthritis	Asia, Africa	*Aedes aegypti*	Monkeys *
O'Nyong-nyong virus	Fever and arthritis	Africa	*Anopheles*	*
Mayaro virus	Fever and arthritis	South America	*Aedes aegypti*	Monkeys
Ross River virus	Epidemic polyarthritis	Australia	*Aedes*	Small animals

Contd...

Ans. 169. **a.** Leukemia 170. **b.** Western blot 171. **c.** Reverse transc... 172. **a.** Endonuclease 173. **b.** Flaviviridae

Contd...

Virus	*Manifestation*	*Distribution*	*Vector*	*Reservoir*
Sindbis virus	Arthralgia, and rash	Africa, Europe, Australia	*Culex*	Birds, mammals
Semliki Forest virus	Fever and arthralgia	Africa	*Aedes*	Birds, rodents
Eastern equine encephalitis virus	Encephalitis	Eastern part of North America	*Aedes, Culex*	Birds
Western equine encephalitis virus	Encephalitis	Western part of North America	*Culex tarsalis, Aedes*	Birds
Venezuelan equine encephalitis virus	Encephalitis	South and central America	*Aedes, Culex*	Horses
Family: Flaviviridae				
Japanese B encephalitis virus	Encephalitis	South East Asia	*Culex tritaeniorhynchus*	Pigs, Birds
St. Louis encephalitis virus	Encephalitis	United States	*Culex*	Wild birds
West Nile encephalitis virus	Encephalitis	East Africa (Uganda), Algeria, Romania	*Culex, Aedes, Anopheles*	Birds
Murray Valley encephalitis virus	Encephalitis	America	*Culex annulirostris*	Birds
Rocio virus	Encephalitis	São Paulo, Brazil	*Culex*	*
Russian spring-summer encephalitis virus	Encephalitis	Central Europe, Russia	Tick	Rodents, other mammals, birds
Powassan virus	Encephalitis	America	Tick	Rodents
Louping-ill virus	Encephalitis	Europe	Tick	Sheep
Dengue virus	Hemorrhagic fever	India	*Aedes aegypti*	*
Yellow fever virus	Hemorrhagic fever	West Africa, Central South America	*Aedes aegypti*	Monkeys
Kyasanur Forest disease virus	Hemorrhagic fever	India (Karnataka)	Tick	Monkeys and rats
Omsk hemorrhagic fever virus	Hemorrhagic fever	Russia	Tick	Small mammals
Family: Bunyaviridae				
California encephalitis virus	Encephalitis	USA	*Aedes triseriatus*	Rodents
Oropouche virus	Rash and aseptic meningitis	Central and South America	*Culicoides paraensis*	Not known
Sandfly fever virus	fever and myalgia	Southern Europe, North Africa, India	Sandfly	Small mammals
Rift Valley fever virus	fever and myalgia	Africa	*Aedes*	Sheep, cattle
Crimean Congo hemorrhagic fever virus	Hemorrhagic fever	Africa	Tick	Small mammals
Ganjam virus	*	India	Tick	Small mammals
Family: Reoviridae				
Colorado tick fever virus	Fever, rarely encephalitis	America (mountains)	Tick	Rodents
Orungo virus	Fever	Sub-Saharan Africa	*Aedes*	*
Kemerovo virus	Fever, meningism	Russia	Tick	*
Family: Rhabdoviridae				
Vesicular stomatitis virus	Oral mucosal vesicles	Indiana	Sandfly	*
Chandipura virus	Encephalitis	India	Sandfly	*

*Not yet identified

174. Only hepatitis virus which can be cultured:

a. HAV b. HBV
c. HCV d. HDV

Hepatitis A virus can be grown in cell culture and sufficient amounts of the virus can be obtained for vaccine production. The virus is propagated in human fibroblasts or human diploid cell cultures, purified from cell lysates, inactivated with formalin, and adsorbed to an aluminum hydroxide adjuvant or a virosome consisting of phospholipids vesicles spiked with influenza haemagglutinin and neuraminidase. 2-phenoxyethanol (2-PE) is included as a preservatives in the formulation of some vaccines.

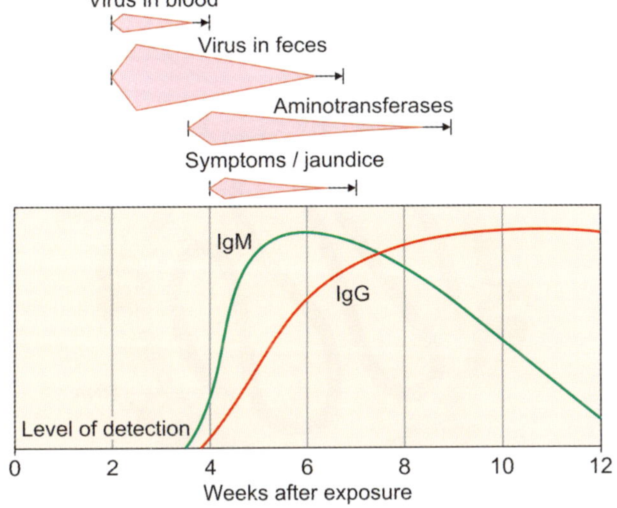

Course of HAV markers with symptoms.

175. NOT a cause of hemorrhagic fever:

a. KFD
b. Dengue hemorrhagic fever
c. Yellow fever
d. Rocky Mountain spotted fever

The family ***Flaviviridae*** include dengue, yellow fever, and two viruses in the tick-borne encephalitis group that cause VHF (viral hemorrhagic fevers): Omsk hemorrhagic fever virus and Kyasanur Forest disease virus.

176. Hepatitis A virus is best diagnosed by:

a. IgM antibodies in serum b. Isolation from stool
c. Culture from blood d. Isolation from bile

Cases of hepatitis A are not clinically distinguishable from other types of acute viral hepatitis. Specific diagnosis is made by the detection of HAV-specific IgM and IgG antibodies in the blood. Additional tests include reverse transcriptase polymerase chain reaction (RT-PCR) to detect the hepatitis A virus RNA, but may require specialised laboratory facilities.

177. Diagnostic of rabies:

a. Guarneri bodies b. Negri bodies
c. Cowdry A body d. Bollinger bodies

The diagnosis can be reliably made from brain samples taken after death. The diagnosis can also be made from saliva, urine, and cerebrospinal fluid samples, but this is not as sensitive and reliable as brain samples. Cerebral inclusion bodies called Negri bodies are 100% diagnostic for rabies infection but are found in only about 80% of cases. If possible, the animal from which the bite was received should also be examined for rabies.

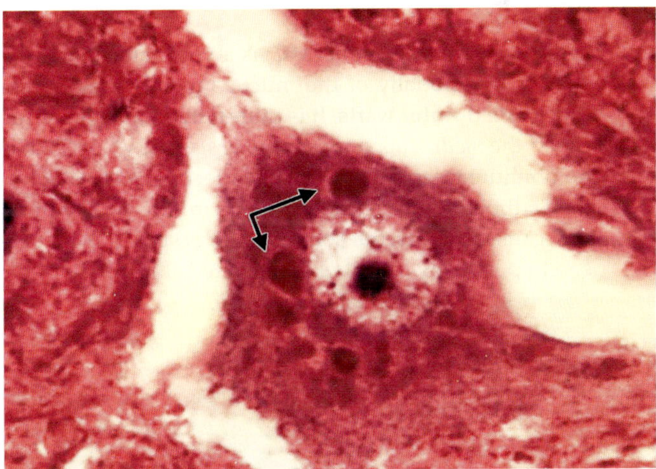

Negri bodies in brain biopsy by H and E stain *(arrow showing).*
Source: Public Health Image Library, ID# 3377//Dr. Daniel P. Perl/ Centers for Disease Control and Prevention (CDC), Atlanta (with permission).

178. Intranuclear and intracytoplasmic inclusion bodies are seen in:

a. Pox virus b. Rabies virus
c. Measles virus d. Herpes virus

Measles virus shows both intracytoplasmic and intranuclear inclusion bodies.

Characteristics of family Paramyxoviridae.

Subfamilies	*Paramyxovirinae*				*Pneumovirinae*	
Genera	*Respirovirus*	*Rubulavirus*	*Morbillivirus*	Henipavirus	*Pneumovirus*	*Metapneumovirus*
Human viruses	Parainfluenza 1, 3	Mumps, Parainfluenza 2, 4a, 4b	Measles	Hendra, Nipah (Zoonotic)	Respiratory syncytial virus	Human metapneumovirus
Nucleocapsid	18 nm	18 nm	18 nm	*	13 nm	13 nm

Contd...

MCQs with Short Explanations

Ans. **174. a.** HAV **175. d.** Rocky Mountain spot... **176. a.** IgM antibodies in... **177. b.** Negri bodies
178. c. Measles virus

Contd...

Subfamilies		Paramyxovirinae				Pneumovirinae	
Large Glycoproteins		HN type	HN type	H type	G type	G type	G type
	Hemagglutinin	+	+	+	–	–	–
	Neuraminidase	+	+	–	–	–	–
Fusion protein		+	+	+	+	+	+
Hemolysin		+	+	+	*	–	–
Inclusions		Cytoplasm	Cytoplasm	Cytoplasm and Nucleus	*	Cytoplasm	*

* Not yet identified

HN: Have both hemagglutinin and neuraminidase activities; H: Have only hemagglutinin activity; G: Do not have both hemagglutinin and neuraminidase activities.

179. Molluscum contagiosum is caused by:

a. Bacteria
b. Fungus
c. Protozoa
d. Virus

Molluscum contagiosum (**MC**) is a viral infection of the skin or occasionally of the mucous membranes, sometimes called **water warts**. It is caused by a DNA poxvirus called the *molluscum contagiosum virus* (MCV). MCV has no nonhuman-animal reservoir (infecting primarily humans, though equids can rarely be infected). The virus that causes molluscum contagiosum is spread from person to person by touching the affected skin.

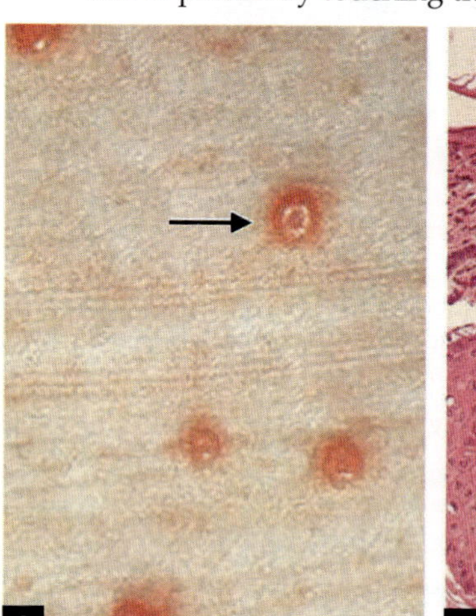

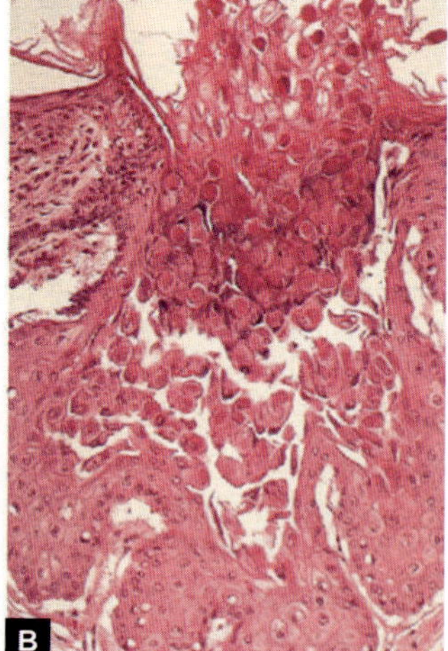

(A) Molluscum contagiosum lesions on skin; (B) Histopathology of skin showing molluscum bodies.
Source: A. CDC/ L. Sperling, MD, Walter Reed Army Medical Center; B. Public Health Image Library, ID# 860/Centers for Disease Control and Prevention (CDC), Atlanta/ Dr. Edwin P. Ewing, Jr (with permission).

180. SSPE is a complication of:

a. Measles
b. Mumps
c. Rubella
d. Rabies

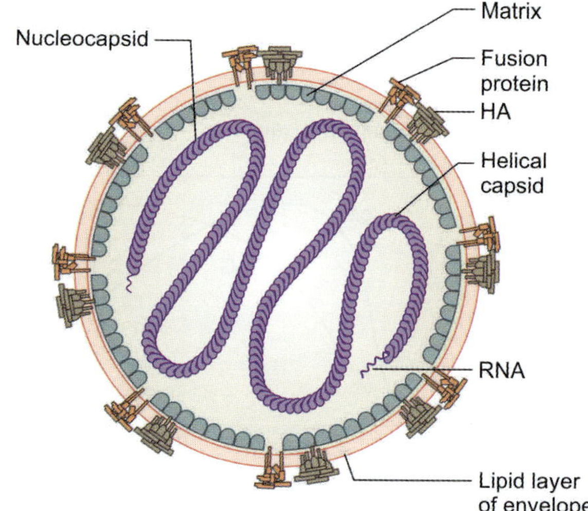

Measles virus (schematic diagram).

181. Which subtype of human papilloma virus has maximum chances of causing carcinoma cervix:

a. HPV 16 and 18
b. HPV 6 and 11
c. HPV 31 and 32
d. HPV 1 and 2

Most HPV infections are subclinical and will cause no physical symptoms; however, in some people subclinical infections will become clinical and may cause benign papillomas (such as warts [verrucae] or squamous cell papilloma), premalignant lesions that will drive to cancers of the cervix, vulva, vagina, penis, oropharynx and anus. In particular, HPV16 and HPV18 are known to cause around 70% of cervical cancer cases

Clinical features of human papillomavirus (HPV) and the types responsible for various types of lesions.

Clinical lesion	Oncogenic potential	HPV types
Plantar warts	Benign	1
Common skin warts	Benign	2, 4, 27, 57
Epidermodysplasia verruciformis	Mostly benign, Rarely progress to malignancy	5, 8, 9, 12, 17

Contd...

Ans. 179. d. Virus **180. a.** Measles **181. a.** HPV 16 and 18

Contd...

Clinical lesion	*Oncogenic potential*	*HPV types*
Anogenital warts Laryngeal papillomas Intraepithelial neoplasia	Low malignant potential	6, 11
Palmar warts seen in butchers	Low malignant potential	7
Carcinomas of cervix and other genital mucosa/larynx/ esophagus	High malignant potential	16, 18, 30, 31, 33 and 45

182. All are DNA viruses EXCEPT:

a. Varicella zoster virus
b. Dengue virus
c. HBV
d. Parvovirus B19

The **dengue virus** (DENV) is the cause of dengue fever. It is a mosquito-borne single positive-stranded RNA virus of the family *Flaviviridae;* genus *Flavivirus.*

Classification of viruses

Family	*Nucleic acid*	*Envelope*	*Symmetry*	*Size (nm)*	*Representative viruses*
DNA Viruses	*DNA*				
herpesviridae	ds, linear	Yes	Icosahedron	150–200	❑ Herpes simplex virus (HSV)-1 ❑ Herpes simplex virus (HSV)-2 ❑ Varicella-zoster virus ❑ Epstein-Barr virus (EBV) ❑ Cytomegalovirus (CMV) ❑ Human herpesvirus 6, 7 and 8
Hepadnaviridae	ds, circular, incomplete	Yes	Icosahedron	40–48	❑ Hepatitis B virus
Parvoviridae	ss, linear	Absent	Icosahedron	18–26	❑ Parvovirus B19
Papovaviridae	ds, circular	Absent	Icosahedron	45–55	❑ Human papillomavirus ❑ JC virus and BK virus
Poxviridae	ds, linear	Yes	Complex	230 × 400	❑ Variola (smallpox) ❑ Molluscum contagiosum virus
Adenoviridae	ds, linear	Absent	Icosahedron	70–90	❑ Human adenovirus
RNA Viruses	*RNA*				
Picornaviridae	ss, +ve sense	Absent	Icosahedron	28–30	❑ Poliovirus ❑ Coxsackievirus ❑ Echovirus ❑ Enterovirus ❑ Rhinovirus ❑ Hepatitis A virus
Caliciviridae	ss, +ve sense	Absent	Icosahedral	27–40	❑ Norwalk agent ❑ Hepatitis E virus
Togaviridae	ss, +ve sense	Yes	Icosahedral	50–70	❑ Rubella virus ❑ Eastern equine encephalitis virus ❑ Western equine encephalitis virus
Flaviviridae	ss, +ve sense	Yes	Icosahedral*	40–60	❑ Yellow fever virus ❑ Dengue virus ❑ St. Louis encephalitis virus ❑ West Nile virus ❑ Hepatitis C virus
Coronaviridae	ss, +ve sense	Yes	Helical	120–160	❑ Coronaviruses
RNA Viruses	RNA				
Rhabdoviridae	ss, -ve sense	Yes	Helical	75 × 180	❑ Rabies virus ❑ Vesicular stomatitis virus
Filoviridae	ss, -ve sense	Yes	Helical	80 × 1000	❑ Marburg virus ❑ Ebola virus
Paramyxoviridae	ss, -ve sense	Yes	Helical	150–300	❑ Parainfluenza virus ❑ Mumps virus ❑ Measles virus ❑ Respiratory syncytial virus (RSV) ❑ Newcastle disease virus ❑ Metapneumovirus
Orthomyxoviridae	ss, -ve sense, 8 segments	Yes	Helical	80–120	❑ Influenza viruses- A, B, and C

Contd...

Ans. 182. **b.** Dengue virus

Contd...

Family	Nucleic acid	Envelope	Symmetry	Size (nm)	Representative viruses
Bunyaviridae	ss, -ve sense, 3 circular segments	Yes	Helical	80–120	❑ Hantavirus ❑ California encephalitis virus ❑ Sandfly fever virus
Arenaviridae	ss, -ve sense 2 circular segments	Yes	Helical*	50–300	❑ Lymphocytic choriomeningitis virus ❑ Lassa fever virus ❑ South American hemorrhagic fever virus
Reoviridae	ds, 10–12 segments	Absent	Icosahedral	60–80	❑ Rotavirus ❑ Reovirus ❑ Colorado tick fever virus
Retroviridae	Two identical copies of +ve sense ss RNA	Yes	Icosahedral (spherical)	80–110	❑ HTLV (Human T Lymphotropic virus) ❑ HIV (Human immunodeficiency virus)

*Doubtful

DNA: Deoxyribonucleic acid; RNA: Ribonucleic acid; ds: Double stranded; SS: Single stranded; +ve: Positive; –ve Negative.

MYCOLOGY

183. India ink preparation is employed for demonstration of capsule of:

a. Cryptosporidium b. Cryptococcus
c. Chromoblastomycese d. Cladosporium

India ink preparation

- Under the microscope, the India ink stain is used for easy visualization of the capsule in cerebral spinal fluid.
- The particles of ink pigment do not enter the capsule that surrounds the spherical yeast cell, resulting in a zone of clearance or "halo" around the cells.
- This allows for quick and easy identification of C. neoformans.

184. Malt Worker's lung is caused by:

a. Micropolyspora faeni b. Pseudomonas
c. Aspergillus fumigatus d. Aspergillus clavatus

Due to the small size of the spores, about 70% of spores of *A. fumigates* are able to penetrate into the trachea and primary bronchi and close to 1% into alveoli. Inhalation of spores of *Aspergillus* is a health risk. *A. clavatus* is allergenic, causing the occupational hypersensitivity pneumonitis known as malt-worker's lung.

185. NOT a dimorphic fungi:

a. Blastomyces b. Cryptococcus
c. Paracoccidioides d. Histoplasma

Cryptococcus (Greek for "hidden sphere") is a genus of fungus. These fungi grow in culture as yeasts. The sexual forms or teleomorphs of *Cryptococcus* species are filamentous fungi in the genus *Filobasidiella*. The name *Cryptococcus* is used when referring to the yeast states of the fungi.

186. Stain used in staining fungal elements:

a. Acid fast stain b. Gram stain
c. Methenamine silver d. All of the above

Gomori methenamine silver/GMS stain is used as alternative to periodic acid Schiff/PAS for detecting fungi. It stains both live and dead fungi, as compared to PAS which stains only live fungi. GMS stains the polysaccharide component of the cell wall. Fungi appear black whereas the background tissues takes pale green colour.

187. The capsule of Cryptococcus neoformans in a CSF sample is best seen by:

a. Grams stain
b. Indian ink preparation
c. Giemsa stain
d. Methenamine-Silver stain

Cryptococcus neoformans, because of its large polysaccharide capsule, can be visualized by the India stain. Organisms that possess a polysaccharide capsule exhibit a halo around the cell against the black background created by the India, stain.

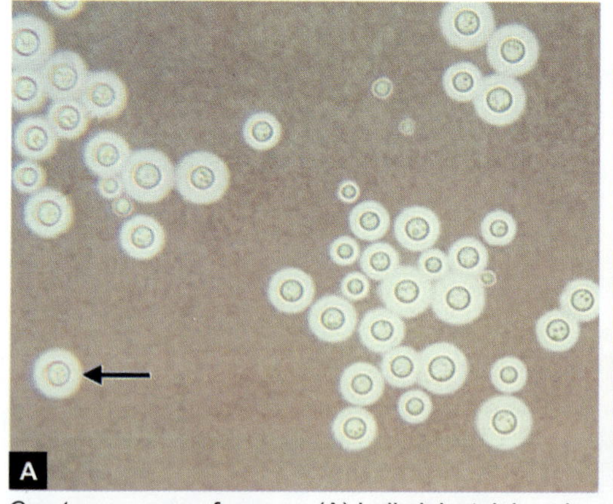

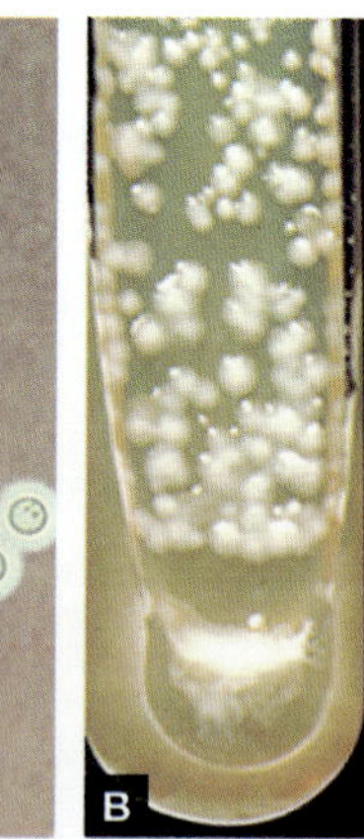

Cryptococcus neoformans. (A) India ink staining shows clear refractile capsules surrounding round budding yeast cells; (arrow showing) (B) Growth on SDA at 37°C—shows creamy white mucoid colonies.
Source: Public Health Image Library/A. Dr. Leanor Haley, ID#:3771 B. Dr. William Kaplan, ID#:3199/Centers for Disease Control and Prevention (CDC), Atlanta (with permission).

188. True regarding Histoplasmosis:

a. In early stages, it is indistinguishable from TB
b. Culture is NOT diagnostic
c. Hyphal forms are infectious forms
d. Person to person spread occurs by droplet infection

Ans. 183. **b.** Cryptococcus 184. **d.** Aspergillus... 185. **b.** Cryptococcus 186. **c.** Methenamine silver
187. **b.** Indian ink... 188. **a.** In early stages, it is indistinguishable from TB

If symptoms of histoplasmosis infection occur, they will start within 3 to 17 days after exposure; the average is 12–14 days. Most affected individuals have clinically silent manifestations and show no apparent ill effects. The acute phase of histoplasmosis is characterized by non-specific respiratory symptoms, often cough or flu-like. Chest X-ray findings are normal in 40–70% of cases. Chronic histoplasmosis cases can resemble tuberculosis; disseminated histoplasmosis affects multiple organ systems and is fatal unless treated.

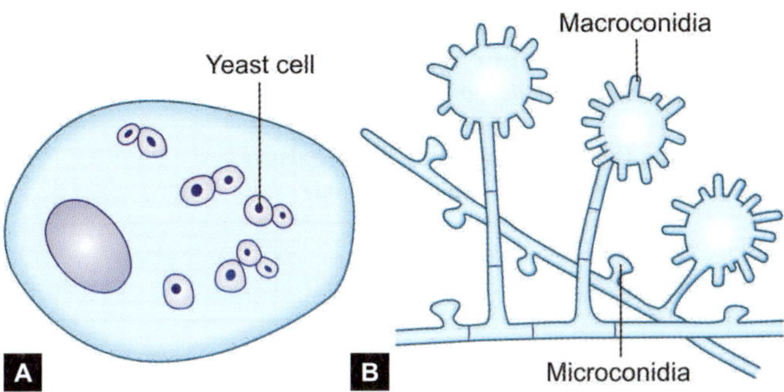

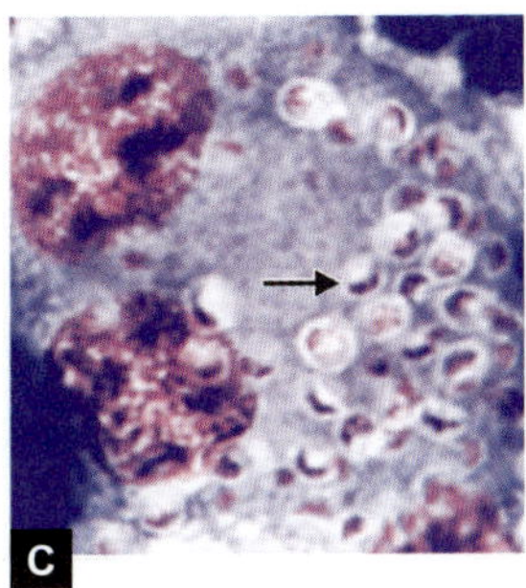

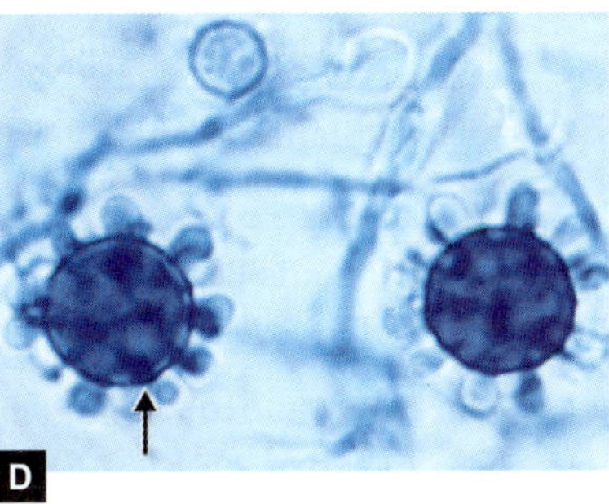

(A and B) *Histoplasma capsulatum* (schematic diagram). A. Yeast form; B. Mycelial form; (C and D) *Histoplasma capsulatum*; C. 2–4 μm yeast cells with narrow based budding (Giemsa stain); D. Mold form, septate thin hyphae with tuberculate macroconidia *(arrows showing)*.
Source: Public Health Image Library/C. Dr. Lucille K. Georg/ID#:15365, D. Dr. Libero Ajello/ID#:15364/Centers for Disease Control and Prevention (CDC), Atlanta (with permission).

MISCELLANEOUS

189. True regarding Cat-scratch disease is:

a. Associated with positive Frei skin test
b. Caused by a DNA virus
c. Associated with regional lymphadenopathy
d. Associated with a positive Hangar-Rose test

Cat-scratch disease (CSD), also known as **cat-scratch fever**, **Teeny's disease**, **inoculation lymphoreticulosis**, and **subacute regional lymph-adenitis**

- It is a common and usually benign infectious disease caused by a bacterium, either Bartonella henselae or Bartonella quintana.
- It is most commonly found in children following a scratch or bite from a cat within about one to two weeks.

Ans. **189.** **c.** Associated with regional lymphadenopathy

ANSWERS WITH REFERENCES

GENERAL MICROBIOLOGY

1. **Ans. (a)** 5%
   Ref: Ananthanarayan's Microbiology, 6/e p10

2. **Ans. (c)** Stationary phase
   Ref: Sastry's Microbiology 1/e p27

3. **Ans. (d)** Louis Pasteur
   Ref: Sastry's Microbiology 1/e p4

4. **Ans. (b)** Robertson's cooked meat medium
   Ref: Sastry's Microbiology 1/e p257

5. **Ans. (a)** Conjugation
   Ref: Sastry's Microbiology 1/e p74

6. **Ans. (b)** Phosphatage
   Ref: Internet resources

7. **Ans. (d)** None of the above
   Ref: Sastry's Microbiology 1/e p72

8. **Ans. (a)** Transposons
   Ref: Internet resources

9. **Ans. (d)** All of the above
   Ref: Sastry's Microbiology 1/e p45

10. **Ans. (b)** Enriched media
    Ref: Sastry's Microbiology 1/e p44

11. **Ans. (c)** Conjugation
    Ref: Sastry's Microbiology 1/e p75

12. **Ans. (c)** Discovery of M. tuberculosis
    Ref: Sastry's Microbiology 1/e p4

13. **Ans. (a)** Koch
    Ref: Sastry's Microbiology 1/e p4

14. **Ans. (c)** C. diphtheriae
    Ref: Sastry's Microbiology 1/e p246

15. **Ans. (c)** Streptococci
    Ref: Sastry's Microbiology 1/e p45

STERILIZATION

16. **Ans. (c)** Glutaraldehyde
    Ref: Sastry's Microbiology 1/e p37

17. **Ans. (c)** Bacillus stearothermophilus
    Ref: Sastry's Microbiology 1/e p40

18. **Ans. (b)** 121 degree C
    Ref: Sastry's Microbiology 1/e p34

19. **Ans. (b)** Anatomy waste
    Ref: Sastry's Microbiology 1/e p32

20. **Ans. (b)** Formaldehyde fumigation
    Ref: Sastry's Microbiology 1/e p37

21. **Ans. (c)** Hot air oven
    Ref: Sastry's Microbiology 1/e p32

22. **Ans. (b)** Ionizing radiation
    Ref: Sastry's Microbiology 1/e p31

23. **Ans. (a)** Blue bag
    Ref: Sastry's Microbiology 1/e p613

24. **Ans. (b)** Steam under pressure
    Ref: Sastry's Microbiology 1/e p33

25. **Ans. (a)** Efficiency of a disinfectant
    Ref: Sastry's Microbiology 1/e p41

26. **Ans. (b)** 15 lb pressure, 120°C temperature for 15 minutes
    Ref: Sastry's Microbiology 1/e p35

27. **Ans. (c)** Glutaraldehyde
    Ref: Sastry's Microbiology 1/e p41

IMMUNITY

28. **Ans. (c)** Thymus
    Ref: Ananthanarayan's Microbiology, 8/e p124

29. **Ans. (a)** Slide flocculation test
    Ref: Sastry's Microbiology 1/e p377

30. **Ans. (d)** Infectious mononucleosis
    Ref: Sastry's Microbiology 1/e p444

31. **Ans. (b)** Produce immunoglobulins
    Ref: Sastry's Microbiology 1/e p150

32. **Ans. (a)** 19S globulin
    Ref: Sastry's Microbiology 1/e p184

33. **Ans. (b)** Activates classical complement
    Ref: Sastry's Microbiology 1/e p113

34. **Ans. (c)** C3
    Ref: Sastry's Microbiology 1/e p141

35. **Ans. (b)** Cell mediated immunity
    Ref: Sastry's Microbiology 1/e p187

36. **Ans. (b) IgE**
Ref: Sastry's Microbiology 1/e p111

37. **Ans. (a) Stevens-Johnson syndrome**
Ref: Sastry's Microbiology 1/e p172

38. **Ans. (d) IgG**
Ref: Sastry's Microbiology 1/e p110

39. **Ans. (b) Type II**
Ref: Sastry's Microbiology 1/e p176

40. **Ans. (b) B cells**
Ref: Sastry's Microbiology 1/e p98

41. **Ans. (c) Arthus reaction**
Ref: Sastry's Microbiology 1/e p177

42. **Ans. (b) Impaired bacteriolysis**
Ref: Sastry's Microbiology 1/e p191

43. **Ans. (a) Agglutination**
Ref: Sastry's Microbiology 1/e p123

44. **Ans. (a) Type I hypersensitivity**
Ref: Sastry's Microbiology 1/e p173

45. **Ans. (a) Ig A**
Ref: Sastry's Microbiology 1/e p114

46. **Ans. (b) Primary response**
Ref: Sastry's Microbiology 1/e p102

47. **Ans. (a) It is less sensitive than precipitation reaction for detecting antibodies**
Ref: Sastry's Microbiology 1/e p126

48. **Ans. (d) Mantoux test**
Ref: Sastry's Microbiology 1/e p179

49. **Ans. (c) Wassermann reaction**
Ref: Sastry's Microbiology 1/e p128

50. **Ans. (c) Agglutination test**
Ref: Sastry's Microbiology 1/e p126

51. **Ans. (d) Phagocytes**
Ref: Sastry's Microbiology 1/e p191

52. **Ans. (a) T-cells**
Ref: Internet resources

53. **Ans. (b) Takes 5 days to appear**
Ref: Sastry's Microbiology 1/e p102

54. **Ans. (d) Opsonization**
Ref: Sastry's Microbiology 1/e p142

55. **Ans. (a) Type I**
Ref: Sastry's Microbiology 1/e p165

56. **Ans. (b) IgM**
Ref: Sastry's Microbiology 1/e p115

57. **Ans. (c) IgG**
Ref: Sastry's Microbiology 1/e p113

58. **Ans. (c) Type III**
Ref: Sastry's Microbiology 1/e p179

59. **Ans. (d) 5**
Ref: Sastry's Microbiology 1/e p111

60. **Ans. (a) NK cells**
Ref: Sastry's Microbiology 1/e p166

61. **Ans. (d) Granuloma**
Ref: Sastry's Microbiology 1/e p180

62. **Ans. (c) C3**
Ref: Sastry's Microbiology 1/e p140

63. **Ans. (b) T cells**
Ref: Sastry's Microbiology 1/e p163

64. **Ans. (a) Antibody to H antigen appears first and persists**
Ref: Sastry's Microbiology 1/e p324

65. **Ans. (b) Raised IgM**
Ref: Sastry's Microbiology 1/e p190

66. **Ans. (a) IgM antibody against Fc fragment of IgG**
Ref: Sastry's Microbiology 1/e p186

67. **Ans. (d) Cases of paternal dispute**
Ref: Internet resources

68. **Ans. (c) Thymus**
Ref: Sastry's Microbiology 1/e p153

69. **Ans. (a) Acts as a mucosa barrier for infection**
Ref: Sastry's Microbiology 1/e p113

70. **Ans. (c) IgG**
Ref: Sastry's Microbiology 1/e p113

71. **Ans. (d) All of the above**
Ref: Sastry's Microbiology 1/e p126

72. **Ans. (d) VDRL**
Ref: Sastry's Microbiology 1/e p123

73. **Ans. (a) Goodpasture syndrome**
Ref: Sastry's Microbiology 1/e p177

74. **Ans. (d) All of the above**
Ref: Sastry's Microbiology 1/e p159

BACTERIOLOGY

75. **Ans. (d)** Pseudomonas
Ref: Ananthanarayan's Microbiology, 6/e p296

76. **Ans. (b and c)** Enterohemorrhagic E. coli and Shigella
Ref: Ananthanarayan's Microbiology, 8/e p277

77. **Ans. (d)** Antibiotic use
Ref: Ananthanarayan's Microbiology, 8/e p263

78. **Ans. (a)** Neisseria gonorrhoeae
Ref: Ananthanarayan's Microbiology, 8/e p224,265

79. **Ans. (d)** Salmonella typhi
Ref: Sastry's Microbiology 1/e p26

80. **Ans. (c)** L. monocytogenes
Ref: Internet resources

81. **Ans. (d)** Myocardial abscess
Ref: Sastry's Microbiology 1/e p596

82. **Ans. (c)** Pneumococci
Ref: Sastry's Microbiology 1/e p232

83. **Ans. (b)** Pseudomonas
Ref: Sastry's Microbiology 1/e p340

84. **Ans. (b)** B. anthrax
Ref: Sastry's Microbiology 1/e p253

85. **Ans. (b)** Rat flea
Ref: Sastry's Microbiology 1/e p390

86. **Ans. (a)** Gram positive bacteria
Ref: Sastry's Microbiology 1/e p294

87. **Ans. (d)** C. burnetii
Ref: Sastry's Microbiology 1/e p394

88. **Ans. (a)** Rickettsia rickettsii
Ref: Sastry's Microbiology 1/e p391

89. **Ans. (d)** Parotitis
Ref: Sastry's Microbiology 1/e p399

90. **Ans. (a)** Elementary body is metabolically active
Ref: Sastry's Microbiology 1/e p398

91. **Ans. (d)** Gram positive, spore forming
Ref: Sastry's Microbiology 1/e p262

92. **Ans. (c)** 10000/mL
Ref: Sastry's Microbiology 1/e p375

93. **Ans. (a)** T. pertunae
Ref: Sastry's Microbiology 1/e p372

94. **Ans. (b)** Differs from L forms
Ref: Sastry's Microbiology 1/e p405

95. **Ans. (a)** They are inhibited by penicillins
Ref: Sastry's Microbiology 1/e p405

96. **Ans. (a)** Inhibit acetylcholine release
Ref: Sastry's Microbiology 1/e p264

97. **Ans. (c)** Diphtheria
Ref: Sastry's Microbiology 1/e p247

98. **Ans. (b)** Mycoplasma
Ref: Sastry's Microbiology 1/e p5

99. **Ans. (c)** Histiocytes
Ref: Sastry's Microbiology 1/e p286

100. **Ans. (c)** Rifampicin
Ref: Sastry's Microbiology 1/e p291

101. **Ans. (a)** 12 days
Ref: Sastry's Microbiology 1/e p285

102. **Ans. (a)** Mycobacterium ulcerans
Ref: Sastry's Microbiology 1/e p283

103. **Ans. (b)** Corynebacterium diphtheria
Ref: Sastry's Microbiology 1/e p243

104. **Ans. (a)** Anthrax
Ref: Sastry's Microbiology 1/e p252

105. **Ans. (d)** Ticks
Ref: Sastry's Microbiology 1/e p90

106. **Ans. (a)** Auramine rhodamine stain
Ref: Sastry's Microbiology 1/e p276

107. **Ans. (a)** Production of niacin
Ref: Sastry's Microbiology 1/e p278

108. **Ans. (b)** LJ media
Ref: Sastry's Microbiology 1/e p277

109. **Ans. (a)** Skin to skin contact
Ref: Sastry's Microbiology 1/e p287

110. **Ans. (b)** Foot pad of mice
Ref: Sastry's Microbiology 1/e p285

111. **Ans. (a)** Borrelia burgdorferi
Ref: Sastry's Microbiology 1/e p382

112. **Ans. (d)** Haemophilus
Ref: Sastry's Microbiology 1/e p346

113. **Ans. (c)** Pasteurella
Ref: Sastry's Microbiology 1/e p314

114. **Ans. (c)** Vi antibody is seen in normal population
Ref: Sastry's Microbiology 1/e p318

115. **Ans. (a) Koch**
Ref: Sastry's Microbiology 1/e p333

116. **Ans. (a) V. cholerae**
Ref: Sastry's Microbiology 1/e p329

117. **Ans. (c) Both of the above**
Ref: Sastry's Microbiology 1/e p272

118. **Ans. (b) Cord factor**
Ref: Internet resources

119. **Ans. (a) Listeria**
Ref: Sastry's Microbiology 1/e p23

120. **Ans. (d) Clostridium difficile**
Ref: Sastry's Microbiology 1/e p266

121. **Ans. (a) Enterotoxigenic E. coli**
Ref: Sastry's Microbiology 1/e p589

122. **Ans. (b) Stool culture**
Ref: Sastry's Microbiology 1/e p306

123. **Ans. (c) Mannitol**
Ref: Sastry's Microbiology 1/e p307

124. **Ans. (b) H antigen**
Ref: Sastry's Microbiology 1/e p318

125. **Ans. (c) BCYE medium**
Ref: Sastry's Microbiology 1/e p366

126. **Ans. (b) Actinomyces israelii**
Ref: Sastry's Microbiology 1/e p293

127. **Ans. (a) Pneumococcus**
Ref: Sastry's Microbiology 1/e p234

128. **Ans. (a) Pneumonic form of anthrax**
Ref: Sastry's Microbiology 1/e p251

129. **Ans. (b) Parasympathetic system**
Ref: Sastry's Microbiology 1/e p93

130. **Ans. (a) Causes acute gastroenteritis in infants**
Ref: Sastry's Microbiology 1/e p302

131. **Ans. (c) P. aeruginosa**
Ref: Sastry's Microbiology 1/e p341

132. **Ans. (a) Pathogenicity correlated with coagulase**
Ref: Sastry's Microbiology 1/e p212

133. **Ans. (a) Vaccine made from capsular polysacchride**
Ref: Sastry's Microbiology 1/e p231

134. **Ans. (a) Glucose**
Ref: Sastry's Microbiology 1/e p236

135. **Ans. (c) Intracytoplasmic gram negative**
Ref: Sastry's Microbiology 1/e p240

136. **Ans. (a) Gram negative**
Ref: Sastry's Microbiology 1/e p17

137. **Ans. (d) Human is the only reservoir**
Ref: Sastry's Microbiology 1/e p362

138. **Ans. (b) Highly sensitive to penicillin**
Ref: Sastry's Microbiology 1/e p241

139. **Ans. (c) Acinetobacter baumannii**
Ref: Sastry's Microbiology 1/e p349

140. **Ans. (b) Brucella melitensis**
Ref: Sastry's Microbiology 1/e p359

141. **Ans. (b) It ferments maltose**
Ref: Sastry's Microbiology 1/e p238

142. **Ans. (c) Yellow**
Ref: Sastry's Microbiology 1/e p293

143. **Ans. (c) Causes continued activation of adenylate cyclase**
Ref: Sastry's Microbiology 1/e p330

144. **Ans. (d) Mycobacterium**
Ref: Sastry's Microbiology 1/e p276

145. **Ans. (d) Mycoplasma**
Ref: Sastry's Microbiology 1/e p407

146. **Ans. (b) Giemsa stain**
Ref: Sastry's Microbiology 1/e p405

147. **Ans. (d) 100,000/mL**
Ref: Sastry's Microbiology 1/e p586

148. **Ans. (d) Clostridium**
Ref: Sastry's Microbiology 1/e p258

149. **Ans. (d) All of the above**
Ref: Sastry's Microbiology 1/e p302

150. **Ans. (a) ADP ribosylation of the G regulatory protein**
Ref: Sastry's Microbiology 1/e p331

151. **Ans. (b) Campylobacter jejuni**
Ref: Sastry's Microbiology 1/e p362

152. **Ans. (d) Streptococcus pyogenes**
Ref: Sastry's Microbiology 1/e p227

153. **Ans. (c) Common with dairy products**
Ref: Sastry's Microbiology 1/e p589

154. **Ans. (a) Leptospirosis**
Ref: Sastry's Microbiology 1/e p386

155. **Ans. (a) Proteus**
Ref: Internet resources

156. **Ans. (c) Secondary attack rate is high in family**
Ref: Sastry's Microbiology 1/e p329

157. **Ans. (b) Uncommon in developing Asian countries**
Ref: Sastry's Microbiology 1/e p364

158. **Ans. (a) Salmonella**
Ref: Sastry's Microbiology 1/e p586

159. **Ans. (a) Clostridium welchii**
Ref: Sastry's Microbiology 1/e p259

160. **Ans. (a) Presynaptic block**
Ref: Sastry's Microbiology 1/e p590

161. **Ans. (b) Streptococcus pneumoniae**
Ref: Sastry's Microbiology 1/e p592

162. **Ans. (b) Widal test**
Ref: Sastry's Microbiology 1/e p321

163. **Ans. (b) Antibiotic associated diarrhea**
Ref: Sastry's Microbiology 1/e p266

VIROLOGY

164. **Ans. (c) Rhabdoviridae**
Ref: Ananthanarayan's Microbiology, 6/e p413

165. **Ans. (a) Polio**
Ref: Sastry's Microbiology 1/e p419

166. **Ans. (b) HBsAg may be present in saliva**
Ref: Sastry's Microbiology 1/e p527

167. **Ans. (d) $CD4^+$ T-cells**
Ref: Sastry's Microbiology 1/e p506

168. **Ans. (d) Rabies**
Ref: Sastry's Microbiology 1/e p421

169. **Ans. (a) Leukemia**
Ref: Sastry's Microbiology 1/e p442

170. **Ans. (b) Western blot**
Ref: Sastry's Microbiology 1/e p511

171. **Ans. (c) Reverse transcriptase PCR**
Ref: Sastry's Microbiology 1/e p504

172. **Ans. (a) Endonuclease**
Ref: Sastry's Microbiology 1/e p504

173. **Ans. (b) Flaviviridae**
Ref: Sastry's Microbiology 1/e p484

174. **Ans. (a) HAV**
Ref: Sastry's Microbiology 1/e p529

175. **Ans. (d) Rocky Mountain spotted fever**
Ref: Sastry's Microbiology 1/e p484

176. **Ans. (a) IgM antibodies in serum**
Ref: Sastry's Microbiology 1/e p529

177. **Ans. (b) Negri bodies**
Ref: Sastry's Microbiology 1/e p499

178. **Ans. (c) Measles virus**
Ref: Sastry's Microbiology 1/e p464

179. **Ans. (d) Virus**
Ref: Sastry's Microbiology 1/e p454

180. **Ans. (a) Measles**
Ref: Sastry's Microbiology 1/e p464

181. **Ans. (a) HPV 16 and 18**
Ref: Sastry's Microbiology 1/e p448

182. **Ans. (b) Dengue virus**
Ref: Sastry's Microbiology 1/e p413

MYCOLOGY

183. **Ans. (b) Cryptococcus**
Ref: Ananthanarayan's Microbiology, 8/e p610

184. **Ans. (d) Aspergillus clavatus**
Ref: Internet resources

185. **Ans. (b) Cryptococcus**
Ref: Sastry's Microbiology 1/e p550

186. **Ans. (c) Methenamine silver**
Ref: Sastry's Microbiology 1/e p551

187. **Ans. (b) Indian ink preparation**
Ref: Sastry's Microbiology 1/e p570

188. **Ans. (a) In early stages, it is indistinguishable from TB**
Ref: Sastry's Microbiology 1/e p563

MISCELLANEOUS

189. **Ans. (c) Associated with regional lymphadenopathy**
Ref: Harrison's Medicine, 18/e p1314

PRACTICE QUESTIONS

GENERAL MICROBIOLOGY

1. **Hanging drop preparation is seen in:**
   a. Light microscopy
   b. Electron microscopy
   c. Naked eye
   d. None of the above
2. **Gram positive cell wall predominantly consists of:**
   a. Lipopolysaccharide
   b. Core polysaccharide
   c. Peptidoglycan
   d. All of the above
3. **Endotoxins are:**
   a. Proteins
   b. Lipids
   c. Lipopolysaccharide
   d. Polysaccharide
4. **Which of the following is true for exotoxin:**
   a. Heat stable
   b. Secreted by Gram negative
   c. Poorly antigenic
   d. Highly potent
5. **Phage mediated transfer of genetic material across bacterium is known as:**
   a. Transformation
   b. Transcription
   c. Translation
   d. Transduction
6. **Dark field microscope is used for visualizing:**
   a. Staphylococcus
   b. Vibrio cholerae
   c. Salmonella
   d. Treponema pallidum
7. **Which of the following is a negative staining method:**
   a. Gram staining
   b. Quellung's reaction
   c. Indian ink preparation
   d. Auramine-rhodamine stain
8. **R-plasmid is transferred by which of the following:**
   a. Transduction b. Transformation
   c. Conjugation d. Transposition
9. **Sporulation occurs in which phase:**
   a. Lag phase b. Stationary phase
   c. Log phase d. Decline phase

STERILIZATION

10. **Bronchoscope is best sterilized by:**
    a. Cidex b. Alcohol
    c. Autoclaving d. Hot air oven

IMMUNITY

11. **Helper T cells subtype 1 secretes:**
    a. IL-1 b. IL-2
    c. IL-3 d. IL-4
12. **Marker for T cell:**
    a. CD1 b. CD2
    c. CD3 d. All of the above
13. **True for Null cells are:**
    a. Agranular WBC
    b. Different from B cells
    c. Develops in bone marrow
    d. All of the above
14. **Which of the following is affected in severe combined immunodeficiency:**
    a. Pre B cell
    b. Pre T cell
    c. Both of the above
    d. None of the above
15. **True regarding IgM:**
    a. Monomer
    b. Pentamer
    c. Both of the above
    d. None of the above

BACTERIOLOGY

16. **A male patient aged 1 year, presented with diarrhoea. Which of the following may be responsible:**
    a. EHEC b. EIEC
    c. EPEC d. ETEC

Ans.
1. a. Light microscopy 2. c. Peptidoglycan 3. c. Lipopolysaccharide 4. d. Highly potent
5. d. Transduction 6. d. Treponema pallidum 7. c. Indian ink preparation 8. c. Conjugation
9. b. Stationary phase 10. a. Cidex 11. b. IL-2 12. c. CD3
13. d. All of the above 14. c. Both of the above 15. c. Both of the above 16. c. EPEC

17. Hemorrhagic uremic syndrome is caused by:
a. Shigella
b. E. coli
c. Salmonella
d. Vibrio cholerae

18. Cholera is caused by:
a. Bacteria
b. Virus
c. Protozoa
d. Helminth

19. Ecthyma gangrenosum is caused by:
a. Shigella
b. Salmonella
c. Pseudomonas
d. E. coli

20. In Clostridium perfringenes, meat color of Robertson cooked meat media will change from yellowish orange to:
a. Pink
b. Black
c. Chocolate
d. Blue

21. Which type of diarrhoea can be managed by giving antimicrobial:
a. Traveller's diarrhoea
b. Rotavirus
c. Secretory diarrhoea
d. Osmotic diarrhoea

22. A child presented with cystic fibrosis and pulmonary infection. Which set of organism may be responsible:
a. Staph aureus, H. influenza, Pseudomonas
b. Streptococcus, H. influenza, Klebsiella
c. Staph aureus, H. influenza, Klebsiella
d. Staph aureus, H. influenza, Streptococcus

23. Organism causing genital TB is best diagnosed by:
a. PCR
b. Mantoux
c. LJ media culture
d. Zeihl-Neelsen staining

24. Gram positive and coagulase positive cocci:
a. Staph aureus
b. Staph saprophyticus
c. Staph lugdunensis
d. Staph epidermidis

25. A patient presenting with complaints of nausea, vomiting and diarrhoea within 6 hours of consuming milk product. Organism responsible is:
a. Bacillus cereus
b. Staph aureus
c. Salmonella paratyphi
d. Salmonella typhi

26. Urease test is done for:
a. Shigella
b. Proteus
c. Klebsiella
d. H. pylori

27. Which of the following stain mycobacterium leprae:
a. Auramine-rhodamine stain
b. Ziehl-Neelsen stain
c. Indian ink preparation
d. Quellung reaction

28. Gram negative diplococcic is:
a. Pseudomonas
b. Treponema pallidum
c. Neisseria
d. Chlamydia trachomatis

29. Coxiella burnetii transmitted by:
a. Mite
b. Tick
c. Louse
d. Mosquito

30. Vincent angina is caused by:
a. B. recurrentis
b. B. burgdorferi
c. B. afzelii
d. B. vincentii

VIROLOGY

31. Measles lead to deficiency of which vitamin:
a. Vitamin K
b. Vitamin C
c. Vitamin A
d. Vitamin D

32. Dane particles is:
a. RNA virus
b. DNA virus
c. Mixed virus
d. None of the above

Ans. **17.** b. E. coli **18.** a. Bacteria **19.** c. Pseudomonas **20.** a. Pink **21.** a. Traveller's... **22.** a. Staph aureus, H. influenza, Pseudomonas **23.** a. PCR **24.** a. Staph aureus **25.** b. Staph aureus **26.** d. H. pylori **27.** b. Ziehl-Neelsen stain **28.** c. Neisseria **29.** b. Tick **30.** d. B. vincentii **31.** c. Vitamin A **32.** b. DNA virus

33. Shape of Ebola virus:
a. Spindle shaped
b. Circular
c. Filamentous
d. Octogonal

34. SARS is related to which virus family:
a. Measles virus
b. Corona virus
c. Respiratory syncytial virus
d. Influenza virus

35. Which of the following converts mRNA to C-DNA:
a. Reverse transcriptase
b. DNA polymerase
c. RNA polymerase
d. DNA ligase

36. Diagnosis of congenital rubella is best established by:
a. IgM against rubella at birth
b. IgM against rubella at 4 months
c. IgG against rubella at birth
d. IgG against rubella at 4 months

37. Henderson Paterson bodies are seen in:
a. Erythema infectiosum
b. Erythema marginatum
c. Molluscum contagiosum
d. Erythema migrans

38. Paramyxovirus is:
a. ssDNA virus
b. dsDNA virus
c. ssRNA virus
d. dsRNA virus

MYCOLOGY

39. Candida can be grown on:
a. SDA
b. Cetrimide agar
c. LJ media
d. BYCE medium

MISCELLANEOUS

40. Citrate test is indicated for:
a. G6PD deficiency
b. Bacteria using glucose
c. Bacteria using citrate
d. Virus using citrate

Ans. **33.** c. Filamentous **34.** b. Corona virus **35.** a. Reverse transcriptase **36.** a. IgM against rubella at...
37. c. Molluscum cont... **38.** c. ssRNA virus **39.** a. SDA **40.** c. Bacteria using citrate

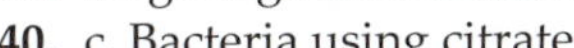

IMAGE-BASED QUESTIONS

1. **Process in which there is transfer of genetic material from one cell to another by mating:**

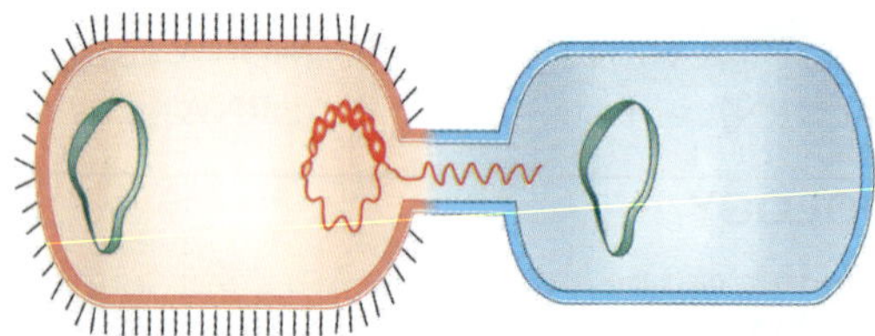

a. Transduction b. Transformation
c. Transposons d. Conjugation

Conjugation is the mating of the two bacterial cells during which DNA is transferred from the donor to the recipient cell.

2. **Identify the organism, which shows swarming growth:**

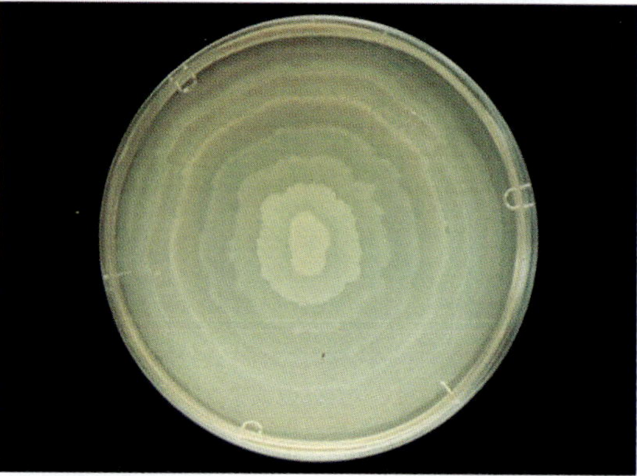

a. Pseudomonas b. Klebsiella
c. Proteus d. H. pylori

Proteus is a highly motile organism and produces a 'swarming' overgrowth on blood agar, which can frustrate efforts to recover pure cultures of other organisms.

3. **Such colonies are suggestive of:**

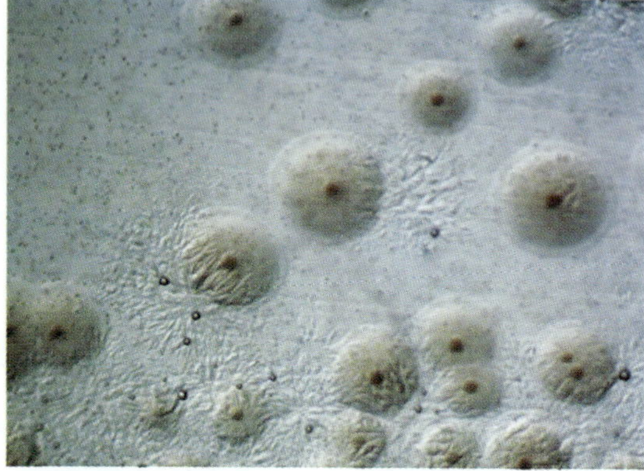

a. Pseudomonas b. Mycoplasma
c. Staphylococcus d. Streptococcus

The colony of mycoplasma frequently has a characteristic 'fried egg' shape, with a raised center and a thinner outer edge.

4. **Identify this Gram positive bacteria:**

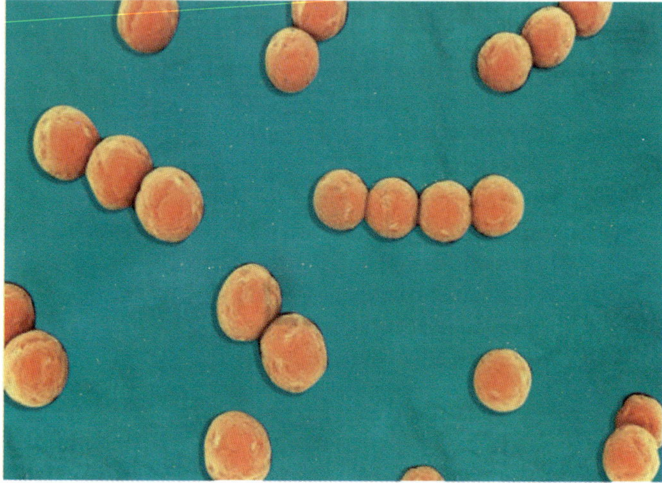

a. Staphylococcus b. Listeria
c. Streptococcus d. Vibrio cholerae

Streptococci are spherical gram positive cocci usually arranged in chains or pairs.

5. **Identify the organism:**

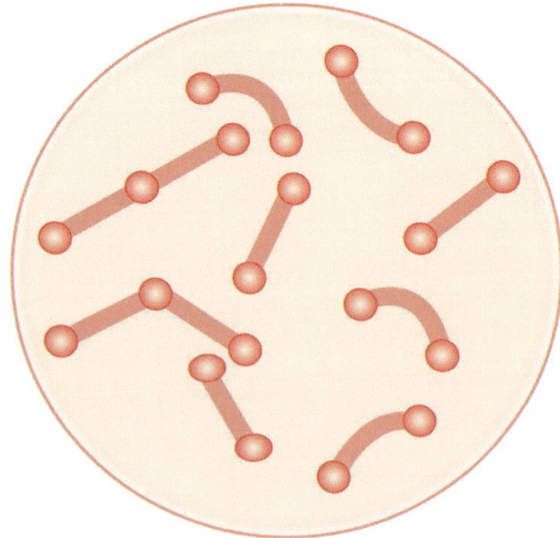

a. Listeria
b. Proteus
c. Pseudomonas
d. Corynebacterium diphtheriae

Corynebacteria are Gram positive rods that appear club-shaped (wider at one end) and are arranged in palisades or in V- or L-shaped formations. The rods have a beaded appearance.

6. **Identify the organism, which shows medusa head appearance:**

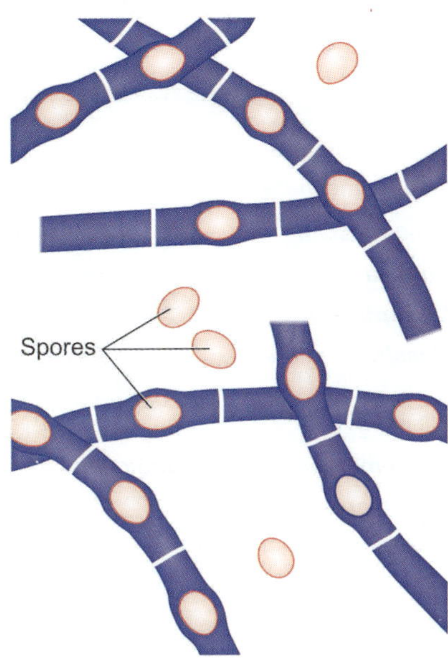

a. Bacillus anthracis
b. Clostridium tetani
c. Clostridium welchii
d. Clostridium perfringenes

B. anthracis is a one of the largest (of pathogenic bacteria) Gram positive rod with square ends. In cultures, the bacilli are arranged end to end in long chains. Spores are central, elliptical or oval in shape, and are of the same width as the bacillary rods.

7. **Identify the organism:**

a. Clostridium tertium
b. Clostridium tetani
c. Clostridium welchi
d. Clostridium perfringens

Oval and terminal spores giving rise to tennis racket appearance is seen in C. Tertium.

8. **Identify the organism:**

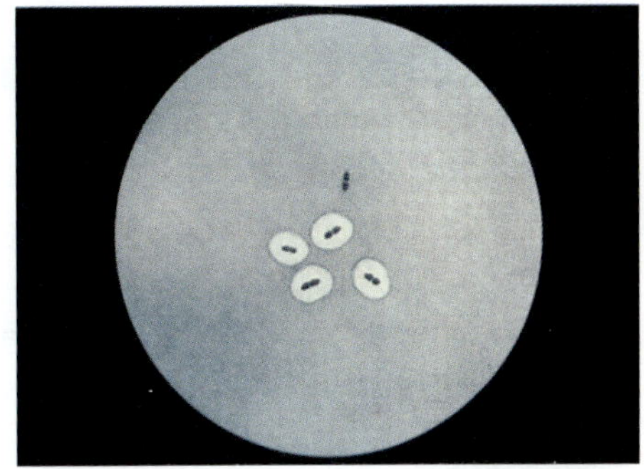

a. Klebsiella
b. Proteus
c. H. pylori
d. Pneumococci

Pneumococci are typicall small (1 micrometer), slightly elongated cocci, with one end broad or rounded and the other pointed, presenting a flame shaped or lanceolate appearance. They occur in pairs (diplococci), with broad ends in apposition, the long axis of the coccus parallel to the line joining the two cocci in a pair.

9. **Identify the organism, which is shown by dark ground microscopy:**

a. Treponema pallidum
b. Clostridium tetani
c. Clostridium welchii
d. Clostridium perfringens

Treponema pallidum morphology and motility can be seen under the dark ground or phase contrast microscopy.

10. **Identify the bacteria, which produces urease enzyme:**

a. Klebsiella
b. Staphylococcus
c. H. pylori
d. Ureaplasma urealyticum

H. pylori is a Gram negative spiral rod, motile by a unipolar tuft of lophotrichous flagella.

MCQ POINTS

S. No.	Question statements	Answers
1.	Stain used for electron microscopy	***Phosphotungstic acid***
2.	Pathology of Wiskot Aldrich syndrome is	***Wasp gene mutation***
3.	Treponema pallidum is stained using which stain	***Fontana stain***
4.	Prions are killed by:	***Autoclaving/ NaOH/ Hypochlorite***
5.	Citron bodies are formed by which clostridial species	***Cl. septicum***
6.	Both intra-cytoplasmic and intra-nuclear inclusion bodies are seen in which virus	***Measles***
7.	Incubation period of gas gangrene	***2-3 days***
8.	Donovanosis is caused by	***Calymmatobacterium granulomatosis***
9.	NNN media is used in	***Leishmania***
10.	Antemortem rabies diagnosis is made commonly from	***Skin biopsy***
11.	Incubation period of yellow fever	***4-6 days***
12.	Another term for Corynebacterium diphtheriae	***Klebs Loeffler bacillus***
13.	Negri bodies are mainly found in which part of brain	***Hippocampus***
14.	Grave's disease is which type of hypersensitivity reaction	***Type II***
15.	Bacillus used to test efficacy of sterilization by autoclave	***Bacillus stearothermophilus***
16.	Causative agent of whooping cough	***B. pertussis***
17.	Mechanism of action of tetanus toxin	***Presynaptic blocking***
18.	MC initial site of involvement in tetanus	***Face***
19.	Charcot Leyden crystal in stool is seen in infection with which bacteria	***Entamoeba histolytica***
20.	Inclusion bodies of trachoma are stained with	***Iodine***
21.	Botulism is most commonly seen after ingestion of which type of food	***Canned foods***
22.	Complement synthesized in liver is	***C3***
23.	Which IL is activator of NK cells	***IL-12***
24.	Hand foot mouth syndrome is caused by which virus	***Coxsackie virus A16***
25.	Phenol test/ Reidel walker test is done to determine	***Efficacy of disinfectant***
26.	In-utero infection leads to which immunoglobulin secretion	***IgM***
27.	Immunoglobulin present in local secretions	***IgA***
28.	Immunoglobulin in Peyer's patches	***IgA***
29.	Charcot leyden crystals are derived from	***Eosinophils***
30.	Which complement factor is responsible for phagocytosis	***C3b***
31.	Which complement fraction is chemo-attractant	***C5a***
32.	Swine flu is caused by which strain	***H1N1 strain***
33.	Ig that is inactive at high temperature	***IgE***
34.	Ig that crosses placenta readily	***IgG***
35.	Antonie van leeuwenhoek is associated with invention of	***Microscope***
36.	Who gave theory of web of causation	***Mcmahon and Pugh***
37.	Compound used for fixation of protozoa found in stool	***Alcohol***
38.	Investigation of choice for amoebiasis	***Microscopy + ELISA***
39.	Widal test is which type of reaction	***Tube agglutination***
40.	Lepra cells are also known as	***Histiocytes***

S. No.	Question statements	Answers
41.	Aschoff bodies is made up of	*Lymphocyte*
42.	Sterilization of fibre-optic is done by	*Glutaraldehyde*
43.	Intermediate host of toxoplasma gondii is	*Humans and Sheep (cat is definitive host)*
44.	Salmonellosis is MC in which type of anemia:	*Sickle cell anemia*
45.	Stain used for degenerated fungi in tissue	*Gomori methenamine silver*
46.	Measles virus belongs to which group	*Paramyxovirus*
47.	Which parasite can pass through intact skin	*Strongyloides*
48.	Number of nucleus present in mature cyst of E. histolytica	*4*
49.	Chagas disease is caused by	*Trypanosoma cruzii*
50.	Food poisoning in canned food is caused by which organism	*Clostridium botulinum*
51.	Intermediate host of malarial parasite	*Humans*
52.	Schizont are NOT seen in peripheral smear of which type of malaria	*Falciparum*
53.	MC cause of dysentery in adults	*Amoebic colitis*
54.	Cause of melioidosis	*B. pseudomallei*
55.	Which parasite causes myocarditis	*Trichinella spiralis*
56.	Metachromatic granules are seen in	*C. diphtheriae*
57.	Skin test useful in Hydatid disease	*Casoni's test*
58.	Weil's disease is caused by which organism	*Leptospira*
59.	Which complement fraction acts as opsonin	*C3b*
60.	MC deep mycosis in India	*Histoplasmosis*
61.	MC cause of Yaws	*T. pertunae*
62.	Cell mediated immunity is due to which cells	*T-helper 1 cells*
63.	Paul Bunnell test is done for which condition	*Infectious mononucleosis*
64.	Color of granules produced by actinomycosis is	*Yellow*
65.	Sclerotic bodies are found in	*Chromoblastomycosis*
66.	Which Ig acts as a receptor on B cell	*IgM*
67.	Wheal and flare reaction is which type of hypersensitivity reaction	*Type I*
68.	Fried egg colonies are produced by	*Mycoplasma*
69.	Ascaris lumbricoides causes deficiency of which vitamin	*Vitamin A*
70.	Nematode which resides in the caecum and appendix	*Enterobius vermicularis*
71.	HIV primarily affects which cells	*CD4*
72.	Ig with a pentameric structure and J chain	*IgM*
73.	Kaposi sarcoma is related to which virus	*HHV-8*
74.	Oral hairy leukoplakia is associated with which virus	*EBV*
75.	Which vessel carries highly oxygenated blood toward fetal heart	*Umbilical vein*
76.	A negative staining technique	*India ink*
77.	Clostridia is gram	*Positive*
78.	Preformed toxin of which organism produces diarrhoea	*Staph. Aureus*
79.	Q fever is caused by	*C. burnettii*
80.	Cerebral malaria is caused by which plasmodia	*Falciparum*
81.	Pathogenicity of legionella is because of	*Defective oxygen burst*
82.	H. pylori is found in	*Mucosa (of stomach)*
83.	Fungus which can not be grown on artificial media	*Rhinosporidium*
84.	Macrophages are a major source of which IL	*IL-1*

S. No.	Question statements	Answers
85.	Furuncle is caused by	***Staph. aureus***
86.	Classification of Ig is based on	***Heavy chain***
87.	SSPE is a rare complication of	***Measles***
88.	Cyclopropagative cycle is seen in	***Malaria in anopheles***
89.	Prausnitz Kustner reaction demonstrates which Ig antibodies	***IgE***
90.	Casoni's test is positive in	***Echinococcosis***
91.	Organism causing pseudo-membranous enterocolitis	***Clostridium difficile***
92.	Sterilization of rubber gloves is done by	***Autoclave***
93.	Autoclaving is done for	***Linen, rubber gloves***
94.	Sterilization of surgical blade is done by	***Hot air oven***
95.	Proctoscope is sterilized by	***Glutaraldehyde***
96.	Which subtype of shigella causes arthritis	***Shigella flexner***
97.	Strain of BCG vaccine is obtained from which mycobacterium	***Mycobacterium bovis***
98.	Tuberculin test is which type of hypersensitivity reaction	***IV***
99.	Treatment of allergic pulmonary aspergillosis	***Steroids***
100.	MC cause of fungal meningitis in AIDS	***Cryptococcus***
101.	Aflatoxin is produced by which fungus	***Aspergillus flavus***
102.	Draughtsman concentric rings on culture is produced by	***Pneumococcus***
103.	Clostridium tetani is gram ….	***Positive***
104.	Eaton agent is	***Mycoplasma***
105.	Lyme's disease is caused by	***B. burgdorferi***
106.	Coating of pathogens by Ig and complement is known as	***Opsonization***
107.	Transmitting agent for prions	***Proteins***
108.	Heterophile antibody test is used to detect	***Infectious mononucleosis***
109.	Paul Bunnell test is done for	***Infectious mononucleosis***
110.	In typhoid carriers, typhoid bacilli is seen in	***Gall bladder***
111.	Pinta is caused by	***T. caratenum***
112.	Risus sardonicus is seen in	***Tetanus***
113.	HLA complex is on chromosome number	***6***
114.	Correct order of Gram staining	***Violet → iodine → red***
115.	Shingle is caused by	***Herpes zoster***
116.	Milk ring test is done for	***Brucella***
117.	Negri bodies are seen in which condition	***Rabies encephalitis***
118.	Schistosomiasis is transmitted by	***Snails***
119.	Necrotizing fasciitis is caused by	***Beta hemolytic streptococci***
120.	Prions is best killed by	***Autoclaving/ NaOH/ Hypochlorite***
121.	Human fibroblast cell line is used for cultivation of	***Poliovirus***
122.	Elcthyma gangrenosum is caused by	***Pseudomonas***
123.	Reynolds Braude phenomenon is shown by which fungus	***Candida***
124.	Serological testing of a patient showed HBsAg, IgM anti-HBc and HBeAg positive. Status of patient	***Acute HBV with high infectivity***
125.	Prozone phenomenon is seen when	***Excess antibody***
126.	Bullous impetigo is caused by	***Staph aureus***
127.	Which organism require cholesterol for growth	***Mycoplasma***

S. No.	Question statements	Answers
128.	Post splenectomy patient is in need of which vaccination	***Pneumococcal***
129.	In nutrient agar, concentration of agar is ...%	***2***
130.	Most virulent dengue fever strain	***Type II***
131.	Tumbling motility is shown by	***Listeria***
132.	Paul Bunnell test is seen in	***Infectious mononucleosis***
133.	Erythrasma is caused by	***C. minutissimum***
134.	All oncogenic viruses containing RNA belongs to which group	***Retroviridae***
135.	Fungus which is NOT cultivable usually	***Rhinosporidium***
136.	MC cause of diarrhoea in children of developing country	***ETEC***
137.	Burkitt's virus is	***EBV***
138.	Painless, genital ulcer in male with everted margins is seen in	***Syphilis***
139.	A child come with fever, cold, cough and membrane over tonsils. Nasal swab is taken. Culture should be done on which medium	***Loeffler's serum slope/ tellurite media***
140.	Diagnosis of rotavirus is done by	***Antigen in stool***
141.	Traveller's diarrhoea is caused by	***ETEC***
142.	Leptospirosis is transmitted by	***Rat urine***
143.	Cellular immunity is induced by	***T-helper cells***
144.	Botulism is most commonly due to	***Canned food/ meat***
145.	Which organism grows at alkaline pH	***Proteus***
146.	Obligate intracellular organism	***Chlamydiae***
147.	Hepatitis C virus belongs to which group	***Flavivirus***
148.	Wheal and flare is which type of hypersensitivity reaction	***Type I***
149.	Yaws is caused by	***T. pertunae***
150.	Most potent chemoattractant leukotriene	***C5a***
151.	Suckling mice is used for isolation of	***Coxsackie virus***
152.	HHV-8 causes which disease	***Kaposi sarcoma***
153.	A child with fever with RBCs and pus in stools. Causative agent	***EHEC***
154.	Staphylococcal scalded skin syndrome is caused by which toxin	***Epidermolytic toxin***
155.	Fish tank granuloma is caused by	***Mycobacterium marinum***
156.	Amplifier host in japanese encephalitis is	***Pigs***
157.	Pentavalent Ig is	***IgM***
158.	Slapped cheek appearance is seen in infections caused by which virus	***Parvovirus***
159.	Colour of granule of actinomycosis is	***Yellow***
160.	MC post-splenectomy infection	***Pneumococcal***
161.	Enterovirus-72 is also known as	***Hepatitis A virus***
162.	Buruli ulcer is caused by	***Mycobacterium ulcerans***
163.	Investigation of choice for cryptococcus	***India ink***
164.	Presentation of botulism	***Descending flaccid paralysis***
165.	Human papilloma virus belongs to which family	***Papova virus***
166.	Diagnosis of polio is made by	***Stool culture***
167.	Cercariae are infective forms of which parasite	***Schistosoma hematobium***
168.	Type I hypersensitivity reaction is mediated by which Ig	***IgE***
169.	Infection/ multiplication of HBsAg is best diagnosed by	***HBeAg and HBV DNA***
170.	ENL is associated with which type of leprosy	***Lepromatous***

S. No.	Question statements	Answers
171.	Which type of plasmodium is associated with renal failure	***Falciparum***
172.	Smallpox belongs to which class of poxvirus	***Orthopox***
173.	Food poisoning case with diarrhoea within 6 hours is due to	***Staph aureus***
174.	Weil felix reaction is used for which organism	***Rickettsia***
175.	Chancroid is caused by	***H. ducreyi***
176.	Antigens are present on which cells	***RBC***
177.	Ig with maximum half life	***IgG***
178.	Ig responsible for opsonization	***IgG***
179.	Most common site of actinomycosis	***Face***
180.	Inclusion bodies are feature of	***Chlamydia***
181.	Hepatitis D virus is ….. stranded, RNA virus	***Single***
182.	Most common oncogenic RNA virus is	***Retrovirus***
183.	Schick test is done in diphtheria to asses	***Susceptibility***
184.	Carry Blair media is used for transporting which	***Vibrio cholera***
185.	Which Ig can cross placenta	***IgG***
186.	Brick shaped virus	***Poxvirus***
187.	Waterhouse Friderichsen syndrome is caused by	***N. meningitides***
188.	Sclerotic bodies are seen in	***Chromoblastomycosis***
189.	MC type of Human papilloma virus associated with cervical cancer	***16***
190.	First antibody to appear in hepatitis B infection	***IgM anti-HBc***
191.	Progressive multifocal leuko-enc aphalopathy is caused by which virus	***JC virus***
192.	Endoscopes are best sterilized by	***Glutaraldehyde***
193.	Phenol coefficient indicates	***Efficacy of disinfectants***
194.	Immunoglobulin involved in atopy	***IgE***
195.	Ig found in fetal serum in case of maternal infections	***IgG***
196.	Transporting media for vibrio cholerae	***Carry Blair, VR media***
197.	Media for tubercle bacilli	***LJ media***
198.	Loeffler's serum slope is used for	***C. diphtheria***
199.	Organism which are bounded by membrane containing sterols	***Mycoplasma***
200.	Test done for infectious mononucleosis	***Paul Bunnell test***
201.	Example of yeast like fungi	***Candida***
202.	Northern blot test is done for	***RNA***
203.	Significant bacteriuria is present if bacterial count in urine is	***> 10^5***
204.	Tennis stick appearance is of clostridium …….	***Clostridium difficile***
205.	Organism seen in dark ground microscopy	***Spirochaetes***
206.	Capsules are detected by	***India ink (cryptococcus), Quellung (pneumococcus)***
207.	Phlyctenular conjunctivitis is type … hypersensitivity reaction	***Type IV***
208.	Traveler's diarrhoea is caused by	***ETEC***
209.	MC cause of diarrhoea in infants	***EPEC***
210.	Antigen (in typhoid) which is absent in normal population	***V_i***
211.	VDRL is a type of ….. test	***Slide flocculation***
212.	Nasopharyngeal Ca is caused by	***EBV***

S. No.	Question statements	Answers
213.	Endotoxin from gram negative are composed of	***Lipopolysaccharide***
214.	MC nosocomial infection is	***E. coli***
215.	Opsonization is defined as	***Coating of antigen for efficient phagocytosis***
216.	Secretory immunoglobulin is which Ig	***IgA***
217.	Immunoglobulin produced after primary immunization	***IgM***
218.	Pneumocystis carinii infection can develop in a HIV patient if CD4-T cell count falls below	***200***
219.	Rat bite fever is caused by	***Spirillum minus***
220.	Lepromin test is type .... hypersensitivity reaction	***IV***
221.	Dorset egg medium is used for	***Mycobacteria***
222.	Draughtsman colonies are seen in culture of	***Pneumococcus***
223.	Tryptophan is an important growth factor for	***Salmonella***
224.	Virulence of mycobacterium TB depends on	***Cord factor***
225.	Bacteria, which is known as Eaton agent	***Mycoplasma***
226.	Metachromatic staining is a feature of	***C. diphtheria***
227.	Cholera red reaction and Indole formation is shown by	***V. cholera***
228.	Motility shown by proteus	***Swarming***
229.	Typical feature of botulinisum	***Descending flaccid paralysis***
230.	Factor responsible for acid fastness of mycobacterium TB	***Mycolic acid in cell wall***
231.	Leptospirosis is transmitted by	***Rat urine***
232.	Sulfur granules in actinomycosis consist of	***Organism***
233.	Q fever is caused by	***C. burnetii***
234.	Swine flu was due to .... strain	***H1N1***
235.	Negri bodies are seen in which disease	***Rabies encephalitis***
236.	Retroviral sequence of HIV virus in host cell	***RNA-DNA-RNA***
237.	MC cause of diarrhoea in AIDS	***Cryptosporidium***
238.	MC cause of meningitis in AIDS	***Cryptococcus***
239.	MC cause of infantile diarrhoea	***Rotavirus/EPEC***
240.	Infective agent of malaria	***Sporozoite***
241.	MC fungal infection in neutropenic patients	***Candida***
242.	Weil Felix reaction detects anti-rickettsial antibodies that can cross react with which bacteria	***Proteus***
243.	Ramsay Hunt is involvement of facial nerve by which virus	***Herpes zoster***
244.	Virus with single stranded DNA	***Parvovirus***
245.	Virus with double stranded RNA	***Rotavirus (reovirus)***
246.	Negri bodies are seen in which part of CNS	***Hippocampus***
247.	Hepatitis which usually have a subclinical course	***HCV***
248.	Pigment which is diagnostic of infection by pseudomonas aeruginosa	***Pyocyanin***
249.	Borrelia burgdorferi causes which disease	***Lyme's disease***
250.	Erythema infectiosum is caused by	***Parvovirus***
251.	Very rare delayed sequel to infection with measles virus	***SSPE***
252.	Culture media for fungus	***Sabouraud's dextrose agar***
253.	Method for detection of capsule of Cryptococcus neoformans	***India ink***
254.	10% KOH mount is used for examining which micro-organism	***Fungus***
255.	Pityrosporum orbiculare causes which skin disease	***Pityriasis versicolor***

S. No.	Question statements	Answers
256.	Microsporum affects which parts of bodies	***Skin and hair***
257.	Etiological agent of mycetoma	***Madurella, actinomycetes***
258.	Sclerotic bodies are suggestive of infection with	***Chromoblastomycosis***
259.	Reynolds Braude phenomenon is shown by	***Candida***
260.	Antigen (in typhoid) which is highly immunogenic	***H***
261.	VDRL is positive in	***Secondary syphilis***
262.	Infectious mononucleosis is caused by	***EBV***
263.	Exotoxin from gram positive bacteria are composed of	***Polypeptide***
264.	Anton test is done for	***Listeria***
265.	Chemotaxis is defined as	***Attraction of phagocytic cells towards antigen***
266.	For HIV, relative risk % per exposure is maximum for which route	***Blood transfusion***
267.	Immunoglobulin produced after boosters of vaccine	***IgG***
268.	Mycobacterium avium infection can develop in a HIV patient if CD4-T cell count falls below	***50***
269.	Rat urine is associated with which disease	***Leptospirosis***
270.	Mantoux test is type .... hypersensitivity reaction	***IV***
271.	Which hepatitis never takes a chronic course	***HAV***
272.	Route of transmission of Hepatitis A virus	***Fecal-oral***
273.	Niacin is produced by which bacteria	***Mycobacterium TB***
274.	AFB positivity of mycobacterium TB depends on	***Mycolic acid in cell wall***
275.	Bacteria, which is known as Friedlander's bacteria	***Klebsiella pneumonia***
276.	Bipolar staining is a feature of which bacteria	***Yersinia pestis***
277.	Mannitol fermentation is used for classifying	***Shigella***
278.	Motility shown by clostridium	***Swarming***
279.	Sardonic grin is a feature of	***Tetanus***
280.	Globi is a histological feature of	***Mycobacterium leprae***
281.	Schistosoma is transmitted by	***Snails***
282.	Habitat of wuchereria bancrofti	***Lymphatic***
283.	Malta fever is caused by	***Brucella***
284.	Avian flu was due to .... strain	***H5N1***
285.	HP bodies are suggestive of infection with	***Chlamydia trachomatis and molluscum contagiosum***
286.	% of HIV transmission with accidental needle prick injury	***0.3%***
287.	MC cause CNS disorder in AIDS	***Dementia (disorder), Cryptococcus (cause)***
288.	Infective protein particles are	***Proteins***
289.	Nuclear and cytoplasmic inclusion bodies are shown by which virus	***Measles***
290.	Infective form of leishmaniasis	***Promastigote***
291.	Maurer's dot are related to which malarial parasite	***Falciparum***

CHAPTER

6

PARASITOLOGY

KEY POINTS

Tests and Parasites

- Sabin-Feldman dye test: Toxoplasmosis
- Casoni test: Hydatid cyst
- Frenkel's skin test: Toxoplasmosis

Diseases and Causative Parasites

- Biliary obstruction: Clonorchis sinensis
- Cirrhosis of liver, Katayama disease: S. japonicum
- Pipestem/periportal cirrhosis: S. mansoni
- Ground itch/Ancylostoma dermatitis: Necator
- Cutaneous larva migrans/cutis and creeping eruptions: Ancylostoma braziliense and A. caninum
- Visceral larva migrans: Toxocara canis
- Ocular larva migrans: Toxocara canis
- Larva currens/hyperinfection syndrome/autoinfection: Strongyloides
- Malignant hydatid disease: Echinococcus multilocularis
- L. donovani causes: Visceral leishmaniasis
- Loa Loa causes: Calabar swelling

Other Names of Parasites

- Oriental liver fluke: C. sinensis
- Oriental lung fluke: P. westermani
- Oriental blood fluke: S. japonicum
- Smallest tapeworm: Echinococcus granulosus
- Dwarf tapeworm: H. nana
- Longest tapeworm: T. saginata
- Largest intestinal fluke/trematode: F. buski

Plasmodium Falciparum

- Resistance: Drug resistance widespread
- CNS involvement: Present
- Anaemia: Present
- Hypnozoites: Absent
- Incubation period: 12 days
- Stages: Only rings and gametocytes
- Special forms: Accole, wing, marginal
- RBC size: Not enlarged
- Dots: Maurer's dots
- Infection: Multiple infections per RBC

Occult Filarias is

- Occult filariasis/Mayers-Kouwenaar syndrome
- Cause: Microfilariae
- Organs involved: Lymphatic system, lungs, Liver and spleen
- Therapeutic response: Responds to DEC
- Microfilaria: Present in affected tissues
- Loa Loa: Microfilariae are detected in blood in daytime.

Classical Filariasis

- Cause: Developing worms and adults
- Organs involved: Lymphatic system
- Therapeutic response: No response
- Microfilaria: Present in blood

MCQs WITH SHORT EXPLANATIONS

1. Which of the following is the intermediate host for schistosoma haematobium?

a. Cat
b. Dog
c. Rat
d. Fresh water snail

Schistosoma haematobium

- It is an important digenetic trematode, and is found in the Middle East, India, Portugal and Africa.
- It is a major agent of schistosomiasis; more specifically, it is associated with urinary schistosomiasis.
- Adults are found in the Venous plexuses around the urinary bladder and the released eggs traverse the wall of the bladder causing haematuria and fibrosis of the bladder.
- The bladder becomes calcified, and there is increased pressure on ureters and kidneys otherwise known as hydronephrosis.
- Inflammation of the genitals due to S. haematobium may contribute to the propagation of HIV.
- Studies have shown the relationship between S. haematobium infection and the development of squamous cell carcinoma of the bladder

Life cycle

- The female fluke lays as many as 30 eggs per day which migrate to the lumen of the urinary bladder and ureters.
- The eggs are eliminated from the host into the water supply with micturition.
- In fresh water, the eggs hatch forming free swimming miracidia which penetrate into the intermediate snail host (Bulinus spp., e.g. B. globosus, B. forskalii, B. nyassanus and B. truncatus).
- Inside the snail, the miracidium sheds it epithelium and develops into a mother sporocyst.
- After two weeks the mother begins forming daughter sporocysts.
- Four weeks after the initial penetration of the miracardium into the snail furcocercous cercariae begin to be released.
- The cercariae cycle from the top of the water to the bottom for three days in the search of a human host.
- Within half an hour the cercariae enter the host epithelium

2. Which of the following is the largest trematode which infest humans?

a. F. hepatica
b. F. buski
c. E. granulosus
d. Clonorchosis sinensis

Fasciolopsis buski

- It is commonly called the giant intestinal fluke, because it is an exceptionally large parasitic fluke, and the largest known to parasitise humans.
- Its size is variable and a mature specimen might be as little as 2 cm long, but the body may grow to a length of 7.5 cm and a width of 2.5 cm.
- It is a common parasite of humans and pigs and is most prevalent in Southern and Southeaster n Asia.
- It is a member of the family Fasciolidae in the order Echinostomida.
- The Echinostomida are members of the class Trematoda, the flukes.
- The fluke differs from most species that parasitise large mammals, in that they inhabit the gut rather than the liver as Fasciola species do.
- Fasciolopsis buski generally occupies the upper region of the small intestine, but in heavy infestations can also be found in the stomach and lower regions of the intestine.
- Fasciolopsis buski is the cause of the pathological condition fasciolopsiasis.

3. Sabin-Feldman test is done for:

a. Multiple myeloma
b. Toxoplasmosis
c. Leptospirosis
d. Syphilis

A **Sabin–Feldman dye test** is a serologic test to diagnose for toxoplasmosis. The test is based on the presence of certain antibodies that prevent methylene blue dye from entering the cytoplasm of *Toxoplasma* organisms. Patient serum is treated with Toxoplasma trophozoites and complements as activator, and then incubated. After incubation, methylene blue is added. If anti-Toxo antibodies are present in the serum, because these antibodies are activated by complements and lyse the parasite membrane, Toxoplasma trophozoites are not stained (positive result); if there are no antibodies, trophozoites with intact membrane are stained and appear blue under microscope (negative result).

Ans. 1. **d.** Fresh water snail 2. **b.** F. buski 3. **b.** Toxoplasmosis

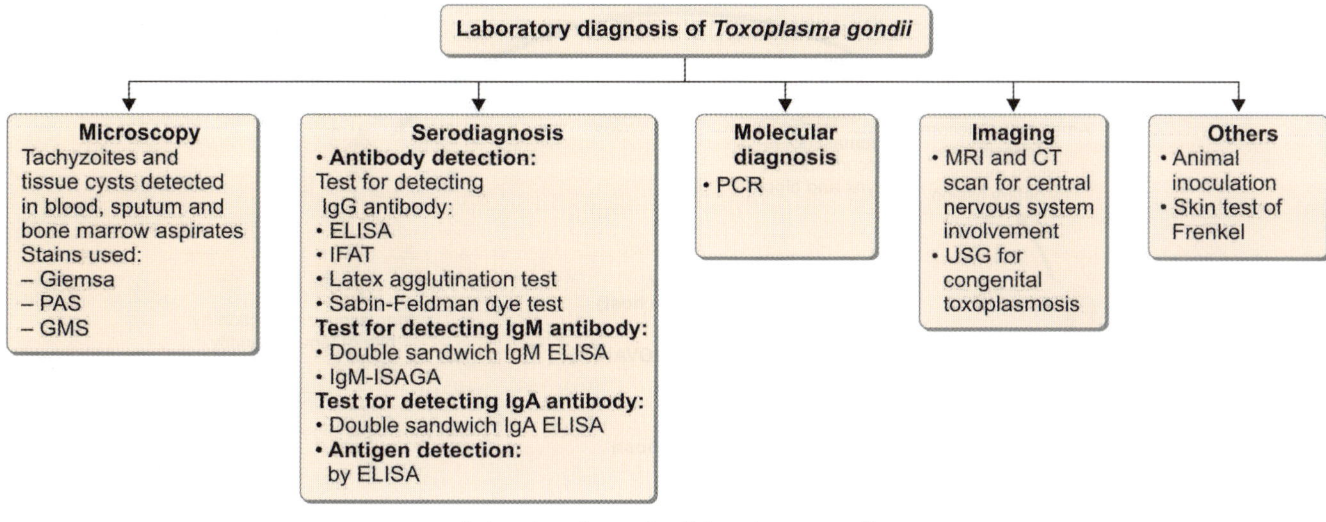

Laboratory diagnosis of *Toxoplasma gondii.*

4. Two nuclei at the tail tip are seen in:

a. Brugia malayi
b. Wuchereria bancrofti
c. Onchocerca volvulus
d. Mansonella ozzardi

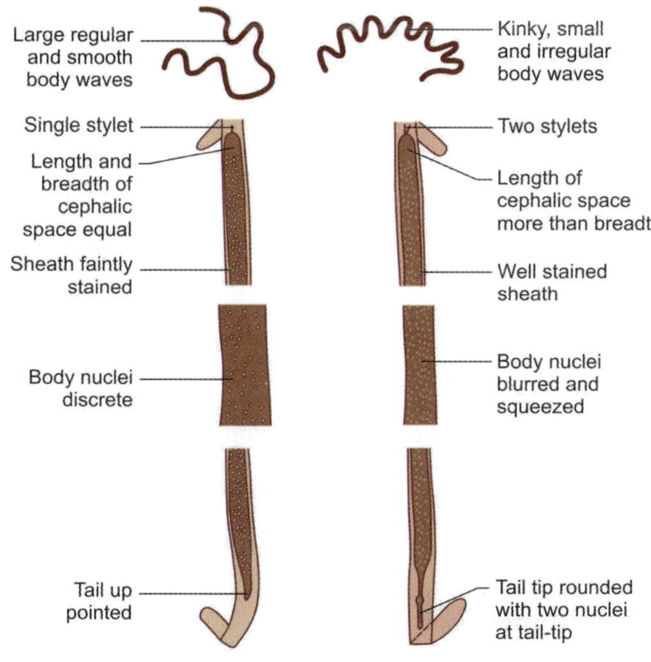

Schematic diagram showing distinguishing features of Microfilariae bancrofti and Microfilariae malayi.

B. malayi microfilariae resemble *W. bancrofti* and *Loa loa* microfilariae with minor differences that can aid in laboratory diagnosis. *B. malayi* microfilariae can be distinguished by the noncontinuous row of nuclei found in the tip of the tail. There are two terminal nuclei that are distinctly separated from the other nuclei in the tail, whereas the tail of *W. bancrofti* contains no nuclei and *Loa loa* microfilariae nuclei form a continuous row in the tail. *B. malayi* microfilariae also have a characteristic cephalic space ratio of 2:1.

5. Highly specific and sensitive test for diagnosing kala-azar:

a. Complement fixation test with WKK antigen
b. Napier's aldehyde test
c. Chopra's antimony test
d. Immunofluorescent antibody test

Indirect fluorescent antibody test (IFAT), a group specific test, detects. antibodies against Leishmania that appear early in the course of the disease and persists as long as six months after cure. This test, therefore, can also be used for monitoring treatment. A titer of 1:20 is significant and 1:28 is strongly suggestive of Kala azar.

6. Promastigote form of Leishmania is found in which part of sandfly:

a. Lymph node
b. GIT
c. Spleen
d. Bone marrow

The **promastigote** form is found in the alimentary tract of sand flies. It is an extracellular and motile form. It is considerably larger and highly elongated, measuring 15-30 μm in length and 5 μm in width. It is spindle-shaped, tapering at both ends. A long flagellum (about the body length) is projected externally at the anterior end. The nucleus lies at the centre, and in front of it are the kinetoplast and the basal body.

Ans. **4. a.** Brugia malayi **5. d.** Immunofluorescent antibody test **6. b.** GIT

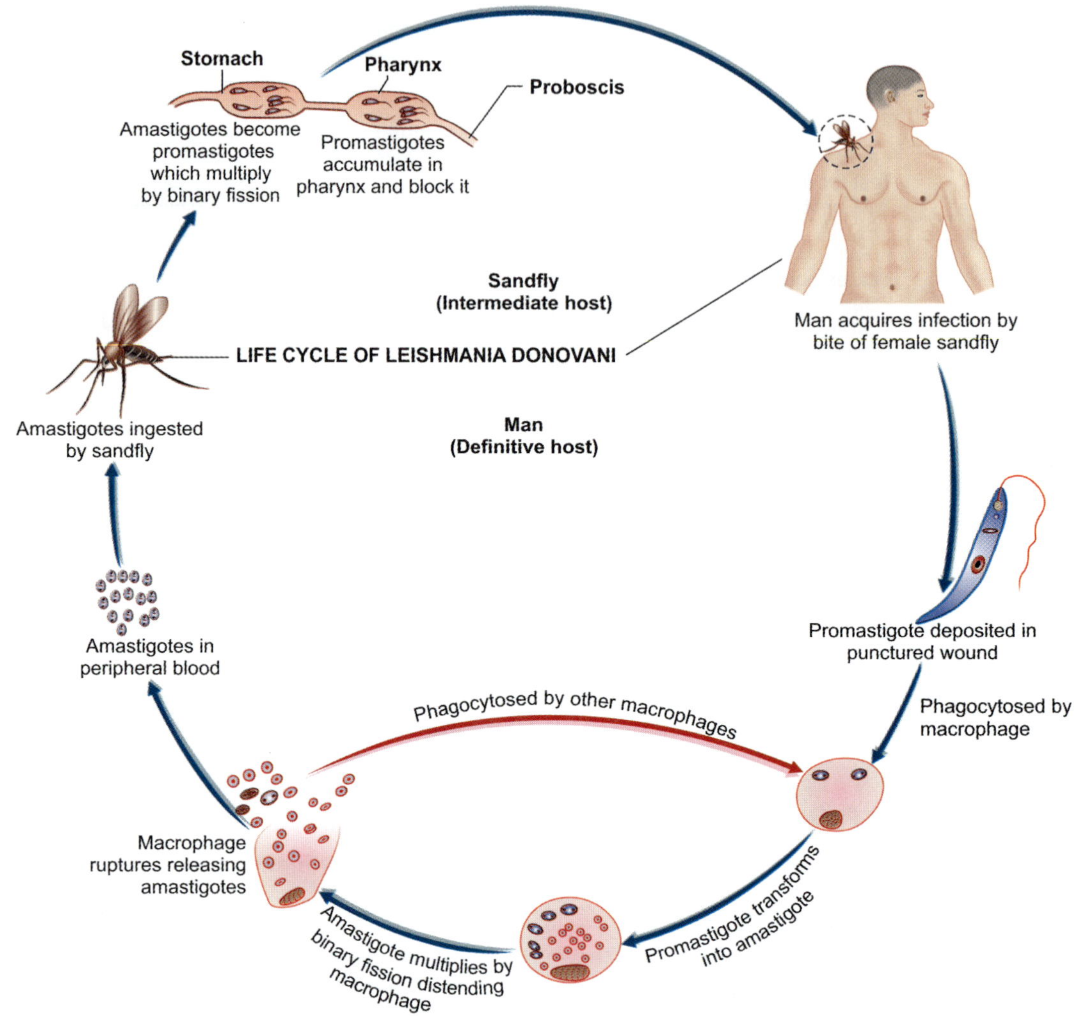

Life cycle of *Leishmania donovani.*

7. Black malarial pigment is seen in:

a. P. vivax
b. P. falciparum
c. P. malariae
d. P. ovlae

In *P. falciparum*, only early (ring-form) trophozoites and gametocytes are seen in the peripheral blood. It is unusual to see mature trophozoites or schizonts in peripheral blood smears, as these are usually sequestered in the tissues. The parasitised erythrocytes are not enlarged, and it is common to see cells with more than one parasite within them (multiply parasitised erythrocytes). On occasion, faint, comma-shaped, red dots called "Maurer's dots" are seen on the red cell surface. The comma-shaped dots can also appear as pear-shaped blotches. *(See Diagram on next page 470)*

8. Microfilaria is NOT seen in:

a. Lymphatics
b. Hydrocoele fluid
c. Chylous urine
d. Blood

The adult worms, which usually stay in one tissue, release early larval forms known as microfilariae into the host's bloodstream. These circulating microfilariae can be taken up with a blood meal by the arthropod vector; in the vector, they develop into infective larvae that can be transmitted to a new host. Microfilaria can be demonstrated in blood, chylous urine, exudates of lymph varix, and hydrocoele fluid. Peripheral blood is the specimen of choice.

9. Cysticercosis cellulosae is seen with:

a. Echinococcus granulosus
b. Taenia solium
c. Taenia saginata
d. All of the above

The cause of human cysticercosis is the egg form of *Taenia solium* (*T. solium* and also called pork tapeworm), which is transmitted through the oral-fecal route. Eggs are accidentally ingested from contaminated water or vegetables.

Ans. **7. b.** P. falciparum **8. a.** Lymphatics **9. b.** Taenia solium

Erythrocyte
Marginal ring form
Young ring stage
Ring forms with double chromation dots
Mature ring and maurer's dots
Trophozite amoeboid stage commencing chromatin division
Nuclear division
Merozoite development
Rarely seen in peripheral circulation
Advanced merozoite development with commencing pigmentation
Schizont mature with centralized pigment
Female gametocyte (crescent)
Male gametocyte (crescent)
Rarely seen in peripheral circulation

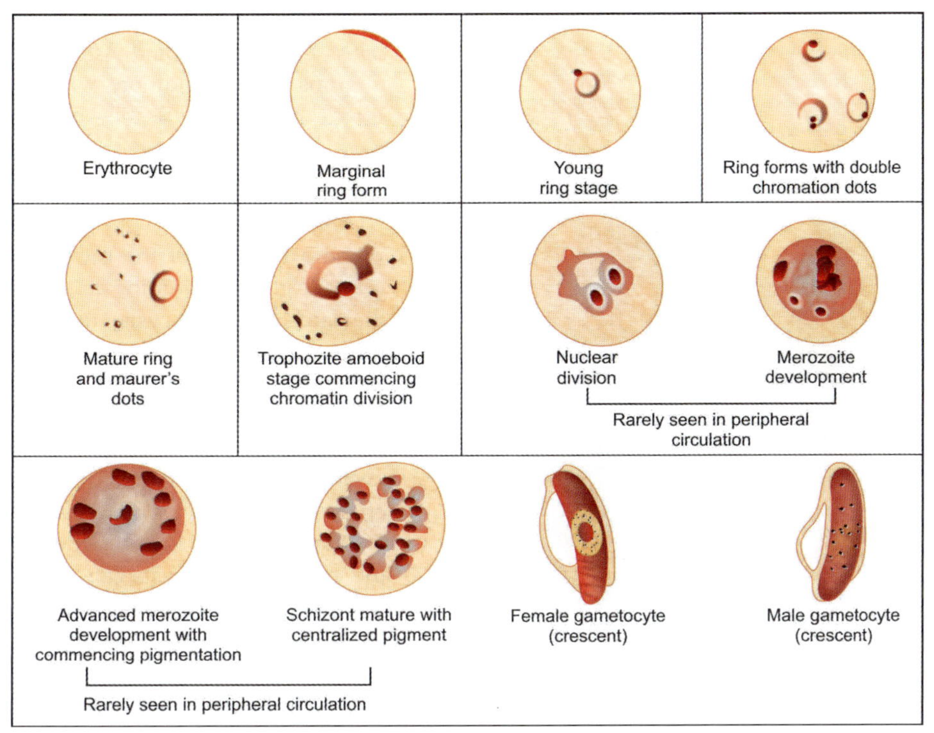

Plasmodium falciparum (Giemsa stain, magn x 2000).

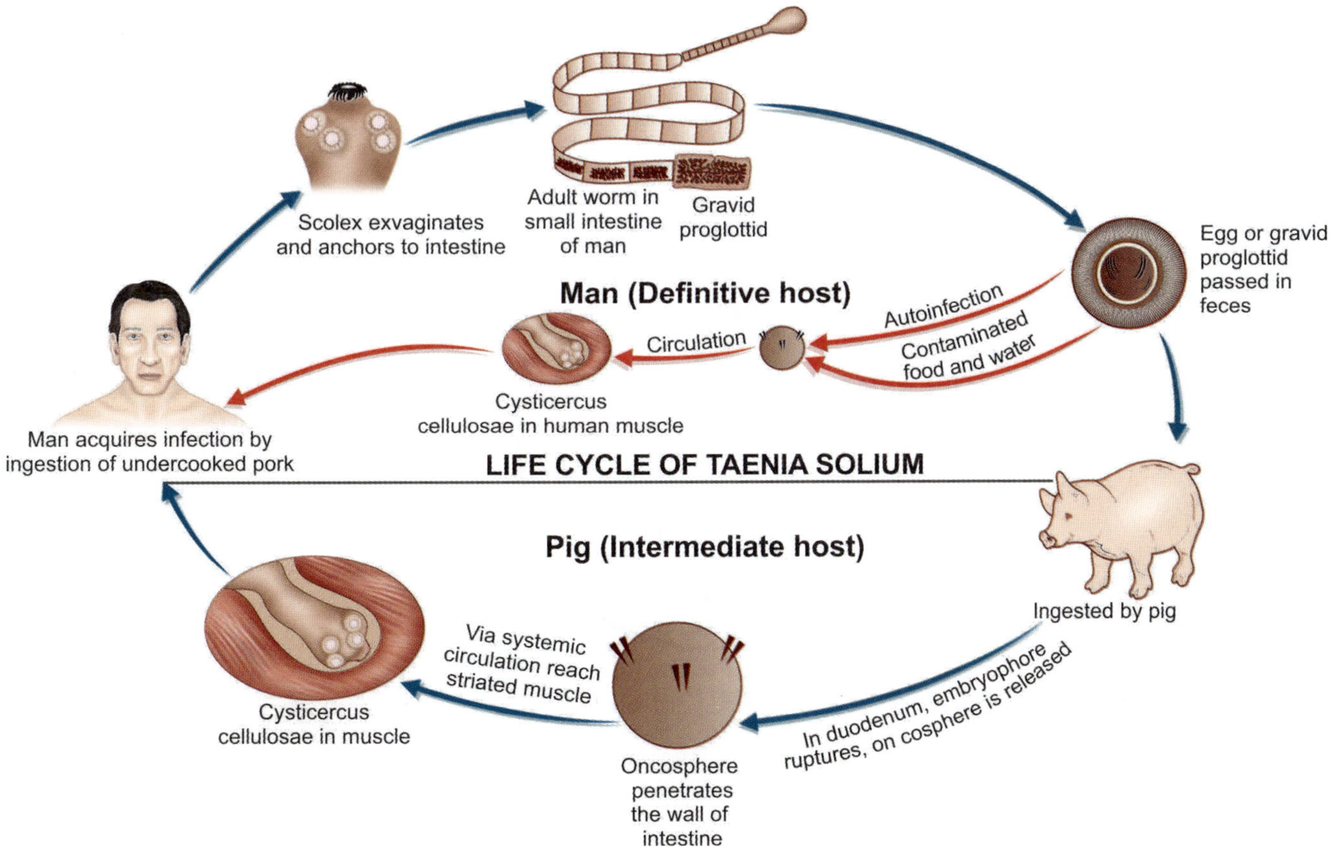

Scolex exvaginates and anchors to intestine
Adult worm in small intestine of man
Gravid proglottid
Egg or gravid proglottid passed in feces
Man (Definitive host)
Autoinfection
Contaminated food and water
Circulation
Cysticercus cellulosae in human muscle
Man acquires infection by ingestion of undercooked pork
LIFE CYCLE OF TAENIA SOLIUM
Pig (Intermediate host)
Ingested by pig
In duodenum, embryophore ruptures, on cosphere is released
Oncosphere penetrates the wall of intestine
Via systemic circulation reach striated muscle
Cysticercus cellulosae in muscle

Life cycle of *Taenia solium.*

10. Visceral larva migrans is due to:

a. Loa Loa
b. Clonorchis sinensis
c. Toxocara canis
d. Ascaris lumbricoides

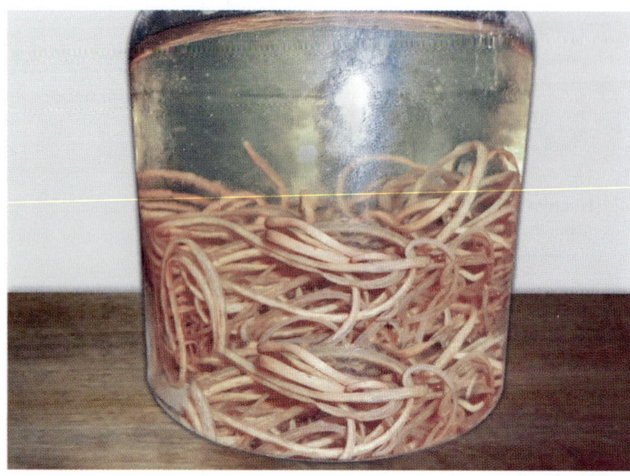

Adult worms of *Toxocara canis.*

Visceral larva migrans is caused by the migratory larvae of certain nematodes, humans being a dead-end host, and was first reported in 1952. Nematodes causing such zoonotic infections are *Baylisascaris procyonis*, *Toxocara canis*, *Toxocara cati*, and *Ascaris suum*. Cutaneous larva migrans is a condition where nematodes such as *Ancylostoma braziliense* migrate to the skin.

11. Route of transmission of toxoplasma from cat to mice:

a. Faeces
b. Urine
c. Blood
d. Food

When a member of the cat family is infected with *T. gondii* (e.g. by consuming an infected mouse laden with the parasite's tissue cysts), the parasite survives passage through the stomach, eventually infecting epithelial cells of the cat's small intestine. Inside these intestinal cells, the parasites undergo sexual development and reproduction, producing millions of thick-walled, zygote-containing cysts known as oocysts. Infected epithelial cells eventually rupture and release oocysts into the intestinal lumen, whereupon they are shed in the cat's feces. Oocysts can then spread to soil, water, food, or anything potentially contaminated with the feces. Mice eat materials contaminated with oocysts shed in cats faeces. Tissue cysts develop in mice. When such mice are eaten by cats, they get infected and again shed oocysts in feces.

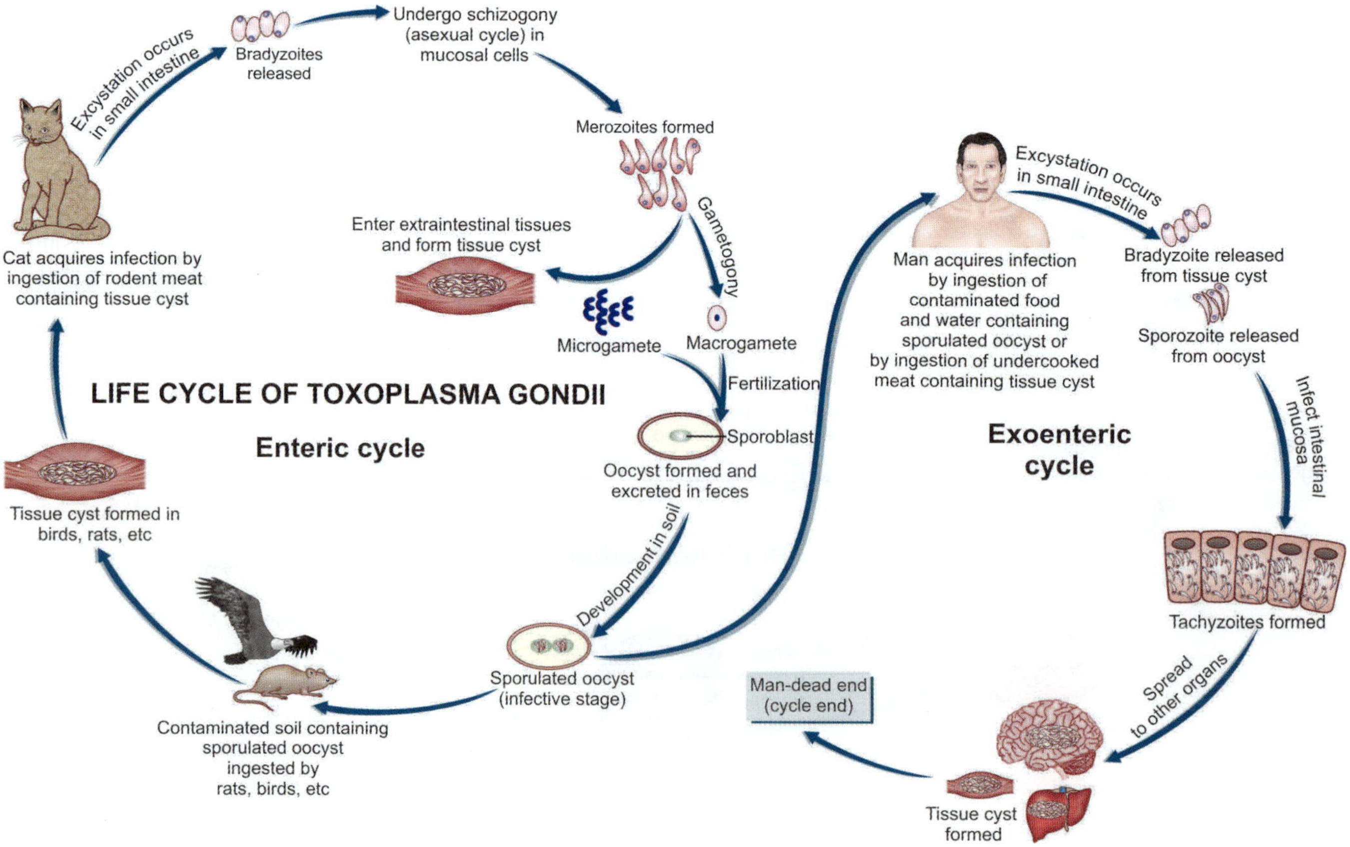

LIFE CYCLE OF TOXOPLASMA GONDII
Enteric cycle
Exoenteric cycle
Excystation occurs in small intestine
Bradyzoites released
Undergo schizogony (asexual cycle) in mucosal cells
Merozoites formed
Gametogony
Enter extraintestinal tissues and form tissue cyst
Microgamete
Macrogamete
Fertilization
Sporoblast
Oocyst formed and excreted in feces
Development in soil
Sporulated oocyst (infective stage)
Contaminated soil containing sporulated oocyst ingested by rats, birds, etc
Tissue cyst formed in birds, rats, etc
Cat acquires infection by ingestion of rodent meat containing tissue cyst
Man acquires infection by ingestion of contaminated food and water containing sporulated oocyst or by ingestion of undercooked meat containing tissue cyst
Excystation occurs in small intestine
Bradyzoite released from tissue cyst
Sporozoite released from oocyst
Infect intestinal mucosa
Tachyzoites formed
Spread to other organs
Tissue cyst formed
Man-dead end (cycle end)

Life cycle of *Toxoplasma gondii.*

Ans. **10. c.** Toxocara canis **11. a.** Faeces

12. Megaloblastic anemia caused by:

a. Taenia saginata
b. Diphyllobothrium latum
c. Taenia solium
d. Echinococcus granulosus

Symptoms of diphyllobothriasis are generally mild, and can include diarrhea, abdominal pain, vomiting, weight loss, fatigue, constipation and discomfort. Approximately four out of five cases are asymptomatic and may go many years without being detected. In a small number of cases, this leads to severe vitamin B_{12} deficiency due to the parasite absorbing 80% or more of the host's B_{12} intake, and a megaloblastic anemia indistinguishable from pernicious anemia. The anemia can also lead to subtle demyelinative neurological symptoms (subacute combined degeneration of spinal cord).

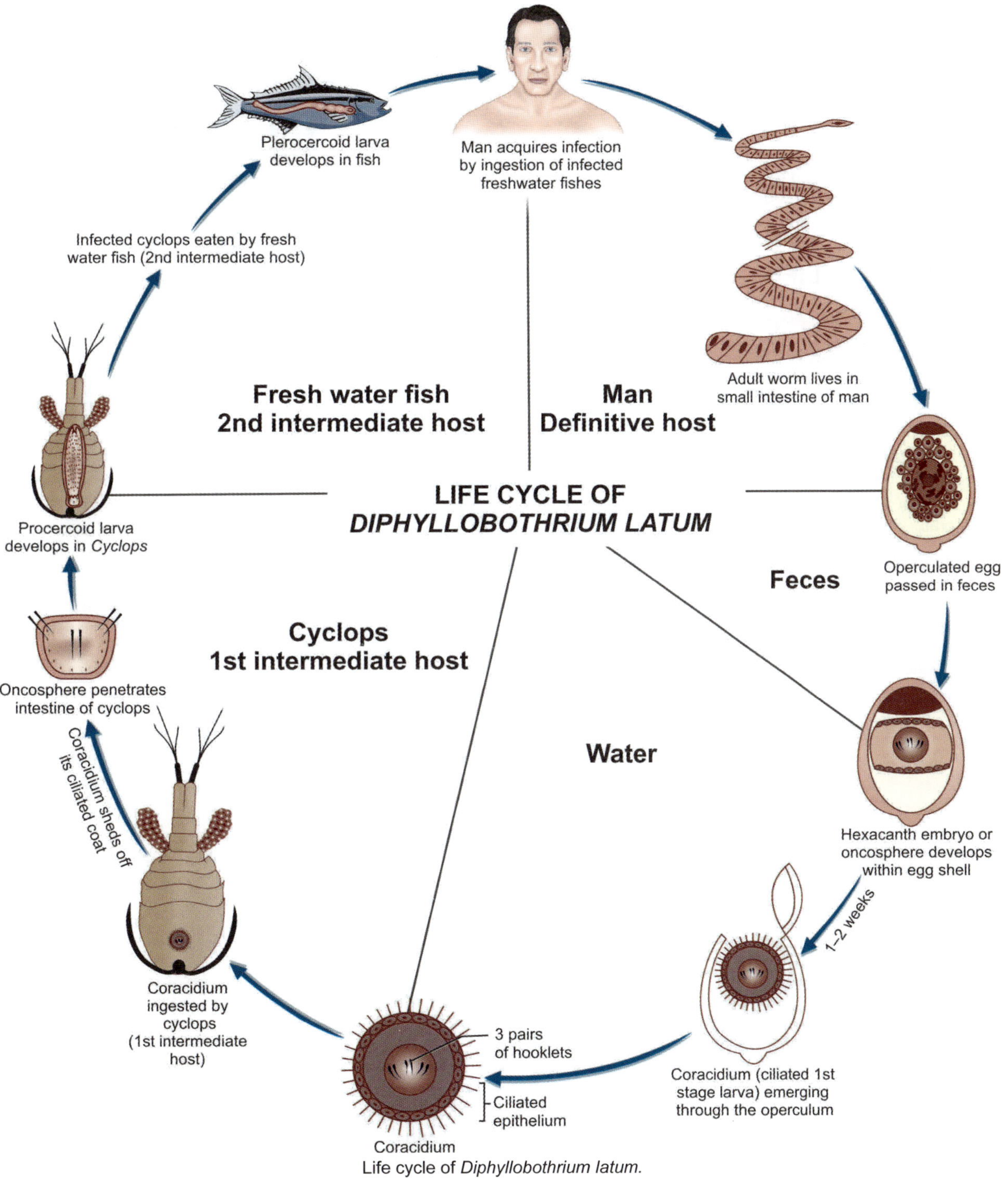

Life cycle of *Diphyllobothrium latum*.

Ans. 12. **b.** Diphyllobothrium latum

13. Paragonimus westermani is commonly called:

a. Lung fluke
b. Tapeworms
c. Intestinal flukes
d. Liver flukes

The most prominent species of Paragonimus in human medicine is *Paragonimus westermani*, an infectious oriental lung fluke originating in eastern Asia. Worldwide, about nine species of *Paragonimus* are known to cause human paragonimiasis in which many of the species reside in East Asia, West Africa, and in North and South America.

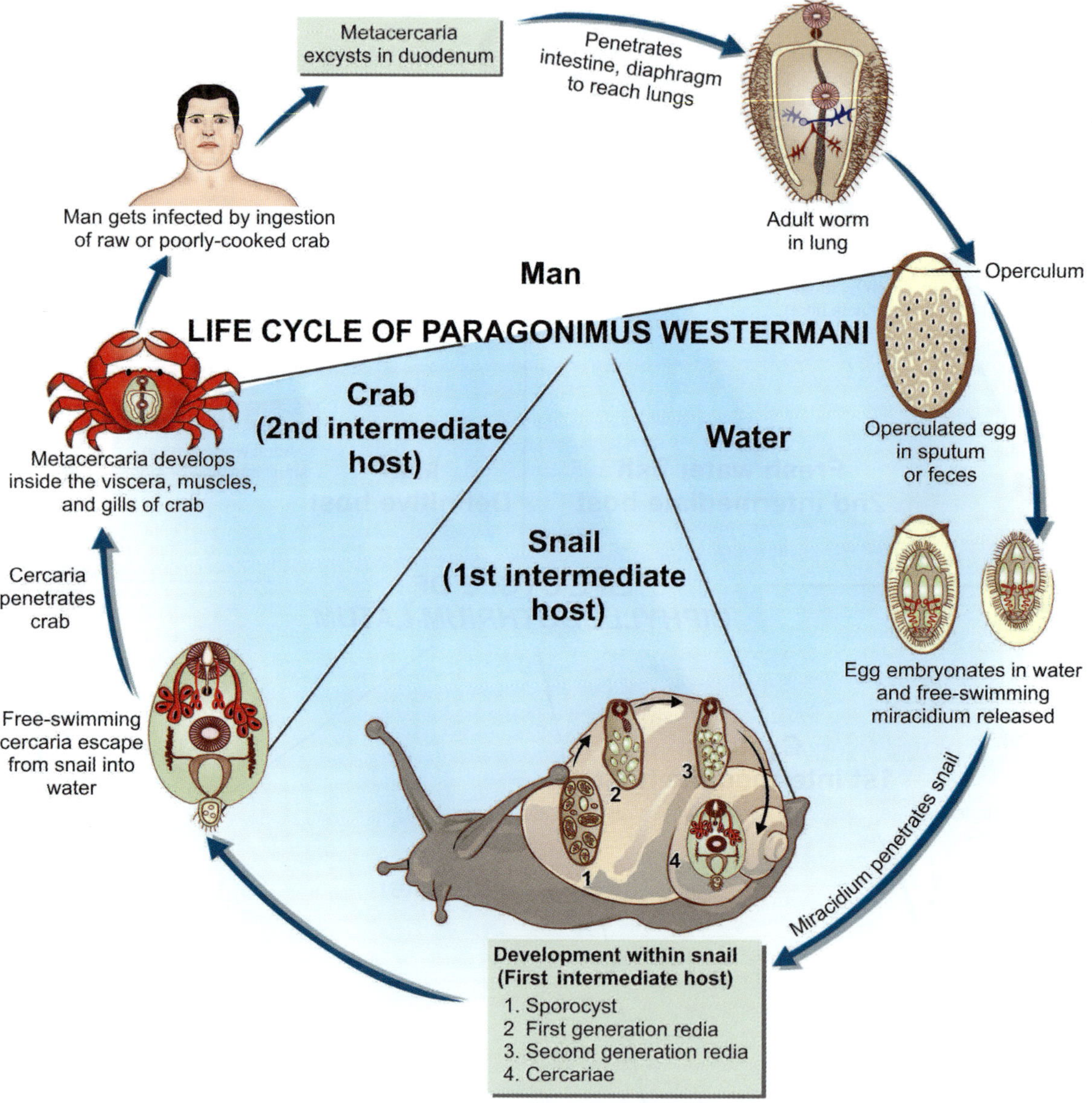

Life cycle of *Paragonimus westermani*.

14. Iron Deficiency anemia is commonly caused by:

a. Enterobius vermicularis
b. Taenia solium
c. Ancylostoma duodenale
d. All of the above

A light infection causes abdominal pain, loss of appetite and geophagy. Heavy infection causes severe protein deficiency or iron deficiency anemia. Protein deficiency may lead to dry skin, edema and potbelly, while iron deficiency anemia might result in mental dullness and heart failure.

Ans. **13. a.** Lung fluke **14. c.** Ancylostoma duodenale

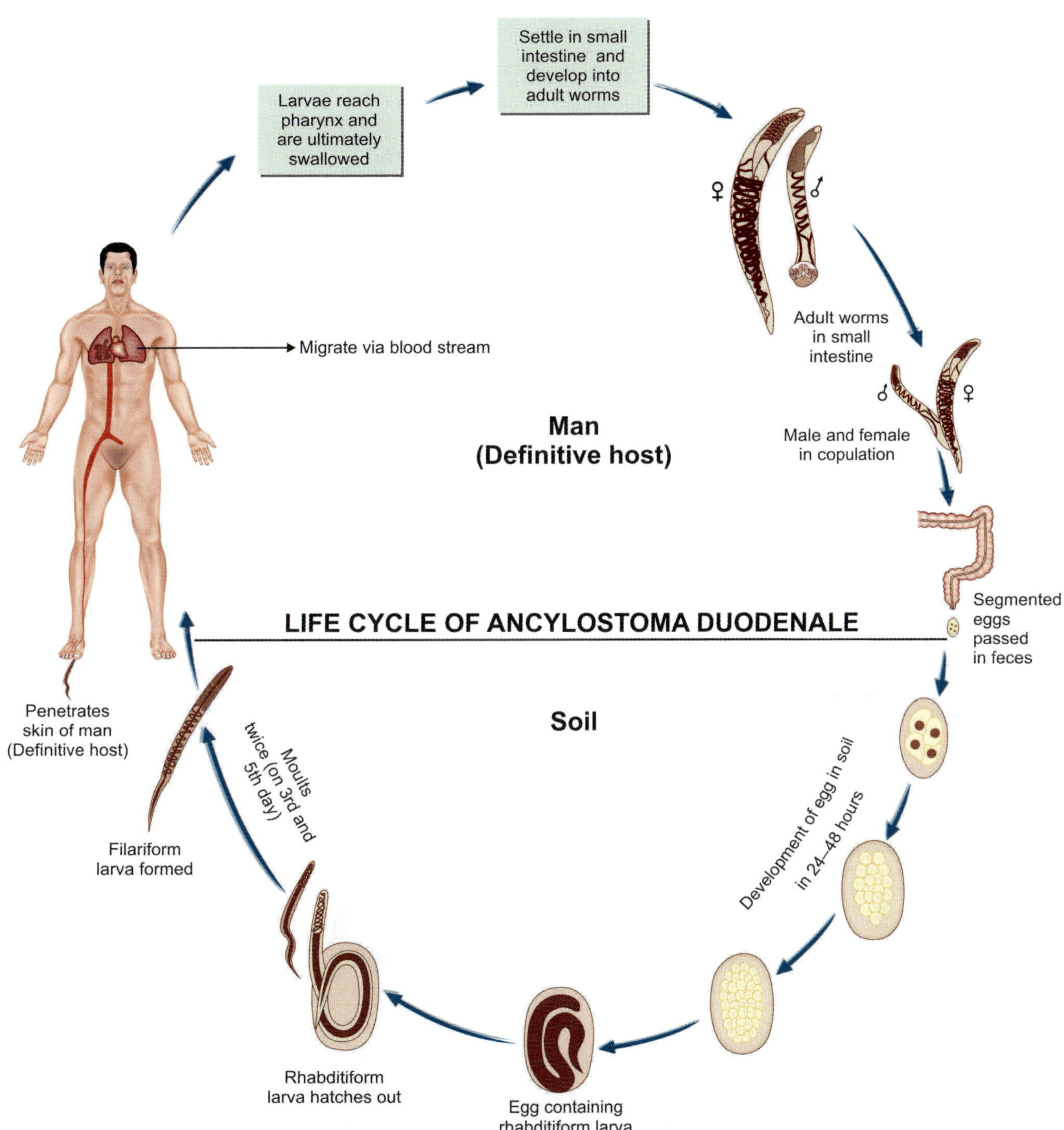

Life cycle of *Ancylostoma duodenale.*

15. True regarding plasmodium falciparum is:

a. Preferentially infects old erythrocytes only
b. Schuffner's dots is characteristic
c. Crescentic macrogametocyte
d. Large schizonts

Gametocyte of P. falciparum are crescent or sausage shape with chromatin in a single mass (macrogametocyte) or diffuse (microgametocyte).

Ans. **15. c.** Crescentic macrogametocyte

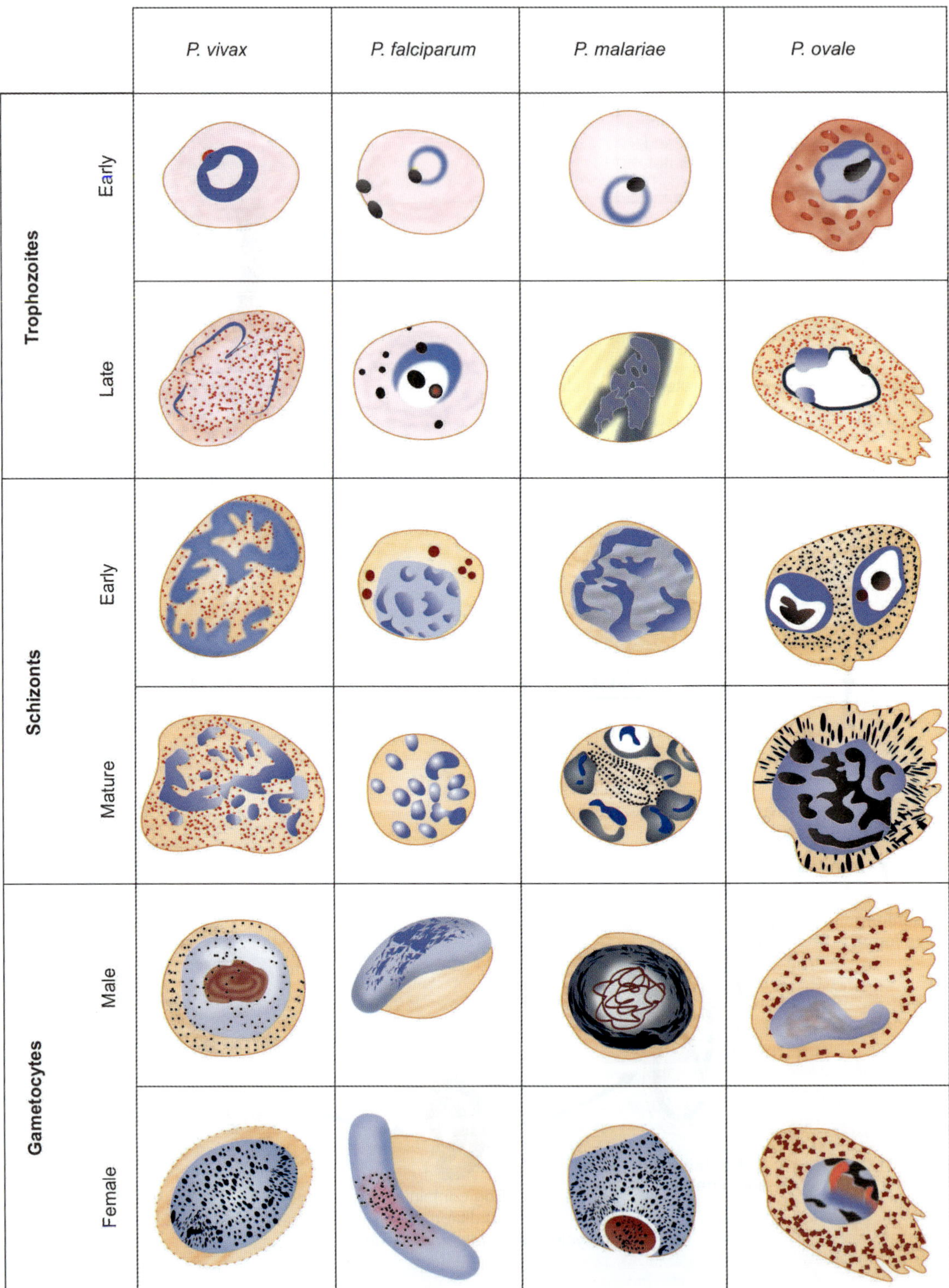

Malaria parasites—Erythrocytic stages of the four species (Giemsa stain. Magn × 2000).

16. Kala azar is transmitted by:

a. Sand fly
b. Tsetse fly
c. Flea
d. Hard tick

Ans. **16. a.** Sand fly

Leishmania species involved in human disease

Species	Disease	Geographical distribution	Vector	Reservoir	Transmission
Leishmania donovani	Visceral leishmaniasis (Kala-azar or dumdum fever)	Middle East, Africa, and Indian Subcontinent	*Phlebotomus argentipes, Phlebotomus orientalis*	Humans	Anthroponotic, occasionally zoonotic
Leishmania infantum	Visceral leishmaniasis, cutaneous leishmaniasis	Mediterranean Coast, Middle East, and China.	*Phlebotomus perniciosus, Phlebotomus ariasi, Phlebotomus papatasi*	Dog, fox, jackal, and wolf	Zoonotic
Leishmania chagasi	Visceral leishmaniasis	Tropical South America	*Lutzomyra longipalpis*	Fox and wild canines	Zoonotic
Leishmania tropica	Cutaneous Leishmaniasis (oriental sore, Baghdad boil)	Middle East and Central Asia	*Phlebotomus sergenti*	Humans	Anthroponotic
Leishmania major	Cutaneous leishmaniasis	Africa, Indian Subcontinent, and Central Asia	*Phlebotomus papatasi, Phlebotomus duboscqi*	Gerbil	Zoonotic
Leishmania aethiopica	Cutaneous and diffuse cutaneous leishmaniasis	Ethiopia and Kenya	*Phlebotomus longipes Phlebotomus pedifer*	Hydraxes	Zoonotic
Leishmania braziliensis complex	Mucocutaneous leishmaniasis (Espundia)	Tropical South America	*Lutzomyra umbratilis*	Forest rodents and peridomestic animals	Zoonotic
Leishmania mexicana complex	Mucocutaneous leishmaniasis (Chiclero's ulcer)	Central America and Amazon basin	*Lutzomyra olmeca, Lutzomyra flairscutellata*	Forest rodents and marsupials	Zoonotic

The life cycle of *Leishmania* is completed in two hosts, humans and sandflies. As the fly bites, the promastigotes are released from the proboscis and introduced locally at the bite site.

17. Cyclops is a part of life cycle of:

a. Toxoplasmosis
b. Echinococcus
c. Leishmaniasis
d. Dracunculiasis

Cyclops is intermediate host of dracunculiasis (guinea-worm disease) and fish tapeworm (*Diphyllobothrium latum*) infection. *(See Diagram on next page)*

18. Largest intestinal protozoa is:

a. Toxoplasma gondii
b. Giardia lamblia
c. Balantidium coli
d. Entamoeba coli

Balantidium coli is the largest protozoan parasite in humans and causes a disease called balantidiasis. It belongs to the ciliophora phylum and is the only protozoan ciliate to infect humans. It goes through two development phases; a cyst and a trophozoite.

MCQs with Short Explanations

Ans. 17. **d.** Dracunculiasis 18. **c.** Balantidium coli

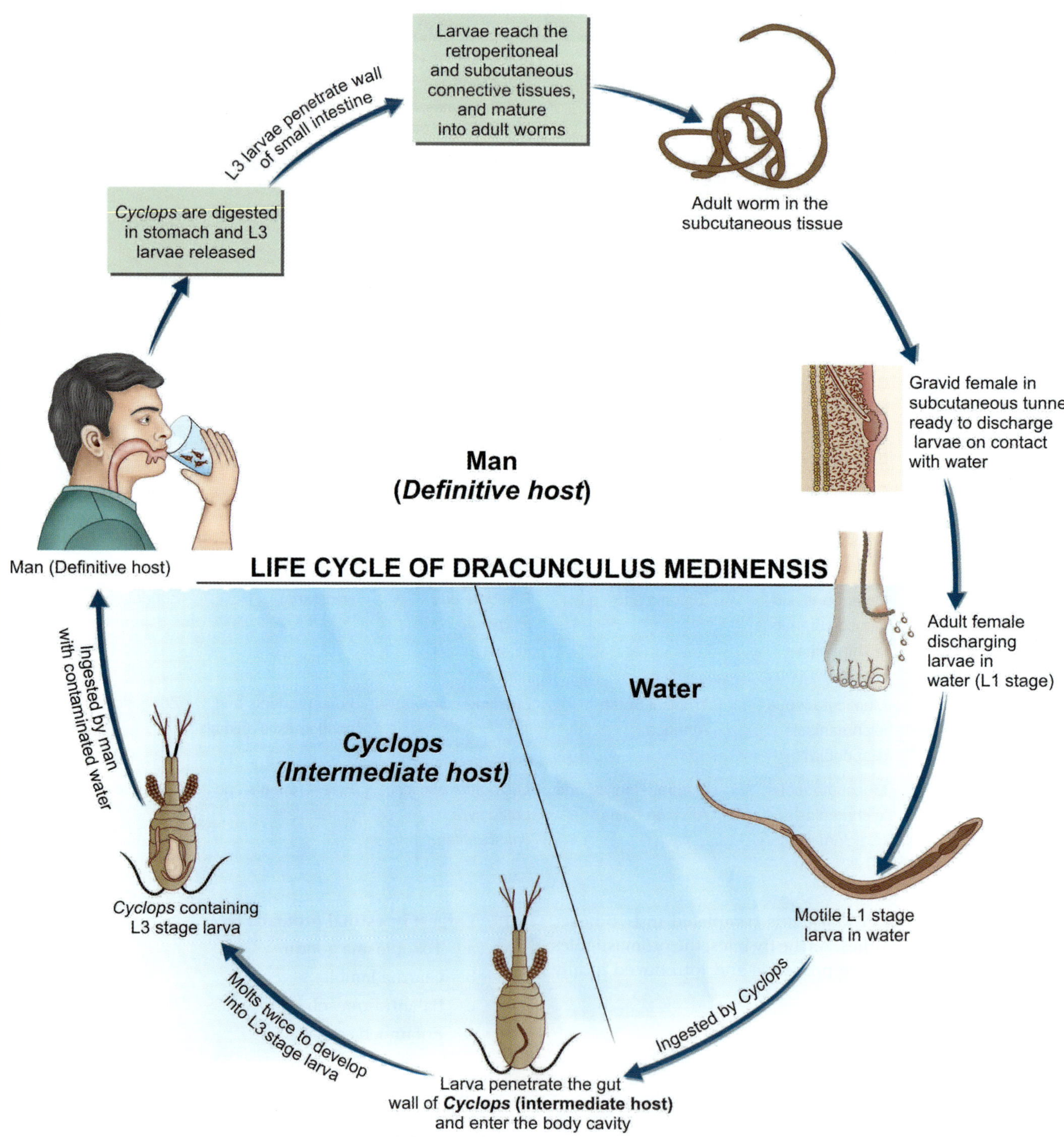

Life cycle of *Dracunculus medinensis*.

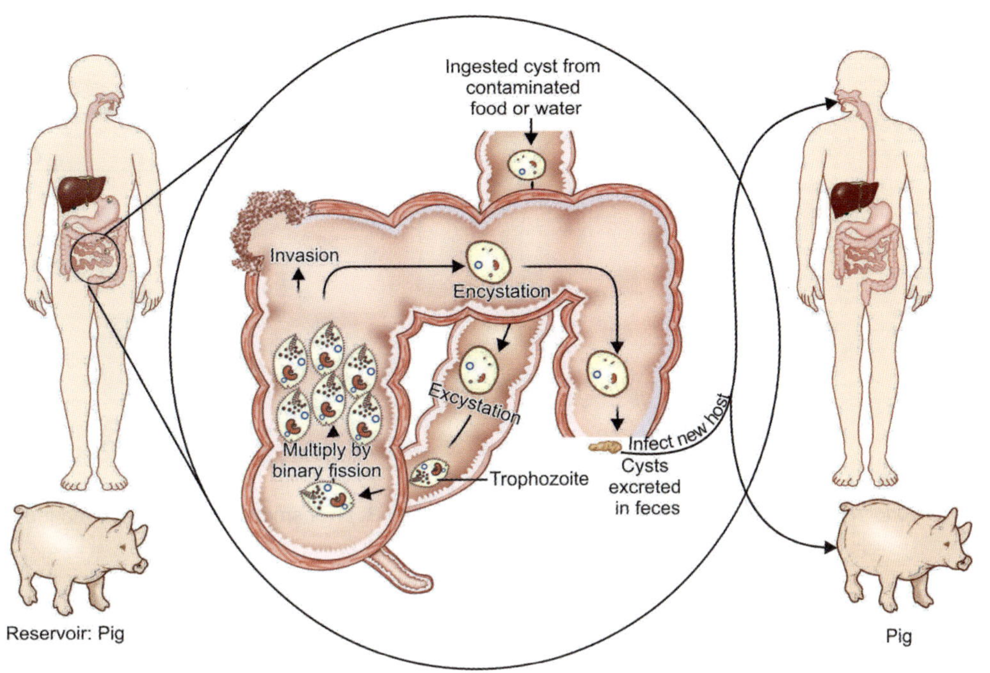

Life cycle of *Balantidium coli*.

19. Aldehyde test is for:

a. Toxocara canis
b. Toxoplasmosis
c. Leishmania
d. Fasciola hepatica

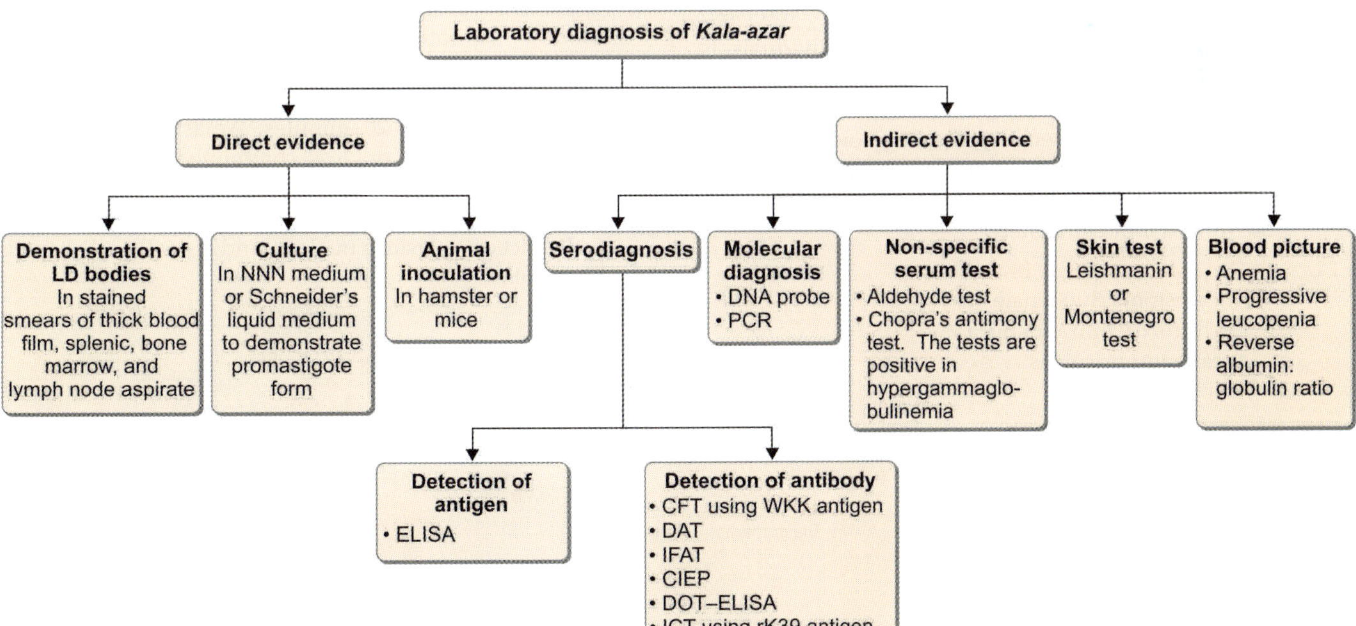

Laboratory diagnosis of Kala-azar.

Napier' aldehyde test, widely used for diagnostic purposes in kala-azar, has a sensitivity of 94% but only in cases with a illness of 3 months or more.

20. Novy-MacNeal-Nicolle [NNN] medium is used for:

a. Giardia lamblia
b. Leishmania donovani
c. Echinococcus
d. Toxoplasma gondii

Ans. **19. c.** Leishmania **20. b.** Leishmania...

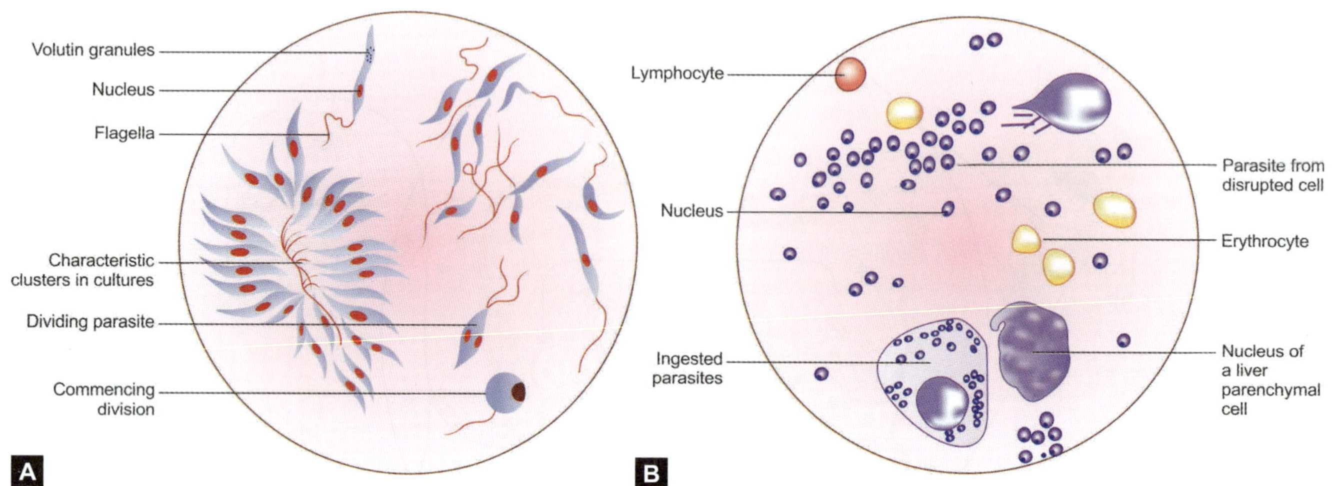

Leishmania donovani. A. Culture form (Giemsa stain, magn. × 1100); B. Liver smear (Giemsa stain, magn. × 1100).

Novy-MacNeal-Nicolle medium (NNN) is a culture medium used to grow Leishmania. It consists of 0.6% sodium chloride (NaCl) added to a simple blood agar slope. NNN can also be used to grow Trypanosoma cruzi.

21. Most common parasitic infection in AIDS:

a. Ancylostoma duodenale
b. Echinococcus granulosus
c. Strongyloides stercoralis
d. Enterobius vermicularis

(Figure on Next page)

Strongyloidiasis in immunocompetent individuals is usually an indolent disease. However, in immunocompromised individuals, it can cause a hyperinfective syndrome (also called disseminated strongyloidiasis) due to the reproductive capacity of the parasite inside the host. This hyperinfective syndrome can have a mortality rate close to 90% if disseminated.

22. Non-bile stained egg is found in:

a. Ancylostoma duodenale
b. Trichuris trichiura trichura
c. Ascaris lumbricoides
d. All of the above

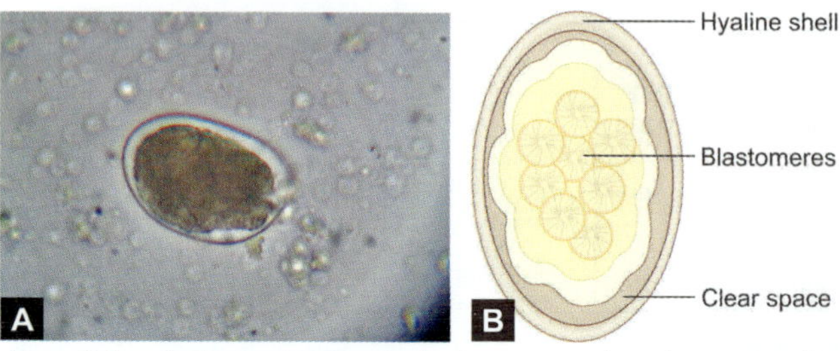

Egg of *Ancylostoma duodenale*. A. As seen under microscope; B. Schematic diagram.

The mnemonic for **non bile stained eggs** is **"A HEN"** laid nonbile-stained eggs

- Ancylostoma duodenale
- Hymenolepis nana
- Enterobius vermicularis
- Necator americanus

23. LD bodies are associated with:

a. Larva migrans
b. Kala azar
c. Malaria
d. Loa loa

Leishmaniasis is diagnosed in the hematology laboratory by direct visualization of the amastigotes (Leishman-Donovan bodies). Buffy-coat preparations of peripheral blood or aspirates from marrow, spleen, lymph nodes, or skin lesions should be spread on a slide to make a thin smear and stained with Leishman stain or Giemsa stain (pH 7.2) for 20 minutes. Amastigotes are seen within monocytes or, less commonly in neutrophils, of peripheral blood and in macrophages of aspirates. They are small, round bodies 2–4 μm in diameter with indistinct cytoplasm, a nucleus, and a small, rod-shaped kinetoplast.

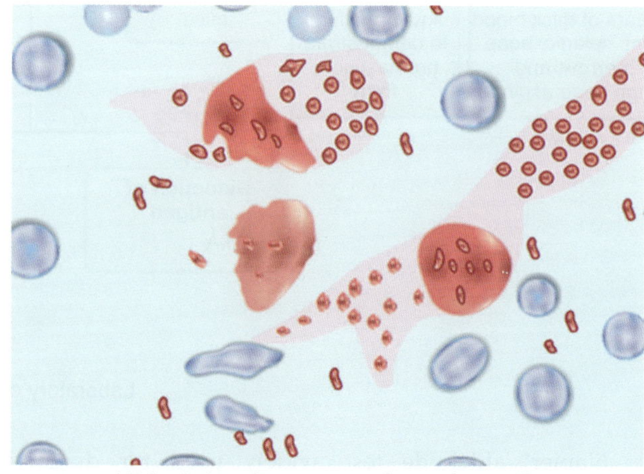

LD body in spleen smear of experimentally infected animal (Giemsa stain).

Ans. **21. c.** Strongyloides... **22. a.** Ancylostoma duode... **23. b.** Kala azar

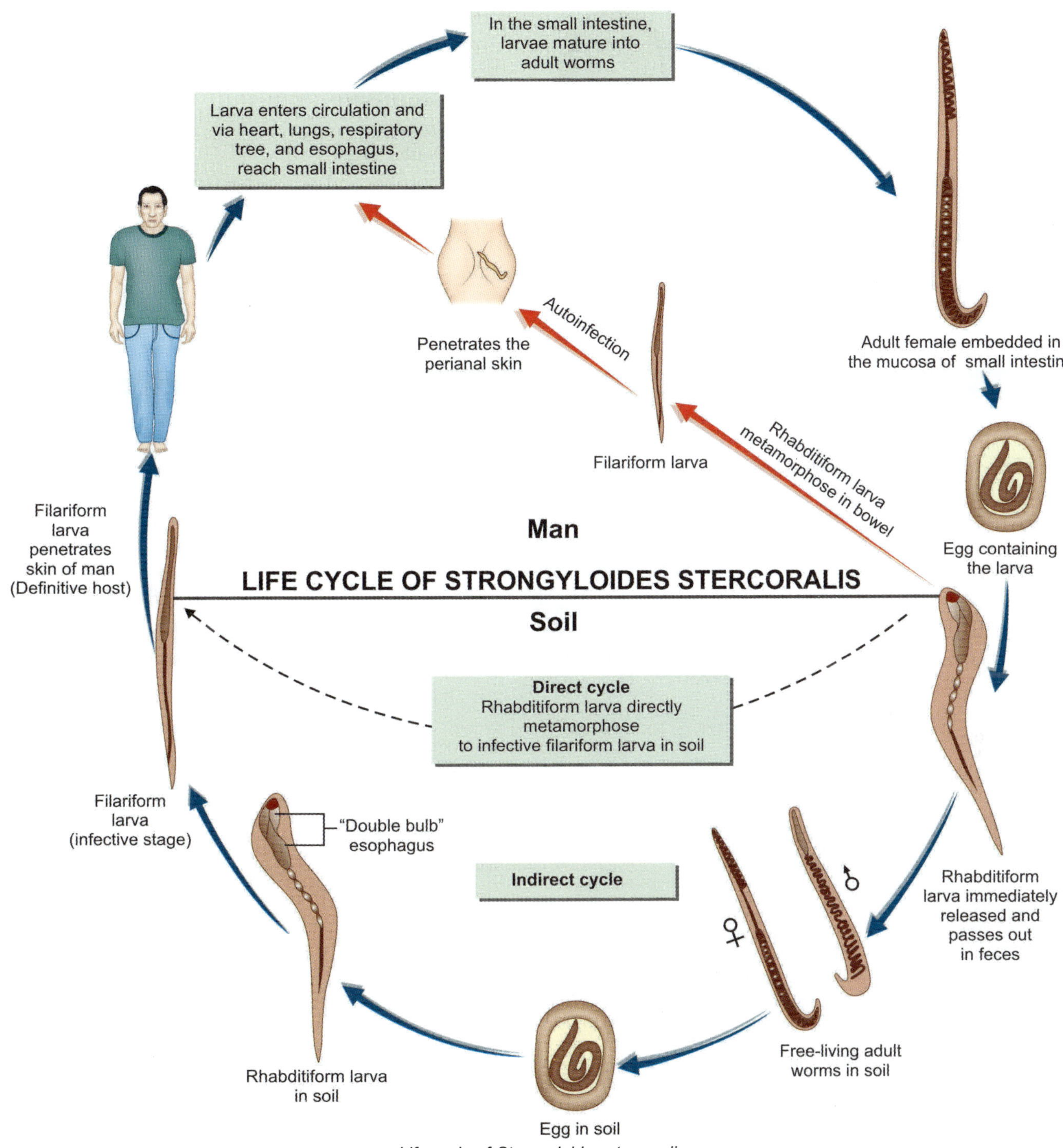

Life cycle of *Strongyloides stercoralis*.

24. Which egg does NOT float in a saturated solution of saline:

a. Trichuris eggs
b. Unfertilized eggs of Ascaris
c. Ancylostoma eggs
d. Fertilized eggs of Ascaris

Females will release unfertilized eggs, which are more elongate than fertilized eggs. Unfertilized eggs may also lack the mammillated layer.

Ans. **24. b.** Unfertilized eggs of Ascaris

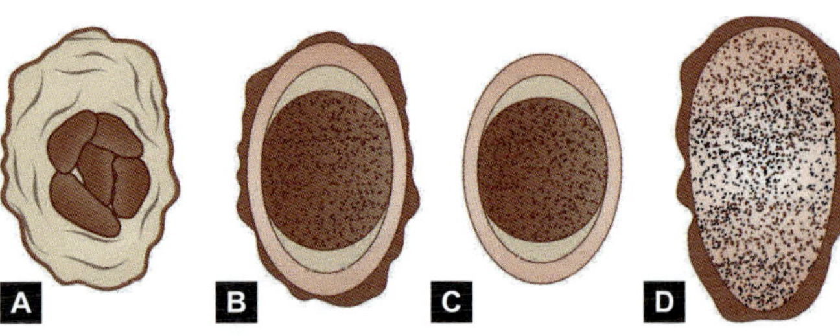

Types of *Ascaris* eggs found in stools. A. Fertilized egg surface focus, showing outer mmamillary coat; B. Fertilized egg, median focus, showing unsegmented ovum surrounded by 3 layers of coats; C. Decorticated fertilized egg, the mammillary coat is absent; D. Unfertilized egg, elongated, with atrophic ovum.

25. Stage of plasmodium falciparum NOT seen in peripheral blood smear (PBS) is:

a. Schizont
b. Gametocyte
c. Ring form
d. Double ring

Trophozoite- and schizont-infected erythrocytes of *P. falciparum* sequester in the microvasculature and are not found in the peripheral circulation.

Comparison of the characteristics of plasmodia causing human malariae

	P. vivax	*P. falciparum*	*P. malariae*	*P. ovale*
Hypnozoites	Yes	No	No	Yes
Erythrocyte preference	Reticulocytes	Young erythrocytes, but can infect all stages	Old erythrocytes	Reticulocytes
Stages found in peripheral blood	Rings, trophozoites, schizonts, gametocytes	Only rings and gametocytes	As in vivax	As in vivax
Ring stage	Large, 2.5 µm, usually single, prominent chromatin	Delicate, small, 1.5 µm, double chromatin, and multiple rings common, Accole forms found.	Similar to vivax, but thicker	Similar to vivax, more compact
Late trophozoite	Large irregular, actively amoeboid, prominent vacuole	Compact, seldom seen in blood smear	Band form characteristic	Compact, coarse pigment
Schizont	Large filling red cell	Small, compact, seldom seen in blood smear	Medium size	Medium size
Number of merozoites	12–24 in irregular grape-like cluster	8–24 grape-like cluster	6–12 in daisy-head or rosette pattern	6–12 irregularly arranged
Microgametocyte	Spherical, compact, pale blue cytoplasm, diffuse nucleus	Sausage or banana-shaped pale blue or pink cytoplasm, large diffuse nucleus	As in vivax	As in vivax
Macrogametocyte	Large, spherical, deep blue cytoplasm, compact nucleus	Crescentic, deep blue cytoplasm, compact nucleus	As in vivax	As in vivax
Infected erythrocyte	Enlarged, pale, with Schuffner's dots	Normal size, Maurer's clefts, sometimes basophilic stippling	Normal, occasionally Ziemann's stippling	Enlarged, oval fimbriated, prominent Schuffner's dots
Duration of schizogony (days)	2	2	3	2
Prepatent period (days)	8	5	13	9
Average incubation period (days)	14	12	30	14
Appearance of gametocyte after parasite patency (days)	4–5	10–12	11–14	5–6
Duration of sporogony in mosquito (25°C) (days)	9–10	10–12	25–28	14–16
Average duration of untreated infection (years)	4	2	40	4

Ans. **25. a.** Schizont

26. Cutaneous larva migrans is due to:

a. Ancylostoma braziliense
b. W. bancrofti
c. B. malayi
d. D. medinensis

Cutaneous larva migrans (abbreviated **CLM**) is a skin disease in humans, caused by the larvae of various nematode parasites of the hookworm family (Ancylostomatidae). The most common species causing this disease in the Americas is *Ancylostoma braziliense*. These parasites live in the intestines of dogs, cats and wild animals and should not be confused with other members of the hookworm family for which humans are definitive hosts, namely *Ancylostoma duodenale* and *Necator americanus*.

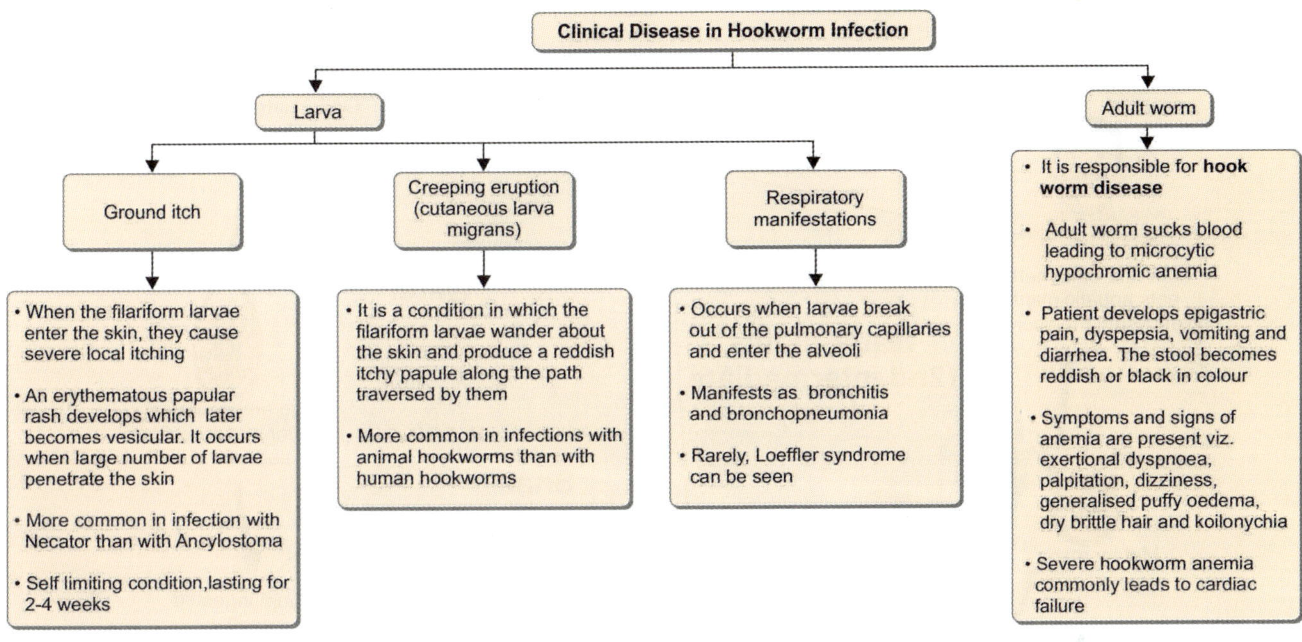

Clinical disease in Hookworm.

27. The largest trematode infecting man is:

a. Fasciolopsis hepatica
b. Fasciolopsis buski
c. Fasciolopsis granulosus
d. Clonorchis sinensis

Fasciolopsis buski is commonly called the giant intestinal fluke, because it is an exceptionally large parasitic fluke, and the largest known to parasitize' humans. Its size is variable and a mature specimen might be as little as 2 cm long, but the body may grow to a length of 7.5 cm and a width of 2.5 cm. It is a common parasite of humans and pigs and is most prevalent in Southern and Southeastern Asia. *(See Diagram on next page)*

28. The most distinctive feature of pathogenic Entamoeba histolytica on fresh stool examination is:

a. Presence of active pseudopodia
b. Erythrophagocytosis
c. Presence of intracytoplasmic vacuoles
d. Presence of two nucleoli

Entamoeba histolytica ingests the destroyed cells by phagocytosis and is often seen with red blood cells (a process known as erythrophagocytosis) inside when viewed in stool samples.

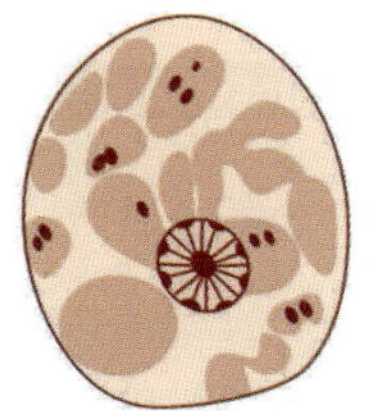
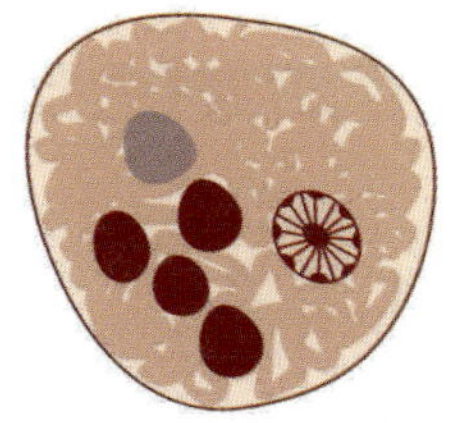

Left–*E. histolytica* trophozoite, minuta form–smaller, no ingested erythrocytes. Right–Trophozoite, magna (tissue invading) form containing ingested erythrocytes.

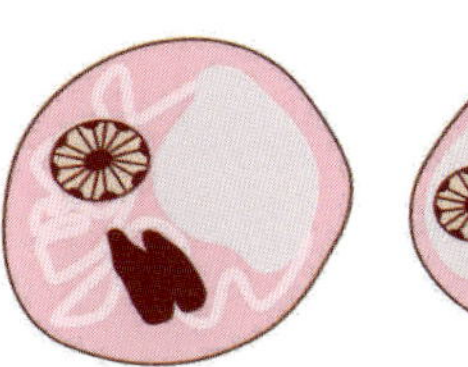
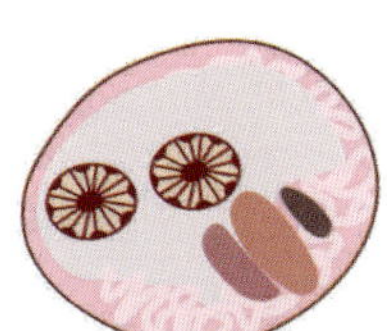
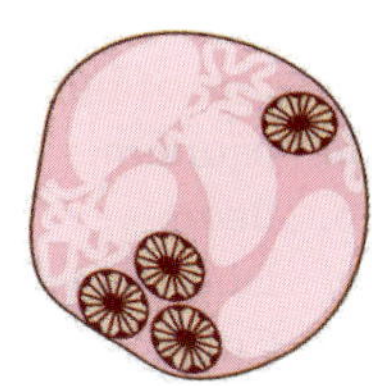

Left–*E. histolytica* uninucleate cyst. Middle–Binucleate cyst Right–quadrinucleate cyst.(Heidenhain's hematoxylin stain. Magn. X 2000)

Entamoeba histolytica as it appears in laboratory specimen.

Ans. 26. **a.** Ancylostoma... 27. **b.** Fasciolopsis buski 28. **b.** Erythrophagocytosis

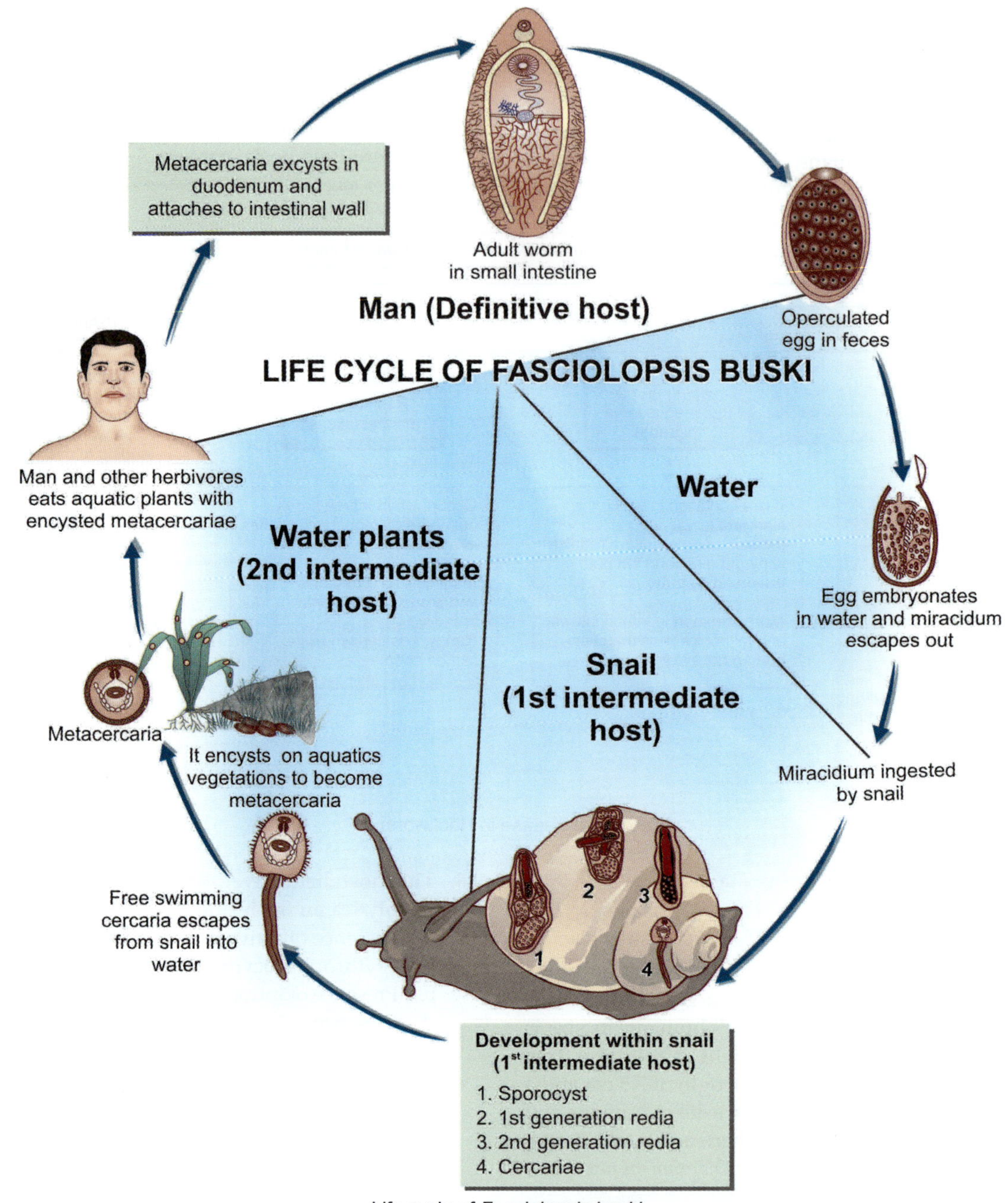

Life cycle of *Fasciolopsis buski.*

29. Habitat of hookworm is:

a. Jejunum
b. Ileum
c. Duodenum
d. Colon

Hookworm infections include ancylostomiasis and necatoriasis. These worms live in the small intestine of their host, which may be a bird or a mammal such as a dog, cat, or human.

Differentiating features of two species of hookworm.

	Ancylostoma duodenale	*Necator americanus*
Adult Worms		
Size	Large and thicker	Small and slender
Shape	Head bent in same direction as body	Head bent in opposite direction
Buccal capsule	4 ventral teeth and 2 dorsal knob like teeth	2 ventral and 2 dorsal chitinious cutting plates

Contd…

Ans. **29. a.** Jejunum

Contd…

	Ancylostoma duodenale	*Necator americanus*
Copulatory bursa	13 rays, two separate spicules, dorsal ray single	14 rays, two spicules fused at the tip, dorsal ray split
Caudal spine in female	Present	Absent
Vulval opening	Situated behind the middle of the body	Situated in anterior to middle part of body
Pathogenicity	More	Comparatively less
Eggs	Similar	Similar
1st and 2nd stage Larvae	Similar	Similar
Egg/day	15,000–20,000	6,000–11,000
Rate of development	Faster	Slower

Contd…

Contd…

	Ancylostoma duodenale	*Necator americanus*
Pulmonary reaction	More common	Less common
Blood loss/worm	0.2 mL/day	0.03 mL/day
Iron loss (mg/day)	0.76 mg	0.45 mg
Male:female ratio	1:1	1.5:1
Life span	2–7 years	4–20 years

30. True about Cryptosporidium parvum:

a. Affect only immunocompromised patient
b. It is one of common opportunistic infection in AIDS
c. Cyst size 12-15 mm
d. Treatment is metronidazole

Cryptosporidium causes cryptosporidiosis, an infection that may present as a diarrhoeal with or without an persistent cough in immunocompetent hosts.

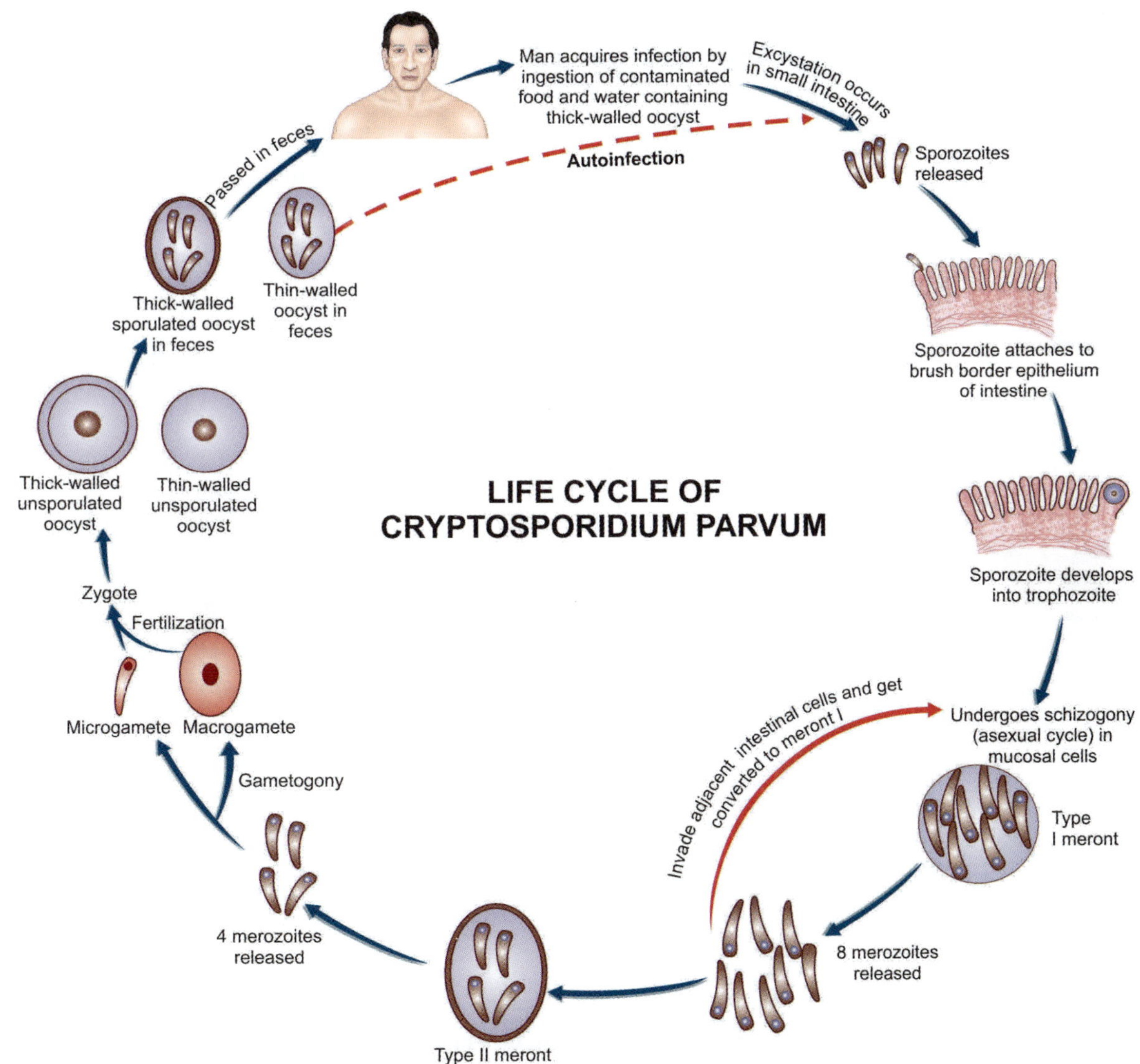

Life cycle of *Cryptosporidium parvum*.

Ans. 30. b. It is one of common opportunistic infection in AIDS

31. Staining technique for Cryptosporidium:
a. Indian ink
b. Modified acid fast
c. Giemsa
d. Methylene blue

Cryptosporidium oocysts are 4-6 μm in diameter and exhibit partial acid-fast staining. They must be differentiated from other partially acid-fast organisms including *Cyclospora cayetanensis*.

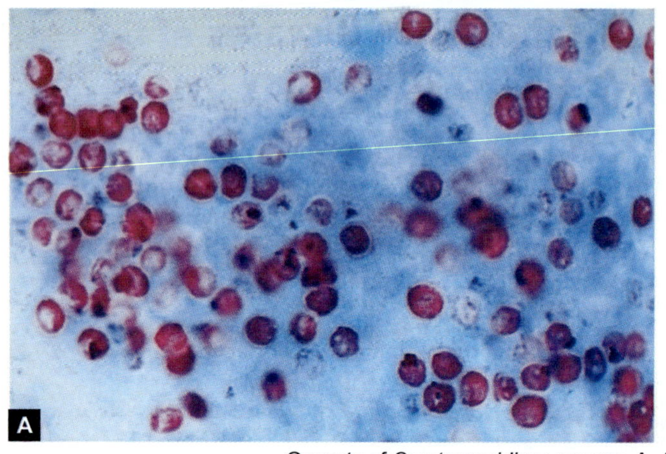

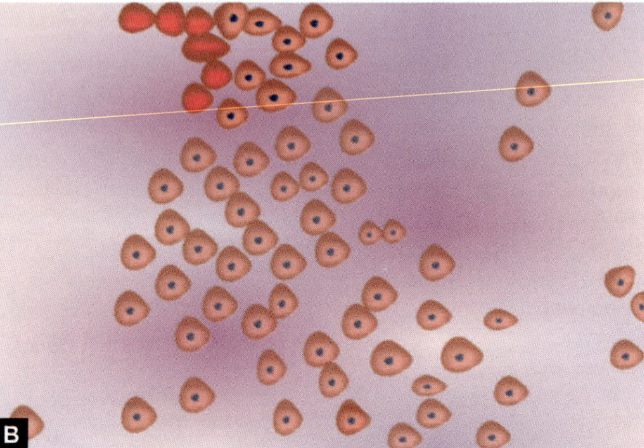

Oocysts of *Cryptosporidium parvum*. A. Acid-fast stain; B. Ziehl-Neelsen stain.

32. The pathogenecity of Entamoeba histolytica is indicated by:
a. Zymodeme pattern
b. Size
c. Nuclear pattern
d. ELISA test

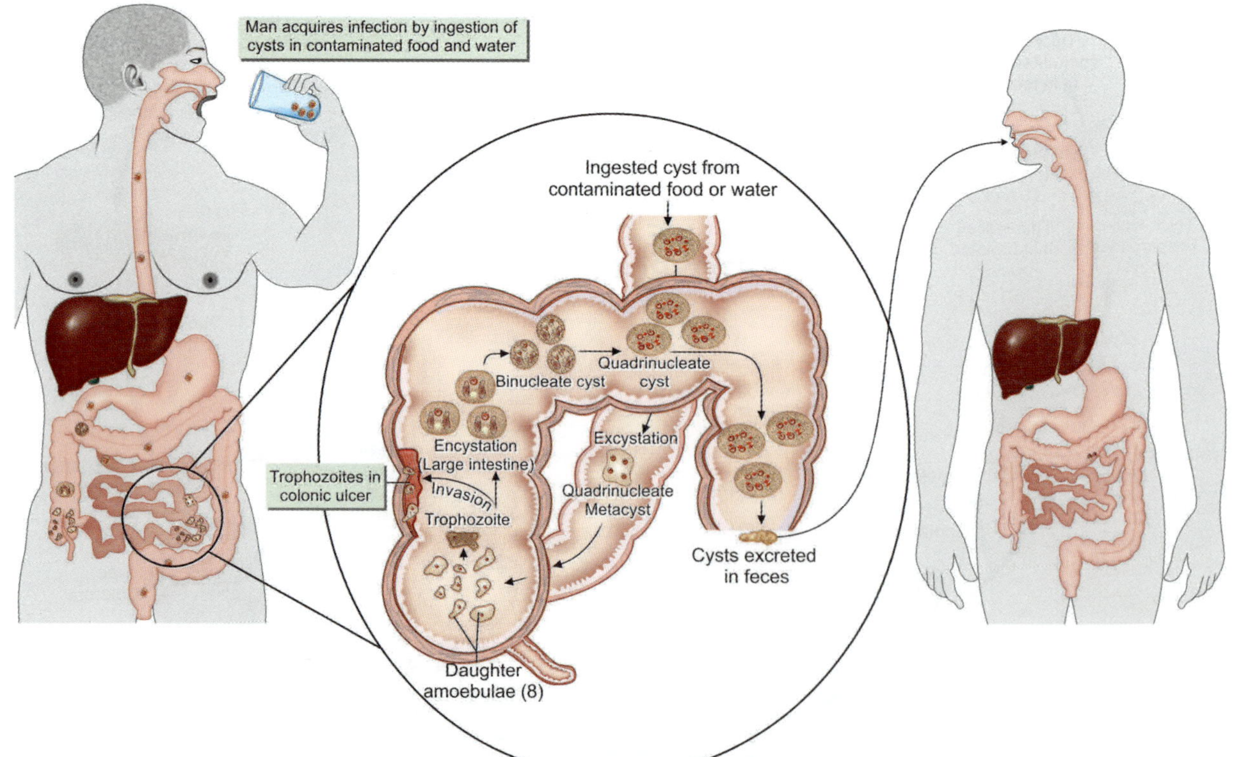

Life cycle of *Entamoeba histolytica*.

Ans. **31. b.** Modified acid fast **32. a.** Zymodeme pattern

ANSWERS WITH REFERENCES

1. **Ans. (d) Fresh water snail**
   Ref: Chatterjee's Parasitology 13/e p177

2. **Ans. (b) F. buski**
   Ref: Chatterjee's Parasitology 13/e p188

3. **Ans. (b) Toxoplasmosis**
   Ref: Paniker's Parasitology 7/e p91

4. **Ans. (a) Brugian malayi**
   Ref: Paniker's Parasitology 7/e p215

5. **Ans. (d) Immunofluorescent antibody test**
   Ref: Paniker's Parasitology 7/e p242

6. **Ans. (b) GIT**
   Ref: Paniker's Parasitology 7/e p53

7. **Ans. (b) P. falciparum**
   Ref: Paniker's Parasitology 7/e p72

8. **Ans. (a) Lymphatics**
   Ref: Paniker's Parasitology 7/e p210

9. **Ans. (b) Taenia solium**
   Ref: Paniker's Parasitology 7/e p124

10. **Ans. (c) Toxocara canis**
    Ref: Paniker's Parasitology 7/e p201

11. **Ans. (a) Faeces**
    Ref: Paniker's Parasitology 7/e p89

12. **Ans. (b) Diphyllobothrium latum**
    Ref: Paniker's Parasitology 7/e p117

13. **Ans. (a) Lung fluke**
    Ref: Paniker's Parasitology 7/e p158

14. **Ans. (c) Ancylostoma duodenale**
    Ref: Paniker's Parasitology 7/e p184

15. **Ans. (c) Crescentic macrogametocyte**
    Ref: Paniker's Parasitology 7/e p68

16. **Ans. (a) Sand fly**
    Ref: Paniker's Parasitology 7/e p50

17. **Ans. (d) Dracunculiasis**
    Ref: Paniker's Parasitology 7/e p222

18. **Ans. (c) Balantidium coli**
    Ref: Paniker's Parasitology 7/e p108

19. **Ans. (c) Leishmania**
    Ref: Paniker's Parasitology 7/e p56

20. **Ans. (b) Leishmania donovani**
    Ref: Paniker's Parasitology 7/e p57

21. **Ans. (c) Strongyloides stercoralis**
    Ref: Paniker's Parasitology 7/e p178

22. **Ans. (a) Ancylostoma duodenale**
    Ref: Paniker's Parasitology 7/e p183

23. **Ans. (b) Kala azar**
    Ref: Paniker's Parasitology 7/e p57

24. **Ans. (b) Unfertilized eggs of Ascaris**
    Ref: Paniker's Parasitology 7/e p196

25. **Ans. (a) Schizont**
    Ref: Paniker's Parasitology 7/e p75

26. **Ans. (a) Ancylostoma braziliense**
    Ref: Paniker's Parasitology 7/e p187

27. **Ans. (b) Fasciolopsis buski**
    Ref: Paniker's Parasitology 7/e p155

28. **Ans. (b) Erythrophagocytosis**
    Ref: Paniker's Parasitology 7/e p21

29. **Ans. (a) Jejunum**
    Ref: Paniker's Parasitology 7/e p185

30. **Ans. (b) It is one of common opportunistic infection in AIDS**
    Ref: Paniker's Parasitology 7/e p96

31. **Ans. (b) Modified acid fast**
    Ref: Paniker's Parasitology 7/e p97

32. **Ans. (a) Zymodeme pattern**
    Ref: Paniker's Parasitology 7/e p17

PRACTICE QUESTIONS

1. Schuffner's dots is related to which plasmodia:
a. Vivax
b. Falciparum
c. Ovale
d. Malariae

2. Microfilariae of the following nematode has 2 terminal nuclei:
a. Wucheria bancrofti b. Brugia malayi
c. Loa loa d. Onchocerca volvulus

3. Which of the following infestations lead to malabsorption:
a. Giardia lamblia
b. Ascaris lumbricoides
c. Necator americana
d. Ancylostoma duodenale

4. Chaga's disease is caused by:
a. Trypanosoma brucei gambiense
b. T. cruzi
c. T. rangeli
d. T. brucei brucei

5. Enterobius commonly inhabit the:
a. Duodenum b. Jejunum
c. Ileum d. Caecum

6. Hydatid cyst is commonly seen in:
a. Lungs b. Liver
c. Spleen d. Heart

7. Two nuclei at the tail tip is seen in:
a. Brugian malayi
b. Wucheria bancrofti
c. Onchocerca volvulus
d. Mansonella ozzardi

8. Highly specific and sensitive test for diagnosing kala-azar:
a. Complement fixation test with WKK antigen
b. Napier's aldehyde test
c. Chopra's antimony test
d. Immunofluorescent antibody test

9. Accidental Intermediate host for hydatid disease is:
a. Cow b. Man
c. Dog d. Pig

10. Investigation for definitive identification of cryptosporodium:
a. ELISA
b. Immunofluorescence test
c. Demonstration of oocyte in feces
d. Fluoroscent staining with auramine

Ans. **1. a.** Vivax **2. b.** Brugia malayi **3. a.** Giardia lamblia **4. b.** T. cruzi
5. d. Caecum **6. b.** Liver **7. a.** Brugian malayi **8. d.** Immunofluor...
9. b. Man **10. b.** Immunofluorescence test

IMAGE-BASED QUESTIONS

1. **Following picture represents the ring form of which plasmodia:**

a. Vivax b. Falciparum
c. Malariae d. Ovale

The trophozoite of plasmodium vivax is actively mobile, as indicated by its name vivax. The ring form is well defined, with a prominent central vacuole. One side of the ring is thicker and the other side thin. Nucleus is situated on the thin side of the ring. The ring is about 2.5-3 microns in diameter, about a third of the size of an erythrocyte. The cytoplasm is blue and the nucleus red in stained films.

2. **Such gametocytes are indicative of which plasmodia:**

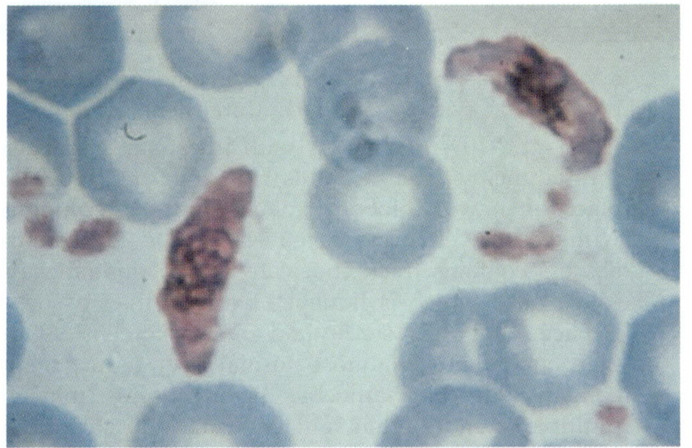

a. Vivax b. Falciparum
c. Malariae d. Ovale

Gametocytes of plasmodium falciparum are seen in circulation about 10 days after the ring stage first appears. The early gametocytes seldom appear in peripheral circulation. The mature gametocytes, which are seen in peripheral smears are curved oblong structures, described as crescentic, sickle, sausage, or banana shaped. They are usually referred to as crescents.

3. **Such a picture is suggestive of:**

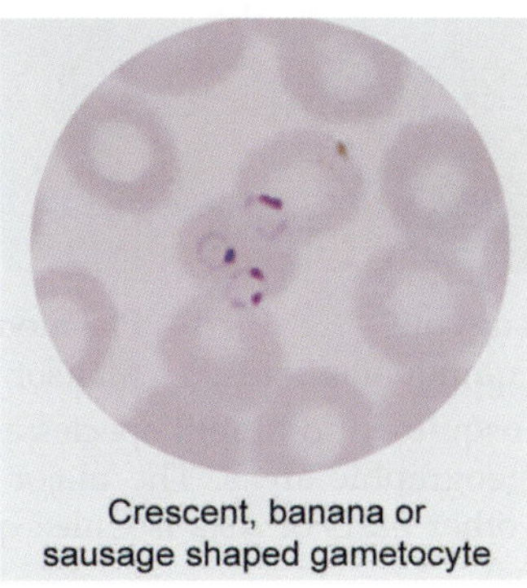

Crescent, banana or sausage shaped gametocyte

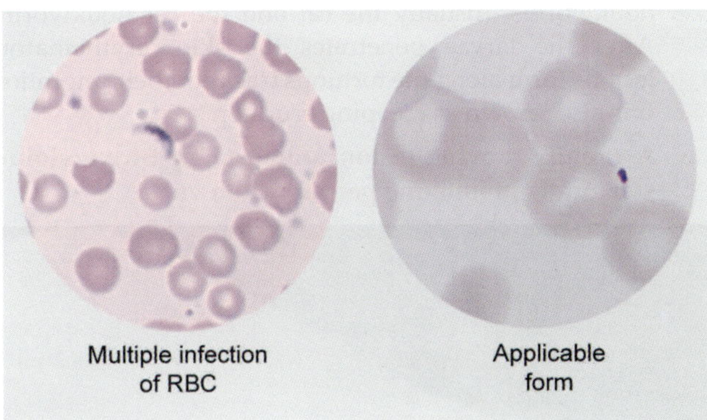

a. Vivax
b. Falciparum
c. Malariae
d. Ovale

The early ring form of the plasmodium falciparum in erythrocyte is very delicate and tiny, measuring only a sixth (1/6) of the red blood cell diameter. Rings are often seen attached along the margin of the red cell, the so called form appliqué or accole. Binucleate rings (double chromatin) are common resembling stereo headphones in appearance. Several rings may be seen within a single erythrocyte.

4. **Which parasite:**

a. Onchocerca volvulus
b. Loa loa
c. Ocular ascaris
d. Ocular ancylostoma

Definitive diagnosis of loa loa (causes calabar swelling) requires the detection of microfilaria in peripheral blood or the isolation of the adult worm from the eye.

5. **Such a presentation is suggestive of:**

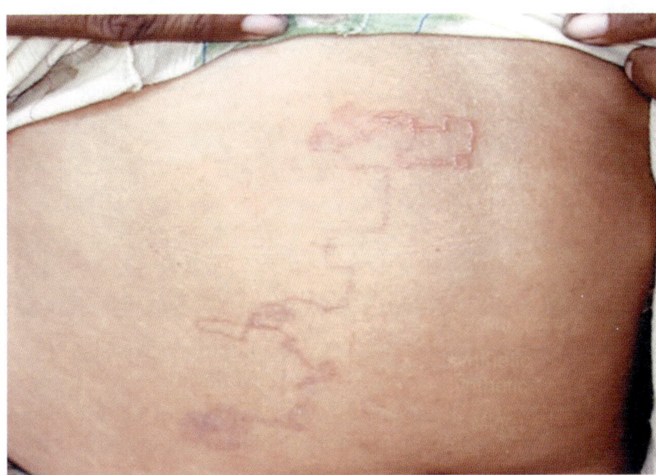

a. Strongyloides stercoralis b. Toxocara
c. Toxoplasma d. Trypanosoma

CLM or cutaneous larva migrans is a serpiginous skin eruption caused by burrowing larvae of animal hookworms, (usually the cat and the cat hookworm). After the larvae penetrates the skin, erythematous lesions form along the tortuous tracks of their migration. It is also known as creeping eruption.

6. A rapidly moving lesion produced by Strongyloides stercoralis in immune person is known as:

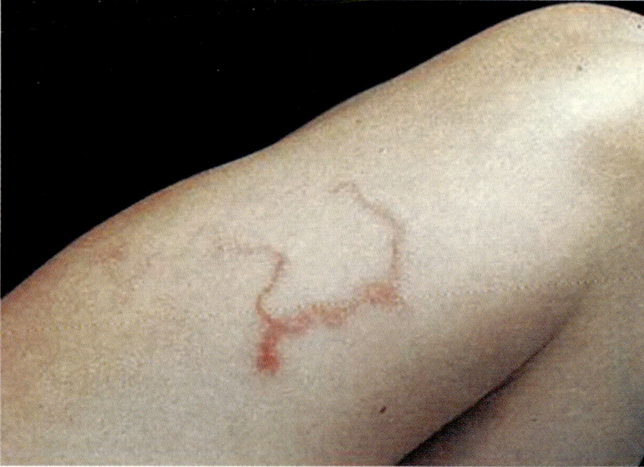

a. Visceral larva migrans b. Larva currens
c. Triple reaction d. Cutaneous ulcers

The term larva currens (meaning 'racing larvae') has been applied to the rapidly progressing linear or serpiginous urticarial tracks caused by migrating filariform larvae. These often follow autoinfection and starts perianally.

7. Scrambled egg appearance of the cyst is suggestive of:

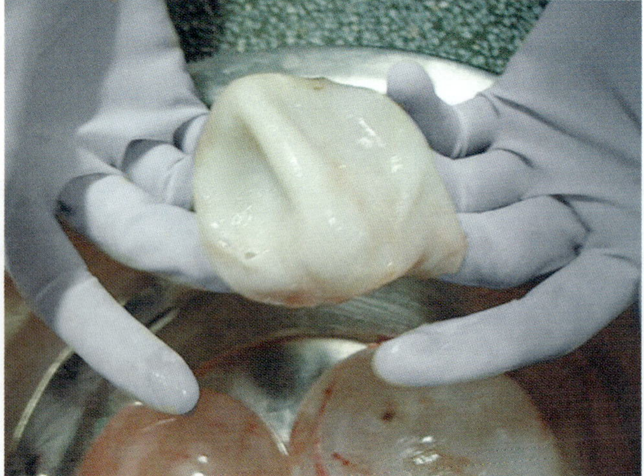

a. Amoebiasis b. Echinococcosisis
c. Kala azar d. Malaria

At the site of deposition, the embryo of echinococcus slowly develops into a hollow bladder or cyst filled with fluid. This becomes the hydatid cyst.

8. In a patient presenting complaining of dysentery with large, foul smelling stools, such a CT suggests the diagnosis of:

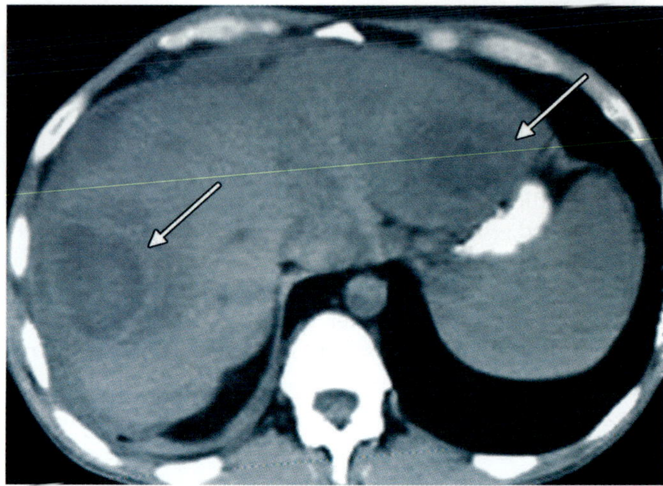

a. Amoebiasis b. Pyogenic liver abscess
c. Hydatid cyst of liver d. Carcinoma liver

In about 5-10% of persons with intestinal amoebiasis (presenting with large, fouls smelling, and brownish black often with blood streaked mucus intermingled with feces), liver abscesses may ensue. The center of the abscess contains thick chocolate brown pus (anchovy sauce pus), which is liquefied necrotic liver tissue. It is bacteriologically sterile and free of amoeba. At the periphery, there is almost normal liver tissue, which contains invading amoeba. Liver abscess may be multiple or more often solitary, usually located in the upper right lobe of the liver.

9. Vector for this condition in India:

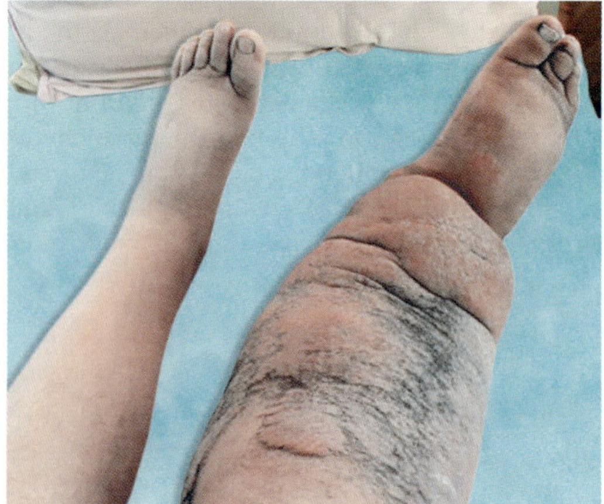

a. Aedes agyptii b. Plasmodium vivax
c. Culex quinquefasciatus d. Mansonides

Female mosquito, of different species acts as vectors in different geographic areas. The major vector in India and most other parts of Asia is Culex quinquefasciatus (C. fatigans).

10. Ophthalmic larva migrans is commonly caused by:

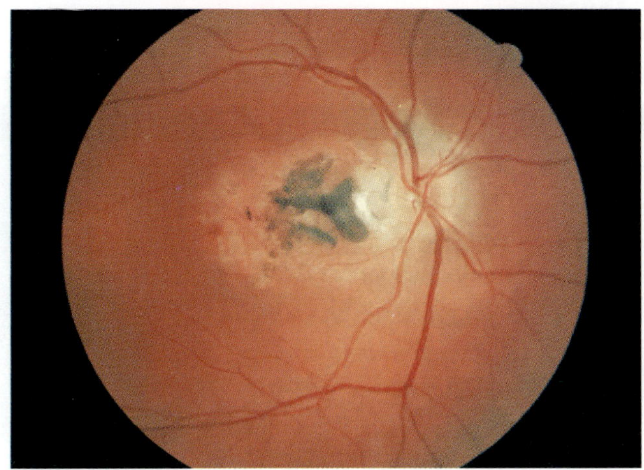

a. Strongyloides stercoralis
b. Toxocara cati
c. Toxocara canis
d. Ancylostoma braziliense

The most common cause of visceral larva migrans is the dog ascarid, Toxocara canis and less often the cat ascarid, Toxocara cati. Patient may develop neurological disturbances (neural larva migrans) or endophthalmitis (ophthalmic larva migrans).

MCQ POINTS

S. No	Question statement	Answer
1.	Intermediate host for schistosoma	***Fresh water snail***
2.	Longest cestode infecting man	***Diphyllobothrium latum***
3.	Definitive host for guinea worm	***Man***
4.	Larval forms of which parasite can be found in muscle biopsy	***Taenia solium***
5.	Sputum examination is commonly done for detecting eggs of	***Paragonismus westermani***
6.	Modified acid fast stain is used in diagnosis of	***Cryptosporidium parvum***
7.	Time of collection of blood is very important for detection of	***Microfilaria***
8.	Filarial form which can be seen in conjunctiva	***Loa loa***
9.	River blindness is the name given to disease caused by	***Onchocerca volvulus***
10.	Fugitive/calabar swelling is seen in infection with	***Loa loa***
11.	In which stage of filariasis, microfilaria are seen in peripheral blood	***Early adenolymphangitis stage***
12.	Loeffler's syndrome may be seen in infection with	***Ascaris lumbricoides***
13.	Which nematode lays eggs containing larvae	***Enterobius vermicularis***
14.	Average blood loss per worm in ancylostomiasis	***0.2 mL/day***
15.	Stage of ancylostoma duodenale infective to human beings	***Filrifirm larvae***
16.	Autoinfection is seen with	***Strongyloides***
17.	Parasite residing in caecum	***Trichuris***
18.	A viviparous parasite	***Trichinella spiralis***
19.	Best site for taking biopsy for diagnosing trichinellosis	***Deltoid***
20.	Which fluke is carcinogenic	***Clonorchis***
21.	Schistosoma japonicum resides in which vessel	***Superior mesenteric vein***
22.	Consumption of uncooked pork is likely to cause which helminthic disease	***Taneia solium***
23.	In humans, cryptosporidiosis clinically presents as	***Diarrhoea***
24.	Oocyst of toxoplasma is found in	***Cat***
25.	Babesiosis is transmitted by	***Ticks***
26.	Which plasmodial infection is more often associated with nephritic syndrome	***Plasmodium malariae***
27.	Crescent-shaped or banana-shaped gametocytes are seen in infection with	***Plasmodium falciparum***
28.	Quartan malaria is caused by	***Plasmodium malariae***
29.	Old RBCs are preferentially infected by which plasmodia	***Plasmodium malariae***
30.	Vector for trypanosoma cruzi	***Reduviid bug***
31.	Mucocutaneous leishmaniasis is caused by	***Leishmania braziliensis***
32.	Normal habitat of giardia is	***Duodenum and jejunum***
33.	Infective form of entamoeba histolytica is	***Quadrinucleate***
34.	Entry of necator americanus in body	***Piercing the skin***

CHAPTER

7

PHARMACOLOGY

KEY POINTS

Some Important Definitions

- Pharmacokinetics: Study of drug movement in the body/ effect of body on the drug
- Side-effects: Unwanted effect at therapeutic doses
- Agonist: Have affinity and maximal efficacy
- Antagonist: Have affinity and NO maximal efficacy
- Clearance: Measure of body's ability to excrete a drug
- Therapeutic window phenomenon: Optimal effect is exerted only over a narrow range of plasma drug concentration, e.g. TCA, clonidine, glipizide
- Therapeutic index: Toxic dose/therapeutic dose (LD50/ ED50)
- Drug efficacy: Maximal effect that a drug may elicit; More important (than efficacy) in determining drug of choice
- Drug potency: Amount of drug required to produce a certain response
- Bioavailability: Fraction of drug that reaches in the blood.

Transport of Drugs

- Active transport of the drug is: Carrier mediated, requires ATP, saturation occurs
- Factors affecting drug absorption: Route of administration, vascularity, solubility
- Absorption of drug from gut is decreased by: Presence of food, first pass metabolism, increased expression of p-glycoprotein.

Effect of pH

- pKa is: Numerically equal to the pH at which the drug is 50% ionized (but for every unit by which pH is changed, the ratio of un-ionized to ionized molecules changes 10 fold)
- If an acidic drug has pKa value of 4.5, then % of ionized drug at pH of 3.5 will be 10%
- Acidic drugs are more ionized at alkaline pH
- Acidic drugs are largely unionized at acidic pH and are absorbed from stomach
- A highly ionized drug is excreted mainly by the kidneys.

Bioavailability (BA)

- BA can be determined from plasma concentration or urinary excretion data
- BA is determined by the area under the plasma concentration-time curve
- BA depends upon extent of absorption and extent of 1st pass metabolism in intestinal wall, portal blood or liver
- Bioavailability by intravenous route is: 100%.

Microsomal Enzyme Inducers

- Phenytoin
- Phenobarbitone
- Rifampicin

Acetylation is the Mode of Metabolism for

- Isoniazid
- Hydralazine

First Pass Effect/First Pass Elimination

- First pass metabolism (metabolism of drug in liver, intestinal wall or portal blood) + excretion of drug into bile is known as first pass elimination
- First pass metabolism is seen with: Oral route, rectal route
- Drug showing high first pass metabolism are: Lignocaine, propranolol, salbutamol.

Volume of Distribution (VOD)

- Calculated as dose administered/plasma concentration
- Factors influencing VOD: Drug plasma protein binding, lipid solubility, degree of blood flow, age, tissue affinity, pKa
- Apparent VOD may exceed total body fluid volume if a drug is: Sequestrated in body tissues.

Blood Brain Barrier

- Drug crossing blood brain barrier: Propranolol, physostigmine.

Placental Barrier

- Maximum transfer of drug across placenta occurs in 1st trimester
- Ion trapping of basic drugs occurs in the placenta
- Drug crossing placental barrier: Warfarin, lithium, morphine
- Heparin and insulin DOES NOT cross placental barrier and hence are agents of choice in pregnancy.

Half Life (t1/2)

- Time taken for amount of drug in the body to decline by 50%
- Amount of drug excreted in 4th t1/2: 93.7%
- t1/2 can determine: Elimination time, steady state plasma concentration, dosing rate, maintenance dose.

Prodrugs

- Enalapril
- Sulindac
- Ticlopidine
- Clopidogrel

Zero Order Reaction

- Constant AMOUNT is excreted
- Rate of elimination INDEPENDENT of plasma concentration
- Variable t1/2
- Phenytoin
- Ethanol
- Salicylates

First Order Reaction

- Constant FRACTION of drug is eliminated
- Rate of elimination is directly DEPENDENT on plasma concentration
- t1/2 is constant.

Miscellaneous

- Drug metabolized in liver are: Phenytoin, erythromycin, cimetidine, diazepam
- Drug metabolized in kidney: Penicillin G
- Duration of action of a drug administered intravenously depends upon: Protein binding, clearance, distribution volume, lipid solubility, drug concentration
- Effect of displacement of protein bound drug: Raises plasma level of that drug
- Drugs bindings sites on protein are: Non-specific (one drug can displace other)
- Drugs bound to albumin: Phenytoin warfarin
- Ionized drugs are mainly excreted by: Kidney
- Basic drugs are absorbed from: Proximal intestine
- Phase II of drug metabolism involves: Conjugation with glucuronide, sulfate, glutathione.

Competitive Antagonist

- Chemically resembles the agonist
- Reduces potency of the agonist
- Binds to the same receptor
- Maximal response can be obtained
- V_{max} is same, Km increases

Drugs and the Enzyme they Inhibit

- 5 fluorouracil: Thymidine synthetase
- Omeprazole: Gastric H ATPase
- Phenelzine: MAO
- Pargyline: MAO
- Acetazolamide: Carbonic anhydrase
- Captopril: Angiotensin convertase
- Penicillin: Transpeptidase
- Aspirin: Cyclo-oxygenase
- Allopurinol: Xanthine oxidase
- Beta aminopropionitrile: Lysyl oxidase
- Sarin: Cholinesterase
- Statins: HMG-CoA reductase

Acetyl-Cholinesterase Inhibitors

- Edrophonium (diagnosis of myasthenia gravis)
- Neostigmine/pyridostigmine (treatment of urinary retention, ileus, reversal of neuromuscular blockade)

Organophosphate Poisoning

- Pupils in organophosphate poisoning: Pin point pupils
- Treatment of organophosphate poisoning: Atropine and pralidoxime (reactivates cholinesterase)

Atropine

- Mydriasis
- Cycloplegia
- Decreases: Respiratory secretions, acid secretion in stomach, motility of gut
- Can cause acute angle closure glaucoma in eyes with narrow angles
- Can cause urinary retention in elderly with BPH
- Can cause hyperthermia in infants

Adrenergic Receptor Location

- Alpha 1: Postjunctional
- Alpha 2: Pre and postjunctional
- Beta 1: Heart
- Beta 2: Bronchi

Thromboxanes

- Platelet aggregator

Actions of Prostaglandins

- PGE_1/PGI_2: Vasodilation, inhibition of platelet aggregation
- PGE_2: Vasodilation, bronchodilation, uterine contraction
- PGF_2 alpha: Uterine contraction, bronchoconstriction, vasoconstriction
- TXA_2: Vasoconstriction, bronchoconstriction, platelet aggregation.

Uses of Prostaglandin Drugs

- PGE_1 (Alprostadil): Causes vasodilation, useful in erectile dysfunction
- PGE_1 analogue (misoprostol): Gastric cytoprotection, useful in preventing peptic ulcers caused due to NSAIDs
- PGE_2 (dinoprostone): Causes contraction of uterus, useful as abortifacient, cervical ripening

Drugs for Raised Intracranial Tension

- Intravenous mannitol
- Frusemide

DOC for Diabetes Insipidus

- Desmopressin (intranasally)

DOC for SIADH

- Demeclocycline

Rapid Acting Insulin

- Insulin aspartate
- Lispro insulin
- Insulin glusuline

Long Acting Insulin

- Protamine zinc insulin
- Insulin glargine

Intermediate Acting Insulin

- Lente/insulin—zinc suspension (7 Ultra Lente + 3 Semilente): 20–24 hours
- NPH: Neutral protamine hagedorn / isophane: 20–24 hours

Anti-Asthmatic Drug

- MOA of sodium cromoglycate (used for prophylaxis): Inhibitor of mast cell degranulation
- Zafirlukast (LTRA) is taken: Once daily
- Zileuton inhibits: 5 lipo-oxygenase
- Anticholinergic bronchodilators:
  - Ipratropium
  - Tiotropium

Procaine Penicillin

- Plasma concentration is more
- Painless injection
- Small dose 0.5–1 MU
- Short duration of action
- Allergic phenomenon common
- Can be fortified with aqueous penicillin G

Benzathine Penicillin

- Plasma concentration is less, so only prophylactic use
- Painful injection
- Allergic phenomenon not common
- Large dose 0.6–2.4 MU
- Very long duration of action
- Not fortified with aqueous penicillin G

1st Generation Cephalosporins

- Parenteral: Cefazolin
- Oral: Cephalexin, Cephradine, Cefadroxil

2nd Generation Cephalosporins

- Parenteral: Cefuroxime
- Oral: Cefaclor, Cefuroxime axetil

3rd Generation Cephalosporins

- Parenteral: Cefotaxime, Ceftizoxime, Ceftriaxone, Ceftazidime, Cefoperazone
- Oral: Cefixime, Cefpodoxime proxetil, Cefdinir, Ceftibuten

4th Generation Cephalosporins

- Parenteral: Cefepime

Pathogenic Agent and Chemoprophylaxis

- Streptococci: Penicillin
- Neisseria meningitides: Rifampicin/ciprofloxacin
- Clostridium perfringens: Metronidazole
- Clostridium tetani: Penicillin
- Yersinia pestis (plague): Tetracycline/cotrimoxazole
- Bordetella pertussis (whooping cough): Erythromycin
- Mycobacterium tuberculosis: Isoniazid and rifampicin
- Leptospira: Doxycycline

Chemoprophylaxis of Vivax and Chloroquine Sensitive Falciparum Malaria

- Chloroquine 300 mg of base once weekly, started one week before exposure and continued for 4 weeks after returning

Chemoprophylaxis of Chloroquine Resistant Falciparum Malaria

- Mefloquine 250 mg base once weekly.

Viral Condition and Drug of Choice

- H. simplex encephalitis: Acyclovir
- Neonatal herpes simplex: Acyclovir
- Herpes simplex keratitis: Trifluridine/vidarabine
- Herpes simplex oro-labialis: Penciclovire

Most Effective Drug for Specific Population of M. tuberculosis

- Spurters: Rifampicin
- Dormant: No drug is effective
- Rapid growers: Isoniazid
- Slow growing: Pyrazinamide

Adverse Reactions of Rifampicin

- Cutaneous syndrome—chills, fever, headache
- Abdominal syndrome—nausea, vomiting, abdominal cramps
- Hepatitis
- Respiratory syndrome—breathlessness

Remember

- S/E of ethambutol: Retrobulbar optic neuritis

Treatment of Paucibacillary Leprosy

- Rifampicin 600 mg monthly and Dapsone 100 mg daily
- Treatment for 6 months
- Follow up for 2 years

Treatment of Multibacillary Leprosy

- Rifampicin 600 mg and clofazimine 300 mg monthly
- Dapsone 100 mg and clofazimine 50 mg daily
- Treatment for 2 years
- Follow-up for 5 years

Arteriolar Dilators

- Hydralazine
- Minoxidil
- Calcium channel openers

Venodilators

- Nitrates
- Glyceryl trinitrate
- Isosorbide dinitrate

Mixed Dilators

- ACE inhibitors
- Losartan
- Prazosin
- Phentolamine
- Nitroprusside

Hypolipidemic Drug and Mechanism of Action

- Statins: Decrease cholesterol synthesis by inhibition of rate limiting HMG-CoA reductase
- Bile acid sequestrants: Decrease bile acid absorption, increased hepatic conversion of cholesterol to bile acids
- Fibric acid derivatives, gemfibrozil: Increased activity of lipoprotein lipase, decreased release of fatty acids from adipose tissue
- Nicotinic acid: Decrease production of VLDL, decrease lipolysis in adipocytes

Mechanism of Action of Antiepileptics

- Phenytoin, carbamazepine, lamotrigine, valproate: Prolongation of Na^+ channel inactivation
- Barbiturates, benzodiazepines, vigabatrin, gabapentin, valproate: Facilitation of GABA-mediated chloride channel opening
- Ethosuximide, trimethadione, valproate: Inhibition of T type of calcium current

Propyl Thiouracil

- Less potent
- Safe in pregnancy
- t½ 1–2 hr.
- No active metabolites
- Peripheral conversion of t4 → t3 prevented
- Useful in thyroid storm

MCQs WITH SHORT EXPLANATIONS

GENERAL PRINCIPLES

1. **An enzyme inducer:**
   a. Isoniazid
   b. Erythromycin
   c. Ketoconazole
   d. Rifampicin

   Microsomal enzyme inducers
   - CYP3A inducers
     - Anticonvulsants (phenobarbitone, phenytoin)
     - Rifampicin
     - Glucocorticoids
   - CYP2E1 inducers
     - Isoniazid
     - Chronic alcohol consumption
   - CYP1A inducers
     - Omeprazole
     - Cigarette smoke

Drugs that inhibit drug metabolizing enzymes.	
Allopurinol	Amiodarone
Omeprazole	Propoxyphene
Erythromycin	Isoniazid
Clarithromycin	Cimetidine
Chloramphenicol	Quinidine
Ketoconazole	Disulfiram
Itraconazole	Diltiazem
Metronidazole	Verapamil
Ciprofloxacin	MAO inhibitors
Sulfonamides	Ritonavir (and other)
Fluoxetine (and other SSRIs)	HIV protease inhibitors

2. **Drug requiring therapeutic dose monitoring/ TDM:**
   a. Propanolol b. Metformin
   c. Warfarin d. Phenytoin

   TDM
   - Drugs with low safety margin
     - Digoxin
     - Anticonvulsants
     - Theophylline
     - Aminoglycosides
     - Lithium
     - TCA
   - If individual variations are large
     - Antidepressants
     - Lithium
   - Potentially toxic drugs in the presence of renal failure
     - Aminoglycosides
     - Vancomycin

3. **Number of patients included in Clinical trial-phase II:**
   a. 20–100 b. 100–500
   c. 500–100 d. 1000–2000

   Phase II of clinical trial is used for establishing the efficacy of the drug, usually against a placebo. It includes testing with a larger group of people (100–300) to see if it is effective and to further evaluate its safety. The gradual increase in test group size, allows less common side effects to be progressively sought.

Stages in new drug development.
- Synthesis/isolation of the compound: (1–2 years)
- Preclinical studies: Screening, evaluation, pharmacokinetic and short-term toxicity testing in animals: (2–4 years)
- Scrutiny and grant of permission for clinical trials: (3–6 months)
- Pharmaceutical formulation, standardization of chemical/biological/immuno-assay of the compound: (0.5–1 year)
- Clinical studies: Phase I, phase II, phase III trials; long-term animal toxicity testing: (3–10 years)
- Review and grant of marketing permission: (0.5–2 years)
- Postmarketing surveillance: (phase IV studies)

4. **Therapeutic index of a drug is an indicator of:**
   a. Potency b. Safety
   c. Toxicity d. Efficacy

   The **therapeutic index (TI)** (also referred to as **therapeutic window** or **safety window** or sometimes as **therapeutic ratio**) is a comparison of the amount of a therapeutic agent that causes the therapeutic effect to the amount that causes toxicity.

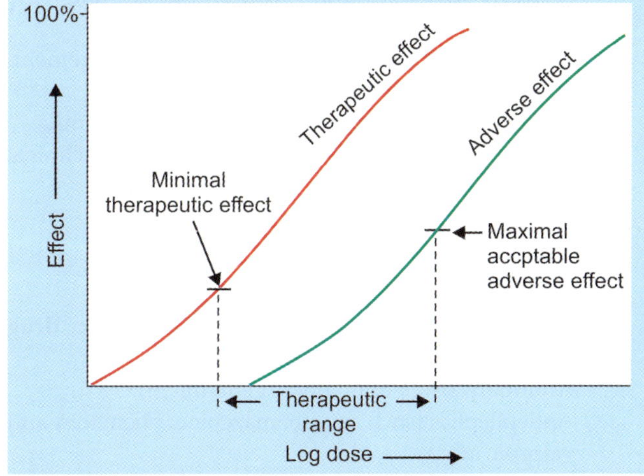

Illustrative dose-response curves for therapeutic effect and adverse effect of the same drug.

5. **Zero order kinetics is seen with:**
   a. Phenytoin b. Phenobarbitone
   c. Erythromycin d. Digoxin

Ans. 1. **d.** Rifampicin 2. **d.** Phenytoin 3. **b.** 100–500 4. **b.** Safety 5. **a.** Phenytoin

The elimination of some drugs approaches saturation over the therapeutic range, kinetics changes from first order to zero order at higher doses. As a result plasma concentration increases disproportionately with increase in dose as occurs in case of phenytoin, tolbutamide, theophylline, warfarin.

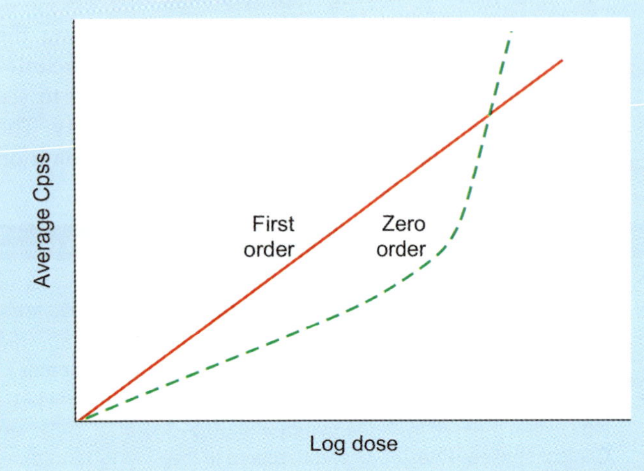

Relationship between dose rate and average steady-state plasma concentration of drugs eliminated by first order and Michaelis-Menten (zero order) kinetics.

6. **MC indication for therapeutic monitoring of the plasma level of a drug is:**
   a. Hit and run drugs
   b. Drugs with irreversible action
   c. Narrow therapeutic range
   d. Failure of responses

Indications for therapeutic drug monitoring include:
- There is an experimentally determined relationship between plasma drug concentration and the pharmacological effect.
- Knowledge of the drug level influences management.
- There is a narrow therapeutic window
- There are potential patient compliance problems.
- The drug dose cannot be optimised by clinical observation alone.

7. **Narrow therapeutic index is seen with:**
   a. Desipramine b. Lithium
   c. Penicillin d. Diazepam

Examples of drugs analysed by therapeutic drug monitoring (narrow therapeutic index)
- Aminoglycoside antibiotics (gentamicin)
- Antiepileptics (such as carbamazepine, phenytoin and valproic acid)
- Mood stabilisers, especially lithium citrate
- Antipsychotics (such as pimozide and clozapine)

8. **Which of the following is a pro-drug:**
   a. Clonidine b. Enalapril
   c. Streptomycin d. Morphine

Pharmacokinetics and Pharmacodynamics of enalapril
- Onset of action: about 1 hour
- Peak effect: 4–6 hours
- Duration: 12–24 hours
- Absorption: ~60%
- Metabolism: Prodrug, undergoes biotransformation to enalaprilat

Prodrug		Active form
Levodopa	—	Dopamine
Enalapril	—	Enalaprilat
a-Methyldopa	—	a-methylnorepinephrine
Dipivefrine	—	Epinephrine
Sulindac	—	Sulfide metabolite
Proguanil	—	Cycloguanil
Prednisone	—	Prednisolone
Bacampicillin	—	Ampicillin
Sulfasalazine	—	5-aminosalicylic acid
Cyclophos-phamide	—	Aldophosphamide, phosphoramide mustard, acrolein
Fluorouracil	—	Fluorouridine monophosphate
Mercaptopurine	—	Methylmercaptopurine ribonucleotide
Acyclovir	—	Acyclovir triphosphate

9. **Pharmacodynamics deals with:**
   a. Mode of excretion of a drug
   b. Mechanism of action of a drug
   c. Transport of drug across the biological membranes
   d. Latency of onset

Pharmacodynamics is the study of the biochemical and physiological effects of drugs on the body or on microorganisms or parasites within or on the body and the mechanisms of drug action and the relationship between drug concentration and effect.

10. **First pass metabolism is maximum with which route:**
   a. Oral b. Subcutaneous
   c. Rectal d. Sublingual

The **first-pass effect** (also known as **first-pass metabolism** or **presystemic metabolism**) is a phenomenon of drug metabolism whereby the concentration of a drug is greatly reduced before it reaches the systemic circulation. It is the fraction of drug lost during the process of absorption which is generally related to the liver and gut wall. Notable drugs that experience a significant first-pass effect are imipramine, morphine, propranolol, buprenorphine, diazepam, midazolam, demerol, cimetidine, and lidocaine.

11. **In higher doses, drugs which shows zero order kinetics:**
   a. Lithium and theophylline
   b. Amiloride and probenecid
   c. Digoxin and propranolol
   d. Phenytoin and warfarin

Ans. 6. **c.** Narrow... 7. **b.** Lithium 8. **b.** Enalapril 9. **b.** Mechanism of... 10. **a.** Oral 11. **d.** Phenytoin and warfarin

At higher doses, metabolism of phenytoin, tolbutamide, theophylline and warfarin changes from first order to zero order.

12. **Elimination of alcohol follows:**
   a. Zero order kinetics   b. First order kinetics
   c. Second order kinetics   d. Third order kinetics

   A few substances are eliminated by zero-order elimination kinetics, because their elimination process is saturated. Examples are Ethanol, Phenytoin, Salicylates, Cisplatin, Fluoxetine, Omeprazole.

13. **Area under time and plasma concentration curve signifies:**
   a. Potency
   b. Extent of absorption of drug
   c. Efficacy
   d. Plasma clearance of a drug

   AUC (area under curve) becomes useful for knowing the average concentration over a time interval, AUC/t. Also, AUC is referenced when talking about elimination.

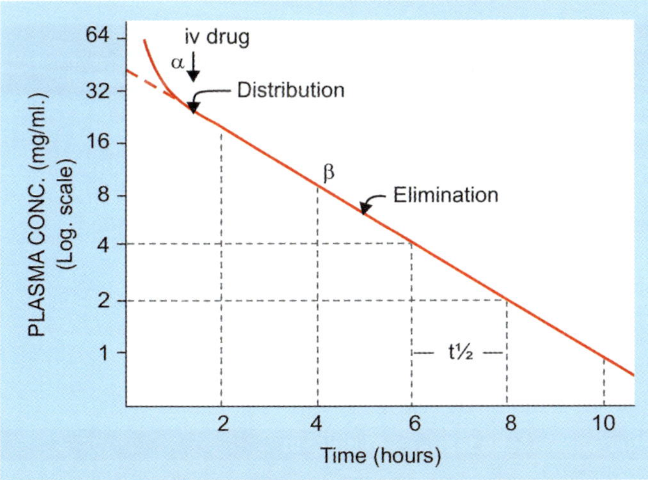

Semilog plasma concentration-time plot of adrug eliminated by first order kinetics after intravenous injection.

14. **First order kinetics is:**
   a. Absorption of the drug is independent of the serum concentration.
   b. Elimination of the drug is independent of the serum concentration.
   c. Elimination of the drug is proportional to the serum concentration.
   d. Absorption of the drug is proportional to the serum concentration.

   First-order reaction

   The reaction proceeds at a rate that is dependent on the concentration of A present in the body. It is assumed that the processes of ADME (absorption, distribution, metabolism, excretion) follow first-order reactions and most drugs are eliminated in this manner.

15. **Steady state concentration of a drug is achieved in:**
   a. 2–3 half lives   b. 3–4 half lives
   c. 4–5 half lives   d. 5–6 half lives

   Steady state refers to the situation where the overall intake of a drug is fairly in dynamic equilibrium with its elimination. In practice, it is generally considered that steady state is reached when a time of 4 to 5 times the half-life for a drug after regular dosing is started.

16. **Orphan drugs are:**
   a. Commercially easy to obtain.
   b. Drugs to treat rare diseases usually
   c. Developed with an intention of monetary gain
   d. All of the above

   "**Orphan drugs**" are medicinal products intended for diagnosis, prevention or treatment of life-threatening or very serious diseases or disorders that are rare. These are drugs or biological products for diagnosis/treatment/prevention of a rare disease or condition, or a more common disease (endemic only in resource poor countries) for which there is no reasonable expectation that the cost of developing and marketing it will be recovered from the sales of that drug.

17. **Therapeutic drug monitoring is required for:**
   a. Sulfonamides   b. Metformin
   c. Cycloserine   d. Gentamycin

   Examples of drugs analysed by therapeutic drug monitoring
   - Aminoglycoside antibiotics (gentamicin)
   - Antiepileptics (such as carbamazepine, phenytoin and valproic acid)
   - Mood stabilisers, especially lithium citrate
   - Antipsychotics (such as pimozide and clozapine)

18. **Pharmacovigilance is for monitoring:**
   a. Cost of drugs
   b. Pharmacy students
   c. Drug safety
   d. Unauthorized drug companies

   Pharmacovigilance is the practice of monitoring the effects of medical drugs after they have been licensed for use, especially in order to identify and evaluate previously unreported adverse reactions.

19. **Elimination after 4 half lives in first order kinetics is:**
   a. 84%   b. 93%
   c. 80.5%   d. 4.75%

   The duration of action of a drug is known as its half life. This is the period of time required for the concentration or amount of drug in the body to be reduced by one-half. After 4 half lives, amount of drug eliminated would be 93.75%.

Half life of some representative drugs.			
Aspirin	4 hrs	Digoxin	40 hrs
Penicillin-G	30 mins	Digitoxin	7 days
Doxycycline	20 hrs	Phenobarbitone	90 hrs

Ans. 12. **a.** Zero order...   13. **d.** Plasma clearance...   14. **c.** Elimination of...   15. **c.** 4–5 half lives
16. **b.** Drugs to treat...   17. **d.** Gentamycin   18. **c.** Drug safety   19. **b.** 93%

20. The maximum effect of a drug is defined by its:

a. Potency b. Efficacy
c. Therapeutic index d. Adversity

Efficacy (E_{max}) is the maximum response achievable from a **drug**. Intrinsic activity is a relative term that describes a **drug's efficacy** relative to a **drug** with the highest observed **efficacy**. Effectiveness refers to the ability of a **drug** to produce a beneficial effect.

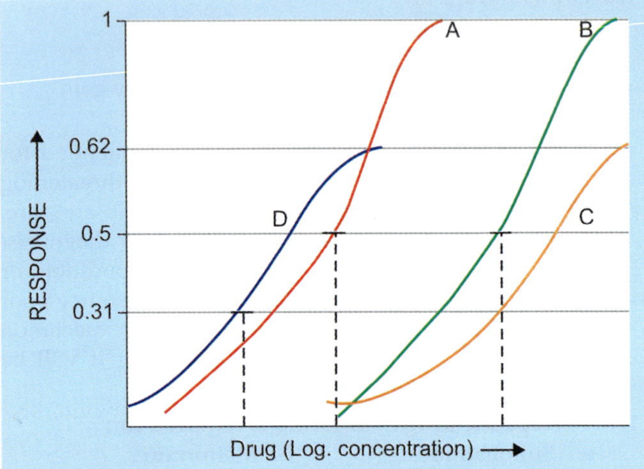

Illustration of drug potency and drug efficacy. Dose-response curve of four drugs producing the same qualitative effect.
Note: Drug B is less potent but equally efficacious as drug A. Drug C is less potent and less efficacious than drug A. Drug D is more potent than drugs A, B, & C, but less efficacious than drugs A & B, and equally efficacious as drug C.

21. True for Phase IV of clinical trials:

a. Done for paediatric drugs
b. Done for rare drugs
c. After-marketing surveillance of drugs
d. Human pharmacology and safety

Phase IV of clinical trials

Studies are done after the drug or treatment has been marketed to gather information on the drug's effect in various populations and any side effects associated with long-term use.

DRUGS ACTING ON CVS

22. A hypertensive patient on medication with beta blockers develops bradycardia and sweating on taking medicines. All of the following are likely responsible agents EXCEPT:

a. Nadolol b. Metoprolol
c. Acebutolol d. Atenolol

Adverse effects of Acebutolol

- The development of anti-nuclear antibodies (ANA) has been found in 10 to 30% of patients under treatment with acebutolol.
- A systemic disease with arthralgic pain and myalgias has been observed in 1%.
- A lupus erythematosus-like syndrome with skin rash and multiforme organ involvement is even less frequent.
- Some few cases of hepatotoxicity with increased liver enzymes (ALT, AST) have been seen.

23. A young hypertensive patient had a past history of myocardial infarction. Which of the following antihypertensive should be used in such a patient:

a. Diuretics
b. ACE inhibitors
c. Beta adrenergic blockers
d. Calcium channel blockers

Indications for ACE inhibitors as antihypertensive agents

- Heart failure
- Post-MI
- High CAD risk
- Diabetes
- Chronic kidney disease
- Recurrent stroke prevention
- Relatively young patients

BP classification	BP (mm Hg)		
	Systolic		Diastolic
1. Normal	<120	and	<80
2. Prehypertension	120–139	or	80–89
3. Hypertension Stage I	140–159	or	90–99
4. Hypertension Stage II	≥ 160	or	≥ 100

24. Mechanism of action of Digitalis:

a. Na^+K^+ ATPase
b. K^+H^+ ATPAse
c. Na^+K^+ cotransporter
d. Na^+H^+ ATPAse

Pharmacokinetic features of digoxin

	DIGOXIN
• Oral absorption	60–80%
• Plasma protein binding	25%
• Time course of action*	
– Onset	15–30 min
– Peak	2–5 hr
– Duration	2–6 days
• Plasma t½	40 hr
• Therapeutic concn.	0.5–1.4 ng/mL
• Toxic concn.	. 2 ng/mL
• Daily maintenance dose	0.125–0.5 mg
• Daily elimination**	35%
• Route of elimination (predominant)	Renal excretion
• Route of administration	Oral, I.V.

*Of full digitalizing dose given I.V;
*Fraction of total amount present in the body

Ans. 20. **b.** Efficacy 21. **c.** After-marketing... 22. **c.** Acebutolol 23. **b.** ACE inhibitors 24. **a.** Na+K+ ATPase

Digitalis works by inhibiting sodium-potassium ATPase. This results in an increased intracellular concentration of sodium ion and thus a decreased concentration gradient across the cell membrane. This increase in intracellular sodium causes the Na/Ca exchanger to reverse potential, i.e., transition from pumping sodium into the cell in exchange for pumping calcium out of the cell, to pumping sodium out of the cell in exchange for pumping calcium into the cell. This leads to an increase in cytoplasmic calcium concentration, which improves cardiac contractility.

25. NOT an inotropic agent:

a. Dobutamine b. Dopamine
c. Diltiazem d. Amrinone

Diltiazem is a nondihydropyridines (non-DHP) calcium channel blocker used in the treatment of hypertension, angina pectoris, and some types of arrhythmia. It relaxes the smooth muscles in the walls of arteries, which opens (dilates) the arteries, allows blood to flow more easily, and lowers blood pressure. Additionally, it lowers blood pressure by acting on the heart itself to reduce the rate, strength, and conduction speed of each beat.

26. Drug of choice for paroxysmal supraventricular tachycardia is:

a. Digoxin b. Propranolol
c. Adenosine d. Diltiazem

In addition to adenosine's endogenous forms, it is also used as a medication, specifically, as an antiarrhythmic agent, to treat a number of forms of supraventricular tachycardia that do not improve with vagal maneuvers. Common side effects include chest pain, feeling faint, shortness of breath along with tingling of the senses . Serious side effects include a worsening dysrhythmia and low blood pressure.

Clinical classification of antiarrhythmic drugs.

Supraventricular arrhythmias only	*Supraventricular and ventricular arrhythmias*		*Ventricular arrhythmias only*
Adenosine	Amiodarone	Procainamide	Lidocaine
Verapamil	β blockers	Disopyramide	Mexiletine
Diltiazem	Propranolol	Quinidine	
Dronedarone	Sotalol	Flecainide	
Digoxin	Esmolol	Propafenone	

27. All of the following are inotropic agents except:

a. Digitalis b. Amiodarone
c. Amrinone d. Dopamine

Amiodarone is a class III antiarrhythmic agent used for various types of cardiac dysrhythmias, both ventricular and atrial. It was discovered in 1961. Despite relatively common side-effects, it is used in arrhythmias that are otherwise difficult to treat with medication.

28. Potassium channel openers are all except:

a. Minoxidil b. Glibenclamide
c. Penacidil d. Nicorandil

Glibenclamide, also known as **glyburide**, is an antidiabetic drug in a class of medications known as sulfonylureas, closely related to sulfonamide antibiotics.

29. Antihypertensive, which is also useful in gout and DM:

a. Diazoxide b. Propranolol
c. Enalapril d. Thiazide

Enalapril is an angiotensin-converting-enzyme (ACE) inhibitor used in the treatment of hypertension, diabetic nephropathy, and some types of chronic heart failure. ACE converts the peptide hormone angiotensin I to angiotensin II.

Selection of first line antihypertensive drugs

Compelling indications	*Suitable for*	*To be avoided in*
	Diuretics	
1. Heart failure	1. Older patients	1. Gout or family history of gout
2. High CAD risk	2. Isolated systolic hypertension	2. Abnormal lipid profile
3. Recurrent stroke prevention	3. Obese with volume overload	3. Pregnancy induced hypertension
4. Diabetes	4. Low cost therapy	
	ACE inhibitors/Ang II receptor blockers	
1. Heart failure	1. Relatively young patients	1. Bilateral renal artery stenosis or that in single kidney
2. Post-MI	2. Patients with left ventricular hypertrophy	2. Pregnancy
3. High CAD risk		
4. Diabetes	3. Gout, PVD, dyslipidemic patients	3. Hyperkalaemia
5. Chronic kidney disease		4. Preexisting dry cough (ACE inhibitor)
6. Recurrent stroke prevention		
	β Adrenergic blockers	
		(especially applicable to nonselective β blockers)
1. Stable heart failure	1. Coexisting anxiety or tachycardia	1. Asthma, COPD

Contd...

Ans. 25. **c.** Diltiazem 26. **c.** Adenosine 27. **b.** Amiodarone 28. **b.** Glibenclamide 29. **c.** Enalapril

Contd...

Compelling indications	*Suitable for*	*To be avoided in*	
2. Post-MI	2. Relatively young patient	2. Bradycardia, conduction defects	
3. High CAD risk	3. Migraine patients	3. Decompensated heart failure	
	4. Low cost therapy	4. PVD	
		5. Abnormal lipid profile	
Calcium channel blockers			
1. Recurrent stroke prevention	1. Older with poor arterial wall compliance	1. Mycardial inadequacy, CHF	Verapamil and diltiazem
	2. Isolated systolic hypertension	2. Conduction defects, sick sinus	
	3. Asthma/COPD patients	3. Receiving β blockers	
	4. Raynaud's (and other PVD) patients	4. Ischaemic heart disease; post MI cases	DHPs
	5. Pregnant hypertensive	5. Males with prostate enlargement	
	6. Diabetics	6. Gastroesophageal reflux	

30. Beta blockers are anti-arrhythmic agents, type:

a. I
b. II
c. III
d. IV

Class II antiarrhythmic: Beta blockers (partial list)

- Propranolol (decreases slope of phase 4)
- Esmolol (decreases slope of phase 4)
- Timolol (decreases slope of phase 4)
- Metoprolol (decreases slope of phase 4)
- Atenolol (decreases slope of phase 4)

Antiarrhythmic drugs.

Class	*Actions*	*Drugs*
I.	Membrane stabilizing agents (Na^+ channel blockers)	
	A. *Moderately decrease dv/dt of 0 phase*	Quinidine, Procainamide, Disopyramide
	B. Little decrease in dv/dt of 0 phase	Lidocaine, Mexiletine
	C. *Marked decrease in dv/dt of 0 phase*	Propafenone, Flecainide
II.	*Antiadrenergic agents* (β *blockers*)	Propranolol, Esmolol, Sotalol (also class III)
III.	*Agents widening AP (prolong repolarization and ERP)*	Amiodarone, Dronedarone Dofetilide, Ibutilide
IV.	*Calcium channel blockers*	Verapamil, Diltiazem
Note: Class IA agents also have Class III property; Propranolol has Class I action as well; sotalol has both Class II and Class III actions.		

In addition

1. *For PSVT* : Adenosine, Digoxin
2. *For A-V block* : Sympathomimetics—Isoprenaline, etc. Anticholinergics—Atropine.
3. Digitalis is used in AF, AFl and PSVT to control ventricular rate.

31. In a patient with concomitant diabetes, anti-hypertensive agent of choice is:

a. Calcium channel blocker
b. Beta adrenergic blocker
c. ACE inhibitor
d. Plasma kinins

Enalapril is used to treat hypertension, symptomatic heart failure, and asymptomatic left ventricular dysfunction. It has been proven to protect the function of the kidneys in hypertension, heart failure, and diabetes, and may be used in the absence of hypertension for its kidney protective effects. It is widely used in chronic kidney failure.

32. Calcium channel blocker causing cerebral vasodilatation is:

a. Nimodipine
b. Felodipine
c. Amlodipine
d. Nitrendipine

Because it has some selectivity for cerebral vasculature, nimodipine's main use is in the prevention of cerebral vasospasm and resultant ischemia, a complication of

Ans. 30. **b.** II 31. **c.** ACE inhibitor 32. **a.** Nimodipine

subarachnoid hemorrhage (a form of cerebral bleed), specifically from ruptured intracranial berry aneurysms irrespective of the patient's post-ictus neurological condition.

33. ACE inhibitors are CONTRAINDICATED in:

a. Hypertension
b. Myocardial infarction
c. Renal artery stenosis
d. Left ventricular dysfunction

Angiotensin-converting enzyme **inhibitors** (ACEIs) are **contraindicated** in patients with bilateral **renal artery stenosis** due to risk of azotemia resulting from preferential efferent arteriolar vasodilation in the **renal** glomerulus due to **inhibition** of angiotensin II.

34. Which does NOT contribute to digoxin toxicity:

a. Hypomagnesemia b. Renal failure
c. Hypercalcemia d. Hyperkalemia

The occurrence of adverse drug reactions is common in digoxin therapy, owing to its narrow therapeutic index (the margin between effectiveness and toxicity). Adverse effects are concentration-dependent, and are rare when plasma digoxin concentration is <0.8 nanograms/l. They are also more common in patients with low potassium levels (hypokalemia), since digoxin normally competes with K^+ ions for the same binding site on the Na^+/K^+ ATPase pump.

35. Digitalis given for atrial flutter often produces:

a. Atrial fibrillation
b. Atrial tachycardia
c. Atrial extrasystole
d. All of the above

Less frequent adverse effects (0.1%–1%) of digitalis include: acute psychosis, delirium, amnesia, convulsions, shortened QRS complex, atrial or ventricular extrasystoles, paroxysmal atrial tachycardia with AV block, ventricular tachycardia or fibrillation, and heart block.

36. Both therapeutic and toxic effects of digitalis are enhanced by:

a. Sodium b. Chloride
c. Calcium d. Potassium

Increased intracellular Ca^{2+} synergises with digitalis and may precipitate its toxicity.

37. Drug of choice for digitalis-induced ventricular arrhythmias:

a. Verapamil b. Lidocaine
c. Quinidine d. Encainide

The primary treatment of digoxin toxicity is Digoxin immune fab (ovine), which is an antibody made up of anti-digoxin immunoglobulin fragments. Other treatment that may be used to treat life-threatening arrhythmias until Fab is acquired are magnesium, phenytoin (dilantin), and lidocaine.

38. Of the following, drug of choice for PSVT:

a. Verapamil b. Digitalis
c. Quinidine d. Diphenylhydantoin

Verapamil is a class-IV antiarrhythmic, more effective than digoxin in controlling ventricular rate

Choice of antiarrhythmics for cardiac arrhythmias.

Arrhythmia	*Clinical objective*	*Drug (s)*
1. Atrial extrasystoles Symptomatic	: Suppression, symptom relief	No drug if asymptomatic or non-disturbing Propranolol (only if disturbing)
2. Paroxysmal supraventricular tachycardia (PSVT)	: Termination of PSVT : Prevention of recurrence	i.v. adenosine/verapamil/diltiazem/esmolol Oral verapamil/diltiazem/propranolol/sotalol
3. Atrial fibrillation (AF)	: Reversal to SR (for paroxysmal/persistent AF) : Maintenance of SR : Ventricular rate control (for permanent AF/during recurrence of AF) : Urgent vent. rate control	Cardioversion i.v. amiodarone Sotalol/propafenone/amiodarone/dronedarone/disopyramide oral verapamil/diltiazem/propranolol ± digoxin i.v. esmolol/verapamil/amiodarone
4. Atrial flutter (AFl)	: Reversal to SR : Ventricular rate control	Cardioversion, radiofrequency ablation, Propafenone (after rate control with verapamil/propranolol) Propranolol/verapamil/diltiazem ± digoxin or amiodarone
5. Wolff-Parkinson-White syndrome (WPW) tachycardia	: Termination : Maintenance – narrow QRS – wide QRS	Radiofrequency ablation, cardioversion Propafenone/procainamide Propafenone + verapamil/propranolol or Amiodarone/sotalol
6. Acute-MI arrhythmia Bradycardia Vent. extrasystoles/tachycardia	: Reversal to normal rate : Abolition to prevent serious arrhythmia	Atropine (i.v.)—no effect—Pacing i.v. Lidocaine/procainamide/amiodarone Cardioversion (if haemodynamically unstable)

Contd...

Ans. 33. c. Renal artery... 34. d. Hyperkalemia 35. d. All of the above 36. c. Calcium
37. b. Lidocaine 38. a. Verapamil

Contd...

Arrhythmia	*Clinical objective*	*Drug (s)*
7. Chronic vent. tachycardia Nonsustained VT Sustained VT	: Suppression : Abolition : Maintenance therapy (prevention of VF/ arrest)	Propranolol/amiodarone (oral) i.v. Amiodarone ± propranolol or cardioversion or propafenone/lidocaine (i.v.) Amiodarone/sotalol Implantable defibrillator
8. Ventricular fibrillation (VF)	: Termination : Recurrence prevention	Defibrillation ± amiodarone (i.v.) Amiodarone (oral)/propranolol

(SR: Sinus rhythm).

39. Antihypertensives act by all of the following mechanism except:

a. Na^+ K^+ ATPase inhibition
b. Alpha adrenergic blockade
c. Beta adrenergic blockade
d. Potassium channel opener

Digoxin's primary mechanism of action involves inhibition of the Na+/K+ ATPase, mainly in the myocardium. This inhibition causes an increase in intracellular sodium levels, resulting in a reversal of the action of the sodium-calcium exchanger, which normally imports three extracellular sodium ions into the cell and transports one intracellular calcium ion out of the cell. The reversal of this exchange causes an increase in the intracellular calcium concentration that is available to the contractile proteins. Increased intracellular calcium lengthens phase 4 and phase 0 of the cardiac action potential, which leads to a decrease in heart rate. Increased amounts of Ca^{2+} also leads to increased storage of calcium in the sarcoplasmic reticulum, causing a corresponding increase in the release of calcium during each action potential. This leads to increased contractility (the force of contraction) of the heart without increasing heart energy expenditure.

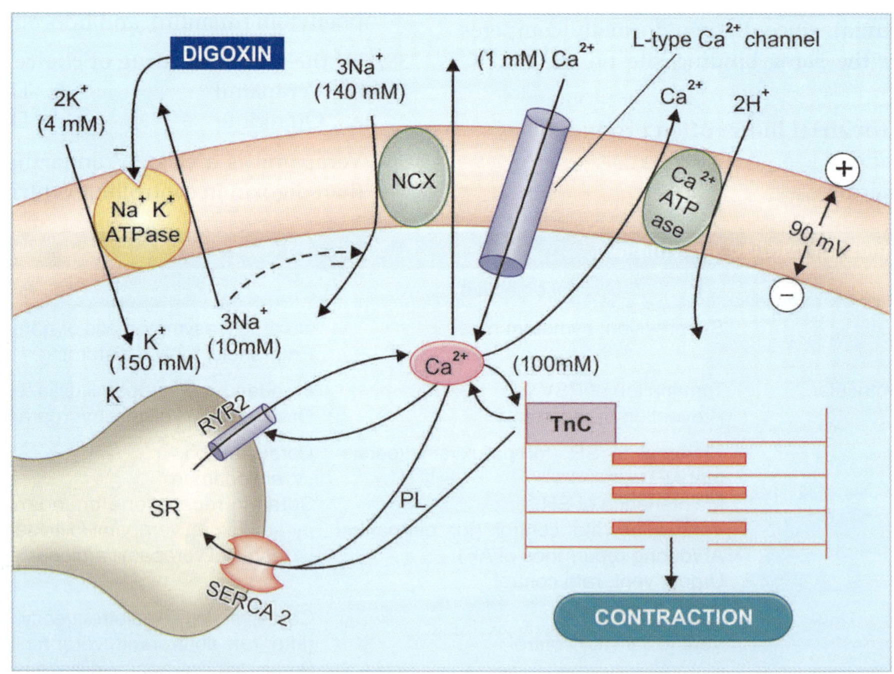

Mechanism of positive inotropic action of cardiac glycosides. SR: Sarcoplasmic reticulum; TnC: Troponin C; NCX: Na^+-Ca^{2+} exchanger; RyR2: Ryanodine receptor calcium channel 2; PL: Phospholamban; SERCA2: Sarcoplasmic-endoplasmic reticulum calcium ATPase 2.

DRUGS ACTING ON RESPIRATORY SYSTEM

40. Which of the following can NOT be used in status asthmaticus:

a. Terbutaline
b. Salmeterol
c. Salbutamol
d. Hydrocortisone

Salmeterol is a long-acting $beta_2$-adrenergic receptor agonist drug used in the maintenance and prevention of asthma symptoms and maintenance of chronic obstructive pulmonary disease (COPD) symptoms.

Ans. **39. a.** Na^+ K^+ ATPase **40. b.** Salmeterol

41. Which of the following is a lipoxygenase inhibitor:

a. Montelukast
b. Thromboxanes
c. Zileuton
d. Sodium cromoglycate

Zileuton is an orally active inhibitor of 5-lipoxygenase, and thus inhibits leukotrienes (LTB_4, LTC_4, LTD_4, and LTE_4) formation. Zileuton is used for the maintenance treatment of asthma.

42. Anti-asthmatic drug, which requires LEAST systemic monitoring:

a. Dexamethasone
b. Hydrocortisone
c. Budesonide
d. Prednisolone

Budesonide is nebulized for maintenance and prophylactic treatment of asthma including patients who require oral corticosteroids and those who may benefit from a systemic dose reduction.

43. Sodium chromoglycate acts by:

a. Antihistaminic action
b. Mast cell stabilization
c. Bronchorelaxation
d. Prevents antigen antibody reaction

Cromoglicic acid (also referred to as **cromolyn**, **cromoglycate**, or **cromoglycate**) is traditionally described as a mast cell stabilizer, and is commonly marketed as the sodium salt **sodium cromoglicate** or **cromolyn sodium**. This drug prevents the release of inflammatory chemicals such as histamine from mast cells.

44. The drug which interferes with metabolism of theophylline:

a. Gentamycin
b. Penicillin
c. Erythromycin
d. Sulfonamide

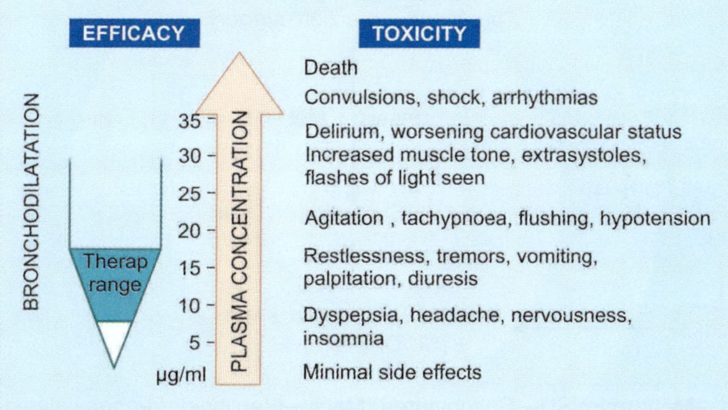

Relationship between efficacy and toxicity of theophylline with its plasma concentration. The depicted concentration ranges are approximate.

The toxicity of theophylline is increased by erythromycin, cimetidine, and fluoroquinolones, such as ciprofloxacin. It can reach toxic levels when taken with fatty meals, an effect called dose dumping. Theophylline toxicity can be treated with beta blockers.

45. Drug of choice for theophylline poisoning:

a. Phenobarbitone
b. Thyroxine
c. Charcoal hemoperfusion
d. Cortisone

Multidose activated charcoal (MDAC) enhances elimination of theophylline. It is a very effective method of elimination, and it is considered the mainstay treatment of theophylline toxicity.

46. Mechanism of action of corticosteroids in asthma is:

a. Decreases mucosal edema by suppressing inflammatory response
b. Mast cell stabilization
c. Causes bronchodilatation
d. Leukotriene antagonist

Steroids are the most potent anti-inflammatory agents. Inhaled forms are topically active, poorly absorbed, and least likely to cause adverse effects.

47. Drug of choice for managing asthmatic patient with hypertension:

a. Timolol
b. Propranolol
c. Metoprolol
d. Amlodipine

Dihydropyridine calcium channel blockers anything that ends in "dipine" such as amlodipine or nifedipine) work to block vascular calcium channels resulting in vascular smooth muscle relaxation and have no specific contraindications.

48. Drug of choice for acute severe asthma is:

a. Short acting beta 2 agonists
b. Long acting beta 2 agonists
c. Oral theophylline
d. Inhaled ipratropium bromide

Quick relief medications are used to relieve acute asthma exacerbations and to prevent exercise-induced asthma (EIA) or exercise-induced bronchospasm (EIB) symptoms. These medications include short-acting beta agonists (SABAs), anticholinergics (used only for severe exacerbations), and systemic corticosteroids, which speed recovery from acute exacerbations.

49. All of the following are true regarding sodium cromoglycate except:

a. Given in acute bronchial asthma
b. Inhibits degranulation of mast cells
c. It is not a bronchodilator
d. It is not absorbed orally

Ans. **41. c.** Zileuton **42. c.** Budesonide **43. b.** Mast cell stabi... **44. c.** Erythromycin **45. c.** Charcoal... **46. a.** Decreases mucosal... **47. d.** Amlodipine **48. a.** Short acting... **49. a.** Given in acute...

Cromolyn sodium was discovered by Roger Altounyan who was himself a lifelong asthma sufferer. It is considered a breakthrough drug in management of asthma, as the patients can be freed from steroids in many cases; however, it is mainly effective as a prophylaxis for allergic and exercise induced asthma, not as a treatment for acute attacks.

50. Beta blocker drug CONTRAINDICATED in asthma patients:

a. Metoprolol
b. Atenolol
c. Propranolol
d. Acebutolol

Propranolol should not be used in those with an already slow heart rate and most of those with heart failure. Quickly stopping the medication in those with coronary artery disease may worsen symptoms. It may worsen the symptoms of asthma.

51. Which of the following agent is NOT used in management of bronchial asthma:

a. Phospho-di-esterase inhibitors
b. Steroids
c. Beta agonists
d. Cholinergic drugs

Cholinergic drugs cause bronchoconstriction and will aggravate the asthmatic symptoms. Anticholinergics are used as an anti-asthmatic agent.

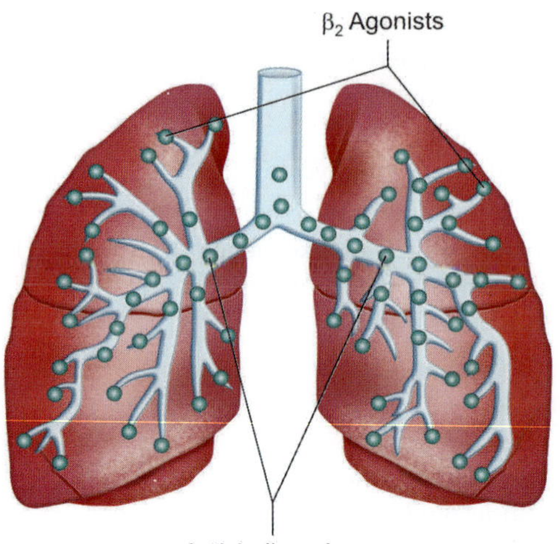

Primary sites of bronchodilator action of inhaled adrenergic β_2 agonists and inhaled anticholinergics. Salbutamol mainly relaxes bronchiolar smooth muscle; Ipratropium blocks bronchoconstriction mainly in the larger airways.

ANTIDIABETIC DRUGS

52. Metformin action:

a. Stimulate hepatic gluconeogenesis
b. Stimulate glycogenolysis
c. Enhance glucose uptake by skeletal muscle
d. Decrease absorption of glucose from intestine

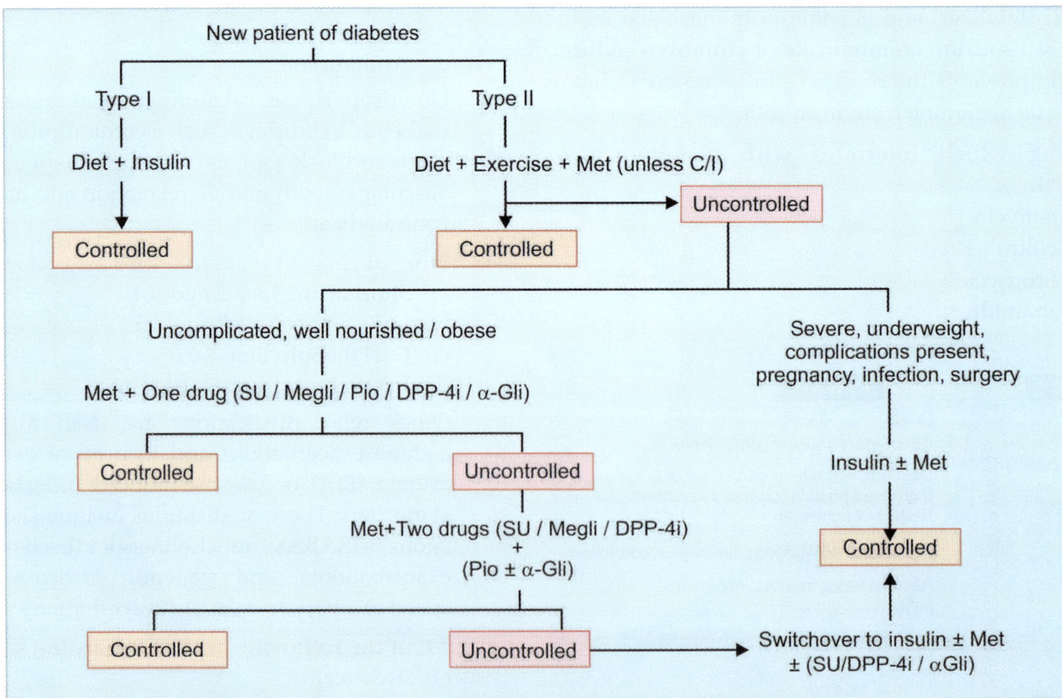

Simplified flow chart of management approaches in diabetes mellitus. Met—Metformin; SU—Sulfonylurea; Megli—Meglitinide/d-phenylalanine analogue; DPP-4i—Dipeptidyl peptidase-4 inhibitor; α Gli—α Glucosidase inhibitor; Pio—Pioglitazone.
Note: A meglitinide drug is indicated only in patients with predominant postprandial hyperglycemia.
An α glucosidase inhibitor can be additional add on drug.

Ans. **50. c.** Propranolol **51. d.** Cholinergic drugs **52. c.** Enhance glucose...

Metformin decreases hyperglycemia primarily by suppressing glucose production by the liver (hepatic gluconeogenesis). In addition to suppressing hepatic glucose production, metformin increases insulin sensitivity, enhances peripheral glucose uptake (by inducing the phosphorylation of GLUT4 enhancer factor), decreases insulin-induced suppression of fatty acid oxidation, and decreases absorption of glucose from the gastrointestinal tract.

53. NOT a side-effect of insulin:

a. Lipodystrophy b. Hypoglycemia
c. Albuminuria d. Edema

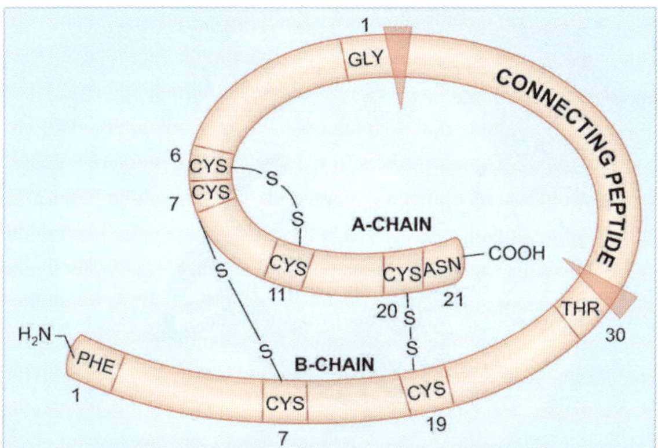

Human proinsulin; simplified structure depicting the main features. The connecting peptide, having 35 amino acids, is split off leaving insulin molecule with two chains joined by two disulfide bridges.

The kidneys normally do not filter large molecules into the urine, so albuminuria can be an indicator of damage to the kidneys or excessive salt intake. It can also occur in patients with long-standing diabetes, especially type 1 diabetes.

54. In the management of diabetes mellitus, lactic acidosis is commonly caused by:

a. Tolbutamide b. Glipizide
c. Pioglitazone d. Metformin

Metformin causes few adverse effects when prescribed appropriately (the most common is gastrointestinal upset) and has been associated with a low risk of having a low blood sugar. Lactic acidosis (a buildup of lactate in the blood) can be a serious concern in overdose and when it is prescribed to people with contraindications, but otherwise, no significant risk exists. It is in the biguanide class.

55. Drug used in diabetes:

a. Salmeterol b. Acetohexamide
c. Benserazide d. Methoxamine

Acetohexamide is a first-generation sulfonylurea medication used to treat diabetes mellitus type 2, particularly in people whose diabetes cannot be controlled by diet alone.

56. Rapidly acting insulin:

a. Lente b. Insulin glargine
c. Ultralente d. Insulin lispro

Insulin lispro is a fast acting insulin analog. It was first approved for use in the United States in 1996, making it the first insulin analog to enter the market.

Types of insulin preparations and insulin analogues

Type	*Appearance*	*Onset (hr)*	*Peak (hr)*	*Duration (hr)*	*Can be mixed with*
Rapid acting					
Insulin lispro	Clear	0.2–0.3	1–1.5	3–5	Regular, NPH
Insulin aspart	Clear	0.2–0.3	1–1.5	3–5	Regular, NPH
Insulin glulisine	Clear	0.2–0.4	1–2	3–5	Regular, NPH
Short acting					
Regular (soluble) insulin	Clear	0.5–1	2–3	6–8	All preparations (except insulin glargine/ detemir)
Intermediate acting					
Insulin zinc suspension or Lente*	Cloudy	1–2	8–10	20–24	Regular
Neutral protamine hagedorn (NPH) or isophane insulin	Cloudy	1–2	8–10	20–24	Regular
Long acting					
Insulin glargine	Clear	2–4	—	24	None
Insulin detemir	Clear	1–4	—	20–24	None

57. True statement regarding mechanism of action of sulfonylureas is:

a. Increased peripheral utilization of glucose
b. Reduce hepatic glucose output
c. Act on SUR receptors on pancreatic beta cell membrane
d. Transcription of genes regulating glucose metabolism

Ans. **53. c.** Albuminuria **54. d.** Metformin **55. b.** Aceto-hexamide **56. d.** Insulin lispro **57. c.** Act on SUR...

Sulfonylureas bind to an ATP-sensitive $K^+(K_{ATP})$ channel on the cell membrane of pancreatic beta cells. This inhibits a tonic, hyperpolarizing efflux of potassium, thus causing the electric potential over the membrane to become more positive. This depolarization opens voltage-gated Ca^{2+}channels. The rise in intracellular calcium leads to increased fusion of insulin granulae with the cell membrane, and therefore increased secretion of (pro)insulin. The K_{ATP} channel is an octameric complex of the inward-rectifier potassium ion channel $K_{ir}6.x$ and sulfonylurea receptor SUR which associate with a stoichiometry of 4:4.

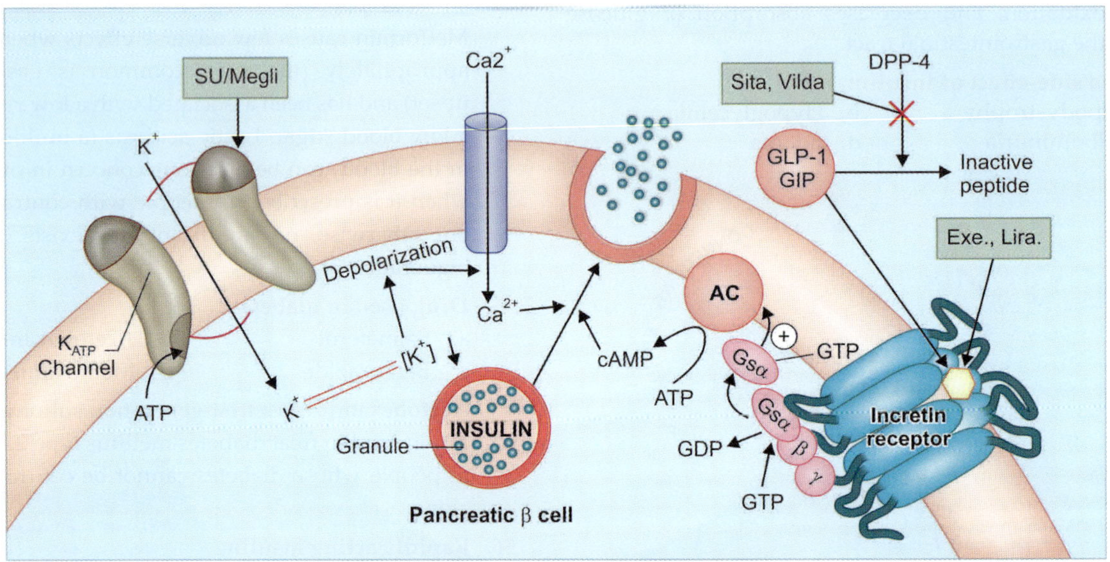

Mechanism of action of insulin secretagogues

The sulfonylureas (SU) and meglitinide analogues (Megli) block the sulfonylurea receptor (SUR1) which constitutes a subunit of the inwardly rectifying ATP-sensitive K^+ channel (K_{ATP}) in the membrane of pancreatic β cells. The inward flow of K^+ ions is thereby restricted, intracellular K^+ concentration falls and the membrane is partially depolarized augmenting Ca^{2+} channel opening as well as release of Ca^{2+} from intracellular stores. The Ca^{2+} ions promote fusion of insulin containing intracellular granules with the plasma membrane and exocytotic release of insulin.

Incretins such as glucagon-like peptide 1 (GLP1) and glucose-dependent insulinotropic polypeptide (GIP) act upon their own G-protein coupled receptors on the β cell membrane to activate adenylyl cyclase and generate cAMP, which also promotes exocytosis of insulin. Exenatide (Exe) and liraglutide (Lira) are GLP1 receptor agonists—produce the same response as GLP1. The incretins GLP1 and GIP are rapidly inactivated by the capillary endothelial enzyme dipeptidyl peptidase-4 (DPP-4). Their action is enhanced by DPP-4 inhibitors sitagliptin (sita) and vildagliptin (vilda). The DPP-4 inhibitors thus markedly accentuate the insulin response to ingested glucose/meal and attenuate postprandial glycaemia.

58. Drug that does NOT cause hypoglycemia:

a. Tolbutamide b. Glibenclamide
c. Metformin d. Chlorpropamide

The most common symptoms following metformin overdose appear to include vomiting, diarrhea, abdominal pain, tachycardia, drowsiness, etc.

Important features of oral hypoglycaemics.

Drug	Preparations	Plasma t½ (hr)	Duration of action (hr)	Clearance route*	Daily dose	No. of doses per day	Remarks
Sulfonylureas							
1. Tolbutamide	RASTINON, 0.5 g tab.	6	6–8	L	0.5–3 g	2–3	Weaker, shorter acting, flexible dosage, safer in elderly and in those prone to hypoglycaemia.
2. Glibenclamide (Glyburide)	DAONIL, EUGLUCON, BETANASE 2.5, 5 mg tab.	2–4	24	L	2.5–15 mg	1–2	Potent but slow acting, higher incidence of hypoglycaemia, single daily dose despite short t½ due to active metabolite and sequestration in β cells.
3. Glipizide	GLYNASE, GLIDE MINIDIAB 5 mg tab	3–5	12	L	5–20 mg	1–2	Fast and shorter acting, higher daily dose to be divided, hypoglycaemia and weight gain less likely, preferable in elderly.

Contd...

Ans. 58. c. Metformin

Contd...

Drug	Preparations	Plasma t½ (hr)	Duration of action (hr)	Clearance route*	Daily dose	No. of doses per day	Remarks
4. Gliclazide	DIAMICRON 80 mg tab. DIAZIDE 20, 80 mg tab GLIZID 30, 40, 80 mg tab	8–20	12–24	L	40–240 mg	1–2	Has antiplatelet action, generates only inactive metabolite, daily dose > 80 mg to be divided.
5. Glimepiride	AMARYL, GLY-PRIDE GLIMER 1, 2 mg tab	5–7	24	L	1–6 mg	1–2	Long acting, only inactive metabolite. Stronger extra-pancreatic action. Lower incidence of hypoglycaemia.
Meglitinide/Phenylalanine Analogues							
1. Repaglinide	EUREPA, RAPLIN REGAN 0.5, 1, 2 mg tab	< 1	3–5	L	1–8 mg	3–4	Given ½ hr before each meal for limiting p.p. hyperglycaemia.
2. Nateglinide	GLINATE, NA-TELIDE 60, 120 mg tab	1.5	2–4	L	180–480 mg	3–4	Stimulates 1st phase insulin secretion, less likely to cause delayed hypoglycaemia.
DPP-4 INHIBITORS							
1. Sitagliptin	JANUVIA 100 mg tab.	~12	24	K	100 mg	1	Non-covalent binding to DPP-4; excreted unchanged in urine. Low risk of hypoglycaemia. Body weight neutral.
2. Vildagliptin	GALVUS, JALRA, ZOMELIS 50 mg cap	2–4	12–24	L,K	50–100 mg	1–2	Covalent binding to DPP-4; Metabolized in liver. Hepatotoxicity reported.
Biguanide							
1. Metformin	GLYCIPHAGE, GLYCOMET 0.5, 0.85 g tab, 0.5 g and 1.0 g SR tabs	1.5–3	6–8	K	0.5–2.5 g	1–2	No hypoglycaemia. Not metabolized. Lactic acidosis rare, only in kidney disease.
Thiazolidinedione							
1. Pioglitazone	PIONORM, PIOR-EST, PIOZONE 15, 30 mg tab	3–5	24	L	15–45 mg	1	May improve lipid profile. Reverses insulin resistance. No hypoglycaemia, C/I in liver and heart disease.

*L: Metabolized in liver; K: Excreted unchanged by kidney; p.p.: postprandial.

59. An oral hypoglycemic agent used to treat obesity is:
a. Tolbutamide
b. Glipizide
c. Gliclazide
d. Metformin

In people with diabetes mellitus type 2, the drug metformin (Glucophage) can reduce weight. Metformin limits the amount of glucose that is produced by the liver as well as increases muscle consumption of glucose. It also helps in increasing our body's response to insulin.

60. Type I diabetes mellitus is initially managed by:
a. Metformin
b. Sulfonylureas
c. Meglitinide
d. None of the above

Patients with type 1 diabetes mellitus (DM) require lifelong insulin therapy. Most require 2 or more injections of insulin daily, with doses adjusted on the basis of self-monitoring of blood glucose levels.

61. All of the following are true regarding adverse effects of chlorpropamide except:
a. Sensitizes the kidney to ADH action
b. Less incidence of hypoglycemia
c. More incidence of weight gain
d. Disulfiram like reaction may occur

Chlorpropamide and other sulfonylureas encourage weight gain, so they are generally not favored for use in very obese patients. The most common side effects of chlorpropamide are skin related, such as rashes, photoallergy and (in rare cases) Stevens-Johnson syndrome. Less common side effects of chlorpropamide include gastrointestinal symptoms such as nausea, vomiting, and diarrhea. It may cause facial flushing after the ingestion of alcohol. In very high doses it can increase secretion of antidiuretic hormone (ADH), which can lead to hyponatremia. It also markedly raises the serum level of alkaline phosphatase. It is one of the Sulfonyl ureas/SUs which has been discontinued because of long duration of action (≥ 2 days) and frequent hypoglycemia.

Ans. 59. **d.** Metformin 60. **d.** None of the above 61. **b.** Less incidence...

62. Which of the following is true of biguanides:

a. Cause little or no hypoglycemia
b. Stimulates pancreatic beta cells
c. Completely metabolized
d. Promotes hepatic gluconeogenesis

The most common side effect of metformin (Biguanide) is diarrhea and dyspepsia, occurring in up to 30% of patients. The most important and serious side effect is lactic acidosis, therefore metformin is contraindicated in renal insufficiency. Renal functions should be assessed before starting metformin. Phenformin and buformin are more prone to cause acidosis than metformin; therefore, they have been practically replaced by it. Though metformin is non-hypoglycemic, however, when metformin is combined with other drugs (combination therapy), hypoglycemia and other side effects are possible.

63. Insulin with peak action at 2–3 hours:

a. Lispro insulin b. Regular insulin
c. Insulin aspart d. Insulin glusuline

Regular Human Insulin which has an onset of action of 1/2 hour to 1 hour, peak effect in 2 to 4 hours, and duration of action of 6 to 8 hours. The larger the dose of regular the faster the onset of action, but the longer the time to peak effect and the longer the duration of the effect.

DRUGS ACTING ON NERVOUS SYSTEM

64. In pregnancy, Phenytoin therapy may lead to deficiency of:

a. Folic acid b. Vitamin B12
c. Vitamin B1 d. Vitamin B6

It has been suggested that phenytoin causes a reduction in folic acid levels, predisposing patients to megaloblastic anemia. Folate is presented in foods as polyglutamate, which is then converted into monoglutamates by intestinal conjugase. Phenytoin acts by inhibiting this enzyme, thereby causing folate deficiency.

Plasma half life, therapeutic and toxic plasma concentration range of some important antiepileptic drugs.

Drug	Half life (hr)	Plasma concentration (μg/mL)	
		Therapeutic	Toxic
Phenobarbitone	80–120	10–30	> 30 mild > 60 severe
Phenytoin	12–36	10–20	> 20 mild > 35 severe
Carbamazepine	10–40	5–10	> 12
Ethosuximide	30–50	50–100*	> 200
Valproate	10–15	40–100*	–
Clonazepam	20–40	0.01–0.1*	–

*Poorly correlated with response.

65. Which of the following is a long acting SSRI:

a. Fluvoxamine b. Fluoxetine
c. Paroxetine d. Sertraline

Fluoxetine, a bicylic compound, is the first SSRI to be introduced and the longest acting. Its plasma $t_{1/2}$ is 2 days, and that of its active demethylated metabolite is 7–10 days.

66. Extrapyramidal side effects are common with all EXCEPT:

a. Fluphenazine b. Chlorpromazine
c. Carbamazepine d. Haloperidol

Side effects of Carbamazepine

- Dose related neurotoxicity (sedation, dizziness etc.)
- Worsening of seizures
- Hypersensitivity reaction (rashes, photosensitivity etc.)
- Agranulocytosis and aplastic anemia
- Water retention and hyponatremia
- Minor fetal malformations

67. Drug to be used CAUTIOUSLY in pseudo-cholinesterase deficiency:

a. Gallamine b. Halothane
c. Scoline d. Barbiturate

Suxamethonium acts as a depolarizing neuromuscular blocker. It acts on nicotinic receptors resulting in persistent depolarization of the motor end plate. It is degraded by butyrylcholinesterase (**pseudocholinesterase**, or **plasma cholinesterase)** into succinic acid and choline. This hydrolysis by butyrylcholinesterase is much slower than that of acetylcholine by acetylcholinesterase.

68. Carisoprodol activation forms:

a. Meprobamate b. Dimethadione
c. Doxylamine d. Amphetamine

Although carisoprodol has significant pharmacological activity, its benefit in therapy is likely due mostly to the meprobamate metabolite as meprobamate remains in the system significantly longer and reaches a higher peak plasma concentration than the parent drug a few hours following administration. This is further evidenced by carisoprodol's ability to maintain relevant benefits when administered 3-4 times a day despite its short half-life of only two hours.

69. Which of the following does NOT interfere with folic acid metabolism:

a. Phenytoin b. Gabapentin
c. Phenobarbitone d. Primidone

Medications can interfere with folate utilization

- Anticonvulsant medications (such as phenytoin, primidone, carbamazepine or valproate)
- Metformin (sometimes prescribed to control blood sugar in type 2 diabetes)
- Methotrexate, an anti-cancer drug also used to control inflammation associated with Crohn's disease, ulcerative colitis and rheumatoid arthritis.

Ans. 62. **a.** Cause little or no... 63. **b.** Regular insulin 64. **a.** Folic acid 65. **b.** Fluoxetine
66. **c.** Carbamazepine 67. **c.** Scoline 68. **a.** Meprobamate 69. **b.** Gabapentin

- Sulfasalazine (used to control inflammation associated with Crohn's disease, ulcerative colitis and rheumatoid arthritis)
- Triamterene (a diuretic)
- Oral contraceptives

70. DOC for delirium tremens:

a. Haloperidol b. Chlorpromazine
c. Diazepam d. Morphine

Delirium tremens due to alcohol withdrawal can be treated with benzodiazepines. High doses may be necessary to prevent death. Pharmacotherapy is symptomatic and supportive. Typically the person is kept sedated with benzodiazepines, such as chlordiazepoxide (DOC for delirium tremens), diazepam, lorazepam, or oxazepam. In some cases, antipsychotics, such as haloperidol may also be used. Older drugs such as paraldehyde and clomethiazole were formerly the traditional treatment but have now largely been superseded by the benzodiazepines.

71. Which of the following does NOT bind to GABA receptor chloride channels:

a. Ethanol
b. Alphaxalone
c. Zolpidem
d. Buspirone

Buspirone functions as a serotonin 5-HT_{1A} receptor partial agonist (IA = 0.465). It is the action that is thought to mediate its anxiolytic and antidepressant effects. Additionally, it functions as a presynaptic dopamine antagonist at the D_2, D_3 and D_4 receptors. Buspirone is also a partial α_1 receptor agonist.

Drugs affecting $GABA_A$-receptor gated chloride channel.	
• GABA	: Endogenous agonist at $GABA_A$ receptor → promotes Cl^- influx
• Muscimol	: Agonist at GAB_{AA} site
• Bicuculline	: Competitive antagonist at $GABA_A$ receptor
• Picrotoxin	: Blocks Cl^- channel noncompetitively; acts on picrotoxin sensitive site
• Barbiturates	: Agonist at an allosteric site; prolong GABA action; and open Cl^- channel
• Alcohol, inhalational • anaesthetics, propofol	: Open Cl^- channel directly; allosteric facilitation of GABA
• Benzodiazepines	: Agonist at an allosteric BZD site → facilitate GABA action
• β-Carboline (DMCM)	: Inverse agonist at BZD site → impede GABA action
• Flumazenil	: Competitive antagonist at BZD site

72. Treatment of choice for myoclonic jerks and absence seizures:

a. Carbamazepine
b. Phenytoin
c. Valproate
d. Ethosuximide

Valproate (**VPA**), also known **valproic acid**, **sodium valproate**, and **divalproex sodium**, is a medication primarily used to treat epilepsy and bipolar disorder and to prevent migraine headaches. It is useful for the prevention of seizures in those with absence seizures, partial seizures, and generalized seizures. It can be given intravenously or by mouth.

Choice of antiseizure drugs.

Type of seizure	*First choice drugs*	*Second choice drugs*	*Alternative/Add-on drugs*
1. Generalised tonic-clonic/simple partial with or without generalization	Carbamazepine, Phenytoin	Valproate, Phenobarbitone	Lamotrigine, Gabapentin, Topiramate, Primidone, Levetiracetam
2. Complex partial with or without generalization	Carbamazepine, Valproate, Phenytoin,	Gabapentin, Lamotrigine, Levetiracetam	Clobazam, Zonisamide, Topiramate
3. Absence	Valproate	Ethosuximide, Lamotrigine	Clobazam, Clonazepam
4. Myoclonic	Valproate	Lamotrigine, Topiramate	Levetiracetam, Clonazepam
5. Atonic	Valproate	Clonazepam, Clobazam	Lamotrigine
6. Febrile seizures	Diazepam (rectal)	—	—
7. Status epilepticus	Lorazepam (i.v.), Diazepam (i.v.)	Fosphenytoin (i.v.) Phenobarbitone (i.v., i.m.)	Gen. anaesthetics

73. Drug which increase GABA level in brain:

a. Diazepam
b. Phenobarbitone
c. Sodium valproate
d. Carbamazepine

Although the mechanism of action of valproate is not fully understood, it has recently been shown to protect against a seizure-induced reduction in phosphatidylinositol (3,4,5)-trisphosphate (PIP3) as a potential therapeutic mechanism. In addition, its anticonvulsant effect has been attributed to the blockade of voltage-dependent sodium channels and increased brain levels of gamma-aminobutyric acid (GABA). The GABAergic effect is also believed to contribute towards the anti-manic properties of valproate.

Ans. 70. c. Diazepam 71. d. Buspirone 72. c. Valproate 73. c. Sodium valproate

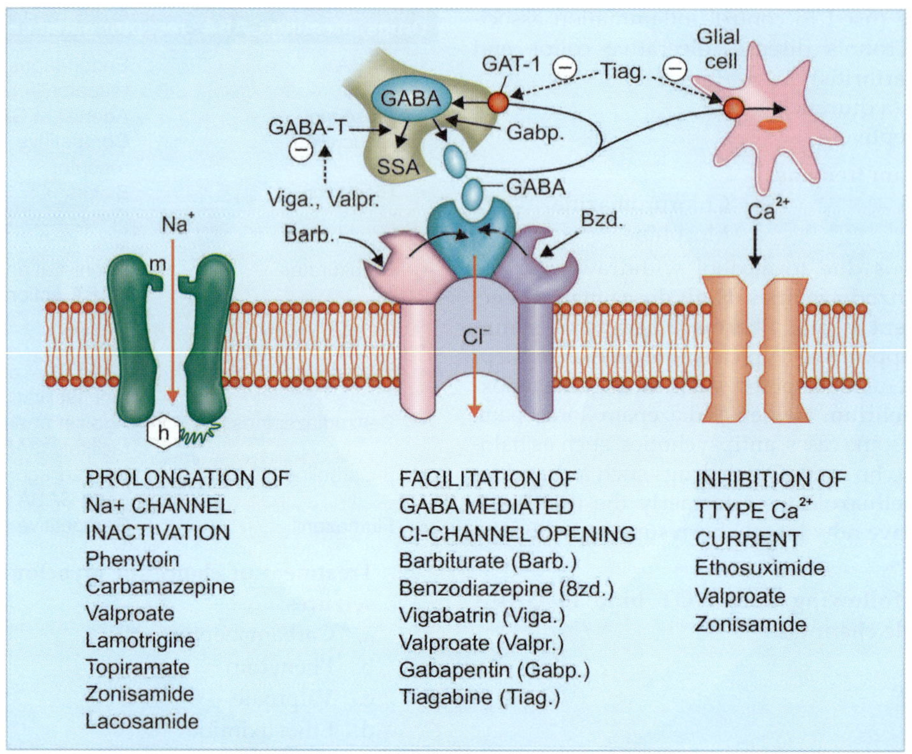

Major mechanisms of anticonvulsant action.
(m: Activation gate; h: Inactivation gate; GABA-T: GABA transaminase; SSA: Succinic semialdehyde; GAT-1: GABA transporter).

74. Vigabatrin is:
a. GABA agonist
b. GABA transaminase inhibitor
c. NMDA agonist
d. Dopa decarboxylase inhibitor

Vigabatrin, also known as gamma-vinyl-GABA, is an antiepileptic drug that inhibits the breakdown of γ-aminobutyric acid (GABA) by acting as a suicide inhibitor of GABA transaminase (GABA-T). It is a structural analog of GABA, but does not bind to GABA receptors.

75. Regarding phenytoin, all are true except:
a. Potent microsomal enzyme inducer
b. Highly protein bound
c. At lower concentration, it follows zero order kinetics
d. With increasing dose, the t1/2 increases

Phenytoin elimination kinetics show mixed-order behaviour at therapeutic concentrations. A small increase in dose may lead to a large increase in drug concentration as elimination becomes saturated. The time to reach steady state is often longer than 2 weeks.

76. Fetal hydantoin syndrome is caused by:
a. Phenytoin
b. Alcohol
c. Tetracycline
d. Sodium valproate

Phenytoin is a known teratogen. The syndrome consists of craniofacial anomalies (broad nasal bridge, cleft lip and palate, smaller than normal head) and a mild form of mental retardation (average IQ = 71). This syndrome resembles the well-described Fetal Alcohol Syndrome and has also been called the "fetal hydantoin syndrome".

77. DOC for drug-induced parkinsonism:
a. Levodopa
b. Benzhexol
c. Amantadine
d. Carbidopa

Trihexyphenidyl is used for the symptomatic treatment of Parkinson's disease in mono- and combination therapy. It is active in postencephalitic, arteriosclerotic, and idiopathic forms. The drug is also commonly used to treat extrapyramidal side effects occurring during antipsychotic treatment. It reduces the frequency and duration of oculogyric crises as well as of dyskinetic movements and spastic contractions. Excessive salivation may also respond. Trihexyphenidyl may improve psychotic depression and mental inertia frequently associated with Parkinson's disease and symptomatic problems caused by antipsychotic treatment.

78. L-dopa is combined with carbidopa in the treatment of parkinsonism due to:
a. Decrease the efficacy of levodopa
b. Inhibit peripheral decarboxylation of levodopa
c. Increase the dose of levodopa required
d. Inhibit conversion of levodopa to dopamine in the CNS

Ans. 74. **b.** GABA... 75. **c.** At lower concent... 76. **a.** Phenytoin 77. **b.** Benzhexol 78. **b.** Inhibit peripheral...

Levodopa is converted to dopamine via the action of a naturally occurring enzyme called DOPA decarboxylase. This occurs both in the peripheral circulation and in the central nervous system after levodopa has crossed the blood brain barrier. Activation of central dopamine receptors improves the symptoms of Parkinson's disease; however, activation of peripheral dopamine receptors causes nausea and vomiting. For this reason, levodopa is usually administered in combination with a DOPA decarboxylase inhibitor (DDCI), in this case carbidopa, which is very polar (and charged at physiologic pH) and cannot cross the blood brain barrier, however prevents peripheral conversion of levodopa to dopamine and thereby reduces the unwanted peripheral side effects of levodopa. Use of carbidopa also increases the quantity of levodopa in the bloodstream that is available to enter the brain.

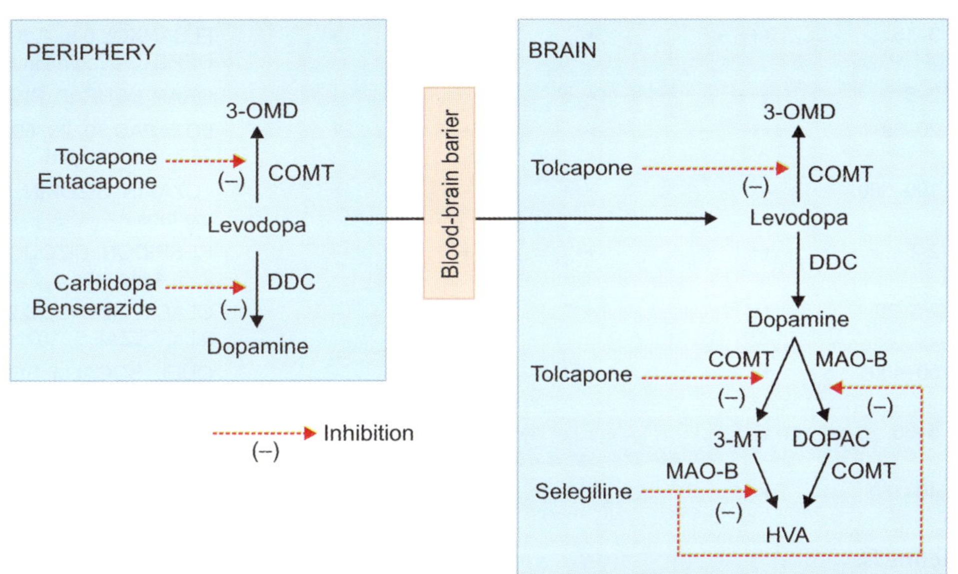

Metabolic pathways of levodopa in the periphery and the brain. (3-OMD: 3-O-methyldopa; COMT: Catechol-O-methyl transferase; MAO: monoamine oxidase; 3-MT: 3-methoxytyramine; DOPAC: 3,4 dihydroxy phenylacetic acid; HVA: Homovanillic acid (3-methoxy-4-hydroxy phenylacetic acid); DDC: Dopa decarboxylase).

79. FALSE statement regarding clozapine:

a. Used in resistant schizophrenia
b. Can cause agranulocytosis
c. Decrease on and off effect
d. Has maximum extra-pyramidal effects

Clozapine may cause side effects. Some are serious and potentially fatal. Common side effects include constipation, bed-wetting, night-time drooling, muscle stiffness, sedation, tremors, orthostatic hypotension, hyperglycemia, and weight gain. The risk of developing extrapyramidal symptoms such as tardive dyskinesia is below that of typical antipsychotics; this may be due to clozapine's anticholinergic effects. Extrapyramidal symptoms may subside somewhat after a person switches from another antipsychotic to clozapine.

Comparative properties and preparations of antipsychotic drugs

Drug	Antipsychotic dose (mg/day)	Relative activity: Extrapyramidal	Sedative	Hypotensive	Antiemetic	Preparations
1. Chlorpromazine	100–800	++	+++	++	++	CHLORPROMAZINE, LARGACTIL 10, 25, 50, 100 mg tab. 5 mg/5 ml (pediatric) & 25 mg/5 ml (adult) Syr., 50 mg/2 ml inj.
2. Triflupromazine	50–200	++±	+++	++	+++	SIQUIL 10 mg tab; 10 mg/ml inj.
3. Thioridazine	100–400	+	+++	+++	±	MELLERIL 25, 100 mg tab, THIORIL 10, 25, 50, 100 mg tab.
4. Trifluoperazine	2–20	+++	+	+	+++	TRINICALM 1, 5 mg tab, NEOCALM 5, 10 mg tab

Contd...

Ans. 79. **d.** Has maximum...

Contd...

Drug	Antipsychotic dose (mg/day)	Relative activity				Preparations
		Extrapyramidal	Sedative	Hypotensive	Antiemetic	
5. Fluphenazine	1–10	+++	+	+	+++	ANATENSOL 1 mg tab, 0.5 mg/ml elixir.
6. Haloperidol	2–20	+++	+	+	+++	SERENACE 1.5, 5, 10, 20 mg tab; 2 mg/ml liq, 5 mg/ml inj., SENORM 1.5, 5, 10 mg tab, 5 mg/ml inj., HALOPIDOL 2, 5, 10, 20 mg tab, 2 mg/ml liq, 10 mg/ml drops
7. Trifluperidol	1–8	+++	+	+	+++	TRIPERIDOL 0.5 mg tab, 2.5 mg/ml inj.
8. Flupenthixol	3–15	+++	+	+	+	FLUANXOL 0.5, 1, 3 mg tab; FLUANXOL DEPOT 20 mg/ml in 1 and 2 ml amp.
9. Pimozide	2–6	+++	+	+	+	ORAP, NEURAP, PIMODAC 2, 4 mg tab.
10. Loxapine	20–50	++	+	++	+	LOXAPAC 10, 25, 50 mg caps, 25 mg/ 5 ml liquid
11. Clozapine	100–300	–	+++	+++	–	LOZAPIN, SIZOPIN, SKIZORIL 25, 100 mg tabs
12. Risperidone	2–8	++	++	++	–	RESPIDON, SIZODON, RISPERDAL 1, 2, 3, 4 mg tabs.
13. Olanzapine	2.5–20	+	+	++	–	OLACE, OLANDUS 2.5, 5, 7.5, 10 mg tabs, OLZAP 5, 10 mg tab
14. Quetiapine	50–400	±	+++	++	–	QUEL, SOCALM, SEROQUIN 25, 100, 200 mg tabs
15. Aripiprazole	5–30	±	±	±	–	ARIPRA, ARILAN, BILIEF 10, 15 mg tabs; ARIVE 10, 15, 20, 30 mg tabs.
16. Ziprasidone	40–160	+	+	+	–	AZONA, ZIPSYDON 20, 40, 80 mg tabs.

80. MOA of fluoxetine is:

a. Serotonin uptake inhibition
b. Serotonin uptake facilitation
c. Dopamine synthesis inhibition
d. Adrenaline synthesis inhibition

Fluoxetine, among others, is an antidepressant of the selective serotonin reuptake inhibitor (SSRI) class. It is used for the treatment of major depressive disorder, obsessive–compulsive disorder, bulimia nervosa, panic disorder, and premenstrual dysphoric disorder. It may decrease the risk of suicide in those over the age of 65. Fluoxetine has also been used to treat premature ejaculation. It is taken by mouth.

Comparative properties and preparations of tricyclic and related antidepressants.

Drug	Sedation	Anti-muscarinic	Hypotension	Cardiac arrhythmia	Seizure precipitation	Daily dose (mg)	Preparations
Tricyclic antidepressants (TCAs)							
1. Imipramine	+	++	++	+++	++	50–200	DEPSONIL, ANTIDEP 25 mg tab, 75 mg SR cap.
2. Amitriptyline	+++	+++	+++	+++	++	50–200	AMLINE, SAROTENA, TRYPTOMER, 10, 25, 75 mg tabs.
3. Trimipramine	+++	+++	++	+++	++	50–150	SURMONTIL 10, 25 mg tab.
4. Doxepin	+++	++	++	+++	++	50–150	SPECTRA, DOXIN, DOXETAR 10, 25, 75 mg tab/cap.
5. Clomipramine	++	+++	++	+++	+++	50–150	CLOFRANIL, 10, 25, 50 mg tab, 75 mg SR tab. CLONIL, ANAFRANIL 10, 25 mg tab.
6. Dothiepin (Dosulpin)	++	++	++	++	++	50–150	PROTHIADEN, DOTHIN 25, 75 mg tab.
7. Nortriptyline	+	++	+	++	+	50–150	SENSIVAL, PRIMOX 25 mg tab.
8. Amoxapine	+	+	++	++	++	100–300	DEMOLOX 50, 100 mg tab.

Contd...

Ans. 80. **a.** Serotonin...

Drug	Sedation	Anti-muscarinic	Hypotension	Cardiac arrhythmia	Seizure precipitation	Daily dose (mg)	Preparations
Selective serotonin reuptake inhibitors (SSRIs)							
1. Fluoxetine	±	—	—	—	±	20–40	FLUDAC 20 mg cap, 20 mg/5 ml susp. FLUNIL 10, 20 mg caps; FLUPAR, PRODAC 20 mg cap.
2. Fluvoxamine	±	—	—	—	—	50–200	FLUVOXIN 50, 100 mg tab.
3. Paroxetine	±	±	—	—	—	20–50	XET 10, 20, 30, 40 mg tabs.
4. Sertraline	±	—	—	—	—	50–150	SERENATA, SERLIN, SERTIL 50, 100 mg tabs.
5. Citalopram	—	—	—	—	—	20–40	CELICA 10, 20, 40 mg tabs.
6. Escitalopram	—	—	—	—	—	10–20	ESDEP, FELIZ-S 5, 10, 20 mg tabs.
Serotonin and noradrenaline reuptake inhibitors (SNRIs)							
1. Venlafaxine	—	—	—	±	—	75–150	VENLOR 25, 37.5, 75 mg tabs, VENIZ-XR 37.5, 75, 150 mg ER caps.
2. Duloxetine	—	—	—	—	—	30–80	DELOK, DULANE, DUZAC, 20, 30, 40 mg caps.
Atypical antidepressants							
1. Trazodone	+++	—	±	±	—	50–200	TRAZODAC 25, 50 mg tab, TRAZONIL, TRAZALON 25, 50, 100 mg tabs.
2. Mianserin	++	+	++	+	++	30–100	TETRADEP 10, 20, 30 mg tab, SERIDAC 10, 30 mg tab.
3. Bupropion	–, -	—	—	—	+++	150–300	SMOQUIT 150 mg tab.
4. Mirtazapine	+++	—	±	—	—	15–45	MIRT 15, 30, 45 mg tabs, MIRTAZ 15, 30 mg tab.

81. Pre-treatment evaluation for lithium therapy should include:

a. Fasting blood sugar b. Serum creatinine
c. LFT d. Platelet count

Lithium is handled by the kidney in much the same way as Na^+. Nearly 80% of the filtered Li^{2+} is reabsorbed in the proximal convoluted tubule. Renal clearance of lithium is 1/5th of creatinine clearance.

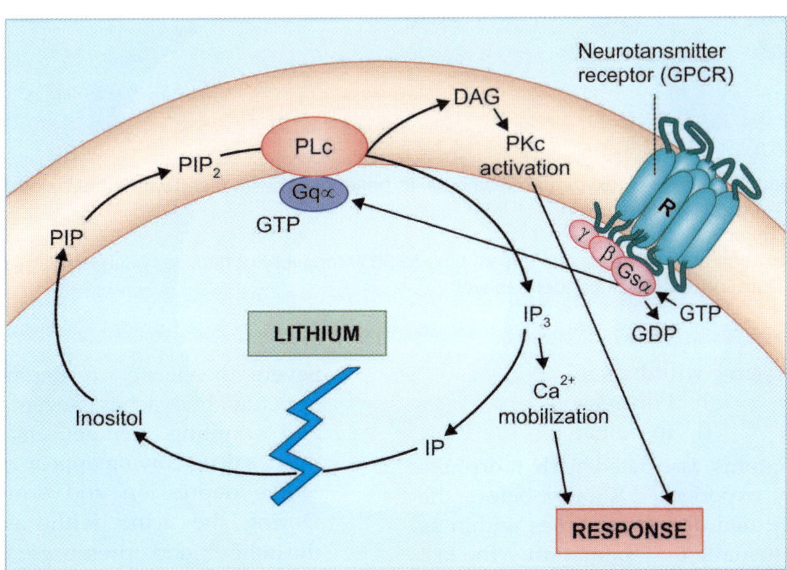

Proposed mechanism of antimanic action of lithium. (PIP: Phosphatidyl inositol phosphate; PIP_2: Phosphatidyl inositol bisphosphate; IP_3: Inositol trisphosphate; IP: Inositol-1-phosphate; PLc: Phospholipase C; DAG: Diacylglycerol; PKc: Protein Kinase C; Gq—Coupling Gq protein; R:Neurotransmitter receptor.

Ans. **81. b.** Serum creatinine

82. Drug of choice for Obsessive Compulsive Disorder:

a. Imipramine b. MAO inhibitor
c. Clonidine d. Fluoxetine

Treatment for OCD involves the use of behavioral therapy and sometimes selective serotonin reuptake inhibitors (SSRIs). The type of behavior therapy used involves increasing exposure to what causes the problems while not allowing the repetitive behavior to occur. Atypical antipsychotics such as quetiapine may be useful when used in addition to an SSRI in treatment-resistant cases but are associated with an increased risk of side effects.

83. FALSE statement regarding phenytoin is:

a. Is highly protein bound
b. Half life decreases with decreasing dose
c. Microsomal enzyme inducer
d. Follows zero order kinetics at lower doses

Phenytoin follows nonlinear (or zero-order) kinetics at therapeutic concentrations, because the rate of metabolism is close to the maximum capacity of the enzymes involved. In nonlinear kinetics, clearance and half-life fluctuate with plasma concentration. As the rate of administration increases, the plasma concentration at steady state increases disproportionately.

84. True about Imipramine:

a. Antiepileptic b. Antidepressant
c. Anxiolytic d. Antipsychotic

Imipramine, also known as **melipramine**, is a tricyclic antidepressant (TCA) of the dibenzazepine group. Imipramine is mainly used in the treatment of major depression and enuresis (inability to control urination).

85. Which of the following is short acting neuromuscular blocking agent:

a. Pancuronium b. Doxacurium
c. Mivacurium d. Vecuronium

Mivacurium chloride is a short-duration non-depolarizing neuromuscular-blocking drug or skeletal muscle relaxant in the category of non-depolarizing neuromuscular-blocking drugs, used adjunctively in anesthesia to facilitate endotracheal intubation and to provide skeletal muscle relaxation during surgery or mechanical ventilation.

Comparative properties of neuromuscular blocking drugs.

Drug	Dose£ (mg/kg)	Onset* (min)	Duration@ (min)	Hist. release	Gang. block	Vagal block
Long Acting						
1. d–Tubocurarine	0.2–0.4	4–6	30–60	+++	++	±
2. Pancuronium	0.04–0.1	4–6	60–120	±	±	+
3. Doxacurium	0.03–0.08	4–8	60–120	+	–	–
4. Pipecuronium	0.05–0.08		2–4 50–100	±	–	–
Intermediate Acting						
5. Vecuronium	0.08–0.1	2–4	30–60	±	–	±
6. Atracurium	0.3–0.6	2–4	20–40	+	–	–
7. Cisatracurium	0.15–0.2	3–6	20–40	–	–	–
8. Rocuronium	0.6–0.9	1–2	25–40	–	–	±
Short Acting						
9. Mivacurium	0.15–0.2	2–4	15–30	+	–	–
10. Succinylcholine	0.5–0.8	1–1.5	5–8	++	St.	St.

£Initial paralysing dose for opioid/nitrous oxide + oxygen anaesthesia. In patients anaesthetised with ether/halothane/isoflurane, the dose may be 1/3–1/2 of the figure given.
*Time to maximal block after i.v. injection.
@Duration of surgical grade relaxation after usual clinical doses; time to 95% recovery of muscle twitch is nearly double of the figure given (especially for long-acting drugs). Duration is dose dependent as well.
(St.: Stimulation).

86. NOT a feature of morphine withdrawal:

a. Constipation b. Piloerection
c. Rhinorrhea d. Insomnia

The withdrawal symptoms associated with morphine addiction are usually experienced shortly before the time of the next scheduled dose, sometimes within as early as a few hours (usually 6–12 hours) after the last administration. Early symptoms include watery eyes, insomnia, diarrhea, runny nose, yawning, dysphoria, sweating, and in some cases a strong drug craving. Severe headache, restlessness, irritability, loss of appetite, bodyaches, severe abdominal pain, nausea and vomiting, tremors, and even stronger and more intense drug craving appear as the syndrome progresses. Severe depression and vomiting are very common. During the acute withdrawal period, systolic and diastolic blood pressures increase, usually beyond premorphine levels, and heart rate increases, which have potential to cause a heart attack, blood clot, or stroke.

Ans. 82. **d.** Fluoxetine 83. **d.** Follows zero order... 84. **b.** Antidepressant 85. **c.** Mivacurium 86. **a.** Constipation

87. **Kaloo, a 43 years male on medication for psychiatric illness for the last 2 weeks, suddenly develops marked rigidity, immobility and fever, fluctuating BP and heart rate. Most likely diagnosis:**
   a. Akathisia b. Parkinsonism
   c. Malignant neuroleptic syndrome
   d. Catatonic schizophrenia

Neuroleptic malignant syndrome (**NMS**) is a life-threatening neurological disorder most often caused by an adverse reaction to neuroleptic or antipsychotic drugs. NMS typically consists of muscle rigidity, fever, autonomic instability, and cognitive changes such as delirium, and is associated with elevated plasma creatine phosphokinase.

88. **Drug of choice for petit mal seizures is:**
   a. Ethosuximide b. Carbamazepine
   c. Phenytoin d. Valproate

Absence seizures are sometimes referred to as **petit mal seizures** (from the French for "little illness", a term dating from the late 18th century). Absence seizures are characterized by a brief loss and return of consciousness, generally not followed by a period of lethargy (without a notable postictal state). Treatment of patients with absence seizures only is mainly with valproic acid or ethosuximide, which are of equal efficacy controlling absences in around 75% of patients.

89. **Malignant neuroleptic syndrome is caused by:**
   a. Antidepressants b. Anxiolytics
   c. Antipsychotics d. Antiepileptics

NMS is usually caused by antipsychotic drug use, and a wide range of drugs can result in NMS. Individuals using butyrophenones (such as haloperidol and droperidol) or phenothiazines (such as promethazine and chlorpromazine) are reported to be at greatest risk. However, various atypical antipsychotics such as clozapine, olanzapine, risperidone, quetiapine, and ziprasidone have also been implicated in cases.

90. **True regarding bupropion is:**
   a. Dopamine reuptake stimulator
   b. It is an antianxiety drug
   c. No precipitation of seizures
   d. Nicotinic receptor antagonist

Bupropion is known to affect several different biological targets, and its mechanism of action is only partly understood. It has been widely described in the literature as a norepinephrine-dopamine reuptake inhibitor (NDRI), and is also a nicotinic antagonist.

91. **Antidote for Restyl/Alprazolam is:**
   a. Protamine sulphate
   b. Flumazenil
   c. EDTA
   d. BAL

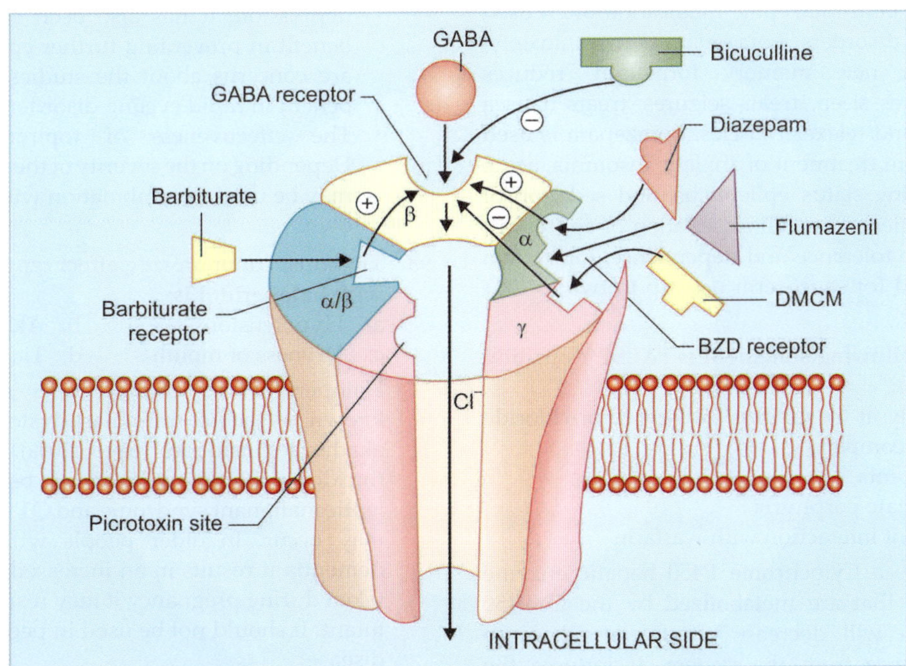

Schematic depiction of GABAA-benzodiazepine receptor-chloride channel complex.
The chloride channel is gated by the primary ligand GABA acting on $GABA_A$ receptor located on the β subunit. The benzodiazepine (BZD) receptor located on the interface of α and γ subunits modulates $GABA_A$ receptor in either direction: agonists like diazepam facilitate, while inverse agonists like DMCM hinder GABA mediated Cl^- channel opening, and BZD antagonist flumazenil blocks the action of both. The barbiturate receptor, located either on α or β subunit also facilitates GABA and is capable of opening Cl^- channel directly as well. Bicuculline blocks $GABA_A$ receptor, while picrotoxin blocks the Cl^- channel directly.

Ans. 87. **c.** Malignant... 88. **d.** Valproate 89. **c.** Antipsychotics 90. **d.** Nicotinic... 91. **b.** Flumazenil

Intravenous flumazenil is primarily used to treat benzodiazepine overdoses and to help reverse anesthesia. Administration of flumazenil by sublingual lozenge and topical cream has also been tested.

92. Treatment of choice in attention deficit hyperactivity disorder is:

a. Haloperidol b. Imipramine
c. Alprazolam d. Methylphenidate

Methylphenidate, among others, is a central nervous system (CNS) stimulant of the phenethylamine and piperidine classes that is used in the treatment of attention deficit hyperactivity disorder (ADHD) and narcolepsy.

93. Baclofen is used in:

a. Parkinsonism
b. Traumatic muscle spasm
c. Spasticity d. Stroke

Baclofen also known as **β-(4-chlorophenyl)-γ-aminobutyric acid** (**β-(4-chlorophenyl)-GABA**) is a central nervous system depressant used as a skeletal muscle relaxant. It is primarily used to treat spasticity.

94. Drug of choice for status epilepticus is:

a. Valproate
b. Phenytoin
c. Lorazepam
d. Carbamazepine

Lorazepam is a benzodiazepine medication often used to treat anxiety disorders. Lorazepam reduces anxiety, interferes with new memory formation, reduces agitation, induces sleep, treats seizures, treats nausea and vomiting, and relaxes muscles. Lorazepam is used for the short-term treatment of anxiety, insomnia, acute seizures including status epilepticus, and sedation of hospitalized patients, as well as sedation of aggressive patients. Due to tolerance and dependence, lorazepam is recommended for short-term use, up to two to four weeks only.

95. Which of the following statement is FALSE regarding phenobarbitone:

a. Act primarily at the GABA: BZD receptor-chloride ion channel complex
b. Crosses placenta
c. May precipitate porphyria
d. No significant interaction with warfarin

Phenobarbital is a Cytochrome P450 hepatic enzyme inducer. Drugs that are metabolized by the CYP450 enzyme system will decrease effectiveness because of faster clearance from the system. It induces the metabolism of warfarin. The dose of anticoagulant determined during therapy with these drugs would be higher: if the same is continued after withdrawing the inducer—marked hypoprothrombinemia can occur—fatal bleeding is on record.

96. Anti-psychotic drugs act through:

a. Dopamine D1 receptor blockade
b. Dopamine D2 receptor blockade
c. Dopamine D3 receptor blockade
d. Dopamine D4 receptor blockade

All antipsychotic drugs tend to block D_2 receptors in the dopamine pathways of the brain. This means that dopamine released in these pathways has less effect.

97. NOT of use in bipolar disorder:

a. Carbamazepine b. Phenytoin
c. Sodium valproate d. Lamotrigine

Four anticonvulsants are used in the treatment of bipolar disorder

- Carbamazepine effectively treats manic episodes, with some evidence it has greater benefit in rapid-cycling bipolar disorder, or those with more psychotic symptoms or a more schizoaffective clinical picture. It is less effective in preventing relapse than lithium or valproate. Carbamazepine became a popular treatment option for bipolar in the late 1980s and early 1990s, but was displaced by sodium valproate in the 1990s.
- Since then, valproate has become a commonly prescribed treatment, and is effective in treating manic episodes.
- Lamotrigine has some efficacy in treating bipolar depression, and this benefit is greatest in more severe depression. It has also been shown to have some benefit in preventing further episodes, though there are concerns about the studies done, and is of no benefit in rapid cycling disorder.
- The effectiveness of topiramate is unknown. Depending on the severity of the case, anticonvulsants may be used in combination with lithium or on their own.

98. The most common side effect reported with treatment with haloperidol is:

a. Hypotension b. Akathisia
c. Dryness of mouth d. Tic disorder

Haloperidol may result in a movement disorder known as acute muscular dystonia (incidence 2%), akathisia (incidence upto 20%), tardive dyskinesia (incidence 10-20%) which may be permanent. Neuroleptic malignant syndrome and QT interval prolongation may occur. In older people with psychosis due to dementia it results in an increased risk of death. When taken during pregnancy it may result in problems in the infant. It should not be used in people with Parkinson's disease.

99. Treatment of absence seizures:

a. Phenytoin b. Diazepam
c. Phenobarbitone d. Ethosuximide

Ethosuximide is a succinimide anticonvulsant, used mainly in absence seizures as an alternative to valproate.

Ans. 92. **d.** Methylphenidate 93. **c.** Spasticity 94. **c.** Lorazepam 95. **d.** No significant... 96. **b.** Dopamine D2... 97. **b.** Phenytoin 98. **b.** Akathisia 99. **d.** Ethosuximide

DRUGS ACTING ON GASTROINTESTINAL TRACT

100. Drug that does NOT interferes with antacids:

a. Tetracycline b. Norfloxacin
c. Azithromycin d. Ranitidine

By raising the gastric pH and forming complexes, the non-absorbable antacids decrease the absorption of many drugs, especially tetracyclines, iron salts, fluoroquinolones, ketoconazole, H_2 blockers, diazepam, phenothiazines, indomethacin, phenytoin, isoniazid, ethambutol and nitrofurantoin.

101. A prokinetic drug with no dopamine antagonism:

a. Chlorpromazine
b. Metaclopramide
c. Domperidone
d. Mosapride

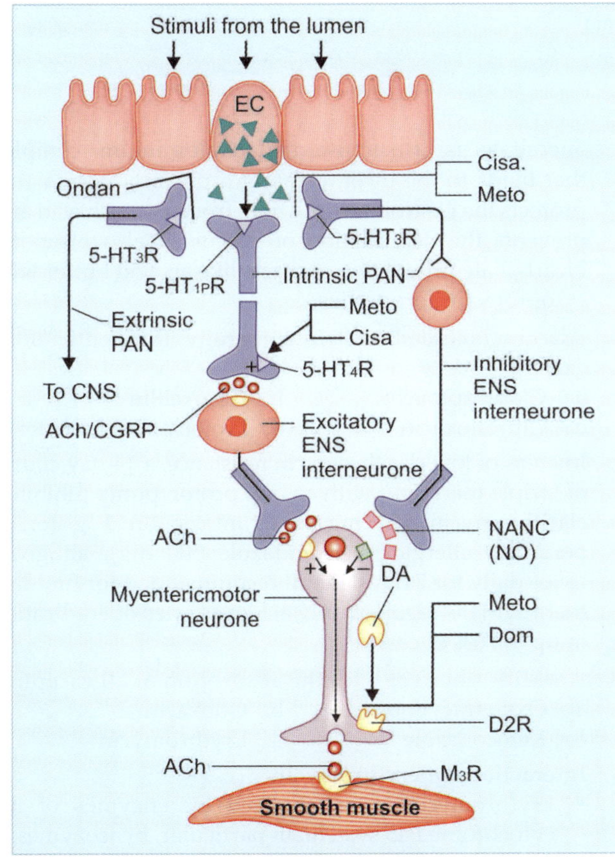

Schematic depiction of seronergic (5-HT) regulation of peristaltic reflex, and sites of action of prokinetic drugs.

Distention and other luminal stimuli trigger 5-HT release from the enterochromaffin cells (EC) located in the enteric mucosa. This stimulates intrinsic and extrinsic primary afferent neurones (PAN) of the enteric nervous system (ENS) through peripheral variant of 5-HT_1 receptor (5-HT_{1P}R) and 5-HT_3 receptor (5-HT3R). The extrinsic PANconvey impulses to the CNS via vagus and dorsal root ganglia and participate in the causation of vomiting when stimulation is strong. Ondansetron (Ondan) acts partly by blocking activation of extrinsic PAN through 5-HT_3R.

The intrinsic PAN interact with excitatory and inhibitory interneurons of the ENS to mediate both contraction (of proximal gut muscles) and relaxation (of distal gut muscles) to coordinate the peristaltic reflex, respectively through release of acetylcholine (ACh)/calcitonin gene related peptide (CGRP) and nonadrenergic–noncholinergic (NANC) transmitter, which mainly is nitric oxide (NO). Cisapride (Cisa.) and metoclopramide (Meto.) activate the prejunctional 5-HT_4 receptors (5-HT_4R) located on the terminals of the intrinsic PAN and promote ACh/CGRP release, and thereby the contractile activity. The weak 5-HT_3 blocking action of Cisa. and Meto., in addition, reduces activity in the inhibitory interneurone (minor action).

Domperidone (Dom) and Meto also block the action of dopamine (DA) on prejunctional D2 receptor (D2R) which normally inhibits ACh release from the myenteric motor neurone, and thus augment smooth muscle contraction elicited through muscarinic M_3 receptor (M_3R).

Mosapride is a gastroprokinetic agent that acts as a selective $5HT_4$ agonist. The major active metabolite of mosapride, known as M1, additionally acts as a $5HT_3$ antagonist. Which accelerates gastric emptying throughout the whole of the gastrointestinal tract in humans, and is used for the treatment of gastritis, gastroesophageal reflux disease, functional dyspepsia and irritable bowel syndrome. It is recommended to be taken on an empty stomach (i.e. at least one hour before food or two hours after food).

102. Treatment for Zollinger-ellison syndrome is:

a. Cimetidine b. Omeprazole
c. Misoprostol d. Aluminium hydroxide

Treatment of ZES can involve surgery or proton pump inhibitors.

103. True about concentration of Oral Rehydration Solution is:

a. Sodium 70 mEq/lit
b. Potassium 20 mEq/lit
c. Bicarbonate 80 mEq/lit
d. Chloride 30 mEq/lit

ReSoMal (Rehydration solution for severely malnourished children) solution contains Sodium 90 mEq/L, 40 mEq/L Potassium and 3 mEq/ L of magnesium. The sodium content is half of the normal WHO-ORS and potassium content is double of the WHO-ORS and is specially designed for severely malnourished as they have high potassium deficit and do not have high sodium losses.

New formula WHO-ORS.

Content		Concentrations	
NaCl	: 2.6 g	Na^+	— 75 mM
KCl	: 1.5 g	K^+	— 20 mM
Trisod. citrate	: 2.9 g	Cl^-	— 65 mM
Glucose	: 13.5 g	Citrate	— 10 mM
Water	: 1 L	Glucose	— 75
Total osmolarity 245 mOsm/L			

(available as ORETRAL-A, ELECTROBION, ELECTRAL 21 g sachet for 1000 ml; WALYTE, RELYTE 4.2 g sachet for 200 ml).

Ans. 100. c. Azithromycin 101. d. Mosapride 102. b. Omeprazole 103. b. Potassium 20 mEq/lit

104. NOT a component of triple drug therapy for Helicobacter pylori:

a. Lansoprazole b. Clarithromycin
c. Amoxicillin d. Cimetidine

The regimen most commonly recommended for first line treatment of *H. pylori* is triple therapy with a PPI (lansoprazole 30 mg twice daily, omeprazole 20 mg twice daily, pantoprazole 40 mg twice daily, rabeprazole 20 mg twice daily, or esomeprazole 40 mg once daily), amoxicillin (1 g twice daily), and clarithromycin (500 mg twice daily) for 7 days.

Anti-H. pylori Regimens*.

Proton pump inhibitor	*Amoxicillin*	*Clarithromycin*	*Metronidazole/Tinidazole*
One week-twice daily			
Omeprazole (20 mg) or	1.0 g	500 mg	—
Esomeprazole (20 mg) or	—	250 mg	400 mg/500 mg
Lansoprazole (30 mg) or	1.0 g	—	400 mg/500 mg
Pantoprazole (40 mg) or			
Rabeprazole (20 mg)			
Two weeks—twice daily			
Omeprazole (20 mg) or	750 mg	—	400 mg/500 mg
Lansoprazole (30 mg) or	—	250 mg	400 mg/500 mg
Pantoprazole (40 mg)	750 mg	500 mg	—

*Adopted from British National Formulary (BNF) Sept. 2010

105. M1 blocker used in peptic ulcer treatment:

a. Probanthine b. Atropine
c. Pyridostigmine d. Pirenzepine

Pirenzepine (**Gastrozepin**), an M_1 selective antagonist, is used in the treatment of peptic ulcers, as it reduces gastric acid secretion and reduces muscle spasm. It is in a class of drugs known as muscarinic receptor antagonists-acetylcholine being the neurotransmitter of the parasympathetic nervous system which initiates the rest-and-digest state (as opposed to fight-or-flight), the result being an increase in gastric motility and digestion. It has no effects on the brain and spinal cord as it cannot diffuse through the blood–brain barrier.

106. NOT an antacid drug:

a. Aluminium hydroxide b. Magnesium sulphate
c. Sodium bicarbonate d. Calcium carbonate

Magnesium salts used as non-systemic antacids are magnesium hydroxide (milk of magnesia) and magnesium trisilicate.

107. Sulfasalazine is used in:

a. Gout b. Irritable bowel disease
c. Ulcerative colitis d. Idiopathic osteoarthritis

Sulfasalazine is used in the treatment of inflammatory bowel disease, including ulcerative colitis and Crohn's disease. It is also indicated for use in rheumatoid arthritis and used in other types of inflammatory arthritis (e.g. psoriatic arthritis) where it has a beneficial effect. It is often well tolerated compared to other DMARDs.

108. Which of the following does NOT change pH of stomach:

a. Sucralfate b. H_2 blocker
c. Omeprazole d. Ranitidine

Sucralfate is a sucrose sulfate-aluminium complex that binds to the ulcer, creating a physical barrier that protects the gastrointestinal tract from stomach acid and prevents the degradation of mucus. It also promotes bicarbonate production and acts like an acid buffer with cytoprotective properties.

109. All are included in triple therapy for peptic ulcer except:

a. Clarithromycin b. Amoxcillin
c. Ciprofloxacin d. Proton pump inhibitor

In areas of low clarithromycin resistance, a 14-day course of "triple therapy, " with an oral proton pump inhibitor, clarithromycin 500 mg, and amoxicillin 1 g (or, if penicillin allergic, metronidazole 500 mg), all given twice daily for 7 days, is still recommended for first-line therapy. This regimen only achieves rates of eradication in up to 70% of cases.

110. Antacids interfere with the absorption of all except:

a. Oxytetracyline b. Ofloxacin
c. Ketoconazole d. Erythromycin

Interactions of erythromycin

- Erythromycin is metabolized by enzymes of the cytochrome P45 system, in particular, by isozymes of the CYP3A superfamily, CYP3A.
- The activity of the CYP3A enzymes can be induced or inhibited by certain drugs (e.g. dexamethasone) which can cause it to affect the metabolism of many different drugs, e.g. erythromycin. If other CYP3A substrates — drugs that are broken down by CYP3A — such as simvastatin, lovastatin, or atorvastatin— are taken concomitantly with erythromycin, levels of the substrates increase, often causing adverse effects.

Ans. **104. d.** Cimetidine **105. d.** Pirenzepine **106. b.** Magnesium... **107. c.** Ulcerative colitis
108. a. Sucralfate **109. c.** Ciprofloxacin **110. d.** Erythromycin

- A noted drug interaction involves erythromycin and simvastatin, resulting in increased simvastatin levels and the potential for rhabdomyolysis.
- Another group of CYP3A4 substrates are drugs used for migraine such as ergotamine and dihydroergotamine; their adverse effects may be more pronounced if erythromycin is associated.
- There is a link between erythromycin, ventricular tachycardia, and sudden cardiac death in patients also taking drugs that prolong the metabolism of erythromycin (like verapamil or diltiazem) by interfering with CYP3A4.
- Hence, erythromycin should not be administered to people using these drugs, or drugs that also prolong the QT interval. Other examples include terfenadine, astemizole, cisapride (withdrawn in many countries for prolonging the QT time) and pimozide.
- Theophylline, which is used mostly in asthma, is also contraindicated.

111. Proton pump inhibitors suppress gastric acid secretion by:

a. H^+/Cl^- ATPase pump
b. H^+/K^+ ATPase pump
c. Na^+/K^+ ATPase pump
d. $Na^+/K^+/Cl^-$ ATPase pump

Proton pump inhibitors act by irreversibly blocking the hydrogen/potassium adenosine triphosphatase enzyme system (the H^+/K^+ ATPase, or, more commonly, the gastric proton pump) of the gastric parietal cells. The proton pump is the terminal stage in gastric acid secretion, being directly responsible for secreting H^+ ions into the gastric lumen, making it an ideal target for inhibiting acid secretion.

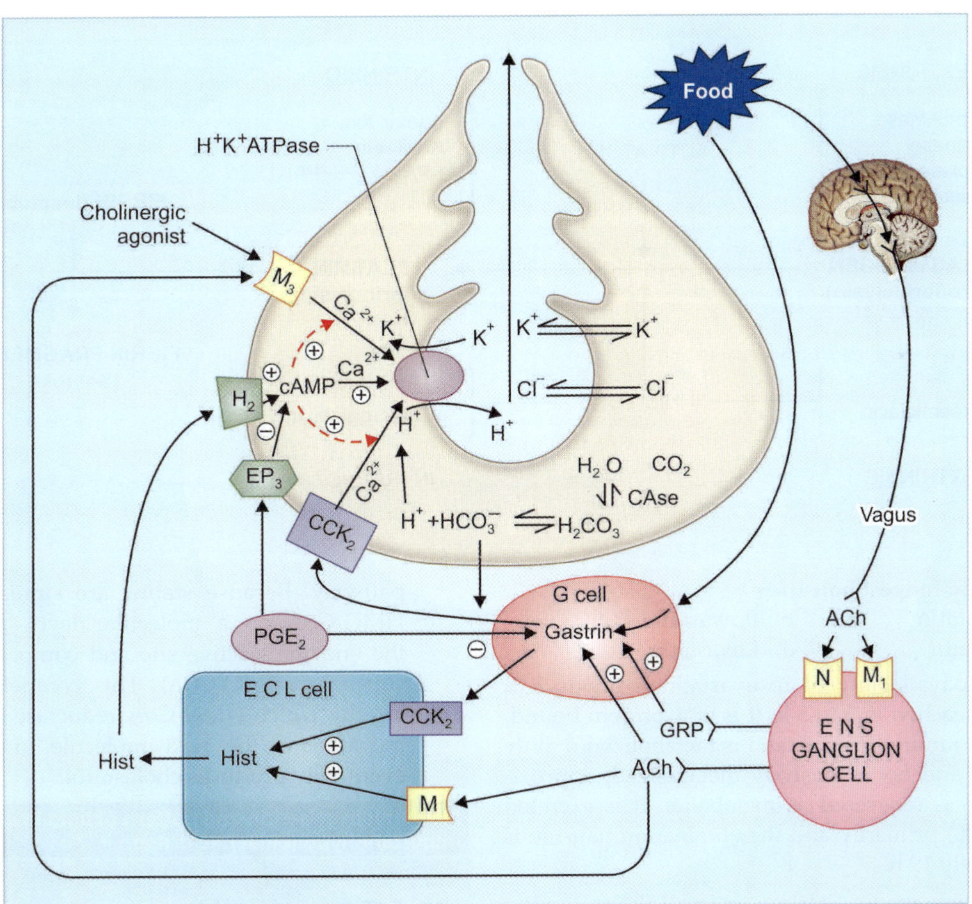

Secretion of HCl by gastric parietal cell and its regulation.
C.Ase.: Carbonic anhydrase; Hist.: Histamine; ACh.: Acetylcholine; CCK_2: Gastrin cholecystokinin receptor; M.: Muscarinic receptor; N: Nicotinic receptor; H_2: Histamine H_2 receptor; EP_3: Prostaglandin receptor; ENS: Enteric nervous system; ECL cell: Enterochromaffin-like cell; GRP: Gastrin releasing peptide; +: Stimulation; –: Inhibition.

112. Prokinetic drug WITHOUT D2 blockade is:

a. Metoclopramide
b. Cisapride
c. Domperidone
d. Chlorpromazine

Cisapride is a gastroprokinetic agent, a drug that increases motility in the upper gastrointestinal tract. It acts directly as a serotonin 5-HT_4 receptor agonist and

Ans. **111. b.** H^+/K^+ ATPase... **112. b.** Cisapride indirectly as a parasympathomimetic. Stimulation of the serotonin receptors increases acetylcholine release in the enteric nervous system.

113. Drug of choice for NSAID-induced gastric ulcer:

a. Proton pump inhibitor b. PGE2
c. Antacids d. H2 antagonists

Commonly, gastric (but not necessarily intestinal) adverse effects of NSAIDs can be reduced through suppressing acid production, by concomitant use of a proton pump inhibitor, e.g. omeprazole, esomeprazole; or the prostaglandin analogue misoprostol. Misoprostol is itself associated with a high incidence of gastrointestinal ADRs (diarrhea).

114. Drugs indicated in drug–induced vomiting are all except:

a. Metoclopramide b. Hyoscine butylbromide
c. Ondansetron d. Chlorpromazine

Hyoscine butylbromide, also known as **scopolamine butylbromide** and sold under the brandname **Buscopan**, is a medication used to treat crampy abdominal pain, renal colic, and bladder spasms. It is also used to improve a death rattle at the end of life.

DRUGS ACTING ON HAEMTOPOIETIC SYSTEM

115. All are anti-platelet drugs EXCEPT:

a. Aspirin
b. Clopidogrel
c. Tranexamic acid
d. Abciximab

Tranexamic acid is an antifibrinolytic that competitively inhibits the activation of plasminogen to plasmin, by binding to specific sites of both plasminogen and plasmin, a molecule responsible for the degradation of fibrin, a protein that forms the framework of blood clots.

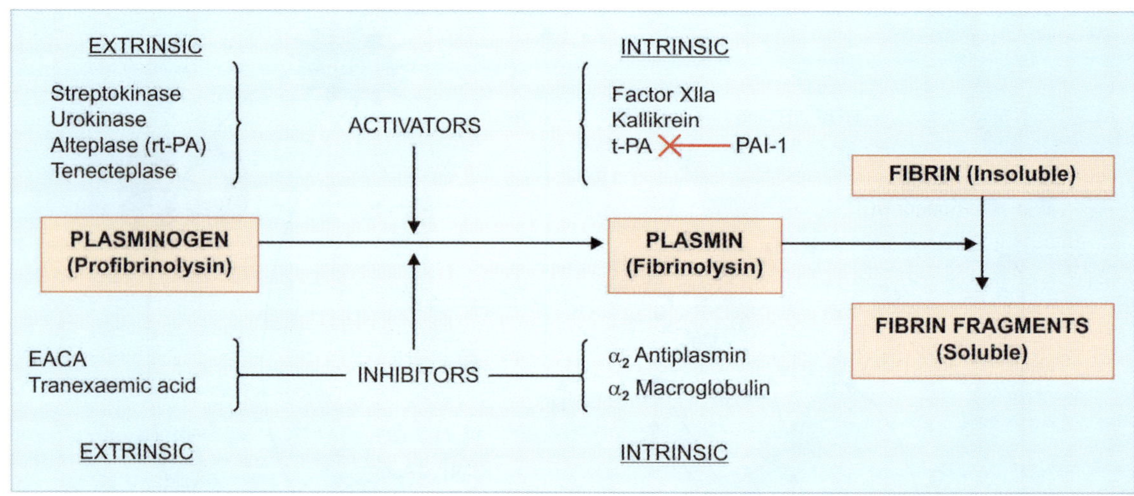

Th

116. Statin having longest half life:

a. Rosuvastatin b. Pravastatin
c. Simvastatin d. Lovastatin

Absolute bioavailability of rosuvastatin is about 20% and C_{max} is reached in 3 to 5 h. It is 88% protein bound, mainly to albumin. Rosuvastatin is metabolized mainly by CYP2C9 and not extensively metabolized; approximately, 10% is recovered as metabolite. It is excreted in feces (90%) primarily and the elimination half-life is approximately 19 h.

117. Lipid lowering agents, Statins, act in all the following ways, except:

a. Decreased hepatic cholesterol synthesis
b. Decreased LDL receptors
c. Inhibiting HMG CoA reductase
d. Decreasing VLDL

Statins act by competitively inhibiting HMG-CoA reductase, the first committed enzyme of the mevalonate pathway. Because statins are similar in structure to HMG-CoA on a molecular level, they will fit into the enzyme's active site and compete with the native substrate (HMG-CoA). This competition reduces the rate by which HMG-CoA reductase is able to produce mevalonate, the next molecule in the cascade that eventually produces cholesterol.

Mechanism of action and pattern of lipid lowering effect of important hypolipidaemic drugs.

Drug (daily dose)	*Mechanism of action*	*Effect on lipids (%)*
HMG-CoA reductase inhibitors		
Lovastatin (10–80 mg)	↓ CH synthesis by inhibition of rate	LDL ↓ 20–55
Simvastatin (5–40 mg)	limiting HMG-CoA reductase	HDL ↑ 5–15
Atorvastatin (10–80 mg)		TG ↓ 10–35
Rosuvastatin (5–20 mg)		

Contd...

Ans. 113. a. Proton pump... **114. b.** Hyoscine... **115. c.** Tranexamic acid **116. a.** Rosuvastatin **117. b.** Decreased LDL...

Contd...

Drug (daily dose)	*Mechanism of action*	*Effect on lipids (%)*
Bile acid sequestrants		
Cholestyramine (4–16 g) Colestipol (5–30 g)	↓ bile acid absorption, ↑ hepatic conversion of CH to bile acids, ↑ LDL receptors on hepatocytes	LDL ↓ 15–30 HDL ↑ 3–5 TG not affected, may ↑ in some
Fibric acid derivatives		
Gemfibrozil (1200 mg)	↑ Activity of lipoprotein lipase,	LDL ↓ 5–20*
Bezafibrate (600 mg)	↓ release of fatty acids from adipose tissue	HDL ↑ 10–20
Fenofibrate (200 mg)		TG ↓ 20–50
Nicotinic acid (2–6 g)	↓ Production of VLDL, ↓ lipolysis in adipocytes	LDL ↓ 15–25 HDL ↑ 20–35 TG ↓ 20–50

*Gemfibrozil may ↑ LDL-CH when TG levels are high; bezafibrate and fenofibrate not likely to raise LDL-CH

118. Warfarin acts by inhibiting all of the following factors except:

a. Factor III b. Factor VII
c. Factor IX d. Factor X

Warfarin inhibits the vitamin K-dependent synthesis of biologically active forms of the calcium-dependent clotting factors II, VII, IX and X, as well as the regulatory factors protein C, protein S, and protein Z. Other proteins not involved in blood clotting, such as osteocalcin, or matrix Gla protein, may also be affected.

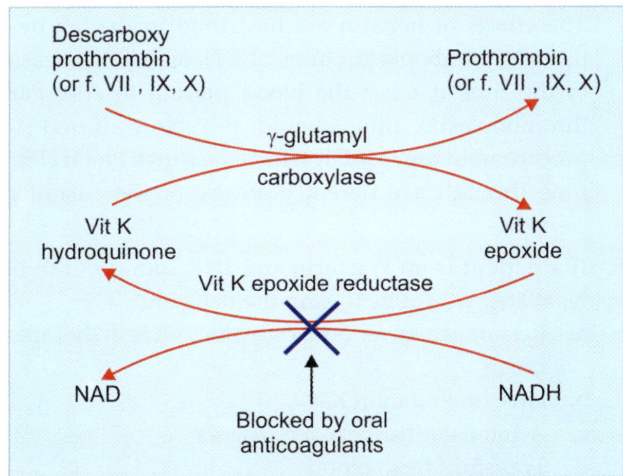

Mechanism of action of oral anticoagulants.
NAD: Nicotinamide adenine dinucleotide; NADH: its reduced form.

119. Warfarin effect is enhanced by:

a. Phenobarbitone b. Ketoconazole
c. Rifampicin d. Chronic alcoholism

Excessive use of alcohol is also known to affect the metabolism of warfarin and can elevate the INR and thus increase the risk of bleeding. Many commonly used antibiotics, such as metronidazole or the macrolides, will greatly increase the effect of warfarin by reducing the metabolism of warfarin in the body. Other broad-spectrum antibiotics can reduce the amount of the normal bacterial flora in the bowel, which make significant quantities of vitamin K_1, thus potentiating the effect of warfarin.

120. Drug which inhibits aggregation of platelets:

a. Tranexamic acid b. EACA
c. Aprotinin d. Aspirin

Low-dose aspirin use irreversibly blocks the formation of thromboxane A_2 in platelets, producing an inhibitory effect on platelet aggregation during the lifetime of the affected platelet (8–9 days). This antithrombotic property makes aspirin useful for reducing the incidence of heart attacks.

Antiplatelet Drugs.	
Aspirin *Dipyridamole*	
$P2Y_{12}$ Receptor Blockers	*$GPII_b/III_a$ Antagonists*
Ticlopidine	Abciximab
Clopidogrel	Eptifibatide
Prasugrel	Tirofiban

121. Anticoagulants are indicated in all of the following conditions except:

a. Pulmonary embolism b. DVT
c. Pericarditis d. Myocardial infarction

The treatment in viral or idiopathic pericarditis is with aspirin, or non-steroidal anti-inflammatory drugs (NSAIDs such as ibuprofen). Colchicine may be added to the above as it decreases the risk of further episodes of pericarditis.

122. Aspirin in very low doses inhibits the formation of:

a. Cyclo-oxygenase 1 b. Thromboxane A2
c. Prostaglandin I2 d. None of the above

Aspirin's ability to suppress the production of prostaglandins and thromboxanes is due to its irreversible inactivation of the cyclooxygenase (COX; officially known as prostaglandin-endoperoxide synthase, PTGS) enzyme required for prostaglandin and thromboxane synthesis. It is possible that at low doses (75-150 mg/day or 300 mg twice weekly), TXA_2 formation by platelets is suppressed, whereas higher doses (>900 mg/day) may decrease both TXA_2 and PGI_2 production.

123. Aspirin is CONTRAINDICATED in patients on:

a. Oral contraceptives
b. Theophylline
c. Warfarin
d. Prednisolone

Ans. **118. a.** Factor III **119. d.** Chronic alcoholism **120. d.** Aspirin **121. c.** Pericarditis **122. b.** Thromboxane... **123. c.** Warfarin

Aspirin is known to interact with other drugs. For example, acetazolamide and ammonium chloride are known to enhance the intoxicating effect of salicylates, and alcohol, and also increases the gastrointestinal bleeding associated with these types of drugs. Aspirin is known to displace a number of drugs from protein-binding sites in the blood, including the antidiabetic drugs tolbutamide and chlorpropamide, warfarin, methotrexate, phenytoin, probenecid, valproic acid (as well as interfering with beta oxidation, an important part of valproate metabolism), and other NSAIDs. Corticosteroids may also reduce the concentration of aspirin. Ibuprofen can negate the antiplatelet effect of aspirin used for cardioprotection and stroke prevention. The pharmacological activity of spironolactone may be reduced by taking aspirin, and it is known to compete with penicillin G for renal tubular secretion. Aspirin may also inhibit the absorption of vitamin C.

124. Aspirin is used for secondary prevention of IHD because:

a. It inhibits TXA2 synthesis by platelets
b. Inhibit prostacyclin synthesis
c. Inhibits release of EDRF
d. Inhibit synthesis of endothelium

Low-dose aspirin use irreversibly blocks the formation of thromboxane A_2 in platelets, producing an inhibitory effect on platelet aggregation during the lifetime of the affected platelet (8–9 days). This antithrombotic property makes aspirin useful for reducing the incidence of heart attacks.

125. A direct thrombin inhibitor:

a. Argatroban
b. Fondaparinux
c. Dalteparin
d. Enoxaparin

Argatroban is an anticoagulant that is a small molecule direct thrombin inhibitor. In 2000, argatroban was licensed by the Food and Drug Administration (FDA) for prophylaxis or treatment of thrombosis in patients with heparin-induced thrombocytopenia (HIT). In 2002, it was approved for use during percutaneous coronary interventions in patients who have HIT or are at risk for developing it.

126. Anticoagulant of choice for prophylaxis of pulmonary thromboembolism is:

a. Heparin sulfate
b. Protamine sulfate
c. Low molecular weight heparin
d. Warfarin

Low-molecular-weight heparin (LMWH) is a class of anticoagulant medications. They are used in the prevention and treatment of venous thromboembolism (deep vein thrombosis and pulmonary embolism) and in the treatment of myocardial infarction.

Some comparative aspects of heparin and oral anticoagulants

	Heparin	*Warfarin*
1. Chemistry	Mucopolysaccharide	Coumarin derivative
2. Source	Hog lung, pig intestine	Synthetic
3. Route of admin	Parenteral (i.v., s.c.)	Oral
4. Onset of action	Immediate	Delayed (1–3 days)
5. Duration of action	4–6 hrs	3–6 days
6. Activity	*In vitro* and *in vivo*	*In vivo* only
7. Mechanism	Blocks action of factor X and thrombin	Inhibits synthesis of clotting factors
8. Antagonist	Protamine sulphate	Vit K
9. Variability in response	Little	Marked
10. Lab. control	aPTT/clotting time (desirable)	Prothrombin time/ INR (essential)
11. Drug interactions	Few and not significant	Many and significant
12. Use	To initiate therapy	For maintenance

127. Parameter which should be tested before starting heparin therapy:

a. Serum bleeding time
b. Serum clotting time
c. Prothrombin time
d. Activated partial thromboplastin time

The effects of heparin are measured in the lab by the partial thromboplastin time (aPTT), one of the measures of the time it takes the blood plasma to clot. Partial thromboplastin time should not be confused with prothrombin time, or PT, which measures blood clotting time through a different pathway of the coagulation cascade.

128. If a patient is on Warfarin and INR comes out to be 8. Next step would be to stop the drug and:

a. Restart at a lower dose once the INR is in therapeutic range
b. Give oral vitamin K1
c. Administer fresh frozen plasma
d. Transfuse fresh blood

Warfarin and related 4-hydroxycoumarin-containing molecules decrease blood coagulation by inhibiting vitamin K epoxide reductase, an enzyme that recycles oxidized vitamin K_1 to its reduced form after it has participated in the carboxylation of several blood coagulation proteins, mainly prothrombin and factor VII. Despite being labeled a vitamin K antagonist, warfarin does not antagonize the action of vitamin K_1,

Ans. **124. a.** It inhibits TXA2... **125. a.** Argatroban **126. c.** Low molecular... **127. d.** Activated partial... **128. b.** Give oral vitamin K_1

but rather antagonizes vitamin K_1 recycling, depleting active vitamin K_1. Thus, the pharmacologic action may always be reversed by fresh vitamin K_1.

Recommended INR for various indications of oral anticoagulants.	
	INR
1. Prophylaxis of deep vein thrombosis and similar indications	2–2.5
2. Treatment of deep vein thrombosis, pulmonary embolism, TIAs, hip surgery	2–3
3. Recurrent thromboembolism, arterial disease (MI), prosthetic heart valves	3–3.5

129. Acute severe bleeding as a result of Warfarin therapy can be controlled by all except:

a. Withhold the anticoagulant
b. Blood transfusion
c. Vitamin K_1
d. Fresh frozen plasma

When administered, Warfarin do not anticoagulate blood immediately. Instead, onset of their effect requires about two to three days before remaining active clotting factors have had time to naturally disappear in metabolism, and the duration of action of a single dose of warfarin is 2 to 5 days. Reversal of Warfarin's effect by discontinuing its use, or by administering vitamin K_1, requires a similar period of time.

130. As compared to unfractionated heparin, low molecular weight heparins/LMWH:

a. Are absorbed more uniformly when given subcutaneously
b. Can be given to patient with heparin induced thrombocytopenia
c. Require more frequent laboratory monitoring
d. A higher risk of osteopenia

Differences of LMWH from heparin (i.e. "unfractionated heparin")

- Average molecular weight: Heparin is about 15 kDa and LMWH is about 4.5 kDa.
- Less frequent subcutaneous dosing than for heparin for postoperative prophylaxis of venous thromboembolism.
- Once or twice daily subcutaneous injection for treatment of venous thromboembolism and in unstable angina instead of intravenous infusion of high dose heparin.
- No need for monitoring of the APTT coagulation parameter as required for high dose heparin.
- Possibly a smaller risk of bleeding.
- Smaller risk of osteoporosis in long-term use.
- Smaller risk of heparin-induced thrombocytopenia, a potential side effect of heparin.
- The anticoagulant effects of heparin are typically reversible with protamine sulfate, while protamine's effect on LMWH is limited.

131. Laboratory monitoring of which of the following is desirable with low molecular weight heparin therapy:

a. aPTT
b. CT
c. PT
d. Anti-factor Xa activity

The effects of LMWHs cannot be acceptably measured using the partial thromboplastin time (PTT) or activated clotting time (ACT) tests. Rather, LMWH therapy is monitored by the *anti-factor Xa* assay, measuring *anti-factor Xa activity*.

DRUGS ACTING ON EXCRETORY SYSTEM

132. Drug CONTRAINDICATED in chronic renal failure:

a. Furosemide
b. Ethacrynic acid
c. Triamterene
d. Bumetanide

Triamterene can also cause kidney stones through direct crystallization or by seeding calcium oxalate stones. Triamterene is best avoided in patients with chronic kidney disease due to the possibility of hyperkalemia

133. Which is the drug of choice (DOC) for SIADH/ syndrome of inappropriate ADH secretion:

a. Demeclocycline
b. Vasopressin
c. Thiazide diuretics
d. Chlorpropamide

Demeclocycline is widely used (though off-label in many countries) in the treatment of hyponatremia (low blood sodium concentration) due to the syndrome of inappropriate antidiuretic hormone (SIADH) when fluid restriction alone has been ineffective. Physiologically, this works by reducing the responsiveness of the collecting tubule cells to ADH. The use in SIADH actually relies on a side effect; demeclocycline induces nephrogenic diabetes insipidus (dehydration due to the inability to concentrate urine).

Comparative features of tetracyclines.

	Tetracycline (T) Oxytetracycline (OxyT)	*Demeclocycline*	*Doxycycline (Doxy) Minocycline (Mino)*
1. Source	Oxy T: *S. rimosus* T: semisynthetic	S. aureofaciens (mutant)	Doxy: semisynthetic Mino: semisynthetic
2. Potency	Low	Intermediate	High (Doxy < Mino)

Contd...

Ans. **129. c.** Vitamin K_1 **130. a.** Are absorbed more... **131. d.** Anti-factor... **132. c.** Triamterene **133. a.** Demeclocycline

Contd...

	Tetracycline (T) Oxytetracycline (OxyT)	*Demeclocycline*	*Doxycycline (Doxy) Minocycline (Mino)*
3. Intestinal absorption	60–80%	60–80%	95–100% no interference by food
4. Plasma protein binding	Oxy T: Low T: Moderate	High	High
5. Elimination	T: } Rapid renal Oxy T: } excretion	Partial metabolism, slower renal excretion	Doxy: Primarily excreted in faeces as conjugate Mino: Primarily metabolized, excreted in urine and bile
6. Plasma t½	6–10 hrs	16–18 hrs	18–24 hrs
7. Dosage	250–500 mg QID or TDS	300 mg BD	200 mg initially, then 100–200 mg OD
8. Alteration of intestinal flora	Marked	Moderate	Least
9. Incidence of diarrhoea	High	Intermediate	Low
10. Phototoxicity	Low	Highest	Doxy: High
11. Specific toxicity	Oxy T: less tooth discolouration	More phototoxic, diabetes insipidus	Doxy: Low renal toxicity. Mino: Vestibular toxicity, less superinfections

134. NOT to be co-administered with spironolactone:

a. Amlodipine
b. ACE inhibitors
c. Beta blockers
d. Chlorothiazide

More pronounced hyperkalemia can occur if spironolactone is given to patients receiving ACE inhibitors /ARBs.

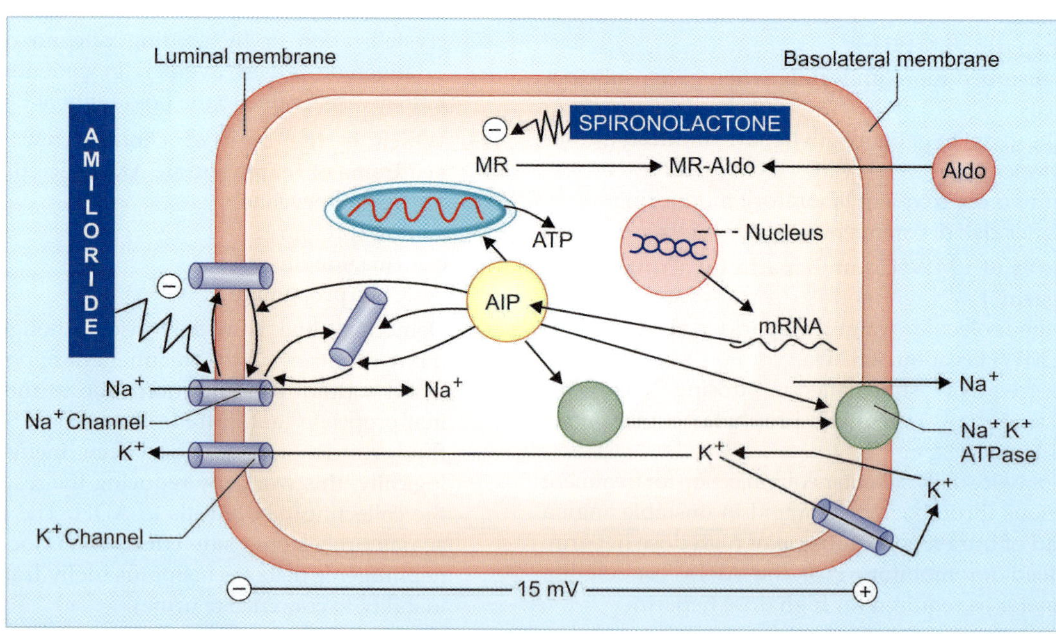

Site and mechanism of action of potassium sparing diuretics on the late distal tubule/collecting duct cell.
Aldosterone (Aldo) penetrates the cell from the interstitial side and combines with the mineralocorticoid receptor (MR). The complex translocates to the nucleus—promotes gene-mediated mRNA synthesis. The mRNA then directs synthesis of aldosterone-induced proteins (AIPs). The AIPs include Na^+K^+ ATPase and renal epithelial (amiloride sensitive) Na^+ channels. More of these proteins are synthesized. The AIPs also activate these Na^+ channels and, translocate them from cytosolic site to luminal membrane. They also translocate Na^+K^+ ATPase to the basolateral membrane. AIPs also increase ATP production by mitochondria. All these changes promote Na^+ reabsorption. More K^+ and H^+ is secreted indirectly. Spironolactone binds to MR, prevents Aldo action and produces opposite effects.

Amiloride approaches the Na^+ channel from the luminal side and blocks it—reducing the lumen negative transepithelial potential difference which governs K^+ and H^+ secretion.

Ans. 134. b. ACE inhibitors

135. Effect of thiazides:
a. Impotence
b. Hypouricemia
c. Hypolipidemia
d. Hypokalemic metabolic alkalosis

Thiazide diuretics, which have been used for decades to treat hypertension, have been known to cause **erectile** dysfunction (**ED**).

Thiazides and related diuretics.

Drug	*Trade name (Tab. strength) (mg)*	*Daily dose (mg)*	*CAse inhibition*	*Duration of action (Hr)*
1. Hydrochlorothiazide	AQUAZIDE, HYDRIDE THIAZIDE (12.5, 25, 50 mg) ESIDREX (50)	12.5–100	+	6–12
2. Chlorthalidone	HYTHALTON (50,100) HYDRAZIDE, THALIZIDE (12.5, 25)	50–100	++	48
3. Metolazone	ZAROXOLYN (5, 10) DIUREM, METORAL (2.5, 5, 10)	5–20	+	12–24
4. Xipamide	XIPAMID (20)	20–40	+	12
5. Indapamide	LORVAS (2.5)	2.5–5	–	12–24
6. Clopamide	BRINALDIX (20)	10–60	±	12–18

136. Inhibitor of carbonic anhydrase enzyme:
a. Spironolactone
b. Thiazides
c. Acetazolamide
d. Triamterene

Acetazolamide is a carbonic anhydrase (type II) inhibitor that is used for the medical treatment of glaucoma, epileptic seizure, idiopathic intracranial hypertension, altitude sickness, cystinuria, periodic paralysis, central sleep apnea, and dural ectasia. Acetazolamide is a diuretic.

137. FALSE regarding mannitol:
a. Reduces GFR
b. Osmotic diuretic
c. Non-electrolyte
d. Renal vasodilator

Mannitol expands extracellular fluid volume (because it does not enter cells, mannitol draws water from the intracellular compartment)—increases GFR and inhibits rennin release.

Urinary electrolyte pattern and natriuretic efficacy of some diuretics.

Diuretic	*Urinary electrolyte excretion* Na^+	K^+	Cl^-	HCO_3^-	*Max. % of filtered* Na^+ *excreted*	*Efficacy*
1. Furosemide	↑↑↑	↑	↑↑	↑,–	25%	High
2. Thiazide	↑↑	↑	↑	↑	8%	Intermediate
3. Acetazolamide	↑	↑↑	↑,–	↑↑	5%	Mild
4. Spironolactone	↑	↓	↑	–,↑	3%	Low
5. Amiloride	↑	↓	↑	–,↑	3%	Low
6. Mannitol	↑↑	↑	↑	↑	20%	High

138. DOC for diabetes insipidus is:
a. Insulin
b. Desmopressin
c. Diazoxide
d. Chlorpropamide

Desmopressin (trade names: **DDAVP**, others) is a synthetic replacement for vasopressin, the hormone that reduces urine production. It may be taken nasally, intravenously, or as an oral or sublingual tablet. It is prescribed most frequently for treatment of diabetes insipidus, bedwetting, or nocturia.

ANTIMICROBIAL DRUGS

139. All of the following antibiotic inhibit cell wall synthesis EXCEPT:
a. Vancomycin
b. Cycloserine
c. Clindamycin
d. Cephalosporin

Clindamycin has a primarily bacteriostatic effect. It is a bacterial protein synthesis inhibitor by inhibiting ribosomal translocation, in a similar way to macrolides. It does so by binding to the 50S rRNA of the large bacterial ribosome subunit.

Ans. **135. a.** Impotence **136. c.** Acetazolamide **137. a.** Reduces GFR **138. b.** Desmopressin **139. c.** Clindamycin

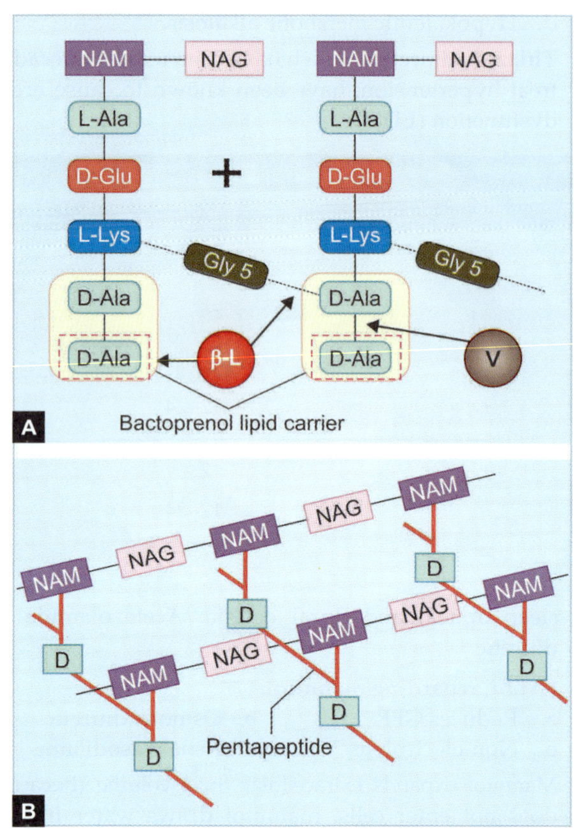

Key features of bacterial cell wall synthesis and cell wall structure, depicting the site of action of β-lactam antibiotics and vancomycin. A. Cross linking of peptidoglycan residues of neighbouring strands by cleavage of terminal D-alanine (D-Ala/D) and transpeptidation with the chain of 5 glycine (Gly5) residues. The β-lactam antibiotics (β-L) block cleavage of terminal D-Ala and transpeptidation. The peptidoglycan units are synthesized within the bacterial cell and are transported across the cell membrane by attachment to a bactoprenol lipid carrier for assembly into strands. Vancomycin (V) binds tightly to the terminal D-Ala-D-Ala sequence and prevents its release from the carrier, so that further transpeptidation cannot take place. B. The highly cross linked peptidoglycan strands in bacterial cell wall
NAM—N-acetyl muramic acid
NAG—N-acetylglucosamine
L-Ala—L-alanine
D-Glu—D-glutamic acid
L-Lys—L-Lysine

140. Which of the following commonly have Neuropsychiatric side effects:

a. Ethosuximide b. Cycloserine
c. Pyrazinamide d. Rifampicin

Reason for limited use of cycloserine is the neurological side effects it causes, since it is able to penetrate into the central nervous system (CNS) and cause headaches, drowsiness, depression, dizziness, vertigo, confusion, paresthesias, dysarthria, hyperirritability, psychosis, convulsions, and shaking (tremors). Overdose of cycloserine may result in paresis, seizures, and coma, while alcohol consumption may increase the risk of seizures.

Standardized TNTCP regimen for MDR–TB*.	
Intensive phase (6–9 months)	*Continuation phase (18 months)*
• Kanamycin (Km)	• Ofloxacin or Levofloxacin
• Ofloxacin (Ofx) or Levofloxacin (Lfx)	• Ethionamide
• Ethionamide (Eto)	• Cycloserine
• Cycloserine (Cs)	• Ethambutol
• Pyrazinamide (Z)	
• Ethambutol (E)	
+ Pyridoxine 100 mg/day	

*Revised National Tuberculosis Control Programme: DOTS-Plus Guidelines (2010); Central TB Division, Directorate General of Heatlh Services, Ministry of Health and family welfare, new Delhi.

141. Hypothyroidism may be a side-effect of:

a. Cycloserine b. Ethionamide
c. INH d. Rifampicin

Ethionamide is structurally similar to methimazole, has been shown to inhibit thyroid hormone synthesis, and was reported to cause hypothyroidism in several TB patients.

142. Drug, which can be given in G-6-PD deficients:

a. Primaquine b. Aminopyrine
c. Probenecid d. Chloroquine

Antimalarial drugs that can cause acute hemolysis in people with G6PD deficiency include primaquine, pamaquine, and chloroquine. There is evidence that other antimalarials may also exacerbate G6PD deficiency, but only at higher doses. Sulfonamides (such as sulfanilamide, sulfamethoxazole, and mafenide), thiazolesulfone, methylene blue, and naphthalene should also be avoided by people with G6PD deficiency as they antagonize folate synthesis, as should certain analgesics (such as aspirin, phenazopyridine, and acetanilide) and a few non-sulfa antibiotics (nalidixic acid, nitrofurantoin, isoniazid, dapsone, and furazolidone).

Drugs with potential* to cause haemolysis in G-6-PD deficient individuals.	
Primaquine	Nalidixic acid
Chloroquine	Fluoroquinolones
Quinine/Quinidine	Chloramphenicol
Proguanil	Nitrofurantoin
Pyrimethamine	Furazolidone
Dapsone	Methyldopa
Sulfonamides	Hydralazine
Cotrimoxazole	Procainamide
Sulfasalazine	Probenecid
Thiazide diuretics	Colchicine
Aspirin	*Methylene blue*

*Drugs carrying higher risk are italicized

Ans. 140. b. Cycloserine **141. b.** Ethionamide **142. b.** Aminopyrine

143. Most phototoxic quinolone is:

a. Pefloxacin b. Norfloxacin
c. Ofloxacin d. Ciprofloxacin

The phototoxicity order reported in humans is: fleroxacin > lomefloxacin, pefloxacin >> ciprofloxacin > enoxacin, norfloxacin and ofloxacin.

Pharmacokinetic characteristics and doses of fluoroquinolones.

	CIPROFL	*NORFL*	*PEFL*	*OFL*	*LEVOFL*	*GEMI*	*PRULI*	*MOXI*
1. Oral bioavailability (%)	60–80	35–45	90–100	85–95	~100	70	90	85
2. Plasma protein binding (%)	20–35	15	20–30	25	25	55–73	45	40
3. Vol. of distribution (L/kg)	3–4	2	2	1.5	1.3	—	—	2
4. Percent metabolized	20	25	85	5–10	5	—	>90	70–80
5. Elimination t½ (hr)	3–5	4–6	8–14	5–8	8	7	10–12	10–15
6. Routes of administration	oral, i.v.	oral	oral, i.v.	oral, i.v.	oral, i.v.	oral	oral	oral, i.v.
7. Dose (mg) : oral	250–750	400	400	200–400	500	320	600	400
	(BD)	(BD)	(BD)	(BD)	(OD)	(OD)	(OD)	(OD)
: iv	100–200	—	400	200	500	—	—	400

144. Antihelminthic drug, also acting as immuno-modulator:

a. Piperazine b. Mebendazole
c. Levamisole d. Albendazole

Levamisole works as a nicotinic acetylcholine receptor agonist that causes continued stimulation of the parasitic worm muscles, leading to paralysis. **Levamisole** is used to treat parasitic worm infections and as a immunomodulator (restores depressed T cell function).

145. Ratio of trimethoprim to sulfa-methoxazole in co-trimoxazole:

a. 1:2 b. 2:1
c. 1:5 d. 5:1

Trimethoprim/sulfamethoxazole (**TMP/SMX**), also known as **co-trimoxazole,** is used to treat a variety of bacterial infections. It consists of one part trimethoprim to five parts sulfamethoxazole. It is used for urinary tract infections, MRSA skin infections, travelers' diarrhea, respiratory tract infections, and cholera, among others. It may be used both to treat and prevent pneumocystis pneumonia in people with HIV/AIDS. It can be given by mouth or intravenously.

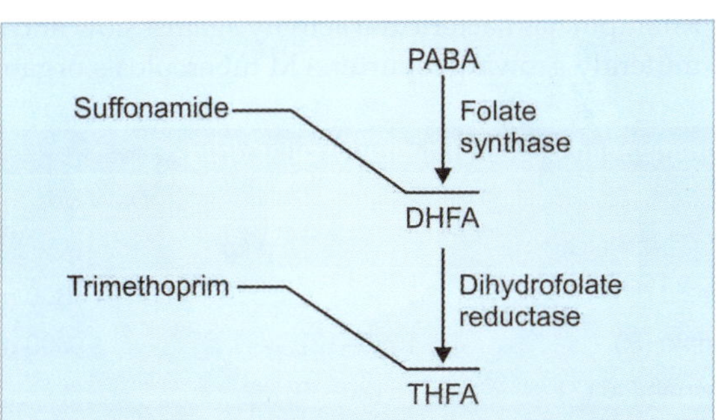

Sequential block in bacterial folate metabolism. (PABA: Para amino-benzoic acid; DHFA: Dihydrofolic acid; THFA: Tetrahydrofolic acid).

146. Resistance to anti-tubercular drug develops by:

a. Mutation b. Transformation
c. Conjugation d. Transduction

DR (drug resistance) is caused by specific mutations in independent genes of M. tuberculosis bacillus. The MC mechanism which confers high level INH resistance is by mutation of the catalase-peroxidase (KatG) gene so that the bacilli do not generate the reactive metabolite of INH. Rifampicin resistance is nearly always due to mutation in the rpoB gene reducing its affinity for the drug.

Alternative grouping of antitubercular drugs*.

Group I	First line oral anti-TB drugs	Isoniazid (INH), Rifampin, Pyrazinamide, Ethambutol
Group II	Injectable anti-TB drugs	Streptomycin, Kanamycin, Amikacin, Capreomycin
Group III	Fluoroquinolones	Ofloxacin, Levofloxacin, Moxifloxacin, Ciprofloxacin
Group IV	Second line oral anti-TB drugs	Ethionamide, Prothionamide, Cycloserine, Terizidone, Para-aminosalicylic acid
Group V	Drugs with unclear efficacy[£]	Thiacetazone, Clarithromycin, Clofazimine, Linezolid, Amoxicillin/clavulanate, Imipenem/cilastatin

*Adopted from: Treatment of Tuberculosis Guidelines; WHO, Fourth edition (2010) and Revised National Tuberculosis Control Programme (RNTCP), DOTS-Plus Guidelines 2010.

£Not recommended by WHO for routine use in MDR-TB patients.

Group I: are the most potent and best tolerated oral drugs used routinely.
Group II: are potent and bactericidal, but injectable drugs.
Group III: include fluoroquinolones (FQs) which are well tolerated bactericidal oral drugs; all patients with drug resistant TB should receive one FQ.
Group IV: are less effective, bacteriostatic/more toxic oral drugs for resistant TB.
Group V: are drugs with uncertain efficacy; not recommended for MDR-TB; may be used in extensively resistant TB (XDR-TB).

Ans. 143. a. Pefloxacin **144. c.** Levamisole **145. c.** 1: 5 **146. a.** Mutation

147. Kalavathi, 22 years, recently married is receiving oral contraceptives. She develops cough with expectoration which is NOT controlled with antibiotics. She was diagnosed to have TB and was put on ATT. Which ATT will result in failure of contraception:

a. INH b. Pyrazinamide
c. Rifampicin d. Streptomycin

Rifampicin is an inducer of many enzymes of the cytochrome P450 superfamily, including CYP 1A2, CYP2B6, CYP2D6, CYP2C8, CYP2C9, CYP2C19, CYP3A4, CYP3A5, and CYP3A7. Thus it will speed up the metabolism of any drug metabolized by any of these enzymes in the body.

148. Most effective anti-tubercular drug against slowly multiplying intra-cellular mycobacteria:

a. Ethambutol b. Pyrazinamide
c. Isoniazid d. Rifampicin

Rifampin has bactericidal activity against slow and intermittently growing (spurters) M tuberculosis organisms. Rifampin inhibits DNA-dependent RNA polymerase activity in susceptible cells. Specifically, it interacts with bacterial RNA polymerase but does not inhibit the mammalian enzyme. Rifampin at therapeutic levels has demonstrated bactericidal activity against both intracellular and extracellular Mycobacterium tuberculosis organisms.

149. Penicillinase resistant penicillin is:

a. Ticarcillin b. Carbenicillin
c. Ampicillin d. Methicillin

Penicillinase resistant Penicillins (MCD)

- Methicillin
- Cloxacillin
- Dicloxacillin

150. DNA dependent RNA synthesis is inhibited by:

a. Chloromycetin b. Colchicine
c. Ethambutol d. Rifampicin

Rifampicin inhibits bacterial DNA-dependent RNA synthesis by inhibiting bacterial DNA-dependent RNA polymerase.

Recommended doses of antitubercular drugs@

DRUG	Daily dose		3 times per week dose	
	mg/kg	maximum	mg/kg	daily maximum
Isoniazid (H)	5 (4–6)	300 mg	10 (8–12)	900 mg
Rifampin (R)	10 (8–12)	600 mg	10 (8–12)	600 mg
Pyrazinamide (Z)	25 (20–30)	—	35 (30–40)	—
Ethambutol (E)	15 (15–20)	—	30 (25–35)	—
Streptomycin (S)*	15 (12–18)	—	15 (12–18)	1000 mg

*Patients over 60 years age—10 mg/kg or 500–750 mg/day (i.m.).
@Adopted from Treatment of Tuberculosis: Guidelines, 4th edition (2010), WHO, Geneva.

151. Drug of choice for Legionnaire's disease:

a. Streptomycin b. Penicillin
c. Erythromycin d. Tetracycline

Legionella multiply within the cell, so any effective treatment must have excellent intracellular penetration. Current treatments of choice are the respiratory tract quinolones (levofloxacin, moxifloxacin, gemifloxacin) or newer macrolides (azithromycin, clarithromycin, roxithromycin). The antibiotics used most frequently have been levofloxacin, doxycycline, and azithromycin.

152. Action of dapsone is antagonized by:

a. Niacin
b. Para-amino-benzoic acid
c. Pyridoxine
d. Folate

As an antibacterial, dapsone inhibits bacterial synthesis of dihydrofolic acid, via competition with para-aminobenzoate for the active site of dihydropteroate synthase. Though structurally distinct from dapsone, the sulfonamide group of antibacterial drugs also work in this way.

Multidrug therapy (MDT) of leprosy

	Multibacillary	Paucibacillary
Rifampin	600 mg once a month supervised	600 mg once a month supervised
Dapsone	100 mg daily self administered	100 mg daily self administered
Clofazimine	300 mg once a month supervised and 50 mg daily self administered	—
Duration	12 months	6 months
Doses to be reduced suitably for children		

Blister packs of tablets for 28-day treatment are made available free of cost to all MBL cases, and 12 such blister packs have to be consumed by each MBL patient. Separate blister packs are given to PBL cases and 6 packs are to be taken by each patient.

153. Drug causing Pseudomembranous colitis:

a. Penicillin b. Vancomycin
c. Metronidazole d. Clindamycin

Ans. 147. c. Rifampicin 148. d. Rifampicin 149. d. Methicillin 150. d. Rifampicin
151. c. Erythromycin 152. b. Para-amino-... 153. d. Clindamycin

Common side effects of clindamycin include nausea, diarrhea, rash, and pain at the site of injection. It increases the risk of *Clostridium difficile* colitis about fourfold.

154. Metrifonate is effective against:

a. Giardiasis b. Schistosomiasis
c. Leishmaniasis d. Amoebiasis

Metrifonate or **trichlorfon** is an irreversible organophosphate acetylcholinesterase inhibitor. It is a prodrug which is activated non-enzymatically into 2,2-dichlorovinyl dimethyl phosphate (DDVP).

It is used as an insecticide. It can be used to treat schistosomiasis caused by *Schistosoma haematobium*, but is no longer commercially available.

155. Drug safer in patient allergic to penicillin:

a. Aztreonam b. Cefepime
c. Imipenem d. Cephalexin

Aztreonam is often used in patients who are penicillin allergic or who cannot tolerate aminoglycosides. **Aztreonam** is a monobactam antibiotic used primarily to treat infections caused by Gram-negative bacteria. It is a synthetic drug based on a simpler monobactam isolated from *Chromobacterium violaceum*. It is resistant to some beta-lactamases, but is inactivated by extended-spectrum beta-lactamases.

156. True regarding imipenem:

a. Used with sulbactam
b. Can be used with cilastatin
c. Easily degraded by beta lactam
d. Narrow spectrum antibiotic

Imipenem is rapidly degraded by the renal enzyme dehydropeptidase 1 when administered alone, and is always coadministered with cilastatin to prevent this inactivation.

157. Voriconazole is useful in all except:

a. Mucormycosis b. Candida tropicalis
c. Candida albicans d. Aspergillosis

If mucormycosis is suspected, amphotericin B therapy should be immediately administered due to the rapid spread and high mortality rate of the disease. Amphotericin B is usually administered for an additional 4–6 weeks after initial therapy begins to ensure eradication of the infection. Posaconazole has been shown to be effective against mucormycosis, perhaps more so than amphotericin B, but has not yet replaced it as the standard of care.

Properties of drugs used for systemic mycoses.

Characteristic	*AMB*	*Caspo*	*5-FC*	*KTZ*	*FLU*	*ITR*	*VORI*
Antifungal spectrum	Broad	Narrow	Narrow	Broad	Broad	Broad	Broad
Absorbed orally	No	No	Yes	Yes	Yes	Yes	Yes
Administered i.v.	Yes	Yes	Yes	No	Yes	Yes	Yes
Resistance *(in vivo)*	No	No	Yes	Limited	Limited	No	No
Nephrotoxicity	Yes	No	No	No	No	No	No
Anaemia	Yes	No	Mild	No	No	No	No
Leucopenia	No	No	Yes	No	No	No	No
Gastrointestinal upset	Yes	Mild	Yes	Mild	Mild	Moderate	Mild
Overall toxicity	High	Low	Medium	Medium	Low	Low	Low

AMB: AmphotericinB; 5-FC: Flucytosine; KTZ: Ketoconazole; FLU: Fluconazole; ITR: Itraconazole; Caspo: Caspofungin, VORI: Voriconazole

158. Dose of chloroquine for prophylaxis against vivax malaria:

a. 150 mg (base) weekly
b. 300 mg (base) weekly
c. 600 mg (base) weekly
d. 900 mg (base) weekly

Both adults and children should take one dose of chloroquine per week starting at least 1 week before traveling to the area where malaria transmission occurs. They should take one dose per week while there, and for 4 consecutive weeks after leaving. The weekly dosage for adults is 300 mg base (500 mg salt).

Comparative properties of antimalarial drugs.

Drug	*Pre-erythro.*		*Erythrocytic phase*			*Hypnozoite*	*Gametes*	*Resistance*	*Toxicity grading*
	Fal.	*Viv.*	*Activity*	*Onset*	*Duration*				
1. Chloroquine	–	–	+	Fast	Long	–	–	Slow	+
2. Mefloquine	–	–	+	Int	Long	–	–	Minor	++
3. Quinine	–	–	+	Int	Short	–	–	Minor	+++
4. Proguanil	+	–	+	Int	Short	–	*	Rapid	±
5. Pyrimethamine	–	–	+	Slow	Long	–	–	Rapid	+

Contd...

Ans. 154. b. Schistosomiasis 155. a. Aztreonam 156. b. Can be used... 157. a. Mucormycosis
158. b. 300 mg (base) weekly

Contd...

Drug	Pre-erythro.		Erythrocytic phase			Hypnozoite	Gametes	Resistance	Toxicity grading
	Fal.	Viv.	Activity	Onset	Duration				
6. Primaquine	+	+	–	–	–	+	+	Minor	++
7. Sulfonamides	–	–	±	Slow	Long	–	–	Minor	+±
8. Tetracyclines	–	–	+	Slow	Short	–	–	Nil	+
9. Clindamycin	–	–	+	Slow	Short	–	–	Nil	+
10. Artemisinin	–	–	+	Fastest	Short	–	+	Nil	+
11. Lumefantrine	–	–	+	Int	Long	–	–	Nil	+

*Do not kill gametes but may inhibit their development in mosquito.
Pre-erythro.: Preerythrocytic stage; Fal.: *P. falciparum*; Viv: *P. vivax*; Int: Intermediate.

159. Dosage and drug of choice for primary syphilis:
a. Amoxicillin (500 mg for 5 days)
b. Benzathine penicillin (2.4 mega units deep IM)
c. Erythromycin (2 gm daily for 2 weeks)
d. Doxycycline (100 mg daily for 2 weeks)

Primary and secondary syphilis
- Benzathine penicillin G 2.4 million units IM for 1 dose
- Retreatment: Benzathine penicillin G 2.4 million units IM once weekly for 3 weeks
- Pediatric dosing: Benzathine penicillin G 50,000 units/kg IM, up to the adult dose of 2.4 million units for 1 dose

160. NOT to be used in renal failure:
a. Cephalothin
b. Penicillin G
c. Erythromycin
d. Doxycycline

Cephalothin has been reported to **cause** proximal tubule damage and acute tubular necrosis at high doses and has caused reversible deterioration in renal function patients with prerenal and renal azotemia.

First generation cephalosporins.	
Parenteral	*Oral*
Cefazolin	Cephalexin
	Cefadroxil
Second generation cephalosporins	
Parenteral	*Oral*
Cefuroxime	Cefaclor
Cefoxitin*	Cefuroxime axetil
	Cefprozil
Third generation cephalosporins	
Parenteral	*Oral*
Cefotaxime	Cefixime
Ceftizoxime	Cefpodoxime proxetil
Ceftriaxone	Cefdinir
Ceftazidime	Ceftibuten
Cefoperazone	Ceftamet pivoxil

Contd...

Contd...

Fourth generation cephalosporins	
Parenteral	
Cefepime	
Cefpirome	

*Not available in India

161. Mechanism of action of clindamycin is inhibition of:
a. Protein synthesis b. DNA gyrase
c. Lysosomal enzyme d. Cell wall synthesis

Clindamycin has a primarily bacteriostatic effect. It is a bacterial protein synthesis inhibitor by inhibiting ribosomal translocation, in a similar way to macrolides. It does so by binding to the 50S rRNA of the large bacterial ribosome subunit.

162. Drug which acts by the release of formaldehyde in the urinary tract is:
a. Ammonium chloride b. Nalidixic acid
c. Nitrofurantoin
d. Methenamine mandelate

As the mandelic acid salt, hexamethylenetetramine (generic methenamine mandelate), it is used for the treatment of urinary tract infection. It decomposes at an acidic pH to form formaldehyde and ammonia, and the formaldehyde is bactericidal; the mandelic acid adds to this effect. Urinary acidity is typically ensured by co-administering vitamin C (ascorbic acid) or ammonium chloride. Its use had temporarily been reduced in the late 1990s, due to adverse effects, particularly chemically-induced hemorrhagic cystitis in overdose, but its use has now been re-approved because of the prevalence of antibiotic resistance to more commonly used drugs. This drug is particularly suitable for long-term prophylactic treatment of urinary tract infection, because bacteria do not develop resistance to formaldehyde. It should not be used in the presence of renal insufficiency.

163. Drug NOT used in TB and leprosy is:
a. Ofloxacin b. Rifampin
c. Ethionamide d. None

Classification of drugs used in leprosy
- Sulfone: Dapsone

Ans. 159. b. Benzathine... 160. a. Cephalothin 161. a. Protein synthesis 162. d. Methenamine... 163. d. None

- Phenazine derivative: Clofazimine
- Antitubercular drugs: Rifampin, Ethionamide
- Other antibiotics: Ofloxacin, Moxifloxacin, Minocycline, Clarithromycin

NLEP (2009) Classification of Leprosy.	
Paucibacillary (PB)	*Multibacillary (MB)*
• 1–5 skin lesions	• 6 or more skin lesions
• No nerve/only one nerve involvement, ± 1–5 skin lesions.	• > 1 nerve involved irrespective of number of skin lesions
• Skin smear negative at all sites	• Skin smear positive at any one site

164. Ivermectin is NOT used for:

a. Onchocerciasis b. Malaria
c. Filariasis
d. Ascariasis

Ivermectin is a broad-spectrum antiparasitic agent, traditionally against parasitic worms. It is mainly used in humans in the treatment of onchocerciasis (river blindness), but is also effective against other worm infestations (such as strongyloidiasis, ascariasis, trichuriasis, filariasis and enterobiasis), and some epidermal parasitic skin diseases, including scabies.

165. Mechanism of action of nitazoxanide:

a. Inhibitor of cell wall synthesis
b. Disruption of cell membrane
c. Inhibitor of PFOR enzyme
d. Inhibitor of motility

The anti-protozoal activity of nitazoxanide is believed to be due to interference with the pyruvate: ferredoxin oxidoreductase (PFOR) enzyme-dependent electron transfer reaction which is essential to anaerobic energy metabolism.

166. Erythromycin combined with which drug may cause ventricular arrhythmias:

a. Tetracycline b. Streptomycin
c. Ebastine d. Cisapride

Cisapride should be avoided with use of agents inhibiting metabolism by cytochrome P450 3A4: macrolide antibiotics (erythromycin, clarithromycin, etc.), azole antifungals (ketoconazole, itraconazole, fluconazole, etc.), protease inhibitors (ritonavir, indinavir, etc.), nefazodone and grapefruit juice.

Selected clinically important drug interactions.		
*Precipitant drug**	*Object drug£*	*Likely interaction and comments*
1. Ampicillin, Amoxicillin	Oral contraceptives Oral anticoagulants	Interruption of enterohepatic circulation of the estrogen → failure of contraception; Advise alternative contraception. Inhibition of gut flora → decreased vit K production in gut → risk of bleeding; Monitor INR and reduce anticoagulant dose if needed.
2. Probenecid	Penicillin, Ampicillin, Cephalosporins	Inhibition of tubular secretion → prolongation of antibiotic action; Desirable interaction utilized for single dose therapy.
3. Allopurinol	Ampicillin 6-Mercaptopurine, Azathioprine Warfarin, Theophylline	Increased incidence of rashes; Avoid concurrent use. Inhibition of metabolism; Reduce dose of 6-MP/azathioprine to 1/3. Inhibition of metabolism; Monitor and reduce dose of object drug.
4. Carbenicillin, Ticarcillin	Aspirin and other antiplatelet drugs	Perturbation of surface receptors on platelets → additive platelet inhibition → risk of bleeding; Avoid concurrent use.
5. Ceftriaxone, Cefoperazone	Oral anticoagulants	Additive hypoprothrombinaemia → bleeding; Monitor INR and reduce dose of anticoagulant.
6. Sulfonamides, Cotrimoxazole	Phenytoin Warfarin Sulfonylureas Thiazide diuretics Oral contraceptives	Displacement$ + inhibition of metabolism → phenytoin toxicity; Avoid concurrent use. Displacement + inhibition of metabolism + decreased production of vit K in gut → risk of bleeding; Monitor INR and reduce dose of warfarin. Displacement + inhibition of metabolism → hypoglycaemia; Avoid concurrent use. Increased incidence of thrombocytopenia; Avoid concurrent use. Interruption of enterohepatic circulation of the estrogen → failure of contraception; Advise alternative contraception.
7. Metronidazole, Tinidazole, Cefoperazone	Alcohol	Possibly accumulation of acetaldehyde → disulfiram-like or bizarre reactions; Warn the patient not to drink alcohol.

Contd...

Ans. **164. b.** Malaria **165. c.** Inhibitor... **166. d.** Cisapride

Contd...

*Precipitant drug**	*Object drug£*	*Likely interaction and comments*
8. Metronidazole Tinidazole	Lithium salts Warfarin	Decreased excretion → Li+ toxicity; Monitor Li+ level and reduce lithium dose. Inhibition of metabolism → risk of bleeding; Avoid concurrent use.
9. Ciprofloxacin Norfloxacin Pefloxacin	Theophylline Warfarin	Inhibition of metabolism → toxicity of object drug; Monitor and reduce dose of object drug.
10. Erythromycin Clarithromycin Ketoconazole Itraconazole Fluconazole Protease inhibitors	Terfenadine Astemizole Cisapride	Inhibition of metabolism by CYP3A4 → rise in blood level of object drug → dangerous ventricular arrhythmia; Concurrent use contraindicated.
	Phenytoin Carbamazepine Warfarin Sulfonylureas Diazepam Theophylline Cyclosporine HIV protease inhibitors	Inhibition of metabolism by CYP3A4 → toxicity of object drug; Avoid concurrent use or readjust dose of object drug.
	Statins	Inhibition of metabolism, higher risk of myopathy; Avoid concurrent use.
11. Gemfibrozil Nicotinic acid	Statins	Increased risk of myopathy; Caution in concurrent use.
12. Tetracyclines	Oral contraceptives Lithium salts	Interruption of enterohepatic circulation of the estrogen → failure of contraception; Advise alternative contraception. Rise in plasma Li⁺ level due to decreased excretion; Avoid use of tetracycline or monitor and reduce dose of lithium.
13. Iron salts Calcium salts Antacids Sucralfate	Tetracyclines Fluoroquinolones	Decreased absorption due to formation of complexes in g.i.t. → failure of antibiotic therapy; Stager drugv administration by 2–3 hours.
14. Furosemide	Minocycline Aminoglycoside antibiotics	Enhanced vestibular toxicity; Avoid concurrent use. Additive ototoxicity and nephrotoxicity; Avoid concurrent use.
15. Diuretics	Tetracycline Lithium Digoxin	Antianabolic effect of tetracycline increases urea production which is retained by the diuretic; Avoid concurrent use. Decreased excretion—rise in Li^+ level—toxicity; Reduce dose of lithium and monitor level. Hypokalaemia caused by diuretic increases digoxin toxicity; Give K^+ sparing diuretic/K^+ supplements.
16. Tetracyclines Chloramphenicol Macrolide antibiotics Clindamycin	Penicillins Cephalosporins	Bactericidal action of penicillins and cephalosporins may be antagonized by the bacteriostatic antibiotics; Avoid antibiotics concurrent use.

Contd...

Contd...

*Precipitant drug**	*Object drug£*	*Likely interaction and comments*
17. Clindamycin	Erythromycin Clarithromycin Azithromycin Chloramphenicol	Mutual antagonism of antibacterial action due to proximal binding sites on bacterial ribosomes; Avoid concurrent use.
18. Phenobarbitone Phenytoin Carbamazepine Rifampin	Metronidazole Doxycycline Chloramphenicol Protease inhibitors Warfarin Corticosteroids Oral contraceptives Sulfonylureas Antidepressants	Induction of metabolism → loss of efficacy of object drug; Avoid concurrent use or increase dose of object drug with monitoring.
19. Chloramphenicol	Warfarin Phenytoin Sulfonylureas	Inhibition of metabolism → toxicity of the object drug. Avoid concurrent use or monitor and reduce dose of object drug.
20. NSAIDs	Ciprofloxacin and other fluoroquinolones	Enhanced CNS toxicity, seizures; Avoid concurrent use.
21. Aspirin and other NSAIDs	Sulfonylureas Phenytoin Valproate Methotrexate Warfarin Heparin ACE inhibitors β blockers Thiazide diuretics Furosemide Alcohol Corticosteroids	Displacement and/or reduced elimination → toxicity of object drug; Avoid concurrent use/substitute NSAID with paracetamol. Enhanced risk of bleeding due to antiplatelet action and gastric mucosal damage; Avoid concurrent use. Reduced antihypertensive effect due to inhibition of renal PG synthesis; Avoid concurrent use. Reduced diuretic action due to PG synthesis inhibition in kidney; Avoid concurrent use. Increased risk of gastric mucosal damage and gastric bleeding; Concurrent use contraindicated.
22. Aspirin	Spironolactone	Reduced K^+ conserving action due to decreased tubular secretion of canrenone (active metabolite of spironolactone); Avoid concurrent use.
23. Chronic alcoholism	Paracetamol	Hepatotoxic dose of paracetamol is reduced; doses ≤ 3 g/day are safe.
24. Chlorpromazine Imipramine and other TCAs	Morphine Pethidine Codeine	Enhanced CNS and respiratory depression; Avoid concurrent use.
25. Chlorpromazine Haloperidol Metoclopramide	Levodopa-carbidopa	Antagonism of antiparkinsonian effect; Concurrent use contraindicated.
26. Levodopa-carbidopa	ACE inhibitors Vasodilators Prazosin	Excessive postural hypotension; Reduce dose of antihypertensives.
27. TCAs	Adrenaline (added to local anaesthetic)	Potentiation due to neuronal uptake inhibition → rise in BP; Use plain local anaesthetic solution.
28. Promethazine Alcohol Opioids Antipsychotics	Diazepam and other benzodiazepines	Additive CNS and respiratory depression, motor impairment; Avoid concurrent use.

Contd...

Contd...

*Precipitant drug**	*Object drug*[£]	*Likely interaction and comments*
29. Cimetidine Isoniazid }	Diazepam and other benzodiazepines	Inhibition of metabolism → exaggerated CNS depression; Avoid concurrent use or reduce benzodiazepine dose.
30. Sildenafil Tadalafil }	Nitrates	Marked potentiation → precipitous fall in BP; Concurrent use contraindicated.
31. Propranolol	Adrenaline (injected with local anaesthetic) Lidocaine	Rise in BP due to blockade of vasodilator action of adrenaline that enters systemic circulation; Avoid adrenaline containing local anaesthetic. Reduced hepatic clearance of lidocaine; Ceiling amount used in local anaesthesia is reduced.
32. Lidocaine	β-blockers Quinidine and other antiarrhythmic drugs	Enhanced bradycardia and hypotension; Avoid concurrent use. Exaggerated cardiac depression, precipitation of arrhythmias; Avoid concurrent use.

*Precipitant drug is the drug, which alters the action/pharmacokinetics of the other drug.
[£]Object drug is the drug whose action/pharmacokinetics is altered.
[$]Displacement of plasma protein bound drug.
NSAIDs: Nonsteroidal antiinflammatory drugs; TCAs: Tricyclic antidepressants.

167. Cephalosporin that does NOT require dose reduction in patient with any degree of renal impairment:
a. Cefuroxime b. Cefoperazone
c. Ceftazidime d. Cefotaxime

Cefoperazone contains an *N*-methylthiotetrazole (NMTT or 1-MTT) side chain. As the antibiotic is broken down in the body, it releases free NMTT, which can cause hypoprothrombinemia (likely due to inhibition of the enzyme vitamin K epoxide reductase) and a reaction with ethanol similar to that produced by disulfiram (Antabuse), due to inhibition of aldehyde dehydrogenase. It is primarily excreted in bile.

168. True for Bacitracin:
a. Polysaccharide b. Systemic antifungal
c. Derived from bacteria
d. Effective against Gram-negative organism

Bacitracin is a mixture of related cyclic peptides produced by organisms of the licheniformis group of *Bacillus subtilis var* Tracy, first isolated in 1945. These peptides disrupt both Gram-positive and Gram-negative bacteria by interfering with cell wall and peptidoglycan synthesis. Bacitracin is primarily used as a topical preparation (as it is can cause kidney damage when used internally).

169. Oral vancomycin may be given in:
a. Plague b. Prostatitis
c. Tularemia
d. Pseudomembranous colitis

Vancomycin is used in treatment of pseudomembranous colitis caused by *Clostridium difficile*; in particular, in cases of relapse or where the infection is unresponsive to metronidazole treatment, which is the agent of choice (for this indication, vancomycin is given orally, rather than by its typical intravenous (IV) route).

170. Drugs indicated in MRSA infection are all except:
a. Vancomycin b. Teicoplanin
c. Linezolid d. Imipenem

Imipenem has a broad spectrum of activity against aerobic and anaerobic, Gram-positive and Gram-negative bacteria. It is particularly important for its activity against *Pseudomonas aeruginosa* and the *Enterococcus* species. Though some MRSA are inhibited, it is not reliable for treating such infections.

171. Nucleoside reverse transcriptase inhibiting drug, which is a guanosine analogue:
a. Ritonavir b. Zidovudine
c. Abacavir d. Acyclovir

Abacavir (**ABC**) is an antiretroviral medication used to prevent and treat HIV/AIDS. It is of the nucleoside analog reverse transcriptase inhibitor (NRTI) type. Viral strains that are resistant to zidovudine (AZT) or lamivudine (3TC) are generally, but not always, sensitive to abacavir.

ANTICANCER AND ANTI-INFLAMMATORY DRUGS

172. Which of the following is NOT a purine antagonist antimetabolite:
a. Fludarabine b. Cytarabine
c. Azathioprine d. 6-Mercaptopurine

Cytarabine is a pyrimidine antagonist antimetabolite, used mainly in the treatment of cancers of white blood cells such as acute myeloid leukemia (AML) and non-Hodgkin lymphoma. It is also known as **ara-C** (**ara**binofuranosyl **c**ytidine). It kills cancer cells by interfering with DNA synthesis.

173. NOT included in managing Hodgkin's lymphoma:
a. Actinomycin-D b. Bleomycin
c. Dacarbazine d. Vincristine

Uses of Actinomycin
- Gestational trophoblastic neoplasia
- Wilms' tumor
- Rhabdomyosarcoma

Ans. **167. b.** Cefoperazone **168. c.** Derived from... **169. d.** Pseudomemb... **170. d.** Imipenem
171. c. Abacavir **172. b.** Cytarabine **173. a.** Actinomycin-D

- Ewing's sarcoma
- Malignant hydatidiform mole

174. Methotrexate acts by:

a. Folic acid antagonism b. Purine antagonism
c. Pyramidine antagonism d. All

Methotrexate competitively inhibits dihydrofolate reductase (DHFR), an enzyme that participates in the tetrahydrofolate synthesis. DHFR catalyses the conversion of dihydrofolate to the active tetrahydrofolate.Folic acid is needed for the *de novo* synthesis of the nucleoside thymidine, required for DNA synthesis. Also, folate is essential for purine and pyrimidine base biosynthesis, so synthesis will be inhibited.

175. Which of the following causes Hemorrhagic cystitis:

a. Azithromycin b. Cyclophosphamide
c. Methotrexate d. Actinomycin D

Adverse drug reactions from cyclophosphamide are related to the cumulative medication dose and include chemotherapy-induced nausea and vomiting, bone marrow suppression, stomach ache, hemorrhagic cystitis, diarrhea, darkening of the skin/nails, alopecia (hair loss) or thinning of hair, changes in color and texture of the hair, and lethargy.

176. Drug of choice in choriocarcinoma:

a. 6-Thioguanine b. Vincristine
c. Actinomycin-D d. Methotrexate

Methotrexate was originally developed and continues to be used for chemotherapy, either alone or in combination with other agents. It is effective for the treatment of a number of cancers including: breast, head and neck, leukemia, lymphoma, lung, osteosarcoma, bladder, and trophoblastic neoplasms (choriocarcinoma).

177. Anti-neoplastic drug, which is also an anti-folate:

a. Cyclophosphamide b. Vincristine
c. Adriamycin d. Methotrexate

Methotrexate (**MTX**) and formerly known as **amethopterin**, is an antimetabolite and antifolate drug.

178. Cyclosporine-A acts on:

a. B-lymphocytes
b. CD8 cells and lymphocytes
c. CD4 cells and lymphocytes
d. CD3 cells and lymphocytes

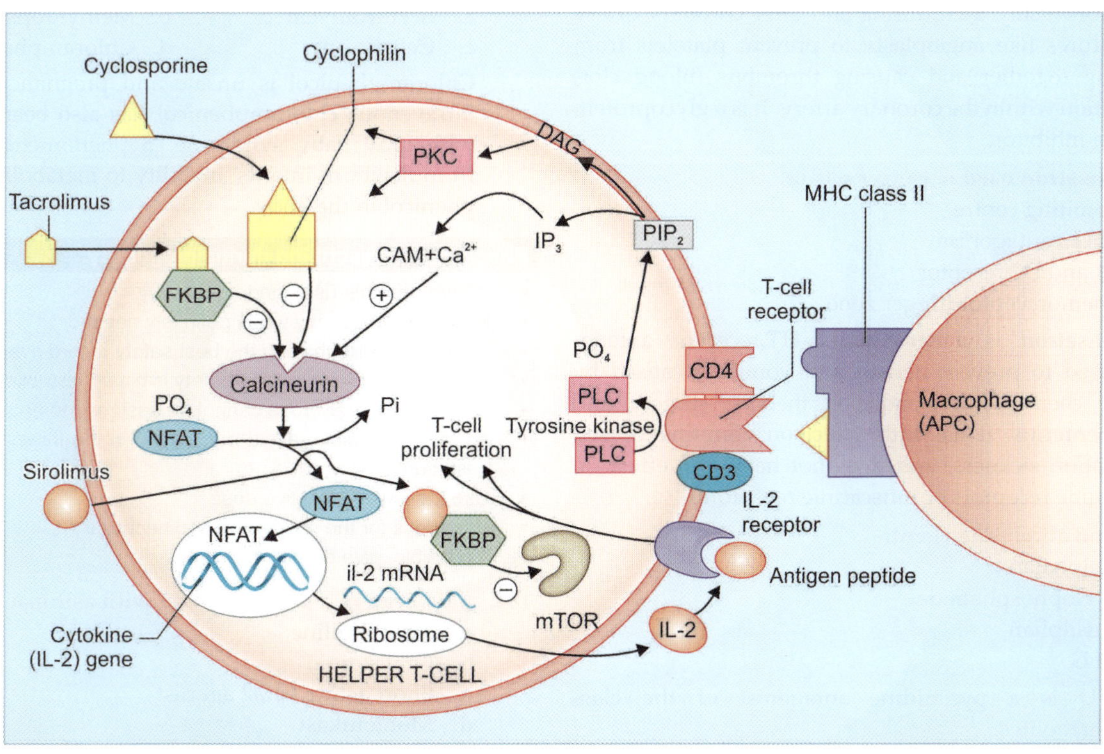

Interaction between macrophage antigen presenting cell (APC) and helper T-cell in the immune response and mechanism of action of cyclosporine, tacrolimus and sirolimus.

Cyclosporine binds to an intracellular protein 'Cyclophilin' and this complex inhibits Ca^{2+}-Calmodulin (Ca^{2+}-CAM) activated phosphatase 'Calcineurin'. Tacrolimus also inhibits calcineurin, but after binding to a different protein FKBP (FK binding protein). Normally, after activation through T-cell receptor, calcineurin dephosphorylates a 'nuclear factor of activated T-cells' (NFAT) which translocates to the nucleus and triggers transcription of cytokine genes resulting in production of IL-2 and other cytokines. IL-2 diffuses out and acts on IL-2 receptor to stimulate T-cell proliferation and other processes, carrying forward the immune response.

Sirolimus also binds to FKBP, but this complex acts at a later stage. It binds to and inhibits a kinase termed m-TOR (mammalian target of rapamycin) which is a key factor for progression of cell proliferation. (PLC: phospholipase C; PIP$_2$: phosphatidylinositol bisphosphate; DAG: Diacyl glycerol; PKC: Protein kinase C).

Ans. **174. a.** Folic acid... **175. b.** Cyclophosphamide **176. d.** Methotrexate **177. d.** Methotrexate
178. c. CD4 cells and lymphocytes

Cyclosporine binds to the cytosolic protein cyclophilin (immunophilin) of lymphocytes, especially T cells. This complex of cyclosporine and cyclophilin inhibits calcineurin, which, under normal circumstances, is responsible for activating the transcription of interleukin 2. In T-cells, activation of the T-cell receptor normally increases intracellular calcium, which acts via calmodulin to activate calcineurin. Calcineurin then dephosphorylates the transcription factor nuclear factor of activated T-cells (NFATc), which moves to the nucleus of the T-cell and increases the activity of genes coding for IL-2 and related cytokines. Cyclosporin prevents the dephosphorylation of NF-AT by binding to cyclophilin. It also inhibits lymphokine production and interleukin release and, therefore, leads to a reduced function of effector T-cells.

179. NOT a tumour necrosis factor blocking agent:

a. Abciximab b. Infliximab
c. Etanercept d. Adalimumab

Abciximab (previously known as **c7E3 Fab**), a glycoprotein IIb/IIIa receptor antagonist, is a platelet aggregation inhibitor mainly used during and after coronary artery procedures like angioplasty to prevent platelets from sticking together and causing thrombus (blood clot) formation within the coronary artery. It is a glycoprotein IIb/IIIa inhibitor.

180. Ondansetron used in cancer acts on:

a. Vomiting centre
b. 5-HT3 antagonism
c. D1 and D2 receptor
d. Chemoreceptor trigger zone

Ondansetron is a serotonin 5-HT_3receptor antagonist used to prevent nausea and vomiting caused by cancer chemotherapy, radiation therapy, surgery and gastroenteritis. It has little effect on vomiting caused by motion sickness, and does not have any effect on dopamine receptors or muscarinic receptors.

181. NOT an alkylating agent:

a. Melphalan
b. Cyclophosphamide
c. Busulphan
d. 5-FU

5-FU is a pyrimidine antagonist of the class antimetabolites.

182. Cytotoxic agent with maximum emetogenic potential:

a. Cisplatin b. Daunorubicin
c. Bleomycin d. Methotrexate

Cisplatin is one of the most emetogenic chemotherapy agents, but this symptom is managed with prophylactic antiemetics (ondansetron, granisetron, etc.) in combination with corticosteroids. Aprepitant combined with ondansetron and dexamethasone has been shown to be better for highly emetogenic chemotherapy than just ondansetron and dexamethasone.

Emetogenic potential of cytotoxic drugs.

High	*Moderate*	*Mild*
Cisplatin	Carboplatin	Bleomycin
Mustine	Cytarabine	Chlorambucil
Cyclophosphamide	Procarbazine	Busulfan
Actinomycin D	Vinblastine	Fluorouracil
Dacarbazine	Doxorubicin	6-Thioguanine
Lomustine	Daunorubicin Ifosfamide 6-Mercapto-purine Paclitaxel	Hydroxyurea Vincristine Methotrexate Etoposide l-Asparaginase

MEDICATIONS IN PREGNANCY AND LACTATION

183. Drug absolutely CONTRAINDICATED in pregnancy:

a. Erythromycin b. Methyldopa
c. Ceftriaxone d. Chloramphenicol

Chloramphenicol is unsafe and pregnancy & Use of intravenous chloramphenicol has also been associated with gray baby syndrome, a phenomenon resulting from newborn infants' inability to metabolize chloramphenicol in the body.

Principles of prescribing during pregnancy.

- Where possible use nondrug therapy
- Prescribe drugs only when definitely needed
- Choose the drug having the best safety record over time
- Avoid newer drugs, unless safety is clearly established
- Over-the-counter drugs cannot be assumed to be safe
- As far as possible, avoid medication in the initial 10 weeks of gestation
- Use the lowest effective dose
- Use drugs for the shortest period necessary
- If possible, give drugs intermittently

184. Safe drug in a pregnant lady with asthma:

a. Theophylline
b. Oral steroid
c. Short acting beta2 agonist
d. Montelukast

Safer antiasthmatic in pregnancy include (inhaled) salbutamol/ salmeterol/ ipratropium bromide/beclomethasone/ budesonide/ sodium cromoglycate

(See the table on next page)

185. Agent of choice for management of malaria in pregnancy:

a. Primaquine b. Chloroquine
c. Quinine d. Artesunate

Ans. 179. **a.** Abciximab 180. **b.** 5-HT3 antagonism 181. **d.** 5-FU 182. **a.** Cisplatin
183. **d.** Chloramph... 184. **c.** Short acting... 185. **b.** Chloroquine

Chloroquine has not been shown to have any harmful effects on the fetus when used for malarial prophylaxis in pregnancy. Small amounts of chloroquine are excreted in the breast milk of lactating women. However, because this drug can be safely prescribed to infants, the effects are not harmful.

Choice of drugs for common problems during pregnancy.

	Drug class (condition)	*Safety uncertain/unsafe*	*Safer alternative*
1.	Antiemetics (morning sickness, other types of vomiting)	Domperidone (X) Ondansetron	Promethazine, Doxylamine Dicyclomine, Prochlorperazine Metoclopramide
2.	Drugs for peptic ulcer and GERD	Cimetidine, Lansoprazole cisapride (X), Mosapride	Ranitidine, Famotidine Omeprazole Pantoprazole,
3.	Laxatives (constipation)	Senna, Bisacodyl, Docusates saline purgatives	Dietary fibre, Ispaghula Lactulose
4.	Antidiarrheals	Diphenoxylate-atropine, Loperamide	Oral rehydration salts
5.	Analgesics (headache, body-ache, joint pain, visceral pain)	Aspirin, Metamizol, NSAIDs COX-2 inhibitors, Codeine Dextropropoxyphene, Morphine (X) Pethidine, Tramadol	Paracetamol Ibuprofen (low dose)
6.	Cold-cough remedies	Codeine, Dextromethorphan Bromhexine, Expectorants	Xylometazoline, Oxymetazoline, Budesonide } Nasal drops
7.	Antiallergics	Cetirizine, Loratadine Fexofenadine, Astemizole (X)	Chlorpheniramine Promethazine
8.	Antibacterials (systemic bacterial infections)	Cotrimoxazole, Fluoroquinolones (X), Tetracycline (X), Doxycycline (X), Chloramphenicol (X), Gentamicin, Streptomycin (X), Kanamycin (X), Tobramycin (X), Clarithromycin, Azithromycin, Clindamycin, Vancomycin, Nitrofurantoin	Penicillin G, Ampicillin, Amoxicillin-clavulanate Cloxacillin, Piperacillin, Cephalosporins, Erythromycin
9.	Antitubercular	Pyrazinamide, Streptomycin (X)	Isoniazid, Rifampicin, Ethambutol
10.	Antiamoebic	Metronidazole, Tinidazole Quiniodochlor	Diloxanide furoate, Paromomycin
11.	Antimalarial	Artemether, Artesunate Primaquine (X)	Chloroquine, Mefloquine, Proguanil Quinine (only in 1st trimester), Pyrimethamine + Sulfadoxine (only single dose)
12.	Anthelmintic	Albendazole (X), Mebendazole (X) Ivermectin, Pyrantel pamoate, Diethylcarbamazine (X)	Piperazine, Niclosamide, Praziquantel
13.	Antifungal (superficial and deep mycosis)	Amphotericin B (X), Fluconazole Itraconazole (X), Ketoconazole (X), Griseofulvin (X), Terbinafine	Clotrimazole, Nystatin, Tolnaftate } Topical
14.	Antiretroviral (HIV-AIDS)	Didanosine, Abacavir, Indinavir Ritonavir, Efavirenz	Zidovudine, Lamivudine, Nevirapine, Nelfinavir, Saquinavir
15.	Antiviral (other than HIV)	Acyclovir, Ganciclovir (X), Foscarnet (X), Amantadine (X), Vidarabine (X), α-interferon (X)	—
16.	Antihypertensives	ACE inhibitors (X), Angiotensin antagonists (X), Thiazide diuretics Furosemide, Propranolol, Nitroprusside	Methyldopa, Hydralazine, Atenolol, Metoprolol, Pindolol, Nifedipine, Prazosin, Clonidine
17.	Antianemic	—	Iron salts (oral), Iron dextran (I.M.) Folic acid, Vit B_{12}
18.	Antidiabetics	Sulfonylureas (X), Metformin (X), Pioglitazone, Repaglinide, Nateglinide, Acarbose (X)	Insulin (preferably human insulin)
19.	Corticosteroids	Betamethasone, Dexamethasone (high dose and prolonged use)	Inhaled corticosteroids Topical corticosteroids Prednisolone oral (low dose)
20.	Thyroid hormone (hypothyroidism)	—	Thyroxine
21.	Antithyroid drugs (thyrotoxicosis)	Carbimazole, Radioactive iodine (X), Iodide	Propylthiouracil

Contd...

Contd...

	Drug class (condition)	*Safety uncertain/unsafe*	*Safer alternative*
22.	Antipsychotic (schizophrenia)	Chlorpromazine, Fluphenazine (X), Clozapine, Olanzapine, Risperidone	Haloperidol Trifluoperazine
23.	Antimanic (bipolar illness)	Lithium carbonate, Valproate Carbamazepine	—
24.	Antidepressants	Trimipramine (X), Dothiepin (X) Sertraline, Paroxetine, Citalopram Trazodone, Venlafaxine, Moclobemide	Amitriptyline, Imipramine, Fluoxetine
25.	Anticoagulants (thromboembolism)	Warfarin (X), Acenocoumarol Phenindione (X)	Heparin (unfractionated) Heparin (LMW)
26.	Antiasthmatic	Theophylline, Ketotifen (X), Montelukast, Zafirlukast, Systemic corticosteroids	Salbutamol/Salmeterol, Ipratropium bromide Beclomethasone/ Budesonide, Sod. cromoglycate } Inhaled

186. Failure of lactation occurs due to:

a. Ergot
b. Bromocriptine
c. Chlorpromazine
d. Metoclopramide

Amenorrhea, female infertility, galactorrhea, hypogonadism, and acromegaly may all be caused by pituitary problems, such as hyperprolactinaemia, and, therefore, these problems may be treated with bromocriptine.

187. Which of the following crosses plasma membrane commonly:

a. Vit-D3 b. Androstene-dione
c. Thyroxine d. Epinephrine

Epinephrine crosses the human placenta and may, in high concentrations, cause both maternal and fetal glycogenolysis and elevated blood glucose concentrations.

Thyroxine is indicated for maternal hypothyroidism.

Risk category of drugs during pregnancy*.

Category		*Examples*
A No risk	Adequate studies in pregnant women have failed to demonstrate a risk to the foetus	Inj. Mag. sulfate, thyroxine
B No evidence of risk in humans	Adequate human studies are lacking, but animal studies have failed to demonstrate a risk to the foetus or Adequate studies in pregnant women have failed to demonstrate a risk to the foetus, but animal studies have shown an adverse effect on the foetus	Penicillin V, amoxicillin, cefactor, erythromycin, paracetamol, lidocaine
C Risk cannot be ruled old	No adequate studies in pregnant women, and animal studies are lacking or have shown an adverse effect on foetus, but potential benefit may warrant use of the drug in pregnant women despite potential risk	Morphine, codeine, atropine, corticosteroids, adrenaline, thiopentone, bupivacaine
D Benefit may out weigh potential risk	There is evidence of human foetal risk, but the potential benefits from use of the drug may be acceptable despite the potential risk	Aspirin, phenytoin, carbamazepine, valproate, lorazepam, methotrexate
X Contraindicated	Studies in animals or humans have demonstrated foetal abnormalities, and potential risk clearly outweighs possible benefit	Estrogens, isotretinoin, ergometrine thalidomide

*As per US-FDA.

188. Safest antimalarial during pregnancy is:

a. Quinine
b. Proguanil
c. Pyrimethamine
d. Mefloquine

Proguanil has a long history of safe use during pregnancy, but it should only be used after seeking medical advice from a doctor. It is recommended that pregnant women who take this medicine also take a daily 5 mg supplement of folic acid.

189. Dose of anti-D immunoglobulin (in microgram) to Rh negative (post partum) mother:

a. 50 b. 150
c. 300 d. 450

The rosette test is a sensitive method to detect fetomaternal hemorrhage of 10 cc or more. A rosette test will be positive if fetal D-positive cells are present in the maternal sample, indicating a significantly large fetomaternal hemorrhage has occurred. A rosette test may be falsely positive if the mother is positive for the

Ans. **186. b.** Bromocriptine **187. d.** Epinephrine **188. b.** Proguanil **189. c.** 300

weak D phenotype and falsely negative if the neonate is weak D. If the rosette test is negative, then a dose of 300 micrograms of RhIG is given (sufficient to prevent alloimmunization after delivery in 99% of cases).

190. Fetal hydantoin syndrome is caused by:
a. Sodium valproate b. Alcohol
c. Phenytoin d. Tetracycline

Fetal hydantoin syndrome, also called **fetal dilantin syndrome** is a group of defects caused to the developing fetus by exposure to the teratogenic effects of phenytoin or carbamazepine. Dilantin is the brand name of the drug phenytoin sodium in the United States, commonly used in the treatment of epilepsy.

It may also be called **congenital hydantoin syndrome**, **Fetal Hydantoin Syndrome**, **Dilantin Embryopathy**, or **Phenytoin Embryopathy**.

Association with EPHX1 has been suggested.

Human teratogenic drugs

Drug	*Abnormality*
Thalidomide	Phocomelia, multiple defects of internal organs
Anticancer drugs (methotrexate)	Cleft palate, hydrocephalus, multiple defects, foetal death
Androgens	Virilization; limb, esophageal, cardiac defects
Progestins	Virilization of female foetus
Stilboestrol	Vaginal carcinoma in teenage female offspring
Tetracyclines	Discoloured and deformed teeth, retarded bone growth
Warfarin	Depressed nose; eye and hand defects, growth retardation
Phenytoin	Hypoplastic phalanges, cleft lip/palate, microcephaly
Phenobarbitone	Various malformations
Carbamazepine	Neural tube defects, assorted abnormalities
Valproate sod.	Spina bifida and other neural tube defects, heart and limb abnormalities
Alcohol	Low IQ baby, growth retardation, foetal alcohol syndrome
ACE inhibitors	Hypoplasia of organs, growth retardation, foetal loss
Lithium	Foetal goiter, cardiac and other abnormalities
Antithyroid drugs	Foetal goiter and hypothyroidism
Indomethacin/aspirin	Premature closure of ductus arteriosus
Isotretinoin	Craniofacial, heart and CNS defects, hydrocephalus

191. A child has phocomelia. This is due to drug taken by mother:
a. Tetracycline b. Thalidomide
c. Warf d. Chloroquine

Phocomelia ("seal (animal)" + "limb") is an extremely rare congenital disorder involving malformation of the limbs (dysmelia). Étienne Geoffroy Saint-Hilaire coined the term in 1836. Although many factors can cause phocomelia, the prominent roots come from the use of the drug thalidomide and from genetic inheritance.

SIDE EFFECTS

192. Photodermatitis and corneal microdeposits are side effects of:
a. Verapamil b. Procainamide
c. Flecainide d. Amiodarone

Corneal micro-deposits (Cornea verticillata, also called vortex or whorl keratopathy) are almost universally present (over 90%) in individuals taking amiodarone longer than 6 months, especially doses greater than 400 mg/day. These deposits typically do not cause any symptoms. Long-term administration of amiodarone (usually more than eighteen months) is associated with a light-sensitive blue-grey discoloration of the skin; such patients should avoid exposure to the sun and use sunscreen that protects against ultraviolet-A and -B.

193. NOT a cause of gynecomastia:
a. Pyrazinamide b. Digitalis
c. Cimetidine d. INH

The most common (approximately 1%) side effect of pyrazinamide is joint pains (arthralgia), but this is not usually so severe that patients need to stop taking the pyrazinamide. Pyrazinamide can precipitate gout flares by decreasing renal excretion of uric acid. The most dangerous side effect of pyrazinamide is hepatotoxicity, which is dose related. It is contraindicated in patients with liver disease. Safety during pregnancy is uncertain.

194. Drug causing retroperitoneal fibrosis:
a. Methysergide b. Cyclosporine
c. Melphalan d. Vincristine

Methysergide (1-methyl-*D*-lysergic acid butanolamide) is a prescription drug formerly used for prophylaxis of cluster headaches/migraine headaches, but is no longer recommended due to retroperitoneal/retropulmonary fibrosis.

Ans. **190. c.** Phenytoin **191. b.** Thalidomide **192. d.** Amiodarone **193. a.** Pyrazinamide **194. a.** Methysergide

195. Hemolysis in G6PD is precipitated by all except:

a. Dapsone b. Cotrimoxazole
c. Quinine d. Penicillin

Many substances are potentially harmful to people with G6PD deficiency. Variation in response to these substances makes individual predictions difficult. Antimalarial drugs that can cause acute hemolysis in people with G6PD deficiency include primaquine, pamaquine, and chloroquine. There is evidence that other antimalarials may also exacerbate G6PD deficiency, but only at higher doses. Sulfonamides (such as sulfanilamide, sulfamethoxazole, and mafenide), thiazolesulfone, methylene blue, and naphthalene should also be avoided by people with G6PD deficiency as they antagonize folate synthesis, as should certain analgesics (such as aspirin, phenazopyridine, and acetanilide) and a few non-sulfa antibiotics (nalidixic acid, nitrofurantoin, isoniazid, dapsone, and furazolidone).

196. Pancreatitis occurs with:

a. Abacavir b. Zidovudine
c. Lamivudine d. Didanosine

The most common adverse events with didanosine are diarrhea, nausea, vomiting, abdominal pain, fever, headache and rash. Peripheral neuropathy occurred in 21-26% of participants in key didanosine trials. Pancreatitis is rarely observed but has caused occasional fatalities, and has black box warning status.

First-line antiretroviral regimens*.
Preferred regimen
1. Lamivudine + Zidovudine + Nevirapine
Alternative regimens
1. Lamivudine + Zidovudine + Efavirenz
2. Lamivudine + Stavudine[1] + Efavirenz
3. Lamivudine + Stavudine + Nevirapine
Other options
1. Lamivudine + Tenofovir[2] + Nevirapine
2. Lamivudine + Tenofovir[2] + Efavirenz
3. Lamivudine[3] + Zidovudine + Tenofovir

* Recommended by NACO

1. Stavudine is substituted for zidovudine if patient is anaemic
2. Tenofovir is included when there is toxicity or other contraindication to both zidovudine and stavudine
3. 3NRTI regimen is only for patients unable to tolerate both nevirapine and efavirenz.

197. NOT a hepatotoxic antitubercular drug:

a. Pyrazinamide b. Rifampicin
c. INH d. Ethambutol

Side effects of ethambutol

- Optic neuritis (hence contraindicated in children below six years of age)
- Red-green color blindness
- Peripheral neuropathy
- Arthralgia
- Hyperuricaemia
- Vertical nystagmus
- Milk skin reaction

Recommended doses of antitubercular drugs.@

DRUG	Daily dose		3 times per week dose	
	mg/kg	*maximum*	*mg/kg*	*daily maximum*
Isoniazid (H)	5 (4–6)	300 mg 10 (8–12)	900 mg	
Rifampin (R)	10 (8–12)	600 mg 10 (8–12)	600 mg	
Pyrazinamide (Z)	25 (20–30)	–	35 (30–40)	–
Ethambutol (E)	15 (15–20)	–	30 (25–35)	–
Streptomycin (S)*	15 (12–18)	–	15 (12–18)	1000 mg

* Patients over 60 years age—10 mg/kg or 500–750 mg/day (i.m.).
@ Adopted from Treatment of Tuberculosis: Guidelines, 4th edition (2010), WHO, Geneva.

198. Drug causing cholestatic jaundice:

a. Ethionamide
b. Pyrazinamide
c. Erythromycin estolate
d. INH

Gastrointestinal disturbances, such as diarrhea, nausea, abdominal pain, and vomiting, are very common because erythromycin is a motilin agonist. Because of this, erythromycin tends not to be prescribed as a first-line drug. It may be useful in treating gastroparesis due to this promotility effect. Intravenous erythromycin may also be used in endoscopy as an adjunct to clear gastric contents. More serious side effects include arrhythmia with prolonged QT intervals including *torsades de pointes*, and reversible deafness. Allergic reactions range from urticaria to anaphylaxis. Cholestasis, Stevens–Johnson syndrome, and toxic epidermal necrolysis are some other rare side effects that may occur.

Ans. 195. d. Penicillin 196. d. Didanosine 197. d. Ethambutol 198. c. Erythromycin estolate

199. Oral hypoglycemic agent causing cholestatic jaundice:
a. Tolbutamide b. Glibenclamide
c. Glipizide d. Chlorpropamide

Drugs such as gold salts, nitrofurantoin, anabolic steroids, chlorpromazine, prochlorperazine, sulindac, cimetidine, erythromycin, estrogen, and statins can cause cholestasis and may result in damage to the liver.

200. Hyperprolactinemia is a side-effect of:
a. Metoclopramide b. Amantadine
c. Levo-dopa d. Bromocriptine

Common adverse drug reactions (ADRs) associated with metoclopramide therapy include restlessness (akathisia), and focal dystonia. Infrequent ADRs include hypertension, hypotension, hyperprolactinaemia leading to galactorrhea, constipation, depression, headache, and extrapyramidal effects such as oculogyric crisis. Rare but serious ADRs associated with metoclopramide therapy include agranulocytosis, supraventricular tachycardia, hyperaldosteronism, neuroleptic malignant syndrome, akathisia and tardive dyskinesia.

201. Cough is an adverse effect of:
a. Prazosin b. Enalapril
c. Nifedipine d. Thiazide

The most common side effects of enalapril include increased serum creatinine (20%), dizziness (2–8%), low blood pressure (1–7%), syncope (2%), and dry cough (1–2%). The most serious common adverse event is angioedema (swelling) (0.68%) which often affects the face and lips, endangering the patient's airway.

Comparative features of some ACE inhibitors.

	Captopril	*Enalapril*	*Lisinopril*	*Fosinopril*	*Perindopril*	*Ramipril*
1. Chemical nature	Sulfhydryl	Carboxyl	Carboxyl	Phosphinate	Carboxyl	Carboxyl
2. Activity status	Active	Prodrug	Active	Prodrug	Prodrug	Prodrug
3. Bioavailability (as active form)	70%	50%	25%	30%	30–50%	60%
4. Time to peak action	1 hr	4–6 hr	6–8 hr	3–5 hr	6 hr	3–6 hr
5. Elimination t½*	2 hr	11 hr	12 hr	12 hr	25–30 hr	8–48 hr
6. Mode of excretion	Renal	Renal	Renal	Renal/hepatic	Renal	Renal
7. Duration of action		6–12 hr	24 hr ≥ 24 hr	24 hr	> 24 hr	>24 hr
8. Daily dose (mg)	25–150	2.5–40	5–40	10–40	2–8	1.25–10

*t½ including that of active metabolite

202. The major toxicity of acetaminophen overdose involves:
a. CNS b. Heart
c. Liver d. Acid-base metabolism

Paracetamol toxicity is caused by excessive use or overdose of the analgesic drug paracetamol (called acetaminophen in North America). Mainly causing liver injury, paracetamol toxicity is one of the most common causes of poisoning worldwide.

203. Pulmonary fibrosis is a side effect of:
a. Methotrexate b. Vincristine
c. Adriomycin d. Busulfan

Toxicity of busulfan may include interstitial pulmonary fibrosis ("Busulfan Lung"), hyperpigmentation, seizures, hepatic (veno-occlusive disease) (VOD), emesis, and wasting syndrome. Busulfan also induces thrombocytopenia, a condition of lowered blood platelet count and activity. Seizures and VOD are serious concerns with busulfan therapy and prophylaxis is often utilized to avoid these effects. Hepatic VOD is a dose-limiting toxicity.

204. Peripheral neuropathy may occur with the use of all of the following except:
a. Vincristine b. Cisplatin
c. L-asparaginase d. Procarbazine

The main side effect of L-asparaginase is an allergic or hypersensitivity reaction; anaphylaxis is a possibility. Additionally, it can also be associated with a coagulopathy as it decreases protein synthesis, including synthesis of coagulation factors (e.g. progressive isolated decrease of fibrinogen) and anticoagulant factor (generally antithrombin III; sometimes protein C and S as well), leading to bleeding or thrombotic events such as stroke. Bone marrow suppression is common but only mild to moderate, rarely reaches clinical significance and therapeutic consequences are rarely required.

Other common side effects include pancreatitis.

205. Maximum propensity for photodermatitis:
a. Oxytetracycline b. Doxycycline
c. Minocycline d. Beta2 agonist

An erythematous rash in sun-exposed parts of the body has been reported to occur in 7.3–21.2% of persons taking doxycycline. The rash resolves upon discontinuation of the drug. Unlike some other members of the tetracycline group, it may be used in those with renal impairment. Doxycycline is contraindicated in the pediatric treatment of acute bacterial rhinosinusitis.

Ans. 199. **d.** Chlorpropamide 200. **a.** Metoclopramide 201. **b.** Enalapril 202. **c.** Liver
203. **d.** Busulfan 204. **c.** L-asparaginase 205. **b.** Doxycycline

206. Gynaecomastia is caused by:

a. Clomiphene citrate b. Tamoxifen
c. Spironolactone d. Testosterone

The most common side effect of spironolactone is urinary frequency. Other general side effects include ataxia, drowsiness, dry skin, and rashes. Because it reduces androgen levels and blocks androgen receptors, spironolactone can, in males, cause breast tenderness, gynecomastia, and physical feminization in general, as well as testicular atrophy, reversible infertility, and sexual dysfunction, including loss of libido and erectile dysfunction. In females, spironolactone can cause menstrual irregularities and breast tenderness and enlargement, likely due to a combination of its progestogenic and indirect estrogenic actions.

207. Pulmonary fibrosis is a side effect of:

a. Mitomycin-C b. Hydroxyurea
c. Bleomycin d. Cisplatin

The most serious complication of bleomycin is pulmonary fibrosis and impaired lung function. It has been suggested that bleomycin induces sensitivity to oxygen toxicity and recent studies support the role of the proinflammatory cytokines IL-18 and IL-1beta in the mechanism of bleomycin-induced lung injury. Any previous treatment with bleomycin should therefore always be disclosed to the anaesthetist prior to undergoing a procedure requiring general anaesthesia.

208. Ototoxicity and nephrotoxicity may be the side effect of:

a. Vancomycin b. Azithromycin
c. Clindamycin d. Penicillin

Common adverse drug reactions (≥1% of patients) associated with IV vancomycin include: local pain, which may be severe, and thrombophlebitis.

Damage to the kidneys and to the hearing were a side effect of the early impure versions of vancomycin, and these were prominent in the clinical trials. Later trials using purer forms of vancomycin found nephrotoxicity is an infrequent adverse effect (0.1–1% of patients), but this is accentuated in the presence of aminoglycosides.

MISCELLANEOUS

209. All of the following are used in drug induced vomiting EXCEPT:

a. Chlorpromazine
b. Hyoscine
c. Metoclopramide
d. Ondansetron

Scopolamine/ Hyoscine exerts its effects by acting as a competitive antagonist at muscarinic acetylcholine receptors, specifically M1 receptors and is useful in motion sickness and post-operative nausea and vomiting.

210. All of the following beta blockers have an intrinsic sympathomimetic activity EXCEPT:

a. Acebutolol b. Pindolol
c. Propanolol d. Celiprolol

Propranolol is a sympatholytic nonselective beta blocker. It is used to treat high blood pressure, a number of heart dysrhythmias, those with thyrotoxicosis, and essential tremors. It is used to prevent migraine headaches, and further heart problems in those with angina or previous myocardial infarction.

211. Lugol's solution is:

a. 5% iodine & 5% potassium iodide
b. 5% iodine & 10% potassium iodide
c. 10% iodine & 5% potassium iodide
d. 10% iodine & 10% potassium iodide

Lugol's solution is available in different potencies of 1%, 2%, or 5% iodine. The 5% solution consists of 5% (wt/v) iodine (I2) and 10% (wt/v) potassium iodide (KI) mixed in distilled water and has a total iodine content of 5 mg/mL.

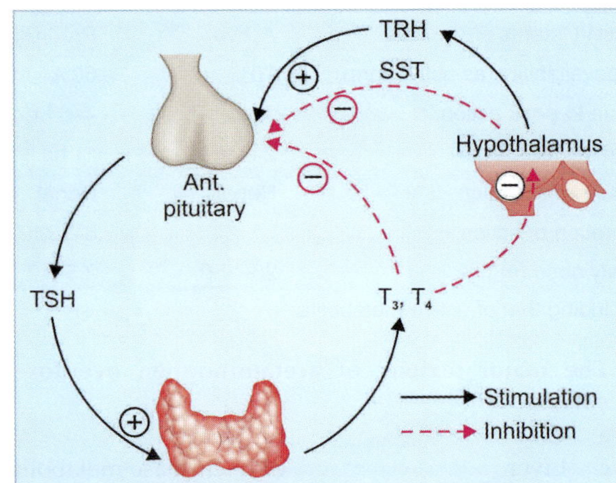

Regulation of thyroid function TSH—Thyroid stimulating hormone; TRH—Thyrotropin releasing hormone; T_3—Triiodothyronine; T_4—Thyroxine; SST—Somatostatin.

212. Which of the following is the treatment of mild drug allergy:

a. Antidote
b. Steroid
c. Stop the offending drug & start symptomatic treatment
d. I/V adrenaline

Treatments for allergies include avoiding known allergens, steroids that modify the immune system in general, and medications such as antihistamines and decongestants which reduce symptoms. Many of these medications are taken by mouth, although epinephrine, which is used to treat anaphylactic reactions, is injected.

213. Which of the following is a PDE-4 inhibitor drug:

a. Amrinone b. Milrinone
c. Sildenafil d. Drotaverine

Ans. **206. c.** Spironolactone **207. c.** Bleomycin **208. a.** Vancomycin **209. b.** Hyoscine **210. c.** Propranolol **211. b.** 5% iodine & 10%... **212. c.** Stop the offending... **213. d.** Drotaverine

Drotaverine is an antispasmodic drug, structurally related to papaverine. Drotaverine is a selective inhibitor of phosphodiesterase 4, and has no anticholinergic effects,

214. Drug increasing gastro-intestinal motility:

a. Fentanyl
b. Neostigmine
c. Atropine
d. Glycopyrrolate

Neostigmine (from greek *neos*, meaning "new," and "-stigmine," in reference to its parent molecule, physostigmine, on which it is based) is a parasympathomimetic compound that acts as a reversible acetylcholinesterase inhibitor. Given that it is a quaternary amine (unlike physostigmine, which is a tertiary amine), it penetrates the central nervous system poorly and has lower propensity to cause side effects there.

Comparative features of physostigmine and neostigmine.

	Physostigmine	*Neostigmine*
1. Source	Natural alkaloid from *Physostigma venenosum* (Calabar bean)	Synthetic
2. Chemistry	Tertiary amine derivative	Quaternary ammonium compound
3. Oral absorption	Good	Poor
4. CNS actions	Present	Absent
5. Applied to eye	Penetrates cornea	Poor penetration
6. Direct action on N_M cholinoceptors	Absent	Present
7. Prominent effect on	Autonomic effectors	Skeletal muscles
8. Important use	Miotic (glaucoma)	Myasthenia gravis
9. Dose	0.5–1 mg oral/parenteral	0.5–2.5 mg i.m./s.c.
	0.1–1.0% eye drops	15–30 mg orally
10. Duration of action	Systemic 4–6 hrs In eye 6 to 24 hrs	3–4 hrs.

215. Mechanism of action of pralidoxime:

a. Direct activation of cholinergic receptors
b. Reactivation of cholinesterase
c. Inactivation of cholinesterase
d. Inhibition of acetylcholine

Pralidoxime is typically used in cases of organophosphate poisoning. The acetylcholinesterase enzyme has two parts to it. An acetylcholine molecule, bound at both ends to both sites of the enzyme, is cleaved in two to form acetic acid and choline. In organophosphate poisoning, an organophosphate binds to just one end of the acetylcholinesterase enzyme (the esteric site), blocking its activity. Pralidoxime is able to attach to the other half (the unblocked, anionic site) of the acetylcholinesterase enzyme. It then binds to the organophosphate, the organophosphate changes conformation, and loses its binding to the acetylcholinesterase enzyme. The conjoined poison/antidote then unbinds from the site, and thus regenerates the enzyme, which is now able to function again.

216. Atropine is CONTRAINDICATED in:

a. Scleritis
b. Corneal ulcer
c. Glaucoma
d. Infants

Atropine is contraindicated in patients pre-disposed to narrow angle glaucoma.

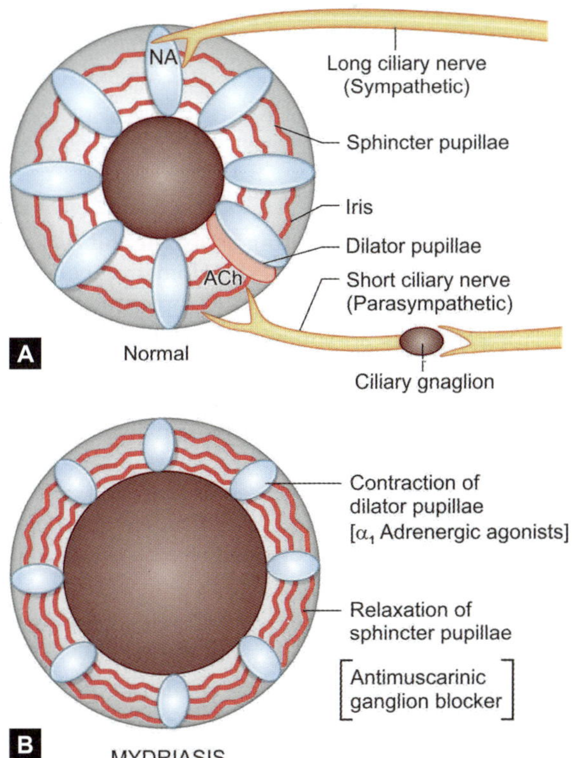

Contd...

Ans. 214. b. Neostigmine **215. b.** Reactivation... **216. c.** Glaucoma

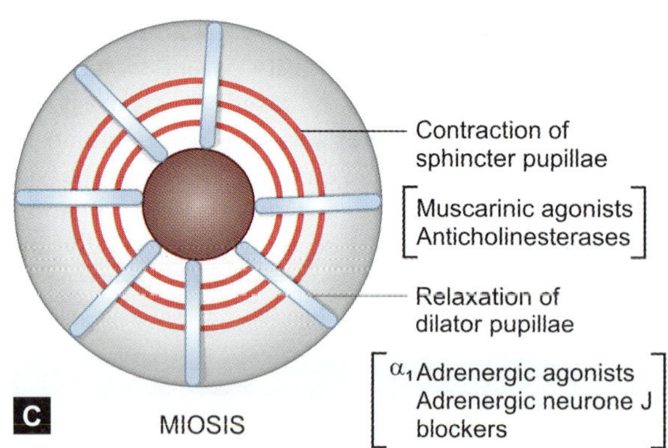

Autonomic control of pupil (A); and site of action of mydriatics (B) and miotics (C).

217. NOT a cardio-selective beta-blocker:

a. Metoprolol b. Pindolol
c. Atenolol d. Acebutolol

Pindolol is a nonselective beta blocker with partial beta-adrenergic receptor agonist activity and also possesses intrinsic sympathomimetic activity. This means that pindolol, particularly in high doses, exerts effects like epinephrine or isoprenaline (increased pulse rate, increased blood pressure, bronchodilation), but these effects are limited.

First generation (older, nonselective)	Second generation (β1 selective)	Third generation (with additional α blocking and/ or vasodilator property)
Propranolol	Metoprolol	Labetalol
Timolol	Atenolol	Carvedilol
Sotalol	Acebutolol	Celiprolol
Pindolol	Bisoprolol	Nebivolol
	Esmolol	Betaxolol

218. Which is the shortest acting mydriatic and cycloplegic:

a. Scopolamine b. Homatropine
c. Cyclopentolate d. Tropicamide

Tropicamide is an antimuscarinic drug that produces short acting mydriasis (dilation of the pupil) and cycloplegia when applied as eye drops. It is used to allow better examination of the lens, vitreous humor, and retina. Due to its relatively short duration of effect (4–8 hours), it is typically used during eye examinations such as the dilated fundus examination, but it may also be used before or after eye surgery.

219. Adrenaline increases all of the following except:

a. Automaticity b. Conduction velocity
c. Refractory period d. Contractility

Epinephrine is a nonselective agonist of all adrenergic receptors, including the major subtypes α_1, α_2, β_1, β_2, and β_3. Stimulation of β_1 receptors by epinephrine and norepinephrine induces a positive chronotropic and inotropic effect on the heart and increases cardiac conduction velocity and automaticity.

Comparative effects of intravenous infusion of adrenaline, noradrenaline and isoprenaline.

	Adr	*NA*	*Iso*
1. Heart rate	↑	↓	↑↑
2. Cardiac output	↑↑	–	↑↑
3. BP—Systolic	↑↑	↑↑	↑
Diastolic	↓↑	↑↑	↓↓
Mean	↑	↑↑	↓
4. Blood flow			
Skin and mm	↓	↓	–
Sk. muscle	↑↑	–, ↓	
Kidney	↓	↓	–
Liver	↑↑	–	↑
Coronary	↑	↑	↑
5. Bronchial muscle	↓↓	–	↓↓
6. Intestinal muscle	↓↓	↓	↓
7. Blood sugar	↑↑	–, ↑	↑

220. Immediate treatment of anaphylaxis is:

a. Hydrocortisone b. Atropine
c. Adrenaline d. Benzyl penicillin

Epinephrine is the drug of choice for treating anaphylaxis. Different strengths, doses and routes of administration of epinephrine are used.

The commonly used epinephrine autoinjector delivers a 0.3 mg epinephrine injection (0.3 mL, 1:1000) and is indicated in the emergency treatment of allergic reactions including anaphylaxis to stings, contrast agents, medicines or people with a history of anaphylactic reactions to known triggers.

221. Decrease in vascular resistance of mesenteric and renal vasculature is caused by:

a. Dopamine b. Dobutamine
c. Ephedrine d. Noradrenaline

Dopamine is a dopaminergic (D1 and D2) as well as alpha and beta1 (not beta2) agonist. The D1 receptors in renal and mesenteric blood vessels are the most sensitive: intravenous infusion of low dose of DA dilates these vessels (by raising intracellular cAMP). This increases GFR.

222. Dopamine is preferred in treatment of shock due to:

a. Renal vasodilatory effect
b. Increased cardiac output
c. Peripheral vasoconstriction
d. Prolonged action

Dopamine stimulates adrenergic and dopaminergic receptors. Its hemodynamic effect depends on the dose. Lower doses primarily stimulate dopaminergic receptors that produce renal and mesenteric vasodilation. Higher doses produce cardiac stimulation and vasoconstriction.

Ans. 217. **b.** Pindolol 218. **d.** Tropicamide 219. **c.** Refractory period 220. **c.** Adrenaline 221. **a.** Dopamine 222. **a.** Renal vasodilatory effect

223. Drug which is alpha as well as beta blocker:

a. Atenolol b. Acebutolol
c. Metoprolol d. Labetalol

Labetalol is a dual alpha (α1) and beta (β1/β2) adrenergic receptor blocker and competes with other Catecholamines for binding to these sites. Its action on these receptors are potent and reversible. Labetalol is highly selective for postsynaptic alpha1-adrenergic, and non-selective for beta-adrenergic receptors. It is about equipotent in blocking both beta1- and beta2- receptors.

Comparative properties of β blockers.

β–BLOCKER	Potency (on β1)	Partial agonistic action	Membrane stabilizing action	Lipid solubility	Daily dose (mg)	Oral bioavailability (%)	First pass metabolism	Major route of elimination	Plasma t½ (hours)
Nonselective									
1. Propranolol	1	–	++	+++	40–480	~30	Yes	Hep.*	3–5
2. Sotalol	1/3	–	–	±	160–480	~60	No	Ren.[I]+Hep.	6–12
3. Timolol	6	–	–	++	10–40	50–75	Partial	Ren.+Hep.	4–5
4. Pindolol	6	+++	±	+	10–30	90	No	Ren.+Hep.	3–4
Cardioselective									
1. Metoprolol	1	–	±	++	100–400	40–50	Yes	Hep.	3–6
2. Atenolol	1	–	–	–	25–100	50–60	No	Ren.	6–9
3. Acebutolol	1/3	+	+	±	400–1200	40–60	Yes	Hep.+Ren.	3–4
4. Bisoprolol	6	–	–	–	2.5–10	80	No	Hep.+Ren.	9–12
α + β Blocker									
1. Labetalol	1/3	+	+	±	300–600	~30	Yes	Hep.	4–6

*Hep: Hepatic metabolism; [I]Ren.: Renal excretion

224. Use of ergotamine is CONTRAINDICATED in:

a. DM
b. Anemia
c. Ischemic heart disease
d. Post partum hemorrhage

Ergotamine produces vasoconstriction peripherally as well as damages the peripheral epithelium. In high doses, ergotamine is conducive to vascular stasis, thrombosis, and gangrene. It can increase uterine contractivity and occasionally is used therapeutically immediately post-partum to decrease uterine bleeding. Ergotamine continues to be prescribed for migraines.

Contraindications include: atherosclerosis, Buerger's syndrome, coronary artery disease, hepatic disease, pregnancy, pruritus, Raynaud's syndrome, and renal disease.

225. ONLY mydriatic action is:

a. Tropicamide b. Homatropine
c. Phenylephrine d. Cyclopentolate

Phenylephrine is used as an eye drop to dilate the pupil to facilitate visualization of the retina. It is often used in combination with tropicamide as a synergist when tropicamide alone is not sufficient. Narrow-angle glaucoma is a contraindication to phenylephrine use. As a mydriatic, it is available in 2.5% and 10% minims. Phenylephrine eye drops are applied to the eye after a topical anestheic is applied.

226. Beta-blockers are used in all of the following except:

a. Essential tremors b. AV block
c. Angina pectoris d. Migraine prophylaxis

The antiarrhythmic effects of beta blockers arise from sympathetic nervous system blockade—resulting in depression of sinus node function and atrioventricular node conduction, and prolonged atrial refractory periods. Propranolol is contraindicated in partial and complete heart block; arrest may occur.

227. Which of the following is the shortest acting beta-blocker:

a. Acebutolol b. Sotalol
c. Bisoprolol d. Esmolol

Esmolol is a cardioselective beta$_1$ receptor blocker with rapid onset, a very short duration of action (half life of <10 minutes; action disappears 15-20 minutes after terminating i.v. infusion), and no significant intrinsic sympathomimetic or membrane stabilising activity at therapeutic dosages.

228. Dopamine is preferred over dobutamine in treatment of renal shock because:

a. Renal vasodilatory effect
b. Increased cardiac output
c. Peripheral vasoconstriction
d. Prolonged action

Ans. 223. **d.** Labetalol 224. **c.** Ischemic heart disease 225. **c.** Phenylephrine 226. **b.** AV block
227. **d.** Esmolol 228. **a.** Renal vasodilatory...

Dopamine is a direct-acting catecholamine with a short half-life that has many advantages in treating visceral hypoperfusion states such as shock and refractory heart failure. Unlike other inotropic drugs, dopamine directly dilates the mesenteric, renal, and cerebral vessels and redirects blood flow to essential viscera. This dopaminergic effect is prominent with doses of 100-700 μg/min in adults and is attenuated by phenothiazines and haloperidol. At doses of 700-1400 μg/min, dopamine also has a significant beta-adrenergic, inotropic effect, increasing myocardial contractility. The inotropic effect is equivalent to that of isoproterenol, epinephrine, and norepinephrine, but tachycardia, tachyarrhythmias, and angina may be less frequent with dopamine. In doses greater than 1400 mug/min, dopamine is a vasoconstrictor with pressor effects usually equivalent to that of norepinephrine. Dopamine does not dilate bronchi, and does not shunt blood from viscera to skeletal muscles as does isoproterenol. Because dopamine increases myocardial contractility, selectively redistributes perfusion to essential viscera and allows a pharmacologic titration of effect, it is a logical first-choice catecholamine for treatment of shock and refractory heart failure.

229. Effects of beta blocker on heart are all of the following except:

a. Decrease in heart rate
b. Decreases duration of systole
c. Decreases cardiac output
d. Precipitates heart failure

Because there is generally some level of sympathetic tone on the heart, beta-blockers are able to reduce sympathetic influences that normally stimulate chronotropy (heart rate), inotropy (contractility), dromotropy (electrical conduction) and lusitropy (relaxation). Therefore, beta-blockers cause decreases in heart rate, contractility, conduction velocity, and relaxation rate. They prolong systole by retarding conduction so that synergy of contraction of ventricular fibres is disturbed. These drugs have an even greater effect when there is elevated sympathetic activity.

230. Features of atropine poisoning are all of the following except:

a. Mydriasis
b. Hypothermia
c. Confusion
d. Hallucinations

Adverse reactions to atropine include ventricular fibrillation, supraventricular or ventricular tachycardia, dizziness, nausea, blurred vision, loss of balance, dilated pupils, photophobia, dry mouth and potentially extreme confusion, dissociative hallucinations and excitation especially amongst the elderly. There is rise in body temperature occurs at higher doses. It is due to both inhibition of sweating as well as stimulation of temperature regulating centre in the hypothalamus.

Relative autonomic tone and effects of ganglionic blockade on organ function.

Organ	*Dominant tone*	*Effect of ganglionic blockade (Side effect)*
1. Heart	Para-symp.	Tachycardia (palpitation)
2. Blood vessels	Symp.	Vasodilatation, abolition of reflexes (postural and exercise hypotension, syncope)
3. Iris	Para-symp.	Mydriasis (photophobia)
4. Ciliary muscle	Para-symp.	Cycloplegia (blurring of near vision)
5. Intestines	Para-symp.	Decreased motility (distension, constipation)
6. Bladder	Para-symp.	Decreased tone (difficulty in micturition)
7. Male sexual function	Para-symp. Symp.	Inhibition of erection Inhibition of ejaculation } (impotence)
8. Salivary glands	Para-symp.	Inhibition of salivation (dryness of mouth, difficulty in swallowing and talking)
9. Sweat glands	Symp. (cholinergic)	Inhibition of sweating (anhydrosis)

231. Drug most useful in cardiogenic shock:

a. Dopamine b. Dobutamine
c. Noradrenaline d. Adrenaline

Cardiogenic shock may be treated with intravenous dobutamine, which acts on $\beta_1$receptors of the heart leading to increased contractility and heart rate.

Adrenergic responses mediated through α and β receptors.

α actions	*β actions*
1. Constriction of arterioles and veins → rise in BP (α_1 + α_2)	Dilatation of arterioles and veins → fall in BP (β_2)
2. Heart—little action, arrhythmia at high dose (α_1)	Cardiac stimulation (β_1), ↑ rate, force and conduction velocity
3. —	Bronchodilatation (β_2)
4. Contraction of radial muscles of iris → mydriasis (α_1), decreased aqueous secretion	No effect on iris, slight relaxation of ciliary muscle, enhanced aqueous secretion

Contd...

Ans. **229. b.** Decreases... **230. b.** Hypothermia **231. a.** Dopamine

Contd...

α actions	*β actions*
5. Intestinal relaxation, contraction of sphincters	Intestinal relaxation (β_2)
6. Bladder trigone—contraction (α_1)	Detrusor—relaxation (β_2)
7. Uterus—contraction (α_1)	Relaxation (β_2)
8. Splenic capsule—contraction (α_1)	Relaxation (β_2) (slight)
9. Neuromuscular transmission facilitated, ↑ ACh release	Active state—prolonged in fast contracting muscle, abbreviated in slow contracting muscle; tremors (β_2)
10. Insulin secretion inhibited (α_2) (dominant)	Augmented insulin (mild) and glucagon secretion (β_2)
11. Liver—glycogenolysis (α in some species)	Liver—glycogenolysis (β_2) → hyperglycaemia Muscle—glycogenolysis (β_2) → hyperlactacidaemia Fat—lipolysis ($\beta_1 + \beta_2 + \beta_3$) → increased blood FFA, calorigenesis
12. —	Renin release from kidney (β_1)
13. Male sex organs—ejaculation (α_1)	—
14. Salivary gland—K^+ and water secretion (α_1)	Ptyalin secretion
15. —	ADH secretion from posterior pituitary (β_1)
16. Nictitating membrane—contraction (in animals)	—

232. Misoprostol is:

a. Prostaglandin E1 analogue
b. Prostaglandin E2 analogue
c. Prostaglandin antagonist
d. Antiprogestin

Misoprostol is a medication used to start labor, cause an abortion, prevent and treat stomach ulcers, and treat postpartum bleeding due to poor contraction of the uterus. For abortions it is often used with mifepristone or methotrexate. By itself effectiveness for this purpose is between 66% and 90%. It is taken either by mouth, under the tongue, or placed in the vagina. It is a synthetic prostaglandin E_1(PGE_1).

233. Which of the following is beneficial in NSAID induced gastric ulcer:

a. PGE1 agonist
b. PGE2 agonist
c. PGD agonist
d. PGF2 agonist

Misoprostol is approved for use in the prevention of NSAID-induced gastric ulcers. It acts upon gastric parietal cells, inhibiting the secretion of gastric acid by G-protein coupled receptor-mediated inhibition of adenylate cyclase, which leads to decreased intracellular cyclic AMP levels and decreased proton pump activity at the apical surface of the parietal cell. Because other classes of drugs, especially H2-receptor antagonists and proton pump inhibitors (drug of choice), are more effective for the treatment of acute peptic ulcers, misoprostol is only indicated for use by people who are both taking NSAIDs and are at high risk for NSAID-induced ulcers, including the elderly and people with ulcer complications. Misoprostol is sometimes coprescribed with NSAIDs to prevent their common adverse effect of gastric ulceration.

A summary of the actions of major prostaglandins, prostacyclin and thromboxane.

Organ	*Prostaglandin E_2 (PGE_2)*	*Prostaglandin $F_{2\alpha}$ ($PGF_{2\alpha}$)*	*Prostacyclin (PGI_2)*	*Thromboxane A_2 (TXA_2)*
1. Blood vessels	Vasodilatation, ↓ BP	Vasodilatation (mostly), veins constrict, little effect on BP larger	Vasodilatation (marked and widespread), ↓ ↓ BP	Vasoconstriction
2. Heart Weak	Weak inotropic, reflex cardiac stimulation		—	—
3. Platelets	Variable effect	—	Antiaggregatory	Aggregation and release reaction
4. Uterus	Contraction (*in vivo*), relaxes non-gravid human uterus *in vitro*, softening of cervix	Contraction (*in vivo* and *in vitro*), softening of cervix	—	—
5. Bronchi	Dilatation, Inhibit histamine release	Constriction	Dilatation (mild), inhibit histamine release	Constriction
6. Stomach	↓ acid secretion, ↑ mucus production	—	↓ acid secretion (weak), mucosal vasodilatation	—

Contd...

Ans. 232. a. Prostaglandin... **233. a.** PGE1 agonist

Contd...

Organ	*Prostaglandin E_2 (PGE_2)*	*Prostaglandin $F_{2\alpha}$ ($PGF_{2\alpha}$)*	*Prostacyclin (PGI_2)*	*Thromboxane A_2 (TXA_2)*
7. Intestine	Contracts longitudinal and relaxes circular muscles, ↑ peristalsis, ↑ Cl^- & water secretion	Spasmogenic, ↑ fluid and electrolyte secretion (weak)	Weak spasmogenic, inhibit toxin-induced fluid secretion	Weak spasmogenic
8. Kidney	Natriuresis, ↓ Cl^- reabsorption, inhibit ADH action, vasodilatation, renin release	—	Natriuresis, vasodilatation, renin release	Vasoconstriction
9. CNS	Pyrogenic, variety of effects on i.c.v. inj.			
10. Release of NA	↑ or ↓	↑ or ↓		
11. Afferent nerves	Sensitize to noxious stimuli → tenderness	—	Same as PGE_2	—
12. Endocrine system	Release of ant. pituitary hormones, steroids, insulin; TSH-like action	Release of gonadotropins & prolactin, luteolysis (in animals)	—	—
13. Metabolism	Antilipolytic, insulin-like action, mobilization of bone Ca^{2+}	—	—	—

234. An uricosuric drug:

a. Allopurinol b. Probenecid
c. Indomethacin d. Aspirin

Probenecid increases uric acid excretion in the urine. It is primarily used in treating gout and hyperuricemia.

235. Drug used in acute gout:

a. Aspirin b. Indomethacin
c. Allopurinol d. All of the above

Treatment with nonsteroidal anti-inflammatory drugs (NSAIDs), steroids, or colchicine improves symptoms of acute gout. While indomethacin has historically been the most commonly used NSAID, an alternative, such as naproxen, piroxicam, diclofenac, etoricoxib or ibuprofen, may be preferred due to its better side effect profile in the absence of superior effectiveness. Once the acute attack subsides, levels of uric acid are usually lowered via lifestyle changes, and in those with frequent attacks, allopurinol or probenecid provides long-term prevention.

236. Mechanism of action of colchicine:

a. Decreased uric acid synthesis
b. Increased uric acid synthesis
c. Suppression of immunity
d. None of the above

Colchicine inhibits microtubule polymerization by binding to tubulin, one of the main constituents of microtubules. Availability of tubulin is essential to mitosis, so colchicine effectively functions as a "mitotic poison" or spindle poison. Apart from inhibiting mitosis (a process heavily dependent on cytoskeletal changes), colchicine also inhibits neutrophil motility and activity, leading to a net anti-inflammatory effect. This has proven useful in the treatment of acute gout flares.

237. Action NOT caused by H1 receptor:

a. Vasoconstriction b. Gastric acid secretion
c. Cardiac stimulation d. Bronchoconstriction

The histamine receptor H_2belongs to the rhodopsin-like family of G protein-coupled receptors. It is an integral membrane protein and stimulates gastric acid secretion. It also regulates gastrointestinal motility and intestinal secretion and is thought to be involved in regulating cell growth and differentiation.

Distinctive features of three types of histaminergic receptors

	H_1	*H_2*	*H_3*
1. Selective agonists (relative selectivity H_1:H_2)	2-Methyl histamine (8:1) 2-Pyridylethylamine (30:1) 2-Thiazolyl ethylamine (90:1)	Dimaprit (1:2000) Impromidine (1:10,000)	(R) α-Methyl histamine (H_1: H_3 1:3000) Imetit
2. Selective antagonists (relative selectivity H_1:H_2)	Mepyramine (6000:1) Chlorpheniramine (15000:1)	Cimetidine (1:500) Ranitidine (I:>500)	Thioperamide (H_1: H_3 1: 23000) Impromidine (H_2 agonist) Tiprolisant
3. Receptor type	Gq-protein coupled	Gs-protein coupled	Gi/Go-protein coupled

Contd...

Ans. 234. b. Probenecid **235. b.** Indomethacin **236. c.** Suppression... **237. b.** Gastric acid secretion

Contd...

	H_1	H_2	H_3
4. Effector pathway	PIP_2 hydrolysis → IP_3/DAG : Release of $Ca2^+$ from intracellular stores; Protein kinase-C activation NO release→cGMP	Adenylyl cyclase activation—cAMP ↑—phosphorylation of specific proteins	a) Restricting Ca^{2+} influx b) K^+ channel activation c) cAMP ↓
5. Distribution in body: actions mediated	a) Smooth muscle (intestine, airway, uterus)—contraction b) Blood vessels i) Endothelium: Release of NO and, PGI_2—vasodilatation. widening of gap junctions—increased capillary permeability ii) Smooth muscle of larger vessels—vasoconstriction. c) Afferent nerve endings—stimulation d) Ganglionic cell—stimulation. e) Adrenal medulla—release of CAs. f) Brain—transmitter.	a) Gastric glands—acid secretion b) Blood vessels (smooth muscle)—dilatation c) Heart Atria: +ive chronotropy Ventricles: +ive inotropy d) Uterus (rat)—relaxation e) Brain—transmitter	a) Brain (presynaptically)—inhibition of histamine release—sedation b) Lung, spleen, skin, gastric mucosa—decrease histamine release c) Ileum—inhibition of ACh release from myenteric plexus neurones d) Certain blood vessels—inhibit NA release—vasodilatation

PIP2: Phosphatidyl inositol bisphosphate; IP3: Inositol trisphosphate; DAG: Diacylglycerols; EDRF: Endothelium dependent relaxing factor; NO: Nitric oxide; PGI_2: Prostacyclin; CAs: Catecholamines; cAMP : Cyclic 3', 5' adenosine monophosphate; ACh: Acetylcholine.

238. Sumatriptan in pharmacological doses is useful in migraine due to action on:

a. 5-HT-1A
b. 5-HT-1B/1D
c. 5-HT-3
d. 5-HT-4

Sumatriptan is structurally similar to serotonin (5HT), and is a 5-HT receptor (types 5-HT_{1D} and 5-HT_{1B}) agonist. The specific receptor subtypes it activates are present on the cranial arteries and veins. Acting as an agonist at these receptors, sumatriptan reduces the vascular inflammation associated with migraines.

Salient features of important 5-HT receptor subtypes.	
5-HT_1:	Autoreceptors; inhibit serotonergic neural activity in brain.
	5-HT_{1A}—present in raphe nuclei and hippocampus; buspirone (antianxiety) may act through these receptors.
	5-$HT_{1D/1B}$—Constricts cranial blood vessels and inhibits release of inflammatory neuropeptides in them; sumatriptan (antimigraine) acts through these receptors.
5-HT_2A :	Previously D type receptor; most important postjunctional receptor mediating direct actions of 5-HT like vascular and visceral smooth muscle contraction, platelet aggregation, neuronal activation in brain; ketanserin blocks these receptors.
5-HT_3:	Previously M type receptor; depolarizes neurones by gating cation channels; elicits reflex effects of 5-HT—emesis, gut peristalsis, bradycardia, transient hypotension, apnoea, pain, itch; ondansetron (antiemetic) acts by blocking these receptors.
5-HT_4:	Mediate intestinal secretion, augmentation of peristalsis. Renzapride (prokinetic) is a selective 5-HT_4 agonist.

239. DOC for Addison disease:

a. Triamcinolone
b. Dexamethasone
c. Betamethasone
d. Hydrocortisone

Treatment for Addison's disease involves replacing the missing cortisol, sometimes in the form of hydrocortisone tablets, or prednisone tablets in a dosing regimen that mimics the physiological concentrations of cortisol. Alternatively, one-quarter as much prednisolone may be used for equal glucocorticoid effect as hydrocortisone. Treatment is usually lifelong. In addition, many patients require fludrocortisone as replacement for the missing aldosterone.

Ans. 238. b. 5-HT-1B/1D **239. d.** Hydrocortisone

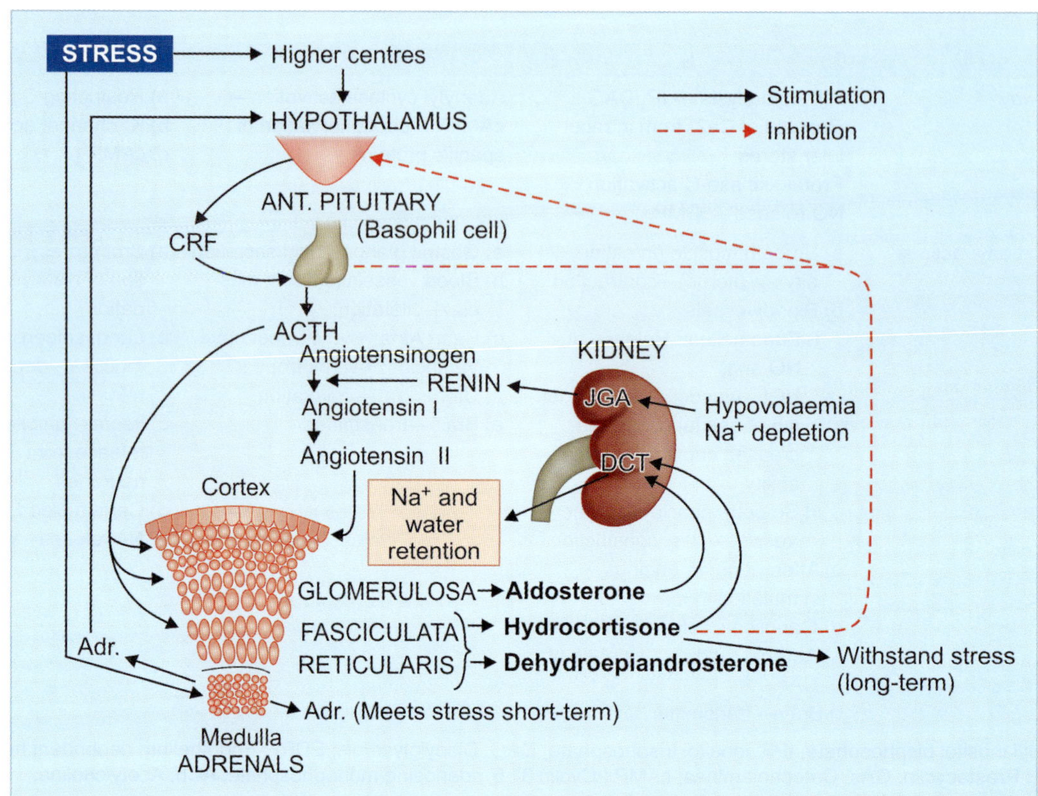

Hypothalamo-pituitary-adrenal (HPA) axis; regulation of corticosteroid production and response to stress which overrides the negative feedback regulation of ACTH release.

240. Steroids are CONTRAINDICATED in:

a. Uveitis b. Spring catarrh
c. Episcleritis
d. Herpetic corneal ulcer

Drugs that are usually contraindicated in corneal ulcer are topical corticosteroids and anesthetics - these should not be used on any type of corneal ulcer because they prevent healing, may lead to superinfection with fungi and other bacteria and will often make the condition much worse.

241. Depot progestins is administered by which route:

a. Subcutaneous route
b. Intravenous route
c. Intramuscular route
d. Both subcutaneous and intramuscular route

Some progestins can be delivered by intra-muscular injection every several months or released over time by diffusion from an subcutaneous implant or an IUD (Intra-Uterine-Device) (intrauterine system) depending on their solubility characteristics.

Effects of different forms of hormonal contraception.

	Oral pills			*Injections*
	Combined E + P	*Minipill only P*	*Postcoital only P*	*Progestin only*
1. FSH inhibition	++	–	–	+
2. LH inhibition	+++	+	+	+++
3. Antiovulatory effect	+++	+	+,–	++
4. Hostile cervical mucus	+++	+++	–	+++
5. Endometrium	Hyper-secretory	Out of phase	Unfavourable	Atrophic
6. Failure rate (pregnancy/100 women years)	0.1–0.3	2–3	2–4%	< 0.5
7. Contraceptive efficacy	++++	+++	++	++++

E: Estrogen; P: Progestin

Ans. 240. d. Herpetic... **241. d.** Both subcutaneous and intramuscular route

242. MOA of clomiphene citrate:
a. Binds to estrogen receptors and causes negative feedback at hypothalamus
b. Binds estrogen receptors and prevents negative feedback at hypothalamus
c. Binds to progesterone receptors
d. Progesterone agonist

Clomifene inhibits estrogen receptors in the hypothalamus, inhibiting negative feedback of estrogen on gonadotropin release, leading to up-regulation of the hypothalamic–pituitary–gonadal axis.

243. OCPs can cause all except:
a. Mastalgia
b. Dysmenorrhea
c. Chloasma
d. Breakthrough bleeding

The most common side effect of OCP is breakthrough bleeding. On the other hand, the pills can sometimes improve conditions such as pelvic inflammatory disease, dysmenorrhea, premenstrual syndrome, reduce symptoms of endometriosis and polycystic ovary syndrome, and decrease the risk of anemia. Use of oral contraceptives also reduces lifetime risk of ovarian cancer.

244. Stress increases all hormones except:
a. ACTH b. Noradrenaline
c. Insulin d. Glucagon

Insulin levels are low in stress conditions as body needs glucose and hence those hormones are elevated which raises blood glucose levels.

245. Viagra like medicine is given in which condition:
a. Pulmonary hypertension
b. Essential hypertension
c. Malignant hypertension
d. Hypertension in pregnancy

Sildenafil, sold as **Viagra** and other trade names, is used to treat erectile dysfunction and pulmonary arterial hypertension.

246. Most potent glucocorticoid:
a. Hydrocortisone
b. Prednisolone
c. Betamethasone
d. Triamcinolone

Betamethasone and Dexamethasone is very potent and highly selective glucocorticoid. They are long acting, causes marked pituitary adrenal suppression, but fluid retention and hypertension are not a problem.

Relative activity of systemic corticosteroids.

		Compound	Gluco	Mineralo	Equiv. dose (antiinflammatory)
Glucocorticoids	Short acting (Biological t½ < 12 hr)	1. Hydrocortisone (cortisol)	1	1	20 mg
	Intermediate acting (Biological t½ 12–36 hr)	2. Prednisolone 3. Methyl-prednisolone 4. Triamcinolone 5. Deflazacort	4 5 5 3–4	0.8 0.5 0 0	5 mg 4 mg 4 mg 6 mg
	Long acting (Biological t½ > 36 hr)	6. Dexamethasone 7. Betamethasone	25 25	0 0	0.75 mg 0.75 mg
Mineralocorticoids					Equiv. salt retaining dose
		8. Desoxycortico-sterone acetate (DOCA) 9. Fludrocortisone 10. Aldosterone	0 10 0.3	100 150 3000	2.5 mg (sublingual) 0.2 mg not used clinically

247. Dose of mifepristone (in mg) for post-coital contraception:
a. 100 b. 200
c. 400 d. 600

One 600-mg dose of mifepristone given within 72 hours of unprotected intercourse was 100 percent effective as an emergency contraceptive.

248. Drug of choice for hyperprolactinemia:
a. Methyl-dopa b. Bromocriptine
c. Metoclopramide d. Maprotiline

Treatment of hyperprolactinemia is usually medication with dopamine agonists such as cabergoline, bromocriptine (often preferred when pregnancy is possible), and less frequently lisuride. A new drug in use is norprolac with the active ingredient quinagolide.

249. Lugol's iodine acts by inhibiting:
a. Peroxidase b. d-Iodinase
c. Iodide uptake d. None of the above

In hyperthyroid patients, strong iodine produces rapid remission of symptoms by inhibiting the release of thyroid hormone into the circulation. The effects of strong iodine on the thyroid gland include reduction of vascularity, a firming of the glandular tissue, shrinkage of the size of individual cells, reaccumulation of colloid in the follicles, and increases in bound iodine. These actions may facilitate thyroidectomy when the medication is given prior to surgery.

Ans. 242. **b.** Binds... 243. **b.** Dysmenorrhea 244. **c.** Insulin 245. **a.** Pulmonary...
246. **c.** Betamethasone 247. **d.** 600 248. **b.** Bromocriptine 249. **d.** None of the above

250. Which is a selective estrogen receptor modulator:

a. Raloxifene b. Mifepristone
c. Danazol d. Anastozole

SERMs are competitive partial agonists of the ER. Different tissues have different degrees of sensitivity to and activity of endogenous estrogens, so SERMs produce estrogenic or antiestrogenic effects depending on the specific tissue in question as well as the percentage of intrinsic activity (IA) of the SERM. An example of a SERM with high IA and thus mostly estrogenic effects is chlorotrianisene, while an example of a SERM with low IA and thus mostly antiestrogenic effects is ethamoxytriphetol. SERMs like clomiphene and tamoxifen are more in the middle in their IA and their balance of estrogenic and antiestrogenic actions in comparison. Raloxifene is a SERM that is more antiestrogenic than tamoxifen; both are estrogenic in bone, but raloxifene is antiestrogenic in the uterus while tamoxifen is estrogenic in this location.

251. Glucocorticoids with mineralocorticoids activity is seen in:

a. Triamcinolone b. Fludrocortisone
c. Dexamethasone d. All of the above

Fluorocortisol (or **9α-fluorohydrocortisone**) is a synthetic corticosteroid with moderate glucocorticoid potency (10) and much greater mineralocorticoid potency (150). Therapeutically, it is used for its mineralocorticoid activity and not for its glucocorticoid activity.

252. Thiocyanates and perchlorates acts by:

a. Inhibiting the uptake of iodide into the acinar cells
b. Inhibiting the conversion of iodide into the acinar cells
c. Inhibiting the synthesis of mono-iodo-tyrosine from iodine
d. Inhibiting the release of T3 and T4 into the blood

Thiocyanate is a potent competitive inhibitor of the thyroid sodium-iodide symporter. Iodine is an essential component of thyroxine. Since thiocyanates will decrease iodide transport into the thyroid follicular cell, they will decrease the amount of thyroxine produced by the thyroid gland. As such, foodstuffs containing thiocyanate are best avoided by hypothyroid patients.

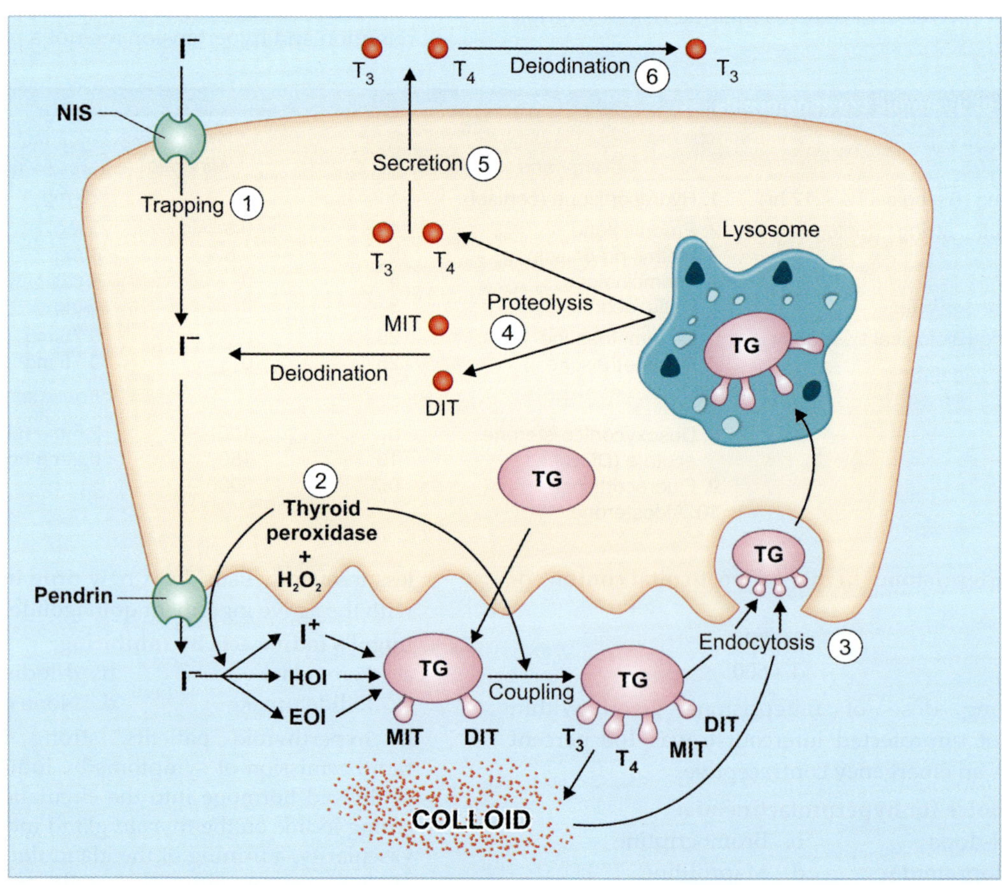

Synthesis, storage and secretion of thyroid hormone. TG: Thyroglobulin; MIT: Monoiodotyrosine; DIT: Diiodotyrosine; T_3: Triiodothyronine; T_4: Thyroxine (Tetraiodothyronine); HOI: Hypoiodous acid; EOI: Enzyme linked hypoiodate; NIS: Na^+-iodide symporter; Thyroid-stimulating hormone (TSH) activates steps 1, 2, 3, 4, and 5; Ionic inhibitors block step 1; Excess iodide interferes with steps 1, 2, 3 and 5 with primary action on step 3 and 5; Propylthiouracil inhibits steps 2 and 6; Carbimazole inhibits step 2 only.

Ans. 250. a. Raloxifene **251. b.** Fludricortisone **252. a.** Inhibiting...

253. People with high risk for developing breast carcinoma, can be prevented by prophylactic administration of:

a. Tamoxifen
b. Amino-glutethimide
c. Di-ethyl-stilbestrol
d. Letrozole

Tamoxifen is currently used for the treatment of both early and advanced ER+ (estrogen receptor positive) breast cancer in pre- and post-menopausal women. Additionally, it is the most common hormone treatment for male breast cancer. It is also approved by the FDA for the prevention of breast cancer in women at high risk of developing the disease. It has been further approved for the reduction of contralateral (in the opposite breast) cancer. The use of tamoxifen is recommended for 10 years.

Comparative properties of tamoxifen (SERM) and letrozole/anastrozole (AIs).

Tamoxifen	*Letrozole/Anastrozole*
1. Estrogen antagonist in breast and blood vessels, but agonist in uterus, bone, liver and pituitary.	1. Inhibits production of estrogens in all tissues. Nearly total estrogen deprivation.
2. Can be used for breast Ca. in premenopausal women as well.	2. Not to be used in premenopausal women.
3. Less effective in delaying recurrence when used as adjuvant therapy after surgery.	3. More effective in delaying recurrence of early stage breast Ca. (adjuvant therapy)
4. Prophylactic use for breast Ca. recurrence limited to 5 years.	4. Continues to exert prophylactic effect beyond 5 years.
5. Less delay in disease progression and lower survival advantage in advanced/metastatic breast Ca. than AIs.	5. Greater delay in disease progression and greater survival advantage in palliative treatment of advanced/metastatic breast Ca.
6. Not effective in failure cases.	6. Effective in tamoxifen failure cases of advanced breast Ca.
7. Causes endometrial hyperplasia, predisposes to endometrial carcinoma	7. No endometrial hyperplasia/cancer predisposition.
8. No bone losss, no increase in fractures or arthritic symptoms	8. Accelerates bone loss, predisposes to fractures, arthritic symptoms.
9. Increases risk of venous thromboembolism	9. No increase in thromboembolic risk
10. Improves lipid profile; small lowering of LDL Ch.	10. No effect on lipid profile.

SERM: Selective estrogen receptor modulate; AIs: Aromatase inhibitors; Ca.: Carcinoma; LDL Ch: Low density lipoprotein cholesterol

254. Mechanism of action of sildenafil is:

a. 5 alpha reductase inhibitor
b. Antiandrogen
c. Phosphodiesterase-5 inhibitor
d. Androgenic

Sildenafil acts by inhibiting cGMP-specific phosphodiesterase type 5 (PDE5), an enzyme that promotes degradation of cGMP, which regulates blood flow in the penis.

255. An old man is having benign prostatic hypertrophy. Drug useful in such a patient would be:

a. Cyproterone acetate
b. Danazol
c. Bicalutamide
d. Finasteride

Finasteride is used for the treatment of benign prostatic hyperplasia (BPH) and male pattern baldness (MPB). It is a type II and type III 5α-reductase inhibitor; 5α-reductase, an enzyme, converts testosterone to dihydrotestosterone (DHT).

256. Treatment of choice of cyanide poisoning:

a. Sodium nitrite followed by thiosulphate
b. NaCl
c. $KMnO_4$
d. $NaHCO_3$

The United States standard cyanide antidote kit first uses a small inhaled dose of amyl nitrite, followed by intravenous sodium nitrite, followed by intravenous sodium thiosulfate.

Haemoglobin
↓ ← Sod. nitrite (10 ml of 3% solution i.v.)
Methaemoglobin
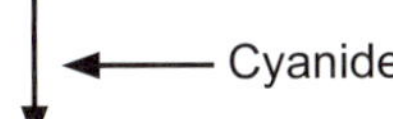
↓ ← Cyanide
Cyanomethaemoglobin
↓ ← Sod. thiosulfate (50 ml of 25% solution i.v.)
Methaemoglobin + Sod. thiocyanate
↓
Excreted in urine

257. Podophylin is used for:

a. Verruca plana
b. Genital wart
c. Plantar wart
d. All of the above

Podophyllin, a natural plant resin very high in podophyllotoxin content, has been used to remove genital warts since its efficacy was first demonstrated in 1942.

Ans. 253. **a.** Tamoxifen 254. **c.** Phosphodiesterase... 255. **d.** Finasteride 256. **a.** Sodium nitrite... 257. **b.** Genital wart

258. N-acetyl-cysteine is antidote for:

a. Heparin b. Acetaminophen
c. Morphine d. Benzodiazepine

When paracetamol is taken in large quantities, a minor metabolite called *N*-acetyl-*p*-benzoquinone imine (NAPQI) accumulates within the body. It is normally conjugated by glutathione, but when taken in excess, the body's glutathione reserves are not sufficient to inactivate the toxic NAPQI. This metabolite is then free to react with key hepatic enzymes, thereby damaging liver cells. This may lead to severe liver damage and even death by acute liver failure.

In the treatment of acetaminophen overdose, acetylcysteine acts to maintain or replenish depleted glutathione reserves in the liver and enhance non-toxic metabolism of acetaminophen. These actions serve to protect liver cells from NAPQI toxicity. It is most effective in preventing or lessening hepatic injury when administered within 8–10 hours after overdose.

259. Drug of choice for dermatitis herpetiformis:

a. Rifampin b. Clofazimine
c. Dapsone d. Metronidazole

Dapsone is commonly used in combination with rifampicin and clofazimine for the treatment of leprosy. It is used to both treat and prevent pneumocystis pneumonia (PCP) and prevent toxoplasmosis in people unable to tolerate trimethoprim with sulfamethoxazole. Dapsone may be used to treat brown recluse spider bites that become necrotic. It, along with a gluten free diet, may also help with dermatitis herpetiformis.

Ans. **258. b.** Acetaminophen **259. c.** Dapsone

ANSWERS WITH REFERENCES

GENERAL PRINCIPLES

1. **Ans. (d) Rifampicin**
   Ref: KD Tripathi's Pharmacology, 7/e p26

2. **Ans. (d) Phenytoin**
   Ref: KD Tripathi's Pharmacology, 7/e p34

3. **Ans. (b) 100-500**
   Ref: KD Tripathi's Pharmacology, 7/e p77

4. **Ans. (b) Safety**
   Ref: KD Tripathi's Pharmacology 7/e p56

5. **Ans. (a) Phenytoin**
   Ref: KD Tripathi's Pharmacology 7/e p32

6. **Ans. (c) Narrow therapeutic range**
   Ref: KD Tripathi's Pharmacology 7/e p34

7. **Ans. (b) Lithium**
   Ref: KD Tripathi's Pharmacology 7/e p34

8. **Ans. (b) Enalapril**
   Ref: KD Tripathi's Pharmacology 7/e p23

9. **Ans. (b) Mechanism of action of a drug**
   Ref: KD Tripathi's Pharmacology 7/e p1

10. **Ans. (a) Oral**
    Ref: KD Tripathi's Pharmacology 7/e p27

11. **Ans. (d) Phenytoin and warfarin**
    Ref: KD Tripathi's Pharmacology 7/e p32

12. **Ans. (a) Zero order kinetics**
    Ref: KD Tripathi's Pharmacology 7/e p391

13. **Ans. (d) Plasma clearance of a drug**
    Ref: KD Tripathi's Pharmacology 7/e p31

14. **Ans. (c) Elimination of the drug is proportional to the serum concentration.**
    Ref: KD Tripathi's Pharmacology 7/e p30

15. **Ans. (c) 4–5 half lives**
    Ref: KD Tripathi's Pharmacology 7/e p32

16. **Ans. (b) Drugs to treat rare diseases usually**
    Ref: KD Tripathi's Pharmacology 7/e p5

17. **Ans. (d) Gentamycin**
    Ref: KD Tripathi's Pharmacology 7/e p34

18. **Ans. (c) Drug safety**
    Ref: KD Tripathi's Pharmacology 7/e p82

19. **Ans. (b) 93%**
    Ref: KD Tripathi's Pharmacology 7/e p32

20. **Ans. (b) Efficacy**
    Ref: KD Tripathi's Pharmacology 7/e p54

21. **Ans. (c) After-marketing surveillance of drugs**
    Ref: KD Tripathi's Pharmacology 7/e p80

DRUGS ACTIN ON CVS

22. **Ans. (c) Acebutolol**
    Ref: KD Tripathi's Pharmacology, 7/e p147

23. **Ans. (b) ACE inhibitors**
    Ref: KD Tripathi's Pharmacology, 7/e p568

24. **Ans. (a) Na+K+ ATPase**
    Ref: KD Tripathi's Pharmacology, 7/e p515

25. **Ans. (c) Diltiazem**
    Ref: KD Tripathi's Pharmacology 7/e p548

26. **Ans. (c) Adenosine**
    Ref: KD Tripathi's Pharmacology 7/e p537

27. **Ans. (b) Amiodarone**
    Ref: KD Tripathi's Pharmacology 7/e p529

28. **Ans. (b) Glibenclamide**
    Ref: KD Tripathi's Pharmacology 7/e p552

29. **Ans. (c) Enalapril**
    Ref: KD Tripathi's Pharmacology 7/e p570

30. **Ans. (b) II**
    Ref: KD Tripathi's Pharmacology 7/e p529

31. **Ans. (c) ACE inhibitor**
    Ref: KD Tripathi's Pharmacology 7/e p570

32. **Ans. (a) Nimodipine**
    Ref: KD Tripathi's Pharmacology 7/e p550

33. **Ans. (c) Renal artery stenosis**
    Ref: KD Tripathi's Pharmacology 7/e p570

34. **Ans. (d) Hyperkalemia**
    Ref: KD Tripathi's Pharmacology 7/e p516

35. **Ans. (d) All of the above**
    Ref: KD Tripathi's Pharmacology 7/e p516

36. **Ans. (c) Calcium**
    Ref: KD Tripathi's Pharmacology 7/e p517

37. **Ans. (b)** Lidocaine
Ref: KD Tripathi's Pharmacology 7/e p516

38. **Ans. (a)** Verapamil
Ref: KD Tripathi's Pharmacology 7/e p538

39. **Ans. (a)** $Na^+ K^+$ ATPase inhibition
Ref: KD Tripathi's Pharmacology 7/e p514

DRUGS ACTING ON RESPIRATORY SYSTEM

40. **Ans. (b)** Salmeterol
Ref: KD Tripathi's Pharmacology, 7/e p233

41. **Ans. (c)** Zileuton
Ref: KD Tripathi's Pharmacology 7/e p229

42. **Ans. (c)** Budesonide
Ref: Internet resources

43. **Ans. (b)** Mast cell stabilization
Ref: KD Tripathi's Pharmacology 7/e p229

44. **Ans. (c)** Erythromycin
Ref: KD Tripathi's Pharmacology 7/e p226

45. **Ans. (c)** Charcoal hemoperfusion
Ref: Internet resources

46. **Ans. (a)** Decreases mucosal edema by suppressing inflammatory response
Ref: KD Tripathi's Pharmacology 7/e p229

47. **Ans. (d)** Amlodipine
Ref: KD Tripathi's Pharmacology 7/e p570

48. **Ans. (a)** Short acting beta 2 agonists
Ref: KD Tripathi's Pharmacology 7/e p223

49. **Ans. (a)** Given in acute bronchial asthma
Ref: KD Tripathi's Pharmacology 7/e p229

50. **Ans. (c)** Propranolol
Ref: KD Tripathi's Pharmacology 7/e p147

51. **Ans. (d)** Cholinergic drugs
Ref: KD Tripathi's Pharmacology 7/e p228

ANTIDIABETIC DRUGS

52. **Ans. (c)** Enhance glucose uptake by skeletal muscle
Ref: KD Tripathi's Pharmacology, 7/e p280

53. **Ans. (c)** Albuminuria
Ref: KD Tripathi's Pharmacology 7/e p259

54. **Ans. (d)** Metformin
Ref: KD Tripathi's Pharmacology 7/e p276

55. **Ans. (b)** Acetohexamide
Ref: Internet resources

56. **Ans. (d)** Insulin lispro
Ref: KD Tripathi's Pharmacology 7/e p263

57. **Ans. (c)** Act on SUR receptors on pancreatic beta cell membrane
Ref: KD Tripathi's Pharmacology 7/e p274

58. **Ans. (c)** Metformin
Ref: KD Tripathi's Pharmacology 7/e p272

59. **Ans. (d)** Metformin
Ref: KD Tripathi's Pharmacology 7/e p276

60. **Ans. (d)** None of the above
Ref: KD Tripathi's Pharmacology 7/e p266

61. **Ans. (b)** Less incidence of hypoglycemia
Ref: KD Tripathi's Pharmacology 7/e p273

62. **Ans. (a)** Cause little or no hypoglycemia
Ref: KD Tripathi's Pharmacology 7/e p276

63. **Ans. (b)** Regular insulin
Ref: KD Tripathi's Pharmacology 7/e p263

DRUGS ACTING ON NERVOUS SYSTEM

64. **Ans. (a)** Folic acid
Ref: KD Tripathi's Pharmacology, 7/e p422

65. **Ans. (b)** Fluoxetine
Ref: KD Tripathi's Pharmacology, 7/e p461

66. **Ans. (c)** Carbamazepine
Ref: KD Tripathi's Pharmacology, 7/e p416

67. **Ans. (c)** Scoline
Ref: KD Tripathi's Pharmacology 7/e p353

68. **Ans. (a)** Meprobamate
Ref: Internet resources

69. **Ans. (b)** Gabapentin
Ref: KD Tripathi's Pharmacology 7/e p420

70. **Ans. (c)** Diazepam
Ref: KD Tripathi's Pharmacology 7/e p408

71. **Ans. (d)** Buspirone
Ref: KD Tripathi's Pharmacology 7/e p404

72. **Ans. (c)** Valproate
Ref: KD Tripathi's Pharmacology 7/e p421

73. **Ans. (c)** Sodium valproate
Ref: KD Tripathi's Pharmacology 7/e p414

74. **Ans. (b)** GABA transaminase inhibitor
Ref: KD Tripathi's Pharmacology 7/e p421

75. Ans. (c) At lower concentration, it follows zero order kinetics
Ref: KD Tripathi's Pharmacology 7/e p413

76. Ans. (a) Phenytoin
Ref: KD Tripathi's Pharmacology 7/e p414

77. Ans. (b) Benzhexol
Ref: KD Tripathi's Pharmacology 7/e p433

78. Ans. (b) Inhibit peripheral decarboxylation of levodopa
Ref: KD Tripathi's Pharmacology 7/e p428

79. Ans. (d) Has maximum extra-pyramidal effects
Ref: KD Tripathi's Pharmacology 7/e p440

80. Ans. (a) Serotonin uptake inhibition
Ref: KD Tripathi's Pharmacology 7/e p458

81. Ans. (b) Serum creatinine
Ref: KD Tripathi's Pharmacology 7/e p448

82. Ans. (d) Fluoxetine
Ref: KD Tripathi's Pharmacology 7/e p461

83. Ans. (d) Follows zero order kinetics at lower doses
Ref: KD Tripathi's Pharmacology 7/e p413

84. Ans. (b) Antidepressant
Ref: KD Tripathi's Pharmacology 7/e p454

85. Ans. (c) Mivacurium
Ref: KD Tripathi's Pharmacology 7/e p352

86. Ans. (a) Constipation
Ref: KD Tripathi's Pharmacology 7/e p473

87. Ans. (c) Malignant neuroleptic syndrome
Ref: KD Tripathi's Pharmacology 7/e p444

88. Ans. (d) Valproate
Ref: KD Tripathi's Pharmacology 7/e p421

89. Ans. (c) Antipsychotics
Ref: KD Tripathi's Pharmacology 7/e p444

90. Ans. (d) Nicotinic receptor antagonist
Ref: KD Tripathi's Pharmacology 7/e p463

91. Ans. (b) Flumazenil
Ref: KD Tripathi's Pharmacology 7/e p403

92. Ans. (d) Methylphenidate
Ref: KD Tripathi's Pharmacology 7/e p487

93. Ans. (c) Spasticity
Ref: KD Tripathi's Pharmacology 7/e p358

94. Ans. (c) Lorazepam
Ref: KD Tripathi's Pharmacology 7/e p424

95. Ans. (d) No significant interaction with warfarin
Ref: KD Tripathi's Pharmacology 7/e p623

96. Ans. (b) Dopamine D2 receptor blockade
Ref: KD Tripathi's Pharmacology 7/e p437

97. Ans. (b) Phenytoin
Ref: KD Tripathi's Pharmacology 7/e p451

98. Ans. (b) Akathisia
Ref: KD Tripathi's Pharmacology 7/e p444

99. Ans. (d) Ethosuximide
Ref: KD Tripathi's Pharmacology 7/e p421

DRUGS ACTING ON GASTROINTESTINAL TRACT

100. Ans. (c) Azithromycin
Ref: KD Tripathi's Pharmacology 7/e p656

101. Ans. (d) Mosapride
Ref: KD Tripathi's Pharmacology 7/e p665

102. Ans. (b) Omeprazole
Ref: KD Tripathi's Pharmacology 7/e p653

103. Ans. (b) Potassium 20 mEq/lit
Ref: KD Tripathi's Pharmacology 7/e p680

104. Ans. (d) Cimetidine
Ref: KD Tripathi's Pharmacology 7/e p657

105. Ans. (d) Pirenzedpine
Ref: KD Tripathi's Pharmacology 7/e p654

106. Ans. (b) Magnesium sulphate
Ref: KD Tripathi's Pharmacology 7/e p649

107. Ans. (c) Ulcerative colitis
Ref: KD Tripathi's Pharmacology 7/e p683

108. Ans. (a) Sucralfate
Ref: KD Tripathi's Pharmacology 7/e p656

109. Ans. (c) Ciprofloxacin
Ref: KD Tripathi's Pharmacology 7/e p657

110. Ans. (d) Erythromycin
Ref: KD Tripathi's Pharmacology 7/e p753

111. Ans. (b) H^+/K^+ ATPase pump
Ref: KD Tripathi's Pharmacology 7/e p648

112. Ans. (b) Cisapride
Ref: KD Tripathi's Pharmacology 7/e p667

113. Ans. (a) Proton pump inhibitor
Ref: KD Tripathi's Pharmacology 7/e p652

114. Ans. (b) Hyoscine butylbromide
Ref: KD Tripathi's Pharmacology 7/e p116

DRUGS ACTING ON HAEMATOPOIETIC SYSTEM

115. **Ans. (c) Tranexamic acid**
Ref: KD Tripathi's Pharmacology, 7/e p626

116. **Ans. (a) Rosuvastatin**
Ref: KD Tripathi's Pharmacology 7/e p637

117. **Ans. (b) Decreased LDL receptors**
Ref: KD Tripathi's Pharmacology 7/e p636

118. **Ans. (a) Factor III**
Ref: KD Tripathi's Pharmacology 7/e p621

119. **Ans. (d) Chronic alcoholism**
Ref: KD Tripathi's Pharmacology 7/e p622

120. **Ans. (d) Aspirin**
Ref: KD Tripathi's Pharmacology 7/e p629

121. **Ans. (c) Pericarditis**
Ref: KD Tripathi's Pharmacology 7/e p624-625

122. **Ans. (b) Thromboxane A2**
Ref: KD Tripathi's Pharmacology 7/e p629

123. **Ans. (c) Warfarin**
Ref: KD Tripathi's Pharmacology 7/e p623

124. **Ans. (a) It inhibits TXA_2 synthesis by platelets**
Ref: KD Tripathi's Pharmacology 7/e p629

125. **Ans. (a) Argatroban**
Ref: KD Tripathi's Pharmacology 7/e p620

126. **Ans. (c) Low molecular weight heparin**
Ref: KD Tripathi's Pharmacology 7/e p624

127. **Ans. (d) Activated partial thromboplastin time**
Ref: KD Tripathi's Pharmacology 7/e p618

128. **Ans. (b) Give oral Vitamin K_1**
Ref: KD Tripathi's Pharmacology 7/e p622

129. **Ans. (c) Vitamin K_1**
Ref: KD Tripathi's Pharmacology 7/e p622

130. **Ans. (a) Are absorbed more uniformly when given subcutaneously**
Ref: KD Tripathi's Pharmacology 7/e p619

131. **Ans. (d) Anti-factor Xa activity**
Ref: KD Tripathi's Pharmacology 7/e p619

DRUGS ACTING ON EXCRETORY SYSTEM

132. **Ans. (c) Triamterene**
Ref: KD Tripathi's Pharmacology, 6/e p571

133. **Ans. (a) Demeclocycline**
Ref: KD Tripathi's Pharmacology 7/e p736

134. **Ans. (b) ACE inhibitors**
Ref: KD Tripathi's Pharmacology 7/e p588

135. **Ans. (a) Impotence**
Ref: KD Tripathi's Pharmacology 7/e p584

136. **Ans. (c) Acetazolamide**
Ref: KD Tripathi's Pharmacology 7/e p586

137. **Ans. (a) Reduces GFR**
Ref: KD Tripathi's Pharmacology 7/e p591

138. **Ans. (b) Desmopressin**
Ref: KD Tripathi's Pharmacology 7/e p597

ANTIMICROBIAL DRUGS

139. **Ans. (c) Clindamycin**
Ref: KD Tripathi's Pharmacology, 7/e p717

140. **Ans. (b) Cycloserine**
Ref: KD Tripathi's Pharmacology, 7/e p776

141. **Ans. (b) Ethionamide**
Ref: KD Tripathi's Pharmacology, 7/e p771

142. **Ans. (b) Aminopyrine**
Ref: KD Tripathi's Pharmacology 7/e p66

143. **Ans. (a) Pefloxacin**
Ref: KD Tripathi's Pharmacology 7/e p711

144. **Ans. (c) Levamisole**
Ref: KD Tripathi's Pharmacology 7/e p852

145. **Ans. (c) 1:5**
Ref: KD Tripathi's Pharmacology 7/e p706

146. **Ans. (a) Mutation**
Ref: KD Tripathi's Pharmacology 7/e p766

147. **Ans. (c) Rifampicin**
Ref: KD Tripathi's Pharmacology 7/e p768

148. **Ans. (d) Rifampicin**
Ref: KD Tripathi's Pharmacology 7/e p767

149. **Ans. (d) Methicillin**
Ref: KD Tripathi's Pharmacology 7/e p721

150. **Ans. (d) Rifampicin**
Ref: KD Tripathi's Pharmacology 7/e p774

151. **Ans. (c) Erythromycin**
Ref: KD Tripathi's Pharmacology 7/e p754

152. **Ans. (b) Para-amino-benzoic acid**
Ref: KD Tripathi's Pharmacology 7/e p785

153. **Ans. (d) Clindamycin**
Ref: KD Tripathi's Pharmacology 7/e p756

154. **Ans. (b) Schistosomiasis**
Ref: Internet resources

155. **Ans. (a) Aztreonam**
Ref: KD Tripathi's Pharmacology 7/e p730

156. **Ans. (b) Can be used with cilastatin**
Ref: KD Tripathi's Pharmacology 7/e p731

157. **Ans. (a) Mucormycosis**
Ref: KD Tripathi's Pharmacology 7/e p794

158. **Ans. (b) 300 mg (base) weekly**
Ref: KD Tripathi's Pharmacology 7/e p818

159. **Ans. (b) Benzathine penicillin (2.4 mega units deep IM)**
Ref: KD Tripathi's Pharmacology 7/e p720

160. **Ans. (a) Cephalothin**
Ref: KD Tripathi's Pharmacology 7/e p726

161. **Ans. (a) Protein synthesis**
Ref: KD Tripathi's Pharmacology 7/e p750

162. **Ans. (d) Methenamine mandelate**
Ref: KD Tripathi's Pharmacology 7/e p760

163. **Ans. (d) None**
Ref: KD Tripathi's Pharmacology 7/e p784

164. **Ans. (b) Malaria**
Ref: KD Tripathi's Pharmacology 7/e p854

165. **Ans. (c) Inhibitor of PFOR enzyme**
Ref: KD Tripathi's Pharmacology 7/e p840

166. **Ans. (d) Cisapride**
Ref: KD Tripathi's Pharmacology 7/e p931

167. **Ans. (b) Cefoperazone**
Ref: KD Tripathi's Pharmacology 7/e p128

168. **Ans. (c) Derived from bacteria**
Ref: KD Tripathi's Pharmacology 7/e p759

169. **Ans. (d) Pseudomembranous colitis**
Ref: KD Tripathi's Pharmacology 7/e p757

170. **Ans. (d) Imipenem**
Ref: KD Tripathi's Pharmacology/ 7th/731

171. **Ans. (c) Abacavir**
Ref: KD Tripathi's Pharmacology 7/e p808

ANTICANCER AND ANTI-INFLAMMATORY DRUGS

172. **Ans. (b) Cytarabine**
Ref: KD Tripathi's Pharmacology, 7/e p858

173. **Ans. (a) Actinomycin-D**
Ref: KD Tripathi's Pharmacology, 7/e p867

174. **Ans. (a) Folic acid antagonism**
Ref: KD Tripathi's Pharmacology, 6/e p823

175. **Ans. (b) Cyclophosphamide**
Ref: KD Tripathi's Pharmacology, 7/e p860

176. **Ans. (d) Methotrexate**
Ref: KD Tripathi's Pharmacology 7/e p863

177. **Ans. (d) Methotrexate**
Ref: KD Tripathi's Pharmacology 7/e p808

178. **Ans. (c) CD4 cells and lymphocytes**
Ref: KD Tripathi's Pharmacology 7/e p880

179. **Ans. (a) Abciximab**
Ref: KD Tripathi's Pharmacology 7/e p631

180. **Ans. (b) 5-HT3 antagonism**
Ref: KD Tripathi's Pharmacology 7/e p668

181. **Ans. (d) 5-FU**
Ref: KD Tripathi's Pharmacology 7/e p858

182. **Ans. (a) Cisplatin**
Ref: KD Tripathi's Pharmacology 7/e p859

MEDICATIONS IN PREGNANCY AND LACTATION

183. **Ans. (d) Chloramphenicol**
Ref: KD Tripathi's Pharmacology, 7/e p962

184. **Ans. (c) Short acting beta2 agonist**
Ref: KD Tripathi's Pharmacology, 7/e p964t

185. **Ans. (b) Chloroquine**
Ref: KD Tripathi's Pharmacology 7/e p963

186. **Ans. (b) Bromocriptine**
Ref: KD Tripathi's Pharmacology 7/e p239

187. **Ans. (d) Epinephrine**
Ref: KD Tripathi's Pharmacology 7/e p90

188. **Ans. (b) Proguanil**
Ref: KD Tripathi's Pharmacology 7/e p963

189. **Ans. (c) 300**
Ref: KD Tripathi's Pharmacology 7/e p885

190. **Ans. (c) Phenytoin**
Ref: KD Tripathi's Pharmacology 7/e p89

191. **Ans. (b) Thalidomide**
Ref: KD Tripathi's Pharmacology 7/e p89

SIDE EFFECTS

192. **Ans. (d) Amiodarone**
Ref: KD Tripathi's Pharmacology 7/e p534

193. **Ans. (a) Pyrazinamide**
Ref: KD Tripathi's Pharmacology 7/e p769

194. **Ans. (a) Methysergide**
Ref: KD Tripathi's Pharmacology 7/e p174

195. **Ans. (d) Penicillin**
Ref: KD Tripathi's Pharmacology 7/e p66

196. **Ans. (d) Didanosine**
Ref: KD Tripathi's Pharmacology 7/e p813

197. **Ans. (d) Ethambutol**
Ref: KD Tripathi's Pharmacology 7/e p774

198. **Ans. (c) Erythromycin estolate**
Ref: KD Tripathi's Pharmacology 7/e p753

199. **Ans. (d) Chlorpropamide**
Ref: KD Tripathi's Pharmacology 7/e p273

200. **Ans. (a) Metoclopramide**
Ref: KD Tripathi's Pharmacology 7/e p666

201. **Ans. (b) Enalapril**
Ref: KD Tripathi's Pharmacology 7/e p501

202. **Ans. (c) Liver**
Ref: KD Tripathi's Pharmacology 7/e p207

203. **Ans. (d) Busulfan**
Ref: KD Tripathi's Pharmacology 7/e p861

204. **Ans. (c) L-asparginase**
Ref: KD Tripathi's Pharmacology 7/e p868

205. **Ans. (b) Doxycycline**
Ref: KD Tripathi's Pharmacology 7/e p736

206. **Ans. (c) Spironolactone**
Ref: KD Tripathi's Pharmacology 7/e p589

207. **Ans. (c) Bleomycin**
Ref: KD Tripathi's Pharmacology 7/e p868

208. **Ans. (a) Vancomycin**
Ref: KD Tripathi's Pharmacology 7/e p757

MISCELLANEOUS

209. **Ans. (b) Hyoscine**
Ref: KD Tripathi's Pharmacology, 7/e p113

210. **Ans. (c) Propranolol**
Ref: KD Tripathi's Pharmacology, 7/e p144, 147

211. **Ans. (b) 5% iodine & 10% potassium iodide**
Ref: KD Tripathi's Pharmacology, 7/e p248

212. **Ans. (c) Stop the offending drug & start symptomatic treatment**
Ref: KD Tripathi's Pharmacology, 7/e p86

213. **Ans. (d) Drotaverine**
Ref: KD Tripathi's Pharmacology, 7/e p118

214. **Ans. (b) Neostigmine**
Ref: KD Tripathi's Pharmacology 7/e p108

215. **Ans. (b) Reactivation of cholinesterase**
Ref: KD Tripathi's Pharmacology 7/e p111

216. **Ans. (c) Glaucoma**
Ref: KD Tripathi's Pharmacology 7/e p114

217. **Ans. (b) Pindolol**
Ref: KD Tripathi's Pharmacology 7/e p144

218. **Ans. (d) Tropicamide**
Ref: KD Tripathi's Pharmacology 7/e p118

219. **Ans. (c) Refractory period**
Ref: KD Tripathi's Pharmacology 7/e p131

220. **Ans. (c) Adrenaline**
Ref: KD Tripathi's Pharmacology 7/e p138

221. **Ans. (a) Dopamine**
Ref: KD Tripathi's Pharmacology 7/e p134

222. **Ans. (a) Renal vasodilatory effect**
Ref: KD Tripathi's Pharmacology 7/e p134

223. **Ans. (d) Labetalol**
Ref: KD Tripathi's Pharmacology 7/e p148

224. **Ans. (c) Ischemic heart disease**
Ref: KD Tripathi's Pharmacology 7/e p176

225. **Ans. (c) Phenylephrine**
Ref: KD Tripathi's Pharmacology 7/e p135

226. **Ans. (b) AV block**
Ref: KD Tripathi's Pharmacology 7/e p147

227. **Ans. (d) Esmolol**
Ref: KD Tripathi's Pharmacology 7/e p149

228. **Ans. (a) Renal vasodilatory effect**
Ref: KD Tripathi's Pharmacology 7/e p134

229. **Ans. (b) Decreases duration of systole**
Ref: KD Tripathi's Pharmacology 7/e p145

230. **Ans. (b) Hypothermia**
Ref: KD Tripathi's Pharmacology 7/e p123

231. **Ans. (a) Dopamine**
Ref: KD Tripathi's Pharmacology 7/e p130

232. **Ans. (a) Prostaglandin E1 analogue**
Ref: KD Tripathi's Pharmacology 7/e p654

233. **Ans. (a) PGE1 agonist**
Ref: KD Tripathi's Pharmacology 7/e p185

234. **Ans. (b) Probenecid**
Ref: KD Tripathi's Pharmacology 7/e p215

235. **Ans. (b) Indomethacin**
Ref: KD Tripathi's Pharmacology 7/e p213

236. **Ans. (c) Suppression of immunity**
Ref: KD Tripathi's Pharmacology 7/e p214

237. **Ans. (b) Gastric acid secretion**
Ref: KD Tripathi's Pharmacology 7/e p160

238. **Ans. (b) 5-HT-1B/1D**
Ref: KD Tripathi's Pharmacology 7/e p172

239. **Ans. (d) Hydrocortisone**
Ref: KD Tripathi's Pharmacology 7/e p283

240. **Ans. (d) Herpetic corneal ulcer**
Ref: KD Tripathi's Pharmacology 7/e p294

241. **Ans. (d) Both subcutaneous and intramuscular route**
Ref: KD Tripathi's Pharmacology 7/e p324

242. **Ans. (b) Binds estrogen receptors and prevents negative feedback at hypothalamus**
Ref: KD Tripathi's Pharmacology 7/e p312

243. **Ans. (b) Dysmenorrhea**
Ref: KD Tripathi's Pharmacology 7/e p327

244. **Ans. (c) Insulin**
Ref: Internet resources

245. **Ans. (a) Pulmonary hypertension**
Ref: KD Tripathi's Pharmacology 7/e p304

246. **Ans. (c) Betamethasone**
Ref: KD Tripathi's Pharmacology 7/e p289

247. **Ans. (d) 600**
Ref: KD Tripathi's Pharmacology 7/e p323

248. **Ans. (b) Bromocriptine**
Ref: KD Tripathi's Pharmacology 7/e p239

249. **Ans. (d) None of the above**
Ref: KD Tripathi's Pharmacology 7/e p255

250. **Ans. (a) Raloxifene**
Ref: KD Tripathi's Pharmacology 7/e p314

251. **Ans. (b) Fludrocortisone**
Ref: KD Tripathi's Pharmacology 7/e p289

252. **Ans. (a) Inhibiting the uptake of iodide into the acinar cells**
Ref: KD Tripathi's Pharmacology 7/e p246

253. **Ans. (a) Tamoxifen**
Ref: KD Tripathi's Pharmacology 7/e p315

254. **Ans. (c) Phosphodiesterase-5 inhibitor**
Ref: KD Tripathi's Pharmacology 7/e p303

255. **Ans. (d) Finasteride**
Ref: KD Tripathi's Pharmacology 7/e p302

256. **Ans. (a) Sodium nitrite followed by thiosulphate**
Ref: KD Tripathi's Pharmacology 7/e p545

257. **Ans. (b) Genital wart**
Ref: KD Tripathi's Pharmacology 7/e p889

258. **Ans. (b) Acetaminophen**
Ref: KD Tripathi's Pharmacology 7/e p207

259. **Ans. (c) Dapsone**
Ref: Internet resources

PRACTICE QUESTIONS

GENERAL PRINCIPLES

1. **True regarding placebo:**
   a. Has pharmacodynamic activity
   b. Same effect everytime
   c. Active moiety
   d. Inert substance
2. **Ratio of mean lethal dose to mean effective dose is:**
   a. Drug potency b. Therapeutic index
   c. Therapeutic efficacy d. Potentiation
3. **Which of the following is associated with tachyphylaxis:**
   a. Dopamine b. Ephedrine
   c. Propranolol d. Haloperidol
4. **Which of the following is NOT a prodrug:**
   a. Aspirin b. Levodopa
   c. Dipivefrin d. Captopril
5. **True statement related to expiry date of a drug:**
   a. Pharmaceutical company is not responsible for adverse effects if drug is consumed after expiry date
   b. Maximum period of expiry is 3 years from the date of manufacture
   c. After expiry period, drug changes to more toxic compounds
   d. After expiry period, there is a fall in efficacy of drug
6. **Which of the following does NOT require therapeutic dose monitoring:**
   a. Lithium b. Streptomycin
   c. Heparin d. Amitriptyline
7. **Pharmacovigilance is concerned with detection of:**
   a. Drug interactions
   b. Drug potency
   c. Drug efficacy
   d. Drug adverse effects

CVS

8. **Which of the following is FALSE for side-effects of amiodarone:**
   a. Bradycardia
   b. Irreversible corneal microdeposits
   c. Hypotension
   d. Pulmonary fibrosis
9. **Esmolol produces:**
   a. Raised BP b. Arrhythmias
   c. Cardiac arrest d. Hypotension
10. **Which of the following is a vasodilator:**
    a. Metoprolol b. Atenolol
    c. Propranolol d. Carvedilol
11. **Which of the following condition is NOT a CONTRAINDICATION to the use of ACE inhibitors:**
    a. Bilateral renal artery stenosis
    b. Diabetics
    c. Pregnancy
    d. Hyperkalemia

RESPI

12. **Mechanism of action of cough syrup:**
    a. Raise threshold of cough centre
    b. Inhibition of respiratory centre
    c. Inhibition of breathing centre
    d. Increase tussal impulses
13. **Noscapine is which class drug:**
    a. Anti-tussive
    b. Anti-emetic
    c. Anti-diarrhoeal
    d. Mucolytic

ANTI-DIABETIC

14. **Drug which reduces both microvascular and macrovascular complications:**
    a. Tolbutamide b. Repaglinide
    c. Pioglitazone d. Metformin
15. **A known case of chronic kidney disease stage 4 is on Insulin. What adjustment in Insulin dosage is required:**
    a. Increase dose of insulin
    b. Decrease dose of insulin
    c. No alteration in dose
    d. Variable

CNS

16. **Gum hypertrophy is a side-effect of:**
    a. Valproate b. Carbamazepine
    c. Phenytoin d. Methotrexate

Ans. 1. **d.** Inert substance 2. **b.** Therapeutic index 3. **b.** Ephedrine 4. **d.** Captopril
5. **a.** Pharmaceutical... 6. **c.** Heparin 7. **d.** Drug adverse... 8. **b.** Irreversible...
9. **d.** Hypotension 10. **d.** Carvedilol 11. **b.** Diabetics 12. **a.** Raise threshold...
13. **a.** Antitussive 14. **d.** Metformin 15. **b.** Decrease dose... 16. **c.** Phenytoin

17. **Which of the following anti-epileptic does NOT act by inhibition of T type calcium current:**
    a. Ethosuximide b. Valproate
    c. Vigabatrin d. Zonisamide

GIT

18. **Which of the following anti-emetic drug has some extra-pyramidal side effects:**
    a. Cyclizine b. Mosapride
    c. Prochlorperazine d. Domperidone

HAEMATO

19. **As compared to warfarin, heparin is:**
    a. Long acting
    b. Having few insignificant drug interactions
    c. Used orally
    d. Used in vivo only
20. **Drug inhibiting HMG-CoA reductase:**
    a. Gemfibrozil
    b. Cholestyramine
    c. Statins
    d. All of the above
21. **To decrease serum triglyceride levels, what can be used:**
    a. Fibrates b. Statins
    c. Ezetimibe d. Niacin

RENAL

22. **Which of the following class of diuretic drugs causes maximum potassium excretion:**
    a. Spironolactone b. Frusemide
    c. Acetazolamide d. Aldosterone

ANTIMICROBIAL

23. **Paediatric dose of Isoniazid on daily basis:**
    a. 5 mg/kg body weight
    b. 10 mg/kg body weight
    c. 15 mg/kg body weight
    d. 20 mg/kg body weight
24. **DOC for Diphyllobothruium latum:**
    a. Albendazole
    b. Mebendazole
    c. Praziquantel
    d. Pyrantel pamoate
25. **Erythromycin is used for:**
    a. UTI b. Hepatitis carriers
    c. Diphtheria carriers d. Meningococcal carriers
26. **NRTI with maximum risk of acute pancreatitis:**
    a. Zidovudine b. Abacavir
    c. Didanosine d. Tenofovir
27. **Mechanism of action of aminoglycoside:**
    a. Inhibits cell wall synthesis
    b. Inhibits mycolic acid synthesis
    c. Inhibits translation
    d. Inhibits transcription
28. **Which of the following is NOT a penicillinase resistant penicillin:**
    a. Cloxacillin b. Dicloxacillin
    c. Methicillin d. Carbenicillin
29. **Mechanism of action of ciprofloxacin in Gram negative bacteria:**
    a. Inhibition of topoisomerase IV
    b. Inhibition of mycolic acid
    c. Inhibition of DNA gyrase
    d. Inhibition of helicase
30. **Treatment of neurocysticercosis:**
    a. Praziquantel b. Pyrantel
    c. Albendazole d. Ivermectin
31. **NO reduction in dose is needed, in renal disease for:**
    a. Streptomycin b. Ethmabutol
    c. Doxycycline d. Ciprofloxacin
32. **Which of the following is NOT indicated in management of AIDS:**
    a. Abacavir b. Ritonavir
    c. Acyclovir d. Zidovudine
33. **Which of the following is NOT true for silver sulfadiazine:**
    a. Concentration of 1%
    b. Used for burns
    c. Safer in pregnancy and infants
    d. Active against Staph aureus
34. **Which of the following drug acts by blocking RNA transcription:**
    a. Rifampicin b. Streptomycin
    c. Chloramphenicol d. Isoniazid
35. **Red green colour blindness is a side effect of which ATT drug:**
    a. INH b. Rifampin
    c. Streptomycin d. Ethambutol

ANTI-CANCER

36. **Which of the following drug is NOT categorized under anti-VGEF agent:**
    a. Sunitinib b. 5-Fluoro Uracil
    c. Bevacizumab d. Ranibizumab

Ans.
17. **c.** Vigabatrin 18. **c.** Prochlorpe... 19. **b.** Having few 20. **c.** Statins
21. **a.** Fibrates 22. **c.** Acetazolamide 23. **a.** 5 mg/kg body weight 24. **c.** Praziquantel
25. **c.** Diphtheria carriers 26. **c.** Didanosine 27. **c.** Inhibits translation 28. **d.** Carbenicillin
29. **c.** Inhibition of... 30. **c.** Albendazole 31. **c.** Doxycycline 32. **c.** Acyclovir
33. **d.** Active against... 34. **a.** Rifampicin 35. **d.** Ethambutol 36. **b.** 5-Fluoro Uracil

37. Drugs which affect DNA synthesis are all EXCEPT:
a. 5-FU b. Bevacizumab
c. Methotrexate d. Doxorubicin

38. Which anti-cancer drug affects DNA as well as RNA:
a. Methotrexate b. 5-FU
c. Actinomycin-D d. Etoposide

39. Which of the following is most emetogenic:
a. Vinblastine b. Bleomycin
c. Cisplatin d. Etoposide

40. A 45 years old was diagnosed with breast carcinoma. She was operated and was put of Tamoxifen therapy for the last 1 year. Now she is complaining of bleeding per vaginum. Most likely cause:
a. Development of bleeding disorder
b. Development of endometrial carcinoma
c. Development of ovarian carcinoma
d. Development of cervical cancer

PREGNANCY AND LACTATION

41. Anti-TB CONTRAINDICATED in pregnancy:
a. INH b. Rifampin
c. Pyrazinamide d. Ethambutol

42. DOC for toxoplasmosis in pregnancy:
a. Erythromycin
b. Tetracycline
c. Chloramphenicol
d. Spiramycin

43. DOC for malaria in pregnancy:
a. Chloroquine b. Artesunate
c. Primaquine d. Artemether

44. Drug used for epilepsy during pregnancy:
a. Valproate
b. Carbamazepine
c. Phenobarbitone
d. Phenytoin

MISCELLANEOUS

45. Maximum glucocorticoid activity:
a. Cortisol b. Prednisolone
c. Aldosterone d. Dexamethasone

46. Night shift workers usually takes which drug:
a. Rivastigmine b. Atomoxetine
c. Modafinil d. Sildenafil

47. Morphine acts strongly on which opioid receptors:
a. Mu b. Kappa
c. Delta d. Equally on all

48. All are used in postmenopausal osteoporosis EXCEPT:
a. Vitamin D b. Calcitonin
c. Glucocorticoid d. Bisphosphonates

49. 5-HT$_1$D/$_1$B agonist drug:
a. Cyproheptadine
b. Sumatriptan
c. Methysergide
d. Ondansetron

50. Which of the following is deposited in retina:
a. Steroids b. Chloroquine
c. Amiodarone d. Ethambutol

51. Dobutamine acts on which of the following receptors:
a. Beta1 adrenergic
b. Beta2 adrenergic
c. Alpha1 adrenergic
d. Alpha2 adrenergic

52. Which of the following is an anticholinergic side effect:
a. Salivation
b. Dryness of mouth
c. Increased GIT motility
d. Sweating

53. Who can sell pharmacological medicines:
a. Businessmen
b. Degree/diploma holders in pharmacy
c. Any citizen of India
d. Manager

54. A newborn born with patent ductus arteriosus. Drug used for closure is:
a. Alprostadil b. Paracetamol
c. Indomethacin d. Celecoxib

55. Side effect of atropine:
a. Sweating b. Miosis
c. Hyperthermia d. Bradycardia

Ans.
37. b. Bevacizumab 38. c. Actinomycin-D 39. c. Cisplatin 40. b. Development of...
41. c. Pyrazinamide 42. d. Spiramycin 43. a. Chloroquine 44. c. Phenobarbitone
45. d. Dexamethasone 46. c. Modafinil 47. a. Mu 48. c. Glucocorticoid
49. b. Sumatriptan 50. b. Chloroquine 51. a. Beta1 adrenergic 52. b. Dryness of mouth
53. b. Degree/diploma... 54. c. Indomethacin 55. c. Hyperthermia

IMAGE-BASED QUESTIONS

1. What does the following picture depicts:

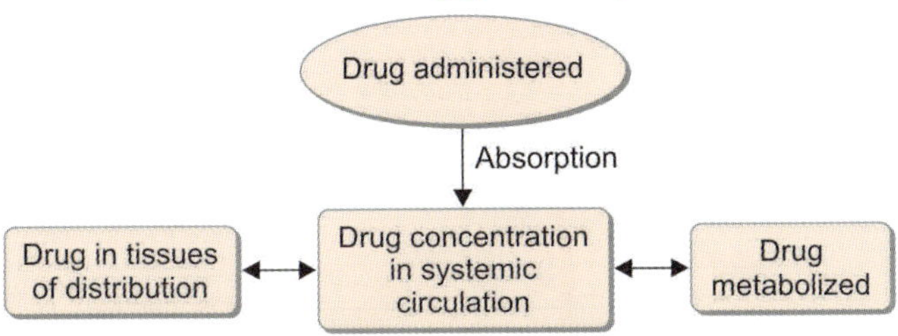

a. Pharmacodynamics b. Pharmacokinetics
c. Pharmacotherapeutics d. Pharmacy

Pharmacokinetics is 'What the body does to a drug'. This refers to movement of the drug in an alteration of the drug by the body; this includes absorption, distribution, binding/localization/storage, biotransformation and excretion of the drug.

2. Effect of which types of adrenergic receptor activation:

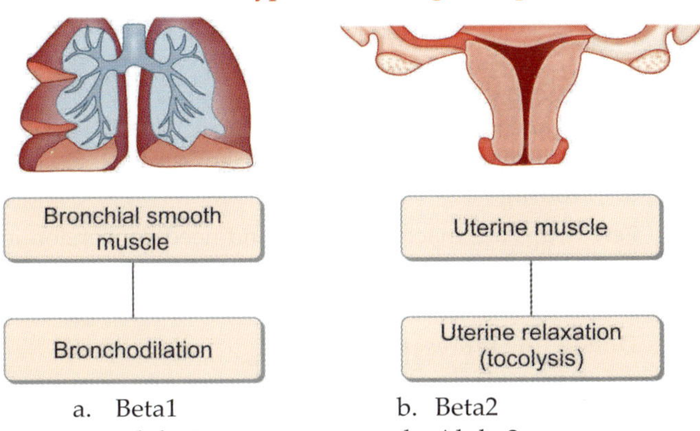

a. Beta1 b. Beta2
c. Alpha1 d. Alpha2

Beta 2 adrenergic receptors are present on bronchi, blood vessels, uterus, liver, GIT, urinary tract and eye.

3. What is being shown in the figure:

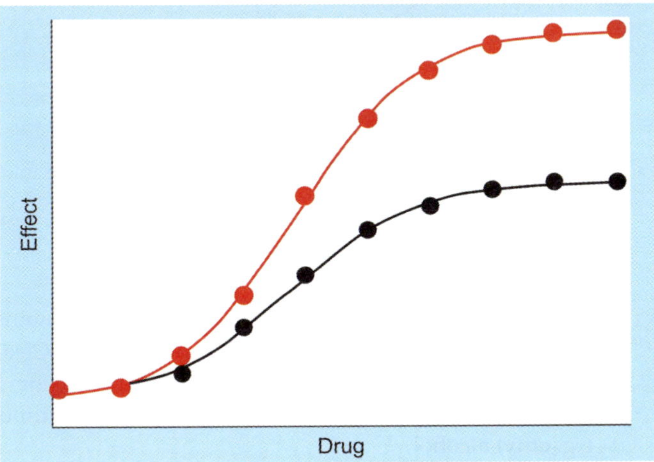

a. Potency b. Efficacy
c. Drug selectivity
d. Therapeutic window phenomenon

The upper limit of the DRC (dose response curve) is the index of drug efficacy and refers to the maximal response that can be elicited by the drug.

4. The following picture depicts potency which is defined as:

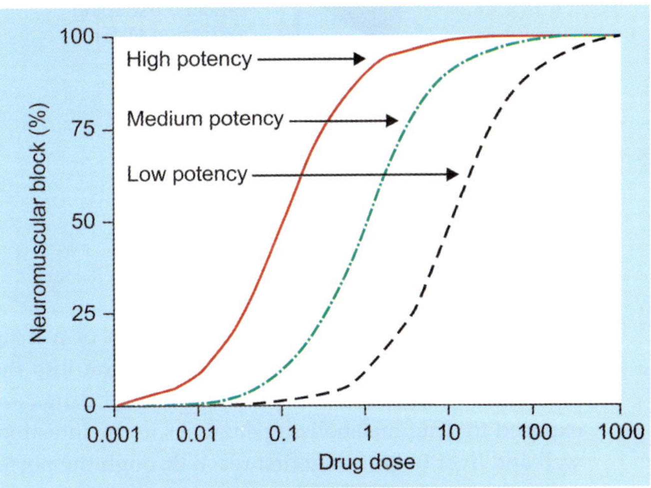

a. Maximal response that a drug can produce
b. Amount of drug required to produce a desired effect
c. Optimum effect of a drug is within a specific plasma range
d. A constant amount of drug is being excreted

The position of the DRC on the dose axis is the index of drug potency which refers to the amount of drug needed to produce a certain response. A DRC positioned rightward indicates lower potency.

5. Which of the following teratogenic drug is responsible for this type of presentation:

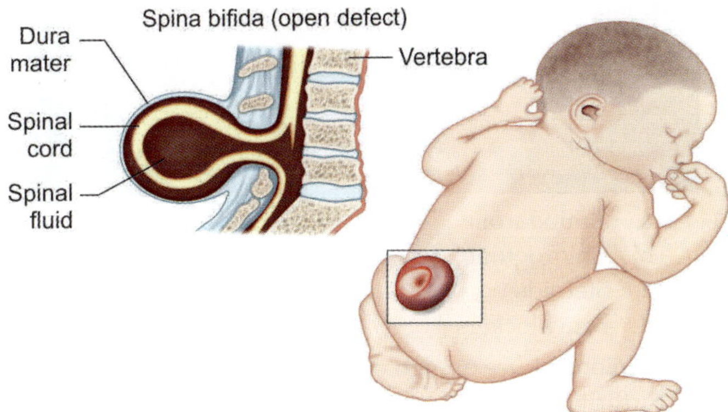

a. Valproate
b. Carbamazepine
c. Phenytoin
d. Ethyl alcohol

Valproate, if taken during pregnancy, may lead to spina bifida and other neural tube defects, heart and limb abnormalities.

6. Following picture depicts which process:

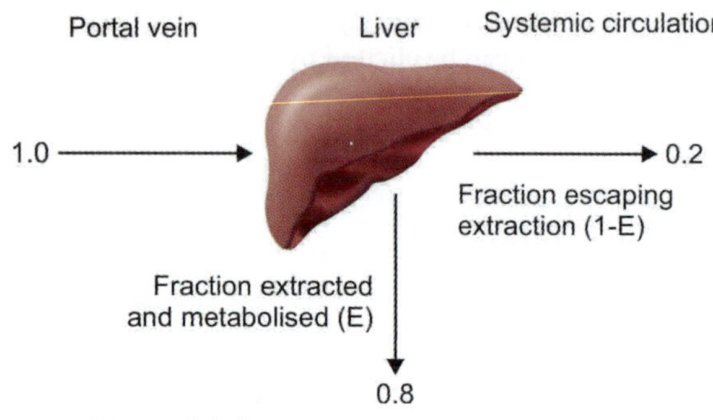

a. Bioavailability
b. Clearance
c. First pass metabolism
d. Microsomal enzyme induction

First pass metabolism refers to metabolism of a drug during its passage from the site of absorption into the systemic circulation. All orally administered drugs are exposed to drug metabolizing enzymes in the intestinal wall and liver (where they first reach through the portal vein).

7. Which of the following drug is responsible for this kind of presentation:

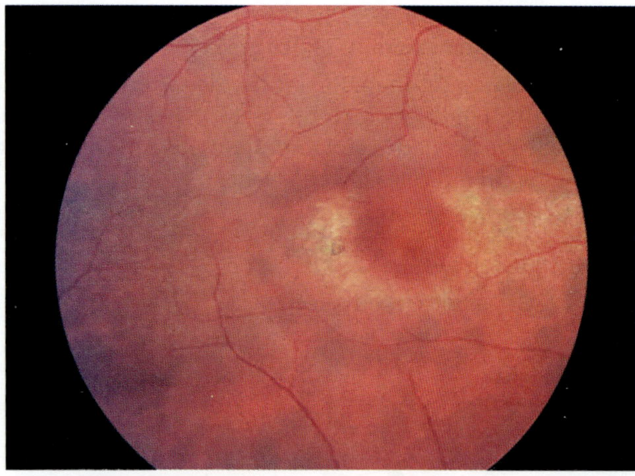

a. Amiodarone
b. Chloroquine
c. Steroids
d. Beta blockers

Prolonged use of high doses (as needed for theumatoid arthritis, DLE etc.) may cause loss of vision due to retinal damage (bulls eye maculopathy). Corneal deposits may also occur and affect vision, but are reversible on discontinuation.

8. Which type of drugs are these:

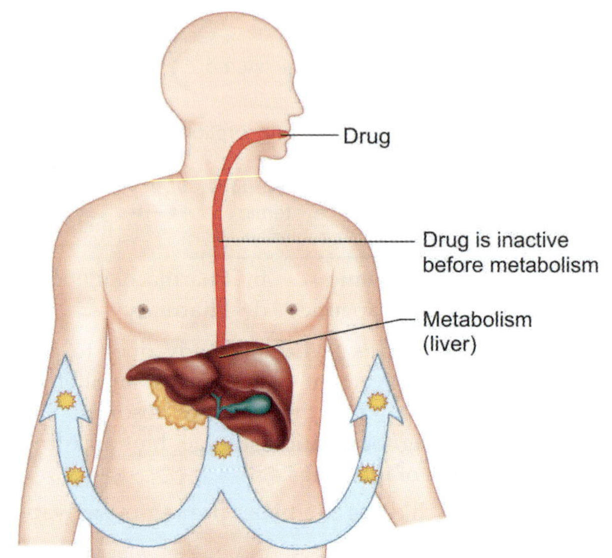

a. Orphan drugs
b. Hit and run drugs
c. Drugs with high first pass metabolism
d. Prodrug

Few drugs are inactive as such and need conversion in the body to one or more active metabolites. Such a drug is called prodrug.

9. Dotted line represents:

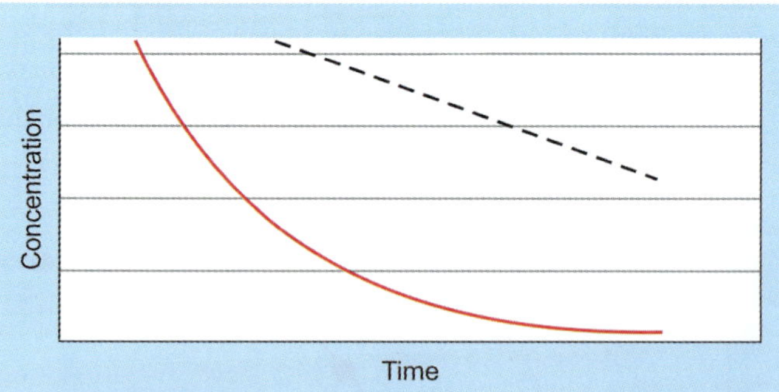

a. Zero order kinetics
b. First order kinetics
c. Steady state plasma concentration
d. Bioavailability

In zero order kinetics, the rate of elimination remains constant irrespective of the drug concentration. Clearance decreases with increase in concentration; or a constant amount of the drug is eliminated in unit time, e.g. ethyl alcohol.

10. Which teratogenic drug is responsible for such a presentation:

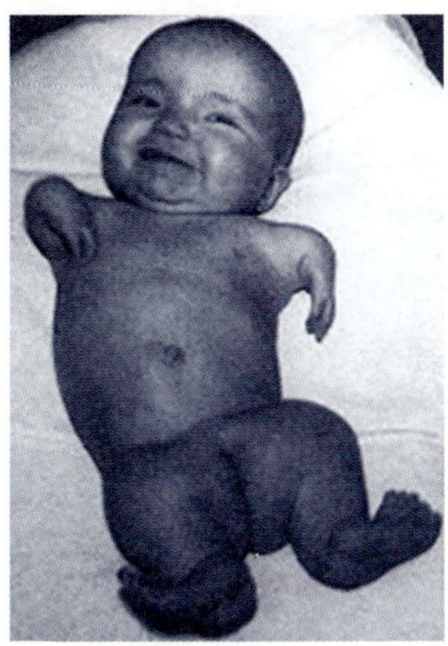

a. Phenytoin
b. Carbamazepine
c. Steroids
d. Thalidomide

Use of thalidomide during pregnancy results in phocomelia and multiple defects of internal organs.

MCQ POINTS

S. No.	Question statements	Answer
1.	Elimination after 4 halves lives in first order kinetics	***93.7%***
2.	Therapeutic index of a drug is an indicator of	***Safety***
3.	Phase II in a clinical trial is done to assess	***Therapeutic efficacy***
4.	Effect of d-tubocurarine can be antagonized by	***Neostigmine, edrophonium***
5.	Mechanism of action of pralidoxime in organophosphrous poisoning	***Choline-esterase reactivator***
6.	Anticholinergic drug that has comparatively specific action on gastric secretion and is useful in peptic ulcer	***Pirenzepine***
7.	Tiotropium is useful in which condition	***Asthma***
8.	Immediate treatment of anaphylaxis is	***I/M adrenaline***
9.	Action of clonidine on adrenegric receptors	***Agonist***
10.	Induction agent that may cause adrenal cortex suppression	***Etomidate***
11.	Mechanism of action of aminophylline	***PDE-4 inhibitor***
12.	Mechanism of action of monteleukast	***Cys-LT1 receptor blocker***
13.	Mechanism of action of sulfonylureas	***Brisk release of insulin from pancreas and Increase in number of receptors***
14.	Metyrapone is useful in congenital adrenal hyperplasia s its inhibits	***11-beta-hydroxylase***
15.	Mechanism of action of clomiphene citrate	***Anti-estrogenic; blocks estrogen receptors and prevent negative feedback on anterior pituitary gland***
16.	Mechanism of action of vigabatrin	***Inhibition of GABA transaminase***
17.	Drug of choice in drug-induced parkinsonism is	***Benzhexol***
18.	Most common side effect reported with treatment with haloperidol	***Akathisia***
19.	Opioid specific antagonist	***Naloxone, Naltrexone***
20.	Opioid derivative which is partial agonist as well as antagonist	***Nalorphine, Pentazocine***
21.	Most commonly used drug in maintenance dose for opioid dependence	***Methadone***
22.	Quinidine exerts its action on heart by inhibiting which channels	***Sodium***
23.	Mechanism of action of dipyridamole	***Phosphodiesterase inhibitor***
24.	Drug for treating heparin-induced thrombocytopenia	***Direct thrombin inhibitors (Argatroban, Lepirudin)***
25.	Cholestyramine increases activity of which enzyme	***Binds bile acids and interrupts their enterohepatic circulation***
26.	Drug of choice for motion sickness	***Transdermal hyoscine (also known as scopolamine)***
27.	Relationship of zero order kinetics to plasma drugs level	***Independent***
28.	Emergence delirium is characteristic of	***Ketamine***
29.	Vitamin deficiency noticed with phenytoin therapy	***Folic acid, vitamin D and vitamin K***
30.	Long post antibiotic effect is seen in which group of drugs	***Fluoroquinolones, aminoglycosides***
31.	Drug used in resistant gonorrhoea	***Spectinomycin***
32.	Which tetracycline can be used in renal failure without any dose adjustment	***Doxycycline***
33.	Penicillinase resistant penicillin is	***Methicillin, cloxacillin, dicloxacillin***
34.	Treatment of Legioairnne's disease	***Azithromycin***
35.	Metrifonate is effective against which parasite	***Schistosomiasis***
36.	Most effective antitubercular drug against slow multiplying intracellular mycobacteria	***Rifampicin***

S. No.	Question statements	Answer
37.	DNA dependent RNA synthesis is inhibited by	***Rifampicin***
38.	Alpha1 adrenergic blocker without any effect on blood pressure	***Tamsulosin***
39.	Anticancer drug causing lung fibrosis	***Busulfan, bleomycin***
40.	Treatment of chronic phase of CML	***Imatinib***
41.	Cyclosporin A acts on which cells	***CD4 T cell***
42.	Galantamine is used for	***Alzheimers disease***
43.	DOC for nocardiosis	***Cotrimoxazole***
44.	DOC for herpes simplex	***Acyclovir***
45.	Corticosteroid with maximum mineralocorticoid action	***Aldosterone***
46.	Mechanism of action of cholestyramine	***Binds to bile acids and prevents enterohepatic circulation***
47.	Half life of digoxin	***36 hours***
48.	Site of action of loop diuretics	***Thick ascending limb of loop of Henle***
49.	Drug of choice in lithium-induced Diabetes insipidus	***Amiloride***
50.	MC cardiac adverse effect of lithium	***Arrhythmia***
51.	Mechanism of action of Dantrolene	***Binds to R_yR_1/ryanodine receptors and prevents release of calcium***
52.	Anti-glaucoma drug which is beta1 selective beta blocker	***Betaxolol***
53.	Drug used for common cold which can cause stroke	***Phenylpropanolamine***
54.	Modafinil is used as an adjunct in the treatment of	***Sleep apnea***
55.	Rizatriptan is a drug used for	***Migraine***
56.	Orally administered anti-Kala azar drug	***Miltefosine***
57.	Febuxostat is used for	***Hyperuricemia/Gout***
58.	Microbial killing by an antibiotic below its "Minimum inhibitory concentration' is known as	***Post antibiotic effect***
59.	Which fluoroquinolone drug is withdrawn in India	***Gatifloxacin***
60.	Drug of choice for prophylaxis of TB	***INH/isoniazid***
61.	Drug of choice for diarrhea in HIV	***Octreotide***
62.	Drug that can cause hypertrophic pyloric stenosis	***Erythromycin***
63.	In anaphylactic shock, epinephrine is given by which route	***Intramuscular***
64.	In the treatment of shock, dobutamine is preferred over dopamine because	***Less renal vasodilatory effect***
65.	Which tetracycline group drug can be used in renal failure without adjustment in dose	***Doxycycline***
66.	Drug used in prophylaxis of meningococcal meningitis	***Rifampicin***
67.	Mechanism of action of Rifampicin	***Inhibition of DNA dependent RNA polymerase***
68.	Fastest acting anti-thyroid drug	***Potassium Iodide***
69.	When a drug binds to the receptor and causes action submaximal to that of agonist. This is called	***Partial agonist***
70.	DOC for systemic aspergillosis	***Amphotericin B***
71.	Amphotericin B toxicity is monitored by	***Serum potassium levels***
72.	Mechanism of action of granisetron	***5-HT_3 antagonist***
73.	Anti-IgE antibodies used in asthma	***Omalizumab***
74.	Most enzyme resistant aminoglycoside	***Amikacin***
75.	Mechanism of action of lovastatin	***HMG CoA reductase inhibition***

S. No.	Question statements	Answer
76.	Drug used in prophylaxis of H. influenzae is	***Rifampicin***
77.	What is a prodrug	***Inactive drug which gets converted to active metabolite within the body***
78.	Chemical used for sclerotherapy for varicose veins	***Ethanolamine oleate, phenol***
79.	Mechanism of action of digitalis	***Inhibition of Na^+ K^+ ATPase inhibition***
80.	Earliest symptom of lithium toxicity	***Fine tremors***
81.	Spina bifida may be a teratogenic effect of	***Valproate***
82.	Steroid with equal mineralocorticoid and glucocorticoid activity	***Hydrocortisone***
83.	Idiosyncrasy is defined as	***Genetically determined abnormal reaction to a chemical***
84.	Antitubercular drug associated with psychosis	***Cycloserine, INH***
85.	Only 1st line antitubercular drug which is bacteriostatic	***Ethambutol***
86.	Red discoloration of the skin is Caused By which antileprotic drug	***Clofazimine***
87.	Mechanism of action of ketotifen	***Mast cell stabilization***
88.	Active form of prodrug 'Sulfasalazine'	***5-amino salicylic acid/5-ASA***
89.	If a constant fraction of drug is excreted, it is known as .... order reaction	***First order***
90.	Drugs causing cardiotoxicity	***Daunorubicin, doxorubicin***
91.	t1/2 of esmolol	***10 minutes***
92.	5-HT_3 antagonist are used in	***Vomiting***
93.	NAC is used in toxicity of	***Acetaminophen/ paracetamol***
94.	Site of action of spironolactone	***Collecting duct and DCT***
95.	DOC for diabetes insipidus	***Intranasal desmopressin***
96.	Anti-diabetic drug which causes lactic acidosis	***Phenformin > metformin***
97.	Side effect of chlorpropamide	***Cholestatic jaundice***
98.	Effect of insulin on potassium	***Promotes intracellular movement of potassium***
99.	Insulin glargine is ……… acting insulin	***Long acting***
100.	Enzyme inhibited by sildenafil	***Phospho-di-esterase 5***
101.	2 drugs which increase theophylline levels	***Erythromycin, Cimetidine***
102.	Side effects of topical steroids	***Glaucoma***
103.	MOA of methotrexate	***Antifolate***
104.	DOC for migraine	***Sumatriptan***
105.	Oral acting drug for scabies	***Ivermectin***
106.	DOC for toxoplasmosis and pneumocytis carinii	***Toxoplasmosis (sulfonamide + pyrimethamine); pneumocystis carinii (co-trimoxazole)***
107.	Which organ is primary site for drug metabolism	***Liver***
108.	DOC for malaria in pregnancy	***Quinine***
109.	Nevirapine belongs to … group	***NNRTI/non-nucleoside reverse transcriptase inhibitor***
110.	Anti TB causing retrobulbar neuritis	***Ethambutol***
111.	Most rapidly acting drug against M. leprae	***Rifampin***
112.	Antihypertensive absolutely contraindicated in pregnancy	***ACE inhibitor***
113.	Orally administered anti-Kala azar drug:	***Miltefosine***
114.	Antibiotic (fluoroquinolone) withdrawn in India:	***Gatifloxacin***
115.	DOC for prophylaxis in TB:	***INH***
116.	Anti-TB drug not given in liver disease:	***INH, pyrazinamide, rifampin***

S. No.	Question statements	Answer
117.	ACE inhibitors should not be used with which diuretic:	***Potassium sparing diuretics***
118.	Drug not useful in treatment of acute asthma:	***Cromolyn sodium, monteleukast***
119.	Effect of food on drug absorption:	***Reduced drug absorption***
120.	DOC for diarrhoea in HIV	***Octreotide***
121.	DOC for absence seizures	***Valproate***
122.	Which mode of biotransformation shows genetic polymorphism:	***Acetylation***
123.	An agent which prevents the action of an agonist on a receptor, but does not have any effect of its own is known as:	***Antagonist***
124.	Opioid having an anti-tussive action:	***Codeine***
125.	Highly albumin bound drug:	***Warfarin, phenytoin***
126.	Loop diuretics act at:	***Thick ascending limb of loop of Henle***
127.	Sibutramine belongs to which group of drugs:	***Anti-obesity***
128.	Allopurinol inhibits which enzyme:	***Xanthine oxidase***
129.	What is the dose of isoniazid in children:	***5-15 mg/ Kg***
130.	Misoprostol is:	***PGE1 analogue***
131.	Anticraving drug used for alcohol intoxication:	***Acamprosate/naltrexone/fluoxetine***
132.	Clozapine is used for:	***Resistant schizophrenia***
133.	Adverse effects/unsuspected drug interactions are studied in which phase of clinical trials:	***IV***
134.	DOC for SIADH	***Demeclocycline***
135.	DOC for mushroom poisoning	***Atropine***
136.	Adrenergic drug used in BPH acts on which receptors	***Alpha 1***
137.	Drug used for closure of ductus arteriosus	***Indomethacin***
138.	MOA of allopurinol	***Inhibition of xanthine oxidase***
139.	DOC for scabies	***5% Permethrin (topical)***
140.	Drugs which inhibits HMG-CoA reductase	***Statins***
141.	Drug which prevents degranulation of mast cell	***Cromolyn sodium, ketotifen***
142.	Antihypertensive agent contraindicated in pregnant lady	***ACE inhibitors***
143.	Drug indicated for malaria during pregnancy	***Quinine***
144.	Hemorrhagic cystitis is a complication of	***Cyclophosphamide***
145.	Folinic acid is given to prevent toxicity of	***Methotrexate***
146.	Retroperitoneal fibrosis is a side effect of	***Methysergide***
147.	Zileuton inhibits	***5-lipoxygenase***
148.	Anti-TB drug unsafe in liver disease	***INH, pyrazinamide, rifampin***
149.	DOC for cerebral malaria	***Quinine/ artesunate***
150.	DOC for herpes simplex	***Acyclovir***
151.	MOA of macrolides	***Binds to 50s subunit and prevent protein synthesis***
152.	DOC for non-gonococcal urethritis	***Azithromycin***
153.	anti-TB drug causing hyperuricemia	***Pyrazinamide and ethambutol***
154.	anti-TB combination safer in patient who develops hepatitis while on ATT	***Ethambutol + streptomycin***
155.	Latanoprost is useful in glaucoma as it	***Increases uveo-scleral outflow***
156.	Vitamin K is an antidote for over-dosage of	***Oral anticoagulants (warfarin)***
157.	INR is used to measure the effects of which drug	***Warfarin***
158.	Treatment of gastrinoma	***Proton pump inhibitors***

S. No.	Question statements	Answer
159.	Drug used for treating spasticity	***Baclofen***
160.	Fomepizole is an antidote for	***Methy lalcohol***
161.	Dopamine is preferred over dobutamine in treatment of renal shock because of	***Renal vasodilatory effect***
162.	DOC for cardiogenic shock	***Dopamine***
163.	DOC for listerial meningitis	***Ampicillin + gentamycin***
164.	Interaction of theophylline with erythromycin	***Increased level of theophylline***
165.	Major side effect of cyclosporine	***Nephrotoxicity***
166.	Main drug for treating inflammatory bowel disease	***Sulfasalazine/5-amino salicylic acid***
167.	DOC for enuresis in children	***Clomipramine/desmopressin***
168.	Longest acting SSRI	***Fluoxetine***
169.	Indicator of safety of a drug	***Therapeutic index***
170.	Intranasal calcitonin is used for	***Postemenopausal osteoporosis***
171.	Selective alpha2 antagonist drug	***Yohimbine, mirtazapine***
172.	DOC for chemotherapy-induced vomiting	***Granisetron***
173.	Stage IV of clinical trials is also known as	***Postmarketing surveillance***
174.	Drug used for prophylaxis of migraine	***Propranolol***
175.	Corticosteroid with maximum mineralo-corticoid activity	***Aldosterone***
176.	Site of action of loop diuretics	***Thick ascending limb of loop of Henle***
177.	DOC for malignant hyperthermia	***Dantrolene sodium***
178.	Protamine Zinc Insulin is …….. acting insulin	***Intermediate***
179.	MOA of penicillin	***Inhibits cell wall synthesis***
180.	Drug for prophylaxis of meningococcal meningitis	***Rifampicin***
181.	A person on Anti-TB drugs complains of deafness and tinnitus. Drug implicated is	***Streptomycin***
182.	MOA of quinolones is	***Inhibits DNA gyraseDNA topo-isomerase IV***
183.	Corticoid with equal mineralocorticoid and glucocorticoid activity	***Hydrocortisone/cortisol***
184.	Site of action of aldosterone	***DCT and collecting duct***
185.	Efficacy of a drug refers to	***Maximum effect produced by a given amount of drug***
186.	Anti-neoplastic drug having very high cardiac toxicity	***Adriamycin/doxorubicin, daunorubicin***
187.	Is ethambutol safe in pregnancy	***Yes***
188.	DOC for maduramycosis	***Itraconazole***
189.	If a constant fraction of drug is excreted, it is known as .... order reaction	***First order***
190.	Anti-glaucoma drug which is selective beta 1 blocker	***Betaxolol***
191.	5-HT_3 antagonist are used in	***Vomiting***
192.	NAC is used in toxicity of	***Paracetamol/acetaminophen***
193.	Site of action of spironolactone	***CD and DCT***
194.	DOC for diabetes insipidus	***Desmopressin***
195.	Anti-diabetic drug which causes lactic acidosis	***Phenformin > metformin***
196.	Side effect of chlorpropamide	***Cholestatic jaundice***
197.	Effect of insulin on potassium	***Increases intracellular entry of potassium***
198.	Enzyme inhibited by sildenafil	***Phosphodiesterase 5***
199.	Side effects of topical steroids	***Glaucoma***
200.	MOA of methotrexate	***Anti-folate (inhibits dihydrofolate reductase)***

S. No.	Question statements	Answer
201.	DOC for migraine	***Sumatriptan***
202.	Oral acting drug for scabies	***Ivermectin***
203.	DOC for toxoplasmosis	***Sulfamethoxazole + pyrimethamine***
204.	Anti TB causing retrobulbar neuritis	***Ethambutol***
205.	Orally administered anti-Kala azar drug:	***Miltefosine***
206.	Drug not useful in treatment of acute asthma:	***Long acting beta 2 agonist***
207.	DOC for absence seizures	***Valproate***
208.	An agent which prevents the action of an agonist on a receptor, but does not have any effect of its own is known as:	***Antagonist***
209.	Sibutramine belongs to which group of drugs:	***Anti-obesity***
210.	What is the dose of isoniazid in children:	***5-15 mg/kg***
211.	Misoprostol is:	***PGE_1 analogue***
212.	Clozapine is used for:	***Resistant schizophrenia***

CHAPTER

8 FORENSIC MEDICINE

KEY POINTS

Types of Inquest

- Police inquest
- Magistrate's Coroner's inquest
- Medical examiner's inquest (best system of inquest).

Magistrate's Inquest is done in

- Prison death
- Police custody death
- Police firing death
- Dowry death
- Exhumation
- Police interrogation death.

Dying Deposition

- Recorded by magistrate
- Recorded under oath
- Presence of accused and its lawyer necessary
- Superior.

Dying Declaration

- Recorded by magistrate or doctor
- No oath necessary
- Presence of accused and its lawyer is not necessary
- Inferior.

Types of Consent

- Implied consent: When he conduct of the person indicated that he has given permission for the act to be done, without expression it verbally or in writing
- Expressed consent: When the person is asked for the consent for an act, then he expresses his consent
- Informed consent: Consent has been given after knowing all the pros and cons of the act for which the consent is being taken.

Tests used for Blood Stains

- Benzidine
- Phenolphthalein (Kestle-Meyer)
- Takayama's hemochromatogen
- Teichmann
- Hemin
- Spectroscopic
- Leucomalachite green
- Luminal.

Tests Used to Detect Seminal Stains

- Barberio's test
- Florence test
- Acid phosphatase test
- Creatinine phosphokinase
- Semen specific glycoprotein
- ELISA (SEMA assay for seminal vesicle specific antigen).

Deciduous Teeth Eruption (in Months)

- Lower central incisor: 6
- Upper central incisor: 7
- Upper lateral incisor: 8
- Lower lateral incisor: 9
- First molar: 12
- Canines: 18
- Second molar: 24.

Permanent Teeth Eruption (in Years)

- First molar: 6
- Central incisor: 7
- Lateral incisor: 8
- First premolar: 9
- Second premolar: 10
- Canines: 11
- Second molar: 12
- Third molar: 17–30.

Accuracy in Sexing Adult Skeletal

- Entire skeleton: 100 percent
- Pelvis: 95 per cent

- Skull alone: 90 per cent
- Pelvis plus skull: 98 per cent
- Long bones alone: 80 per cent.

Postmortem Lividity (Color and Cause)

- Cherry red: Carbon monoxide
- Pinkish: HCN
- Bright red: Cold
- Dark brown: Phosphorus
- Brown: Potassium cyanide, sodium cyanide
- Brown: Aniline, carbon dioxide
- Greenish blue: Hydrogen sulphide
- Red: Drowning.

Postmortem Caloricity is Seen in

- Sunstroke
- Cholera
- Septicemia
- Tetanus
- Alcohol poisoning
- Strychnine poisoning
- Rabies.

Cadavers Spasm/Instantaneous Rigor

- Stiffening of muscles immediately after death without being preceded by primary relaxation
- Seen when the muscles of the body were in a state of strong contraction immediately before death.

Color Changes in Bruise (Time, Color and Cause)

- 0: Red (Blood)
- Few hours—3 days: Blue
- 4 days: Bluish-black to brown (hemosiderin)
- 5–6 days: Green (hematoidin)
- 7–12 days: Yellow (bilirubin)
- 14 days: Normal.

Grievous Hurt (Sec 320 IPC)

- Emasculation
- Permanent privation/loss of sight of either eye
- Permanent privation/loss of heating of either ear
- Privation of any member of any joint
- Destruction or permanent impairing of power of any member of joint
- Permanent disfiguration of head or face
- Fracture or dislocation of bone or tooth
- Any hurt which endangers the life or which causes the sufferer to severe bodily pain makes him unable to follow his ordinary pursuits for a period of 20 days.

Bullets

- Tandem bullets/Piggyback bullet: Bullets ejected one after another, as the previous one was stuck in the barrel.
- Dumdum bullet: Nose cut off
- Ricochet: Before striking the aim, strikes some other object, to get rebound and hit the target.
- Frangible bullets: Designed to fragment upon impact, often to the point of disintegration.

Entry Wound

- Smaller than the diameter of bullet
- Inverted edge
- Abrasion present
- Grease collar present
- Burning, stinging, tattooing, blackening present in close shot wounds
- Bleeding and tissue extrusion are less.

Exit Wound

- Larger than diameter of bullet
- Everted edge
- Abrasion absent
- Grease collar absent
- Burning, stinging, tattooing, blackening absent
- Bleeding and tissue extrusion are more.

Heat Injuries

- Heat cramps/miners cramps/Stokers cramps/Fireman's cramps:
  - Caused by rapid dehydration of body
  - Through the loss of water and salt in the sweat
  - Seen in workers in high temperature
  - There is profuse sweating
- Heat prostration/heat exhaustion/heat syncope/heat collapse:
  - Condition of collapse without increase in body temperature
  - Follows exposure to excessive heat
  - Precipitated by muscular work and unsuitable clothing
- Heat hyperpyrexia/heat stroke:
  - Hyperpyrexia is fever above 41.5°C
  - Heat stroke is rectal temperature greater than 41°C and neurological disturbances.

Hemodialysis is not Useful in Poisoning by Following

- Digoxin
- Kerosene
- Benzodiazepines
- OPC.

Contraindication for Emesis

- Corrosive
- Irritant
- Convulsive
- Volatile
- Comatose
- Heart disease
- Pregnant women.

Contraindication for Gastric Lavage

- Very old
- Corrosive
- Convulsants
- Unconsciousness
- Heart disease
- Peptic ulcer.

Antidotes of Some Poisons

- Acids: Weak noncarbonated alkalies
- Alkalies: Weak vegetable acids—citric acid, acetic acid
- Silver nitrate: Sodium chloride
- Mercuric chloride: Egg albumin
- Arsenic poisoning: Freshly prepared ferric oxide
- Opium: Potassium permanganate, naloxone
- Dhatura: Neostigmine
- Strychnine: Barbiturate
- Oxalic acid: Calcium gluconate
- Phenol/carbolic acid: 20 per cent alcohol for gastric lavage
- Aspirin: Stomach wash with magnesium oxide
- Yellow phosphorus: Stomach was with 0.1 percent solution of copper sulphate
- Lead: Stomach wash with magnesium or sodium sulphate, calcium disodium EDTA I/V
- Mercury: Egg albumin, BAL or penicillamine I/V
- OPC: Atropine, oximes.

Poisons and Active Principle

- Abrus precatorius/Rati: Abrin (Used by jewelers in olden days to measure gold and silver; Local effect similar to viper snake bite)
- Ricinus communis/Castor: Ricin [Castor oil (Erandel oil)]
- Croton tiglium/purging croton/jamalgota: Crotin and Crotonoside (purgative)
- Semecarpus anacardium/Marking nut: Semicarpol and Bhilawanol (used in laundries for making on clothes)
- Calotropis/madar: Calotropin, calotoxin, gigantin, uscharin
- Capsicum annum: Capsicin, capsaicin
- Aconite/Mitha vish: Aconitine [pupils show hippus reaction (alternate constriction and dilatation)].

Colloquial/Street Names of Some Substances of Abuse

- Mitha vish (sweet poison): Aconite
- Siddhi/Bhang: Leaves and stems of cannabis sativa (2% cannabinol)
- Majun: Sweetmeat preparation of Bhang
- Ganja: Flowering tops of female plants of C. sativa (5-10% cannabinol)
- Reefer: Cigarette preparation of Ganja
- Charas: Resinous extract from leaves and flowers of C. sativa (20–50% cannabinol)
- Speed ball/Brown sugar/Smack: Heroin.

Viscera Preservation

- Saturated solution of salt: All poisonings, including carbolic acid, except acids
- Rectified spirit: Acid poisoning (except carbolic acid)
- 10 per cent formalin: Preservation for histopathological examination
- Potassium oxalate + sodium fluoride: Blood preservation in alcohol poisoning case
- Sodium citrate + sodium fluoride: Blood preservation in oxalic acid, ethylene glycol
- Potassium oxalate + sodium nitrite: Blood preservation in fluoride poisoning case.

Signs and Symptoms of Acute Dhatura Poisoning

- Flushed skin (red as beet)
- Hyperthermia (hot as hare)
- Inhibition of secretions (dry as bone)
- Dilation of pupils with loss of accumulation (blind as bat)
- Restlessness, delirium (mad as wet hen).

Epidemic Dropsy

- Adulteration of mustard oil with argemone oil (which contains sanguinarine and dihydrosanguinarine)
- Features:
  - Diarrhea
  - Marked edema/generalized anasarca
  - Glaucomas.

Criteria of Rape in India

- Unlawful intercourse by a man
- With his wife under age of 15 years
- With any woman under 16 years
- With any other woman above 16 years, against her will
- In case of rape—semen sample should be collected within 2 days.

Sexual Offences

- Indecent assault:
  - Offence committed on a female with the intention or knowledge to outrage her modesty
  - Such assaults are punishable under Sec. 354 IPC

- Incest:
  - Sexual intercourse by a man with a woman who is closely related to him by blood
  - In India, incest as such, is not an offence.

Cannabis Sativa

- Active content: THC/tetra-hydro-cannabinol
- Distorted perceptions (during trip)
- Run amok: Depression followed by impulse to murder.

Hydrogen Cyanide Poisoning

- Characteristic bitter almonds smell
- Postmortem staining: Cherry-red color
- Mechanism of action of HCN: Inhibition of cytochrome oxidase and carbonic anhydrase which leads to histotoxic/cytotoxic hypoxia
- Management:
  - Amyl nitrate
  - Sodium nitrite (converts hemoglobin to methaemoglobin)
  - Sodium thiosulphate
  - Hydroxycobalamin

MCQs WITH SHORT EXPLANATIONS

INJURIES

1. Gutter fracture is due to:

a. Osteoporosis
b. Fall from height
c. Sharp weapon
d. Oblique bullet wound

Skull fracture

- Depressed fracture—Crushing of the skull with depression of a portion in towards the brain
- Basilar fracture—Fracture near the floor or base of the skull
- Linear fracture—Break resembling a thin line without obvious distortion
  - Diastatic—Passing through suture lines
  - Hinge—Separates the floor of the skull into two halves
- Ring fracture—Around the foramen magnum, the largest opening in the base of the skull
- Pond fracture—A shallow depressed fracture
- Comminuted fracture—A fracture with many divisions
- Mosaic fracture—A comminuted depressed fracture
- Gutter fracture—A long, narrow fracture of the skull, caused by a gunshot wound

2. Tail of wound indicates:

a. Depth of wound
b. Direction of wound
c. Age of wound
d. Size of wound

Characteristics of incised wound

- Injury varies in sharpness according to the characters of weapon
- Margins are clean cut
- No bruising of wound edges occurs
- Wound is usually linear
- Length of wound is greater than its depth
- All tissues are clearly divided and there is no tissue bridging
- As the vessels are cut, bleeding is profuse even in small incised wounds
- At the commencement, the tissues are more deeply cut and tails off at the end. This indicates the direction of the wound.
- If sharp weapon enters obliquely, one margin of wound is beveled and the other overhangs, indicating the direction

3. Feature of suicidal cut wound:

a. Uses small weapon
b. Over accessible parts of body
c. Hesitation marks
d. All of the above

Small, multiple, superficial and skin deep incised wounds seen at the commencement of a main suicidal incised wound. They usually merge with the main wound. Incised wounds with such hesitation cuts are suicidal.

Difference between suicidal and homicidal cut-throat wounds.

	Trait	*Suicidal wounds*	*Homicidal wounds*
1	Situation:	Left side of the neck and passing across the front of the throat; rarely on both sides.	Usually on both sides.
2	Level :	High; above the thyroid cartilage.	Low; on or below the thyroid cartilage.
3	Direction:	Above downwards and from left to right in right–handed person. Sometimes horizontal cuts across the front of the neck are seen which do not show variation in depth at either end.	Transverse or from below upwards. If attacked from the right side of victim, the wound runs from left to right; if from behind, it may resemble suicidal wound.
4	Number of wounds:	Multiple, may be 20 to 30, superficial, parallel and merged with the main wound; rarely single.	Multiple, cross each other at a deep level; not repeated in depths of the main wound.
5	Edges :	Usually ragged due to overlapping of multiple superficial incisions.	Sharp and clean-cut; bevelling may be seen.
6	Hesitation cuts :	Present.	Absent.
7	Tailing :	Present.	Absent.
8	Severity:	Usually less severe. One wound may be extremely deep, extending up to cervical vertebrae, but sometimes 2 or 3.	More severe; all the tissues including the vertebrae may be cut.
9	Wounds in other parts of the body :	Often present across wrists, groin, thighs, ankles, or knees; and rarely on the back of neck.	No wounds on wrists, etc. but severe injuries usually on the head and neck.
10	Defence wounds:	Absent; unintentional cuts may be found on the fingers if a blade has been used.	Present.

Contd...

Ans. 1. **d.** Oblique bullet wound 2. **b.** Direction of wound 3. **d.** All of the above

Contd...

	Trait	Suicidal wounds	Homicidal wounds
11	Hands:	Weapon may be firmly grasped due to cadaveric spasm.	Fragments of clothing, hair, etc., may be grasped.
12	Weapon:	Usually present.	Usually absent.
13	Vessels:	As head is thrown back, carotid artery is drawn beneath sternomastoid and against the spine and usually escapes injury.	Jugular vein and carotid artery are likely to be cut.
14	Blood stains:	If standing, stains on the mirror and on front of body and clothes running from above downwards and splashes on feet.	If asleep, blood runs down on both sides of the neck and collects behind the neck and shoulder; stains found on both palms, for the victim attempts to cover the wound.
15	Clothes:	Not cut or damaged.	May be cut corresponding in position to those in the body; disarrangement, tears and loss of buttons.
16	Circumstantial evidence:	Quiet place, such as bedroom or locked bath-room; usually stands in front of a mirror in order to direct the hand better; suicidal note or farewell letter may be found.	Disturbance at the scene, such as disarrangement of furniture in a room; trampling and crushing of vegetable matter and shrubs, or confused foot prints outside.

4. Lesion with intact skin but tearing of subcutaneous tissue is:
- a. Scalds
- b. Laceration
- c. Contusion
- d. Abrasion

Extravasation of blood into the tissues due to rupture of capillaries, venules and small arterioles usually as a result of trauma, is called a bruise.

Difference between hypostasis and bruise.

	Trait	Hypostasis	Bruise
1	Cause:	Due to distension of vessels with blood in the dermis.	Due to ruptured vessels which may be superficial or deep.
2	Site:	Occurs over extensive area of the most dependent parts.	Occurs at the site of and surrounding the injury; may appear anywhere on the body.
3	Appearance:	No elevation of the involved area.	Often swollen because of extravasated blood and oedema.
4	Epidermis:	Not abraded.	May be abraded.
5	Margins:	Clearly defined.	Merge with surrounding area.
6	Colour:	Uniform bluish-purple in colour.	Old bruises are of different colour. Fresh bruises may appear more intense than the adjacent hypostatic area.
7	Incision:	On incision blood is seen in blood vessels, which can be easily washed away. Subcutaneous tissues are pale.	Shows extravasation of blood into the surrounding tissues, which is firmly clotted and cannot be washed by gentle stream of water. Subcutaneous tissues are deep reddish-black.
8	Effect of pressure:	Absent in areas of the body which are even under slight pressure.	Little lighter over the area of pressure or support.

5. NOT a grievous injury:
- a. Multiple scars of face
- b. Fracture of femur
- c. Emasculation
- d. Contusion of breast

The following kinds of hurt only are designated as "Grievous:"
- Emasculation
- Permanent privation of the sight of either eye
- Permanent privation of the hearing of either ear
- Privation of any member or joint
- Destruction or permanent impairing of the powers of any member or joint
- Permanent disfiguration of the head or face
- Fracture or dislocation of a bone or tooth
- Any hurt which endangers life or which causes the sufferer to be during the space of twenty days in severe bodily pain, or unable to follow his ordinary pursuits.

6. Abrasion collar is seen in:
- a. Abrasions over neck
- b. Bullet injury
- c. Punctured wounds
- d. Lacerated wounds

Ans. **4. c.** Contusion **5. d.** Contusion of... **6. b.** Bullet injury

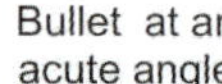

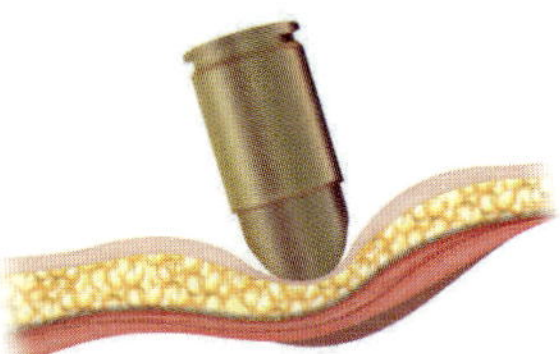

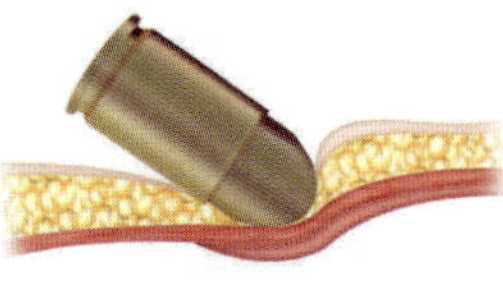

Abrasion collar of an entrance bullet wound.

Close range gunshot wounds

1. Almost always circular in shape
2. Edges are inverted
3. Collar of abrasion
4. 'Metal fouling'
5. Burning effects (within a few centimeters)
6. Tattooing around (or stippling)

7. Bevelling of the skull is seen in:

a. Depressed fracture of the skull
b. Exit point of bullet
c. Inner table of the entry point in bullet injury
d. Outer table of the entry point in bullet injury

Entrance wounds into skull bone typically produces bevelling, or coning, of the bone at the surface away from the weapon on the inner table. In thin areas such as the temple, this may not be observed. Sternum, iliac crest, scapula, or rib may show similar features.

8. Rupture of the skin and subcutaneous tissue is:

a. Incised wound b. Abrasions
c. Lacerated wound d. Contusion

Lacerations are tears or splits of skin, mucous membranes, muscle or internal organs produced by application of blunt force to broad area of the body, which crushed or stretched tissues beyond the limits of their elasticity.

9. In case of bullet shot injury, singeing of hairs & charring of skin indicates a distance of:

a. 1″
b. 3″
c. 6″
d. 9″

Shotgun near contact wound (or close range wound approx. 6 inches)

- Singeing of hair, 'clubbed hair'
- Skin burns due to flame/hot gases
- Smoke/soot soiling around the wound
- Tattooing around the wound
- Partly burnt/unburnt flakes or grains of propellant on the surrounding skin
- Wound is circular or elliptical, depending upon the angle of fire
- Edges are nibbled or irregular due to individual pellets
- Distant bruising around wound due to gas pressure trauma

10. Most common organ affected in blast injury:

a. Liver b. Lung
c. Nervous tissue d. Skeletal system

Unique patterns of injury are found in all blast types. The **lungs**, bowel, and middle ear are most susceptible to primary **blast injuries** (PBIs).

11. True statement regarding postmortem wounds is:

a. Signs of spurting of arterial blood on the body
b. Firmly coagulated blood in the wounds and tissues present
c. Edges of the wound does not gape
d. Increased activity of enzymes

The edges of postmortem wounds are closely approximated.

Difference between antemortem and postmortem wounds.

	Trait	*Antemortem wounds*	*Postmortem wounds*
1	Edges:	The edges are swollen, everted, retracted, and wound gapes.	Edges do not gape, but are closely approximated.
2	Haemorrhage:	Abundant and usually arterial.	Slight or more and venous.
3	Spurting:	Signs of spurting of arterial blood on the body, clothing or in its vicinity present.	No spurting of blood.
4	Extravasation:	Staining of the edges of the wound and extravasation in neighbouring subcutaneous and interstitial tissues which cannot be removed by washing.	Edges and cellular tissues are not deeply stained. The stain can be removed by washing.
5	Coagulation:	Firmly coagulated blood in wounds and tissues present.	No clotting or soft, friable clot.
6	Vital reaction:	Signs of vital reaction present, i.e., inflammation and repair.	No signs of vital reaction.
7	Enzyme histochemistry:	Increased activity of esterases, adenosine triphosphate, aminopeptidase, acid and alkaline phosphatase.	Diminished or no enzyme activity.

Ans. **7. c.** Inner table of the... **8. c.** Lacerated wound **9. c.** 6″ **10. b.** Lung **11. c.** Edges of the...

12. **Hanging results in which type of abrasions:**
    a. Scratch b. Graze
    c. Linear d. Pressure

Pressure abrasion/crushing/friction abrasions
- They are caused by crushing of the superficial layers of the epidermis
- They are associated with a bruise of the surrounding skin
- The ligature mark in cases of hanging and strangulation and the teeth bitemarks are the examples.

13. **Teeth bitemarks are a type of:**
    a. Contusion b. Pressure abrasion
    c. Graze d. Linear abrasion

Types of abrasions
- Linear abrasions (Scratches: Caused by relative movement of a pointed object on the skin. For example nail, thorn, point of sword or knife
- Grazed abrasions: Caused by relative movement of a rough surface on a wide area of skin. For example falls, a victim being dragged on the ground, road traffic accidents
- Imprint abrasions (patterned abrasions, crushing abrasion: Caused by the impact of a rigid hard rough surface over a localized area of the skin without any movement. For example fingernail, tyre, grills, bicycle chain, bitemarks
- Friction abrasions: Caused by pressure upon the skin with an agent with a smooth surface accompanied by movement. For example ligature marks around the neck in hanging, lashes with a whip

14. **True for contrecoup brain injury:**
    a. Located beneath the area of impact
    b. Commoner in stationary head
    c. Commoner in moving head
    d. Seen in brain only

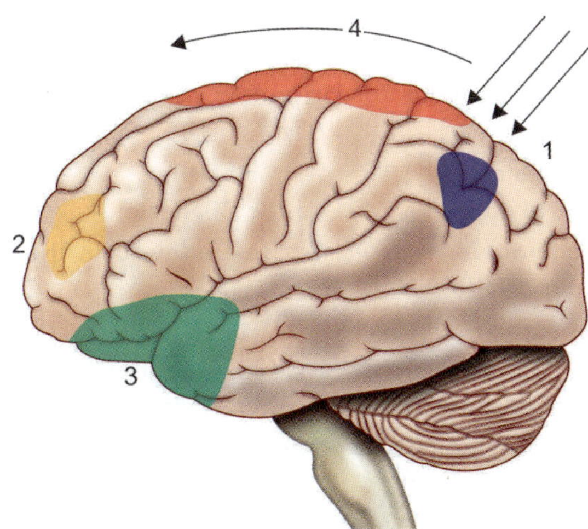

Contusion and laceration of the brain. (1) Coup injury. (2) Contrecoup injury. (3) Dashboard injury in the region of the sphenoidal ridge. (4) Avulsion injury along the superior border of the hemisphere (the rotary vein).

A coup-contrecoup injury is a term applied to head injuries and most often cerebral contusions. It refers to the common pattern of injury whereby damage is located both at the site of impact (often less marked) and on the opposite side of the head to the point of maximum external trauma.

15. **The extent of muscle damage by a bullet depend primary on the:**
    a. Size b. Shape
    c. Velocity d. All of the above

The damage is a result of the energy transferred into the target, therefore how much damage happens depends on how much kinetic energy the bullet has. **Bullet velocity** and mass will **affect** the nature of wounding.

16. **Stellate wound is produced with firearm in:**
    a. Contact shot b. Close shot
    c. Range within 60 cm d. Distant shot

Contact Wounds
- Wound is circular and smaller (may be stellate-shaped over scalp)
- Burning/blackening of immediate wound edges
- Soot within the tissues may be found (usually is less)
- Muzzle mark/imprint
- Inverted margins of the wound
- 'Back spatter,' i.e. blood is sucked up into barrel of the weapon (not common)

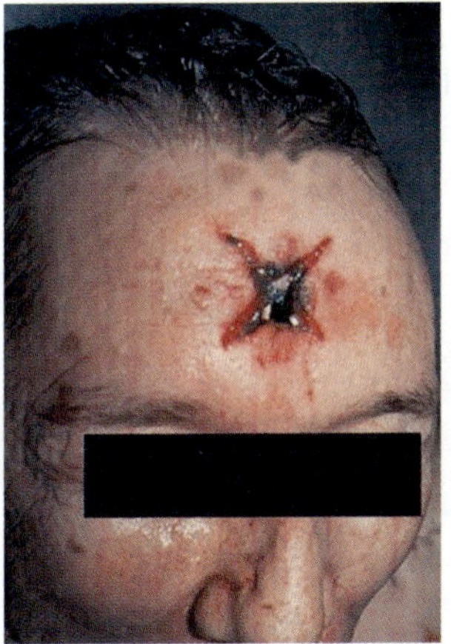
Cruciate injury of the scalp caused by contact shot from a pistol

17. **'Fracture–a-la signature' is:**
    a. Fissured fracture
    b. Depressed fracture
    c. Separation of suture lines
    d. Ring fracture

Fracture-a-la-signature derives its name from forensic medicine because the size and shape of a depressed skull fracture may give information on the type of weapon used. It can be a sign of non-accidental injury in children although it should be noted that these fractures may be accidental.

Ans. 12. **d.** Pressure 13. **b.** Pressure abrasion 14. **c.** Commoner in... 15. **c.** Velocity
16. **a.** Contact shot 17. **b.** Depressed fracture

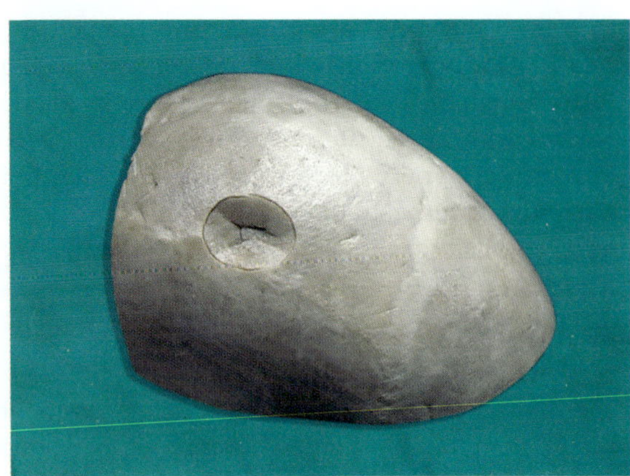
Depressed fracture skull.

18. 'Ewing's postulates' are for:

a. Congenital anomalies cause by drugs
b. Role of disease in modification of effects of trauma
c. Complication resulting from trauma
d. Relationship between malignancy and trauma

Certain criteria, known as '**Ewing's postulates**', must be satisfied before any connection can be maintained between injury and tumor (though, even then, there is no scientific way of proving anything other than a possibility.

19. The effective range of shot gun is:

a. 10–15 meters b. 20–30 meters
c. 30–40 meters d. 60–80 meters

Effective range of the **shotgun** with standard buckshot is limited to about **30–40 meters** with a full stock (depending on the sights on the **gun**.

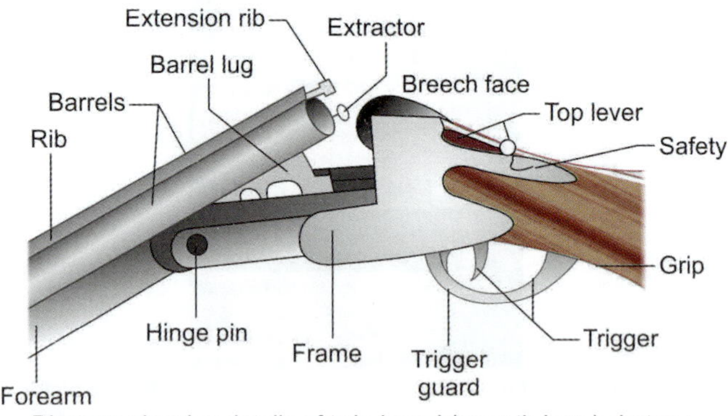

Diagram showing details of twin-barrel (smooth-bore) shotgun.

LAW AND FORENSIC MEDICINE

20. All of the following constitutional articles are related to children EXCEPT?

a. 21A b. 23
c. 24 d. 42

Article 42: Provision for just and humane conditions of work and maternity relief. The state shall make provision for securing just and humane conditions of work and for maternity relief.

21. Locard is associated with which of the following?

a. Body measurement as a mean of personal identification
b. Stature estimation formula
c. Study of fingerprints
d. Exchange theory

Locard's Exchange Principle: When any two objects come into contact, there is always a transfer of material from each object on the other. Traces from the scene may be carried away on the person or tools of the criminal, and at the same time, traces, from all or any of these may be left at the scene.

22. Which of the following defines McNaughten's rule?

a. IPC 84 b. IPC 48
c. CrPC 84 d. CrPC 48

McNaughten rule (the right or wrong test; the legal test) has also been accepted in India as the law of criminal responsibility and is included in Sec. 84, IPC which is as follows: "Nothing is an offence which is done by a person, who at the time of doing it, by reason of unsoundness of mind, is incapable of knowing the nature of the act, or that he is doing what is either wrong or contrary to law".

23. Perjury is dealt under:

a. 190 IPC b. 191 IPC
c. 192 IPC d. 193 IPC

False affidavit is guilty of **perjury** punishable under Section **193 IPC**.

24. In India, magistrate inquest is done in all cases EXCEPT:

a. Exhumation cases
b. Dowry death within 5 years of marriage
c. Murder cases
d. Death of a person in police cases

Police inquest is done in murder cases.

25. Coroner's court was present in:

a. Mumbai b. Delhi
c. Madras d. Bangalore

In India *coroner's inquest* **was followed in the city of** *Mumbai* **till 1999.**

26. In case of death in lock-up, the inquest is held by:

a. A police officer b. Magistrate
c. Panchayat officer d. District attorney

Cases in which magistrate's inquest is held:

- Dowry death
- Exhumation
- Death in police custody
- Death in a psychiatric hospital
- Death in jail
- Death as a result of police shooting

Ans. 18. **d.** Relationship... 19. **c.** 30–40 meters 20. **d.** 42 21. **d.** Exchange theory 22. **a.** IPC 84 23. **d.** 193 IPC 24. **c.** Murder cases 25. **a.** Mumbai 26. **b.** Magistrate

27. Which carries more weight in a court of law:

a. Dying declaration
b. Dying deposition
c. Both carry same weight
d. Both are not significant

Difference between dying declaration and dying deposition

- The former may be recorded by anyone (doctor, police officer or any other) when the latter is recorded only by magistrate.
- Oath is not necessary in the former when it is in the latter.
- Presence of the accused in not essential in the former when presence of the accused/his lawyer is essential in the latter.
- Cross examination is not allowed in the former, when it is allowed in the latter.
- Evidential value of dying declaration is less than dying deposition.
- The former is followed in India when the latter isn't.

28. Criminal responsibility under IPC is NOT applicable if age is below:

a. 5 years b. 7 years
c. 12 years d. 18 years

The age of **criminal responsibility in India is 7 years**. Hence, a child below the age of *7 years* cannot be considered a child in conflict with law (Sec. 82, IPC.

29. Female can give consent for sex if she is above:

a. 12 years b. 16 years
c. 18 years d. 21 years

The legal age of consent for sex in India is 18. It was 16 earlier, but recently the age of consent for sex has been set at 18 years. Any sexual activity with a girl below 18, even with her consent amounts to rape.

30. Police inquest is required in all EXCEPT:

a. Suicide b. Accidental death
c. Dowry death d. Murder

Magistrate inquest is done in dowry death

31. Dying deposition is recorded by:

a. Doctor b. Magistrate
c. Police officer d. Lawyer

A dying declaration is a statement made by a deceased person to anybody who happens to be present when it is made, whereas a dying deposition has to be made before a Magistrate and in the presence of the accused.

32. The power of amnesty for capital punishment is vested with:

a. The president b. Supreme court
c. High court d. The governor

The president of India has the power to grant pardons, remissions of punishments and commutation of death sentence.

33. Who amongst the following is an expert witness:

a. Medical officer
b. Chemical expert
c. Firearm expert
d. All of the above

An **expert witness**, **professional witness** or **judicial expert** is a witness, who by virtue of education, training, skill, or experience, is believed to have expertise and specialized knowledge in a particular subject beyond that of the average person, sufficient that others may officially and legally rely upon the witness's specialized (scientific, technical or other) opinion about an evidence or fact issue within the scope of his expertise, referred to as the expert opinion, as an assistance to the fact-finder.

34. Perjury is defined as:

a. Willful utterance of falsehood
b. Act committed within court premises
c. Failure to sign summons
d. Failure to appear as witness

Perjury, also known as forswearing, is the intentional act of swearing a false oath or of falsifying an affirmation to tell the truth, whether spoken or in writing, concerning matters material to an official proceeding.

35. In India, inquest is carried out by:

a. Police b. Coroner
c. Doctor d. Magistrate

In **India**, normally the **inquest** is conducted by a officer-in-charge (usually sub-inspector) of a police station (S. 174, CrPC).

36. The enquiry into the circumstances of death is called:

a. Homicide enquiry
b. Inquest report
c. Open verdict
d. Adjourned verdict

An **inquest** is a judicial inquiry in common law jurisdictions, particularly one held to determine the cause of a person's death.

37. Exhumation is generally done in the:

a. Early morning b. Evening
c. Night d. Any time

The exhumation commences as early as possible in the morning to ensure maximum privacy and the procedure is carried out in daylight.

38. The time limit for ordering an exhumation in India is:

a. 1 year b. 10 years
c. 20 years d. No limit

Exhumation is the digging out of an already buried body from the grave. There is no time limit for **exhumation** in **India**.

MCQs with Short Explanations

Ans.
27. **b.** Dying deposition 28. **b.** 7 years 29. **c.** 18 years 30. **c.** Dowry death
31. **b.** Magistrate 32. **a.** The president 33. **d.** All of the above 34. **a.** Willful uttera...
35. **a.** Police 36. **b.** Inquest report 37. **a.** Early morning 38. **d.** No limit

39. Leading questions are permitted only in:

a. Examination in chief b. Cross examination
c. Dying declaration d. Re examination

Leading questions may often be answerable with a yes or no (though not all yes-no questions are leading). The propriety of leading questions generally depends on the relationship of the witness to the party conducting the examination. An examiner may generally ask leading questions of a hostile witness or on cross-examination (to elicit testimony which the witness might be reluctant to volunteer), but not on direct examination (to "coach" the witness to provide a particular answer.

40. Husband/relative of husband cruel behavior towards wife come under which IPC section:

a 354 b. 498 A
c. 304 B d. 304 A

Passed by Indian Parliament in 1983, Indian Penal Code 498A, is a criminal law (not a civil law) which is defined as follows:

"Whoever, being the husband or the relative of the husband of a woman, subjects such woman to cruelty shall be punished with imprisonment for a term which may extend to three years and shall also be liable to fine. The offence is Cognizable, non-compoundable and non-bailable.

41. Which of the following defines conduct money:

a. Money paid to the witness to behave properly in the court
b. Money paid to the victim to behave properly in the court
c. Travel expenses for witness
d. Travel expenses for victim

Conduct money is **money** paid in some legal systems to a person under the compulsion of a summons to witness (subpoena) to pay for their expenses to attend in court.

42. Which of the following sections of IPC are concerned with dowry death:

a. 300 b. 302
c. 304A d. 304B

304B. Dowry death

- Where the death of a woman is caused by any burns or bodily injury or occurs otherwise than under normal circumstances within seven years of her marriage and it is shown that soon before her death she was subjected to cruelty or harassment by her husband or any relative of her husband for, or in connection with, any demand for dowry, such death shall be called "dowry death", and such husband or relative shall be deemed to have caused her death.

  Explanation—For the purpose of this sub-section, "dowry" shall have the same meaning as in section 2 of the Dowry Prohibition Act, 1961 (28 of 1961).
- Whoever commits dowry death shall be punished with imprisonment for a term which shall not be less than seven years but which may extend to imprisonment for life.

43. Subpoena is a kind of:

a. Document b. Designation
c. Cout tribunal d. Decomposed body tissue

A **subpoena** is a writ issued by a government agency, most often a court, to compel testimony by a witness or production of evidence under a penalty for failure. Sections 61 to 69 of CrPC deal with summons.

44. First class magistrate can order a maximum punishment of:

a. 1 year jail and ₹ 1000 fine
b. 2 years jail and ₹ 5000 fine
c. 3 years jail and ₹ 5000 fine
d. 4 years jail and ₹ 10000 fine

According to Section 29 of the CrPc., a Judicial Magistrate of First Class may pass a sentence of imprisonment for a term not exceeding three years, or of fine not exceeding five thousand rupees or of both.

Powers of Magistrates (S.29, CrPc.).

Class of Magistrate	*Imprisonment*	*Fine*
Chief Judicial Magistrate	Up to Seven years.	Unlimited (S.63, I.P.C.)
I Class Judicial Magistrate	Up to Three years.	10,000 rupees.
II Class Judicial Magistrate	Up to One year	5,000 rupees.

45. Contributory negligence, if proved, is beneficial to:

a. Nurse b. Patient
c. Treating doctor d. Pharmacist

Indian Courts recognise the concept of contributory negligence. Contributory negligence means the failure by a person to use reasonable care for the safety of either of himself or his property, so that he becomes blameworthy in part as an "author of his own wrong". In the absence of reasonable care on the part of the claimant, courts are likely to reduce the liability of the injurer. "The rule of negligence with the defense of contributory negligence holds an injurer liable if and only if he was negligent and the victim was not. In India, this rule requires proportional sharing of liability when both parties were negligent. That is, the compensation that the victim receives gets reduced in proportion to his or her negligence."

46. Power of a chief judicial magistrate is:

a. Imprisonment up to 7 years
b. Imprisonment up to 5 years
c. Imprisonment up to 3 years
d. Death sentence

Ans. **39. b.** Cross examination **40. b.** 498 A **41. c.** Travel expenses... **42. d.** 304B
43. a. Document **44. c.** 3 years jail and... **45. c.** Treating doctor **46. a.** Imprisonment up to 7...

The Court of a Chief Judicial Magistrate may pass any sentence authorised by law except a sentence of death or of imprisonment for life or of imprisonment for a term exceeding seven years.

MEDICOLEGAL ASPECT OF DEATH

47. What kind of smell emanates from a mummified body?

a. Offensive b. Pungent
c. Putrid d. No smell

Mummification is a modification of putrefaction. Dehydration or drying and shrivelling of the cadaver occurs from the evaporation of water, but the natural appearances of the body and general facial features are preserved. A mummified body is practically odourless.

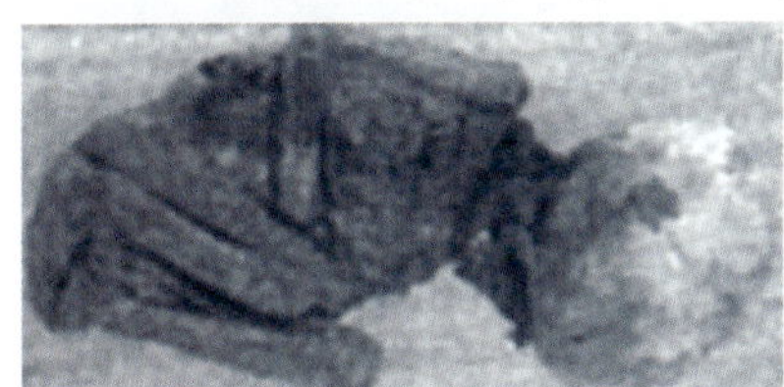

Mummified foetus.

48. Timing of fusion of basi-occiput with basi-sphenoid (in years):

a. 12–14 b. 15–17
c. 18–21 d. 23–25

The basioccipital fuses with the basisphenoid at about 18 to 21 years.

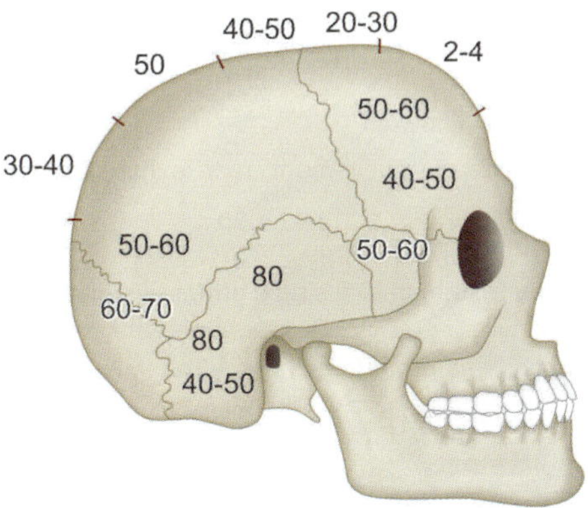

Age of closure of cranial vault.

49. From the given list, which of the following organ putrefies first?

a. Kidney
b. Prostate
c. Heart
d. Brain

As a general rule, the organs show putrefactive changes in the following order. (1) Larynx and trachea. (2) Stomach, intestines, pancreas and spleen. (3) Liver, lungs. (4) Brain. (5) Heart. (6) Kidneys, bladder. (7) Prostate, uterus. (8) Skin, muscle and tendons. (9) Bones.

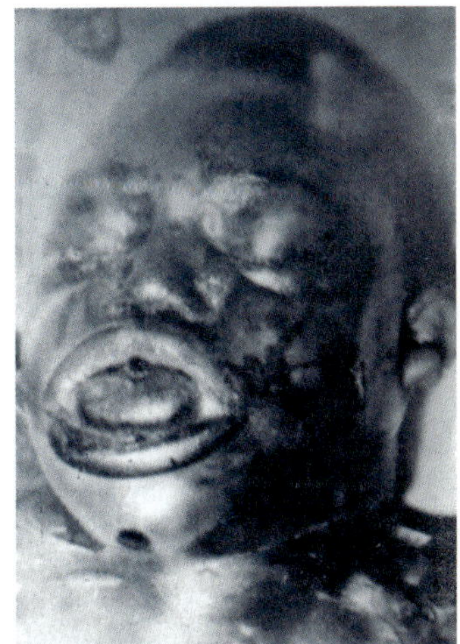

Advanced decomposition showing marked gaseous swelling of face, eye balls and tongue.

50. Which of the following defines posthumous child?

a. Child abandoned by parents
b. Child born after death of father
c. Child born after death of mother
d. Child born after death of mother and father

Posthumous child is a child born after the death of its father, the mother being conceived by the said father.

51. First change in a dead body:

a. Maggot formation
b. Putrefaction
c. Greenish discoloration of right iliac fossa
d. Mummification

Putrefaction timeline

- 2–3 days: Discoloration appears on the skin of the abdomen. The abdomen begins to swell due to gas formation.
- 3–4 days: The discoloration spreads and discolored veins become visible.
- 5–6 days: The abdomen swells noticeably and the skin blisters.
- 2 weeks: The abdomen is bloated; internal gas pressure nears maximum capacity.
- 3 weeks: Tissues have softened. Organs and cavities are bursting. The nails fall off.
- 4 weeks: Soft tissues begin to liquefy and the face becomes unrecognizable.

52. Spalding sign occurs because of:

a. Drowning b. Hanging
c. Maceration d. Mummification

Ultrasound features of intrauterine fetal death

- Absent fetal heart beat
- Absent fetal movements
- Occasional findings
  - Overlapping of skull bones (Spalding sign)
  - Gross distortion of fetal anatomy (maceration)

Ans. 47. **d.** No smell 48. **c.** 18–21 49. **d.** Brain 50. **b.** Child born after death...
51. **c.** Greenish discol... 52. **c.** Maceration

- Soft-tissue oedema: Skin >5 mm
- Echogenic amniotic fluid (fetal demise fragments
- Uncommon findings
  - Thrombus in fetal heart
  - Gas shadow in fetal heart (Robert sign)

53. Pugilistic attitude in fireburns is due to:

a. Coagulation of blood in the vascular channels
b. Splitting of soft parts
c. Tight clothing
d. Coagulation of protein of the muscles

The 'pugilist' attitude—differential heat-related contraction of the limbs results in a characteristic position of the limbs; the arms are flexed at the elbows and wrists for example. The condition generally occurs several hours after death and is caused by a coagulation of muscle proteins when the bosy is exposed to extremely high temperatures.

54. Marbling is noticed by:

a. 18 hours b. 24 hours
c. 36 hours d. 48 hours

36 to 48 hours after death, a process called 'marbling' begins. During this process, parts of the body such as thighs, arms, shoulders and chest show long purple to greenish-colored streaks. These streaks are distended veins, caused by bacteria tracking though the superficial blood vessels causing pigment changes in the blood.

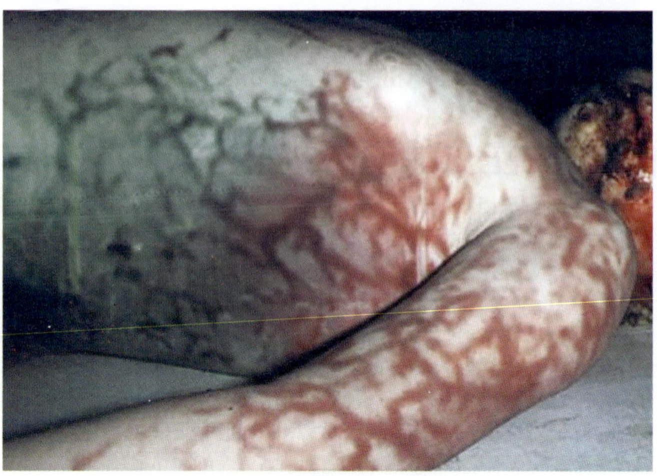

Putrefactive network (marbling).

55. Postmortem stiffening is called:

a. Putrefaction
b. Rigor mortis
c. Livor mortis
d. Mummification

Rigor mortis (Latin: **rigor** "stiffness", **mortis**"of death)" is one of the recognizable signs of death, caused by chemical changes in the muscles after death, causing the limbs of the corpse to stiffen.

Difference between rigor mortis and cadaveric spasm.

Trait	*Rigor mortis*	*Cadaveric spasm*
1. Production	Freezing and exposure to temperature above 65°C will produce rigor	Cannot be produced by any method after death
2. Mechanism	Known. Reduction of ATP	Not clearly known
3. Predisposing factors	Nil	Sudden death, excitement, fear, exhaustion, nervous tension, etc.
4. Time of onset	1–2 hours after death	Instantaneous
5. Muscles involved	All the muscles of the body, both voluntary and involuntary	Usually restricted to a single group of voluntary muscles
6. Muscle stiffening	Not marked; moderate force can overcome it	Marked; very great force is required to overcome it
7. Molecular death	Occurs	Does not occur
8. Body heat	Cold	Warm
9. Electrical stimuli	Muscles do not respond	Muscles respond
10. Muscular reaction	Acidic	Alkaline
11. Medicolegal importance	Indicates time of death	Indicates mode of death, i.e. suicide, homicide or accident

56. Cutis anserine is seen in:

a. Electrocution
b. Lust murder
c. Suffocation
d. Drowning

Signs of immersion

- The skin becomes somewhat opaque and wrinkled, known as 'washerwoman's fingers', develop after a few hours in cold water.
- After a few days, this macerated skin will begin to separate and,
- Usually within 1–2 weeks the skin will peel off the hands and feet.
- Another early sign of immersion is cutis anserina or 'gooseflesh', due to contraction of the erector pili muscles.
- However, this is partly due to cold (and may be seen in refrigerated bodies) and partly due to rigor mortis.

Ans. 53. **d.** Coagulation... 54. **c.** 36 hours 55. **b.** Rigor mortis 56. **d.** Drowning

- Cutis anserina is not a specific sign of immersion.
- In average temperate conditions, a body immersed in water will decompose at about half the speed of one left in air.
- After about a week, the body will be bloated and the face, abdomen and genitals will be distended with gas.
- As the body is moved by the flow of the water, contact with rocks, piers and many other underwater obstructions can cause damage.

57. True about hydrocution are all EXCEPT:

a. Electrocution in water
b. Death results from cardiac arrest
c. Results from falling in the water feet first
d. Emotionally tense individuals are prone for this

Hydrocution/immersion syndrome/submersion inhibition

- This condition is usually found in temperate and cold zones.
- Death here is attributed to cardiac arrest due to vagal inhibition, which results from stimulation of vagal nerve endings and in case of drowning, this may be brought about by several ways:
  - A sudden entry of water into the nasopharynx or larynx
  - Falling or diving into water in a manner so that it suddenly strikes the abdomen, especially the epigastric region.
  - Sudden in-rush of cold water into the ears.

58. The period of mixed dentition is:

a. 2–5 years b. 6–11 years
c. 12–14 years d. 15–17 years

Mixed dentition stage starts when the first permanent molar appears in the mouth, usually at five or six years, and lasts until the last primary tooth is lost, usually at ten, eleven, or twelve years. Permanent teeth in the maxillae erupt in a different order from permanent teeth on the mandible.

Difference between temporary and permanent teeth.

	Trait	Temporary teeth	Permanent teeth
1	Size:	Smaller, lighter, narrower, except temporary molars which are longer than permanent premolars replacing them.	Heavier, stronger, broader, except permanent premolars replacing temporary molars which are smaller.
2	Direction:	Anterior teeth are vertical.	Anterior teeth are usually inclined a little forward.
3	Crown:	China-white colour.	Ivory-white colour.
4	Neck:	More constricted.	Less constricted.
5	Root:	Roots of molar are smaller and more divergent.	Roots of molars are larger and less divergent.
6	Ridge:	A ridge or thick edge at the junction of the crown with the fangs present.	No ridge.

59. First permanent tooth to appear is:

a. Incisor b. Canine
c. Premolar d. Molar

First permanent molar appears in the mouth, usually at five or six years .

Calcification and eruption of permanent teeth.

Tooth	Calcification begins	Eruption	Calcification complete
First molar	At birth	6 to 7 years	9 to 10 years
Central incisor	3 to 4 months	6 to 8 years	10 years
Lateral incisor	1 year	7 to 9 years	11 years
First bicuspid	1½ years	9 to 11 years	12 to 13 years
Second bicuspid	2 years	10 to 12 years	12 to 14 years
Canine	4 to 5 months	11 to 12 years	12 to 13 years
Second molar	2 ½ to 3 years	12 to 14 years	14 to 16 years
Third molar	8 to 10 years	17 to 25 years	18 to 25 years

60. Cheiloscopy is the study of:

a. Foot prints b. Palatal prints
c. Finger prints d. Lip prints

Cheiloscopy is a forensic investigation technique that deals with identification of humans based on lips traces. The aim of this study is to establish the uniqueness of lip prints which aids in personal identification.

61. MC pattern of fingerprint is:

a. Arch b. Loop
c. Whorl d. Composite

Loops

- 60-65% of the population has **loops**.
- Must have one or more ridges entering from one side of the print, curving and exiting from the same side.

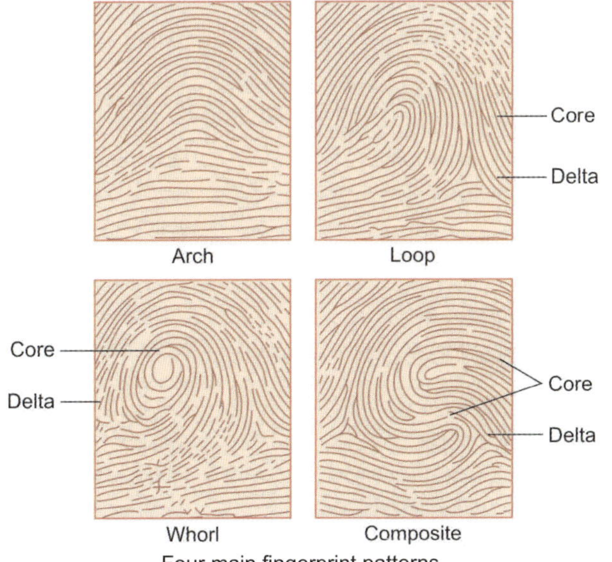

Four main fingerprint patterns.

62. Cephalic index is used for determination of:

a. Race b. Age
c. Sex d. Pelvic abnormality

Ans. 57. **a.** Electrocution in 58. **b.** 6-11 years 59. **d.** Molar 60. **d.** Lip prints
61. **b.** Loop 62. **a.** Race

The **cephalic index** or cranial **index** is the ratio of the maximum width of the head of an organism (human or animal) multiplied by 100 divided by its maximum length (i.e. in the horizontal plane, or front to back).

Racial difference in the skull.		
Type of Skull	*Cephalic Index*	*Race*
1. Dolichocephalic (long-headed)	70 to75	Pure Aryans, Aborigines and Negroes.
2. Mesaticephalic (medium-headed)	75 to 80	Europeans Chinese and Indians.
3. Brachycephalic (short-headed)	80 to 85	Mongolian.

63. Most reliable method of identification of a person is by:

a. Scars
b. Anthropometry
c. Finger printing
d. Photography

Fingerprints remain constant throughout life. In over 140 years of fingerprint comparison worldwide, no two fingerprints have ever been found to be alike, not even those of identical twins.

64. Ischiopubic index is significantly more in:

a. Advanced age
b. Males
c. Females
d. Caucasian

Ischium is longer in males, pubis in females and pubo-ischial index was also more in females.

Traits diagnostic of sex from skeleton.			
	Trait	*Male*	*Female*
	PELVIS		
1	Bony framework:	Massive, rougher, marked muscle sites. Stands higher and more erect.	Less massive, slender, smoother.
2	General:	Deep funnel.	Flat bowl.
3	Ilium:	Less vertical; curve of iliac crest reaches higher level and is more prominent.	More vertical; distance between iliac crests is less; iliac fossae shallow; curves of crest well marked.
4	Preauricular sulcus: (attachment of anterior sacroiliac ligament).	Not frequent; narrow, shallow.	More frequent, broad and deep.
5	Acetabulum:	Large, 52 mm in diameter; directed laterally; wider, deeper.	Small, 46 mm. in diameter; directed anterolaterally; narrower.
6	Obturator foramen:	Large, often oval with base upwards.	Small, triangular with apex forwards.
7	Greater sciatic notch:	Smaller, narrower, deeper.	Larger, wider, shallower.
8	Illeo-pectineal line:	Well marked and rough.	Rounded and smooth.
9	Ischial tuberosity:	Inverted.	Everted; more widely separated.
10	Body of pubis:	Narrow, triangular, thick.	Broad, square; pits on posterior surface if borne children.
11	Ramus of pubis:	It is like continuation of body of pubis.	Has a constricted or narrowed appearance and is short and thick.
12	Ischiopubic rami:	More everted, thicker and roughter.	Less everted, thinner and smoother.
13	Symphysis:	Higher, bigger and narrow in width. Margins of pubic arch everted.	Lower, wider and rounded. Margins of pubic arch not everted; distance between two pubic tubercles greater. The dorsal border is irregular and shows depressions or pits (scars of parturition).
14	Subpubic angle:	V-shaped, sharp angle 70° to 75°.	U-shaped, rounded, broader angle, 90 to 100°.
15	Pelvic brim or inlet:	Heart-shaped.	Circular or elliptical; more spacious; diameters longer.
16	Pelvic cavity:	Conical and funnel-shaped.	Broad and round.
17	Pelvic outlet:	Smaller.	Larger.
18	Sacroiliac articulation:	Large, extends to 2½ to 3 vertebrae.	Small, oblique, extends to 2 to 2½ vertebrae.
19	Sacroiliac joint surface:	Large and less sharply angulated.	L-shaped and elevated anteriorly.
20	Sacrum:	Longer, narrower, with more evenly distributed curvature; promontory well marked. Body of first sacral vertebra larger.	Shorter, wider; upper half almost straight, curve forward in lower half; promontory less marked. Body of first sacral vertebra small.
21	Coccyx:	Less movable.	More movable.

Contd…

Ans. **63. c.** Finger printing **64. c.** Females

Contd...

	Trait	*Male*	*Female*
22	Ischiopubic index: $\frac{\text{Pubic length in mm}}{\text{Ischial length in mm}} \times 100$	73 to 94.	91 to 115.
23	Sciatic notch index: $\frac{\text{Width of sciatic notch}}{\text{Depth of sciatic notch}} \times 100$	4 to 5.	5 to 6.
24	Pubic ramus ratio:	1: 1.	2: 1 or greater.
	THORAX		
1	General:	Longer and narrower.	Shorter and wider.
2	Sternum:	Body longer and more than twice the length of the manubrium; upper margin is in level with lower part of the body of second thoracic vertebra; breadth more. Length more than 149 mm. (Ashley's rule).	Shorter and less than twice the length of the manubrium; upper margin in level with lower part of the body of third thoracic vertebra; breadth less. Length less than 149 mm. (Ashley's rule).
	Sternal index: $\frac{\text{Length of manubrium}}{\text{Length of body}} \times 100$	46.2	54.3
3	Ribs:	Thicker; larger; heavier; lesser curvature and are less oblique.	Thinner; shorter; greater curvature and more oblique.
4	Clavicle:	Longer (151 to 153 cm.) broader, heavier, less curved.	Smaller, narrower (138 cm lighter, more curved).
	VERTEBRAL COLUMN		
1	Atlas, breadth:	7.4 to 9.9 cm. mean 8.3 cm	6.5 to 7.6 cm. (mean 7.2 cm)
2	Length of vertebral column:	70 to 73 cm.	60 cm.
3	Corporobasal index of sacrum: $\frac{\text{Breadth of first sacral vertebra}}{\text{Breadth of the base of sacrum}} \times 100$	45	40.5
	FEMUR		
1	Head:	Larger and forms about 2/3 of a sphere. Vertical diameter more than 47 mm.	Smaller and forms less than 2/3 of a sphere. Vertical diameter less than 45 mm.
2	Neck:	Obtuse angle with the shaft, about 1250.	Less obtuse angle with the shaft.
3	Bicondylar width:	74 to 89 mm.	67 to 76 mm.
4	Angulation of shaft with condyles:	Around 80°	Around 76°
	HUMERUS		
	Diameter of head:	More than 47 mm.	Less than 43 mm.
	RADIUS		
1	Diameter of head:	More than 24 mm.	Less than 21 mm.
2	Circumference of head:	More than 69 mm.	Less than 55 mm.
	SCAPULA		
1	Height:	More than 157 mm.	Less than 144 mm.
2	Glenoid cavity:	Height greater (39.2 mm.	Height less (32.6 mm).

65. True for carbon mono-oxide poisoning:

a. Blue postmortem staining
b. Chcoclate-coloured postmortem staining
c. Pink postmortem staining
d. Cherry red postmortem staining

Deaths from carbon monoxide poisoning often result in a cherry red/pink coloration to the skin, lips and internal body organs.

66. Most informative test in parental identification:

a. HLA
b. Parental likeness
c. Developmental defects
d. DNA finger printing

DNA fingerprinting is a test to identify and evaluate the genetic information-called **DNA** (deoxyribonucleic acid) in a person's cells.

Ans. **65. d.** Cherry red... **66. d.** DNA finger printing

67. Superimposition technique is used for:

a. Skull b. Pelvis
c. Femur d. Ribs

Forensic superimpositions are created by superimposing a photograph of an individual suspected of belonging to the unidentified skeletal remains over an X-ray of the unidentified skull. If the skull and the photograph are of the same individual, then the anatomical features of the face should align accurately. Few points of comparison are: 1. The eyes within the orbital plates, 2. The nasion, 3. The prosthion in the central line, 4. The nasal spine in the centre, 5. The lower border of the nose, 6. The lower border of the upper jaw, 7. The zygomas below the eyes, etc.

68. Total number of teeth at the age of 12 years:

a. 12 b. 20
c. 24 d. 30

At the age 12, there are 24 permanent teeth: 4 canines, 8 incisors, 8 premolars and 4 first molars.

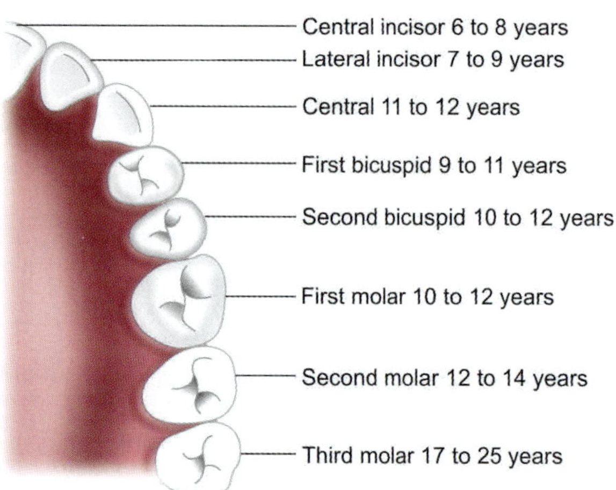

Eruption of permanent teeth.

69. Test used to detect blood group of blood stain:

a. Benzidine test b. Takayama test
c. Luminol test d. Absorption elution test

Absorption elution test

- It can be used to confirm the presence of subgroups in the ABO system. Suspect RBCs are incubated with >A or >B.
- An elution is performed on the RBCs following an elution is performed on the RBCs following incubation.
- The eluate is tested for presence of >A or >B that had adsorbed to the red blood cell antigens during incubation.

70. DNA can be taken as sample from all of the following EXCEPT:

a. Hair roots
b. Semen
c. CSF
d. Buccal mucosa

Developed by Professor of Genetics Sir Alec Jeffrey's, the DNA finger printing process begins with a sample of an individual's DNA (typically called a "reference sample)". The most desirable method of collecting a reference sample is the use of a buccal swab, as this reduces the possibility of contamination. When this is not available (e.g. because a court order is needed but not obtainable) other methods may need to be used to collect a sample of blood, saliva, semen, hair or other appropriate fluid or tissue from personal items (e.g. a toothbrush, razor) or from stored samples (e.g. banked sperm or biopsy tissue).

71. Ossification centre appearing just before birth:

a. Lower end of femur b. Lower end of tibia
c. Upper end of humerus d. Scaphoid

Distal femoral epiphysis and proximal tibial epiphysis is present at birth.

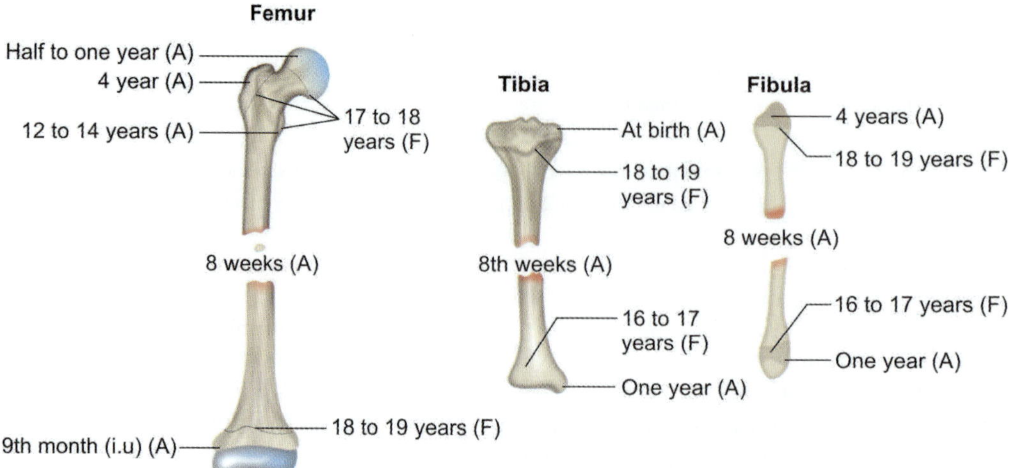

Appearance and fusion of epiphyses in femur, tibia and fibula.

Ans. 67. a. Skull 68. c. 24 69. d. Absorption elution 70. c. CSF
71. a. Lower end of femur

72. **Eruption of temporary teeth will be completed by:**
   a. 1–1.5 years
   b. 2–2.5 years
   c. 3–4 years
   d. 4–5 years

Teething age of primary teeth
- Central incisors: 6–12 months
- Lateral incisors: 9–16 months
- First molars: 13–19 months
- Canine teeth: 16–23 months
- Second molars: 22–33 months

Calcification and eruption of deciduous teeth.

Tooth	*Calcification begins*	*Eruption*	*Calcification of root completed*	*Resorption of root begins*
Central incisor:				
Lower:	5 to 6 months	6 to 8 months	1½ to 2 years	4th year
Upper:	"	7 to 9 months	1½ to 2 years	5th year
Lateral incisor:	"			
Upper:	"	7 to 9 months	1½ to 2 years	5th year
Lower:	"	10 to 12 months	1½ to 2 years	5th year
First molar:	"	12 to 14 months	2 to 2½ years	6th year
Canine:	"	17 to 18 months	2½ to 3 years	8th year
Second molar:	"	20 to 30 months	3 years	7th year

73. **Putrefaction is retarded by:**
   a. Oxalic acid
   b. Organophosphoric acid
   c. HCl
   d. Phenol

Substances which delay putrefaction
- Carbolic acid
- Arsenic and antimony
- Strychnine
- Zinc chloride, $ZnCl_2$

74. **Order of onset of rigor mortis:**
   a. Eyelids → lower limb → thorax
   b. Thorax → lower limb → eyelids
   c. Eyelids → thorax → lower limb
   d. Lower limb → thorax → eyelids

Rigor mortis begins within two to six hours of death, starting with the eyelids, neck, and lower jaw and passes upwards to the muscles of the face, and downwards to the muscles of the chest, upper limbs, abdomen and lower limbs and lastly in the fingers and toes. This sequence may be due to the difference in lactic acid levels among different muscles, which corresponds to the difference in glycogen levels and to the different types of muscle fibers. The onset of rigor mortis is more rapid if the environment is cold and if the decedent had performed hard physical work just before death.

75. **Total number of deciduous teeth in a 14 yrs old child:**
   a. 0
   b. 5
   c. 10
   d. 20

The process of shedding primary teeth and their replacement by permanent teeth is called exfoliation. This may last from age six to age twelve. By age twelve, there usually are only permanent teeth remaining.

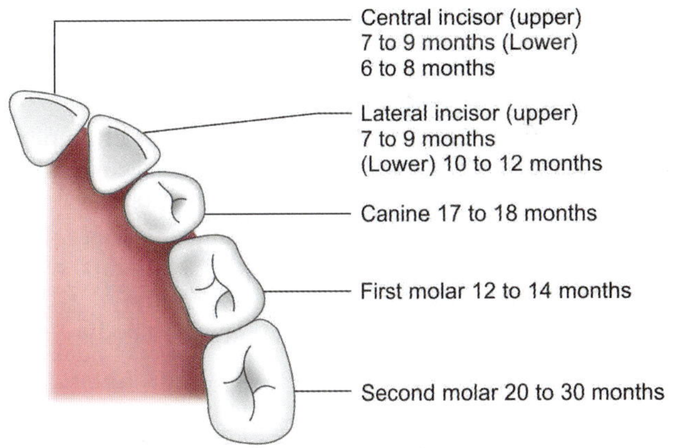

Eruption of temporary teeth.

76. **After death, livor mortis is caused because of:**
   a. Muscle of the body began to relax
   b. Muscle of the body began to stiffen
   c. Discolouration as a result of capillo-venous distension in the dependent parts of the body
   d. Putrefaction of the body tissues

Livor mortis (Latin: *livor*—"bluish color," *mortis*—" of death"), **postmortem lividity** (Latin: *postmortem*—"after death", *lividity*—"black and blue"), **hypostasis** (Greek: *hypo*, meaning "under, beneath"; *stasis*, meaning "a standing") or **suggillation**, is one of the signs of death. Livor mortis is a settling of the blood in the lower (dependent) portion of the body, causing a purplish red discoloration of the skin.

Ans. 72. **b.** 2–2.5 years 73. **d.** Phenol 74. **c.** Eyelids → thorax... 75. **a.** 0 76. **c.** Discolouration...

Difference between postmortem hypostasis and congestion.

Trait	Hypostasis	Congestion
(1) Redness	Irregular and occurs on a dependent part	Uniform all over the organ
(2) Mucous membranes	Dull and lusterless	Normal
(3) Exudate	No inflammatory exudate	Exudate may be seen
(4) Hollow viscus	Stomach and intestine when stretched show alternate stained and unstained areas according to the position of coils	Uniform staining

77. Preservation of CSF is done in:

a. Alcohol poisoning b. Arsenic poisoning
c. Copper poisoning
d. Organophosphorous poisoning

The **cerebrospinal fluid** is **preserved** in suspected **alcohol poisoning**.

78. Pearson's formula is employed for:

a. Cephalic index b. Stature
c. Race d. Age

The stature of a normal European may be estimated within an error of one to two centimetres from certain long bones, especially the femur, humerus, tibia or radius, by using the following formulae compiled by Karl Pearson (1899).

79. Pure Aryans have which type of skull:

a. Brachycephalic b. Mesaticephalic
c. Dolichocephalic d. All of the above

A dolichocephalic skull is relatively long skull (typically with the breadth less than 80% or 75% of the length). It is seen in pure Aryans, aborigines and negroes.

80. Sex can be determined by examining hair root cells for the presence of:

a. Medullary index b. Golgi body
c. Barr body d. Davidson body

Inactivated X chromosomes seen in female somatic cells are called Barr-bodies which are present adjacent to the nuclear membrane. Condensed state of densely stained chromatin signifies that in such cases DNA replication occurred at the later stage of S phase of cell cycle. They generally appear as basophilic structures with varying morphology which can be either spherical, rectangular, planoconvex, biconvex, or triangular measuring 0.8 × 1.1 microns. It also resembles various alphabetical letters in electron microscope as V, W, S, or X. Barr body can also be obtained from buccal smear, pulp tissue, vaginal smears, and hair follicle.

81. Rate of cooling of dead body in normal conditions of temperature and atmosphere:

a. 1. 0 F/hour b. 1.5 F/hour
c. 2.0 F/hour d. 2.5 F/hour

The **dead body cools** at an average **rate** of **1.5°F** per **hour** in a temperate climate and 0.75 °F per hour in tropical climate.

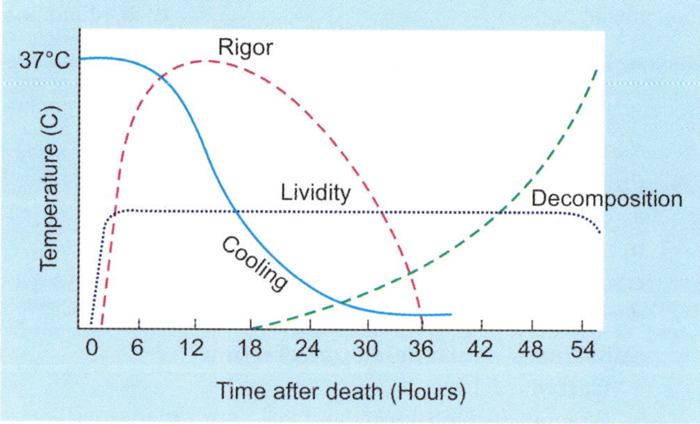

Chart showing the major changes to estimate time since death.

82. Most useful for age determination amongst the following secondary changes in tooth:

a. Root transparency b. Root resorption
c. Secondary dentine deposition d. Attrition

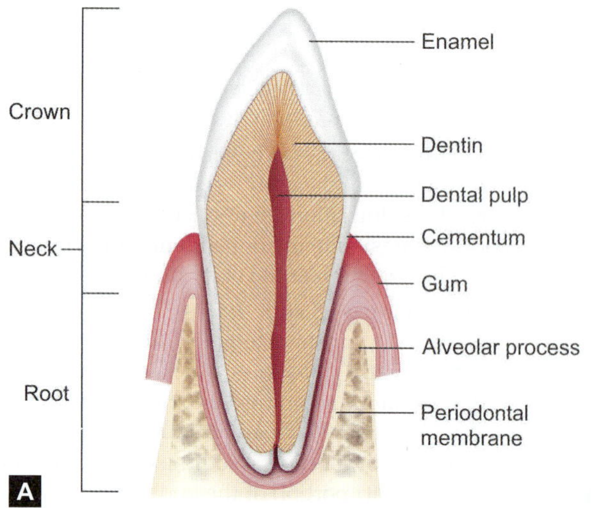

(A) Vertical section of an incisor tooth. (B) Physiological age-processes in teeth.

Ans. 77. **a.** Alcohol poisoning 78. **b.** Stature 79. **c.** Dolichocephalic
80. **c.** Barr body 81. **b.** 1.5 F/ hour 82. **a.** Root transp...

Gustafson's method for age determination from teeth is based on the evaluation of ground sections of teeth. Six age-associated parameters are evaluated in the ground section and are compared to a regression curve of age versus the age-associated changes. Two of these changes, transparency of radicular dentin and secondary dentin, have the highest correlation with age.

83. Brain death is said to occur if there is:

a. Absent spinal reflexes
b. Cortical death following widespread brain injury
c. Absence of brainstem reflexes
d. Core temperature of the body is below 35 degree C

A brain-dead individual has no clinical evidence of brain function upon physical examination. This includes no response to pain and no cranial nerve reflexes. Reflexes include pupillary response (fixed pupils), oculocephalic reflex, corneal reflex, no response to the caloric reflex test, and no spontaneous respirations.

84. First permanent teeth to erupt is:

a. First premolar b. Second premolar
c. First molar d. Second molar

The first of the permanent teeth to erupt are the permanent first molars, right behind the last 'milk' molars of the primary dentition. These first permanent molars are important for the correct development of a permanent dentition. Up to the age of thirteen years, twenty-eight of the thirty-two permanent teeth will appear.

85. Rigor mortis is occurs due to:

a. Muscle of the body began to relax
b. Capillo-venous distension in the most dependent body parts
c. Muscle of the body began to stiffen
d. Mummification of the body tissues

Rigor mortis (Latin: *rigor* "stiffness", *mortis* "of death") is one of the recognizable signs of death, caused by chemical changes in the muscles after death, causing the limbs of the corpse to stiffen. Rigor mortis occurs three to four hours after death.

Rigor related to time of death (hpm).

Stage	*Lower limit*	*Upper limit*
Beginning	0.5	7
Maximum	2.0	20
Re-establishment after breaking	2.0	8

Computed by Mallach from literature data.

86. Lungs are preserved in:

a. Alcohol poisoning b. HCN poisoning
c. CO poisoning d. All of the above

Special Preservations

- Liver is the **most important tissue** because it concentrates many substances
- Heart: Strychnine, Digitalis.
- Spleen: It is the best organ for Cyanide poisoning. (? Supposedly best specimen for DNA)
- Brain: Alkaloids, organophosphates, volatile organic poisons.
- Bile: Narcotic drugs, cocaine, methadone, Glutathione, Barbiturates, Tranquilizers, Opiates and acetaminophen
- Vitreous: Alcohol, Chloroform [Vitreous Humour is preserved by keeping at 4°C for 48 hours, normally preservative is of no value, though could be preserved with sodium fluoride (10 mg/ml]
- Lung: Gaseous poison, HCN, Alcohol, Chloroform.
- Bone: Arsenic, Antimony, Thallium, Radium.
- Skin: Cases of hypodermic injections (10 cm radius about site with muscle and fat), snake bite.
- Hair, Nails, Uterus, spinal card–When indicated.
- CSF: (in 10 mg NaF/ml of fluid) in Alcohol intoxication.
- Body Fat: Endrin, DDT (Organo Chlorines).

87. Most common characteristic of heat rupture:

a. Vessel rupture b. Clot in the wound
c. Smooth and well defined margin
d. Irregular margin

Heat Ruptures: If the heat applied is very great, skin contracts and **heat ruptures** occur, either before or after death. They are produced by splitting of the soft parts. They have **irregular margins**.

88. Causes of death in drowning are all EXCEPT:

a. Vagal hyperactivity b. Asphyxia
c. Ventricular fibrillation d. Laryngospasm

Causes of death in drowning include laryngeal spasm, **vagal inhibition**, ventricular fibrillation, asphyxia, injury including head injury, exhaustion, biting and eating by animals, secondary pulmonary infections and electrolyte imbalance.

89. Inward compression fracture of hyoid bone is indicative of:

a. Throttling b. Suffocation
c. Choking d. Hanging

Manual strangulation (also known as "throttling") is strangling with the hands, fingers, or other extremities and sometimes also with blunt objects, such as batons. Depending on how the strangling is performed, it may compress the airway, interfere with the flow of blood in the neck, or work as a combination of the two. Consequently, manual strangulation may damage the larynx, and fracture the hyoid or other bones in the neck.

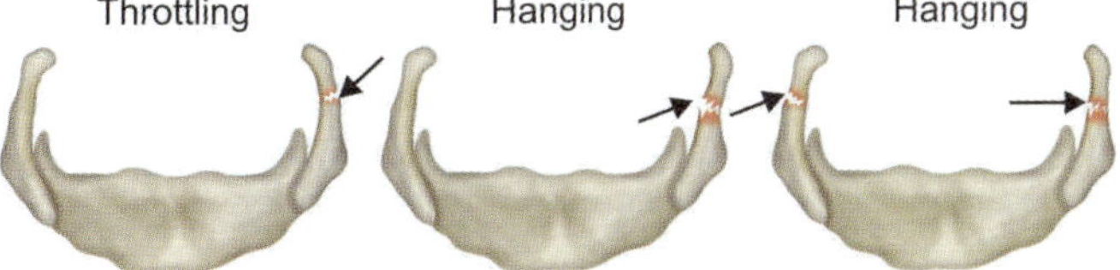

Fracture hyoid bone in throttling and hanging.

Ans. 83. c. Absence of brainst... 84. c. First molar 85. c. Muscle of the body...
86. b. HCN poisoning 87. d. Irregular... 88. a. Vagal hyperactivity 89. a. Throttling

90. In atypical hanging, commonly the knot comes to rest at the:

a. Occiput b. Chin
c. Angle of mandible d. Below the cheek

In typical **hanging**, the **knot** is situated over the nape of the neck, ligature runs from midline above the level of thyroid cartilage symmetrically upwards from both sides of the neck to the occipital region. Other **position of knot** is called Atypical **Hanging**.

91. Identical twins may NOT have the:

a. Same DNA
b. Same finger prints sequence
c. Same blood group
d. Same HLA system

Quetelet's rule that every nature-made object shows infinite variations of forms, and in the world's crime records, no two identical fingerprint patterns have been reported.

92. NOT a feature of antemortem burns:

a. Vesicle with hyperemic base
b. Air vesicle
c. Pus formation
d. Inflammatory red line

The three main points to differentiate between antemortem and post-mortem burns are: 1. Line of redness. 2. Vesication. 3. Reparative processes.

Difference between antemortem burns and postmortem burns.

Trait	Antemortem burns	Postmortem burns
Line of redness:	Present.	Absent.
Blister:	Contains serous fluid with proteins and chlorides. Base is red and inflamed .	Contains air and thin clear fluid. Base is dry, hard and yellow.
Vital reaction:	Marked cellular exudation and reactive changes in the tissue cells present.	Absent.
Enzymes:	Peripheral zone of burn shows increase in enzyme reaction.	Peripheral zone does not show increase in enzyme reaction.

93. Post-mortem rigidity first starts in:

a. Lower limbs
b. Upper limbs
c. Neck
d. Eyelids

Rigor mortis does not start in all muscle simultaneously (Hysten's rule). It **first** appears in involuntary muscles; the myocardium becomes **rigid** in an hour. It **begins** in the **eyelids**, neck and lower jaw and passes upwards to the muscles.

94. Arborescent burns are seen in:

a. Flame burns b. Lightning stroke
c. Heat stroke d. Electrocution

Arborescent/Filigree burns (Lichtenberg flowers seen in the most characteristic of lightning stroke.

95. Pugilistic attitude is seen in:

a. Burns b. Electrocution
c. Drowning d. Strangulation

A 'defensive' position fancifully likened to that adopted by pugilists (boxers), which is typically seen in severely burned bodies, characterised by flexion of elbows, knees, hip, and neck, and clenching of hand into a fist; it is caused by high temperatures in fires, resulting in muscle stiffening and shortening; it occurs even if the person was dead before the fire.

96. Which of the following is NOT seen in death due to starvation:

a. Translucent intestine walls
b. Contracted and empty stomach
c. Large bowel may contain faecolith
d. Shrunken gallbladder

In starvation, gall bladder remains distended with bile as bile is not used in process of digestion.

97. Burking is:

a. Suicidal b. Accidental
c. Homicidal d. None of the above

In homicidal cases, the term burking is often ascribed to a killing method that involves simultaneous smothering and compression of the torso. The term "burking" comes from the method William Burke and William Hare used to kill their victims during the West Port murders. They killed the usually intoxicated victims by sitting on their chests and suffocating them by putting a hand over their nose and mouth, while using the other hand to push the victim's jaw up. The corpses had no visible injuries, and were supplied to medical schools for money.

98. Sweating is ABSENT in:

a. Heat cramps b. Heat stroke
c. Heat fatigue d. Heat exhaustion

Heat stroke generally presents with a hyperthermia of greater than 40.6°C (105.1°F in combination with disorientation and a lack of sweating. However, in exertional heat stroke, the affected person may sweat excessively. Young children, in particular, may have seizures. Eventually, unconsciousness, organ failure, and death will result.

99. In heat stroke, skin will be:

a. Warm b. Normal
c. Cold d. Cyanosis

Heat stroke occurs when thermoregulation is overwhelmed by a combination of excessive metabolic production of heat (exertion), excessive environmental heat, and insufficient or impaired heat loss, resulting in an abnormally high body temperature.

Ans. **90. c.** Angle of mandible **91. b.** Same finger... **92. b.** Air vesicle **93. d.** Eyelids
94. b. Lightning... **95. a.** Burns **96. d.** Shrunken gall bladder
97. c. Homicidal **98. b.** Heat stroke **99. a.** Warm

100. DNA finger printing is done with all EXCEPT:

a. WBC
b. RBC
c. Saliva
d. Spermatozoon

Because all cells in the body contain exactly the same DNA, samples can be taken from almost anywhere in the body, including skin, hair follicles, blood and other bodily fluids.

101. Aseptic autolysis is seen in:

a. Adipocere
b. Maceration
c. Putrefaction
d. Mummification

Dead birth:

- Is a child which has died in utero and shows one of the following signs after complete birth:
- Rigor mortis at delivery
- Maceration (aseptic autolysis after 3-4 days in uterus filled with amniotic fluid and no air). The earliest sign of maceration is skin slippage, which can be seen in 12 hours after death in utero. The body of the macerated fetus is soft, flaccid, and flattens out when placed on a level surface. It has a sweetish disagreeable odor. Spalding's sign is the loss of alignment and overriding of the bones of the cranial vault.
- Mummification: Is the condition in which the fetus dries up, shriveled in the uterus. It occurs when fetus dies from deficient supply of blood, when the liquor amnii is scanty and when no air enters the uterus.

102. Gettlers test is positive in:

a. Hanging
b. Poisoning
c. Strangulation
d. Drowning

Gettler's test is done to measure amount of chloride in each chamber of heart. It is done to distinguish between freshwater **drowning** and saltwater **drowning**. A 25% difference in chloride is significant. The test is of doubtful value.

Difference in lungs between fresh water and sea water drowning.

	Trait	*Fresh water drowning*	*Sea water drowning*
1	Size and weight:	Ballooned but light.	Ballooned and heavy.
2	Colour:	Pale pink.	Purplish or bluish.
3	Consistency:	Emphysematous.	Soft and jelly-like.
4	Shape after removal from the body:	Retained; do not collapse.	Not retained; tend to flatten out.
5	Sectioning:	Crepitus is heard. Little froth and no fluid.	No crepitus. Copious fluid and froth.

103. In autopsy, preservative used for vitreous is:

a. Fluoride
b. HCl
c. Phenol
d. Xylol

Approximately 2-5 mL of vitreous fluid can be aspirated from each eye; even 1 mL can be procured from a newborn. The vitreous should be placed in a sterile tube. If alcohol or drug analysis is to be performed, then sodium fluoride preservative should be in the tube. The specimen should be clear and colorless. If small flecks of black-brown retina are in the sample, then the sample is deemed inadequate.

104. Bluish green hypostasis is seen in poisoning due to:

a. CO
b. Aniline dye
c. H_2S
d. Arsenic

Colour of post mortem lividity (hypostasis)

- Normal—bluish pink which later turns into bluish purple
- Carbon monoxide—bright cherry red
- Cyanide—pink
- Phosphorous—dark brown
- Nitrates—reddish brown
- Chlorates—chocolate brown
- Hydrogen sulphide—bluish Green
- Aniline—Deep blue
- Opiates—black

105. Substance commonly used for organ/tissue preservation for histopath examination:

a. 10% formalin
b. Normal saline
c. Alcohol
d. Salt solution

For histology the standard preferred fixative is **10%** neutral buffered **formalin** (NBF or 95% alcohol.

106. Burn (heat) hematoma is seen between:

a. Brain and arachnoid
b. Skull and dura
c. Arachnoid and pia
d. Pia and dura

Heat haematoma

- An often bilateral pool of blood seen in theextradural space that occurs in response to severe heating of the skull in a fire.
- It is often accompanied by burning of the scalp, and simulates antemortem extradural/epidural haematomas.
- In heat haematomas, the brain itself may show heat-related changes and the hematoma is friable rather than jelly-like as in a proper extradural haematoma.

Ans. **100. d.** Spermatozoon **101. b.** Maceration **102. d.** Drowning **103. a.** Fluoride **104. c.** H_2S **105. a.** 10% formalin **106. b.** Skull and dura

Difference between extradural haematoma due to burns and due to blunt force.			
	Trait	*Epidural haematoma due to burns*	*Epidural haematoma due to blunt force*
1	Cause:	Charring of the skull due to intense heat.	Blunt force to the head.
2	Situation:	Anywhere. Usually bilateral.	Usually adjacent to sylvian fissure.
3	Distribution:	Diffuse.	Localised.
4	Characters:	Thin, granular, soft, friable clot of light Chocolate colour, honeycomb appearance: evenly distributed or sickle-shaped.	Discoid shape; localised, more rubbery consistency, reddish-purple.
5	Skull:	May be fractured.	Associated fracture in temporal area.
6	CNS:	No injury.	Frequently injured.
7	Carboxyhaemoglobin:	Present.	Absent.

107. Diatoms in bone marrow of long bones are suggestive of death due to:

a. Burns
b. Hanging
c. Drowning
d. Firearm injuries

The main goal of diatom analysis in forensics is to differentiate a death by submersion from a post-mortem immersion of a body in water. Laboratory tests may reveal the presence of diatoms in the body. Since the silica-based skeletons of diatoms do not readily decay, they can sometimes be detected even in heavily decomposed bodies. As they do not occur naturally in the body, if laboratory tests show diatoms in the corpse that are of the same species found in the water where the body was recovered, then it may be good evidence of drowning as the cause of death. Further matching of diatoms from bone marrow and drowning site can strengthen this supportive evidence and a positive conclusion can be drawn whether a person was living or not when submerged.

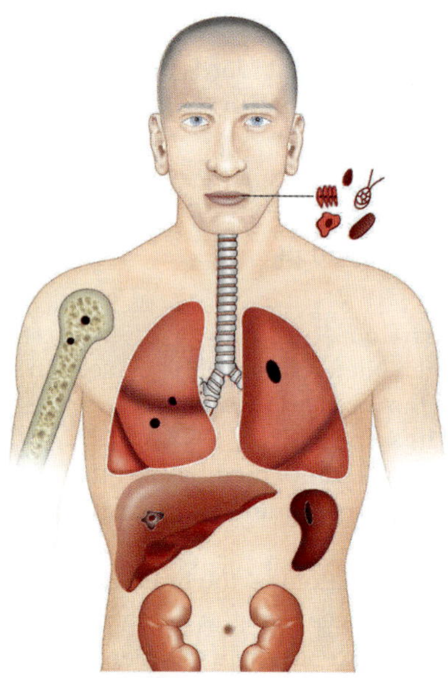

Diatoms in drowning.

108. Rigor mortis appears last in:

a. Eyelids
b. Neck
c. Lower limb
d. Toes

Rigor mortis passes off in the same sequence as it has **appeared**. The small muscles of the finger and **toes** are **last** affected by **rigor mortis**.

SEXUAL OFFENCES

109. Female patient with loss of interest in sex is known as:

a. Vaginismus
b. Impotency
c. Sterility
d. Frigidity

Frigidity, in psychology, the inability of a woman to attain orgasm during sexual intercourse.

110. Florence test done on dry seminal stain shows dark-brown crystals due to:

a. Sperm
b. Dye
c. Spermine
d. Choline

Florence Test

- Basis: Choline is detected in this method.
- Procedure: A few drops of watery solution of the stain is extracted and taken on a slide and a drop of Florence reagent (8%) W/V solution of Iodine in water containing 5% W/V of potassium Iodide is poured and allowed to mix slowly under a cover slip. Dark brown crystals of choline periodide, generally needle shaped, formed with a few minutes.
- Non-specifics and false negative results are common.

111. Masochism means:

a. Sexual intercourse with dead body
b. Sexual pleasure by contact with articles of opposite sex
c. Sexual pleasure by the suffering of pain
d. Sexual pleasure by self stimulation

Sexual masochism disorder, medical condition in which pain is required for sexual arousal, causing distress or impairment.

Ans. **107. c.** Drowning **108. d.** Toes **109. d.** Frigidity **110. d.** Choline **111. c.** Sexual pleasure...

112. All are tests for seminal stains EXCEPT:
a. Florence test
b. Creatine phosphate test
c. Takayama test
d. Barberio test

Many different tests have been used to confirm that a stain contains blood. The oldest is chemical confirmation of the presence of hemoglobin or its derivatives by the formation of specific crystals. For example, the **Takayama** or hemochromogen **test**, in which ferrous iron from hemoglobin reacts with pyridine to produce red feathery crystals of pyridine ferroprotoporphyrin.

TOXICOLOGY

113. Saturnine gout formation is associated with which of the following metal toxicity?
a. Mercury b. Beryllium
c. Lead d. Cadmium

One manifestation of chronic lead toxicity from moonshine or other forms of chronic lead poisoning is the rheumatology entity known as saturnine gout.

114. Which of the following is associated with proximal tubule proteinuria?
a. Lead b. Gold
c. Mercury d. Cadmium

Cadmium is a potent nephrotoxicant that impairs the reabsorptive and secretory functions of the renal proximal tubule, leading to albuminuria.

115. Which of the following metal poisoning cause painful micturition and nephropathy?
a. Lead b. Mercury
c. Cadmium d. Arsenic

Renal effects of arsenic poisoning include oliguria, uraemia; urine contains albumen, red cells and casts, pain during micturition.

Difference between arsenic poisoning and cholera

	Trait	*Arsenic poisoning*	*Cholera*
(1)	Pain in throat :	Before vomiting.	After vomiting.
(2)	Purging :	After vomiting.	Before vomiting.
(3)	Stools:	Dark-coloured and bloody, later rice-watery.	Rice-watery, not bloody and passed in continuous involuntary jet.
(4)	Tenesmus and anal irritation :	Present.	Absent.
(5)	Vomited matter :	Contains mucus, bile and blood.	Watery without mucus, bile and blood.
(6)	Voice:	Not affected.	Rough and whistling.
(7)	Conjunctivae :	Inflamed.	Not inflamed.
(8)	Analysis of excreta :	Arsenic present.	Cholera vibrio present.
(9)	Circumstantial evidence :	Of arsenic poisoning may be present.	Other cases of cholera in locality.

116. Ingestion of which of the following results in turquoise-bluish discoloration of gastric mucosa?
a. Arsenic b. Amytal sodium
c. Cadmium d. Mercury

The capsules of certain barbiturates leave characteristic traces in the mouth, oesophagus and stomach. The colour varies with the manufacturer, but the turquoise-blue of sodium amytal capsules may stain the stomach contents and even be visible through the wall of the intestine when the abdomen is opened.

117. Pin point pupils are seen in all of the following conditions EXCEPT:
a. Organophosprous poisoning
b. Opioid poisoning
c. Cerebellopontine hemorrhage
d. Dhatura poisoning

Due to the potent combination of anticholinergic substances it contains, *Dhatura* intoxication typically produces effects similar to that of an anticholinergic delirium (usually involving a complete inability to differentiate reality from fantasy); hyperthermia; tachycardia; bizarre, and possibly violent behavior; and severe mydriasis (dilated pupils) with resultant painful photophobia that can last and several days. Pronounced amnesia is another commonly reported effect.

118. Hairs are preserved in which poisoning:
a. Arsenic b. Manganese
c. Phosphorous d. Alcohol

Hair is a potential bioindicator for arsenic exposure due to its ability to store trace elements from blood. Incorporated elements maintain their position during growth of hair. Thus for a temporal estimation of exposure, an assay of hair composition needs to be carried out with a single hair which is not possible with older techniques requiring homogenization and dissolution of several strands of hair. This type of biomonitoring has been achieved with newer microanalytical techniques like Synchrotron radiation based X-ray fluorescence (SXRF) spectroscopy and Microparticle-induced X-ray emission (PIXE).

119. All of the following are features of Datura poisoning EXCEPT:
a. Dryness of mouth
b. Delirium
c. Dilated pupil
d. Bradycardia

Initial signs and symptoms of Datura poisoning
- Dry mucous membranes and skin
- Dysphagia and dysarthria
- Photophobia
- Blurred vision
- Tachycardia
- Urinary retention

Ans. 112. c. Takayama test 113. c. Lead 114. d. Cadmium 115. d. Arsenic
116. c. Cadmium 117. d. Datura poisoning 118. a. Arsenic 119. d. Bradycardia

120. Gastric wash is CONTRAINDICATED in:

a. Datura b. Opiate
c. Sulphuric acid d. Oxalic acid

Gastric lavage is contraindicated in corrosive acid poisoning (EXCEPT oxalic acid and phenol) and kerosene poisoning.

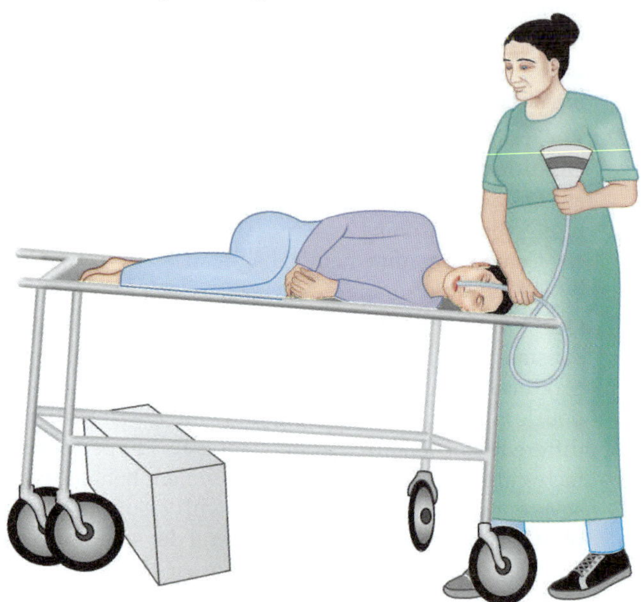

Position of patient for gastric lavage.

121. Cyanides act by binding to:

a. Histamine
b. Alpha2 adrenergic receptors
c. Acetyl-cholinesterase
d. Cytochrome oxidase

Inside cells, cyanide attaches itself to ubiquitous metalloenzymes, rendering them inactive. Its principal toxicity results from inactivation of cytochrome oxidase (at cytochrome a3), thus uncoupling mitochondrial oxidative phosphorylation and inhibiting cellular respiration, even in the presence of adequate oxygen stores. Cellular metabolism shifts from aerobic to anaerobic, with the consequent production of lactic acid. Consequently, the tissues with the highest oxygen requirements (brain and heart) are the most profoundly affected by acute cyanide poisoning.

122. Magnan's phenomenon is a feature of addiction of:

a. Opiates b. LSD
c. Cocaine d. Alcohol

Magnan's sign is a clinical sign in which people with cocaine addiction experience paraesthesia which feels like a constantly moving foreign body, such as fine sand or powder, under the skin.

123. Macewen sign is seen in:

a. Arsenic poisoning b. Lead poisoning
c. Alcoholism d. Cyanide poisoning

If the person intoxicated with alcohol is comatose, to differentiate this person with that of other comatose conditions, Mcewan's sign should be observed.

According to this sign, pinching skin of face or neck would cause transient dilation of the pupils with slow return.

124. NOT an aryl phosphate:

a. Paraoxon b. Malathion
c. Tik-20 d. Parathion

Malathion is an organophosphate parasympathomimetic which binds irreversibly to cholinesterase. Malathion is an insecticide of relatively low human toxicity. It belongs to alkyl phosphate group.

125. Toxin in mushroom poisoning principally affects:

a. Liver b. Lung
c. Bladder d. Nerves

Among the mushrooms that most commonly cause poisoning are *Amanita muscaria, A. phalloides,* and the four white *Amanita* species called destroying angels. The ingestion of *A. muscaria* (fly agaric), which contains muscarine and other toxic alkaloids, is soon followed by nausea, vomiting, diarrhea, excessive salivation, perspiration, watering of the eyes, slowed and difficult breathing, dilated pupils, confusion, and excitability. Illness usually begins within a few hours after eating the mushrooms, and recovery usually occurs within 12 hours.

126. Drug NOT given in organophosphate poisoning:

a. Atropine
b. Pralidoxime
c. Activated charcoal
d. Physostigmine

Pyridostigmine is used to treat muscle weakness in people with myasthenia gravis and to combat the effects of curariform drug toxicity.

127. A 10 years old boy consumes stain remover. He presented with 'coffee-coloured' vomiting and restlessness. Most likely diagnosis:

a. Oxalic acid
b. Diluted HCl
c. Kerosene
d. Carbolic acid

Colour of vomitus in oxalic acid poisoning is coffee ground. (Contains altered blood, mucus-appears greenish brown or black resembling coffee ground)

128. Hooch tragedy was due to consumption of:

a. Cannabis
b. Methyl alcohol
c. Ethyl alcohol
d. Datura

Ans. 120. **c.** Sulphuric acid 121. **d.** Cytochrome... 122. **c.** Cocaine 123. **c.** Alcoholism
124. **b.** Malathion 125. **d.** Nerves 126. **d.** Physostigmine 127. **a.** Oxalic acid
128. **b.** Methyl alcohol

Hooch is a colloquial term for alcoholic beverages (also spelled hootch).

129. The chief compound in cannabis is:

a. 9-tetra-hydro-cannabinol
b. 6-tetra-hydro-cannabinol
c. 5-tetra-hydro-cannabinol
d. 4-tetra-hydro-cannabinol

The two cannabinoids usually produced in greatest abundance are cannabidiol (CBD) and/or Δ^9-tetrahydrocannabinol (THC), but only THC is psychoactive.

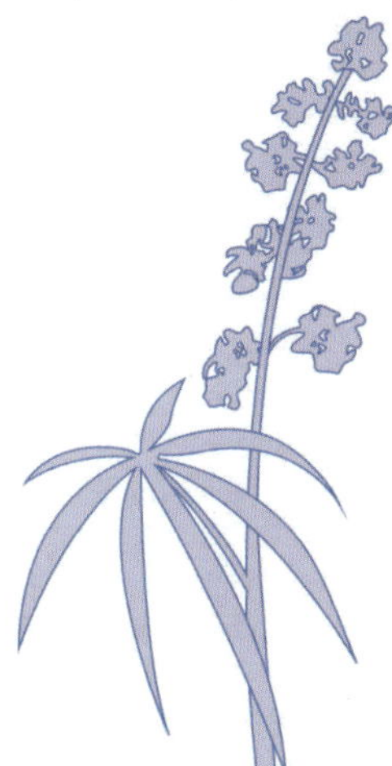

Cannabis indica.

130. Mee's lines are seen in poisoning with:

a. Cadmium b. Lead
c. Mercury d. Arsenic

Symptoms of arsenic poisoning begin with headaches, confusion, severe diarrhea, and drowsiness. As the poisoning develops, convulsions and changes in fingernail pigmentation called leukonychia striata, Mees' lines, or Aldrich-Mees' lines may occur.

131. Rain drop pigmentation is seen in:

a. Arsenic poisoning
b. Phosphorous poisoning
c. Mercury poisoning
d. All of the above

Symptoms of chronic arsenic intoxication include general pigmentation or focal "raindrop" pigmentation of the skin and the appearance of hyperkeratosis of the palms of the hands and soles of the feet.

132. Formication and delusion occurs together in:

a. Cocaine b. LSD
c. Cannabis d. Amphetamine

Cocaine increases alertness, feelings of well-being and euphoria, energy and motor activity, feelings of competence and sexuality. Common side effects include anxiety, increased temperature, paranoia, restlessness, and teeth grinding. With prolonged use, often accompanied by lack of sleep, the drug can cause itching, tachycardia, tactile hallucinations (formication, and paranoid delusions.

133. Oximes are used in poisoning for all EXCEPT:

a. Baygon
b. Tik 20
c. Malathion
d. Parathion

Oxime compounds are used as antidotes for nerve agents. A nerve agent inactivates acetylcholinesterase molecules by phosphorylation of the molecule. Oxime compounds can reactivate acetylcholinesterase by attaching to the phosphorus atom and forming an oxime-phosphonate, which then splits away from the acetylcholinesterase molecule.

134. A patient with history of prolonged intake of some unknown poison presents with digestive disturbances, anorexia, dilated pupils, hallucinations and blackened teeths and tongue. Most likely agent is:

a. Strychnos nux vomica b. Datura
c. Opium d. Cocaine

Tactile hallucinations (Magnan's symptoms or cocaine bugs), visual hallucinations, black staining of tongue and teeth, and ulceration of the nasal septum due to sniffing is seen in cocaine poisoning.

135. Antidote for cyanide poison is:

a. Sodium bicarbonate
b. Sodium chloride
c. Sodium thiosulphate
d. All of the following

Sodium thiosulphate is used as an antidote to cyanide poisoning. Thiosulfate serves as a sulfur donor for the conversion of cyanide to thiocyanate (which can then be safely excreted in the urine), catalyzed by the enzyme rhodanese.

MISCELLANEOUS

136. Regarding medical termination of pregnancy, all of the following are true EXCEPT:

a. Professional secrecy has to be maintained
b. Woman has the right to abort his fetus without consent of husband
c. In an emergency, termination of pregnancy can be done by a single doctor
d. Termination of pregnancy up to 20 weeks by medical practitioner without consulting specialist

Rules of MTP

- If the pregnancy is below 12 weeks period, it can be terminated by on the opinion of single doctor
- If the period of pregnancy is between 12 to 20 weeks, two doctors must agree that there is indication
- In an emergency, pregnancy can be terminated by a single doctor, even without required training (even after 20 weeks), without consulting a second doctor, in a private hospital which is not recognized.

Ans. **129. a.** 9-tetra-hydro-cannabinol **130. d.** Arsenic **131. a.** Arsenic poisoning
132. a. Cocaine **133. a.** Baygon **134. d.** Cocaine **135. c.** Sodium...
136. d. Termination...

ANSWERS WITH REFERENCES

INJURIES

1. **Ans. (d)** Oblique bullet wound
Ref: Reddy's Forensic Medicine 33/e p246

2. **Ans. (b)** Direction of wound
Ref: Reddy's Forensic Medicine 33/e p193

3. **Ans. (d)** All of the above
Ref: Reddy's Forensic Medicine 33/e p195

4. **Ans. (c)** Contusion
Ref: Reddy's Forensic Medicine 33/e p188

5. **Ans. (d)** Contusion of breast
Ref: Reddy's Forensic Medicine 33/e p292

6. **Ans. (b)** Bullet injury
Ref: Reddy's Forensic Medicine 33/e p224

7. **Ans. (c)** Inner table of the entry point in bullet injury
Ref: Reddy's Forensic Medicine 33/e p225

8. **Ans. (c)** Lacerated wound
Ref: Reddy's Forensic Medicine 33/e p190

9. **Ans. (c)** 6"
Ref: Reddy's Forensic Medicine 33/e p217

10. **Ans. (b)** Lung
Ref: Reddy's Forensic Medicine 33/e p239

11. **Ans. (c)** Edges of the wound does not gape
Ref: Reddy's Forensic Medicine 33/e p312

12. **Ans. (d)** Pressure
Ref: Reddy's Forensic Medicine 33/e p182

13. **Ans. (b)** Pressure abrasion
Ref: Reddy's Forensic Medicine 33/e p182

14. **Ans. (c)** Commoner in moving head
Ref: Reddy's Forensic Medicine 33/e p250

15. **Ans. (c)** Velocity
Ref: Reddy's Forensic Medicine 33/e p215

16. **Ans. (a)** Contact shot
Ref: Reddy's Forensic Medicine 33/e p221

17. **Ans. (b)** Depressed fracture
Ref: Reddy's Forensic Medicine 33/e p245

18. **Ans. (d)** Relationship between malignancy and trauma
Ref: Reddy's Forensic Medicine 33/e p315

19. **Ans. (c)** 30-40 meters
Ref: Reddy's Forensic Medicine 33/e p208

LAW AND FORENSIC MEDICINE

20. **Ans. (d)** 42
Ref: Internet resources

21. **Ans. (d)** Exchange theory
Ref: Reddy's FM & T, 33/e p475

22. **Ans. (a)** IPC 84
Ref: Reddy's FM & T, 33/e p493

23. **Ans. (d)** 193 IPC
Ref: Reddy's Forensic Medicine 33/e p55

24. **Ans. (c)** Murder cases
Ref: Reddy's Forensic Medicine 33/e p7

25. **Ans. (a)** Mumbai
Ref: Reddy's Forensic Medicine 33/e p7

26. **Ans. (b)** Magistrate
Ref: Reddy's Forensic Medicine 33/e p7

27. **Ans. (b)** Dying deposition
Ref: Reddy's Forensic Medicine 33/e p11

28. **Ans. (b)** 7 years
Ref: Reddy's Forensic Medicine 33/e p82

29. **Ans. (c)** 18 years
Ref: Reddy's Forensic Medicine 33/e p83

30. **Ans. (c)** Dowry death
Ref: Reddy's Forensic Medicine 33/e p7

31. **Ans. (b)** Magistrate
Ref: Reddy's Forensic Medicine 33/e p11

32. **Ans. (a)** The president
Ref: Reddy's Forensic Medicine 33/e p8

33. **Ans. (d)** All of the above
Ref: Reddy's Forensic Medicine 33/e p12

34. **Ans. (a)** Willful utterance of falsehood
Ref: Reddy's Forensic Medicine 33/e p13

35. **Ans. (a)** Police
Ref: Reddy's Forensic Medicine 33/e p6

36. **Ans. (b)** Inquest report
Ref: Reddy's Forensic Medicine 33/e p6

37. **Ans. (a) Early morning**
Ref: Reddy's Forensic Medicine 33/e p132

38. **Ans. (d) No limit**
Ref: Reddy's Forensic Medicine 33/e p132

39. **Ans. (b) Cross examination**
Ref: Reddy's Forensic Medicine 33/e p14

40. **Ans. (b) 498 A**
Ref: Reddy's Forensic Medicine 33/e p295

41. **Ans. (c) Travel expenses for witness**
Ref: Reddy's Forensic Medicine 33/e p9

42. **Ans. (d) 304B**
Ref: Reddy's Forensic Medicine 33/e p295

43. **Ans. (a) Document**
Ref: Reddy's Forensic Medicine 33/e p8

44. **Ans. (c) 3 years jail and ₹ 5000 fine**
Ref: Reddy's Forensic Medicine 33/e p8

45. **Ans. (c) Treating doctor**
Ref: Reddy's Forensic Medicine 33/e p39

46. **Ans. (a) Imprisonment up to 7 years**
Ref: Reddy's Forensic Medicine 33/e p7

MEDICOLEGAL ASPECT OF DEATH

47. **Ans. (d) No smell**
Ref: Reddy's FM & T, 33/e p172 (Figure 7-8)

48. **Ans. (c) 18–21**
Ref: Reddy's FM & T, 33/e p79 (Figure 4-41)

49. **Ans. (d) Brain**
Ref: Reddy's FM & T, 33/e p166 (Figure 7-5)

50. **Ans. (b) Child born after death of father**
Ref: Reddy's FM & T, 33/e p396

51. **Ans. (c) Greenish discoloration of right iliac fossa**
Ref: Reddy's Forensic Medicine 33/e p164

52. **Ans. (c) Maceration**
Ref: Reddy's Forensic Medicine 33/e p437

53. **Ans. (d) Coagulation of protein of the muscles**
Ref: Reddy's Forensic Medicine 33/e p322

54. **Ans. (c) 36 hours**
Ref: Reddy's Forensic Medicine 33/e p165

55. **Ans. (b) Rigor mortis**
Ref: Reddy's Forensic Medicine 33/e p162

56. **Ans. (d) Drowning**
Ref: Reddy's Forensic Medicine 33/e p368

57. **Ans. (a) Electrocution in water**
Ref: Reddy's Forensic Medicine 33/e p366

58. **Ans. (b) 6–11 years**
Ref: Reddy's Forensic Medicine 33/e p68

59. **Ans. (d) Molar**
Ref: Reddy's Forensic Medicine 33/e p71

60. **Ans. (d) Lip prints**
Ref: Reddy's Forensic Medicine 33/e p88

61. **Ans. (b) Loop**
Ref: Reddy's Forensic Medicine 33/e p86

62. **Ans. (a) Race**
Ref: Reddy's Forensic Medicine 33/e p59

63. **Ans. (c) Finger printing**
Ref: Reddy's Forensic Medicine 33/e p86

64. **Ans. (c) Females**
Ref: Reddy's Forensic Medicine 33/e p62

65. **Ans. (d) Cherry red postmortem staining**
Ref: Reddy's Forensic Medicine 33/e p159

66. **Ans. (d) DNA finger printing**
Ref: Reddy's Forensic Medicine 33/e p466

67. **Ans. (a) Skull**
Ref: Reddy's Forensic Medicine 33/e p89

68. **Ans. (c) 24**
Ref: Reddy's Forensic Medicine 33/e p70

69. **Ans. (d) Absorption elution test**
Ref: Reddy's Forensic Medicine 33/e p454

70. **Ans. (c) CSF**
Ref: Reddy's Forensic Medicine 33/e p464

71. **Ans. (a) Lower end of femur**
Ref: Reddy's Forensic Medicine 33/e p74

72. **Ans. (b) 2–2.5 years**
Ref: Reddy's Forensic Medicine 33/e p71

73. **Ans. (d) Phenol**
Ref: Reddy's Forensic Medicine 33/e p170

74. **Ans. (c) Eyelids → thorax → lower limb**
Ref: Reddy's Forensic Medicine 33/e p161

75. **Ans. (a) 0**
Ref: Reddy's Forensic Medicine 33/e p70

76. **Ans. (c) Discoloration as a result of capillo-venous distension in the dependent parts of the body**
Ref: Reddy's Forensic Medicine 33/e p158

77. **Ans. (a) Alcohol poisoning**
Ref: Reddy's Forensic Medicine 33/e p125

78. **Ans. (b) Stature**
Ref: Reddy's Forensic Medicine 33/e p129

79. **Ans. (c) Dolicocephalic**
Ref: Reddy's Forensic Medicine 33/e p59

80. **Ans. (c) Barr body**
Ref: Reddy's Forensic Medicine 33/e p95

81. **Ans. (b) 1.5 F/ hour**
Ref: Reddy's Forensic Medicine 33/e p158

82. **Ans. (a) Root transparency**
Ref: Reddy's Forensic Medicine 33/e p71

83. **Ans. (c) Absence of brainstem reflexes**
Ref: Reddy's Forensic Medicine 33/e p134

84. **Ans. (c) First molar**
Ref: Reddy's Forensic Medicine 33/e p71

85. **Ans. (c) Muscle of the body began to stiffen**
Ref: Reddy's Forensic Medicine 33/e p160

86. **Ans. (b) HCN poisoning**
Ref: Reddy's Forensic Medicine/ 33rd/e p125

87. **Ans. (d) Irregular margin**
Ref: Reddy's Forensic Medicine 33/e p323

88. **Ans. (a) Vagal hyperactivity**
Ref: Reddy's Forensic Medicine 33/e p366

89. **Ans. (a) Throttling**
Ref: Reddy's Forensic Medicine 33/e p357

90. **Ans. (c) Angle of mandible**
Ref: Internet resources

91. **Ans. (b) Same finger prints sequence**
Ref: Reddy's Forensic Medicine 33/e p86

92. **Ans. (b) Air vesicle**
Ref: Reddy's Forensic Medicine 33/e p326

93. **Ans. (d) Eyelids**
Ref: Reddy's Forensic Medicine 33/e p161

94. **Ans. (b) Lightning stroke**
Ref: Reddy's Forensic Medicine 33/e p334

95. **Ans. (a) Burns**
Ref: Reddy's Forensic Medicine 33/e p322

96. **Ans. (d) Shrunken gallbladder**
Ref: Reddy's Forensic Medicine 33/e p336

97. **Ans. (c) Homicidal**
Ref: Reddy's Forensic Medicine 33/e p364

98. **Ans. (b) Heat stroke**
Ref: Reddy's Forensic Medicine 33/e p319

99. **Ans. (a) Warm**
Ref: Reddy's Forensic Medicine 33/e p319

100. **Ans. (d) Spermatozoon**
Ref: Reddy's Forensic Medicine 33/e p465

101. **Ans. (b) Maceration**
Ref: Reddy's Forensic Medicine 33/e p437

102. **Ans. (d) Drowning**
Ref: Reddy's Forensic Medicine 33/e p371

103. **Ans. (a) Fluoride**
Ref: Reddy's Forensic Medicine 33/e p124

104. **Ans. (c) H_2S**
Ref: Reddy's Forensic Medicine 33/e p159

105. **Ans. (a) 10% formalin**
Ref: Reddy's Forensic Medicine 33/e p123

106. **Ans. (b) Skull and dura**
Ref: Reddy's Forensic Medicine 33/e p324

107. **Ans. (c) Drowning**
Ref: Reddy's Forensic Medicine 33/e p372

108. **Ans. (d) Toes**
Ref: Reddy's Forensic Medicine 33/e p161

SEXUAL OFFENCES

109. **Ans. (d) Frigidity**
Ref: Reddy's Forensic Medicine 33/e p382

110. **Ans. (d) Choline**
Ref: Reddy's Forensic Medicine 33/e p434

111. **Ans. (c) Sexual pleasure by the suffering of pain**
Ref: Reddy's Forensic Medicine 33/e p431

112. **Ans. (c) Takayama test**
Ref: Reddy's Forensic Medicine 33/e p451

TOXICOLOGY

113. **Ans. (c) Lead**
Ref: Reddy's FM & T, 33/e p545

114. **Ans. (d) Cadmium**
Ref: Internet resources

115. **Ans. (d) Arsenic**
Ref: Reddy's FM & T, 33/e p539 (Table 27-1)

116. **Ans. (c) Cadmium**
Ref: Internet resources

117. **Ans. (d) Dhatura poisoning**
Ref: Reddy's Forensic Medicine 33/e p599

118. **Ans. (a) Arsenic**
Ref: Reddy's Forensic Medicine 33/e p541

119. **Ans. (d) Bradycardia**
Ref: Reddy's Forensic Medicine 33/e p599

120. **Ans. (c) Sulphuric acid**
Ref: Reddy's Forensic Medicine 33/e p515

121. **Ans. (d) Cytochrome oxidase**
Ref: Reddy's Forensic Medicine 33/e p627

122. **Ans. (c) Cocaine**
Ref: Reddy's Forensic Medicine 33/e p603

123. **Ans. (c) Alcoholism**
Ref: Reddy's Forensic Medicine 33/e p572

124. **Ans. (b) Malathion**
Ref: Reddy's Forensic Medicine 33/e p520

125. **Ans. (d) Nerves**
Ref: Reddy's Forensic Medicine 33/e p639

126. **Ans. (d) Physostigmine**
Ref: Reddy's Forensic Medicine 33/e p523

127. **Ans. (a) Oxalic acid**
Ref: Reddy's Forensic Medicine 33/e p533

128. **Ans. (b) Methyl alcohol**
Ref: Internet resources

129. **Ans. (a) 9-tetra-hydro-cannabinol**
Ref: Reddy's Forensic Medicine 33/e p601

130. **Ans. (d) Arsenic**
Ref: Reddy's Forensic Medicine 33/e p540

131. **Ans. (a) Arsenic poisoning**
Ref: Reddy's Forensic Medicine 33/e p540

132. **Ans. (a) Cocaine**
Ref: Reddy's Forensic Medicine 33/e p603

133. **Ans. (a) Baygon**
Ref: Internet resources

134. **Ans. (d) Cocaine**
Ref: Reddy's Forensic Medicine 33/e p603

135. **Ans. (c) Sodium thiosulphate**
Ref: Reddy's Forensic Medicine 33/e p628

MISCELLANEOUS

136. **Ans. (d) Termination of pregnancy up to 20 weeks by medical practitioner without consulting specialist**
Ref: Reddy's Forensic Medicine 33/e p401

PRACTICE QUESTIONS

INJURIES

1. At what place, lacerated wound would NOT look like a incised wound:
a. Thigh
b. Head
c. Shin
d. Pelvis

2. All of the following are associated with stabbing injury EXCEPT:
a. Point wound
b. Puncture wound
c. Perforation
d. Chopping

3. All of the following are contents of black gun powder of bullet EXCEPT:
a. Sulphur
b. Charcoal
c. Potassium
d. Nitrocellulose

LAW AND FORENSIC MEDICINE

4. Doctor is a:
a. Common witness
b. Hostile witness
c. Expert witness
d. Occurrence witness

5. IPC 386 is related to:
a. Extortion
b. Infanticide
c. Domestic violence
d. Dowry death

6. Magistrate inquest for:
a. Road accidents death
b. Drowning death
c. Custodial death
d. Death due to poisoning

MEDICOLEGAL ASPECTS OF DEATH

7. Bluish discoloration in putrefaction is first noticed externally in:
a. Left iliac fossa
b. Right hypochondrium
c. Left hypochondrium
d. Right iliac fossa

8. Vagus nerve is inhibited in:
a. Immersion syndrome
b. Dry drowning
c. Wet drowning
d. Typical drowning

9. Which is responsible for death of a subject, who is sitting in his car with exhaust pipe communicating with interior of car:
a. CO_2 poisoning
b. CO poisoning
c. Cardiac failure
d. Respiratory failure

10. Mechanism of death in overlaying:
a. Strangulation
b. Suffocation
c. Mugging
d. Choking

11. Which of the following is NOT a kind of strangulation:
a. Burking
b. Throttling
c. Garrotting
d. Mugging

12. What is the cause of death in case of drowning in cold water:
a. Vagal stimulation
b. Vagal inhibition
c. Hypervolemia
d. Ventricular arrhythmias

13. As compared to oxygen, affinity of CO for haemoglobin is:
a. 25 times
b. 100 times
c. 300 times
d. 500 times

14. In drowning, washerman's hand is seen after:
a. 1–2 hours
b. 4–8 hours
c. 8–14 hours
d. 18–24 hours

SEXUAL OFFENCES

15. Sexplay by using objects of other gender is:
a. Sadism
b. Masochism
c. Paraphilia
d. Fetichism

16. Buccal coitus is also known as:
a. Active algolagnia
b. Passive algolagnia
c. Sin of Gomorrah
d. Greek love

Ans.
1. **a.** Thigh
2. **d.** Chopping
3. **d.** Nitrocellulose
4. **c.** Expert witness
5. **a.** Extortion
6. **c.** Custodial...
7. **d.** Right iliac fossa
8. **a.** Immersion...
9. **b.** CO poisoning
10. **b.** Suffocation
11. **a.** Burking
12. **b.** Vagal inhibition
13. **c.** 300 times
14. **d.** 18–24 hours
15. **c.** Paraphilia
16. **c.** Sin of Gomorrah

17. **Nature of hymen in false virgin:**
   a. Annular b. Elastic
   c. Imperforate d. Semilunar
18. **All of the following are illegal in India EXCEPT:**
   a. Bestiality
   b. Female homosexuality
   c. Buccal coitus
   d. Indecent assault
19. **What will you call a person who enjoys satisfaction by watching others indulge in sexual act:**
   a. Voyeurism b. Frotteurism
   c. Fetichism d. Exhibitionsim

TOXICOLOGY

20. **Which of the following is known as junk or smack:**
   a. Cocaine b. LSD
   c. Heroin d. Chloral hydrate
21. **Important in managing a case of strychnine poisoning:**
   a. N-acetyl cysteine
   b. Diazepam
   c. Amyl nitrite
   d. Freshly prepared ferric oxide
22. **Hippus is a feature of:**
   a. Morphine overdose
   b. Organophosphate poisoning
   c. Datura poisoning
   d. Aconite
23. **A patient with unknown poisoning presented with flushed face, dilated pupils, dry skin and delirium. Likely poisoning is:**
   a. Opium
   b. Organophosphate
   c. Datura
   d. Cannabis
24. **True regarding strychnine poisoning:**
   a. Active component is THC
   b. Quickly disappears from body
   c. Mimics tetanus
   d. Rare in India
25. **Artificial bruises can be produced by:**
   a. Abrin b. Atropine
   c. Bhilawanol d. Crotin

MISCELLANEOUS

26. **Two ovum were released in same menstrual cycle and were fertilized by two separate acts of coitus. This will result in:**
   a. Superfoetation
   b. Pseudocyesis
   c. Superfecundation
   d. Supposititious child
27. **Lungs of a newborn, who had NOT breathed, will:**
   a. Sink in water b. Float in water
   c. Both d. None

Ans. 17. **b.** Elastic 18. **b.** Female homosexuality 19. **a.** Voyeurism 20. **c.** Heroin
21. **b.** Diazepam 22. **d.** Aconite 23. **c.** Datura 24. **c.** Mimics tetanus
25. **c.** Bhilawanol 26. **c.** Superfecundation 27. **a.** Sink in water

IMAGE-BASED QUESTIONS

1. Such measurements are helpful in assessing:

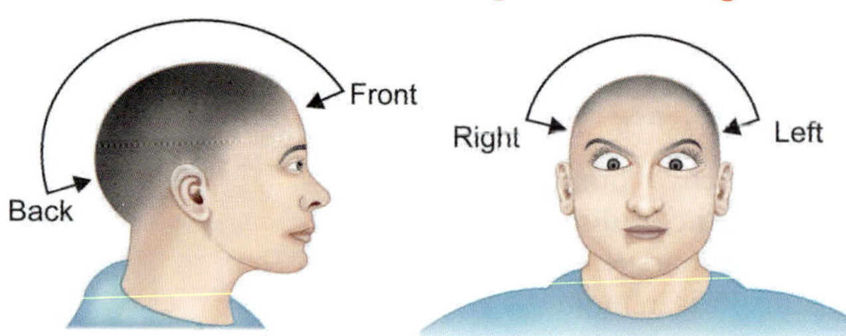

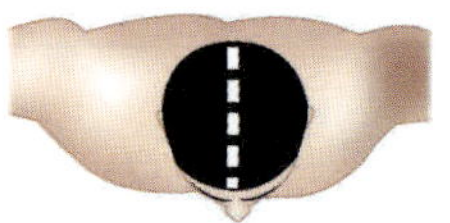

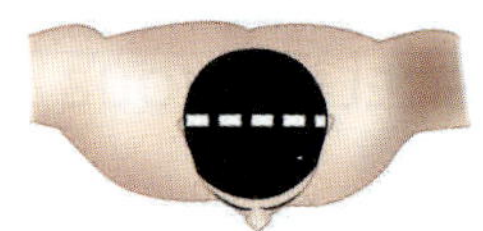

a. Stature
b. Gender
c. Age
d. Race

Cephalic index is being calculated as maximum breadth × 100/maximum length of skull. It is used for determining race.

2. Process behind such postmortem changes:

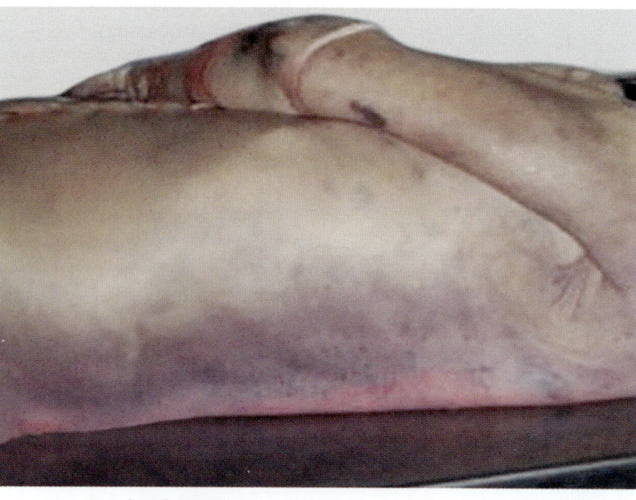

a. Lack of ATP
b. Decomposition by bacteria
c. Hydrolysis of body fats
d. Due to stoppage of circulation

Postmortem hypostasis is caused by stoppage of circulation, the stagnation of blood in blood vessels, and its tendency to sink by the force of gravity.

3. What is the importance of such lines:

a. Estimating time since death
b. Wound gaping
c. Sex determination
d. Age determination

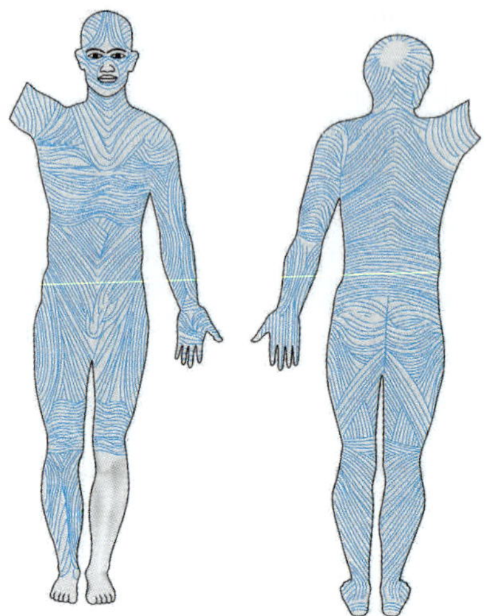

Stab wounds and incised wounds are slit-shpaed with two acute angles, or gape open depending on their location and their orientation, with regard to the so called cleavage lines of Langer.

4. Mechanism behind such postmortem change:

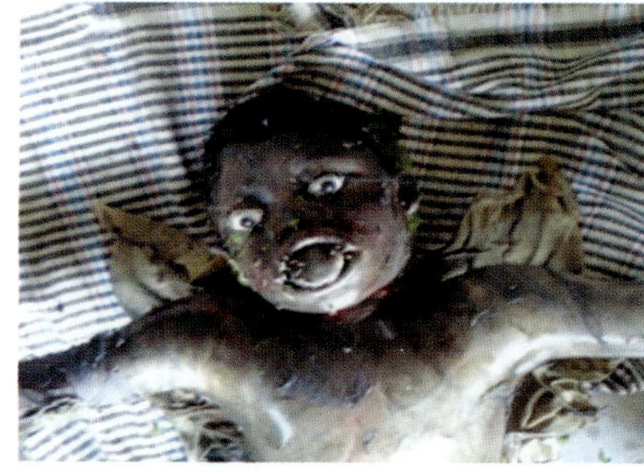

a. Stasis of blood
b. Hydrolysis of body fats
c. Dehydration
d. Destruction of body tissues by bacterial enzymes

After death, the protective agencies of the body are absent, the bacteria spread through the blood vessels using the proteins and carbohydrates of the blood as culture media. Putrefaction is the final stage following death, in which destruction of the soft tissues of the body occurs. Destruction is caused mainly by the action of bacterial enzymes, mostly anaerobic organisms derived from the intestines.

5. Mechanism behind such postmortem change:

a. Bacterial infection
b. Vesication of skin
c. Hydrolysis and hydrogenation of body fats
d Mummification

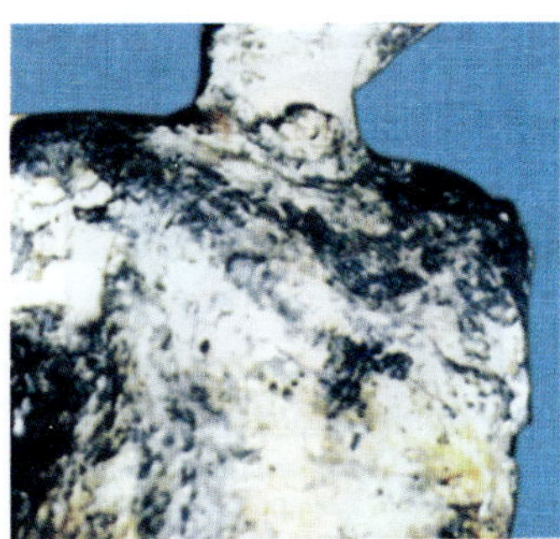

In adipocere formation, there is gradual hydrolysis and hydrogenation of pre-existing fats, such as olein, into higher fatty acids, which combine with calcium and ammonium ions to form insoluble soaps, which being acidic, inhibit putrefactive bacteria.

6. **Identify the postmortem change:**

a. Rigor mortis b. Adipocere formation
c. Hypostasis d. Dehydration

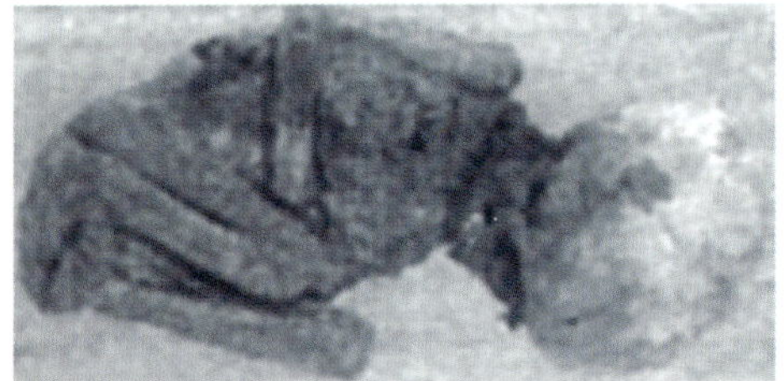

Mummification/dehydration or drying and shrivelling of the cadaver occurs from the evaporation of water, but the natural appearances of the body and general facial features are preserved.

7. **Type of injury seen on the fingers:**

a. Gunshot b. Brush burns
c. Incised wounds d. Insect bites

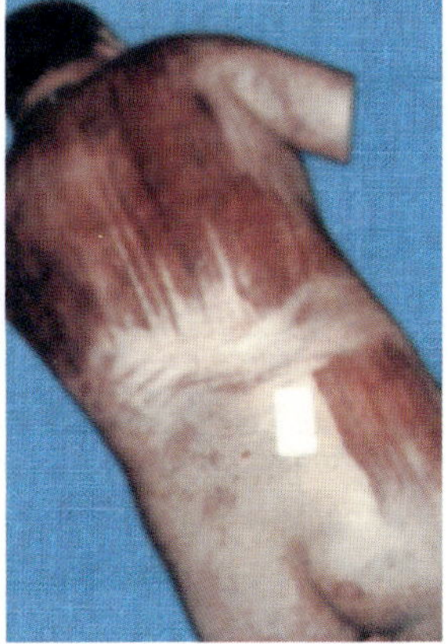

An abrasion caused by a violent lateral (tangential) rubbing against a surface as in dragging over the ground is called brush burn/gravel rash.

8. **Nature of such kind of injuries:**

a. Suicidal b. Accidental
c. Homicidal d. All of the above

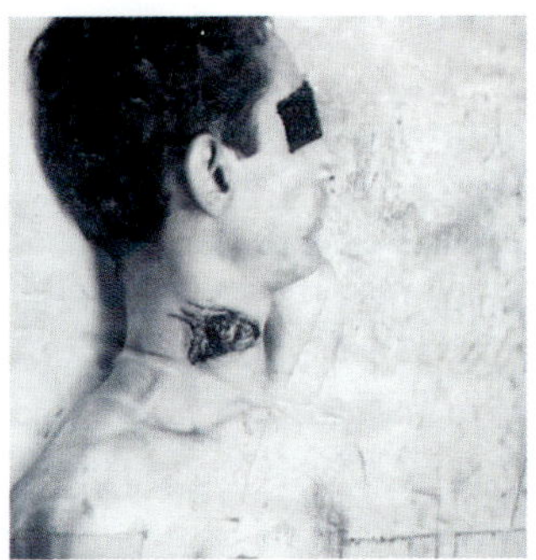

Hesitation marks or tentative cuts or trial wounds are cuts which are multiple, small and superficial often involving only the skin and are seen at the beginning of the self inflicted incised wound.

9. **Identify the type of injury:**

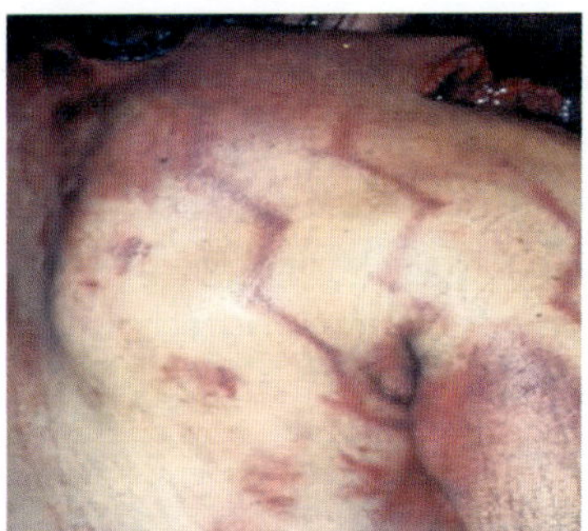

a. Pressure abrasion b. Friction burn
c. Patterned abrasion d. Brush burn

Impact abrasions and pressure abrasions reproduce the pattern of the object causing it and are called patterned abrasions.

10. **Which type of injury:**

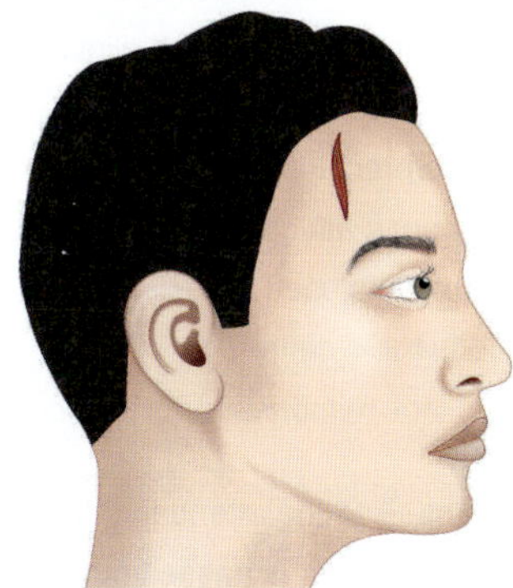

a. Incised wound b. Laceration
c. Chop wound d. Stab wound

Lacerations produced without excessive skin crushing may have relatively sharp margins. Blunt force on areas where the skin is close to bone, and the subcutaneous tissues are scanty, may produce a wound which by linear splitting of the tissues (as the skin is easily stretched during impact), may look like incised wound.

MCQ POINTS

S. No.	Question statements	Answer
1.	A female consumed 20 tablets of Crocin. Best antidote for this case:	***N-acetyl-cysteine***
2.	MC type of fingerprints	***Loops***
3.	If the angle of mandible is obtuse, it belong to which age group	***Infant or old***
4.	In tandem bullet, total numbers of bullets coming out of the gun are	***2 bullets***
5.	A patient came with cuts at wrist. Feature which will suggest suicidal nature of injury:	***Hesitation marks/ tentative cuts***
6.	Grievous injuries are dealt under IPC	***IPC 320***
7.	Entry point of gunshot may show	***Dirt collar/grease collar***
8.	Cause of death in café coronary	***Asphyxia/reflex cardiac arrest***
9.	Le facies sympathique is because of stimulation of …… by knot	***Cervical sympathetic ganglion***
10.	Which substance is estimated in Gettlers test	***NaCl***
11.	Pugilistic attitude is suggestive of	***Burns***
12.	Widmark formula is employed for	***Alcohol***
13.	'Erethism' is associated with which poison	***Mercury***
14.	Poison which retards putrefaction	***Arsenic and carbolic acid***
15.	'Saturnism' is related to which poison	***Chronic lead poisoning***
16.	Burtonian line is associated with which poison	***Lead poisoning***
17.	Sea snake venom is	***Myotoxic***
18.	Last organ to putrefy in males	***Prostate***
19.	Location of knot in typical hanging	***Angle of mandible***
20.	Formication is seen with which poison	***Cocaine***
21.	Inquest in death is carried out by	***Police (in India)***
22.	Leading questions are defined as	***The answer is either Yes or No***
23.	Pattern, in a case of burn due to lightening injury	***Arborescent/ Lichtenbery/Filigree***
24.	Ill effect of methanol on eye is due to formation of	***Formic acid***
25.	Arsenic poisoning mimics which clinical condition	***Gastroenteritis***
26.	Study of finger prints is known as	***Dactylography***
27.	Toxin of abrus precatorius	***Abrin***
28.	Toxicity of aconite affects which organ	***Heart***
29.	Pearson formula is used for estimating	***Height***
30.	Res ipsa loquitur is defined as	***Things speaks for themselves***
31.	A person is not responsible for his crime, if he is not of sound mind. This is …………. rule	***McNaughton's rule***
32.	Document impelling the attendance of witness in court under penalty is	***Summon/sunpoena***
33.	For exhumation, order is passed out by whom	***First class judicial magistrate***
34.	Best method to detect paternity	***DNA finger printing***
35.	Rule of Haase is used for calculating	***Fetal age***
36.	Period of mixed dentition is between ……. and …… years	***6–11 years***
37.	Most reliable criteria (Gustafson method) for dental age estimation	***Transparency of root***
38.	Preauricular sulcus in females is present in which bone	***Pelvis***
39.	CSF is preserved in which poisoning	***Alcohol***
40.	Bruise is greenish in colour on …….. days	***6th day***

S. No.	Question statements	Answer
41.	Pond fracture is seen on which bone	***Skull***
42.	Tangential bullet injury produces which type of fracture	***Gutter fracture***
43.	Contrecoup injury means	***Injury on the opposite side of impact of a moving head***
44.	Lucid interval is seen in which type of skull hemorrhage	***Extradural hemorrhage***
45.	Ricochet bullet is defined as	***Bullet which before striking aims at some intervening object first, rebounds and then hits the object***
46.	Sexual offence which is not a crime in India	***Incest***
47.	Privation of any member of a joint comes is which type of injury	***Grievous***
48.	Absolute proof of life during fire burns (antemortem burns)	***Soot in upper respiratory tract***
49.	Cause of death in electrocution	***Ventricular fibrillation***
50.	Branching tree pattern burn are seen in	***Lightening***
51.	Rigor mortis is delayed by which poison	***Arsenic***
52.	Biochemical basis of adipocere formation	***Hydrolysis and hydrogenation of body fats***
53.	Muscle which develops rigor mortis lastly	***Small muscles of toes and fingers***
54.	Algor mortis may be observed in	***Frostbite, Barbiturate poisoning***
55.	Colour of postmortem lividity in CO poisoning	***Cherry red***
56.	Organ to putrefy last in body	***Bone***
57.	Aseptic autolysis is known as	***Maceration***
58.	Position of knot in typical hanging	***Near the angle of mandible***
59.	Le facies sympathique is term associated with death due to	***Hanging***
60.	Sure sign of death due to hanging	***Dribbling of saliva along the angle of mouth***
61.	Hyoid bone fracture strongly suggest which mode of asphyxia	***Manual strangulation/ throttling***
62.	Repeated slapping on the sides of the head is known as	***Telefona***
63.	Most characteristic external sign of death due to drowning	***Fine, copious, frothy discharge from the mouth and nostrils***
64.	Dermal nitrate test detects	***Gunpowder residues***
65.	When a group of muscles of a dead body were in state of strong contraction immediately prior to death and remain so even after death. This is	***Cadaveric rigidity***
66.	Florence test for seminal stain detects which substance	***Choline iodide***
67.	Gastric lavage is not done in …….. poisoning	***Kerosense and corrosive (except carbolic acid)***
68.	Appearance of pupil in opium poisoning	***Pinpoint***
69.	Morbid jealousy is a feature of which poisoning	***Alcohol***
70.	Run amok is a feature of which poisoning	***Cannabis***
71.	Knock out drops is another term for	***Chloral hydrate***
72.	Metallic poison which may cause necrosis of PCT of kidney	***Mercury***
73.	Metal fume fever is associated with poisoning of	***Zinc***
74.	Poison which inhibits action of cytochrome oxidase	***Cyanide***
75.	Mercuria lentis is associated with which poison	***Mercury***

CHAPTER

9

PREVENTIVE AND SOCIAL MEDICINE

KEY POINTS

Indicator of Health

- Morbidity indicators: Incidence and prevalence, notification rates, attendance rates of hospital, admission and readmission rates, discharge rates, duration of hospital stay, spell of sickness, etc.
- Disability indicators: Sullivan's index (expectation of life free of disability), disability adjusted life year/DALY (measures burden of disease in a defined population and effectiveness of interventions), health adjusted life expectancy/HALE

Physical Quality of Life Index (PQLI)

- Includes literacy rate, infant mortality rate and life expectancy at the age of 1 year

Human Development Index (HDI)

- Includes life expectancy at birth (longevity), adult literacy rate and mean years of schooling (knowledge) and real GDP per capita in purchasing power parity in US dollars (income real)
- Value ranges between 0 and 1
- HDI value in India is 0.619
- Measures average achievements in basic dimensions of human development

Concept of Disease Causation

- Components of epidemiological triad: agent, host and environment
- Determinants of disease behaviour in a community: Infectiousness, density of aggregation of population, standard of hygiene and size of reservoir of infection

Iceberg Diseases

- Waterline in iceberg diseases represents the demarcation between apparent and inapparent cases
- Submerged portion of the iceberg: Constitutes latent, inapparent, presymptomatic, carriers and undiagnosed cases
- Diseases showing iceberg phenomenon: Rubella, polio, Japanese encephalitis, influenza, mumps, hepatitis A and B, diphtheria, etc.
- Iceberg phenomenon is NOT seen in: Rabies, tetanus, measles

Levels of Prevention

- Primary prevention: Has 2 main components – health promotion and specific protection
- Health promotion includes: Health education, environmental modifications, nutritional interventions, lifestyle and behavioral changes (Process of advising a patient to change his lifestyles in order to prevent any risk factor for a disease)
- Specific protection example include: Vitamin A prophylaxis; Iron and folic acid supplementation
- Primary prevention in coronary artery disease include: Changing harmful lifestyles by education to prevent coronary artery disease; exercise in high-risk area, BP monitoring, salt restriction
- Immunization, chemoprophylaxis, marriage counseling are primary level of prevention
- Primordial prevention in myocardial infarction include: Maintenance of normal body weight, change in lifestyle, change in nutritional habits
- Primordial prevention is done in population which has not developed risk factor
- Secondary level of prevention example include: Sputum for AFB, amniocentesis in early pregnancy and Pap smear (screening test) (early diagnosis and treatment), benzathine penicillin prophylaxis for rheumatic fever
- Example of disability limitation (tertiary prevention): Resting affected limb in neutral position

Surveillance

- Epidemiological surveillance: Set of questions are constructed in such a way that it takes into account all the important epidemiological factors of a given disease

- Sentinel surveillance: Detects missing/hidden cases (to find the total amount of disease in a population)
- Active surveillance: Calculates true morbidity
- Diseases under WHO/international surveillance: Rabics, polio, salmonella, louse borne typhus fever, malaria, relapsing fever, human influenza, etc.

International Classification of Disease/ICD

- Denoted as ICD-10
- Done every 10 years
- ICD-10 is arranged in 21 major chapters
- Conducted by WHO
- Poisoning is included in chapter XIX
- Each chapter has 3 character categories
- First character code is a letter
- Accepted for national and international use
- Provides the basis for use in other health fields

Case Fatality Rate (CFR)

- Good index of the severity/lethality of an acute disease
- Represents killing power of a disease
- Closely related to virulence
- Very useful for acute diseases (NOT chronic diseases)
- CFR is calculated as: Total number of deaths due to disease × 100/Total number of cases of the disease
- It is a proportion

Incidence

- Increases in new cases in a community indicates: Increase in incidence rates
- Calculated as: Number of new cases in a given period × 1000/Population at risk during that period
- Incidence is a rate

Prevalence

- In a stable situation: Prevalence = Incidence × duration
- Prevalence: Describes the balance between incidence, mortality and recovery
- If prevalence is very low as compared to the incidence for a disease, it indicates: Either the disease is very fatal or easily curable
- Factor increasing prevalence of a disease: Longer duration of illness
- If a disease has 4 times more incidence in females as compared to males, but the prevalence is same; it implies: Increase fatality in females OR less fatality in males
- Calculated as = Incidence × Duration
- It is a proportion
- Numerator is a part of the denominator

Epidemic

- First thing to be done in an epidemic is: Confirmation of the diagnosis
- Search for new cases in epidemic is done till: Twice the incubation period of the disease since occurrence of the last case

Point Source/Single Exposure Epidemic

- A type of common source epidemic
- All cases occur abruptly and simultaneously (explosive epidemic)
- All cases occurs within a specified period (in one incubation period)
- Rapid rise and rapid fall
- One single peak only
- Explosive
- NO secondary waves and NO plateau phase
- Bhopal gas tragedy is an example

Propagated Epidemic

- Spread depends upon herd immunity
- Person to person transmission occurs
- Secondary waves are SEEN
- Slow rise

Trend of Disease

- Secular trend means: Changes in pattern of the disease over a long period of time
- Seasonal trend is shown by: Measles, varicella (chicken pox), rubella, gastroenteritis, cerebral meningitis
- Cyclical trend is related to: Herd immunity variations, antigenic variations, build up of susceptibles (NOT related to environmental conditions)
- Cyclic trend is shown by: Measles

Cross-Sectional Studies

- Observational study
- Not expensive
- All cases seen at one point of time (for example, many populations participating in the examination at the same time to calculate/identify some particular feature)
- Follow-up is not a necessary feature
- More useful for chronic diseases
- It tells about the distribution of a disease (NOT etiology, so cause and effect relationship cannot be establishes)
- Prevalence can be calculated

Longitudinal Studies

- Measure incidence
- Identifies risk factor
- Studies natural history of the disease

Case Control Studies/Retrospective Study

- A type of analytical study
- Rapid/quick results are obtained
- Proceeds from effect to cause so one can study multiple causal associated factors at a time
- Useful in rare diseases
- Inexpensive, cost effective
- No risk to subjects
- Risk factor can be identified
- Problem of bias is common
- Odds ratio/cross product ratio can be estimated (NOT relative risk)
- Calculated as = ad/bc (where 'a' is number of cases with risk factor present, 'b' is control with risk factors, 'c' is cases with no risk factors and 'd' is control with absent risk factors)
- Odd's ratio (in case control study) measures association between disease and risk factor

Cohort Study/Prospective Study

- Type of analytical study
- Measures incidence rate, relative risk (risk ratio), attributable risk (risk difference) and population attributable risk
- Best design (amongst epidemiological studies) to test the association between risk factors and disease is: Cohort study (though most reliable study is randomized controlled trial)
- In cohort study, non-smokers were found to have carcinoma lung. This indicates: Etiology of lung carcinoma is multifactorial
- Expensive
- Bias is unlikely to invalidate cohort studies used to assess risk of exposure because: Exposure is usually determined prior to disease occurrence

Relative Risk (RR)

- Relative risk can be calculated as: Incidence of the disease among the exposed/incidence of disease among non-exposed
- RR of more than 1: indicates positive association; 0 is no association and -1 hints towards no association between the factor and the disease
- RR is a direct measure of the strength of association between suspected cause and effect

Attributable Risk (AR)

- Attributable risk can be calculated as: Incidence of disease in exposed – incidence of disease among the unexposed × 100/incidence of disease in exposed
- AR measures the extent which is attributed by risk factor to disease
- AR means potential of prevention

Population Attributable Risk (PAR)

- Calculated as = Incidence in total population – incidence in non-exposed × 100/Incidence in total population
- Community physician takes action based on: PAR

Randomized Trial

- Essential purpose of randomization in randomized control trials is: To eliminate the selection bias and confounding factors
- In a controlled trial to compare 2 treatments, the main purpose of randomization is to ensure that: The two groups will be similar in prognostic factors
- Methods of randomization: Computer drawn randomization, lottery, random number table
- While analyzing a data, allocation into similar groups is done to ensure: Comparability
- Non-biased study is: Randomized controlled trials

Nonrandomized Trials

- Degree of comparability is low (NOT high)
- Experiment can serve as its own control or can utilize a natural control
- Several trials may be needed before evaluation is considered conclusive
- Prepost-clinical trials: They use patients as his/her own control

Bias

- Berksonian bias is: Selection bias
- Basic types of bias in epidemiological study: Investigation bias, subject bias, analyzer bias
- Interviewer bias can be reduced by: Allowing equal interview time
- Recall/memory bias is more common with: Case control studies
- Hawthorne effect/attention bias is seen in: Cohort study
- Bias can be eliminated by: Matching, blinding, randomization

Double Blinding

- In double blind clinical drug trials: Study subjects and the investigators are not aware of the treatment study subjects are receiving
- Purpose of double blinding in clinical trials is to: Avoid observer and subject bias

Incubation Period (IP)

- IP of less than 6 hours is seen in: Staphylococcal food poisoning, B. cereus (emetic form)
- Proxy measure of IP are: Latent period, serial interval, generation time (NOT period of communicability)

- IP helps in determining: Period of quarantine, identification of source of infection, immunization (NOT period of isolation)
- Disease highly transmitted during IP is: Pertussis, measles, chicken pox

Secondary Attack Rate (SAR)

- Denominator while calculating secondary attack rate is: All susceptible amongst close contact
- Calculated as: Number of exposed persons developing disease within the range of the IP × 100/total number of exposed or susceptible contact
- SAR is a measure of: Communicability

Modes of Transmission

- Vertical transmission is by: Placenta
- Biological transmission of filarial parasite in culex mosquito is: Cyclodevelopmental
- Transovarian transmission is a feature of: Scrub typhus
- Type of transmission in the case of plague in rate flea: Propagative
- Vector transmits agent by: Contamination of body fluids with vectors, scratching-in of infected faeces, regurgitation

Host Defence

- Active and passive immunity should be given together in: Tetanus, rabies, hepatitis-B
- Postexposure active immunization is done for: Rabies, measles, hepatitis-B, diphtheria, tetanus
- Congenital passive immunity/maternal passive immunity is found in: Polio, measles, rubella, mumps

Vaccines

- Toxoid is prepared from: Exotoxin
- Killed vaccines are: DPT, IP (Salk-inactivated polio vaccine), hepatitis-B
- Vaccine administered through subcutaneous route: Measles
- Vaccine with highest efficacy: Measles (90% after a singe dose)
- Vaccine not to be given in immunodeficient state: Rubella, trivalent oral polio vaccine
- Vaccine contraindicated in a patient on intensive chemotherapy: MMR, BCG
- Dose of OPV, given at birth, in case of institutional deliveries is: Zero dose of OPV

Vaccines and Strains

- Mumps: Jeryl Lynn strain
- Measles: Edmonston Zagreb strain (commonest), Schwarz strain
- Chicken pox: OKA strain
- OPV and IPV: P1, P2, P3 strains (monovalent or trivalent)
- Rubella: RA 27/3
- BCG: Danish 1331

Vaccines and Preservatives/Stabilizers

- Thiomersal is preservative in: DPT, influenza, pneumococcal
- Kanamycin is preservative in: Measles
- BCG has no preservative at all
- Stabilizer in oral polio vaccine: Magnesium chloride

Pregnancy and Immunization

- Vaccine contraindicated in pregnancy: Live viral or bacterial vaccines (MMR, yellow fever, BCG, varicella)
- Vaccine which can be given: Inactivated viral vaccines (Influenza, hepatitis A and B)

Herd Immunity (HI)

- HI provides protection to: Non-immunized persons
- Depends on clinical and subclinical cases
- Influenced by immunization
- Depends on the presence of alternative host
- HI is NOT constant
- % of HI necessary to prevent epidemic spread of diphtheria is: 70%
- HI is not useful in: Tetanus (HI is only relevant for contagious diseases)
- HI is affected by the presence and distribution of alternative animal hosts

Immunoglobulin

- When an antigen is administered for the 1st time to animal or a human being, who has never been exposed to it, the first antibody to develop is: IgM
- Secondary response is mediated by: IgG
- Binary exposure to an antigen results in sudden increase in: IgG

Cold Chain

- Vaccine which requires most stringent conditions for storage/most heat sensitive: OPV
- Vaccine which must be stored in the freezer compartment of the fridge: OPV, measles, BCG, yellow fever
- Vaccines not to be frozen are: DPT, TT
- Frozen DPT vaccine should be: Discarded
- Reverse cold chain is used for: Carrying stool samples of polio patients from a PHC to the laboratory
- Vaccine which can be stored at –10°C temperature: Polio, measles

Isolation

- Isolation period should be: Period of communicability
- Isolation is strictly recommended for: Pneumonic plague, diphtheria, cholera
- Isolation is also done for (though less effective): Polio, typhoid, hepatitis A, mumps
- In salmonellosis, isolation is recommended till: 3 consecutive stool cultures are negative

Quarantine

- Quarantine is related to: Maximum incubation period
- It is NOT synonymous with isolation
- Absolute quarantine is restriction during the incubation period
- Exclusion of children form schools is an example of modified quarantine
- Quarantine should not be longer than the longest incubation period
- Internationally quarantinable disease is: Plague, cholera, yellow fever

Disinfection

- Phenol coefficient indicates: Efficacy of a disinfectant
- Disinfectant used for blood spills: Sodium hypochlorite
- Best disinfectant for cholera stools: Cresol
- Amount of bleaching powder necessary to disinfect choleric stools: 50 gm/litre
- Disinfection of sputum is done by: Boiling, autoclaving, burning
- Pasteurization is: Precurrent/prophylactic disinfection
- Disinfection by autoclaving is NOT recommended for: Sharp instruments, glass syringes

Definitions (Cases)

- Primary case: First case of communicable disease introduced into the population
- Index case: First case to come to the attention of investigators
- Secondary case: Cases developing from contact with primary case

Sensitivity and Specificity

- Specificity of a test refers to ability of a test to detect: True negative
- Sensitivity means the ability to detect: True positive
- Sensitivity is inversely proportional to specificity
- Usefulness of a screening test in a community depends upon: Sensitivity
- When a diagnostic test is used in series mode then: Specificity increases but sensitivity decreases
- Sensitivity can be calculated as: True positives/true positive + false negative
- Specificity can be calculated as: True negative/true negative + false positive

Biological Transmission

- Malaria: Cyclopropagative
- Filaria: Cyclodevelopmental
- Plague: Propagative
- Yellow fever: Propagative

Cleans of Safe Delivery

- For elimination of neonatal tetanus
- Clean delivery surface,
- Clean hands (birth attendants),
- Clean cord cut (blade/instrument),
- Clean cord tie,
- Clean cord stump (no applicant)

Causes of Maternal Mortality (in Descending Order)

- Hemorrhage
- Anemia
- Sepsis
- Obstructed labor

Baby Friendly Hospital Initiative

- Have a written breastfeeding policy that is routinely communicated to all healthcare staff
- Train all healthcare staff in skills necessary to implement this policy.
- Inform all pregnant women about the benefits and management of breastfeeding.
- Help mothers initiate breastfeeding within one half-hour of birth.
- Show mothers how to breastfeed and maintain lactation, even if they should be separated from their infants.
- Give newborn infants no food or drink other than breast milk, unless medically indicated.
- Practice rooming in-that is, allow mothers and infants to remain together 24 hours a day.
- Encourage breastfeeding on demand
- Give no artificial teats or artificial (also called dummies or soothers) to breastfeeding infants.
- Foster the establishment of breastfeeding support groups and refer mothers to them on discharge from the hospital or clinic

Live Attenuated Vaccines

- BCG
- Plague

- Typhoral
- OPV
- Yellow fever
- MMR
- Epidemic typhus
- Chicken pox
- Influenza

Killed Vaccines

- Typhoid
- Cholera
- Pertussis
- Rabies
- IPV
- Influenza
- Hepatitis B
- Plague

Rabies Categorization and Preventive Measures

- Category 1: Touching/licking intact skin
- Category 2: Minor scratches/abrasion, lick on broken skin (Only vaccine)
- Category 3: Bites, scratches, contamination of mucus with licks (Immunoglobulin and vaccine)

Diseases Subject to International Health Regulations

- Paralytic polio
- Malaria
- Louse borne typhus fever
- Relapsing fever
- Viral influenza

Vaccines Contraindicated in HIV/AIDS Patient

- OPV
- Varicella
- Rotavirus
- MMR
- BCG

Zoonoses

- Anthropozoonoses: Infection transmitted from vertebrate animal to man (Rabies, plague, anthrax)
- Zooanthroponosis: Infection transmitted form man to vertebrate animals (Human TB in cattle)
- Amphixenosis: Infection maintained in both man and lower vertebrate animals that may be transmitted in either directions (T. cruzi, S. japonicum)

Characteristic of Zoonoses

- Direct: Direct transmission from animal to human with/without mechanical vector/fomite
- Cyclozoonoses: More than one vertebrate host present
- Metazoonoses: Transmitted biologically via invertebrate vector
- Saprozoonoses: Transmitted via non-animal reservoir
- Anthropozoonoses: Transmitted via vertebrate vector

Mosquitos, Breeding Place and Diseases Transmitted

- Anopheles (Clean stagnant water): Malaria
- Culex (Polluted stagnant water): Bancroftian, Japanese encephalitis, West Nile fever, viral arthritis.
- Aedes (Artificial collections of water): Dengue, Yellow fever, Chikungunya
- Mansonites (Ponds with aquatic plants): Malayan filariasis, Chikungunya.

National Malaria Eradication Program (API > 2)

- Routine spraying: Done
- Entomological assessment: Done
- Active and passive surveillance: Done
- Presumptive and radical treatment: Given
- Follow-up smear after 1 year: Not done

National Malaria Eradication Program (API <2)

- Routine spraying: Not done
- Entomological assessment: Not done
- Active and passive surveillance: Done
- Presumptive and radical treatment: Given
- Follow-up smear after 1 year: Done

Leprosy Survey (Prevalence, Rate and Survey Type)

- Low (<1/1000): Contact
- Moderate (1/1000): Group
- High (> 10/1000): Mass

Disease and Vector

- R. prowazekii: Epidemic typhus, Brill-Zinsser disease (Louse)
- R. typhi, R. felis: Endemic typhus (Rat flea/Cat flea)
- R. rickettsii: Rocky mountain, Spotted fever (Tick)
- Orientia tsutsugamushi: Scrub typhus (Trombiculid mite)
- R. Quintana: Trench fever (Louse)
- R. akari: Rickettsialpox (Mite)
- Coxiella burnettii: Q-fever

Characteristics of Waste

- Sullage: Waste water from domestic sources not containing human excreta
- Sewage: Waste containing human excreta

- Market refuse: Solid waste matter from markets containing putrid vegetable and animal matters

Important Terms

- Net protein utilization = Digestibility coefficient × Biological value/100 = Nitrogen retained × 100/Nitrogen intake
- Protein energy ratio: Energy from protein/Total energy in diet
- Protein efficiency ratio: Weight gain per unit protein consumed
- Amino acid score: mg of amino acid per gram of protein (mg of same amino acid per gram of egg protein)

Vitamin A Prophylaxis

- Newborn: 50,000 IU at birth
- Children below 12 months: 10,0000 IU at 9 Months with MMR and then after every 6 months
- Children more than 12 months: 20,0000 IU till 3 years of age
- Pregnant and lactating women: 5000 IU everyday

Food Toxicity

- Neurolathyrism: BOAA-Lathyrus sativus (kesari dal)
- Aflatoxins: Hepatotoxicity-Aspergillus flavus, Aspergillus Parasiticus infection of groundnut, tapioca, cereals
- Ergotism: Cereals and millets, infected by field fungus claviceps fusiformis
- Epidemic dropsy: Mustard oil adulterated with argemone oil. Toxins are benzophenanthridine alkaloids-sanguinarine and dihydrosanguinarine. Leg edema with diarrhea
- Endemic ascites: Panicum miliare (gondhli) contaminated with weed seeds of crotalaria (jhunjhunia)-ascites with jaundice
- Fusarium toxin: Rice, Sorghum, Fusarium incarnatum.

SAFE Strategy for Trachoma

- S-Trichiasis surgery
- A-Antibiotic treatment
- F-Facial cleanliness
- E-Environmental improvement.

Suggested Norms

- Primary centre: 1/30,000 population in general areas, 1/20,000 population tribal, hilly and backward areas.
- Subcentre: 1/5000 in general areas, 1./3000 in tribal, hilly and backward areas
- Community centre: 1/80,000 to 1.2 lakhs population
- Dai: 1 per village
- Anganwadi worker: 1 per 1000 population
- Village health guide: 1/1000 population or village

Statistic Variables

- Variance = SD2= Sum of squares/n-1
- Coefficient of variation= SD× 100/mean
- Standard error of mean= SD/Square root of 'n'

Characteristic of Data

- Nominal: Cannot be quantified, but divided into qualitative categories, e.g. male-female
- Ordinal: Data can be arranged in a meaningful order, but difference between the value is not constant, e.g. ranking n a class
- Discrete: Variables which can take place only certain values but not between them, e.g. number of children immunized in a village.
- Interval: Data can be arranged in meaningful order and the difference between them is meaningful
- Continuous: Variables can take any value, e.g. weight
- Median: Middle observation when the data is arranged in an ascending or descending order
- Mean: Average value of an observation
- Mode: Most commonly occurring value

Area under Normal Distribution Curve

- Mean + 1 SD: 68.3 percent
- Mean + 2 SD: 95.4 percent
- Mean + 3 SD: 99.7 percent

Skewing

- Positive skewing: Mean > median
- Negative skewing: Median > mode

Factory: An Establishment Employing

- 10 or more workers where power is used
- 20 or more where power is not used
- A minimum of 500 cubic feet of space has been prescribed for each worker
- Prohibits employment of children below 14 years
- Maximum of 48 working hours per week, not exceeding 9 hours per day, with rest for atleast ½hour after 5 hours of continuous work
- Total number of hours in a week (including overtime) shall not exceed 60 hours.

Organization and Location

- ILO, WHO, IRC: Geneva
- UNICEF, UN: New York
- FAO: Rome

UNICEF'S GOBI-FFF Program

- Growth monitoring
- Oral rehydration
- Breastfeeding
- Immunization
- Female education
- Family spacing
- Food supplements

Demographic Cycle

- First stage-high stationary: High birth rate and a high death rate which cancel each other and the population remain stationary
- Second stage-early expanding: Death rate begins to decline while birth rate remains remains unchanged
- Third stage-late expanding: Death rate decline still further and the birth rate tends to fall, population continues to grow as births exceed deaths
- Fourth stage-low stationary: This stage is characterized by low birth and low death rate the population becomes stationary

Population Growth

- Stationary population: No growth
- Slow growth: < 0.5
- Moderate growth: 0.5–1
- Rapid growth: 1–1.5
- Very rapid growth: 1.5–2
- Explosive growth: > 2

MCQs WITH SHORT EXPLANATIONS

GENERAL CONCEPTS

1. **Kuppuswamy scale for upper class:**
   a. 26–29 b. 16–25
   c. 16–26 d. 26–30

Kuppuswamy scale (Score & class)
- 26–29: Upper (I)
- 16–25: Upper middle (II)
- 11–15: Lower middle (III)
- 5–10: Upper lower (IV)
- <5: Lower (V)

2. **All of the following are components of epidemiological triad EXCEPT:**
   a. Environment b. Agent
   c. Host d. Pathogenesis

The germ theory of disease has many limitations. For example, it is well known, that not everyone exposed to tuberculosis may develop TB. The same exposure, however, in an undernourished or otherwise susceptible person may result in clinical diseases. There are other factors relating to the host and the environment which are usually important to determine whether or not disease will occur in the exposed host. This demanded a broader concept of disease causation that synthesized the basic factors of agent, host & environment.

3. **Which of the following is a true statement regarding Cohort studies?**
   a. Disease to risk factor study
   b. Effect to cause
   c. Not associated with attributable risk
   d. Associated with antecedent causation

Cohort study
- Proceeds from 'cause to effect'
- Starts with people exposed to risk factor or suspected cause
- Tests whether disease occurs more frequently in those exposed, than in those not similarly exposed.
- Yields incidence rate, relative risk as well as attributable risk

4. **Which of the following indicates secular trend?**
   a. Seasonal changes b. Periodical changes
   c. Long term changes d. Short term changes

The term 'secular trend' implies changes in the occurrence of disease (i.e., a progressive increase or decrease) over a long period of time, generally several years or decades. Examples include coronary heart disease, lung cancer and diabetes which have shown a consistent upward trend in the developed countries during the past 50 years or so, followed by a decline of such diseases as TB, typhoid, diphtheria and polio.

5. **Iceberg phenomenon with a value of 12 above surface, 20 at surface and 50 beneath surface is best represented by which of the following condition?**
   a. Hypertension b. Measles
   c. Rabies d. Tetanus

A concept closely related to the spectrum of the disease is the concept of the iceberg phenomenon of disease. According to this concept, disease in a community may be compared with an iceberg. The floating tip of the iceberg represents what the physician sees in the community, i.e., clinical cases. The vast submerged portion of the iceberg represents the hidden mass of disease, i.e., latent, inapparent, presymptomatic and undiagnosed cases and carriers in the community. The waterline represents the demarcation between apparent and inapparent diseases. In some disease (e.g., hypertension, diabetes, anaemia, malnutrition, mental illness) the unknown morbidity (i.e., the submerged portion of the iceberg) far exceeds the known morbidity.

6. **Formula for calculating Predictive value indicating positive test:**
   a. TP/ TP + FP b. TN/ TN + FN
   c. TP/ TP + FN d. TN/ FP + TN

Screening test result by diagnosis

Screening test results	Diseased	Not diseased	Total
Positive	A (TP)	B (FP)	A+B
Negative	C (FN)	D (TN)	C+D
Total	A+C	B+D	A+B+C+D

Predictive value of a positive test = A/ (A+B) × 100

7. **PQLI consists of:**
   a. IMR, life expectancy at 1 year of age and literacy rate
   b. MMR, IMR and life expectancy
   c. MMR, life expectancy and literacy
   d. IMR, life expectancy and literacy

The Physical Quality of Life Index (PQLI) is an attempt to measure the quality of life or well-being of a country. The value is the average of three statistics: basic literacy rate, infant mortality, and life expectancy at age one, all equally weighted on a 0 to 100 scale. PQLI does not depend upon per capita GNP, unlike standard of living, showing thereby that 'money is not everything'.

8. **A new drug does NOT prevent a disease from occurring, does NOT cure that disease fully, but reduce death due to that disease. Which of the following is true:**
   a. It will increase the incidence and prevalence
   b. It will decrease the incidence and prevalence

Ans. 1. **a.** 26–29 2. **d.** Pathogenesis 3. **d.** Associated... 4. **c.** Long term changes
5. **a.** Hypertension 6. **a.** TP/ TP + FP 7. **a.** IMR, life expec... 8. **c.** Prevalence is...

c. Prevalence is increased
d. Incidence is increased

Prevalence is a statistical concept referring to the number of cases of a disease that are present in a particular population at a given time (new cases plus old cases), whereas incidence refers to the number of new cases that develop in a given period of time. If a new drug prevents death without curing, it will increase the total number of cases (prevalence) as new cases are also adding to the total number of cases.

Increased by	Decreased by
❑ Longer duration of the disease	❑ Shorter duration of the disease
❑ Prolongation of life of the patients without care.	❑ Improved cure rate of the disease.
❑ Increase in number of new cases (i.e. increased incidence)	❑ Decrease in number of new cases (i.e. decreased incidence)
❑ Immigration of new cases	❑ Emigration of new cases.
❑ Emigration of healthy people.	❑ Immigration of healthy people.
❑ Immigration of susceptible people.	❑ Emigration of susceptible people.
❑ Better reporting of cases.	❑ Under reporting of cases.

9. Test which detects true negative is said to have:

a. Relative risk
b. Odd's ratio
c. Sensitivity
d. Specificity

The specificity of a clinical test refers to the ability of the test to correctly identify those patients without the disease.

$$\text{Specificity} = \frac{\text{True negatives}}{\text{True negatives + False positives}}$$

Therefore, a test with 100% specificity correctly identifies all patients without the disease. A test with 80% specificity correctly reports 80% of patients without the disease as test negative (true negatives) but 20% patients without the disease are incorrectly identified as test positive (false positives).

Diagnosis (Screening test result).			
	Diseased	*Not Diseased*	*Total*
Positive	(True positive)	(False positive)	(Total positives)
	a	b	a + b
Negative	(False negative)	(True negative)	(Total negatives)
	c	d	c + d
Total	(Total diseased)	(Total nondiseased)	(Grand total)
	a + c	b + d	a + b + c + d

10. Disease usually NOT seen in a country but brought from abroad is:

a. Endemic
b. Epidemic
c. Zoonotic
d. Exotic

An **Exotic** Disease is one which does not usually occur in or is foreign to a region or country. For example, yellow fever in India, rabies in UK and Australia.

11. Surveillance is:

a. Monitoring of activity of health workers
b. Continuous monitoring of occurrence and distribution of a disease
c. Monitoring of trends of a disease
d. Related to the virulence of the organism

Disease surveillance: The ongoing systematic collection and analysis of data and the provision of information which leads to action being taken to prevent and control a disease, usually one of an **infectious** nature.

12. A Patient is made to walk early after Surgery. This is for:

a. Treating the patient
b. Reducing disability
c. Specific protection
d. Rehabilitation

Rehabilitation is a treatment or treatments designed to facilitate the process of recovery from injury, **illness**, or **disease** to as normal a condition as possible. Rehabilitation is given for those who have undergone surgery such as amputation of leg, colostomy, mastectomy, etc. and are rehabilitated with a prosthesis and training, later placed in a suitable job.

❑ Physical rehabilitation	Restoration of function
❑ Vocational rehabilitation	Restoration of earning capacity
❑ Social rehabilitation	Restoration of relationship in the society
❑ Psychological rehabilitation	Restoration of personal dignity and confidence

13. Relative risk can be obtained from:

a. Case study
b. Cohort study
c. Case control study
d. Experimental study

Relative risk or **risk** ratio (RR) is the ratio of the probability of an event occurring (for example, developing a disease, being injured) in an exposed group to the probability of the event occurring in a comparison, nonexposed group.

In epidemiological research, the odds ratio is commonly used for case-control studies, as odds, but not probabilities, are usually estimated. Relative risk is used in randomized controlled trials and cohort studies

Ans. 9. **d.** Specificity 10. **d.** Exotic 11. **b.** Continuous... 12. **d.** Rehabilitation 13. **b.** Cohort study

Differences between relative risk and attributable risk.	
Relative risk (RR)	*Attributable risk (AR)*
It is the extent to which exposed persons are relatively at a greater risk of developing the disease than the unexposed persons.	It is the extent to which the suspected cause is attributed as the cause of the disease.
It is the ratio of the incidence of the disease among exposed persons (IE) and the incidence of the disease among unexposed persons (IO). $RR = \frac{IF}{IO}$	It is the ratio of risk difference (RD) and the incidence of the disease among the exposed (IE) RD = IE – IO $AR = \frac{RD}{IE} \times 100$
It is expressed in absolute numbers.	It is often expressed in percentage.
It measures the strength of the association between the suspected cause and the disease (e.g. Smoking and Lung cancer)	It suggests the extent to which the disease can be prevented, if suspected cause is removed.
Higher the RR, stronger is the association between the cause and the effect.	Higher the AR, greater the reduction in the incidence of the disease by elimination of the risk factor.
If RR is 20, that means smokers (exposed persons) are relatively twenty times at a greater risk of developing the disease (lung cancer) than non-smokers (unexposed).	If AR is 60%, that means, 60% of lung cancer (disease) can be prevented if smoking (cause) is eliminated.
RR does not give any information on the prevention of the disease.	AR does give the information about prevention of the disease.
Thus, RR is not of public health importance.	Thus, AR is of much public health importance.

14. A useful index to measure the lethality of an acute infectious disease is:

a. Attack rate b. Incidence rate
c. Case fatality rate d. All of the above

A **case fatality rate** (CFR) or **case fatality risk**, **case fatality ratio** or just **fatality rate**—is the proportion of deaths within a designated population of "cases" (people with a medical condition), over the course of the disease. A CFR is conventionally expressed as a percentage and represents a measure of risk. CFRs are most often used for diseases with discrete, limited time courses, such as outbreaks of acute infections.

Differences between CFR and CDR.	
Case fatality rate (CFR)	*Crude death rate (CDR)*
It is the percentage of the cases dying.	It is the number of deaths per 1000 mid year population, in a given area, during a given period.
Period during which cases are dying is not taken into consideration.	Period considered is usually one year.
Numerator is the number of deaths due to specific illness.	Numerator is the number of deaths due to all causes.
Denominator is the total number of the cases of specific illness.	Denominator is the total mid year population, including both sick and healthy persons.
$CFR = \frac{\text{No. of deaths due to specific disease}}{\text{Total no. of cases of that specific disease}} \times 100$	$CDR = \frac{\text{No. of deaths from all causes during of given year}}{\text{MYP of the area}} \times 1{,}000$
It depends upon factors like age, sex, treatment taken etc.	It does not depend upon such factors.
It reflects the killing power of the disease.	It reflects the health status of that area.
This can be compared with that of other diseases.	This cannot be compared with other diseases.

15. Checking for sputum AFB comes under:

a. Primary prevention b. Secondary prevention
c. Tertiary prevention d. Quaternary prevention

Secondary prevention is concerned with detecting a disease in its earliest stages, before symptoms appear, and intervening to slow or stop its progression: "catch it early." The assumption is that earlier intervention will be more effective, and that the disease can be slowed or reversed. It includes the use of screening tests or other suitable procedures to detect serious disease as early as possible so that its progress can be arrested and, if possible, the disease eradicated.

Ans. **14. c.** Case fatality rate **15. b.** Secondary prevention

A classification of Preventive strategies

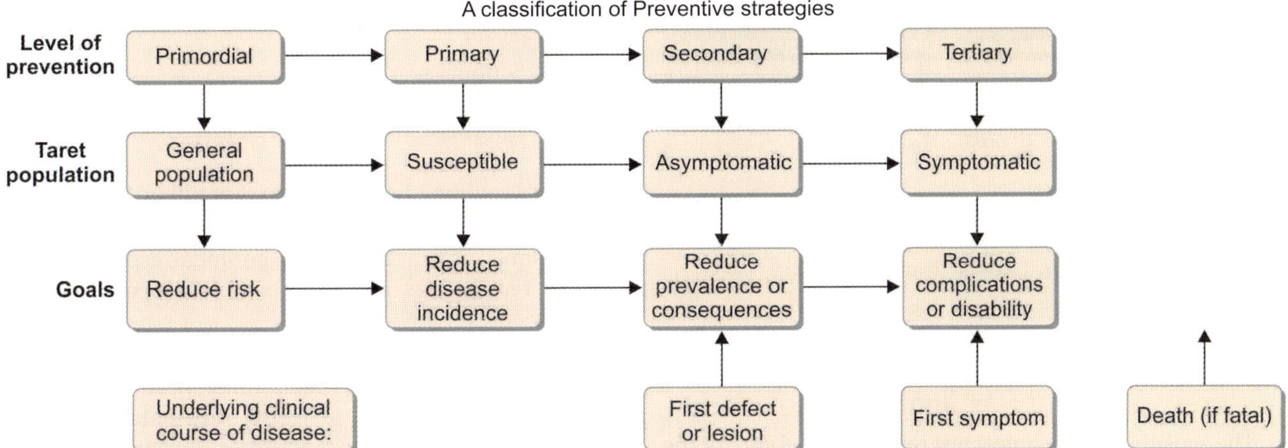

16. Prevalence is a:

a. Rate
b. Ratio
c. Proportion
d. Mode

Prevalence is the proportion of a population found to have a condition (typically a disease or a risk factor such as smoking or seat-belt use). It is arrived at by comparing the number of people found to have the condition with the total number of people studied, and is usually expressed as a fraction, as a percentage or as the number of cases per 10,000 or 100,000 people.

Differences between incidence and prevalence.

Incidence	*Prevalence*
Refers to occurrence of new cases only in a given area, during a given year.	Refers to existence of both old and new cases in a given area, during a given period/ point of time.
Incidence rate is expressed per 1,000 population at risk	Prevalence rate is expressed per 100 population at risk
Estimated from longitudinal studies.	Estimated from cross-sectional studies.
Estimation requires exact knowledge of time of onset of disease.	Such knowledge is not required.
Refers to acute cases having short incubation period.	Refers to chronic cases having long incubation period
Ex: Rabies, measles, Act GE, etc.	Ex: Tuberculosis, leprosy, etc.
Not influenced by duration of illness.	Influenced by not only duration of illness but also by incidence of illness. P = I × D
Related terms are attack rate and secondary attack rate.	Related terms are point prevalence and period prevalence
Incidence rate is an ideal measure to study the etiology of a disease	Prevalence is not an ideal measure to study the etiology of a disease
Incidence rate is more useful in formulation and testing the etiological hypothesis	Prevalence rate is useful to know the magnitude of the problem
Incidence rate helps to evaluate the control measures	Prevalence rate helps for health planning.

17. Essential purpose of randomization in randomized clinical trials:

a. To decrease the sample size
b. To eliminate selection bias
c. To decrease the follow up period
d. To produce double blinding

Selection bias is the selection of individuals, groups or data for analysis in such a way that proper randomization is not achieved, thereby ensuring that the sample obtained is not representative of the population intended to be analyzed. It is sometimes referred to as the **selection effect**. The phrase "selection bias" most often refers to the distortion of a statistical analysis, resulting from the method of collecting samples. If the selection bias is not taken into account, then some conclusions of the study may not be accurate. To eliminate selection bias, randomization is done.

18. Which of the following is secondary level of prevention:

a. Prophylactic drug administration
b. Admitting disabled child in special schools
c. Vaccination
d. Cervical pap smear checking

An example of secondary level of prevention is the Pap test to screen for cancer of the cervix, or a PSA blood test for prostate cancer; other instances include teaching people about the early signs of disease that they should watch for, and what type of treatment to seek.

Screening procedures	Diseases diagnosed early
❑ Periodical recording of weight of a child	Malnutrition
❑ Contact tracing	STDs
❑ Cluster testing	STDs
❑ Blood and urine exam	Diabetes mellitus
❑ Periodical examinations of industrial workers	Pneumoconiosis

Contd...

Ans. 16. **c.** Proportion 17. **b.** To eliminate... 18. **d.** Cervical pap...

Contd...

Screening procedures	Diseases diagnosed early
❑ Screening of blood donors	HIV/AIDS, hepatitis B, syphilis, malaria
❑ Recording of blood pressure	Hypertension
❑ Pap smear of cervix	Cancer cervix
❑ Reading Snellen's chart	Refractive errors
❑ Self-examination of breasts by woman	Ca-Breast

19. Sensitivity of a screening test indicates:

a. False positive b. False negative
c. True positive d. True positive

The sensitivity of a clinical test refers to the ability of the test to correctly identify those patients with the disease.

$$\text{Specificity} = \frac{\text{True positives}}{\text{True positives + False negatives}}$$

A test with 100% sensitivity correctly identifies all patients with the disease. A test with 80% sensitivity detects 80% of patients with the disease (true positives) but 20% with the disease go undetected (false negatives). A high sensitivity is clearly important where the test is used to identify a serious but treatable disease (e.g. cervical cancer). Screening the female population by cervical smear testing is a sensitive test. However, it is not very specific and a high proportion of women with a positive cervical smear who go on to have a colposcopy are ultimately found to have no underlying pathology.

20. Incubation period knowledge helps in all of the following EXCEPT:

a. Isolation
b. Quarantine
c. Detecting source of infection
d. Vaccination

Comparison chart

	Isolation	*Quarantine*
Used for	People who are ill with contagious diseases	People who have been exposed to a contagious disease, but are not sick
Process	Receive care for the disease, with precautions put into place (such as protective clothing for doctors) to prevent the spread of the disease.	Individuals are separated from others who have not been exposed to the disease, and can receive vaccinations, antibiotics, early diagnostic testing and symptom monitoring.
Length	Period of infectiousness for the disease.	Incubation period of the disease.
Location	Hospital, care facility or patient's home.	Home, designated emergency facility or a specialized hospital.

21. Associated with surveillance are all of the following EXCEPT:

a. Sentinel search
b. Randomization
c. Information regarding trends of health status of population
d. Providing timely warnings of public health disasters

Randomization is done to order or select in a random manner, as in a sample or experiment, especially in order to reduce bias and interference caused by irrelevant variables

22. The ratio of development of disease in those exposed minus unexposed to that of unexposed is expressed as:

a. Relative risk b. Attributable risk
c. Linear risk d. Contributable risk

Attributable risk is the difference in rate of a condition between an exposed population and an unexposed population. Attributable risk is mostly calculated in cohort studies, where individuals are assembled on exposure status and followed over a period of time. Investigators count the occurrence of the diseases. The cohort is then subdivided by the level of exposure and the frequency of disease is compared between subgroups. One is considered exposed and another unexposed. The formula commonly used in epidemiology books for Attributable risk is Ie = Iu = AR, where Ie = Incidence in exposed and Iu = incidence in unexposed. Once the AR is calculated, then the AR percent can be determined.

23. In a cohort study, nonsmokers are found having Ca lung, it indicates:

a. Smoking does not cause lung cancer
b. Multifactorial cause of Ca lung
c. Smoking is the only cause of lung Ca
d. All of the above

Advantages of cohort study

- The temporal dimension, whereby exposure is seen to occur before outcome, gives some indication of causality
- Can be used to study more than one outcome
- Good for the study of rare exposures
- Can measure the change in exposure and outcome over time
- Incidence of outcome can be measured

24. Incidence is best measured by:

a. Cross sectional study b. Cohort study
c. Case control study d. Double blind study

A cohort study is often undertaken to obtain evidence to try to refute the existence of a suspected association between cause and effect; failure to refute a hypothesis often strengthens confidence in it. Crucially, the cohort is identified before the appearance of the disease under investigation. The study groups follow a group of people who do not have the disease for a period of time and see who develops the disease (new incidence).

Ans. 19. **d.** True positive 20. **a.** Isolation 21. **b.** Randomization 22. **b.** Attributable risk
23. **b.** Multifactorial... 24. **b.** Cohort study

Differences between case control study and cohort study	
Case-control study	*Cohort study*
❑ It involves the study between the cases and controls	It involves the study between the study cohort (experimental cohort) and the control cohort
❑ The study starts with the disease	Study starts with the people exposed to risk factor
❑ Study proceeds backwards from effect to cause (Retrospective study)	Study proceeds forwards from cause to effect (Prospective study)
❑ Thus, exposure and disease have already occurred at the time of initiation of study	Exposure has already occurred but the effect (disease) has not occurred at the initiation of the study
❑ Study is done to find the frequency of exposure (exposure rate)	Study is done to find the frequency of disease (incidence rate).
❑ Study is easy and cheap	Study is difficult and expensive
❑ Yields results quickly	Yields delayed results
❑ Involves less number of people	Involves more number of people
❑ Techniques are crude	Techniques are refined
❑ Strength of the association is estimated by Odd's ratio.	Strength of the association is estimated by relative risk and attributable risk.
❑ Results are less reliable.	Results are more reliable
❑ Suitable for study of rare diseases	Not suitable
❑ Study cannot yield information about diseases other than that selected for study.	Study can yield information about other outcomes (diseases) also other than the disease under study

25. If a new effective treatment is initiated and all other factors remain the same; which of the following is most likely to happen:

a. Incidence will not change
b. Prevalence will not change
c. Both will not change
d. Both will change

The **incidence rate** is the number of new cases per population at risk in a given time period. Initiation of a new effect treatment is initiated, it will reduce the total number of cases (prevalence).

26. First thing to do in an epidemic:

a. Notification
b. Immunization
c. Isolation
d. Verification of diagnosis

Most outbreak investigations involve the following steps:

- Confirmation of the epidemic
- Confirmation of the diagnosis
- Collection of other relevant, ecological information: Such as fair or mela, season, atmospheric temperature and humidity, which often favor the onset of an epidemic.
- Studying the distribution of the epidemic with reference to time, place and person.
- Rapid search is made by the area health worker by door to door survey to detect many more such new cases.
- Anaylsis of data: Conducting descriptive epidemiology to determine the personal characteristics of the cases, changes in disease frequency over time, and differences in disease frequency based on location.
- Formulating/Developing hypotheses about the cause or source
- Testing/Evaluating the hypotheses and refining the hypotheses and conducting additional studies, if necessary
- Implementing control and prevention measures
- Communicating the findings/Submission of the report

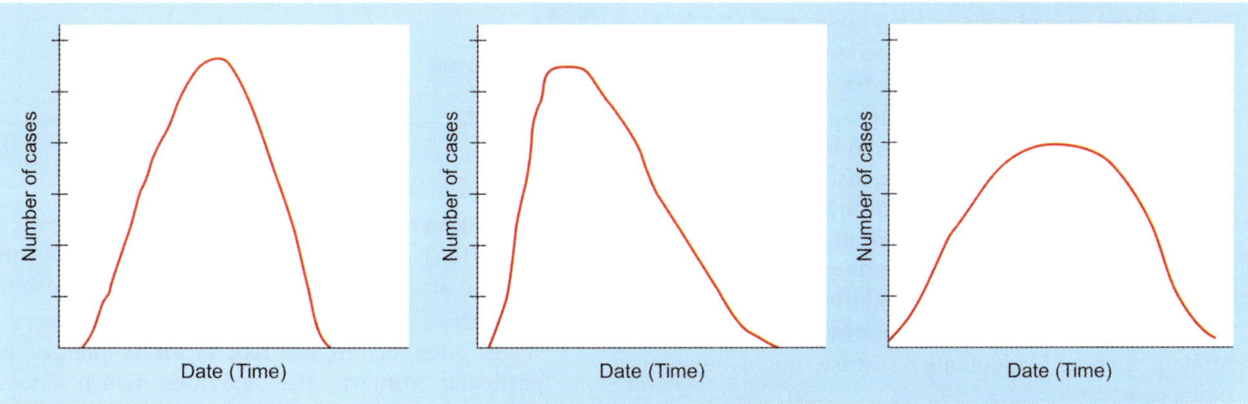

'Sudden rise and sudden fall' of the epidemic curve. This indicates 'common-source, single exposure' epidemic. For example, food poisoning.

'Sudden rise and sudden gradual fall' of the epidemic curve. This indicates 'common source, repeated exposure' epidemic. For example, cholera.

'Gradual rise and gradual fall' of the epidemic curve. This indicates 'propagated epidemic'. For example, viral hepatitis A.

Different types of epidemic curves.

Ans. **25. a.** Incidence will... **26. d.** Verification of...

27. True regarding cohort's study are all of the following EXCEPT:

a. Most reliable mean of showing an association between a suspected risk factor and subsequent disease
b. It can be retrospective or prospective
c. Odd's ratio can be calculated
d. Exposure rates can be calculated

The odds ratio is the measure of association for a case-control study. It tells us how much higher the odds of exposure is among cases of a disease compared with controls. The odds ratio compares the odds of exposure to the factor of interest among cases to the odds of exposure to the factor among controls (The odds is the probability that an event will happen divided by the probability that it won't happen.)

28. Prevention of developing risk factors in CAD comes under:

a. Primary prevention b. Secondary prevention
c. Primordial prevention d. Tertiary prevention

Primordial prevention consists of actions to minimize future hazards to health and hence inhibit the establishment factors (environmental, economic, social, behavioural, cultural) known to increase the risk of disease. It addresses broad health determinants rather than preventing personal exposure to risk factors, which is the goal of primary prevention. Thus, outlawing alcohol in certain countries would represent primordial prevention, whereas a campaign against drinking and would be an example of primary prevention.

Examples of primordial include improving sanitation (such that exposure to infectious agents does not occur), establishing healthy communities, promoting a healthy lifestyle in childhood (for example, through prenatal nutrition programs and supporting early childhood development programmes)

29. First noticed case of a disease is known as:

a. Primary case b. Secondary case
c. Tertiary case d. Index case

The term primary case can only apply to infectious diseases that spread from human to human, and refers to the person who first brings a disease into a group of people—a school class, community, or country. The index case, however, is the patient in an outbreak who is first noticed by the health authorities, and who makes them aware that an outbreak might be emerging. Even outbreaks of disease that is not spread from human to human, such as Legionnaire's disease, might have an index case.

For many outbreaks, the primary case will never be known—the worldwide HIV epidemic is one example. In an outbreak that goes unnoticed, no index case is present, but for all outbreaks that are discovered, there will always be one (or more).

30. Of all the different epidemiological study designs available to test the association between risk factor and disease, the best design is:

a. Case control study b. Ecological study
c. Cohort study d. Cross sectional study

The advantage of prospective cohort study data is that it can help determine risk factors for contracting a new disease because it is a longitudinal observation of the individual through time, and the collection of data at regular intervals, so recall error is reduced.

31. If the prevalence is very low as compared to the incidence for a disease, it implies:

a. Disease is very fatal and/or easily curable
b. Disease is non-fatal
c. Calculation of prevalence and incidence is wrong
d. Nothing can be said as they are independent

Prevalence is the total number of cases. Incidence is number of new cases. If a disease is fatal or easily curable, then the prevalence will be less.

32. Bhopal gas tragedy is an example of:

a. Point source epidemic b. Continuous epidemic
c. Propagated epidemic c. Slow epidemic

Point Source Outbreak: Persons are exposed to the same **source** over a brief time, such as through a single meal or at an event. The number of cases rises rapidly to a peak and falls gradually. Most cases occur within one incubation period.

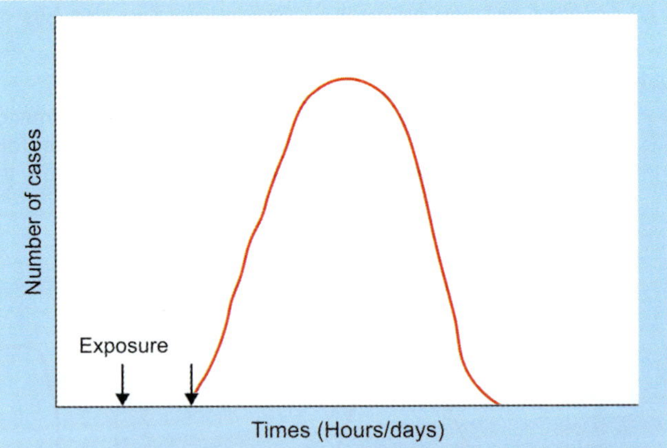

Epidemic curve (Point source).

33. Prevention of emergence of risk factor is known as:

a. Tertiary prevention b. Secondary prevention
c. Primary prevention d. Primordial prevention

Primordial prevention—seeks to prevent at a very early stage, often before the risk factor is present in the particular context, the activities which encourage the emergence of lifestyles, behaviours and exposure patterns that contribute to increased risk of disease. For example, a child seeing their parents smoke cigarettes may wrongly consider this a good lifestyle choice for later in life: advising parents to quit smoking in such circumstances can be considered primordial prevention.

Ans. 27. c. Odd's ratio can... 28. c. Primordial... 29. d. Index case 30. c. Cohort study
31. a. Disease is very... 32. a. Point source... 33. d. Primordial prevention

34. The analytical study where population is the unit of study:

a. Cross-sectional b. Case-control
c. Ecological d. Cohort

Ecological studies are studies of risk-modifying factors on health or other outcomes based on populations defined either geographically or temporally. Both risk-modifying factors and outcomes are averaged for the populations in each geographical or temporal unit and then compared using standard statistical methods.

Ecological studies have often found links between risk-modifying factors and health outcomes well in advance of other epidemiological or laboratory approaches.

35. NOT a proxy measure for incubation period:

a. Generation time b. Serial interval
c. Period of communicability
d. Latent period

The '**period of communicability**' refers to the time during which an infectious agent can be transmitted directly or indirectly from an infected person to another person, from an infected animal to humans, or from an infected person to animals.

Incubation period is the time elapsed between exposure to a pathogenic organism, a chemical or radiation, and when symptoms and signs are first apparent. In a typical infectious disease, incubation period signifies the period taken by the multiplying organism to reach a threshold necessary to produce symptoms in the host.

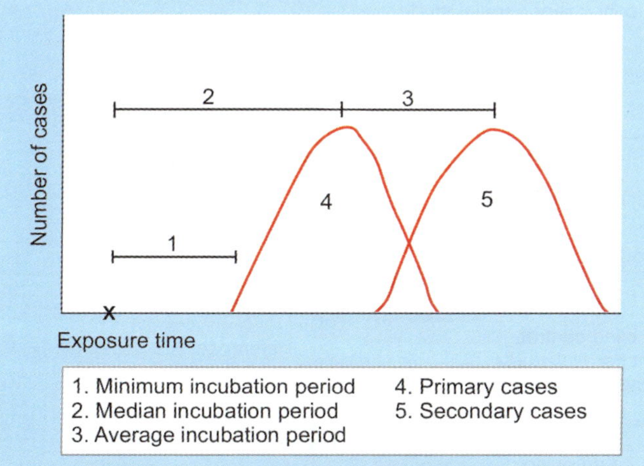

Showing incubation period.

Source: Rothman, Greenland and Lash. Modern epidemiology Lippincott Williams and Wilkins—a Wolters Kluwer Business. Third Edn. 2012.

36. Relative risk can be calculated by:

a. Incidence of disease amongst exposed/incidence of disease amongst non-exposed
b. Incidence of disease amongst non-exposed/incidence of disease amongst exposed
c. Incidence of disease amongst exposed/total population of that area
d. Incidence of disease amongst non-exposed/total population of that area

Relative risk can be calculated from a 2 × 2 table using the following formula: **Relative Risk = [A/(A+B)]/[C/(C+D)]**.

	Disease Yes	*Disease No*	*Total*
Exposure Yes	A	B	A + B
Exposure No	C	D	C + D
Total	A + C	B + D	A + B + C + D

37. Sentinel surveillance is used to detect:

a. New cases b. Missed cases
c. Old cases d. Reference cases

Instead of attempting to gather surveillance data from all health care workers, a sentinel surveillance system selects, either randomly or intentionally, a small group of health workers from whom to gather data. These health workers then receive greater attention from health authorities than would be possible with universal surveillance.

Sentinel surveillance also requires more time and resources, but can often produce more detailed data on cases of illness because the health care workers have agreed to participate and may receive incentives. It may be the best type of surveillance if more intensive investigation of each case is necessary to collect the necessary data.

38. Cohort study is associated with:

a. Prevalence b. Odd's ratio
c. Relative risk d. Exposure rates

Relative risk is calculated using cumulative incidence data to measure the probability of developing disease. Therefore, relative risk can only be calculated if the study was designed in such a way that incidence data can be calculated. For example, study designs such as cohort studies and clinical trials allow the researcher to calculate incidence, whereas case-control studies do not. Thus, relative risk can be calculated for cohort studies and clinical trials, but not for case-control studies. Odds ratios can be used to estimate relative risk for a case-control study.

Relative risk is:

(Cumulative incidence in the exposed)/(Cumulative incidence in the unexposed)

39. High false positives cases in a community signify that disease has:

a. High prevalence and low incidence
b. High incidence and low prevalence
c. Low prevalence and low incidence
d. High incidence and high prevalence

Ans. **34. c.** Ecological **35. c.** Period of commun... **36. a.** Incidence... **37. b.** Missed cases
38. c. Relative risk **39. c.** Low prevalence...

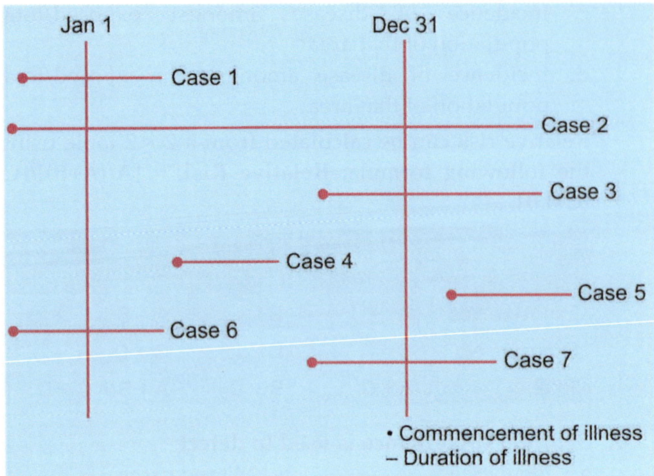

Incidence of the disease during the year = cases 3, 4 and 7.
Point prevalence on January 1 = cases 1, 2 and 6.
Point prevalence on December 31 = cases 2, 3 and 7.
Period prevalence during the year (Jan-Dec) = cases 1, 2, 3, 4, 6 and 7.
Terms incidence and prevalence.

When the incidence, the proportion of those who have a given condition, is lower than the test's false positive rate, even tests that have a very low chance of giving a false positive *in an individual case* will give more false than true positives *overall*.

So, in a society with very few infected people—fewer proportionately than the test gives false positives—there will actually be more who test positive for a disease incorrectly and don't have it than those who test positive accurately and do.

40. NOT an analytical study:

a. Field trials b. Ecological studies
c. Cohort study d. Case control study

A field trial involves evaluation of whether an agent or procedure reduces the risk of developing disease among those free from that condition at enrolment. Because these trials involve healthy rather than diseased people, they tend to be logistically more difficult to carry out than clinical trials. They generally have to be conducted in the 'field' rather than in hospitals or clinics. Moreover, whereas the adverse consequences of a given disease (e.g. disease recurrence, death) may occur with high probability during a relatively short time, typically the risk of contracting a disease among people who are initially free of it is small. This is particularly true for rare diseases such as cancer. Consequently, field trials usually require a greater number of subjects followed up for longer periods than clinical trials.

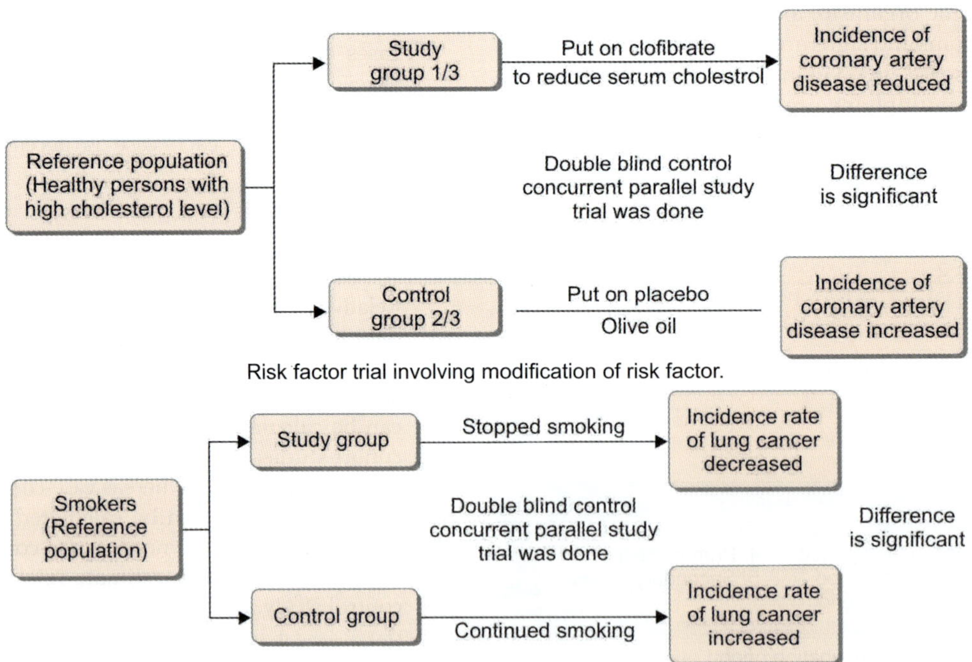

Risk factor trial involving modification of risk factor.

Risk factor trial showing elimination of risk factor (Cessation experiment).

41. True regarding case control study are all of the following EXCEPT:

a. Possibilty of bias
b. Odd's ratio can be derived
c. Relatively inexpensive
d. Attributable risk can be known

The ***Attributable Risk*** (derived from cohort studies) indicates the number of cases of a disease *among exposed individuals* that can be attributed to that exposure: Incidence(exposed)—Incidence (unexposed)
(This shows how much extra disease has been caused by this exposure)

Ans. **40. a.** Field trials **41. d.** Attributable risk can...

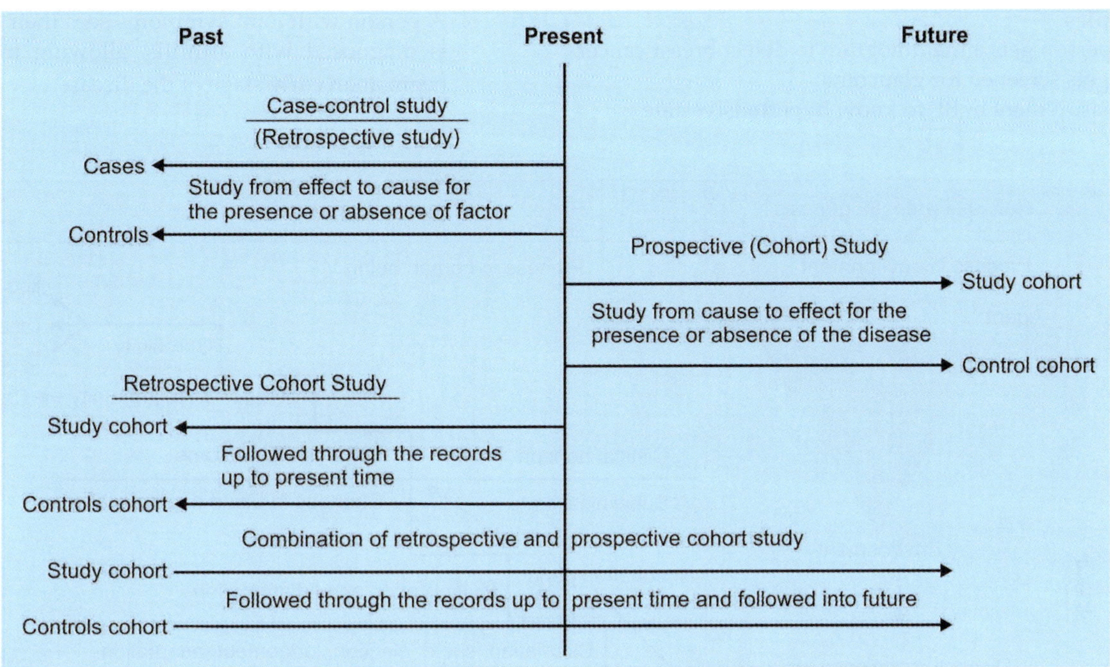

Schematic representation of case-control study and Cohort studies.

This can also be expressed *as a fraction* of all exposed: [Incidence (exposed)−Incidence (unexposed)] ÷ Incidence (exposed).

42. Correct statement regarding longitudinal studies is:

a. Short duration study
b. Inferior to cross-sectional studies
c. Observation is taken only once
d. Helps in identifying risk factors of a disease

A **longitudinal** study is an observational research method in which data is gathered for the same subjects repeatedly over a period of time. **Longitudinal** research projects can extend over years or even decades. In a **longitudinal** cohort study, the same individuals are observed over the study period. This design is used to uncover predictors of certain diseases.

The differences between longitudinal and cross-sectional studies.

Longitudinal studies	*Cross-sectional studies*
❑ Observations are repeated by means of follow-up examinations, in a population	❑ Observations are done only once in the population
❑ Carried over a long period of time (minimum one year)	❑ Carried over a given point of time or period of time
❑ This is compared to a running cine film	❑ This is compared to a still photograph
❑ This helps to find out the occurrence of new cases (Incidence rate).	❑ This helps to find out the existence of both old and new cases (Prevalence rate)
❑ This helps to study the natural history of the disease and the risk factors.	❑ This does not help to study the natural history of the disease and the risk factors
❑ This study is time consuming, difficult and costly.	❑ This is not time consuming, not difficult and cheap

43. True statement for confounding factors:

a. Associated with either the exposure or the disease
b. Confounding can be eliminated by selecting a small group
c. It is a risk factor for the disease
d. Found equally between study and the control groups

A **confounding variable** is a **variable** (say, pollution) that can cause the disease under study (cancer) and is also associated with the exposure of interest (smoking).

44. Primordial prevention in myocardial infarction are all EXCEPT:

a. Maintenance of normal body weight
b. Change in lifestyle
c. Change in nutritional habits
d. Screening for hypertension

Secondary prevention attempts to identify a disease at its earliest stage so that prompt and appropriate management can be initiated. Successful secondary prevention reduces the impact of the disease.

Ans. **42. d.** Helps in ident... **43. c.** It is a risk factor for... **44. d.** Screening...

Examples:

a. A person gets a mammogram to detect breast cancer or gets screened for glaucoma.
b. Measurement of BP to know hypertensivestate
c. A person with joint symptoms sees their doctor and is diagnosed with arthritis, allowing treatment to begin at an early stage of the disease.

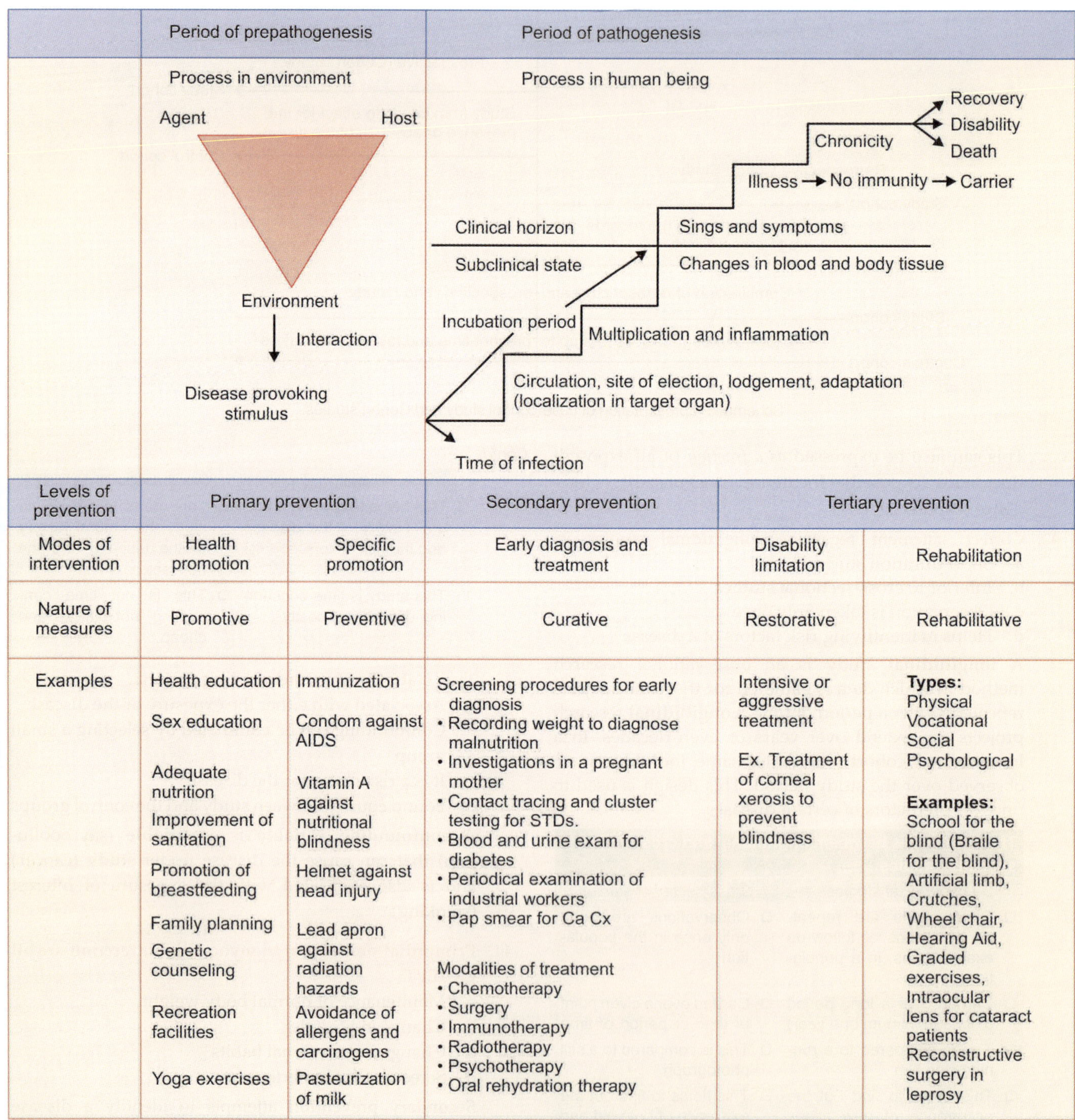

Levels of prevention	Primary prevention		Secondary prevention	Tertiary prevention	
Modes of intervention	Health promotion	Specific promotion	Early diagnosis and treatment	Disability limitation	Rehabilitation
Nature of measures	Promotive	Preventive	Curative	Restorative	Rehabilitative
Examples	Health education Sex education Adequate nutrition Improvement of sanitation Promotion of breastfeeding Family planning Genetic counseling Recreation facilities Yoga exercises	Immunization Condom against AIDS Vitamin A against nutritional blindness Helmet against head injury Lead apron against radiation hazards Avoidance of allergens and carcinogens Pasteurization of milk	Screening procedures for early diagnosis • Recording weight to diagnose malnutrition • Investigations in a pregnant mother • Contact tracing and cluster testing for STDs. • Blood and urine exam for diabetes • Periodical examination of industrial workers • Pap smear for Ca Cx Modalities of treatment • Chemotherapy • Surgery • Immunotherapy • Radiotherapy • Psychotherapy • Oral rehydration therapy	Intensive or aggressive treatment Ex. Treatment of corneal xerosis to prevent blindness	**Types:** Physical Vocational Social Psychological **Examples:** School for the blind (Braile for the blind), Artificial limb, Crutches, Wheel chair, Hearing Aid, Graded exercises, Intraocular lens for cataract patients Reconstructive surgery in leprosy

Natural history of a communicable disease and application of preventive measures.

45. Recall bias is associated with:
a. Cross sectional study
b. Case control study
c. Cohort study
d. Cohort-case control study

Recall bias is a systematic error caused by differences in the accuracy or completeness of the recollections retrieved ("recalled") by study participants regarding events or experiences from the past. Sometimes also referred to as **response bias**, **responder bias** or **reporting bias**, this type of measurement bias can be a methodological issue in research that involves interviews or questionnaires (potentially leading to differential misclassification of various types of exposure). Recall bias can be a particular concern in retrospective studies that use a case-control design to investigate the etiological causes of a disease or psychiatric condition. For example, in studies of risk factors for breast cancer, women who have had the disease may search their memories more thoroughly than unaffected controls to try to recall exposure to factors that have been mentioned in the press, such as use of oral contraceptives.

46. Case-control study is an example of:
a. Experimental analytical study
b. Longitudinal study
c. Analytical study
d. Descriptive epidemiological study

The essence of an **analytic** study is that groups of subjects are compared in order to estimate the magnitude of association between exposures and outcomes. The two main types of **analytic** study design are the cohort study and the case-control study, although there are several variations on these general designs.

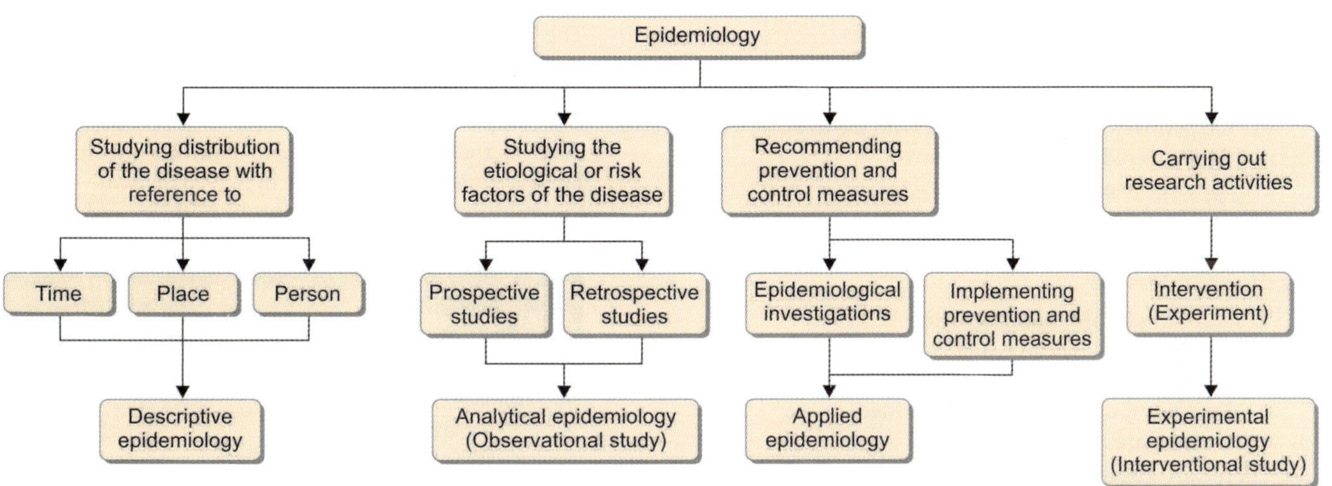

The various scopes of epidemiology.

47. Sullivan index:
a. Measures life expectancy
b. Measures life expectancy adjusted without disability
c. Measures life expectancy adjusted with disability
d. Measures disability

Sullivan's index: It is a measure of expectation of life free of disability. The index is obtained by subtracting from the expectation of life the days of disability

48. True about sentinel surveillance is:
a. Continuous oversight of activities
b. Supplements routine notification system
c. Beneficial for malaria surveillance
d. Keeps a check over health in border regions

A sentinel surveillance system is used when high-quality data are needed about a particular disease that cannot be obtained through a passive system. Selected reporting units, with a high probability of seeing cases of the disease in question, good laboratory facilities and experienced well-qualified staff, identify and notify on certain diseases. Whereas most passive surveillance systems receive data from as many health workers or health facilities as possible, a sentinel system deliberately involves only a limited network of carefully selected reporting sites. For example, a network of large hospitals might be used to collect high-quality data on various diseases and their causative organisms, such as invasive bacterial disease caused by Haemophilus influenzae type b, meningococcus or pneumococcus.

Data collected in a well-designed sentinel system can be used to signal trends, identify outbreaks and monitor the burden of disease in a community, providing a rapid, economical alternative to other surveillance methods. Because sentinel surveillance is conducted only in selected locations, however, it may not be as effective for detecting rare diseases or diseases that occur outside the catchment areas of the sentinel sites.

Ans. 45. **b.** Case control... 46. **c.** Analytical study 47. **b.** Measures life... 48. **b.** Supplements routine...

49. Primordial prevention for CAD is:
a. Screening
b. Regular checkups
c. Preserving traditional lifestyle
d. Treatment for raised BP

The purpose of primordial prevention is to reduce the incidence of disease by preventing the emergence of increased risk. Primordial prevention may relate to the whole population or only its selected groups. In its procedures include creating optimal living conditions. These include measures relating to proper diet, adequate physical activity, relaxation and the fight against smoking and other addictions to drugs. Efficiency is increasing application of these principles since childhood.

50. FALSE about case fatality rate:
a. Represents the killing power of disease
b. Denominator is mid-year population
c. Indicates virulence power of causative agent
d. Not much useful for chronic diseases

Assume 9 deaths among 100 people in a community all diagnosed with the same disease. This means that among the 100 people formally diagnosed with the disease, 9 died and 91 recovered. The CFR, therefore, would be 9%. CFR is proportion of death.

CFR = Number of deaths due to particular disease (Measles) × 100/Total number of cases of that particular disease (Measles)

51. True about simple randomization is:
a. Every person has an equal chance of selection
b. Also known as systemic randomization
c. Less number of samples is obtained
d. Groups are not distributed

There are two processes involved in randomizing patients to different interventions. First is choosing a *randomization procedure* to generate an unpredictable sequence of allocations; this may be a simple random assignment of patients to any of the groups at equal probabilities, may be "restricted," or may be "adaptive." A second and more practical issue is *allocation concealment*, which refers to the stringent precautions taken to ensure that the group assignment of patients are not revealed prior to definitively allocating them to their respective groups.

52. Which of the following is a false statement regarding longitudinal studies:
a. Studies natural history of disease
b. Helps in identifying risk factors
c. Less time consuming
d. Incidence rate can be calculated

A **longitudinal** study, like a cross-sectional one, is observational. So, once again, researchers do not interfere with their subjects. However, in a **longitudinal** study, researchers conduct several observations of the same subjects over a period of time, sometimes lasting many years

53. ICD (International Classification of Diseases) are revised once in how many years:
a. 5 years
b. 10 years
c. 15 years
d. 20 years

In 1898, the American Public Health Association (APHA) recommended that the registrars of Canada, Mexico, and the United States also adopt it. The APHA also recommended revising the system every ten years to ensure the system remained current with medical practice advances. As a result, the first international conference to revise the International Classification of Causes of Death took place in 1900, with revisions occurring every ten years thereafter.

54. Which of the following is NOT a part of Kuppuswamy's socioeconomic status scale:
a. Education
b. Occupation
c. Income
d. Housing

The most widely used scale for urban populations is Kuppuswamy's socioeconomic scale, which was devised by Kuppuswamy in 1976. Kuppuswamy scale is a composite score of education and occupation of the head of the family along with monthly income of the family, which yields a score of 3-29. This scale classifies the study populations into high, middle, and low SES (socioeconomic status)

Socioeconomic status scale of Kuppuswamy (Urban, 1976) Updated for June 2012.		
	Score card	
A.	Education 1. Professional or honors 2. Graduate or postgraduate 3. Intermediate, post-high school diploma 4. High school certificate 5. Middle school certificate 6. Primary school or literate 7. Illiterate	Score 7 6 5 4 3 2 1
B.	Occupation 1. Profession 2. Semi-profession 3. Clerical, shop-owner, farmer 4. Skilled worker 5. Semiskilled worker 6. Unskilled worker 7. Unemployed	Score 10 6 5 4 3 2 1
C.	Family Income per month (in Rs)* (updated for June 2012) 1. >30,375 2. 15188–30374 3. 11362–15187 4. 7594–11361 5. 4556–7593 6. 1521–4555 7. <1520	Source 12 10 6 4 3 2 1

Contd...

Ans. 49. c. Preserving... 50. b. Denominator... 51. a. Every person has... 52. c. Less time consuming 53. b. 10 years 54. d. Housing

Contd...

Score card		
Total score		Socioeconomic class
26 to 29		Upper (I)
16 to 25	Middle	Upper middle (II)
11 to 15		Lower middle (III)
5 to 10	Lower	Upper lower (IV)
< 5		Lower (V)

Source: Indian Journal of Pediatrics. 2003;70:3 This is to be updated for the current year.

55. Human Development Index is measured by all EXCEPT:

a. Under-5 mortality b. Literacy
c. Life expectancy at birth d. Per capita income

The **Human Development Index** (**HDI**) is a composite statistic of life expectancy, education, and income per capita indicators, which are used to rank countries into four tiers of human development. A country scores higher HDI when the life expectancy at birth is longer, the education period is longer, and the income per capita is higher. The HDI was developed by Pakistani economist Mahbub ul Haq, often framed in terms of whether people are able to "be" and "do" desirable things in their life, and was published by the United Nations Development Programme.

HDI	Grade (of human development category)
> 0.8	High
0.79 to 0.50	Medium
< 0.5	Low

56. All are true about Cohort studies EXCEPT:

a. Prospective b. Useful for rare diseases
c. Necessary for incidence d. Costly

The case-control study design is often used in the study of rare diseases or as a preliminary study where little is known about the association between the risk factor and disease of interest.

Cohort group	*Development of disease*		*Total*
	Yes	*No*	
Study cohort (exposed to suspected factor)	a	b	a + b
Control cohort (Not exposed to suspected factor)	c	d	c + d

57. Changes in the occurrence of disease over a long period of time is known as:

a. Seasonal trend b. Cyclic trend
c. Secular trend d. Geographical trend

Secular trend: Changes over a long period of time, generally years or decades.

58. Prevention of the emergence or development of risk factors in community is known as:

a. Primordial prevention
b. Primary prevention
c. Secondary prevention
d. Tertiary prevention

Primordial prevention is defined as **prevention** of risk factors themselves, beginning with change in social and environmental conditions in which these factors are observed to develop, and continuing for high risk children, adolescents and young adults.

59. Serial interval measures:

a. Incubation period of the disease
b. Sensitivity
c. Specificity
d. Positive predictive value

The **serial interval**, in the epidemiology of communicable (infectious) diseases, refers to the time between successive cases in a chain of transmission. Related but distinct quantities include: the 'average transmission interval' sum of average latent and infectious period; the 'incubation period' between infection and disease onset; the 'latent period' between infection and infectiousness.

Differences between intrinsic and extrinsic incubation period

Intrinsic incubation period	*Extrinsic incubation period*
It is with reference to human being.	It is with reference to arthropod (vector).
It is the period between the entrance of the pathogen in a person and the appearance of the first sign or symptom.	It is the period between the entrance of the pathogen/parasite inside the body of vector, till the agent reaches an optimum number or full development.
During this period the pathogen reaches the target organ, gets adapted, multiplies, causes damage of the target organ.	During this period, the parasite undergoes biological transmission inside the vector (i.e. multiplication or development or both).
This period varies from few hours/days to few months/years.	This period varies from 10 to 14 days.
This is influenced by virulence, infective dose and individual susceptibility.	This is influenced by atmospheric temperature and humidity.
Usually, the person is not infective during this period, except in diseases like measles, mumps, chickenpox, diphtheria, pertussis.	Usually, the vector is never infective during this period and it becomes infective only after this period.
The infected person never remains infective throughout the life.	The infective vector remains infective throughout its life.
Uses: Intrinsic incubation period is used for making diagnosis, finding out the source of infection, for immunization purposes and also for assessing the prognosis.	Extrinsic incubation period is utilized for control of vectors.

Ans. **55. a.** Under-5 mortality **56. b.** Useful for rare diseases **57. c.** Secular trend **58. a.** Primordial prevention **59. a.** Incubation period of the disease

60. Bhopal gas tragedy is an example of:
a. Point source epidemic
b. Continuous epidemic
c. Propagated epidemic
d. Slow epidemic

Bhopal gas tragedy and minamata disease in Japan are example of Common source or **point source epidemic.**

61. What is Berksonian bias:
a. Misclassification of disease
b. Recall bias
c. Selection bias
d. Non-response bias

Berksonian bias: Selection bias that arises from evaluating data on biased patients and hospital records only.

62. The major purpose of Randomization in clinical trials is to:
a. Facilitate double blinding
b. Help ensure that the study subjects are NOT representative EOF general population
c. Ensure that the groups are comparable on baseline characteristics
d. Reduce selection bias in allocation of treatment

Randomization as a method of experimental control has been extensively used in human clinical trials and other biological experiments. It prevents the selection bias and insures against the accidental bias. It produces the comparable groups and eliminates the source of bias in treatment assignments. Finally, it permits the use of probability theory to express the likelihood of chance as a source for the difference of end outcome.

63. Most important component of level of living is:
a. Health
b. Education
c. Occupation
d. Housing

Subjective component of well-being relates to quality of life, which is determined by a combination of factors such as health, happiness, education, social and intellectual attainments, freedom of action, justice and expression.

64. The installation and usage of sanitary latrines by general public constitutes which level of prevention:
a. Health promotion
b. Specific protection
c. Early diagnosis and treatment
d. Disability limitation and rehabilitation

The primary means of health promotion occur through developing healthy public policy that addresses the prerequisites of health such as income, housing, food security, employment, and quality working conditions.

65. True for epidemiological triad:
a. Time, place, person
b. Agent, host, environment
c. Disease, prevention, treatment
d. Agent, man, disease

A traditional model of infectious disease causation is known as the Epidemiologic Triad. The triad consists of an external **agent**, a **host** and an **environment** in which host and agent are brought together, causing the disease to occur in the host.

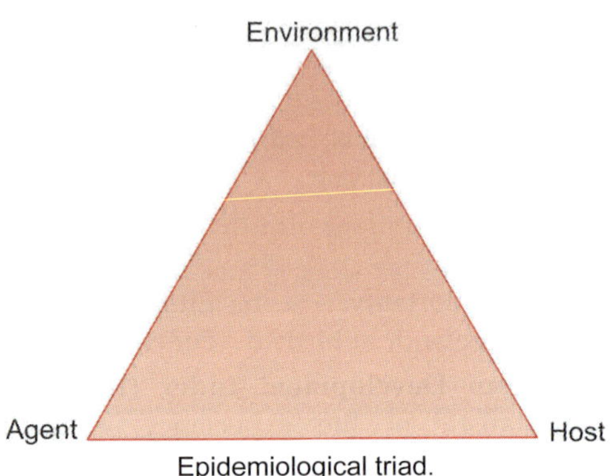

Epidemiological triad.

66. Pap smear is an example of ...... of prevention:
a. Primary level
b. Secondary level
c. Tertiary level
d. Primordial level

Secondary prevention—the application of available measures to detect early departures from health and to introduce appropriate treatment and interventions. Screening is a major component of secondary prevention for example, cervical screening for women to detect early changes which may go on to lead to cancer of the cervix.

67. What is the actual intention of doing sentinel surveillance:
a. To know the total number of cases
b. For health planning
c. To know the natural history of the disease
d. To prevent the disease

Sentinel surveillance is surveillance system in which a designated group of reporting sources—hospitals, agencies—agrees to report all cases of one or more notifiable conditions

68. PQLI is measured by all EXCEPT:
a. Infant mortality
b. Life expectancy at age 1
c. Latency
d. Per capita income

The **Physical Quality of Life Index** (PQLI) is an attempt to measure the quality of life or well-being of a country. The value is the average of three statistics: basic literacy rate, infant mortality, and life expectancy at age one, all equally weighted on a 0 to 100 scale.

69. Which of the following is an example of disability limitation:
a. Reducing occurrence of polio by immunization
b. Arranging for schooling of child suffering from post polio residual paralysis
c. Resting affected limbs in neutral position
d. Providing calipers for walking

Ans. **60. a.** Point source... **61. c.** Selection bias **62. d.** Reduce selection... **63. a.** Health
64. a. Health promotion **65. b.** Agent, host... **66. b.** Secondary level **67. a.** To know the...
68. d. Per capita income **69. c.** Resting affected limbs in neutral position

Disability limitation: Intervention if the patient presents in late pathogenic phase, to prevent the disease go into handicap stage. Such as, resting the limbs in neutral position, while applying casts.

	Disease	*Impairment*	*Disability*	*Handicap*
1.	Accident	Loss of foot	Inability to walk	Loss of job
2.	Vitamin 'A' deficiency	Corneal xerosis	Blurring of vision	Blindness and loss of job
3.	Leprosy	Involvement of nerves	Inability to work because of claw hand	Unemployment

70. True for randomized control trials:

a. Evaluation of health services
b. Before and after comparison studies
c. Preventiv e trials
d. Clinical trials

Most clinical trials today invoke a procedure in which individual patients, upon entering the study, are randomized to treatment.

Randomization is effective in reducing bias because it guarantees that treatment assignment will not be based on patient's prognostic factors. Thus, investigators cannot favor one treatment group over another by assigning patients with better prognoses to it, either knowingly or unknowingly. Procedure selection bias has been documented to have a very strong effect on outcome variables.

VACCINES

71. Live attenuated vaccines should NOT be administered to:

a. Children up to 8 years of age
b. HIV patients
c. Patients on steroids
d. Patients on radiation

Live vaccines should not be administered to persons with immune deficiency diseases or to persons whose immune response may be suppressed because of leukemia, lymphoma or malignancy because of therapy with corticosteroids, alkylating agents, antimetabolic agents, or radiation. Pregnancy is another contraindication unless the risk of infection exceeds the risk of harm to the foetus of some live vaccines.

72. Yellow fever vaccine provides immunity after:

a. 5 days of vaccination b. 10 days of vaccination
c. 15 days of vaccination d. 20 days of vaccination

Vaccination is recommended for those traveling to affected areas of Yellow fever, because non-native people tend to suffer more severe illness when infected. Protection begins by the 10th day after vaccine administration in 95% of people, and lasts for at least 10 years.

73. Measle vaccine is NOT administered before:

a. 9 months b. 12 months
c. 15 months d. 18 months

Immunization for measles is not recommended for children before 9 months of age because the vaccine will be rendered ineffective by the maternal antibodies, which will protect the child upto 9 months.

74. Injectable tetanus toxoid is an example of:

a. Reactive immunity b. Active immunity
c. Passive immunity d. Herd immunity

Indication of tetanus toxoid As Tetanus can occur in cases of even minor injuries it is advisable to actively immunize every person in general.

The differences between active and passive immunization.

Active immunization	*Passive immunization*
This consists of administration of antigens. For example BCG, DPT, MV, OPV, etc.	This consists of administration of antibodies. For example ADS, ATS, etc.
Immunity is produced after sometime (10-15 days)	Immunity is produced instantaneously
Reticuloendothelial cells are educated. So it is an active process	Reticuloendothelial cells are not educated. So passive process
Immunity lasts longer	Immunity lasts shorter
Usually not associated with reactions	Often associated with reactions
Usually it is given before exposure to the disease	Usually it is given after exposure to the disease
This procedure is never used for treatment purposes	This is often used as a part of treatment, as in tetanus, diphtheria
This is more useful	This is less useful

With this aim in view, it is desirable: To actively immunize all children from the age of 6 weeks onwards.

- To protect infants against the risks of tetanus neonatorum by immunizing pregnant mothers.
- To actively immunize civil population particularly those who are exposed to occupational risks such as road workers, athletes agricultural workers, industrial workers, etc.
- To actively immunize civil and defense personnel, home guards and police personnel.

75. Toxoid is prepared from:

a. Exotoxin b. Endotoxin
c. Both of the above d. None

A **toxoid** is a bacterial toxin (usually an exotoxin) whose toxicity has been inactivated or suppressed either by chemical (formalin) or heat treatment, while other properties, typically immunogenicity, are maintained. Thus,

Ans. 70. **d.** Clinical trials 71. **b.** HIV patients 72. **b.** 10 days of... 73. **a.** 9 months
74. **b.** Active immunity 75. **a.** Exotoxin

when used during vaccination, an immune response is mounted and immunological memory is formed against the molecular markers of the toxoid without resulting in toxin-induced illness.

76. Zero dose of polio vaccine is given:

a. Before giving DPT
b. At birth
c. When child is having polio
d. When child is having diarrhoea

In polio-endemic countries and in countries at high risk for importation and subsequent spread, WHO also recommends an OPV dose at birth (also called 'zero dose'), followed by the primary series of 3 OPV doses and at least 1 IPV dose.

Current national immunization schedule for infants, children and pregnant women (NRHM).

Vaccine	*When to give*	*Dose*	*Rate*	*Site*
For pregnant women:				
TT-1	Early in pregnancy	0.5 mL	IM	Upper arm
TT-2	4 weeks after TT-1*	0.5 mL	IM	Upper arm
TT-Booster	1 dose if TT is given in last 3 years*	0.5 mL	IM	Upper arm
For infants:				
BCG	At birth or as early as possible till one year of age	0.1 mL (0.05 mL until one month of age)	ID	Left upper arm
Hepatitis B-O	At birth or as early as possible within 24 hours	0.5 mL	IM	Anterolateral side of mid thigh
OPV-O	At birth or as early as possible within first 15 days	2 drops	Oral	Oral
OPV-1, 2 and 3	At 6 weeks, 10 weeks and 14 weeks	2 drops	Oral	Oral
DPT-1, 2 and 3	At 6 weeks, 10 weeks and 14 weeks	0.5 mL	IM	Anterolateral side of mid thigh
Hepatitis B-1, 2 and 3	At 6 weeks, 10 weeks and 14 weeks	0.5 mL	IM	Anterolateral side of mid thigh
Measles – 1	9 completed months – 12 months	0.5 mL	Subcutaneous	Right upper arm
Vitamin – A (1st dose)	At 9 months with measles vaccine	1.0 mL	Oral	Oral
For Children:				
DPT Booster-1	16-24 months	0.5 mL	IM	Anterolateral side of mid thigh
OPV Booster	16-24 months	2 drops	Oral	Oral
Measles – 2	16-24 months	0.5 mL	Subcutaneous	Right upper arm
Japanese encephalitis**	16-24 months with DPT/OPV booster	0.5 mL	Subcutaneous	Left upper arm
Vitamin A, 2nd dose	With DPT/OPV booster	2.0 mL	Oral	Oral
Vitamin A, 3rd to 9th dose	One dose every 6 months up to the age of 5 years	2.0 mL	Oral	Oral
DPT Booster-2	5-6 years	0.5 mL	IM	Upper arm
TT Booster	10 years and 16 years	0.5 mL	IM	Upper arm

* Give TT-2 or booster dose preferably before 36 weeks of pregnancy.

** JE vaccine in selected endemic districts.

Note: In select states, pentavalent vaccine (DPT + Hib + Hep B) 1, 2 and 3 dose replaces DPT 1, 2 and 3 dose and Hepatitis B1, 2 and 3 doses. During the first phase, (2011) Kerala and Tamil Nadu states were selected. During 2012-13, in the second phase, Delhi, Jammu and Kashmir, Haryana, Gujarat, Goa, Puducherry and Karnataka have been selected. It is proposed to cover the entire country in the next phase. Thus pentavalent vaccine has been introduced by Govt. of India in a phased manner.

Source: Vipin M Vashistha. Key statements of IAPCOI and IAP immunization time table for the year 2012. Pediatric infectious disease. 2012;4(3):112-24.

Ans. **76. b.** At birth

77. A live vaccine:

a. Tetanus toxoid b. DPT
c. Salk d. BCG

Examples of "live" (example attenuated) vaccines include:

- Viral: measles vaccine, mumps vaccine, rubella vaccine, Live attenuated influenza vaccine (the seasonal flu nasal spray and the 2009 H1N1 flu nasal spray), chicken pox vaccine, oral polio vaccine (Sabin), rotavirus vaccine, and yellow fever vaccine. Rabies vaccines are now available in two different attenuated forms, one for use in humans, and one for animal usage.
- Bacterial: BCG vaccine, typhoid vaccine and epidemic typhus vaccine.

78. Which vaccine is contraindicated in pregnancy:

a. Cholera vaccine
b. Typhoid vaccine
c. Meningococcal vaccine
d. Polio vaccine

Meningococcal vaccines are prepared from purified groups of A, C, Y and W135 organisms. Immunization is recommended for high risk group and not for mass prophylaxis. It is contraindicated for pregnant mothers.

79. NOT a live attenuated vaccine:

a. Influenza b. Measles
c. Yellow fever d. Oral polio

Some vaccines contain inactivated, but previously virulent, micro-organisms that have been destroyed with chemicals, heat, radiation, or antibiotics. Examples are influenza, cholera, bubonic plague, polio, hepatitis A, and rabies.

80. True for 'Ring vaccination':

a. Given around a mile of a case detected
b. Given around 100 yards of a case detected
c. Given to produce a ring shaped lesion
d. Given by a ring shaped machine

The idea is to form a buffer of immune individuals to prevent the spread of the disease. **Ring vaccination** was used to control smallpox until the last naturally occurring case in 1977. When an infection was diagnosed, all people who were or may have been exposed were identified and **vaccinated**.

81. Immunoglobulin is used for all of the following diseases EXCEPT:

a. Measles b. Rabies
c. Typhoid d. Chickenpox

Two typhoid vaccines are licensed for use for the prevention of typhoid: the live, oral Ty21a vaccine and the injectable typhoid polysaccharide vaccine. Both are recommended for travellers to areas where typhoid is endemic.

82. Secondary immune response is mediated by:

a. IgG
b. IgM
c. IgE
d. IgA

Primary immune response is mediated by IgM and secondary immune response by IgG.

83. When an antigen is administered for the first time to animal or human being who has never been exposed to it, the first antibody to develop:

a. IgG
b. IgM
c. IgE
d. IgA

Immunoglobulin M, or **IgM** for short, is a basic antibody that is produced by B cells. IgM is by far the physically largest antibody in the human circulatory system. It is the first antibody to appear in response to initial exposure to an antigen. The spleen, where plasmablasts responsible for antibody production reside, is the major site of specific IgM production.

84. All are live vaccines EXCEPT:

a. Measles
b. BCG
c. OPV
d. Hepatitis B

Hepatitis B vaccine is a recombinant vaccine. These are genetically engineered recombinant DNA vaccines, the sub-unit of the virus (antigen) is inserted into the genome of another avirulent virus and vaccine is prepared.

85. Use of which of the following vaccine is contra-indicated in pregnancy:

a. Yellow fever
b. Rabies
c. Cholera
d. Hepatitis-B

Pregnancy is a precaution for yellow fever vaccine administration. The safety of yellow fever vaccination during pregnancy has not been studied in a large prospective trial. However, a recent study of women who were vaccinated with yellow fever vaccine early in their pregnancies found no major malformations in their infants. A slight increased risk was noted for minor, mostly skin, malformations in infants. A higher rate of spontaneous abortions in pregnant women receiving the vaccine was reported but not substantiated.

86. Vaccine which should NOT be kept in freezer:

a. DPT
b. Measles
c. OPV
d. All of the above

DPT vaccine is stored at 2 to 8 degree C (35 to 46 degree F). Do not freeze.

Ans. **77. d.** BCG **78. c.** Meningococcal... **79. a.** Influenza **80. b.** Given around...
81. c. Typhoid **82. a.** IgG **83. b.** IgM **84. d.** Hepatitis B
85. a. Yellow fever **86. a.** DPT

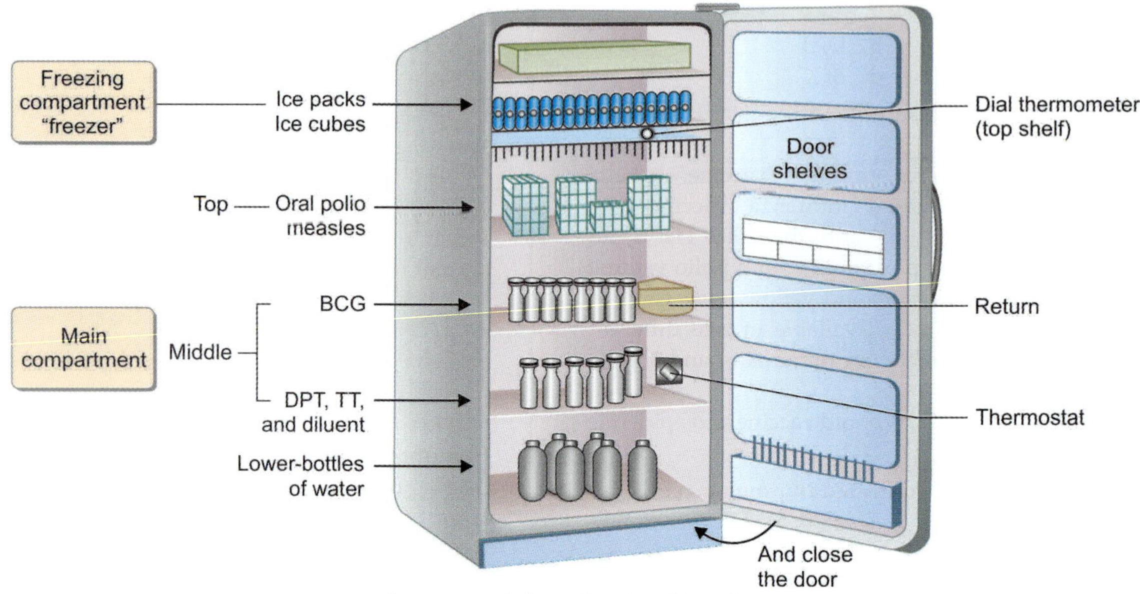

Arrangement of vaccines in refrigerator.
Source: NRHM Bulletin. 2012;7(4).

87. Oral cholera vaccine is effective for:

a. 6 months b. 12 months
c. 2 years d. 3 years

Vaccine with killed whole cell vibrio cholera 01 in combination with a recombinant B-subunit of cholera toxin (WC/rBS) is given orally in 2 doses with 10 to 15 days apart. It confers 50-60% protection. Immunity lasts for 3 years.

88. All are true of OPV EXCEPT:

a. It is a killed vaccine
b. Stored at subzero temperature
c. Induces intestinal and humoral immunity both
d. Residual neurovirulence is a problem

OPV

- Poliovirus vaccine—Live oral trivalent
- Storage requirements:
  - Maintain continuously in the frozen state: –14°C (7°F) or lower.
  - The vaccine may be refrozen.
  - A maximum of 10 freeze-thaw cycles are permissible provided the total cumulative duration of thaw does not exceed 24 hours, and provided the temperature does not exceed 8°C (46°F) during the period of thaw.
- Shelf Life: Up to 1 year
- Instructions for Reconstitution or Use
  - Thaw before using—may be rubbed between hands for rapid thawing.
  - Vaccine in liquid state in unopened dispettes may be used for up to 30 days provided it has been stored at 2–8°C (35–46°F). A maximum of 10 freeze- thaw cycles are permissible provided the total cumulative duration of thaw does not exceed 24 hours and provided the temperature does not exceed 8°C (46°F) during the period of thaw.
- Color Change
  - This vaccine contains phenol red as a pH indicator. The usual color of the vaccine is pink, although some containers of vaccine shipped or stored in dry ice may exhibit a yellow coloration due to the very low temperature or possible absorption of carbon dioxide. The color of the vaccine prior to use (red-pink-yellow) has no effect on the virus or efficacy of the vaccine.

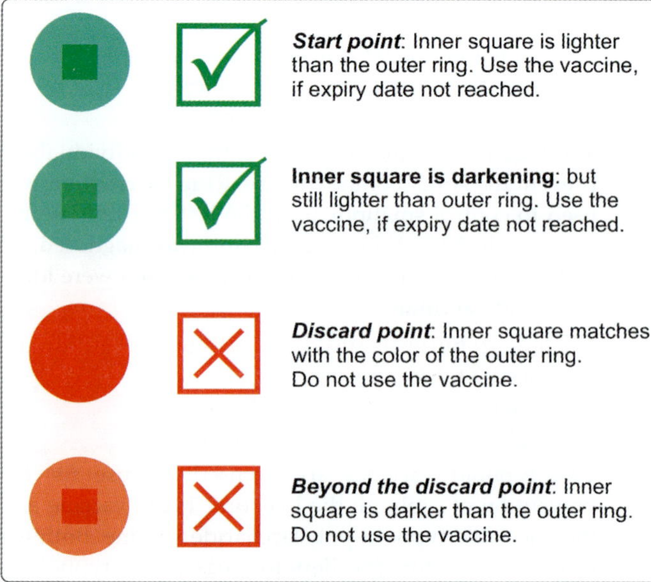

The stages of the VVM.

Ans. 87. **d.** 3 years 88. **a.** It is a killed vaccine

89. Adjuvant used in DPT vaccine:

a. Magnesium b. Copper
c. Aluminium d. Zinc

Aluminum is used in vaccines as an adjuvant. An adjuvant is vaccine component that boosts the immune response to the vaccine. Adjuvants allow for lesser quantities of the vaccine and fewer doses. The adjuvant effects of aluminum were discovered in 1926. Aluminum adjuvants are used in vaccines such as **hepatitis A**, **hepatitis B**, **diphtheria-tetanus-containing vaccines**, hemophilus influenza type **b**, and **pneumococcal vaccines**, but they are not used in the live, viral vaccines, such as **measles, mump, rubella**, **varicella** and **rotavirus**.

90. Hepatitis B vaccine should be given as per which schedule:

a. 0, 1, 6 days
b. 0, 1, 6 weeks
c. 0, 1, 6 months
d. 0, 1, 6 years

The vaccination schedule most often used for HBV in adults and children has been three intramuscular injections, the second and third administered 1 and 6 months after the first.

91. BCG should be given:

a. Immediately after birth
b. At the age of 1 month
c. At the age of 6 months
d. At the age of 1 year

The Advisory Committee on Immunization Practices (ACIP) recommends that all children receive their first dose of Hepatitis B vaccine at birth and complete the vaccine series by age 6–18 months.

IAP immunization time table 2012.

1. IAP recommended vaccine for routine use		
Age (Completed weeks/months/years)	*Vaccines*	*Comments*
Birth	BCG OPV Hep. B-1	Hepatitis B: Administer Hep.B vaccine to all newborns before hospital discharge.
6 weeks	DTP-1* Hib-1* Hep. B-2*	* These three are together available as Pentavalent vaccine (Easy five) *Polio:* ❑ All doses of IPV may be replaced with OPV, if IPV is unavailable/unaffordable.
	IPV-1 Rotavirus-1 Pneumococcal conjugate vaccine (PCV)-1	❑ Additional doses of OPV on all supplementary immunization activities. ❑ Minimum age to start IPV is 6 weeks. ❑ If IPV is started at 8 weeks, only two doses with 8 weeks interval. ❑ IPV catch-up schedule : 2 doses at 2 months apart followed by a booster dose after 6 months. *Rotavirus:* Two doses of RV-1 (Rotarix) or three doses of RV-5 (Rotateq). (Only RV-1 is recommended). Maximum age for the first dose is 14 weeks and not to be initiated after 15 weeks. *Pneumococcal vaccine:* Minimum age 6 weeks for PCV and 2 years for pneumococcal polysaccharide vaccine (PPSV).
10 weeks	DTP-2 Hib-2 IPV-2 Rotavirus-2 PCV-2	DTP and Hib are together available as Tetravalent Vaccine (Easy four)
14 weeks	DTP-3 Hib-3 IPV-3 Rotavirus-3 PCV-3	
6 months	OPV-1 Hep-B-3	*Hepatitis B:* The third dose of HBV should not be administered before 24 weeks of age.
9 months	OPV-2 Measles vaccine	
12 months	Hep. A-1	*Hepatitis A:* For both killed and live hepatitis A vaccines, two doses are recommended with 6-18 months interval.
15 months	MMR-1 Varicella-1 PCV-Booster	*Varicella vaccine:* Second dose may be administered before age 4 years, provided at least 3 months have elapsed since the first dose.

Contd...

Ans. **89. c.** Aluminium **90. c.** 0, 1, 6 months **91. a.** Immediately...

Contd...

Age (Completed weeks/months/years)	*Vaccines*	*Comments*
16 to 18 months	DTP-Booster IPV-Booster 1 Hib-Booster-1	The first booster (4th dose) may be administered as early as 12 months, provided at least 6 months have elapsed since the third dose.
18 months	Hep A-2	
2 years	Typhoid – 1	*Typhoid:* Typhoid revaccination every 3 years, if Vi-polysaccharide vaccine is used.
4½ to 5 years	DTP-Booster 2 OPV-3 MMR-2 Varicella-2 Typhoid-2	*MMR:* The 2nd dose can be given at any time 4-8 weeks after the 1st dose. Varicella: The 2nd dose can be given at anytime months after the first dose.
10-12 years	Tdap HPV	*Tdap:* This is preferred to Td followed by Td every 10 years. Human papilloma virus vaccine: Only for females, 3 doses at 0, 1-2 (depending upon the brands) and 6 months.

Source: Vipin M Vashistha. Key statements of IAPCOI and IAP immunization time table for the year 2012. Pediatric infectious disease. 2012;4(3):112-24.

Note:

1. This time table/schedule includes recommendations in effect as of April 2012. Any dose not administered at the recommended age should be administered at a subsequent visit, when indicated and feasible. Use of a combination vaccine is generally preferred over separate injections of its equivalent component vaccines.
2. The current rotavirus vaccines have been associated with a risk of intussusceptions (about 1-2 per 1,00,000 infants vaccinated). Therefore history of intussusceptions in the past is an absolute contraindication for rotavirus vaccine (RV1 and RV5) administration.
3. Prematurity and very low birth weight infants constitute a high risk category for pneumococcal vaccination because they are at a high risk of invasive pneumococcal diseases compared to full term babies.
4. The sequential schedule with IPV followed by OPV considerably decreases the risk of vaccine associated polio paralysis and also induces immunity against all the three sero types of polio viruses.
5. Changes in polio immunization schedule has become inevitable because of the following reasons.
   - India is polio free for >2 years !!
   - Type 2 wild polio virus has been eradicated in 1999.
   - Vaccine associated polio paralysis (VAPP) cannot be overlooked anymore!
   - New 'end game strategy' announced in November 2011.

92. Cell culture Rabies vaccine is given at:

a. Medial part of thigh b. Deltoid muscle
c. Anterior abdomen d. Lateral part of thigh

Intramuscular regimens:

Both a five-dose and a four-dose i.m. regimen are recommended for post-exposure vaccination of rabies; the five dose regimen is the more commonly used:

- The five-dose regimen is administered on days 0, 3, 7, 14 and 28 into the deltoid muscle.
- The four-dose regimen is administered as two doses on day 0 (one dose in the right and one in the left arm (deltoid muscles), and then one dose on each of days 7 and 21 into the deltoid muscle.

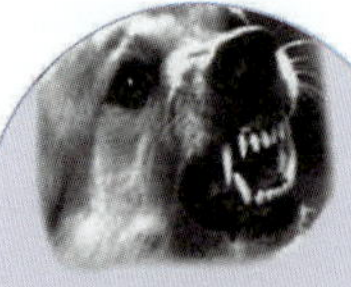

For postexposure prophylaxia, one injection each on day:

0	3	7	14	30

Note: Day 0 is the day of the first injection, preferably the day of the bite. Day 3,7, etc. are to be counted from day 0. WHO category III bites require passive immunization also.

Essen schedule.

Ans. **92. b.** Deltoid muscle

93. BCG vaccine is diluted with:

a. Normal saline b. Distilled water
c. Dextrose d. Colloids

BCG vaccine is stable at ambient temperature in a tropical climate for up to one year, if kept away from sunlight and stored in a cool environment (preferably refrigerated at a temperature of 10°C). Sunlight directly kills the bacilli; the vaccine should be protected from light during storage by wrapping it in a black cloth. Normal saline is recommended as a diluent for reconstituting the vaccine, as distilled water is hypotonic and may cause rupture of bacterial cells. The reconstituted vaccine must be used within 3 hours, and the leftover vaccine should be discarded.

94. For post-exposure prophylaxis, dose of human rabies immunoglobulin is:

a. 10 IU/kg b. 20 IU/kg
c. 30 IU/kg d. 40 IU/kg

Rabies immunoglobulin (RIG) should be given for all category III exposures, irrespective of the interval between exposure and beginning of treatment. Two kinds of rabies antibody preparations may be used: human rabies immunoglobulin (HRIG) and equine rabies immunoglobulin (ERIG). A skin test must be performed prior to the administration of ERIG. As much as possible of the recommended dose (20 IU/kg of body weight of HRIG or 40 IU/kg of body weight of ERIG) should be infiltrated around the wounds, if anatomically feasible. The remainder should be administered intramuscularly (into gluteal region) in a single dose and followed by a complete course of vaccine.

95. Human papilloma vaccine is:

a. Bivalent
b. Quadrivalent
c. Bivalent and quadrivalent
d. Monovalent

Two HPV vaccines are licensed by the Food and Drug Administration (FDA). The bivalent HPV vaccine (Cervarix) prevents the two HPV types, 16 and 18, which cause 70% of cervical cancers. The quadrivalent HPV vaccine (Gardasil) prevents four HPV types: HPV 16 and 18, as well as HPV 6 and 11, which cause 90% of genital warts. Quadrivalent vaccine has also been shown to protect against cancers of the anus, vagina and vulva.

96. How many doses of MMR are given:

a. 1 b. 2
c. 3 d. 4

Children should get 2 doses of MMR vaccine:

- First Dose: 12-15 months of age
- Second Dose: 4-6 years of age (may be given earlier, if at least 28 days after the 1st dose)

Some infants younger than 12 months should get a dose of MMR. if they are traveling out of the country, (This dose will not count toward their routine series).

97. MMR vaccine is a:

a. Killed vaccine b. Toxoid
c. Live attenuated vaccine d. Immunoglobulin

The **MMR vaccine** is an **immunization vaccine** against **measles**, mumps, and rubella (German **measles**). It is a mixture of **live attenuated** viruses of the three diseases, administered via injection. It was first developed by Maurice Hilleman while at Merck.

98. Postexposure vaccination for measles should be done in:

a. 1 day of exposure b. 2 days of exposure
c. 3 days of exposure d. 7 days of exposure

Young susceptible children coming in contact with an active case of measles can be protected from measles by the vaccine, if given within 3 days of exposure, because the incubation period in artificial infection is 7 days whereas in natural infection, it is 10 days.

Passive immunization for measles is done by human normal immunoglobulin. It is gamma globulin. It is given for those young children who have come in contact with a case of measles and are not immunized. It either prevents or modifies the attack of measles, if given within a week of exposure.

99. All are true regarding killed polio vaccine EXCEPT:

a. Produces circulatory antibody
b. Does NOT require stringent refrigeration
c. Immunity against paralytic and wild strains
d. NOT effective in an epidemic

IPV prevents the disease but does not prevent the re-infection of the gut by wild polio virus.

Differences between IPV and OPV.

IPV	*OPV*
❑ Salk-vaccine—A killed vaccine	Sabin-vaccine—A live vaccine
❑ Given IMly	Given orally
❑ Provides only systemic immunity	Provides both local and systemic immunity
❑ Prevents the disease but does not prevent the re-infection of the gut by wild polio virus	Not only prevents the disease but also prevents the intestinal re-infection by wild polio virus
❑ Does not help in the development of herd immunity	Helps in the development of herd immunity
❑ Neither useful in controlling the epidemics of polio nor in the eradication of polio	Not only useful in controlling the epidemics but also in the eradication of poliomyelitis
❑ Administration is costly	Administration is easy, cheap
❑ Requires the services of a trained person	Does not require the services of a trained person
❑ Immunity is shorter (about 5 yrs)	Immunity is lifelong with multiple doses
❑ Vaccine associated paralysis does not occur	Vaccine associated paralysis can occur
❑ Stringent conditions are not required to maintain cold-chain	Stringent conditions are required to maintain cold-chain

Ans. 93. **a.** Normal saline 94. **b.** 20 IU/kg 95. **c.** Bivalent and... 96. **b.** 2
97. **c.** Live attenuated... 98. **c.** 3 days of exposure 99. **c.** Immunity against...

100. For the prevention of Yellow fever, a single vaccination with 17D non-pathogenic strain of virus gives full protection to the individual for at least:

a. 10 years
b. 12 years
c. 15 years
d. 18 years

Protective effect of yellow fever vaccine starts 10th post vaccination day and lasts for 10 years.

101. HAV vaccine is NOT to be given below the age of:

a. 1 year b. 3 years
c. 5 years d. 10 years

Hepatitis A is a liver disease caused by the hepatitis A virus (HAV). Hepatitis A can affect anyone. Vaccines are available for long-term prevention of HAV infection in persons 1 year of age and older. Good personal hygiene and proper sanitation can also help prevent the spread of hepatitis A.

Differences between viral hepatitis A (VHA) and B (VHB).

	VHA	*VHB*
Synonyms	Acute infectious hepatitis Epidemic jaundice. MS_1 hepatitis	Serum hepatitis. Homologous serum jaundice MS_2 hepatitis
Causative agent	RNA-virus	DNA-virus
Infective material	Mainly stools Often blood in acute stage of viremia	Mainly blood and blood products Often saliva, semen and vaginal secretions
Period of infectivity	Several weeks	Several months to years
High-risk groups	Those who consume fecal contaminated water, food and milk	Commercial sex workers, surgeons, dentists, IV drug abusers, Homosexuals, Blood-bank workers, Hemophiliacs
Seasonal and cyclic trend	Observed	Not observed
Age incidence	Common among children	Common among adults
Mode of transmission	Feco-oral route (by blood also in acute phase of viremia)	Parental route, percutaneous route, sexual and perinatal route
Incubation period	15–50 days	50–150 days
Onset	Sudden	Insidious
Fever	Common	Uncommon
Illness	Not protracted	Protracted
Epidemics	Common	Uncommon
Carrier state	By feces for several weeks	By blood for several months to years
Complications	Acute fulminant hepatitis	Cirrhosis and hepatocellular carcinoma
Virus demonstration	Demonstrable in stools in acute phase	Virus not demonstrable, but antigens and antibodies are demonstrable (HBV – markers)
Prevention and control	By construction of sanitation barrier (i.e. Sanitary latrines) supplemented by chlorination of water	By avoiding multiple sexual partners, homosexuals (by adopting safe sex by condoms) By using disposable syringes and needles By screening of blood donors By avoiding sharing of razors, blades and brushes
Immunization Active	By inactivated, purified cell – culture vaccine (HAVRIX) and by live vaccine (Biovac)	By plasma derived vaccine and yeast cell Derived DNA recombinant vaccine
Passive	By human normal immunoglobulin	By human specific immunoglobulin

102. Vaccines are available against group .... meningococcus:

a. A b. B
c. C d. A and C

Internationally marketed meningococcal polysaccharide vaccines are bivalent (A and C), trivalent (A, C and W-135) or tetravalent (A, C, Y and W-135). The vaccines are purified, heat-stable, lyophilized capsular polysaccharides from meningococci of the respective serogroups.

103. The vaccine NOT to be given during pregnancy is:

a. MMR
b. Rabies
c. Hepatitis B
d. Diphtheria

Some vaccines, such as the measles, mumps, rubella (MMR) vaccine, should be given a month or more before pregnancy.

Ans. 100. a. 10 year **101. a.** 1 year **102. d.** A and C **103. a.** MMR

104. What is the correct recommended schedule (in days) for post-exposure treatment of person who had been vaccinated for rabies previously with HDC:

a. 0, 3 and 7
b. 0, 3, 7 and 14
c. 0, 3, 7, 14 and 28
d. 0, 7 and 28

For post-exposure prophylaxis of rabies, one dose of the vaccine should be administered on days 0, 3, 7, 14 and 28. A booster may be needed on day 90. If the subject has been previously vaccinated, he needs only first 3 doses (only first 2 doses of titre is adequate). All intramuscular injections must be given into the deltoid region or, in small children, into the anterolateral area of the thigh muscle. Vaccine should never be administered in the gluteal region.

COMMUNICABLE AND NON-COMMUNICABLE DISEASES

105. All of the following are used while evaluating a pneumonia patient at PHC EXCEPT:

a. Respiratory rate
b. Temperature
c. Oxygen saturation
d. Chest indrawing

Physical examination of a patient with pneumonia

- Count the breaths in one minute
- Look for chest indrawing
- Look and listen for stridor
- Look for wheeze
- See if the child is abnormally sleepy or difficult to wake
- Feel for fever or low body temperature
- Check for severe malnutrition
- Cyanosis

106. All of the following are caused by virus EXCEPT:

a. Rocky mountain spotted fever
b. KFD
c. Dengue
d. Yellow fever

Rocky Mountain Spotted Fever

- Agent: R. rickettsi
- Insect vector: Tick
- Mammalian reservoir: Rodents, dogs

107. According to prevalence criteria by WHO, which of the following is true for determining xerophthalmia problem in an endemic area?

a. Bitot spot >0.5%
b. Conjunctival xerosis 1%
c. Conjunctival ulcers 0.05%
d. Night blindness 0.5%

Prevalence criteria for determining the xerophthalmia problem

Criteria	Prevalence in population at risk (6 months to 6 years)
Corneal ulcer	More than 0.05%
Corneal xerosis/corneal ulceration/ keratomalacia	More than 0.01%
Bitots spots	More than 0.5%
Night blindness	More than 1%
Serum retinol (less than 10 mcg/dl)	More than 5%

108. Hookworm problem is of no significance, if Chandler's index is less than:

a. 100
b. 200
c. 250
d. 300

Average number of hookworm eggs/gram of stool

- <200: No significance
- 200–250: Potential danger
- 250–300: Minor (public health problem)
- >300: Important/ major (public health problem)

109. To eradicate measles, % of population to be vaccinated should be at least:

a. 70
b. 80
c. 90
d. 95

When rates of vaccination within a population are greater than 93% outbreaks of measles typically no longer occur; however, they may occur again, if rates of vaccination decrease.

110. A 'Case' in TB is defined as:

a. X-ray positive
b. Sputum positive
c. Mantoux positive
d. History of cough

For the purpose of tuberculosis control, a 'case' is defined by WHO as a patient whose sputum is positive for tubercle bacilli, and such cases are the target of case finding.

111. Inclusion body in neuron is seen in:

a. Japanese encephalitis
b. Yellow fever
c. Diphtheria
d. Rabies

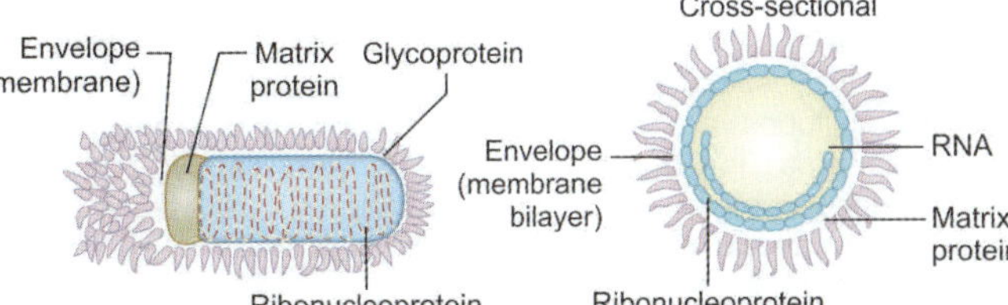

Rabies virions are bullet-shaped with 10 nm spike-like glycoprotein peplomers covering the surface. The ribonucleoprotein is composed of RNA encased in nucleoprotein, phosphorylated or phosphoprotein and polymerase

MCQs with Short Explanations

Ans. **104. a.** 0, 3 and 7 **105. c.** Oxygen saturation **106. a.** Rocky mountain... **107. a.** Bitot spot >0.5%
108. b. 200 **109. d.** 95 **110. b.** Sputum positive **111. d.** Rabies

Negri bodies are eosinophilic, sharply outlined, pathognomonic inclusion **bodies** (2–10 μm in diameter) found in the cytoplasm of certain nerve cells containing the virus of rabies, especially in Ammon's horn of the hippocampus.

112. Disease spread by hard tick is:

a. Rocky mountain spotted fever
b. Epidemic typhus
c. Murine typhus
d. Scrub typhus

In the case of Rocky Mountain spotted fever, ticks are the natural hosts, serving as both reservoirs and vectors of *R. rickettsii*. Ticks transmit the organism to vertebrates primarily by their bites. Less commonly, infections may occur following exposure to crushed tick tissues, fluids, or tick feces.

Diseases having different reservoir and source of infection.

Diseases	*Reservoir*	*Source*
Ancylostomiasis	Human being	Soil containing larvae
Tetanus	Herbivorous animal	Soil containing spores
Plague	Rodents	Rat flea
Japanese encephalitis	Pigs	Female culex mosquito
Kyasanur forest disease	Monkeys	Hard tick

113. Spread by aedes mosquitoes:

a. Loa Loa
b. Malaria
c. Dengue
d. Japanese encephalitis

Dengue is transmitted by several species of mosquito within the genus *Aedes*, principally *A. aegypti*.

Comparative features of the mosquitoes in their life cycle.

Anopheles	*Culex*	*Aedes*	*Mansonia (or monsonioides)*
Egg stage			
❑ Breeds in clean, fresh water. Eggs are laid in singles. ❑ Each egg is boat (spindle) shaped. ❑ Egg floats with lateral floats containing air.	❑ Breeds in dirty, organically contaminated water collections like pits, pools, drains, sewage farms, etc. ❑ Eggs are laid in clusters of 150–200, which are cemented together, in the form of boat shaped mass called 'Egg raft'. Raft helps in floating. ❑ Each egg is cigar shaped. ❑ Eggs have no lateral floats ❑ Exception: Culex vishnui group of mosquitoes breed in water containing aquatic plants.	❑ Breeds in peridomestic artificial collections of water such as broken pots, bottles, tyres, tins, flower pots, flower jars, air-coolers, coconut shells, tree-holes, etc. ❑ Eggs are laid in singles. ❑ Eggs are black in color and do not possess lateral floats. But they possess small air bubble like cavities on the surface, with which they float.	❑ Breeds in water bodies containing certain aquatic plants like pistia plant and water hyacinth. Eggs are laid in 'star' shaped clusters, attached to under-surface of leaves of water plants. Presence of aquatic plants and organic pollution of water are the two important conditions for breeding of this mosquito. ❑ Each egg is black in color, flask shaped and has pointed ends.
Larva stage			
❑ Larva floats horizontally parallel to the water surface, with the help of palmate hairs. ❑ Respiratory apparatus (Siphon tube is absent) consists of two openings, in direct contact with the surface of water. ❑ Feeds on the things present on the surface of the water. ❑ Hence it is called 'surface feeder.'	❑ Larva floats with the head downwards, obliquely from the surface of the water (So it feeds on the things present inside the water. Hence it is called 'bottom-feeder'). ❑ Palmate hairs are scanty. ❑ Siphon tube is long and narrow. ❑ It opens at the surface of the water for respiration.	❑ Larva remains suspended in the water obliquely with the head downwards like culex larva (So bottom feeder). ❑ Palmate hairs are scanty. ❑ Larva is black in color. ❑ Siphon tube is short and barrel shaped, opens at the surface for respiration.	❑ Larva floats with the head downwards, like culex larva but it is attached to the roots and rootlets of the acquatic plant with the help of spines of the siphon tube (It utilizes the stored air in the roots and rootlets of acquatic plant). ❑ It goes to the bottom of water for feeding purpose and then again gets attached to the roots. ❑ Palmate hairs are scanty.
Pupa stage			
❑ 'Comma' shaped structure. ❑ Pupa are suspended in water. ❑ Siphon tubes are short and broad, a pair in number, found on cephalothorax. ❑ Caudal paddles and hairs are seen on the tip of last abdominal segment.	❑ 'Comma' shaped structure. ❑ Suspended in water. ❑ Siphon tubes, a pair in number, long and narrow, open on the surface of the water.	❑ 'Comma' shaped structure. ❑ Similar to culex pupa. ❑ Black in color	❑ 'Comma' shaped structure. ❑ Similar to culex pupa, but attached to the roots and rootlets of the acquatic plants, with the help of spines of the siphon tubes. ❑ Pupa gets detached from the acquatic plants and comes to the water surface only at the time of emergence of the imago, (i.e. young adult).

Contd...

Ans. 112. a. Rocky mountain...**113. c.** Dengue

Contd...

Anopheles	*Culex*	*Aedes*	*Mansonia (or monsonioides)*
Adult stage			
❑ In the resting position, the body (head, thorax and abdomen) is in a line and is inclined at an angle to the resting surface (except Anopheles culicifacies). It is called 'Tail in the air' posture.	❑ In the resting position, the head and thorax are held in an inclined plane pointing downwards and the body is held in horizontal plane parallel to the resting surface, giving a 'Hunch back' appearance.	❑ In the resting position, aedes mosquito also gives 'hunch back' appearance like culex mosquito. ❑ It appears like culex mosquito in all respects except that it is black in color with alternate white bands.	❑ In resting position, the mansonia mosquito also exhibits 'hunch-back' appearance. ❑ There are some white dots on the head and dorsum of thorax and white bands on the abdomen and legs.
❑ Wings are spotted (i.e. the veins in the wings posses alternate band of white and dark fringe scales over them). ❑ Scutellum on the thorax is crescent shaped with long hairs at regular intervals. ❑ Maxillary palpi are long in both the sexes, but the tip is club shaped in males and not club shaped in females. ❑ Antennae are bushy and more hairy in males and less hairy in females. ❑ Mosquito makes no noise while flying. ❑ Scales on the abdomen are arranged in a scattered manner.	❑ Wings are strong and unspotted (i.e. no fringe scales over the veins). ❑ Scutellum is trilobed, each lobe with a group of hairs. ❑ Maxillary palpi are long in males (longer than proboscis) and bent outwards (i.e. acuminate type), the tip being pointed. Palpi are short in females. ❑ Antennae are bushy and more hairy in males and less hairy in females. ❑ Mosquito makes humming noise while flying.	❑ Hence it is called 'Tiger mosquito' (Silver spotted mosquito). Legs are also banded. ❑ Wings are unspotted. ❑ Scutellum is trilobed, each lobe with a tuft of hairs. ❑ Dorsum of thorax reveals two 'Lyre' like pattern, white marked, i.e. two outer curved lines (bracket shaped) and two median parallel lines. ❑ Maxillary palpi are long in males and short in females. ❑ Antennae are bushy in males and less hairy in females.	❑ Wings are unspotted. But veins have dark fringe scales scattered in an indiscriminate fashion, like pepper powder thrown on white background. ❑ Scutellum is trilobed, each lobe with a tuft of hairs. ❑ Maxillary palpi are long in males and short in females. ❑ Antennae are more hairy in males and less hairy in females. ❑ Makes no noise while flying and bites are also not painful.
	❑ Bites are painful and often causes irritation. ❑ Scales on the abdomen are arranged close together overlapping each other.	❑ Antennae are also black with white bands (stripes). ❑ Mosquito does not make any noise while flying and the bites are also not painful. Female mosquito bites during day time mainly.	
Important species			
❑ *Anopheline culicifacies* ❑ *Ano. fluviatilis.* ❑ *Ano. sundaicus.* ❑ *Ano. stephensi.* ❑ *Ano. minimus.* ❑ *Ano. philippinensis*	❑ *Culex quinquefasciatus* ❑ *Cu. vishnui* ❑ *Cu. pseudo vishnui* ❑ *Cu. gelidus* ❑ *Cu. tritaenyrhincus*	❑ *Aedes aegypti* ❑ *Aedes albopictus* ❑ *Aedes vittatus.*	❑ *Mansonioides annulifera* ❑ *M. uniformis* ❑ *M. Indiana* ❑ *M. longipalpis*
Diseases transmitted (by infective female mosquito)			
❑ Malaria	❑ Filariasis caused by Wuchereria bancrofti and transmitted by Cu. quinquefasciatus ❑ Japanese encephalitis by Cu. vishnui and tritaeniorhynchus	❑ Yellow fever ❑ Dengue fever ❑ Chikungunya fever	❑ Filariasis, caused by Brugia malayi
Control measures (antilarval measures)			
❑ Filling and drainage of breeding places. ❑ Overhead tanks are kept clean and dry for one day in a week. ❑ Malarial oil was used to destroy the larvae and pupae. ❑ Paris green is used to destroy the larvae of anopheline mosquito because they are surface feeders.	❑ Proper drainage and disposal of sewage and waste water. ❑ Oiling of breeding places once in a week by using diesel oil. ❑ Paris green can be used to kill bottom feeders, when used in the form of pellets or granules	❑ Artificial containers are turned upside down to drain away the water. Waste containers are collected and disposed off in a far off place. ❑ Oiling is not useful. ❑ Paris green not necessary.	❑ Physical removal of acquatic plants or use of herbicides. ❑ Oiling is not useful. ❑ Paris green can be used in the form of pellets or granules.

114. Causative agent for oriental sore is:

a. Onchocerca volvulus
b. Leishmania donovani
c. Leishmania tropica
d. Brugia malayi

L. donovani, which attacks the liver, spleen, bone marrow, and other viscera, causes kala-azar in Africa, Europe, and Asia. *L. tropica* causes oriental sore in Africa, Europe, and the East; lesions that range from pimples to large ulcers are formed on the skin of the hands, feet, legs, and face.

115. Larvae of which of the following lies parallel to surface of water:

a. Anopheles
b. Culex
c. Aedes
d. Sandfly

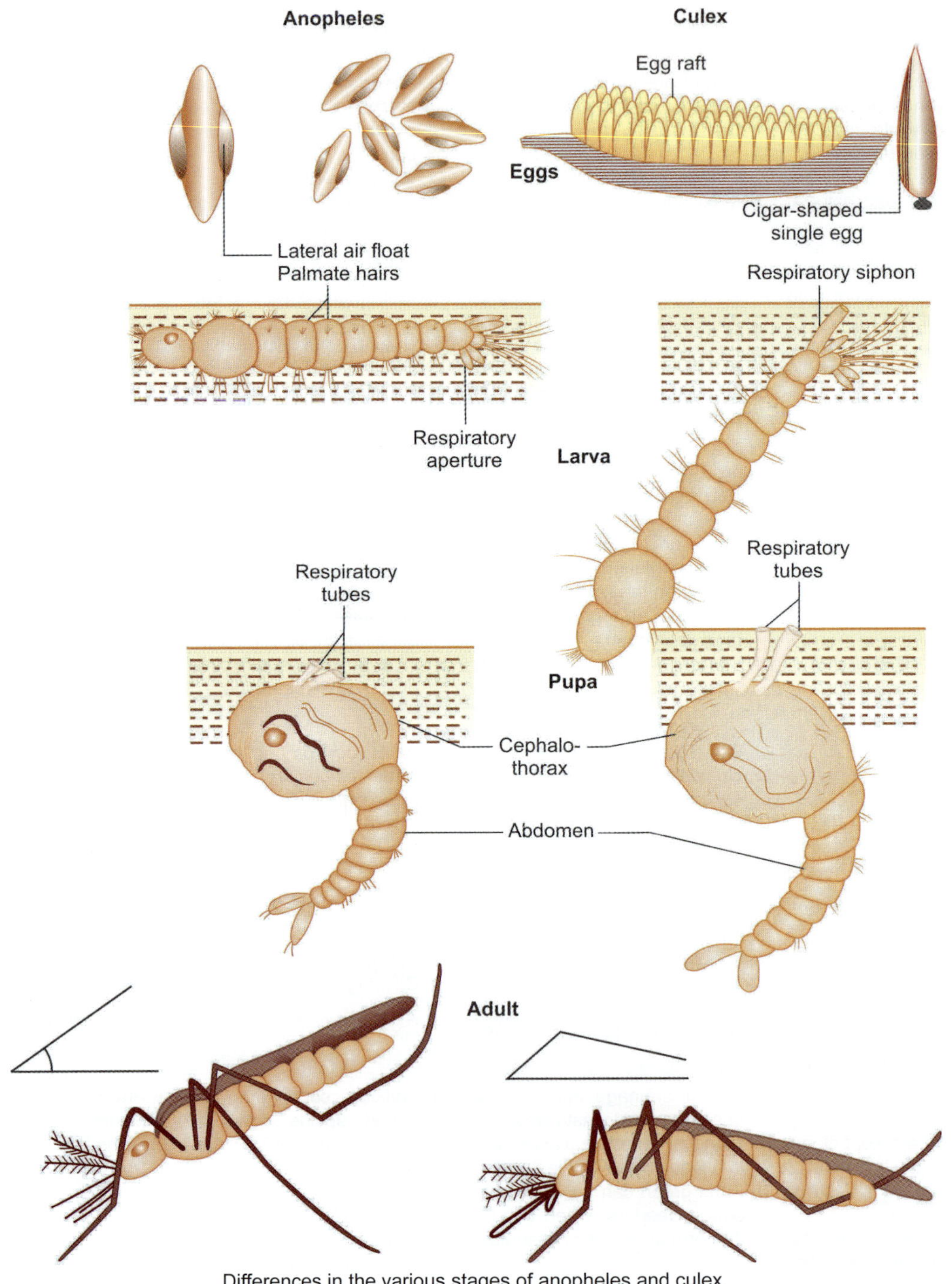

Differences in the various stages of anopheles and culex.
Source: Ratnaswamy GK. A Handbook of Medical Entomology and Elementary Parasitology. 1st edn, 1974.

Ans. 114. c. Leishmania... **115. a.** Anopheles

The mosquito larva has a well-developed head with mouth brushes used for feeding, a large thorax and a nine-segment abdomen. It has no legs. In contrast to other mosquitoes, the*Anopheles* larva lacks a respiratory siphon, so it positions itself so that its body is parallel to the surface of the water. In contrast, feeding larva of a nonanopheline mosquito species attaches itself to the water surface with its posterior siphon, with their body pointing downwards.

116. Method used for HIV pretest counseling:

a. Mass media b. Group approach
c. Individual approach d. All of the above

Individual pre-test counselling is mainly carried out to help a person make an informed decision about whether to take an HIV test.

117. 1 tuberculin unit corresponds to:

a. 0.0001 mg b. 0.00002 mg of PPD
c. 0.1 mg of BCG d. None of the above

Test material for tuberculin/Mantoux/PPD test is 'Tuberculin', a protein derived from the body of RT-23 strain of TB bacilli, which is purified and standardized. It is called PPD-S (purified protein derivative standardized). Tuberculin 1 unit of PPD-S contains 0.00002 mg of tuberculin antigen, which is routinely used for the test.

118. Malarial parasite ABSENT in India:

a. P. malariae b. P. ovale
c. P. falciparum d. P. vivax

P. ovale is primarily concentrated in sub-Saharan Africa and islands in the western Pacific.

119. Plaque is transmitted by:

a. Flea b. Soft tick
c. Mites d. Hard tick

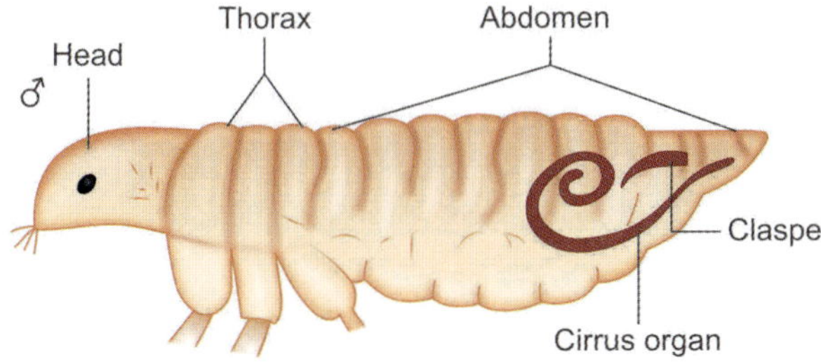

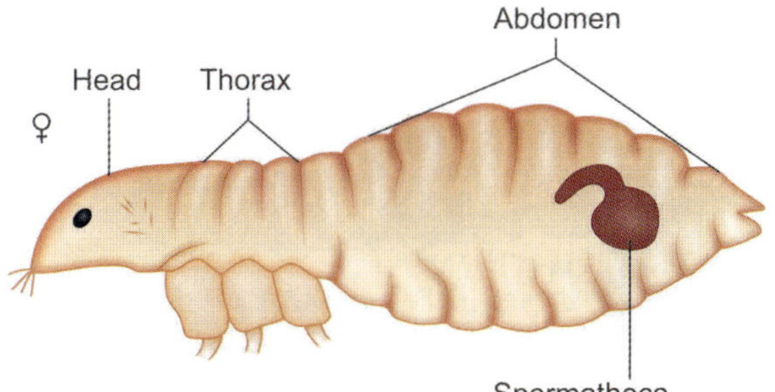

Differences between ♂ and ♀ rat flea

Source: Ratnaswamy GK. A Handbook of Medical Entomology and Elementary Parasitology. 1st edn, 1974

The **Oriental rat flea** (*Xenopsylla cheopis*), also known as the **tropical rat flea**, is a parasite of rodents, primarily of the genus *Rattus*, and is a primary vector for bubonic plague and murine typhus. This occurs when the flea has fed on an infected rodent, and then bites a human.

120. True regarding elimination of neonatal tetanus/NNT in village:

a. Rate more than 1/1000 live births
b. Attended deliveries less than 50%
c. Attended deliveries more than 50%
d. Rate less than 0.1/1000 live births

- NNT High risk district:
  - Neonatal death incidence rate > 1/1000 live births OR
  - 2 doses of tetanus toxoid (TT_2) coverage < 70% OR
  - Deliveries attended by trained dais < 50%
- Medium risk district/NNT control districts:
  - Neonatal death rate < 1 /1000 live births
  - 2 doses of tetanus toxoid coverage > 70%
  - Deliveries attended by dais > 50%
- **Low risk district/NNT elimination districts:**
  - NNT <0.1/1000 Live Birth
  - 2 Doses of T.T Coverage >90%
  - Delivery attended by Trained Dais >75%

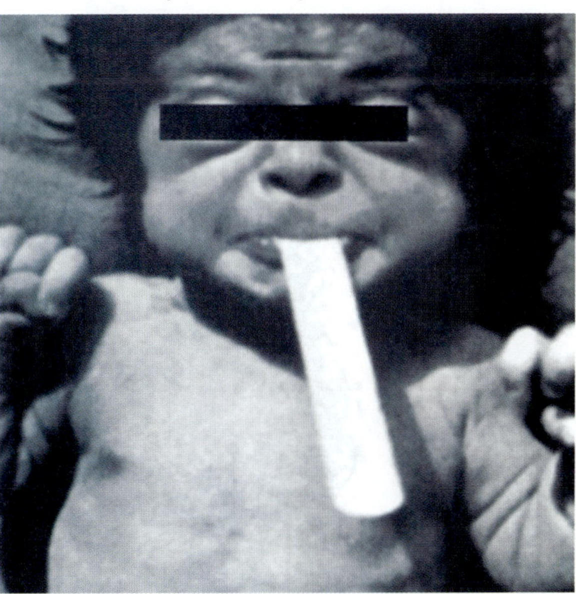

Neonatal tetanus with tongue depressor.

121. Chandler's index is associated with:

a. Round worm
b. Hook worm
c. Pin worm
d. Tape worm

Chandlers **index** is used to identify the importance of hookworm/ancylostoma infestation as a public health problem in a community.

Ans. **116. c.** Individual... **117. b.** 0.00002 mg of PPD **118. b.** P. ovale **119. a.** Flea
120. d. Rate less than... **121. b.** Hook worm

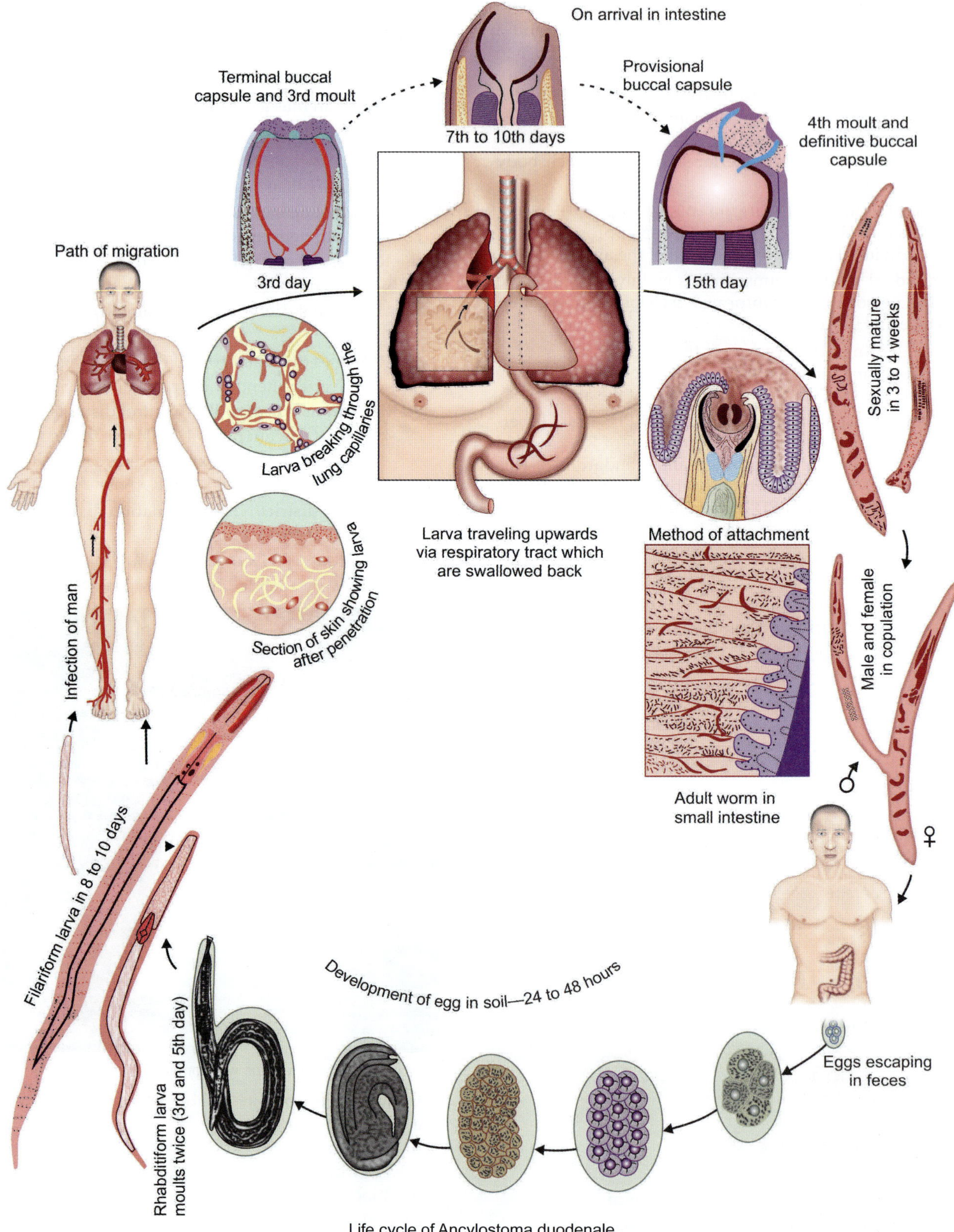

Life cycle of Ancylostoma duodenale.

122. Natural reservoir of chikungunya virus in India is:

a. Monkey b. Guinea pig
c. Aedes d. None of the above

The chikungunya virus is passed to humans by two species of mosquito of the genus *Aedes*: *A. albopictus* and *A. aegypti*. There is no animal reservoir. There is no carrier state also.

123. Cyclopropagative life cycle is seen in:

a. Malaria b. Plague
c. Filaria d. Yellow fever

Biological transmission

Propagative	Pathogens undergo multiplication inside the body of the vector	Plague bacilli in rat flea Yellow fever virus in aedes mosquito
Cyclopropagative	Pathogens undergo not only multiplication but also cyclic development inside the body of the vector	Malarial parasite in female anopheles mosquito
Cyclodevelopmental	Pathogens undergo only developmental changes and no multiplication inside the body of the vector	Wuchereria bancrofti microfilariae inside female culex mosquito Guinea worm embryo in Cyclops

124. Guinea worm infestation is commoner in:

a. Cotton mill workers b. Field workers
c. Textile workers d. Step well-workers

Guinea worm disease is caused by drinking water contaminated by water fleas that host the D. medinensis larvae. Guinea worm disease has a history of being very common in some of the world's poorest areas, particularly those with limited or no access to clean water. In these areas, stagnant water sources may still host copepods, which can carry the larvae of the guinea worm.

125. Rabies free country:

a. India b. China
c. Russia d. Australia

Rabies is a virus. Although rabies itself does not currently occur in Australia, another virus, called Australian bat lyssavirus, does occur in Australia and is treated the same way as rabies. While animal rabies has never been reported in Australia or New Zealand there is the potential for the virus to be introduced into Australia from other countries.

126. Incubation period of Plasmodium vivax:

a. 1-7 days b. 7-10 days
c. 10-14 days d. 15-30 days

Incubation period

Plasmodium vivax	14 days
Plasmodium falciparum	12 days
Plasmodium malariae	28 days
Plasmodium ovale	17 days

127. Mitsuda reaction is read at:

a. 3rd day b. 10th day
c. 21st day d. 45th day

Positive mitsuda reaction means. A) 10 mm or more induration after 48 hrs B) 5 mm or above nodule after 21 days. An extract sample of inactivated Hansen's Bacillus is injected just under the skin, usually on the forearm, so that a small lump pushes the skin upward. The lump indicates that the antigen has been injected at the correct depth. The injection site is labeled and examined at 48 hours (early; Fernandez reaction) and 21 days (late; Mitsuda reaction) later to see, if there is a reaction.

128. Chandlers index is:

a. No. of eggs/gm of soil
b. No. of eggs/gm of stool
c. No. of eggs/100 gm of soil
d. No. of eggs/100 gm of stool

Chandler index is calculated based on average number of hookworm eggs/gram of stool.

Average no. of eggs/g of stools	Public health importance of hookworm infection
< 200	Not of much importance
200–250	Indicates potential danger
250–300	Indicates minor public health problem
> 300	Major public health problem

129. All of the following are true for measles EXCEPT:

a. Maximum incidence is 6 month to 3 year age group
b. Best age for immunization is 9 months
c. Secondary attack rate is 30%
d. Koplik spots seen

SAR of measles is about 80% among the susceptible contact.

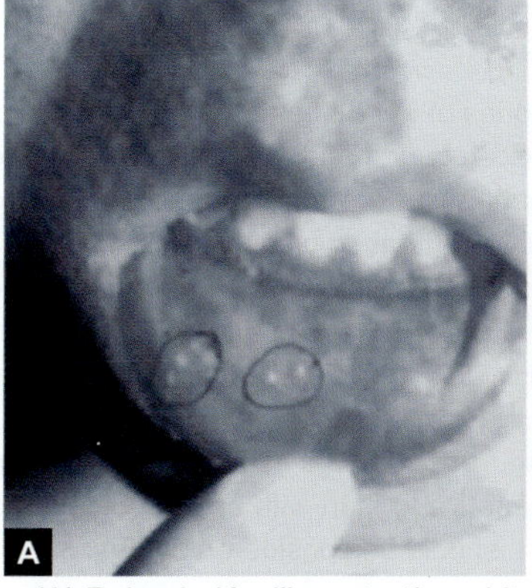

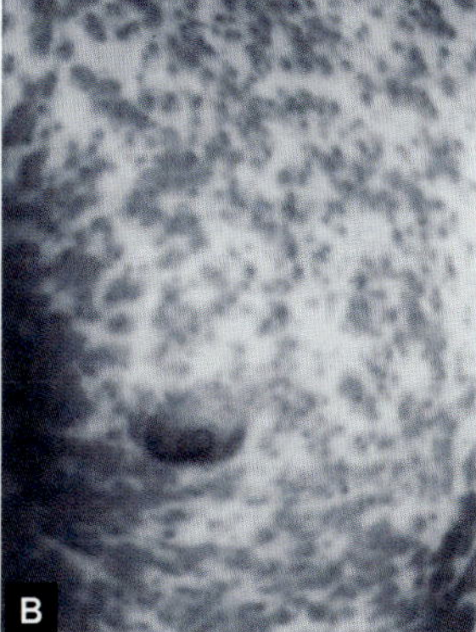

(A) Rubeola-Koplik spots: tiny white papules on oral mucosa; (B) Rubeola—intense morbilliform eruption.

Ans. 122. **d.** None of the above 123. **a.** Malaria 124. **d.** Step well workers 125. **d.** Australia
126. **c.** 10-14 days 127. **c.** 21st day 128. **b.** No. of eggs/gm... 129. **c.** Secondary attack rate...

130. All of the following are true about congenital rubella EXCEPT:

a. It is diagnosed when the infant has IgM antibodies at birth

b. It is diagnosed when IgG antibodies persist for more than 6 months

c. MC congenital defects are deafness, cardiac malformations and cataract

d. Infection after 16 weeks of gestation results in major congenital defects

Congenital rubella syndrome (CRS) can occur in a developing fetus of a pregnant woman who has contracted rubella, usually in the first trimester. If infection occurs 0–28 days before conception, the infant has a 43% chance of being affected. If the infection occurs 0–12 weeks after conception, the chance increases to 51%. If the infection occurs 13–26 weeks after conception, the chance is 23% of the infant being affected by the disease. Infants are not generally affected if rubella is contracted during the third trimester, or 26–40 weeks after conception. Problems rarely occur when rubella is contracted by the mother after 20 weeks of gestation and continues to disseminate the virus after birth.

Stage of gestation	*Risk of damage to the fetus (%)*
4 to 8 weeks	80
8 to 12 weeks	25
12 to 16 weeks	10
> 17 weeks	00

131. A patient was put on ATT for 5 months. Sputum examination is positive for AFB. The likely diagnosis is:

a. Defaulter
b. Relapse
c. Treatment failure
d. Absentee

Relapse is defined as a TB patient who was declared cured or treatment completed by a physician, but who reports back to the health service and is now found to be sputum smear positive. Failure, by definition, is any TB patient who is smear positive at 5 months or more after starting treatment.

Color coded boxes, categories/groups, type of TB patients, the regimens and their follow-up.

Categorization of TB Patients (wef January 2010) Treatment regimen					*Sputum examination*			
Color of the box	*Treatment group*	*Type of patient*	*Intensive phase†*	*Continuation phase†*	*Pre-treatment*	*Test at month*	*If result is*	*→ Then*
Red	New* (category I)	Sputum smear positive Sputum smear negative Extrapulmonary	$2(HRZE)_3$	$4(HR)_3$	+	2	–	Start continuation phase, test sputum again at 4 and 6 months*
					–	2	+	Continue intensive phase for one more month. Test sputum again at 3, 5 and 7 months.*
Blue	Previously treated** (category (II))	Smear positive relapse Smear positive failure Smear positive Treatment after default Others***	$2(HRZES)_3$ $1(HRZE)_3$	$5(HRE)_3$	+	3	–	Start continuation phase. Test sputum again at 5 and 8 months
							+	Continue intensive phase for one more month. Test sputum again at 4, 6 and 9 months

* 'New' includes former categories of I and III and the box is Red colored.

** 'Previously treated' is former category II and the box is Blue colored.

*** 'Others' includes those patients who are sputum smear negative (pulmonary or extrapulmonary), and have recurrence or nonresponse (relapse or failure), diagnosis being based on culture or histological evidence of current active TB. They are given treatment as Cat. II

† The number before the letters refers to the number of months of treatment. Suffix number refers to the number of doses per week (i.e. thrice a week)

Dose (thrice week). H = INH 600 mg; R = Rifampicin 450 mg; Z = Pyrazinamide 1500 mg; E = Ethambutol 1200 mg and S = Streptomycin 750 mg.

Patients weighing less than 30 kg, receive drugs as per pediatric weight band boxes according to body weight.

* Patients whose sputum is negative to start with and becomes positive during continuation phase or whose sputum remains positive at the end of the treatment in Cat. I, should be considered as 'Failure' and put on Cat. II treatment afresh.

Note: It is very importa□

risk of acquiring drug resistance and to prescribe appropriate treatment.

Ans. 130. d. Infection after... **131. c.** Treatment failure

132. Anopheles species most commonly found in coastal region:

a. Anopheles minimus b. Anopheles fluviatilis
c. Anopheles stephensi
d. Anopheles philippinensis

In rural areas, the larvae of A. stephensi may exist in many aquatic habitats, such as: ponds, streams, swamps, marshes, and other sources of standing water. They may also occupy smaller environments, such as: tree holes, leaf axils, and man-made containers. Though larvae of A. stephensi mysorensis exclusively prefer to occupy stone pots and earthenware containers. This species is also able to endure high amounts of salinity, and have been found to breed readily in water where the salinity is equal to or even surpassing that of sea water.

133. Mineral oil is used in mosquito control measures as:

a. Space spray b. Adulticide
c. Larvicide
d. Personal protection methods

Oils and films disperse as a thin layer on the surface of the water which cause larvae and pupae to drown.

- Mineral Oils
- Monomolecular films

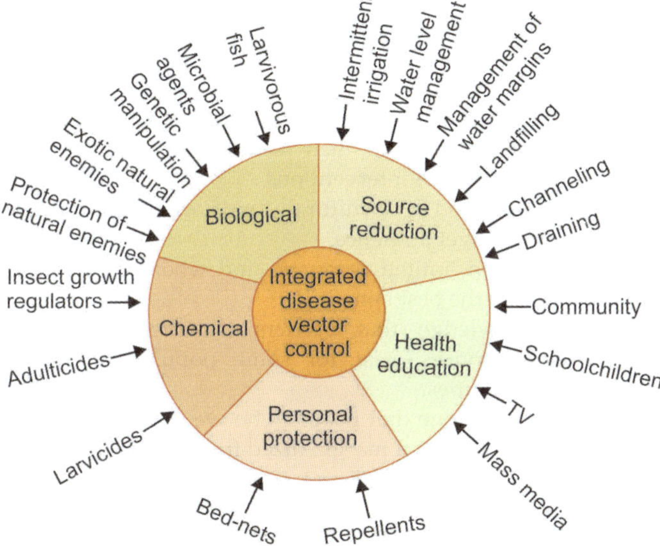

Integration of various potential methods for control of disease vectors.

134. All are true statements about filariasis EXCEPT:

a. Extrinsic incubation period of 10-14 days
b. Man is the intermediate host
c. Adults live in the lymphatics of host
d. No multiplication in the mosquito

Human filarial nematode worms have complicated lifecycles, which primarily consists of five stages. After the male and female worms mate, the female gives birth to live microfilariae by the thousands. The microfilariae are taken up by the vector insect/mosquito (intermediate host) during a blood meal. In the intermediate host, the microfilariae molt and develop into third-stage (infective) larvae. Upon taking another blood meal, the vector insect injects the infectious larvae into the dermis layer of the skin. After about one year, the larvae molt through two more stages, maturing into the adult worms. Man is a definitive host.

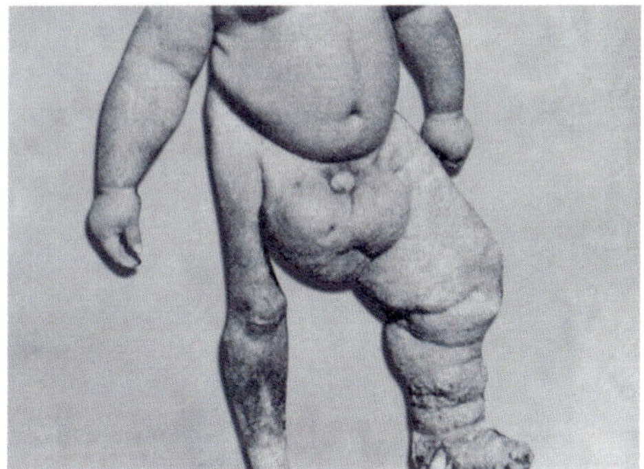
Chronic filariasis.

135. For the treatment of class III dog bite, all of the following are correct EXCEPT:

a. Give immunoglobulins for passive immunity
b. Give ARV/antirabies vaccine
c. Immediately stitch wound under antibiotic coverage
d. Immediately wash wound with soap and water

For category I no treatment is required, whereas for category II immediate vaccination and for category III immediate vaccination and administration of rabies immune globulin are recommended in addition to immediate washing and flushing of all bite wounds and scratches.

Category	*Type of contact with a suspect or confirmed rabid animal or animal not traceable*	*Recommended treatment*
I (No risk)	Touching or feeding of animals. Licks on intact skin	Nothing required
II (Low risk)	Nibbling of uncovered skin, Scratch or abrasion without bleeding; Licks on broken skin.	Administer ARV immediately; Stop treatment if the animal is found healthy for 10 days after the bite or if the animal is euthanized and found to be negative for rabies by laboratory techniques.

Contd...

Ans. 132. c. Anopheles... 133. c. Larvicide 134. b. Man is the inter... 135. c. Immediately stitch...

Contd...

Category	Type of contact with a suspect or confirmed rabid animal or animal not traceable	Recommended treatment
III (High risk)	Single or multiple transdermal bites or scratches with bleeding; Contamination of mucous membrane with saliva, Licks on mucous membrane	Administer both ARV and Rabies Immunoglobulin (RIG) immediately. Stop treatment if the animal is found healthy for 10 days after the bite or if the animal is euthanized and found to be negative for rabies by lab. techniques.

136. FALSE statement about Japanese encephalitis:
  a. Human are incidental host
  b. Birds are involved in life cycle
  c. Pigs manifest disease
  d. Transmitted by culex

Domestic pigs and wild birds (especially herons) are reservoirs of the virus; transmission to humans may cause severe symptoms. Amongst the most important vectors of this disease are the mosquitoes Culex tritaeniorhynchus and Culex vishnui. This disease is most prevalent in Southeast Asia and East Asia.

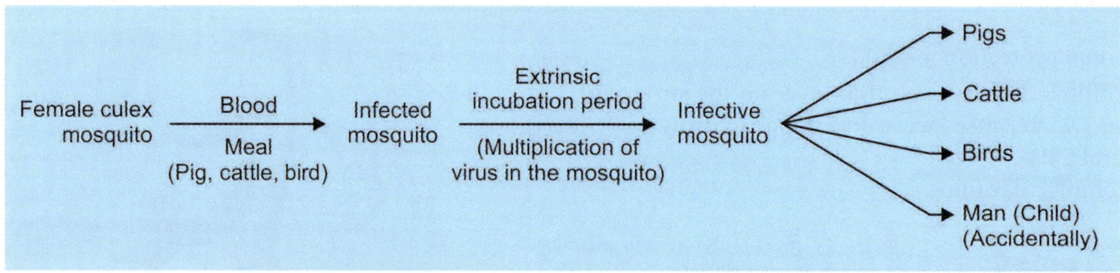

Course of events in the mosquito following flood meal.

137. Shortest incubation period is of:
  a. Influenza b. Rubella
  c. Hepatitis B d. Hepatitis A

The typical incubation period for influenza is 1-4 days (average: 2 days). Adults can be infectious from 1 day before onset of symptoms to 5-7 days after illness onset

138. Targeted intervention for HIV is NOT done for:
  a. Industrial workers b. Street children
  c. Migrant labors d. Commercial sex workers

Targeted interventions

- Are for people within the community who are most at risk of HIV and STI infection.
- Are targeted to behavior and practices not the identity
- Involve them and their issues within the broader frame work of interventions
- Are adapted to be culturally and socially appropriate to the target audience.
- Focus on limited resources and where they can be used to the best benefit.
- Acknowledge that barriers to accessing healthcare services exist for some populations within communities.
- Acknowledge that people who are at risk of HIV infection are often marginalized from the broader community, stigmatized and discriminated against.

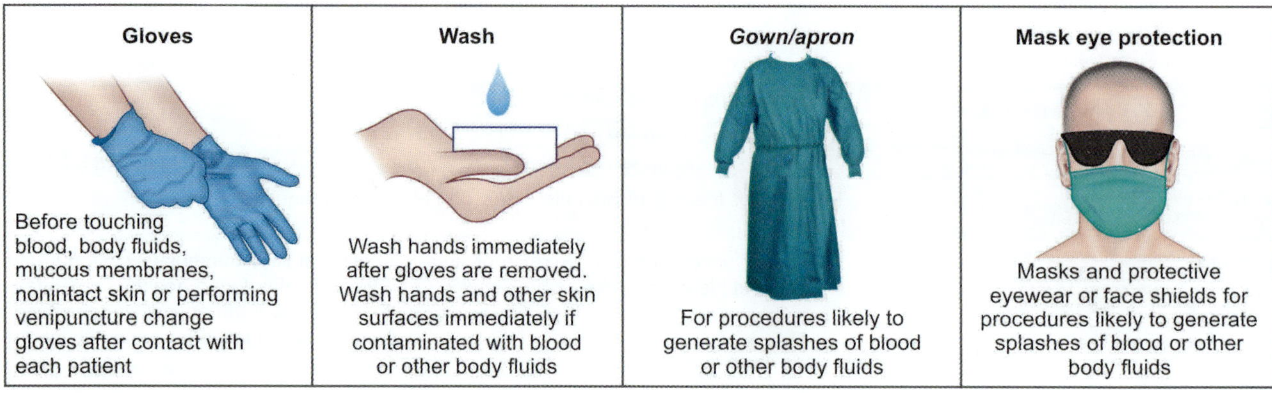

Contd...

Ans. **136. c.** Pigs manifest... **137. a.** Influenza **138. a.** Industrial workers

Contd...

Sharps	Do not recap by hand	Resuscitation	Waste/linen
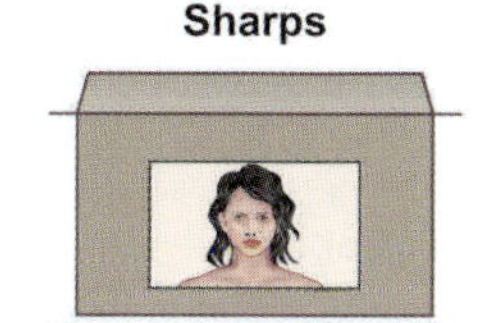 Dispose of needles with syringes and other sharp items in puncture-resistant container near point-of-use	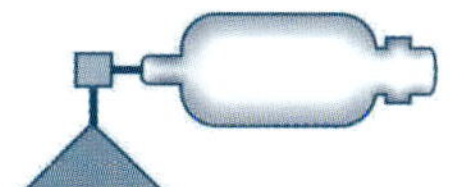 Do not recap needles or otherwise manipulate by hand before disposal	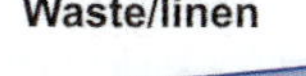 Mouthpieces of resuscitator bags should be available to minimize need for emergency mouth to mouth resuscitation	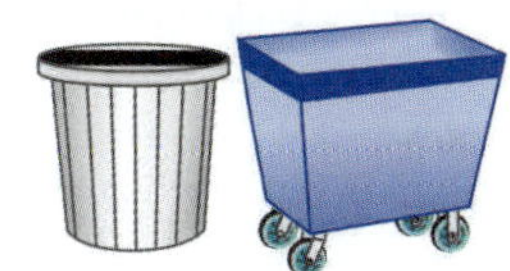 Waste and soiled lined should be handled in accordance with disposal policy and local law

Standard precautions against HIV.

Source: Govt. of Karnataka. India Canada Collaborative HIV/AIDS Project and Karnataka State AIDS Prevention Society. Participant's Manual 2005.

139. Which of the following is NOT included in the SAFE strategy:
- a. Supplementation of vitamins
- b. Antibiotics
- c. Face washing
- d. Improvement of the environment

S in SAFE strategy (of trachoma) stands for surgery.

140. Following procedures EXCEPT one, prevents neonatal tetanus, advised by family welfare program:
- a. Giving TT vaccine between age group 10-15 years girls
- b. Immunise pregnant mothers during 16-36 weeks only
- c. Trained dais conducting deliveries
- d. Single dose of TT to mothers who already received immunization in previous pregnancy

The spores which cause tetanus are present everywhere, so the only prevention is immunization. Three properly spaced doses of tetanus toxoid vaccine are recommended for women of childbearing age, either before or during pregnancy; this will protect their future babies from neonatal tetanus after delivery.

141. Which of the following statements about lepromin test is NOT true:
- a. It is negative in most children in 1st 6 months of life
- b. It is a diagnostic test
- c. It is an important aid to classify type of leprosy disease
- d. BCG vaccination may convert lepra reaction from negative to positive

The lepromin skin test is used to determine what type of leprosy a person has. It involves the injection of a standardized extract of the inactivated "leprosy bacillus", (Mycobacterium leprae or "Hansen's Bacillus") under the skin. It is not recommended as a primary mode of diagnosis.

142. Which of the following is NOT true about Yaws:
- a. Spread by sexual transmission
- b. Caused by T. pertenue
- c. Has cross immunity with syphilis
- d. Cannot be differentiated serologically from T. pallidum

Yaws is spread by direct contact with the fluid from a lesion of an infected person. The contact is usually of a non-sexual nature. The disease is most common among children, who spread it by playing together.

143. Mode of transmission of Q fever:
- a. Mosquito
- b. Louse
- c. Ticks
- d. Mites

Coxiella burnetii is found everywhere except New Zealand. The bacterium is extremely sustainable and virulent: a single organism is able to cause an infection. The common way of infection is inhalation of contaminated dust, contact with contaminated milk, meat, or wool, and particularly birthing products. Ticks can transfer the pathogenic agent to other animals. Transfer between humans seems extremely rare and has so far been described in very few cases.

Differences between hard and soft ticks.

Hard ticks	*Soft ticks*
❑ They belong to the family Ixodidae.	❑ They belong to the family argasidae.
❑ Capitulum is anterior in position.	❑ Capitulum is ventral in position.
❑ Scutum is present.	❑ Scutum is absent.
❑ Dorsally sexual dimorphism is well marked, i.e. scutum covers the entire dorsal surface in male and covers only a small portion in the female.	❑ Sexual dimorphism is absent dorsally.
❑ Spiracles exist behind the fourth pair of legs.	❑ Spiracles exist between the third and the fourth pair of legs.
❑ Festoons are present in some hard ticks.	❑ Festoons are absent.

Contd...

Ans. **139. a.** Supplement... **140. a.** Giving TT vaccine... **141. b.** It is a diagnostic test **142. a.** Spread by sexual... **143. c.** Ticks

Contd...

Hard ticks	Soft ticks
❑ They cannot resist starvation. So they are always found on the body of the host (Day and night) (like lice)	❑ They can resist starvation for months. Therefore they are found on the body of the host only while feeding blood (i.e. only during night times) (like bedbugs).
❑ They require continuous blood meal.	❑ They require intermittent blood meal.
❑ They are always found on the body of their hosts.	❑ They are found in cracks and crevices during day time and on the body of the host during night times.
❑ Gravid female lays hundreds or thousands of eggs at one sitting.	❑ Eggs are laid in batches of 20-100 over a long period of time.
❑ Nymphal stage is one.	❑ Nymphal stages are five.
❑ Important species are Dermacentor andersoni, Haemaphysalis spinigera.	❑ Important specimen is Ornithodoros moubata
❑ Diseases transmitted are Tick typhus, (Africa) Tick paralysis, Tularemia, Viral encephalitis, Hemorrhagic fever (KFD) Human babesiosis. Rocky Mountain Spotted fever (USA), Q-fever (in US and Australia)	❑ Disease transmitted is Endemic Relapsing fever, caused by Borrelia duttoni, a spirochete.

144. Virus causing rabies in man is:

a. Domestic virus b. Street virus
c. Fixed virus d. All of the above

Rabies virus

- Rabies virus street/field virus: An isolate from a naturally infected animal, for example a dog or fox.
- Fixed/seed rabies virus: A rabies virus that has been passaged in tissue culture or animals. Fixed rabies virus has lost its pathogenicity on human beings but retains its antigenicity. The term fixed indicates only that the incubation period and virulence has been stabilized.
- Pathogenic rabies virus: A strain that typically causes rabies after peripheral inoculation.
- Attenuated rabies virus: A strain with a greatly reduced ability to cause rabies after inoculation into an animal.
- Neurotropic rabies virus: A strain that preferentially infects primary neurons or neuronal cell lines.
- Non-neurotropic rabies virus: A strain that infects neuronal cells at a level less than or equal to other cell types.

145. Quarantine period for yellow fever is:

a. 1 day b. 2 days
c. 6 days d. 10 days

Any person, Foreigner or Indian, (excluding infants below six months) arriving by air or sea without a vaccination certificate of yellow fever will be kept in quarantine isolation for a period up to 6 days

146. Which of the following shows "cyclodevelopmental" type of biological transmission:

a. Filarial parasite b. Malarial parasite
c. Plague bacilli d. All of the above

Biological transmission

- Propagative in plague and yellow fever
- Cyclopropagative in malaria
- Cyclodevelopmental in filariasis

147. Causative agent for kala-azar/visceral leishmaniasis:

a. Leishmania donovani b. Leishmania tropica
c. Leishmania braziliensis d. None of the above

Leishmaniasis

L. donovani	Visceral leishmaniasis/kala-azar
L. tropica	Cutaneous leishmaniasis/oriental sore
L. braziliensis	Mucocutaneous/nasopharyngeal leishmaniasis/espundia

148. Amplifier host for Japanese encephalitis is:

a. Man b. Pig
c. Donkey d. Culex mosquito

Japanese encephalitis

- Japanese encephalitis is a vector borne disease.
- Several species of mosquitoes are capable of transmitting JE virus.
- JE is a zoonotic infection. Natural hosts of JE virus include water birds of Ardeidae family (mainly pond herons and cattle egrets). Pigs play an important role in the natural cycle and serve as an amplifier host since they allow manifold virus multiplication without suffering from disease and maintain prolonged viraemia.
- Due to prolonged viraemia, mosquitoes get opportunity to pick up infection from pigs easily.
- Man is a dead end in transmission cycle due to low and short-lived viraemia. Mosquitoes do not get infection from JE patient.

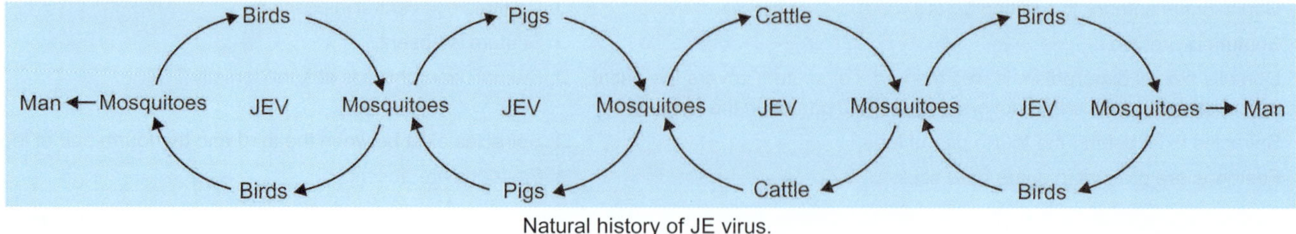

Natural history of JE virus.

Ans. 144. **b.** Street virus 145. **c.** 6 days 146. **a.** Filarial parasite 147. **a.** Leishmania...
148. **b.** Pig

149. Does NOT come under enzootic diseases:

a. Endemic typhus b. Brucellosis
c. Anthrax d. Influenza

Diseases normally present in an area are referred to as endemic, or enzootic, diseases, and they usually reflect a relatively stable relationship between the causative agent and the animals affected by it.

150. Man is dead-end for:

a. Rabies, tetanus b. Tetanus, yellow fever
c. Measles, yellow fever d. Tetanus, measles

A dead-end host or incidental host is an intermediate host that does generally not allow transmission to the definitive host, thereby preventing the parasite from completing its development. For example, humans are dead-end hosts for Echinococcus canine tapeworms, tetanus, rabies, etc.

151. Leprosy commonly spreads by:

a. Mosquitoes b. Water
c. Droplet d. Milk

Transmission of leprosy occurs during close contact with those who are infected. Transmission is believed to be by nasal droplets. *(See Diagram on next page)*

152. Drug of choice for typhoid carriers is:

a. Clindamycin b. Cotrimoxazole
c. Chloramphenicol d. Ampicillin

A chronic carrier is one who continues to discharge S typhi in either urine or stool for longer than 1 year. About 1-4% of patients who develop chronic carriage of Salmonella following enteric fever, can be treated for 6 weeks with an appropriate antibiotic. Treatment is done with amoxicillin/ampicillin and trimethoprim-sulphamethoxazole. Management of Typhoid Fever are effective in eradication of long-term carriage, with cure rates of greater than 80% after 6 weeks of therapy.

153. Scrub typhus is transmitted by:

a. Mosquito b. Tick
c. Mite d. Flea

Scrub typhus is transmitted by some species of trombiculid mites ("chiggers", particularly Leptotrombidium deliense), which are found in areas of heavy scrub vegetation. The bite of this mite leaves a characteristic black eschar that is useful for making the diagnosis.

The rickettsial diseases, their causative agents, their vectors and their reservoirs.

Diseases	*Rickettsial agent*	*Vector*	*Reservoir*
❑ Typhus group			
– Epidemic typhus	*Rickettsia prowazekii*	Louse	Humans
– Endemic typhus	*R. typhi*	Rat flea	Rodents
– Scrub typhus	*R. tsutsugamushi*	Mite*	Rodents
❑ Spotted fever group			
– Indian tick typhus	*R. conorii*	Tick*	Rodents, dogs
– Rocky mountain spotted fever	*R. rickettsii*	Tick*	Rodents, dogs
– Rickettsial pox	*R. akari*	Mite*	Mice
❑ Others			
– Trench fever	*R. quintana*	Louse	Humans
– Q-fever	*Coxiella burnetii*	Nil	Cattle, sheep, goats

* These vectors also serve as arthropod reservoir, by maintaining the rickettsiae through ovarian transmission.

154. After the appearance of rash, prophylactic isolation of measles case is necessary for a minimum of:

a. 2 days b. 5 days
c. 7 days d. 9 days

Infected people with measles should be isolated for four days after they develop a rash. Healthcare providers should follow respiratory etiquette and airborne precautions in healthcare settings.

155. All of the following diseases are reported to WHO EXCEPT:

a. Plague b. Yellow fever
c. Polio d. Cholera

The World Health Organization's International Health Regulations 1969 require disease reporting to the organization in order to help with its global surveillance and advisory role. The current (1969) regulations are rather limited with a focus on reporting of three main diseases: cholera, yellow fever and plague.

156. Culex mosquito spreads all of the following disease EXCEPT:

a. Viral arthritis b. West Nile fever
c. Yellow fever d. Bancroftian filariasis

Yellow fever virus is mainly transmitted through the bite of the yellow fever mosquito Aedes aegypti, but other mostly Aedes mosquitoes such as the tiger mosquito (Aedes albopictus) can also serve as a vector for this virus.

157. Viral infection, transmitted by tick:

a. Yellow fever b. Kyasanur forest disease
c. Dengue fever d. Japanese encephalitis

Kyasanur forest disease (KFD) is a tick-borne viral hemorrhagic fever endemic to South Asia. The disease is caused by a virus belonging to the family Flaviviridae, which also includes yellow fever and dengue fever.

Ans. **149. d.** Influenza **150. a.** Rabies, tetanus **151. c.** Droplet **152. d.** Ampicillin
153. c. Mite **154. b.** 5 days **155. c.** Polio **156. c.** Yellow fever
157. b. Kyasanur forest disease

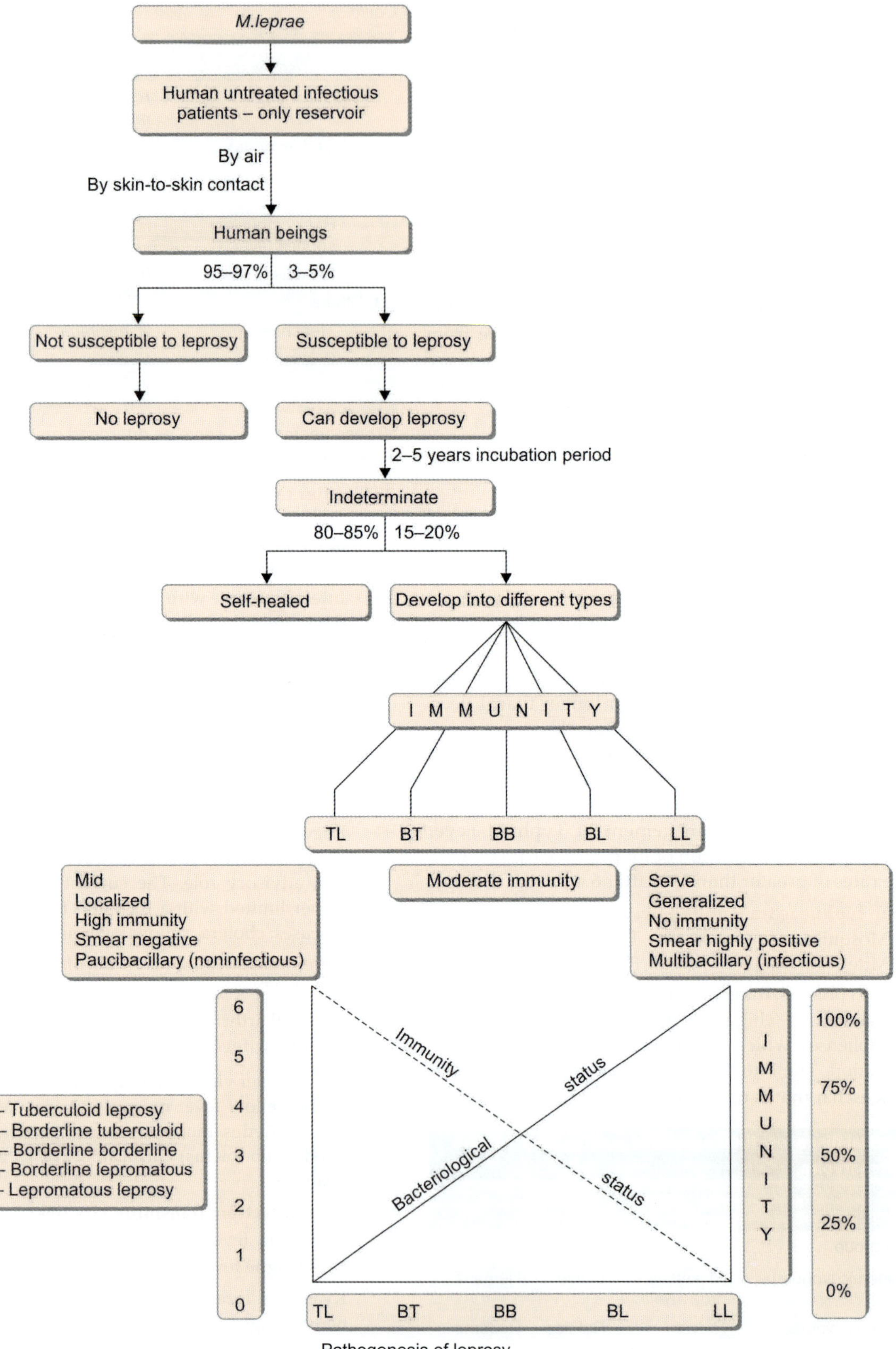

Pathogenesis of leprosy.

Source: Karnataka State Leprosy Society. Manual of Prevention of Deformity. DHFWS, Bangalore.

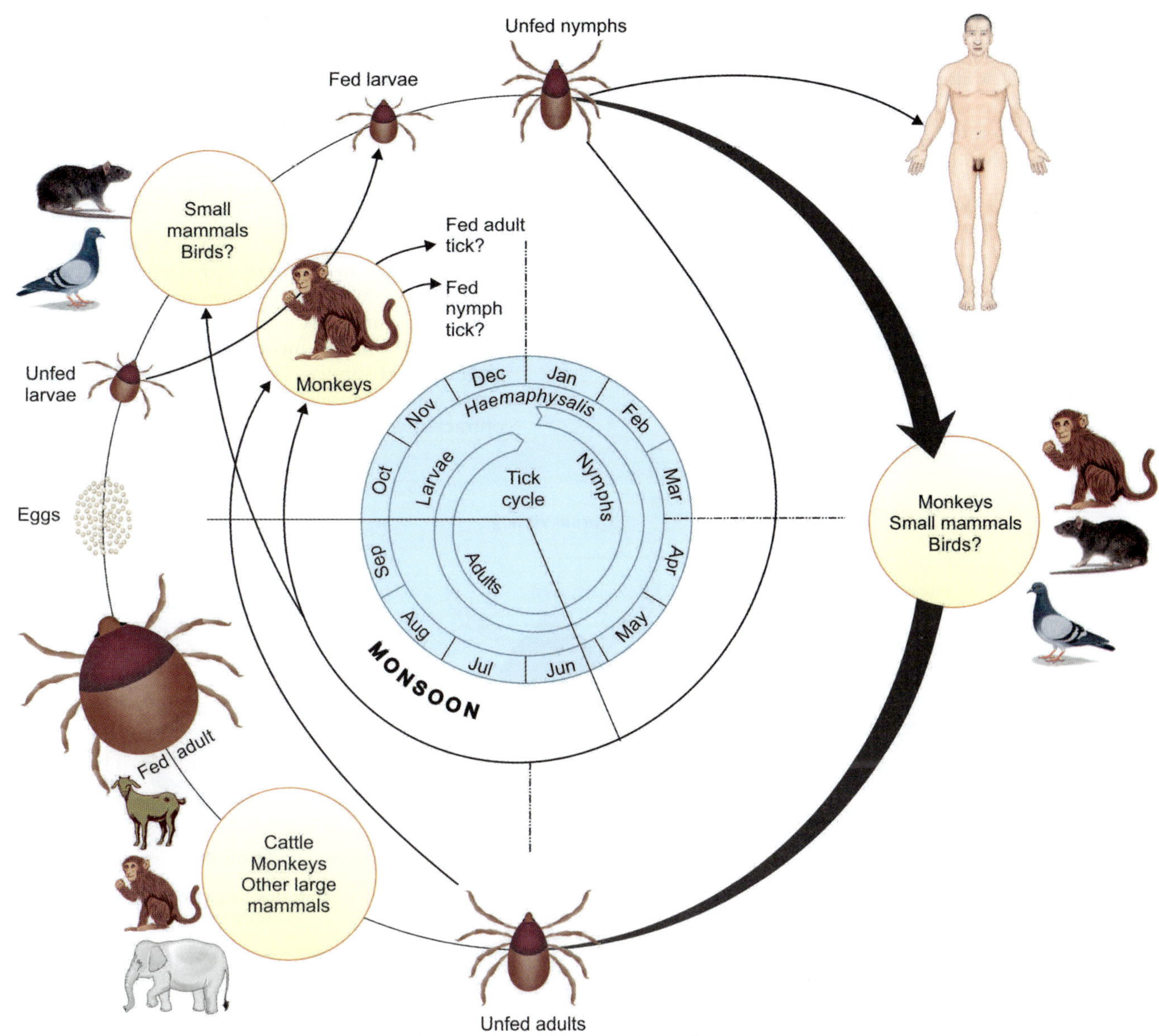

Natural cycle of Kyasanur forest disease.

158. Most appropriate test to assess the prevalence of TB infection in a community:

a. Clinical examination
b. Tuberculin test
c. Sputum examination
d. Mass miniature radiography

The Mantoux test or Mendel-Mantoux test (also known as the Mantoux screening test, tuberculin sensitivity test, Pirquet test, or PPD test for purified protein derivative) is a screening tool for tuberculosis (TB). It is one of the major tuberculin skin tests used around the world, largely replacing multiple-puncture tests such as the Tine test. The Heaf test was used until 2005 in the UK, when it was replaced by the Mantoux test.

159. Herd Immunity is a feature of all of the following diseases EXCEPT:

a. Diphtheria b. Polio
c. Tetanus d. Measles

Herd immunity does not apply to all diseases, just those that are contagious, meaning that they can be transmitted from one individual to another. Tetanus, for example, is infectious but not contagious, so herd immunity does not apply.

160. Clinical goal for prevention of coronary heart disease aims at lowering the ratio of cholesterol/HDL below:

a. 1.5 b. 2.5
c. 3.5 d. 4.5

Clinical goal for prevention of CAD

Ans. 158. b. Tuberculin test **159. c.** Tetanus **160. c.** 3.5

- Total cholesterol/HDL ratio: The goal is to keep this ratio below 5:1, with the ideal being below 3.5:1.
- LDL/HDL ratio: The goal is to keep this ratio below 5:1, with the ideal being below 3.5:1.
- HDL/LDL ratio: The goal is to keep the ratio above 0.3, with the ideal HDL/LDL ratio being above 0.4.

161. Incubation period of measles is:

a. 5 days b. 10 days
c. 15 days d. 20 days

IP of measles is 10 days between the onset of infection and the onset of fever and it is 14 days between the infection and the appearance of rash.

162. Vector for Yellow fever is:

a. Aedes b. Culex
c. Anopheles d. Mansonoides

Some species of Aedes genus transmit serious diseases, including dengue fever, yellow fever, the Zika virus, and chikungunya.

163. Kyasanur forest disease is transmitted by:

a. Mite b. Tick
c. Mosquito d. None of the above

The disease was first reported from Kyasanur Forest of Karnataka in India in March 1957. The disease first manifested as an epizootic outbreak among monkeys killing several of them in the year 1957. Hence the disease is also locally known as Monkey Disease or Monkey Fever. There are a variety of animals thought to be reservoir hosts for the disease, including porcupines, rats, squirrels, mice and shrews. The vector for disease transmission is Haemaphysalis spinigera, a forest tick. Humans contract infection from the bite of nymphs of the tick.

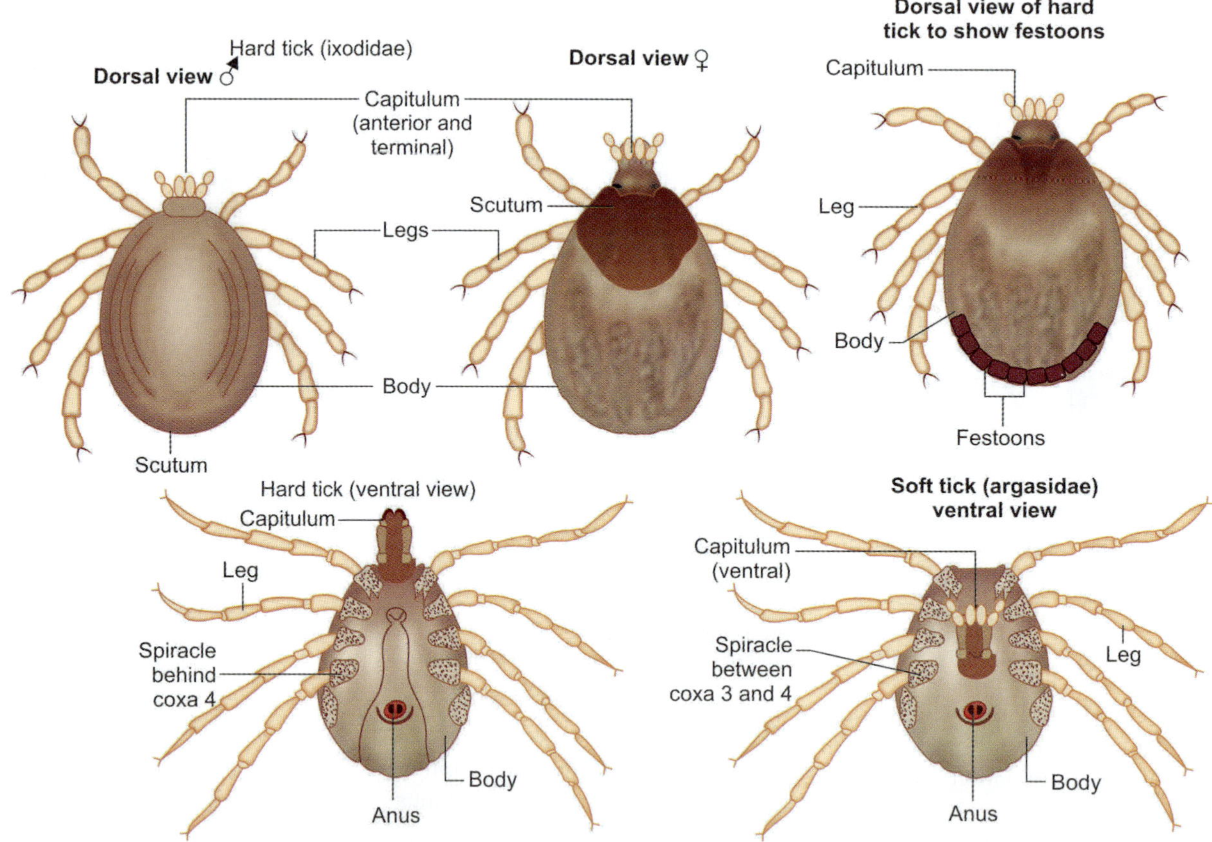

Dorsal and ventral views of hard and soft ticks.
Source: Ratnaswamy GK. A Handbook of Medical Entomology and Elementary Parasitology. 1st edn, 1974.

164. The definitive host for echinococcus granulosus is:

a. Man
b. Sheep
c. Hound
d. Dog

The lifecycle of E. granulosus involves dogs and wild carnivores as a definitive host for the adult tapeworm. Definitive hosts are where parasites reach maturity and reproduce. Wild or domesticated ungulates, such as sheep, serve as an intermediate host.

165. Which is NOT a complication of chicken pox:

a. Pancreatitis b. Pneumonia
c. Encephalitis d. Thrombocytopenia

Ans. **161. b.** 10 days **162. a.** Aedes **163. b.** Tick **164. d.** Dog **165. a.** Pancreatitis

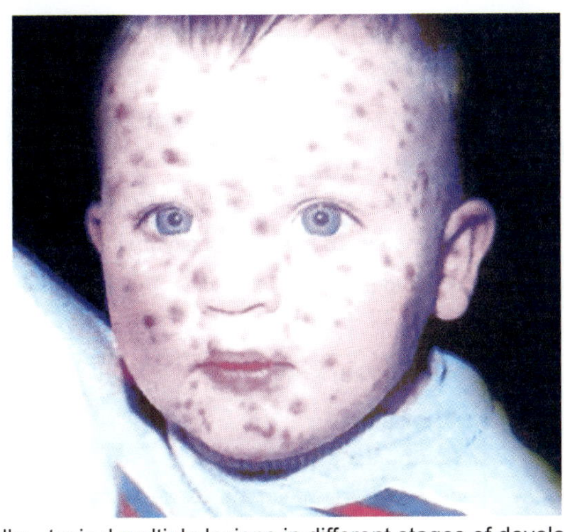
Varicella—typical multiple lesions in different stages of development.

In adults, the disease is more severe, though the incidence is much less common. Infection in adults is associated with greater morbidity and mortality due to pneumonia (either direct viral pneumonia or secondary bacterial pneumonia), bronchitis (either viral bronchitis or secondary bacterial bronchitis), hepatitis, and encephalitis.

166. Nongonococcal urethritis is caused by:

a. Chlamydia
b. Hemophilus
c. Treponema
d. Gardnerella vaginalis

The most common bacterial cause of NGU is Chlamydia trachomatis, but it can also be caused by Ureaplasma urealyticum, Haemophilus vaginalis, and Mycoplasma genitalium.

The syndromes in STI.

	Common clinical signs	*Most common causes*	*Etiology*
Genital ulcer in males or females	Genital ulcer on penis or scrotum in men; on labia, vagina or cervix in women	Syphilis Chancroid Genital herpes Lymphogranuloma-venereum Donovanosis	*Treponema pallidum* *Haemophilus ducreyi* *Herpes simplex virus* *Chlamydia trachomatis (L1-L3)* *Calymmatobacterium granulomatis*
Urethral discharge, dysuria in males	Urethral discharge on milking urethra	Gonorrhea Nongonococcal urethritis	*N. gonorrhoea* *C trachomatis or Ureaplasma*
Vaginal discharge	Abnormal vaginal and/or cervical discharge Vaginal inflammation Cervical friability	Cervicitis Gonorrhea Chlamydial infection	*N. gonorrhoea* *C trachomatis*
	Cervical motion tenderness	Vaginitis Trichomoniasis Bacterial vaginosis Candidiasis	*Trichomonas vaginalis* *Gardnerella vaginalis, anaerobes* *Candida albicans*
Lower abdominal pain in women	Adnexal + cervical motion tenderness	Gonorrhea Chlamydial infection	*N. gonorrhoea* *C. trachomatis*
Dyspareunia, irregular bleeding	Vaginal or cervical discharge Fever (sometimes)	Anaerobes	Anaerobes
Inguinal swelling or bubo in males or females	Inguinal lymphadenopathy with or without ulceration	Lymphogranuloma venereum	*C. trachomatis (L1-L3)*
Scrotal swelling or pain in males	Red + Edematous scrotum Urethral signs	Gonorrhea Nongonococcal urethritis	*N. gonorrhoea* *C. trachomatis or Ureaplasma Urealyticum*

167. Smoking predisposes to all of the following cancers EXCEPT:

a. Carcinoma larynx
b. Carcinoma bladder
c. Carcinoma stomach
d. Lymphoma

Smoking is a leading cause of cancer and death from cancer. It causes cancers of the lung, esophagus, larynx, mouth, throat, kidney, bladder, liver, pancreas, stomach, cervix, colon, and rectum, as well as acute myeloid leukemia

Ans. 166. a. Chlamydia **167. d.** Lymphoma

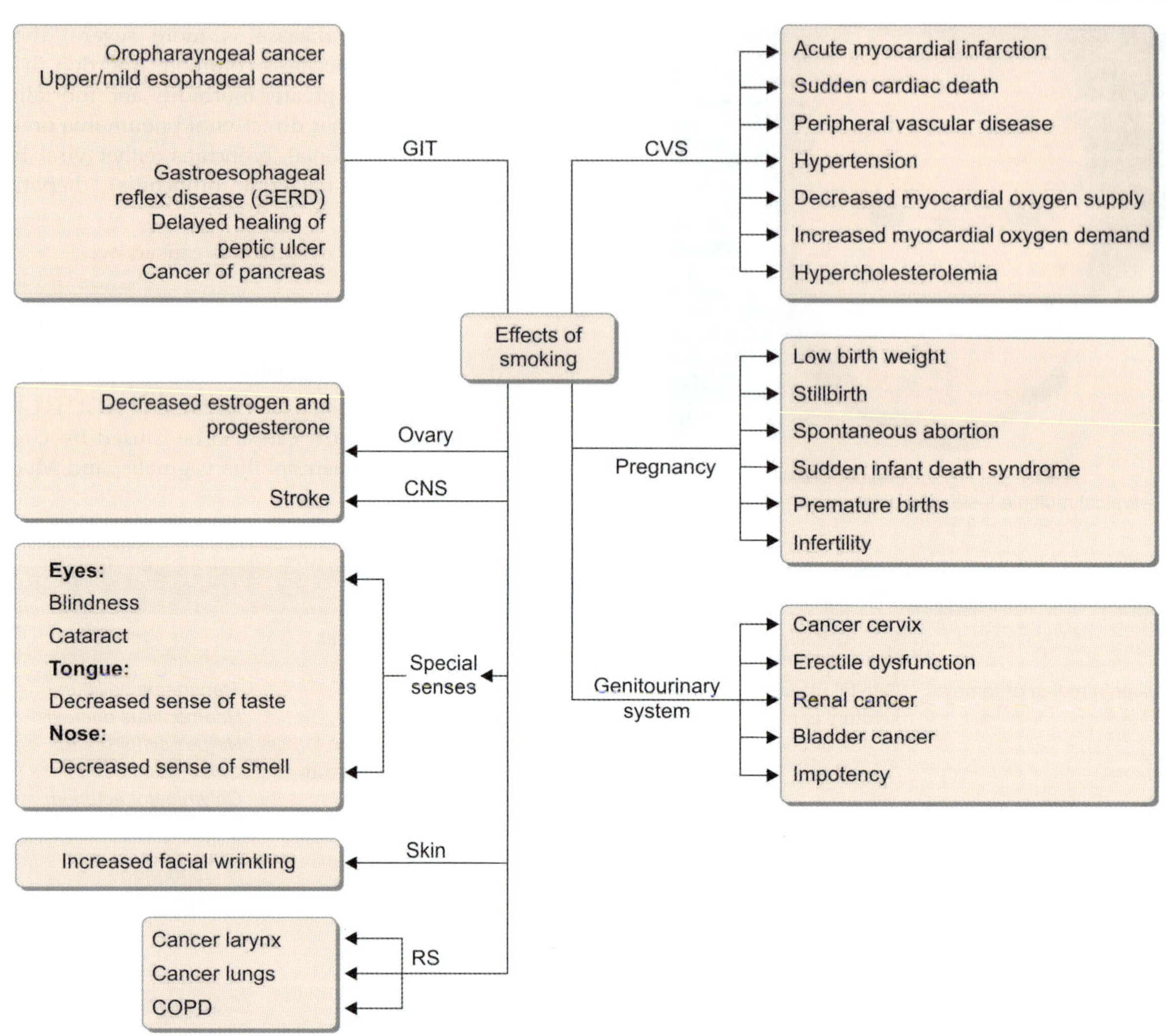

Summary of tobacco related diseases.

168. The mass treatment of trachoma is undertaken if the prevalence in community is:

a. 3% b. 10%
c. 5% d. 6%

If assessment at the subdistrict or community level is undertaken in subdistricts or communities where the prevalence of follicular trachoma in 1- to 9-year-old children is 10% or more, conduct mass treatment of all people with antibiotics.

169. Adult HIV prevalence in India is:

a. 0.2% b. 0.3%
c. 0.4% d. 0.5%

The adult HIV prevalence in India is declining from estimated level of 0.41% in 2000 through 0.36% in 2006 to 0.31% in 2009. Adult HIV prevalence at a national level has declined notably in many states, but variations still exist across the states.

170. Incidence rate of Neonatal tetanus under NT control districts is:

a. Less than 1/1000 live births
b. More than 1/1000 live births
c. Less than 0.1/1000 live births
d. More than 0.1/1000 live births

In 1989 the World Health Congress called for the elimination of neonatal tetanus. UNICEF took the lead, assisted by other United Nations agencies, individual governments, and non-profit organizations. By 2000 the disease was declared as eliminated from 104 of 161 developing countries. "NNT Control district" is defined as incidence rate less than 1 case per 1,000 live births in every district of the country.

171. Cyclopropagative transmission is seen in:

a. Plague bacilli in rate flea
b. Malarial parasite in anopheline mosquito
c. Filarial parasite in culex mosquito
d. Guineaworm embryo in cyclops

Ans. **168. b.** 10% **169. b.** 0.3% **170. a.** Less than 1/1000... **171. b.** Malarial parasite...

Cyclopropagative biological transmission: Disease agent undergoes cyclical change and multiplies in the body of the arthropod, e.g. malaria parasite in anopheline mosquito.

172. Life span of housefly in summer:

a. 5 days b. 15 days
c. 25 days d. 35 days

The average life span of the housefly is 2–3 months but during summer, it is reduced to 2–3 weeks

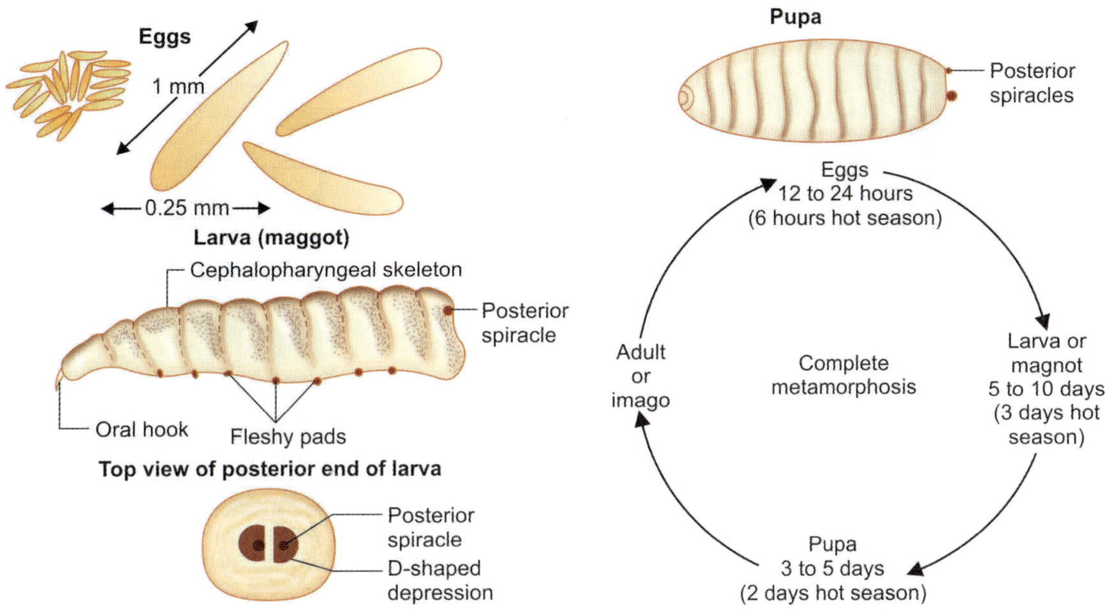

Eggs
1 mm
0.25 mm
Larva (maggot)
Cephalopharyngeal skeleton
Posterior spiracle
Oral hook
Fleshy pads
Top view of posterior end of larva
Posterior spiracle
D-shaped depression
Pupa
Posterior spiracles
Eggs 12 to 24 hours (6 hours hot season)
Larva or magnot 5 to 10 days (3 days hot season)
Pupa 3 to 5 days (2 days hot season)
Adult or imago
Complete metamorphosis

Life cycle of housefly.
Source: Ratnaswamy GK. A Handbook of Medical Entomology and Elementary Parasitology. 1st edn, 1974.

173. Diseases transmitted by louse:

a. Epidemic typhus b. Scrub typhus
c. Q fever
d. Rocky mountain spotted fever

Epidemic typhus (also called "camp fever", "jail fever", "hospital fever", "ship fever", "famine fever", "putrid fever", "petechial fever", "Epidemic louse-borne typhus," and "louse-borne typhus") is a form of typhus so named because the disease often causes epidemics following wars and natural disasters. The causative organism is *Rickettsia prowazekii*, transmitted by the human body louse (*Pediculus humanus humanus*).

Differences between head and body louse.

	Head louse	*Body louse*
Nomenclature	❑ It is pediculus *humanus* capitis	It is pediculus *humanus corporis*
Habitat	❑ It is found on hairs of scalp	Found on body hairs and seams of clothes
Oviposition	❑ Eggs are laid in occipital region. About 150 eggs are laid at the rate of 5–6 daily	Eggs are laid on body hairs and clothes. About 300 eggs are laid at the rate of 8–10 daily
Longevity	❑ Four weeks	Six weeks
Mode of spread	❑ Usually spreads from person to person when they are in close contact or through common items like combs	Usually it spreads through the medium of clothes, combs, caps, towels, bed-sheets or pillow covers, etc.

174. Incubation period of mumps is:

a. 4–5 days b. 7–15 days
c. 12–24 days d. 50 days

Symptoms of mumps typically occur 16 to 18 days after exposure and resolve after 7 to 10 days. Symptoms in adults are often more severe than in children. About a third of people have mild or no symptoms.

175. Life cycle of filaria is:

a. Cyclodevelopmental b. Cyclopropagative
c. Propagative d. Transovarian

Cyclodevelopmental transmission of an arthropod *transmitted* disease wherein the causal organism undergoes cyclical changes but does not multiply in the body of the arthropod. It is seen in filariasis.

Ans. 172. b. 15 days **173. a.** Epidemic typhus **174. c.** 12–24 days **175. a.** Cyclodevelopmental

176. All are transmitted by soft tick EXCEPT:

a. KFD b. Tularemia
c. Q fever d. Relapsing fever

Tularemia (or *tularaemia*; also known as *Pahvant Valley plague, rabbit fever, deer fly fever*, and *Ohara's fever*) is a serious infectious disease caused by the intracellular bacterium *Francisella tularensis*. The primary vectors are hard ticks and deer flies, but the disease can also be spread through other arthropods. The disease is named after Tulare County, California.

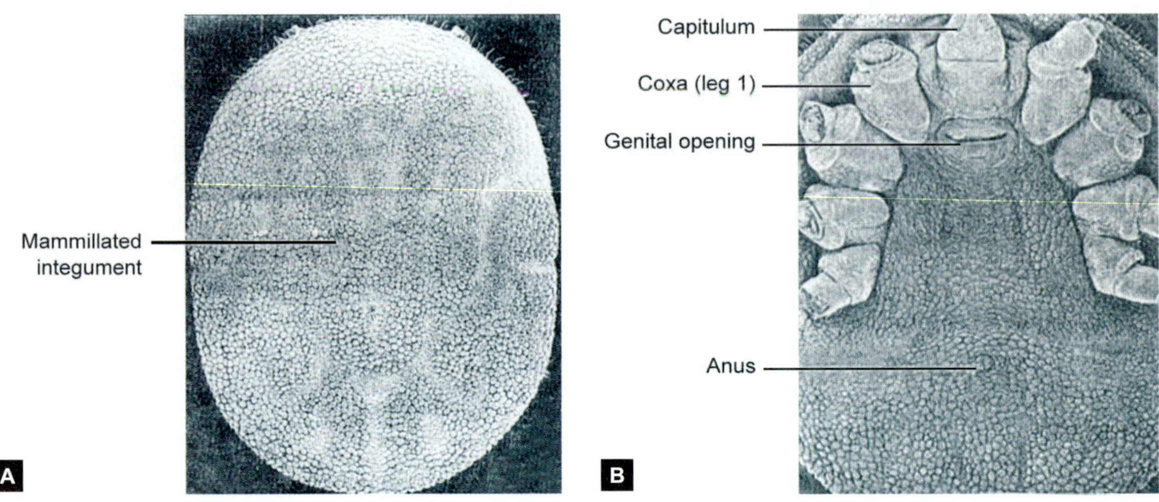

(A) Dorsal view of adult female *Ornithodorus moubata* (soft tick); (B) Ventral view of adult female *Ornithodorus moubata*.
Source (A): Manson Bhar, Bell DR. Manson's Tropical Diseases. ELBS, 19th edn, 1987.

177. Endemic typhus is transmitted by:

a. Flea b. Mite
c. Tick d. Louse

Murine typhus (also called *endemic typhus*) is a form of typhus transmitted by fleas (Xenopsylla cheopis), usually on rats. (This is in contrast to epidemic typhus, which is usually transmitted by lice.) Murine typhus is an under-recognized entity, as it is often confused with viral illnesses. Most people who are infected do not realize that they have been bitten by fleas.

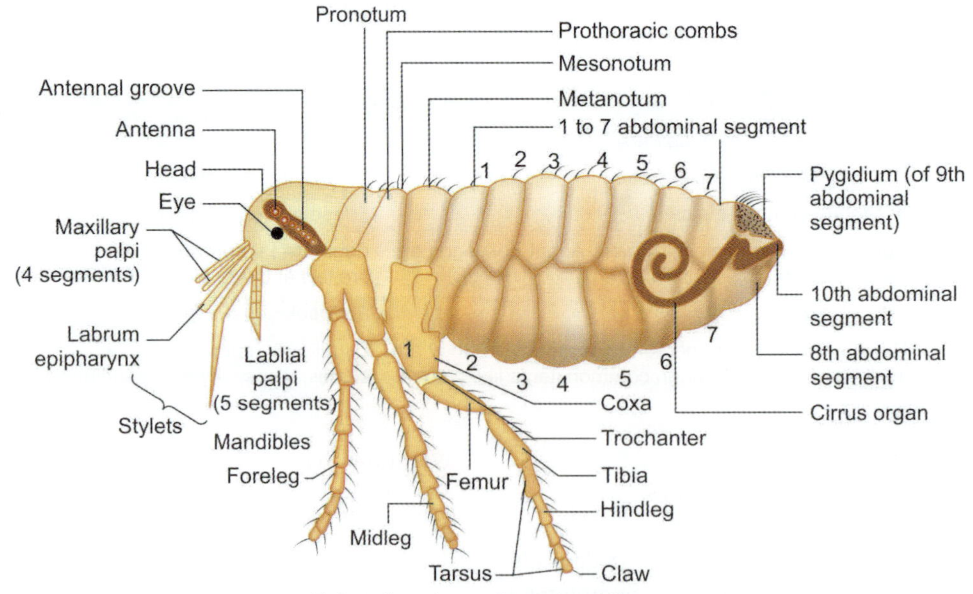

External anatomy of a male rat flea.
Source: Ratnaswamy GK. A Handbook of Medical Entomology and Elementary Parasitology. 1st edn, 1974.

Ans. **176. b.** Tularemia **177. a.** Flea

178. 'DOTS' indicates:
a. Short term treatment under supervision
b. Short term treatment without supervision
c. Long term treatment under supervision
d. Long term treatment without supervision

DOTS (directly observed treatment, short-course.), is the name given to the tuberculosis control strategy recommended by the World Health Organization. According to WHO, "The most cost-effective way to stop the spread of TB in communities with a high incidence is by curing it. The best curative method for TB is known as DOTS." DOTS has five main components:

- Government commitment (including political will at all levels, and establishment of a centralized and prioritized system of TB monitoring, recording and training).
- Case detection by sputum smear microscopy.
- Standardized treatment regimen directly of six to nine months observed by a healthcare worker or community health worker for at least the first two months.
- A drug supply.
- A standardized recording and reporting system that allows assessment of treatment results.

Differences between DOTS and DOTS-plus.

DOTS	*DOTS-plus*
❑ This strategy is to control tuberculosis	❑ This strategy is to control MDR-TB
❑ Launched in India during 1993	❑ Launched in India during 2007
❑ Diagnosis is confirmed by two sputum smear examination done in microscopy center/laboratory (since April 1, 2009)	❑ Diagnosis is confirmed by sputum culture and susceptibility test done in intermediate reference laboratory (IRL)
❑ Patients are categorized as I, II only (since January 2010)	❑ Patients are categorized as resistant cases only
❑ Treatment is by intermittent regimen with first-line of drugs	❑ Treatment is by daily regimen with second-line of drugs
❑ Patients are usually not admitted in the hospital	❑ Patients are admitted and treated in the RNTCP designated sites only
❑ The entire course of intensive phase (IP) and the first dose of the week of continuation phase is provided by DOTS provider	❑ Entire course of treatment during both intensive phase and continuation phase is given by DOTS-provider
❑ Total duration of treatment is for 6 to 9 months only	❑ Total duration of treatment is minimum 2 years
❑ IP is for 2 months in Cats I and for 3 months in Cat II, CP is for 4 to 6 months	❑ IP is for 6 to 9 months CP is for 18 months

179. All of the following are true for Kyasanur Forest Disease EXCEPT:
a. Caused by Arbovirus
b. Transmitted by bite of infective ticks
c. Incubation period of 1 week
d. Man to man transmission is seen

The disease was first noted at Kyasanur village near Sagar in Shivamogga district of Karnataka. The virus has been detected in monkeys in parts of Bandipur National Park (Chamarajnagar) and parts of the Nilgiris. Human infection occurred in Bandipur through handling of dead monkeys that were infected. Man is only an accidental host. Since the human reservoir have a very short period of viremia, affected persons do not act as a source of infection. Thus, human reservoirs play no part in virus transmission.

Treatment regimens under the RNTCP.

Category oftreatment	*Type of patient*	*Regimen*
Category I	New sputum smear-positive Seriously ill sputum smear-negative Seriously ill extrapulmonary	2 $(HRZE)_3$/ 4$(HR)_3$
Category II	Previously treated Sputum smear-positive relapse Sputum smear-positive failure Sputum smear-positive treatment Others	2 $(HRZES)_3$/ 1 $(HRZE)_3$/ 5 $(HRE)_3$

180. Which of the following is true for DOTS:
a. Treatment under supervision
b. Every patient is given the same treatment
c. Streptomycin is given to all the patients
d. Daily regimen

DEMOGRAPHY AND PREVENTIVE HEALTH

181. While calculating dependency ratio, Numerator is:
a. Population of >10 years & <65 years
b. Population <15 years & >65 years
c. Population of <10 years & >65 years
d. Population of >15 years & <60 years

Ans. **178. a.** Short term... **179. d.** Man to man transm... **180. a.** Treatment... **181. b.** Population <15...

Total dependency ratio
- Numerator: Children 0-14 years age + population more than 65 years of age
- Denominator: Population of 15-64 years

182. All are beneficiaries of ICDS scheme EXCEPT:
a. Adolescent females
b. Adolescent males
c. Pregnant females
d. Lactating females

Beneficiaries in ICDS
- Pregnant woman
- Nursing mothers
- Other women 15-45 years
- Children less than 3 years
- Children in age group 3-6 years
- Adolescent girls 11-18 years

183. ICDS scheme does NOT include:
a. Children in the age group of 0–6 years
b. Primary school children
c. Pregnant women d. Lactating women

Integrated Child Development Services (ICDS) is an Indian government welfare programme which provides food, preschool education, and primary healthcare to children under 6 years of age and their mothers. These services are provided from *Anganwadi* centres established mainly in rural areas and staffed with frontline workers. In addition to fighting malnutrition and ill health, the programme is also intended to combat gender inequality by providing girls the same resources as boys.

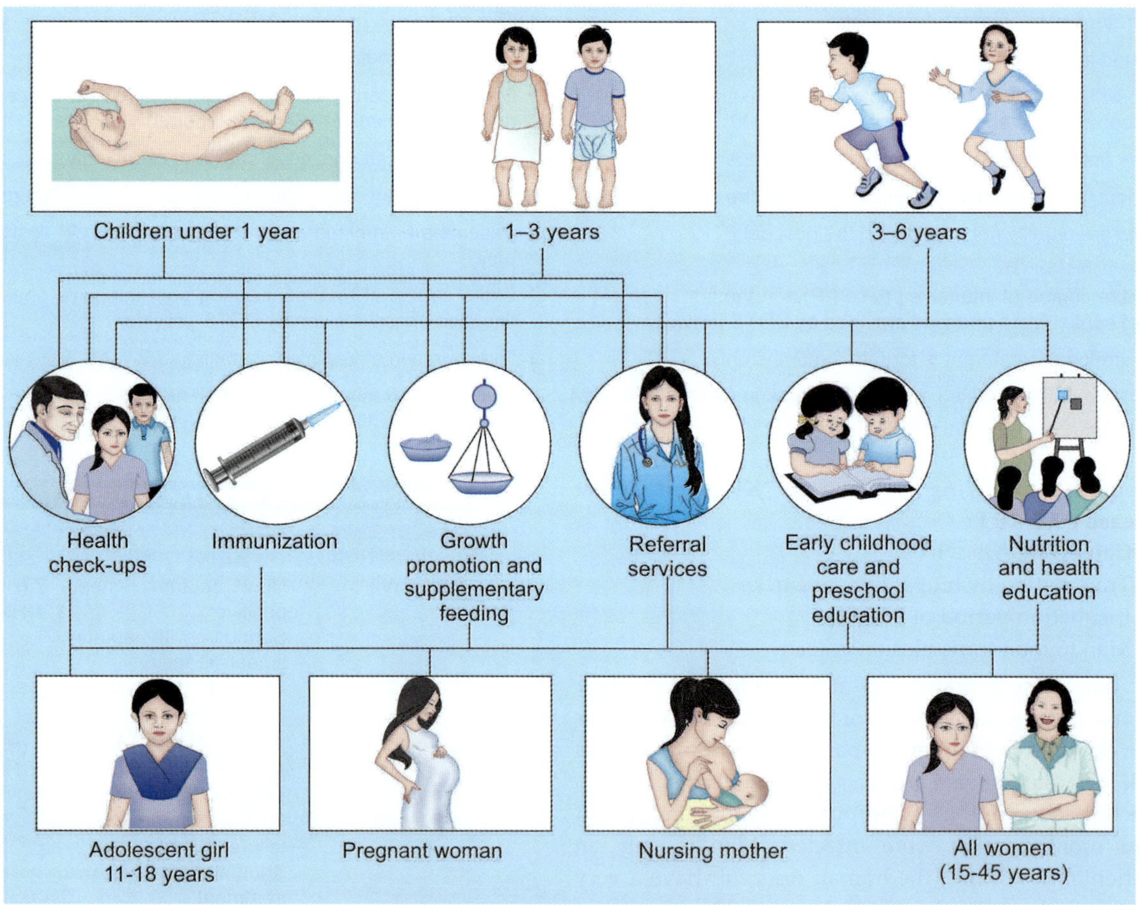

Services and beneficiaries of ICDS.
Source: UNICEF. Integrated Child Development Services. Regional Office, New Delhi 1984.

184. Upper line in road-to-health card corresponds to what percentile of WHO chart:
a. 95th percentile
b. 90th percentile
c. 50th percentile
d. 30th percentile

The **lines** used on growth charts vary greatly and it is important to determine what is being plotted. For the WHO growth chart, the **upper** curve represents the 50th percentile. It is considered 100% standard in growth charts used in India.

Ans. 182. b. Adolescent... **183. b.** Primary school... **184. c.** 50th percentile

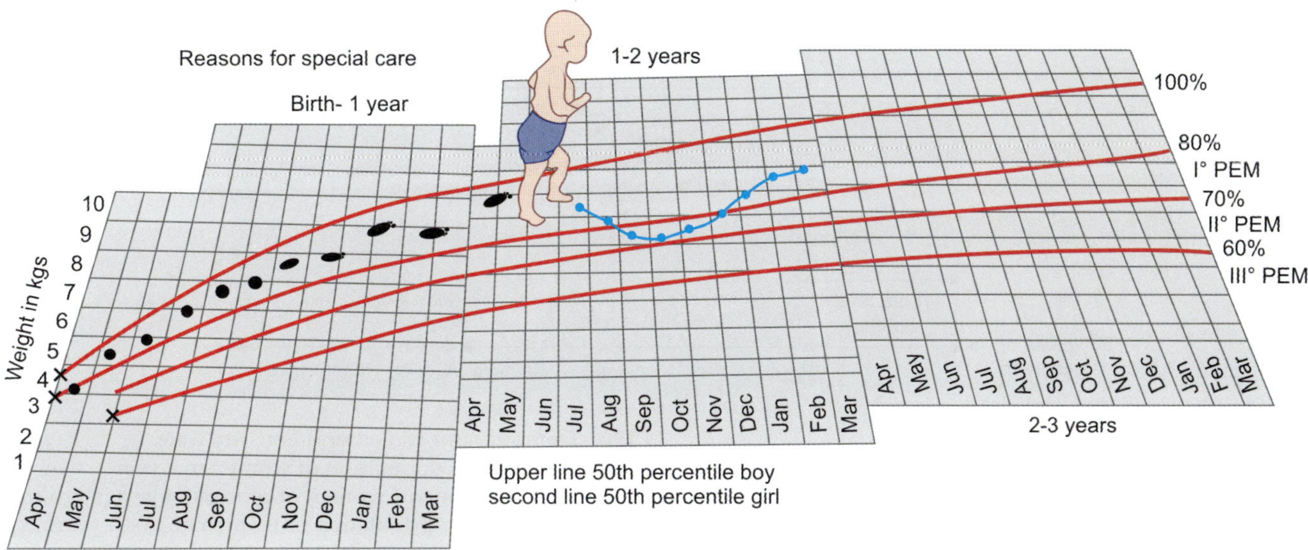

The road to health chart.

185. As per WHO, anemia is considered to exist in pregnancy, if the hemoglobin level is below:

a. 11 gm%
b. 14 gm%
c. 12 gm%
d. 13 gm%

Hemoglobin levels in WHO cut off criteria for anemia (in venous blood)

Adult male	13 g/dL
Adult woman (non-pregnant)	12 g/dL
Adult woman (pregnant)	11 g/dL
Child above 6 years	12 g/dL
Child below 6 years	11 g/dL

186. NOT a parameter in evaluation of the efficacy of acceptance of family planning method:

a. Annual general marriage rate
b. Spacing between first and second child
c. Annual birth rate
d. Number of children born

The **general marriage rate** is the number of **marriages** per 1,000 un-married population aged 16 years and over.

187. Regarding baby friendly UNICEF plan, all are true EXCEPT:

a. Mother and child are left together 24 hours a day
b. Feeding on demand
c. No food/water given other than breast milk
d. Feeding started with 4 hours of birth

Ten steps to successful breastfeeding.

- Have a written breastfeeding policy that is routinely communicated to all health care staff.

Contd...

Contd...

- Train all health care staff in skills necessary to implement this policy.
- Inform all pregnant women about the benefits and management of breastfeeding.
- Help mothers initiate breastfeeding within one half-hour of birth.
- Show mothers how to breastfeed and maintain lactation, even if they should be separated from their infants.
- Give newborn infants no food or drink other than breastmilk, unless medically indicated.
- Practice rooming in—that is, allow mothers and infants to remain together 24 hours a day.
- Encourage breastfeeding on demand.
- Give no artificial teats or pacifiers (also called dummies or soothers) to breastfeeding infants.
- Foster the establishment of breastfeeding support groups and refer mothers to them on discharge from the hospital or clinic.

188. Sensitive parameter of combined obstetric and pediatric care in the country is:

a. Post neonatal mortality rate
b. Infant mortality rate
c. Neonatal mortality rate
d. Perinatal mortality rate

Perinatal mortality rate (PNMR) is defined as the number of stillbirths (SB; 28th week of gestation onwards) and the first week death (FWD) per thousand total births. It is the most sensitive index of maternal and neonatal care and the socioeconomic standard of a particular area. In developed countries, the PNMR has fallen to 10–20 per thousand total births as compared to an alarmingly high rate of 60–120/1000 total births in developing countries. High risk pregnancies have higher PNMR and comprise the majority of perinatal death.

Ans. **185. a.** 11 gm% **186. a.** Annual general... **187. d.** Feeding started... **188. d.** Perinatal mortality rate

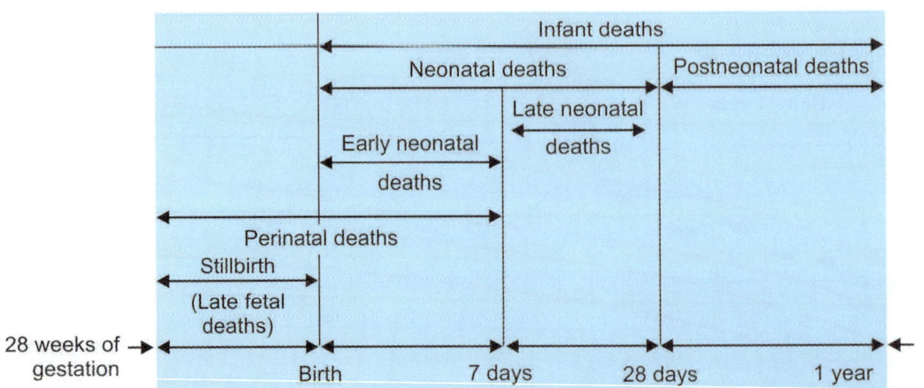

189. Perinatal death includes death:

a. After 28 weeks of pregnancy
b. 7 days after birth
c. Both
d. None

Perinatal mortality rate is the sum of the number of resident fetal deaths of 28 or more weeks gestation plus the number of resident newborns dying under 7 days of age in a specified geographic area (country, state, county, etc.) divided by the sum of the number of resident live births plus the number of resident fetal deaths of 28 or more weeks gestation for the same geographic area (for a specified time period, usually a calendar year) and multiplied by 1,000.

190. Denominator in General Fertility Rate:

a. Average population of women in a year
b. Population of women of reproductive age group
c. Mid-year population of women of 15–44 years age
d. None of the above

Number of live births per 1,000 women ages 15–49 in a given year is general fertility rate.

191. Infant mortality does NOT include:

a. Early neonatal mortality
b. Perinatal mortality
c. Post neonatal mortality
d. Late neonatal mortality

The infant mortality rate (IMR) is the number of **deaths** of **infants** under one year old per 1,000 live births. This **rate** is often used as an indicator of the level of health in a country.

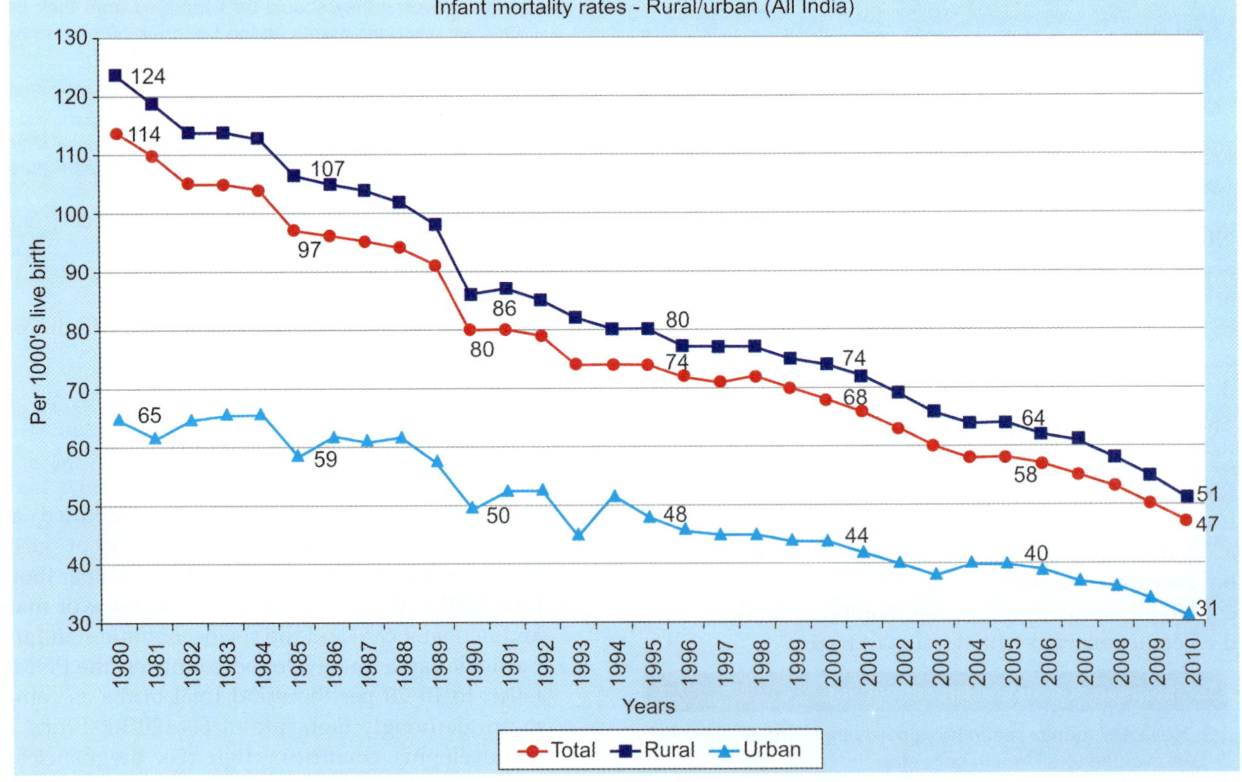

Infant mortality rate.
Source: Government of India. MOHFW. Family Welfare Statistics in India. 2011.

Ans. 189. c. Both **190. c.** Mid-year population... **191. b.** Perinatal mortality

192. Mortality rates are taken into account while calculating:

a. General fertility rate
b. NRR
c. Total fertility rate
d. Gross reproduction rate

The **net reproduction rate** (NRR) is the average number of daughters that would be born to a female (or a group of females) if she passed through her lifetime conforming to the age-specific **fertility** and mortality **rates** of a given year.

193. For international comparisons, perinatal mortality rate is calculated as late fetal deaths (28 weeks gestation or more) plus early neonatal deaths (first week) [weighing over 1 kg at birth] in a year per:

a. 100 live births [weighing over 1 kg at birth]
b. 1,000 live births [weighing over 1 kg at birth]
c. 10,000 live births [weighing over 1 kg at birth]
d. 1,00,000 live births [weighing over 1 kg at birth]

Great variation exists both between and within countries on how the stillbirth component of perinatal mortality is recorded, particularly for early stillbirths that occur at 22- to 27-week gestation. For international comparisons, WHO suggests including only deaths of fetuses weighing at least 1000 g, or of 28-week gestation or more if weight is unavailable (i.e. total live births and not total live- and stillbirths). Presentations of the PMR should include a clear statement of the definition of perinatal mortality used. In practice, in most developing countries accurate data on birth weight or gestational age are difficult to obtain.

194. Which fertility indicator gives the approximate magnitude of completed family size:

a. General fertility rate
b. Age-specific fertility rate
c. Total fertility rate
d. Gross reproduction rate

Total fertility rate: The number of children who would be born per woman (or per 1,000 women) if she/they were to pass through the childbearing years bearing children according to a current schedule of age-specific **fertility rates**.

195. Growth rate of population is calculated as:

a. Crude birth rate + crude death rate
b. Crude birth rate – crude death rate
c. Crude birth rate/crude death rate
d. Crude death rate/crude birth rate

Crude Birth Rate (CBR) is annual number of live births per **1,000 people** in a given area. Crude Death Rate (CDR) is annual number of deaths per **1,000 people** in a given area.

Demographic profile of India.

		1991	*2001*	*2011*
1.	Population (in million)	846	1028	1211
2.	Crude birth rate (per 1,000 MYP)	29.5	25.4	20.97
3.	Crude death rate (per 1,000 MYP)	9.8	8.4	7.48
4.	Growth rate (BR – DR)	19.7	17.0	13.49
5.	Infant mortality rate (per 1,000 LB)	80	66	47.5
6.	Maternal mortality rate (per 1,000 LB)	3.98	3.01	2.12
7.	Literacy rate female (percent)	-	53	65.5
8.	Sex ratio (females per 1,000 males)	927	933	940
9.	Couple protection rate (percent)	44.1	45.6	40.4
10.	Expectation of life at birth (years) Male	60.6	61.8	63
	Female	61.7	63.5	64.2

Source: GOI. MOHFW. Family Welfare Statistics in India 2011.

196. Population of more than 65-year-old as per SRS estimates, 2007:

a. 5.0%
b. 6.3%
c. 7.4%
d. 8.5%

Age structure

0–14 years: 30.8%; male: 188,208,196, female: 171,356,024

15–64 years: 64.3%; male: 386,432,921, female: 364,215,759

65+ years: 4.9%; male: 27,258,259, female: 30, 031, 289 (2007 est.).

197. MC cause of infant mortality in India:

a. Low birth weight
b. Birth injury
c. Sepsis
d. Congenital anomalies

The lack of decrease in **infant** and neonatal **mortality rates** in recent years is due in large part to the increasing proportion of preterm and **low birth weight infants.** Preterm birth is the most common direct cause of newborn mortality. Preterm birth and being small for gestational age (SGA), which is the reason for low-birth-weight (LBW), are also important indirect causes of neonatal deaths. LBW contributes to **60%** to **80%** of all neonatal deaths.

Birth weight	*Grade*
> 3500 g	Obese
3500–2500 g	Normal birth wt (Av = 2.7 to 2.9 kg)
2500–2000 g	LBW
2000–1000 g	Very low birth weight
< 1000 g	Extremely LBW

Ans. **192. b.** NRR **193. b.** 1,000 live births **194. c.** Total fertility rate **195. b.**Crude birth rate... **196. a.** 5.0% **197. a.** Low birth weight

198. Denominator while calculating maternal mortality rate in developed countries:
a. 1,00,000 live births
b. 1,00,000 women of reproductive age
c. 10,000 live births
d. 10,000 women of reproductive age

Maternal death is the death of a woman while pregnant or within 42 days of termination of pregnancy, irrespective of the duration and site of the pregnancy, from any cause related to or aggravated by the pregnancy or its management but not from accidental or incidental causes. In developed countries, it is estimated per 1,00,000 live births because MMR is very low.

199. Under Reproductive and Child Health (RCH) programme, which one of the following interventions is done only in selected district:
a. Medical termination of pregnancy at PHC level
b. High quality of training at all levels
c. Screening and treatment of RTI at district level
d. Transport facility for referral of pregnant women during pregnancy

RCH Program objectives
- Promotion of MCH to ensure safe mother hood and child survival
- Reduction of maternal and child morbidity and mortality
- Attainment of population stabilization

Services provided in tribal areas under RCH-II.

Tier	Services
Community level	Community based worker/ASHA to work as social mobilizer, educator and provider of non-clinical services and to work as Depot holder for contraceptives. To act as DOTS provider for the revised National TB Control Program, to take malaria slides, store and distribute anti-malaria drugs, create awareness about sanitation, safe drinking water and participate in the other health care programs.
Subcenter	ANC and PNC services, IFA distribution, delivery by skilled attendant, referral for institutional delivery, contraceptive distribution and referral for terminal methods, immunization, management of childhood illness, deworming, nutrition and health education for mothers, treatment of minor aliments including RTI/STI, services under national program like DOTS, NMCP, counseling services.
PHC	All above + dispense ayurvedic, homeopathic, unani and tribal system of medicines.
Block PHC/ CHC	All above + Terminal method of FP EOC + elective abortion 1st trimester, MVA, screening and clinical based services for sickle cell anemia, Thalassemia, G-6 PD deficiency and Lab services.

200. Sample registration system is done once in:
a. 6 months b. 1 year
c. 2 years d. 5 years

Half-yearly survey is carried out independently in each sample unit by a fulltime supervisor. The supervisor belonging to the statistical cadre of the State Census Directorates (either a Compiler or a Sr. Compiler or Statistical Investigator or any suitable official) visits each household in the sample unit and records the particulars of births and deaths in Forms 9 and 10 respectively in respect of all the usual residents and visitors (only those occurring within the sample unit) which had occurred during the halfyearly period (January–June or July–December) under reference. Simultaneously, he updates the house-list, the household schedule and the pregnancy status of women by making entries of changes, if any. While carrying out this survey he does not have access to the birth and death records of the enumerator for the same periods which are withdrawn from the field before the supervisor's visit for the half yearly survey.

201. National Family Health Survey has completed how many rounds:
a. 1 round b. 2 rounds
c. 3 rounds d. 4 rounds

In 2014–2015, India implemented the fourth National Family Health Survey (NFHS-4)

202. The number of live births per 1,000 women in the reproductive age group in a year refers to:
a. Gross reproduction rate
b. Total fertility rate
c. Net reproduction rate
d. General fertility rate

The **general fertility rate** (GFR) is the total number of live births per 1,000 women of reproductive age (ages 15 to 49 years) in a population.

NUTRITION

203. All are an essential fatty acids EXCEPT:
a. Linoleic acid b. Linolenic acid
c. Arachidonic acid d. Glutamic acid

Essential fatty acids and richest source
- Linoleic acid: Safflower oil
- Arachidonic acid: Meats, eggs
- Linoleic acid: Soyabean oil
- Eicosapentaenoic acid: Fish oil

204. Folic acid deficiency is characterized by all of the following EXCEPT:
a. Howell–Jolly bodies
b. Hypersegmentation of neutrophils
c. Microcytes
d. None of the above

Folic acid deficiency leads to megaloblastic anemia.

Ans. **198. a.** 1,00,000 live... **199. d.** Transport facility... **200. a.** 6 months **201. d.** 4 rounds
202. d. General fertility... **203. d.** Glutamic acid **204. c.** Microcytes

205. The following tests are used to check the efficiency of pasteurization of milk EXCEPT:

a. Phosphatase test
b. Standard plate count
c. Coliform count
d. Methylene blue reduction test

Methylene Blue Dye Reduction Test, commonly known as MBRT test is used as a quick method to assess the microbiological quality of raw and pasteurized milk. This test is based on the fact that the blue colour of the dye solution added to the milk get decolourized when the oxygen present in the milk get exhausted due to microbial activity. The sooner the decolourization, more inferior is the bacteriological quality of milk assumed to be. This test is widely used at the dairy reception dock, processing units and milk chilling centres where it is followed as acceptance/rejection criteria for the raw and processed milk.

Comparison between pasteurization and sterilization.

	Pasteurization	*Sterilization*
Method	Milk is just heated and not boiled. There are three methods: a. Holder process (65°C × 30') b. HTST process (72°C × 15") c. UHT process (88°C × few secs, then at 125°C × few secs)	Milk is heated to boiling. Only one method. 100°C × 20 to 30'
Bacteriological changes	90% of pathogens and 90% of lactobacilli are destroyed. Remaining 10% of lactobacilli take time to multiply and cause fermentation by converting lactose to lactic acid. Thus souring of milk is delayed or postponed. Spores are not destroyed.	100% of the pathogens and lactobacilli are destroyed. Therefore, souring of the milk is totally prevented. Spores are also destroyed.
Chemical changes		
Proteins	Only 5% lactalbumin is lost.	100% lactalbumin and 100% lactoglobulin are lost.
Fats	No scum (cream) is formed and so calcium and phosphorus are not taken up.	Scum is formed and so calcium and phosphorus are taken-up.
Carbohydrates	Lactose is not charred or caramalized (so no change in color)	Lactose is completely charred or caramalized (so milk becomes brownish)
Vitamins	Vitamin C is reduced	Vitamin C is lost
Minerals	Proportion of insoluble calcium salts is increased by 6%. Other salts are not affected	Calcium and magnesium salts are precipitated
Physical changes	There are no changes in the color, composition, taste, smell and flavor	Color becomes slightly brownish, taste is altered, smell is slightly changed, composition is also affected as above
Souring of milk	This is delayed or postponed	This is prevented completely

206. Highest protein content:

a. Milk b. Egg
c. Soybean
d. Mutton

Soybeans are considered by many agencies to be a source of complete protein. A complete protein is one that contains significant amounts of all the essential amino acids that must be provided to the human body because of the body's inability to synthesize them. For this reason, soy is a good source of protein, amongst many others, for vegetarians and vegans or for people who want to reduce the amount of meat they eat.

Nutritive value of pulses (values per 100 g).

Pulse	*Protein (g)*	*Fat (g)*	*CHO (g)*	*Calcium (mg)*	*Iron (mg)*	*Thiamine (mg)*	*Riboflavin (mg)*	*Niacin*	*Vitamin C*	*Energy (kcals)*
Bengal gram	17.1	5.3	60.9	202	4.6	0.3	0.1	2.9	3	360
Red gram	22.3	1.7	57.6	73	2.7	0.4	0.1	2.9	0	335
Soybean	43.2	19.5	20.9	240	10.4	0.7	0.3	3.2	0	432

Source: ICMR (1989).

Ans. 205. d. Methylene blue... **206. c.** Soybean

207. Lysine is NOT present in:

a. Wheat b. Pulse
c. Both d. None

Lysine is found in particularly low concentrations in the proteins of cereals; wheat gluten, for example, is relatively poor in lysine. This deficiency in lysine is the reason for the failure of diets in some parts of the world that employ cereal protein as a sole source of essential amino acids to support growth in children and general well-being in adults.

Nutritive value of cereals (values per 100 g).

Name of the cereal	*Protein (g)*	*Fat (g)*	*Carbohydrate (g)*	*Thiamine (mg)*	*Niacin (mg)*	*Riboflavin (mg)*	*Iron (mg)*	*Energy (kcal)*
Rice, raw-milled	6.8	0.5	78.2	0.06	1.9	0.06	0.6	345
Wheat flour	12.1	1.7	71.2	0.45	5.0	0.17	1.5	346
Maize	11.1	3.6	66.2	0.42	1.8	0.10	1.5	342

Source: ICMR (1989).

208. Amino acid NOT present in rice:

a. Lysine b. Methionine
c. Both d. None

Rice contains about 6 to 9% of the proteins and rice protein is rich in lysine and therefore, rice protein is considered of better quality (than wheat protein). Limiting amino acids are threonine and to some extent methionine.

209. Deficiency seen in a child exclusively fed on cow milk:

a. Thiamine b. Vitamin A
c. Riboflavin
d. Iron

Cow's milk consumption has long been associated with iron deficiency and iron deficiency anemia in children. Because cow's milk is a staple in the diet of most toddlers, they are at particular risk for these conditions.

Nutritive value of milk (per 100 g).

Milk	*Protein (g)*	*Fat (g)*	*CHO (g)*	*Iron (mg)*	*Calcium (mg)*	*Carotene (μg)*	*Thiamine (mg)*	*Riboflavin (mg)*	*Energy (kcals)*
Human	1.1	3.4	7.4	0.2	28	137	0.02	0.02	65
Cow	3.2	4.1	4.4	0.2	120	174	0.05	0.19	67
Buffalo	4.3	6.5	5.1	0.2	210	160	0.04	0.10	117
Cheese	21.4	25.1	6.3	2.1	–	273	–	–	348

Source: ICMR (1989).

210. Maximum biological value is of:

a. Pulses b. Soybean
c. Milk d. Egg

Biological value (BV) is a measure of the proportion of absorbed protein from a food which becomes incorporated into the proteins of the organism's body. It captures how readily the digested protein can be used in protein synthesis in the cells of the organism.

- Whey protein concentrate: 104
- Whole egg: 100
- Cow milk: 91
- Beef: 80
- Casein: 77
- Soy: 74
- Wheat gluten: 64

211. Linoleic acid is maximum in:

a. Coconut oil b. Mustard oil
c. Safflower oil d. Ground nut oil

Unsaturated fatty acids are primarily derived from vegetable sources. These are further divided into monounsaturated (MUFA, e.g. Oleic acid) and polyunsaturated fatty acids (PUFA, e.g. Linoleic acid). Former can be synthesized in the body, whereas the later cannot.

Fatty acids content of different fats (Percent).

	Fats	*Saturated fatty acids*	*Unsaturated fatty acids*
Animal fats	Butter	60	20.0
	Meat	10–20	0.5
	Egg	13.3	0.3
	Buffalo milk	7.5	0.5
	Cow's milk	3.8	0.5
	Fish oil	2.0	10.0
Vegetable oils	Groundnut oil	20	40
	Mustard oil	08	15
	Safflower oil	10	45
	Sunflower oil	08	45
	Coconut oil	92	04
	Palm oil	46	25

Source: ICMR (1990).

Ans. 207. **a.** Wheat 208. **b.** Methionine 209. **d.** Iron 210. **d.** Egg
211. **c.** Safflower oil

212. Earliest feature of vitamin A deficiency:

a. Hyphema
b. Keratomalacia
c. Nyctalopia
d. Dryness of conjunctiva

Nyctalopia (night blindness) is one of the **first** signs of VAD (vitamin A deficiency). The classical complaint by the mother is that her child cannot find her or dashes against the wall as the dark sets in.

Criteria of vitamin A deficiency.

Criteria	*Prevalence (among children 6 months to 6 years)*
Night blindness	> 1%
Bitot's spots	> 0.5%
Corneal xerosis	> 0.01%
Corneal ulcer/keratomalacia	> 0.05%

Source: WHO. TRS. No. 672, 1982.

213. Lathyrism is due to:

a. Sanguinarine
b. Pyruvic acid
c. BOAA
d. Aflatoxin

The consumption of large quantities of *Lathyrus* grain containing high concentrations of the glutamate analogue neurotoxin β-oxalyl-L-α,β-diaminopropionic acid (ODAP, also known as β-*N*-oxalyl-amino-L-alanine, or BOAA) causes paralysis, characterized by lack of strength in or inability to move the lower limbs, and may involve pyramidal tracts producing signs of upper motor neuron damage.

Examples of food adulteration.

Food materials	*Common adulterant*
Cereals (Rice, wheat)	Stone, sand, grit
Dals (Bengal gram)	Kesari dal (Lathyrism)
Milk	Addition of water, removal of cream, addition of starch (water borne disease)
Ghee	Addition of vanaspati
Butter	Starch, animal fat
Turmeric powder	Lead chromate powder (metanil yellow) (lead poisoning)
Black pepper	Dried seeds of papaya
Chilli powder	Brick powder
Tea leaves	Husk of blackgram, reuse of tea leaves
Coffee seeds	Tamarind seeds
Baking powder	Citric acid
Honey	Sugar, jaggery
Sugar	Chalk
Mustard seeds	Seeds of prickly-poppy (Epidemic dropsy)
Edible oil	Mineral oil
Ice-cream	Starch, cellulose, washing powder
Asafoetida	Resins, gums
Jaggery solution	Honey (or vice-versa)
Coffee powder	Chicory
Nonalcoholic beverages	Nonpermitted colors, saccharin, dulcin, lead, arsenic, copper, dirt and filth.

214. Best parameter to assess chronic malnutrition:

a. Height for age
b. Weight for height
c. Weight for ag
d. Height for weight

The term "stunting" is used to describe a condition in which children fail to gain sufficient height, given their age. Stunting is an extremely low "height-for-age" (H/A) score. Stunting is often associated with long-term factors such as chronic malnutrition, especially protein-energy malnutrition, and frequent illness. It is therefore an indicator of past growth failure and is often used for long-term planning of policies and intervention programs in non-emergency situations. Stunting is very sensitive to socio-economic inequalities.

Master chart of classification of PEM.

Grade/Degree	*(Weight for age in percentage)*			*Waterlow*	
	Gomez	*Jelliffe*	*IAP*	*Height for age (stunting)*	*Weight for height (wasting)*
Normal	90–110	> 90	100–80	> 95%	> 90%
Mild (1°)	89–75	90–81	79–70	94–87.5	90–80
Moderate (2°)	74–60	80–71	69–60	87.4–80	80–70
Severe (3°)	< 60	70–61	59–50	< 80	< 70
Very severe (4°)	–	< 60	< 50	–	–

215. Protein quality indicator adopted by ICMR in recommending dietary protein requirement is:

a. Protein efficiency ratio
b. Biological value
c. Net protein utilization
d. Amino acid score

The **net protein utilization**, or NPU, is the ratio of amino acid converted to proteins to the ratio of amino acids supplied. This figure is somewhat affected by the salvage of essential amino acids within the body, but is profoundly affected by the level of limiting amino acids within a foodstuff.

Ans. 212. c. Nyctalopia **213. c.** BOAA **214. a.** Height for age **215. c.** Net protein utilization

Safe dietary intakes of protein.

Age groups	*Safe protein allowance (g/d)*
Infants	
0–6 months 6–12 months	1.16 g/kg/d 1.69 g/kg/d
Children	
1–3 years 4–6 years 7–9 years 10–12 yrs-boys 10–12 yrs-girls 13–15 yrs-boys 13–15 yrs-girls 16–18 yrs-boys 16–18 yrs-girls	15.7 20.3 29.6 39.3 40.4 54.2 51.9 61.5 52.1
Adults	
Men Women Pregnant women* Lactating women 0–6 months 6–12 months	60.0 55.0 82.2 (55 + 27.2) 77.9 (55 + 22.9) 70.2 (55 + 15.2)
*For weight gain of 10 kg in pregnant women	

216. Highest net protein utilization is in:

a. Fish
b. Milk
c. Wheat
d. Egg

Egg contains all the nutrients, except carbohydrate and vitamin C. Egg protein is biologically a complete protein (it contains all the essential amino-acids) and the net protein utilization is 100 (i.e. high biological value and high digestibility coefficient). Therefore, egg protein is called a 'Reference protein'.

217. Daily extra calorie requirement if first trimester of pregnancy is:

a. 50
b. 150
c. 350
d. 450

The overall **caloric need** increases by only about 15%, amounting to about an **extra 150 kcal**/day during the **first trimester** and an **additional** 350 kcal/day for the remainder of the pregnancy, for a total of about 2200 to 2900 kcal.

Recommended energy requirement.

Age groups	*Category*	*Requirements kcal/day*	*Difference from 1989 RDA kcal/day*
Man	Sedentary work Moderate work Heavy work	2318 2727 3485	– 107 – 148 – 315
Woman	Sedentary work Moderate work Heavy work Pregnant woman* Lactating woman	1899 2234 2854 + 350	+ 24 – 9 – 71 + 50
Infants	0–6 months 6–12 months 0–6 months 6–12 months	+ 600 + 520 92 kcal/kg/day 79 kcal/kg/day	+ 50 + 120 – 16 kcal/kg/day – 19 kcal/kg/day
Children	1–3 years 4–6 years 7–9 years 10–12 years	1036 1350 1691 2189	– 204 – 340 – 259 —
Boys	13–15 years 16–18 years 10–12 years	2748 3017 2008	+ 298 + 377 + 48
Girls	13–15 years 16–18 years	2328 2070	+ 268 + 10

*For weight gain of 10 kg in pregnant women.

218. Clinical symptoms of lead toxicity are noted with blood levels of:

a. 30 microgram/100 mL of blood
b. 40 microgram/100 mL of blood
c. 50 microgram/100 mL of blood
d. 70 microgram/100 mL of blood

In adults, symptoms can occur at levels above 40 μg/dL, but are more likely to occur only above 70 μg/dL. Symptoms begin to appear in children generally at around 60 μg/dL.

Ans. 216. d. Egg **217. b.** 150 **218. d.** 70 microgram/100 mL of blood

Diagnosis of lead poisoning.		
Material	*Normal level*	*Dangerous level*
Blood lead	25–40 mcg per 100 mL	> 70 mcg per 100 mL
Urinary lead	0.2–0.8 mg per liter	> 0.8 mg per liter
Urinary amino levulinic acid (ALA)	6 mg per liter	60 mg per liter
Urinary co-proporphyrin*	<150 mcg per liter	>250 mcg per liter

*In plumbism, coproporphyrin is excreted in the urine because lead combines with Sulfhydryl (SH) group of the enzymes concerned with the synthesis of RBCs, releasing coproporphyrin.

219. Indian reference man has a weight of:

a. 55 kg b. 60 kg
c. 65 kg d. 70 kg

An Indian reference man is between 18 and 30 years of age and weighs **60 kg**.

Reference body weight of Indians (NNMB)*.		
Groups	*Age (years)*	*Weight (kg)*
Infants	0–6 months 6–12 months	5 8
Children	1–3 years 4–6 years 7–9 years	12 18 25
Boys	10–12 years 13–15 years 16–18 years	34 47 55.5
Girls	10–12 years 13–15 years 16–18 years	35.0 46.6 52.1
Adults		
Men	18–30 years	60.0 Height 172 cm BMI 20.3
Women	18–30 years	55.0 Height 161 cm BMI 22.2

*National Nutrition Monitoring Bureau.

220. Tomatoes are rich in:

a. Formic acid b. Acetic acid
c. Citric acid d. Oxalic acid

Tomatoes contain a moderate amount of **oxalic acid**

221. Toxin responsible for epidemic dropsy:

a. Sanguinarine b. Aflatoxin
c. Pyrrolizidine alkaloids d. BOAA

Epidemic dropsy is a clinical state resulting from use of edible oils adulterated with *Argemone mexicana* seed oil. Sanguinarine and dihydrosanguinarine are two major toxic alkaloids of argemone oil, which cause widespread capillary dilatation, proliferation and increased capillary permeability.

222. Endemic ascites is associated with:

a. Sanguinarine b. Aflatoxin
c. Pyrrolizidine alkaloids d. BOAA

Endemic ascites was noticed in the Kusmi block of Sarguja district of Madhya Pradesh during the years 1973 and 1976. There was an outbreak of rapidly progressing ascites and jaundice among the tribals. Mortality rate was 40%. Investigation by the National Institute of Nutrition concluded that this outbreak was due to intake of Millet seeds contaminated with Crotalaria seeds which form their main diet. Crotalaria occured as a weed in areas of millet (Panicum miliare) cultivation. Crotalaria seeds contain pyrrolizidine alkaloids which are hepatotoxic. The methods suggested for preventing this were deweeding of farmlands and sieving of millet seeds before use, as Crotalaria seeds were much smaller.

223. Cereals provided in mid-day meals:

a. 50 grams b. 75 grams
c. 100 grams d. 125 grams

Food stuff	*Quantity (gram/day/child)*
Cereals and millets	75
Pulses	30
Leafy vegetables	30
Non leafy vegetables	30
Oils and fats	8
Milk	150 mL

224. Vitamin least in human milk:

a. Vitamin A b. Vitamin C
c. Vitamin D d. Vitamin K

Milk is a very wholesome food, because it contains almost all the nutrients, except iron and vitamin C.

225. Dates are rich source of:

a. Iron b. Calcium
c. Carotene d. Vitamin C

Fruits are not good source of iron, calcium and phosphorous. However dry fruits like dates, grapefruit are fair sources of iron and calcium.

Nutritive value of some common fruits (values for 100 g of edible portion).						
Fruit	*CHO (g)*	*Iron (mg)*	*Calcium (mg)*	*Carotene (μg)*	*Vitamin C (mg)*	*Energy (kcals)*
Apple	13.4	0.6	0	0	1	59
Banana	27.2	0.5	10	78	7	110
Grapes	16.5	1.5	20	0	1	71
Guava	11.2	0.3	10	0	212	51
Mango	16.9	1.3	14	2210	16	74
Papaya	7.2	0.5	17	2740	57	32
Dates		7.3	120	44	03	317

Source: ICMR (1989)

Ans. **219. b.** 60 kg **220. d.** Oxalic acid **221. a.** Sanguinarine **222. c.** Pyrrolizidine alkaloids
223. b. 75 grams **224. b.** Vitamin C **225. b.** Calcium

226. True regarding comparison values of cow and human milk are all EXCEPT:

a. Human milk has comparatively less of protein
b. Human milk has comparatively less of calcium
c. Human milk has comparatively less of minerals
d. Human milk has comparatively less of lactose

Lactose is the primary carbohydrate found in **human milk**. Milk is the only natural source of lactose.

ENVIRONMENT AND SANITATION

227. Which pneumoconiosis may lead to lung mottling?

a. Byssinosis
b. Bagassosis
c. Asbestosis
d. Anthracosis

Chest X-ray of a patient with bagassosis may show mottling/ shadows

228. Following are true regarding chlorination EXCEPT:

a. Residual chlorine: 0.5 mg/lit
b. Contact period: 30 minutes
c. Water should not be turbid
d. Chlorine demand should be estimated

Contact period is the time period required for the chlorine to disinfect the water. For optimum disinfection, the presence of free chlorine for a contact period of one hour is essential. The free chlorine that remains at the end of one hour is called is 'free residual chlorine' (i.e. after breakpoint chlorination).

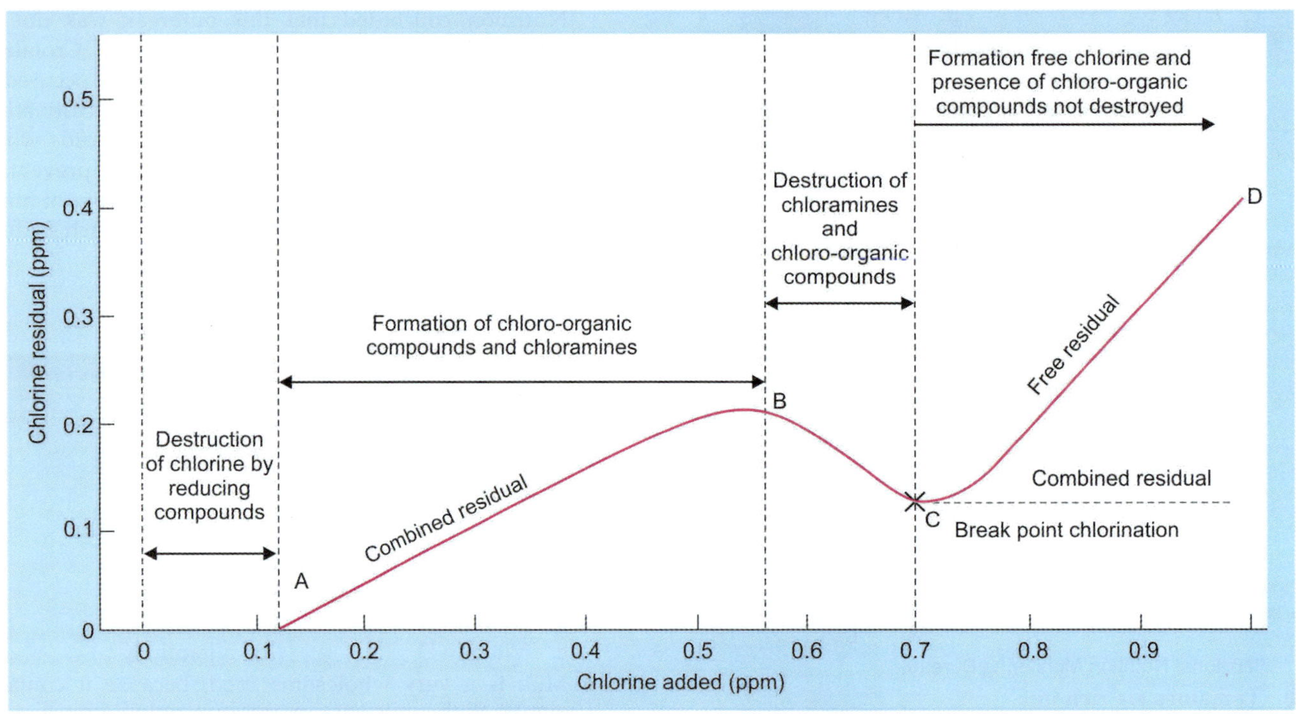

Phases of break-point chlorination.
Source: Dhaar GM, Robbani I. Foundations of Community Medicine. Elsevere, 1st edn, 2006.

229. Number of air changes in one hour in a drawing room should be at least:

a. 2
b. 3
c. 4
d. 5

Air changes per hour, or air change rate, abbreviated ACH or ac/h, is a measure of the air volume added to or removed from a space (normally a room or house) divided by the volume of the space. If the air in the space is either uniform or perfectly mixed, air changes per hour is a measure of how many times the air within a defined space is replaced.

Basement Parking	15–30
Commercial kitchens and toilets	15–30
Smoking rooms	10–15
Laboratories	6–12
Classrooms	3–4
Warehousing	1–2
Living rooms	2–3
Work rooms and assemblies	4–6

230. Mode of disposal of sewage ground water:

a. Activated sludge process
b. Soakage pit
c. Oxidation pond
d. All of the above

The **activated sludge** process is a process for treating sewage and industrial waste waters using air and a biological floc composed of bacteria and protozoa.

Ans. **226. d.** Human milk... **227. b.** Bagassosis **228. b.** Contact period:... **229. b.** 3
230. a. Activated sludge process

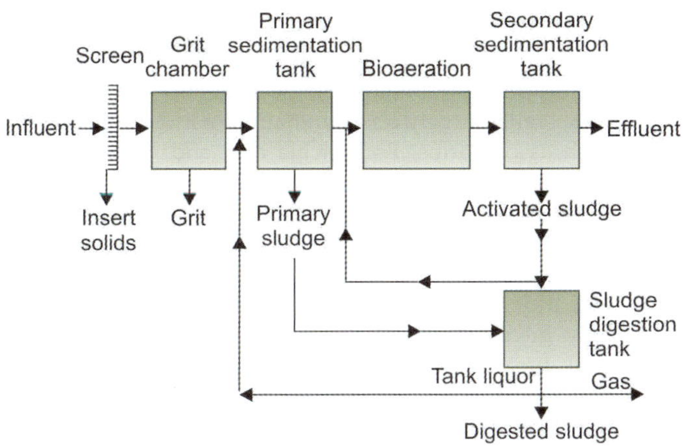

Flow diagram of modern sewage treatment.

231. Best parameter to measure air pollution:

a. N_2 b. CO
c. CO_2 d. SO_2

Sulfur dioxide is a noticeable component in the atmosphere, especially following volcanic eruptions. Sulfur dioxide is a major air pollutant and has significant impacts upon human health. Sulfur dioxide emissions are a precursor to acid rain and atmospheric particulates.

232. Strength of sewage is expressed in terms of:

a. Biological oxygen demand
b. Chemical oxygen demand
c. Suspended solids
d. E. coli count

Biochemical oxygen demand (BOD) is the amount of dissolved oxygen needed (i.e. demanded) by aerobic biological organisms to break down organic material present in a given water sample at certain temperature over a specific time period. The BOD value is most commonly expressed in milligrams of oxygen consumed per litre of sample during 5 days of incubation at 20°C and is often used as a surrogate of the degree of organic pollution of water.

BOD can be used as a gauge of the effectiveness of wastewater treatment plants.

233. WHO accepted chloride levels in water:

a. 0.2 mg/L b. 0.5 mg/L
c. 45 mg/L d. 200 mg/L

Potable **water** should not exceed 200 mg/L of **chloride.**

Substances and their prescribed upper limit.

Substances	*Prescribed upper limit*
Substances affecting the color	5 units (by colorimeter) or 15 true color units (TCU)
Substances affecting the odor	3 units (by threshold odor test)
Substances affecting the taste	Unobjectionable
Optimum – pH	7.5 (range of pH = 7 to 8)
Total dissolved solids (affecting turbidity)	1000 mg/L (< 600 mg/L is very safe)
Total hardness	3 mEq/L (1 to 3 mEq/L of $CaCO_3$) (50 to 150 mg of $CaCO_3$/L)
Iron	0.3 mg/L.
Calcium	75 mg/L.
Magnesium	30 mg/L.
Sulfate	200 mg/L.
Chlorides	200 mg/L.
Zinc	5 mg/L.
Copper	0.05 mg/L.
Manganese	0.05 mg/L.
Phenolic substances	0.001 mg/L.

234. Permanent loss of hearing can occur if exposed to noise above:

a. 85 dB b. 90 dB
c. 100 dB d. 160 dB

Noise level values

Whispering	20–30 dB
Normal conversation	30–65 dB (maximum upper limit is 85 dB)
Street traffic	60–80 dB
Shouting	About 100 dB
Motor car horn, boiler factories	About 120 dB
Train, aeroplane engine	About 120 dB
Threshold of pain	About 140 dB
Jet plane	About 150 dB
Mechanical damage	150–160 dB

235. Emporiatrics deals with:

a. Mine workers b. Industrial worker
c. Travellers d. Farmers

Travel medicine or **emporiatrics** is the branch of medicine that deals with the prevention and management of health problems of international travelers.

236. % of para-para isomer in DDT is:

a. 20–30% b. 40–50%
c. 60–70% d. 70–80%

Active ingredient of DDT is para-para—isomer. It is present to the extent of 70–80% in DDT.

237. True for global warming:

a. KYOTO protocol set the target of net reduction of 20 greenhouse gas emission
b. CFC increases the zone of stratosphere
c. Stratosphere ozone layer is harmful
d. CO_2 is the major greenhouse gas

The primary greenhouse gases in Earth's atmosphere are water vapor, carbon dioxide, methane, nitrous oxide, and ozone. Without greenhouse gases, the average temperature of Earth's surface would be about 15°C (27°F) colder than the present average of 14°C (57°F).

Ans. 231. **d.** SO_2 232. **a.** Biological oxygen... 233. **d.** 200 mg/L 234. **d.** 160 dB
235. **c.** Travellers 236. **d.** 70–80% 237. **d.** CO_2 is the major...

238. Among the following, which of the following is the greatest contributor to global warming as a consequence of human activities and life style:

a. CO_2 b. Chlorofluorocarbons
c. Methane d. Ozone

The Intergovernmental Panel on Climate Change (IPCC) reported in 2014 that scientists were more than 95% certain that global warming is mostly being caused by increasing concentrations of greenhouse gases (GHG) and other human (anthropogenic) activities.

239. Which amongst the following biological agents carries the highest potential for use as biological weapons for microbial bioterrorism:

a. Plague (Yersinia pestis)
b. Small pox (Variola major)
c. Botulism (Cl. botulinum)
d. Brucellosis (Brucella sp.)

Plague is a disease caused by the *Yersinia pestis* bacterium. Rodents are the normal host of plague, and the disease is transmitted to humans by flea bites and occasionally by aerosol in the form of pneumonic plague. The disease has a history of use in biological warfare dating back many centuries, and is considered a threat due to its ease of culture and ability to remain in circulation among local rodents for a long period of time. The weaponized threat comes mainly in the form of pneumonic plague (infection by inhalation). It was the disease that caused the Black Death in Medieval Europe.

240. Value of free residual chlorine should be:

a. 0.2 mg/L b. 0.3 mg/L
c. 0.4 mg/L d. 0.5 mg/L

A free chlorine level of 0.5 mg/L of free chlorine will be enough residual to maintain the quality of water through the distribution network, but is most likely not adequate to maintain the quality of the water when this water is stored in the home in a bucket or jerry can for 24 hours.

241. Content of 'available chlorine' in freshly prepared bleaching powder:

a. 23% b. 33%
c. 43% d. 53%

Bleaching powder is an unstable compound that releases **chlorine** rapidly on storage; fresh **bleaching powder** contains **33%** of available **chlorine**.

242. Which of the following is NOT a greenhouse gas:

a. Carbon mono-oxide b. Methane
c. Nitrous oxide d. Water vapour

In the atmosphere, CO is spatially variable and short lived, having a role in the formation of ground-level ozone.

243. The following organism because of its easy culture methods is widely used as bacteriology indicator of water pollution:

a. Faecal streptococci b. Escherichia coli
c. Clostridium perfringens d. Salmonella typhi

Monitoring the microbiological quality of drinking water relies largely on examination of indicator bacteria such as coliforms, Escherichia coli, and Pseudomonas aeruginosa. E. coli is a member of the faecal coliform group and is a more specific indicator of faecal pollution than other faecal coliforms. Two key factors have led to the trend toward the use of E. coli as the preferred indicator for the detection of faecal contamination, not only in drinking water, but also in other matrices as well: first, the finding that some faecal coliforms were non faecal in origin, and second, the development of improved testing methods for E. coli.

244. Vital layer in slow sand filter is seen in:

a. Top of the water b. On the sand bed
c. Near filter d. None

The **vital layer** is heart of the **slow sand filters** and removes organic matter, filters bacteria and oxidizes ammoniacal nitrogen into nitrates and helps in yielding bacteria free water.

	Slow sand filters	*Rapid sand filters*
1. Area (900 m^2)	Requires large area	Requires small area.
2. Sand bed	Height is 1.2 m.	Height is 1.0 m.
3. Effective size of the sand	0.15 to 0.3 mm	0.6 to 2.0 mm
4. Preliminary storage	It is necessary	Not necessary
5. Preliminary treatment	It is not necessary	is a must
6. Rate of filtration/ hour	0.1 to 0.4 m^3/m^2/hour	5-15 m^3/m^2/hour
7. Mechanism of action	It is mainly biological	is by physical and chemical
8. Operation	It is less skilled	is highly skilled
9. Suitability for turbid water	Not suitable	Suitable
10. Loss of hydraulic head allowed	2 to 4 feet	8 to 10 feet
11. Filter run	3 weeks to 3 months	1 to 3 days
12. Cleaning	By scraping the sand bed	By back-washing
13. Wasting of water	Water is not wasted during cleaning	2 to 3 percent of filter is wasted
14. Cost	Capital cost is high but cost of operation is low	Capital cost is low but cost of operation is high

Contd...

Ans. **238. a.** CO_2 **239. a.** Plague (Yersinia pestis) **240. d.** 0.5 mg/L **241. b.** 33%
242. a. Carbon mono... **243. b.** Escherichia coli **244. b.** On the sand bed

Contd...

		Slow sand filters	Rapid sand filters
15.	Use of sludge	Sludge obtained after scraping is used as manure	Sludge is not obtained and wash water also is not of economic use
16.	Removal of turbidity	Is by vital layer	Is by alum coagulant
17.	Removal of color	Fair	Good
18.	Removal of bacteria	99.99%	99%
19.	Post-treatment chlorination	It is not necessary	Is a must

245. With reference to healthful school environment, which one of the following statements is NOT correct:

a. In the classroom, desks should be of minus type
b. Per capita space per student should be 6 sq. feet
c. Combined window and door area should be 25% of the floor space
d. One urinal should be provided for 60 students

The minimum floor space per student should be 15 sq. feet. The height should be minimum 12 feet.

246. Minimum distance between bore hole latrine and source of water should be at least:

a. 10 metres b. 15 metres
c. 50 metres d. 100 metres

15 meters is safe **distance between** drinking well and earth pit deep **latrine.**

247. Estimation of free chlorine of water is done by:

a. Ortho-tolidine test
b. Horrock's apparatus
c. Paterson's chloronome
d. Kata thermometer

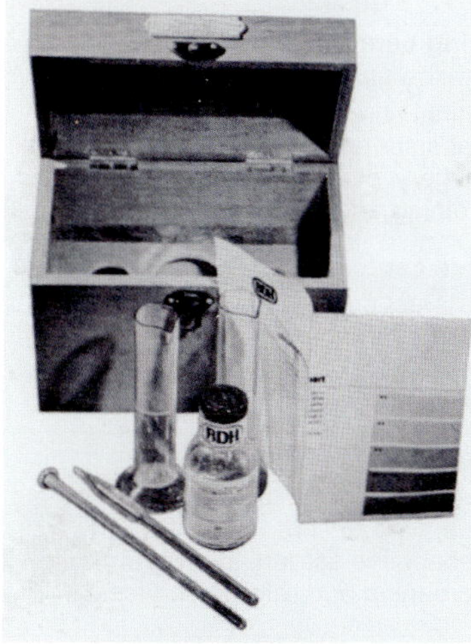

Chlorotex apparatus.

Ortho-tolidine test is a test done to measure rapidly, the free chlorine in the water. The apparatus used for this purpose is called chloroscope (or chlortex apparatus).

248. Preferred bacteriological indicator of faecal contamination of water:

a. Faecal streptococci b. Cl. prefringens
c. Faecal staphylococci d. E. coli

Interpretation of results of disinfected water

No coliforms in 100 cc of water	Excellent water
1–3 coliforms in 100 cc of water	Satisfactory water
4–10 coliforms in 100 cc of water	Suspicious water
More than 10 coliforms in 100 cc of water	Unsatisfactory water

249. Soiling index determines:

a. Contraception failure b. Air pollution
c. Number of hookworm eggs
d. Ratio of mucus secreting glands to thickness of wall of airways

The soiling index/smoke index or coefficient of haze (COH) is an indication of the soiling or darkening potential of fine particulates in the atmosphere, usually resulting from combustion. The particles may remain suspended in the air as dust, smoke, fumes, aerosols, soot, or mist. These particulates, usually in the size range from 0.1 to 1 micron (fine particles) in solid or liquid form, can become trapped in the lungs during breathing. They can cause soiling, decrease visibility, aggravate respiratory problems, and may cause long term effects on the lungs. The soiling index or coefficient of haze (COH) is an indication of the soiling or darkening potential of fine particulates in the atmosphere, usually resulting from combustion. The particles may remain suspended in the air as dust, smoke, fumes, aerosols, soot, or mist. These particulates, usually in the size range from 0.1 to 1 micron (fine particles) in solid or liquid form, can become trapped in the lungs during breathing. They can cause soiling, decrease visibility, aggravate respiratory problems, and may cause long term effects on the lungs.

250. Maximum permissible level of chloride in drinking water is:

a. 200 mg litre b. 300 mg litre
c. 600 mg litre d. 800 mg litre

Chloride greater than **600 mg**/litre would markedly impair the potability of the water.

NATIONAL POLICIES AND HEALTH CARE

251. All are elements of primary health care EXCEPT:

a. Water chlorination b. Maternal health care
c. Sanitation d. Equity of distribution

Elements of primary health care (ELEMENTS)

- Essential drugs
- Locally endemic disease prevention & control
- Extended programme of immunization
- Maternal & child health care including family planning

Ans. **245. b.** Per capita space... **246. b.** 15 metres **247. a.** Ortho-tolidine test **248. d.** E. coli
249. b. Air pollution **250. c.** 600 mg litre **251. d.** Equity of distribution

- Education
- Nutrition
- Treatment of common ailments
- Safe water supply & sanitation

252. Under Suraksha (AIDS programme), patient coming with vaginitis, should be treated with a kit of colour code:

a. White b. Yellow
c. Green d. Grey

Prepacked STI/ RTI colour coded kits

Kit	Colour	Indication
Kit 1	Grey	Urethral discharge, ano-rectal discharge & cervicitis
Kit 2	Green	Vaginitis
Kit 3	White	Genital ulcers
Kit 4	Blue	Genital ulcers
Kit 5	Red	Genital ulcers
Kit 6	Yellow	Lower abdominal pain
Kit 7	Black	Scrotal swelling

253. True about ASHA are all EXCEPT:

a. One per 1,000 rural population
b. Mobilizer of antenatal care
c. Female voluntary worker
d. Skilled birth attendant

Accredited Social Health Activist/ASHAs are local women trained to act as health educators and promoters in their communities. The Indian MoHFW describes them as: health activist(s) in the community who will create awareness on health and its social determinants and mobilize the community towards local health planning and increased utilization and accountability of the existing health services.

Their tasks include motivating women to give birth in hospitals, bringing children to immunization clinics, encouraging family planning (e.g., surgical sterilization), treating basic illness and injury with first aid, keeping demographic records, and improving village sanitation. ASHAs are also meant to serve as a key communication mechanism between the healthcare system and rural populations.

254. Vision 2020 includes all EXCEPT:

a. Onchocerciasis b. Epidemic conjunctivitis
c. Cataract d. Trachoma

Globally, five conditions have been identified for immediate attention for achieving the goals of Vision 2020. They are: Cataract, Trachoma, Onchocerciasis, Childhood blindness and Refractive Errors and Low Vision.

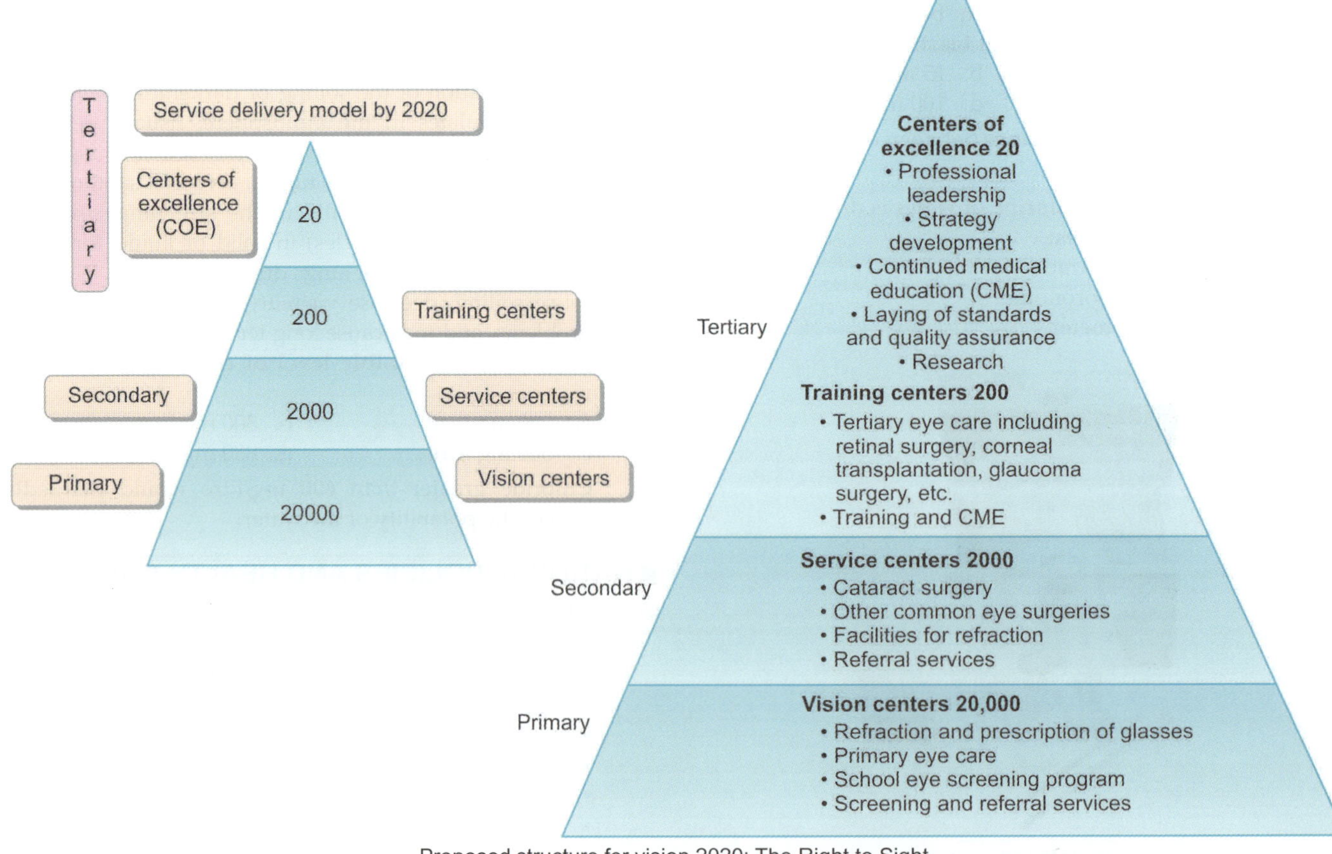

Proposed structure for vision 2020: The Right to Sight.

Ans. **252. c.** Green **253. d.** Skilled birth... **254. b.** Epidemic...

255. Panchayati raj at village level does NOT consist of:
a. Panchayat samiti
b. Gram panchayat
c. Nyay panchayat
d. Zilla parishad

The Panchayati raj is a three tier structure of rural, local, self-government in India, consisting of three institutions namely Gram panchayat (the executive body at the village level), Panchayat samiti (at the block level) and Zilla panchayat/Parishad at the district levels.

256. An ideal subcentre for a rural population caters to a population of:
a. 1,000
b. 2,000
c. 5,000
d. 10,000

Subcenter level
- The subcentre is the peripheral outpost of the Indian healthcare system
- One subcentre caters to the healthcare needs of 5,000 population in general and 3000 population in hilly, tribal and backward areas

Services provided by subcentre:
- Antenatal, natal, postnatal
- Family planning and counselling
- Treatment of common illnesses like respiratory tract infections, diarrhoea, fever, worm infestation
- Prevention of malnutrition
- Implementation of various national health programmes

Staff pattern of subcentre:
- 1 female health worker—Auxiliary nurse midwife
- 1 male health worker—Multipurpose worker
- Voluntary worker to help the Auxiliary nurse midwife
- 1 Female Health Assistant (Lady Health Visitor) and 1 Male Health Assistant at the PHC level are given the supervision of 6 sub-centers

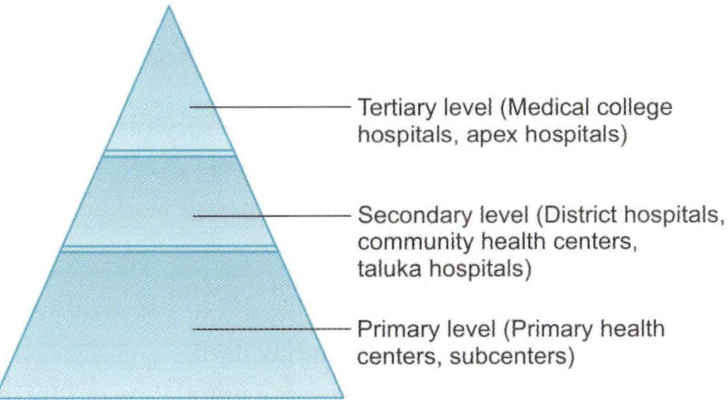

Three-tier system of healthcare.

Funding of subcentre:
- The central government gives salary to the Lady Health Visitor and the Auxiliary Nurse Midwife in addition to contingency fund, drug and equipment supply
- The state government gives salary to the Multipurpose worker
- The voluntary worker is paid from the contingency fund of the Auxiliary Nurse Midwife

257. Best indicator for monitoring the impact of Iodine Deficiency Disorders Control Programme/NIDDCP:
a. Iodine level in soil
b. Neonatal hypothyroidism
c. Urinary iodine levels among pregnant women
d. Prevalence of goiter among school children

Neonatal Hypothyroidism
- Sensitive indicator of environmental iodine deficiency.
- Effective indicator of monitoring the impact of NIDDCP

258. Under the National Polio Eradication programme, a case of Acute Flaccid Paralysis is confirmed as polio, under the following circumstances EXCEPT:
a. If a case is lost to follow-up
b. If a case could not be confirmed because the patient dies before that
c. If a wild strain of polio virus is isolated from stools
d. If a patient develops paralysis within 30 days diagnosis of AFP

Compatible case is reviewed for 60 days by an expert committee, consisting of a paediatrician, a virologist and a neurologist, to decide whether to confirm or discard as polio case. *(See Diagram on next page)*

259. NOT an indicator for effective leprosy control programme:
a. Decreased type 2 disability
b. Increasing number of children affected
c. High new case detection rate
d. None of the above

Proxy indicators of quality in leprosy program
- The treatment completion rate. It measures whether patients have attended for treatment as required (but this does not mean that the patient also took his treatment as prescribed); it is simple to measure and is closely correlated with the cure of the disease (however, there is no direct measurement of cure—bacteriological—in leprosy; and even after completion of treatment the patient may develop immunological reactions).
- The proportion of Disability Grade 2 amongst new cases is a well-established indicator of case-finding efficiency. If patients report late to or are diagnosed late by the health services, a greater proportion will have impairments at the time of diagnosis.
- Proportion of new cases correctly diagnosed. Those not diagnosed correctly are so called false-positives.

Ans. **255. c.** Nyay panchayat **256. c.** 5,000 **257. b.** Neonatal... **258. d.** If a patient develops... **259. b.** Increasing...

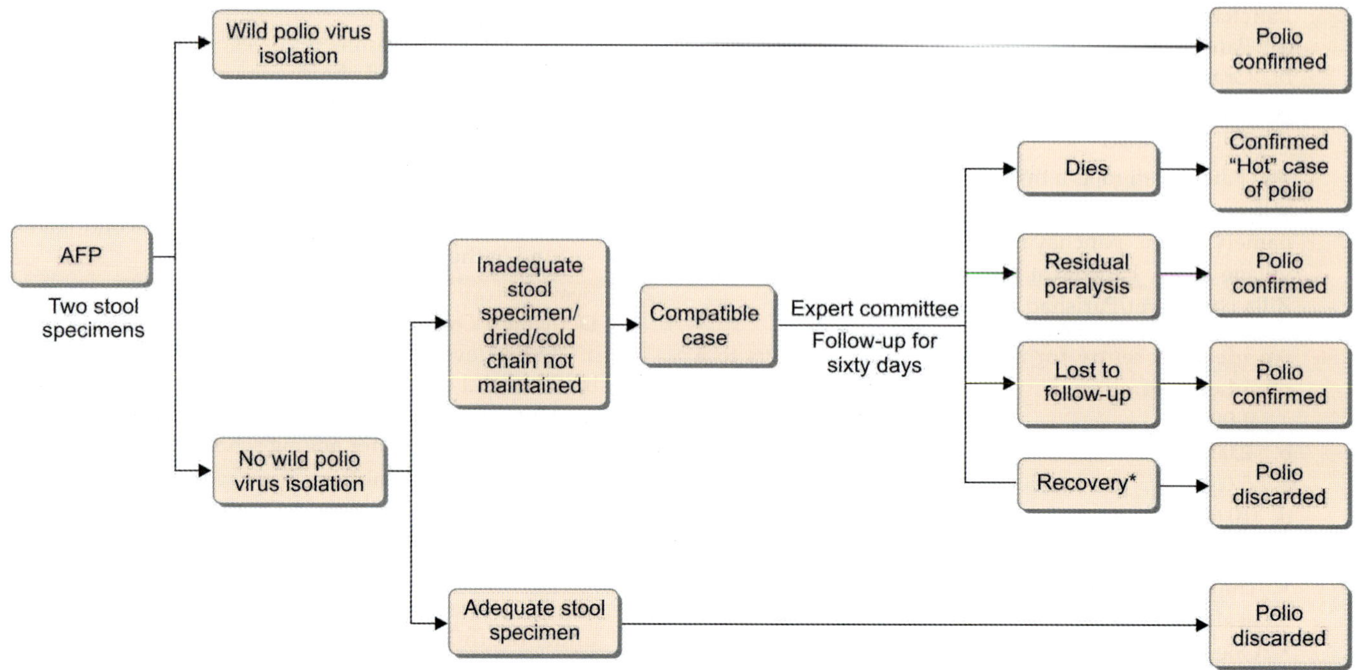

AFP case classification and follow-up of compatible case.
*Recovery from paralysis occurs in cases of Guillian Barre Syndrome, transverse myelitis and traumatic neuritis.

More difficult to measure (and actually even more important) are the false-negatives: leprosy patients who present themselves to the health services, but are not diagnosed by the health services as suffering from leprosy.

- The proportion of contacts examined. Could be an important indicator if implemented properly. In most programmes contact examination does not get the attention it deserves. Especially in declining endemicity, more new patients will be from contacts and fewer from the general population. Contact examination is also an important health education tool: it sensitizes the patient's family to understand the disease and support the patient. Contact examination should not be restricted to the persons within the household, but include the households in the direct neighborhood. Declining endemicity contact examination could assume greater importance as part of a chemoprophylaxis program (including BCG re-vaccination).
- Gender: equality of access is not easy to measure, but the gender balance in new case detection should be monitored. One could estimate what should be the male/female ratio from well-run programmes in the area. One could also implement a Health Systems Research study in health seeking behavior of new leprosy (male and female) patients. In general, males dominate in the MB group, and as such we see more disabilities among male patients. However, the disabled (poor, non-educated, single) female patients are the most (socially) disadvantaged.

260. NOT an objective of National Rural Health Mission (NRHM):

a. Formulation of family planning and welfare societies
b. Formulation of state and district health programme
c. Recruitment of ASHA
d. Implementation of JSY

Basic objectives for implementation of NRHM

- To reduce infant mortality rate and maternal mortality rate
- To ensure population stabilization
- To prevent and control of communicable and non-communicable diseases
- To upgrade AYUSH (Aurvedic Yoga Unani Siddh and Homopath) for promotion of healthy life style
- To provide services through the appointment of ASHA in each village
- To decentralize village and district level health planning and management
- To provide improved health care services under JSY for the below poverty line families.

261. Which is FALSE regarding Anganwadi worker:

a. Part time worker
b. Undergoes 4 month training
c. 1 for 1,000 children
d. Selected from the community itself

An Anganwadi normally covers a **population** of 1,000 in both rural and urban areas.

Ans. 260. b. Formulation... **261. c.** 1 for 1000 children

262. A female multipurpose worker does NOT do:

a. Distribution of condoms
b. Malaria surveillance
c. Birth death statistics
d. Immunization of mothers

Health worker male/HWM detects cases of malaria by active surveillance.

263. In a hospital, ideal bed space should be:

a. 5 feet b. 7 feet
c. 8 feet d. 12 feet

Bed space is an important yet complicated area of **hospitals** as it is occupied by the patients. It was increased to 8.2 m^2 in the 1980s and 1990s to just below **12** m^2 in the 2000s.

264. The World Health Organization day is:

a. 7th April
b. 21st May
c. 2nd August
d. 31st December

In 1948, the WHO held the First World Health Assembly. The Assembly decided to celebrate 7 April of each year, with effect from 1950, as the **World Health Day**.

Month	Date	Event
January	1 30	New Year Day Anti-Leprosy Day
February	1 4 28	Deaf and Dumb Day World Cancer Day National Science Day
March	1 8 9 10 15 16 22 24	World Science Day International Women's Day Anganwadi Worker's Day World Kidney Day World Consumer Rights Day World Immunization Day/Measles Day; World Glaucoma Day World Water Day World Tuberculosis Day
April	7 17 25 30	World Health Day Hemophilia Day World Malaria Day Child Labor Day
May	1 12 13 15 17 31	World Labor Day (May Day) Red Cross Day Mother's Day International Day of the Family World Hypertension Day World No Tobacco Day
June	5 14 26	World Environment Day World Blood Donors' Day International Day of Drug Abuse and Illicit Trafficking

Contd...

Contd...

Month	Date	Event
July	1 8 11	Doctor's Day (India) World Zoonotic Day World Population Day
August	1 1-7 15 20	World Breastfeeding Day World Breastfeeding Week Independence Day (India) World Mosquito Day
September	1-7 5 8 10 20 21 28	National Nutrition Week Teachers' Day International Literacy Day World Suicide Prevention Day International Peace Day Alzheimer's Day World Rabies Day; World Heart Day
October	1 3 8 10 11 13 14 16 29	Blood Donation Day; World Elders Day World Habitat Day World Sight Day World Mental Health Day (Second Thursday) National No Tobacco Day Anti-Natural Disaster Day World Standards Day World Food Day World Stroke Day
November	2 9 11 14 16 18 19 24 25	Red Cross Flag Day Legal Service Day National Filaria Day World Diabetes Day World Day of Remembrance for Road Traffic Victims World Epilepsy Day World Chronic Obstructive Pulmonary Disease Day; National Integration Day NCC Day International Day for the Elimination of Violence against Women
December	1 2 3 8 10 11	World AIDS Day; International Pollution Prevention Day National Pollution Prevention Day World Disabled Day National Day for the Mentally Retarded World Human Rights Day UNICEF Day

265. According to National Leprosy Elimination Programme, elimination of leprosy is defined as prevalence of Leprosy less than or equal to:

a. 1 per 1,000 population
b. 1 per 10,000 population
c. 1 per 1,00,000 population
d. 2 per 10,000 population

Ans. **262. b.** Malaria... **263. d.** 12 feet **264. a.** 7th April **265. b.** 1 per 10,000 population

Access to information, diagnosis and treatment with multidrug therapy (MDT) remain key elements in the strategy to eliminate the disease as a public health problem, defined as reaching a prevalence of less than 1 leprosy case per 10,000 population. Prevalence rate in 2011 was 0.69 per 10,000 population. So leprosy is now said to be eliminated.

266. Each Community development block consists of:

a. 100 villages and a population of ten thousand
b. 100 villages and a population of one lakh
c. 1000 villages and a population of ten thousand
d. 1000 villages and a population of one lakh

The **Community development block** (C.D. block) is a rural area earmarked for administration and development in India. The area is administered by a Block Development Officer. A community development block covers several gram panchayats, local administrative unit at the village level. Currently, C.D. blocks are administrative units of 3rd level in some states of India (equal to tehsils in other states). Under Community development program, the rural India has been organised into community development blocks, each block comprising of 100 villages, covering a population of about 1 lakh (80,000-1,20,000 population).

267. All of the following are duties of a Health worker female/HWF EXCEPT:

a. Detect malpresentation
b. Detect oligohydramnios
c. Diagnose renal diseases
d. Detect anemia

Primary responsibilities health workers female/HWF (now designated as multipurpose worker/MPW) may include treating minor illnesses, looking after pregnant women and caring for children. Additional duties may involve family planning services, promotion of sanitation and hygiene, screening for communicable diseases, performing health education activities, collecting statistics, maintaining records and providing health care referrals.

268. All of the following are components of Child Survival and Safe Motherhood Programme EXCEPT:

a. Medical termination of pregnancy
b. Advice of food, nutrition and rest
c. Detection and referral of high risk pregnancies
d. Birth spacing

India launched a major programme in 1992 called the Child Survival and Safe Motherhool (CSSM) programme with assistance from World Bank, UNICEF and other donors. The child survival component of the programme was a continuation and expansion of previous child survival activities such as immunisation, ARI and diarrhoea management. While the design of the Safe Motherhood programme based on major new understanding of preventing maternal mortality through Emergency Obstetric Care (EOC), early diagnosis and management of complications associated with pregnancy (and their referral). It also includes services for eligible couples like promotion of contraceptive methods and services for medical termination of pregnancy.

269. Number of postnatal visits by female health worker in her area should be atleast:

a. 1
b. 2
c. 3
d. 4

HWF will pay at least 3–5 visits after delivery, where she gives advice on early ambulation, nutrition, breastfeeding, personal hygiene and also motivates the mother for family planning.

BIOSTATISTICS

270. A diagnostic test for a particular disease has a sensitivity of 0.90 and a specificity of 0.80. A single test is applied to each subject in the population in which the diseased population is 30%. What is the probability that a person, negative to this test, has no disease:

a. Less than 50%
b. 70%
c. 95%
d. 72%

Diseased population (total diseased): 30% (300 out of 1000)

Normal population is 70% (700 out of 1000)

Sensitivity is 90% (true positives): 270 (90% of 300)

False negative is total diseased – true positives: 300-270 = 30

Specificity is 80% (true negatives): 560 (80% of 700)

Negative predictive value = TN/TN+FN = 560 × 100/ 560 + 30

271. Sex and age is best represented on:

a. Bar diagram
b. Pyramid
c. Both
d. None

An **age-sex graph**, commonly referred to as a **population pyramid** even though the graph for some countries is not actually a pyramid shape, displays a population's age and sex composition. Horizontal bars represent the numbers or proportions of males and females in each age group, or cohort. The sum of all the age-sex cohorts in the population pyramid equals 100 percent of the population.

Ans. **266. b.** 100 villages... **267. c.** Diagnose renal... **268. b.** Advice of food... **269. c.** 3 **270. c.** 95% **271. c.** Both

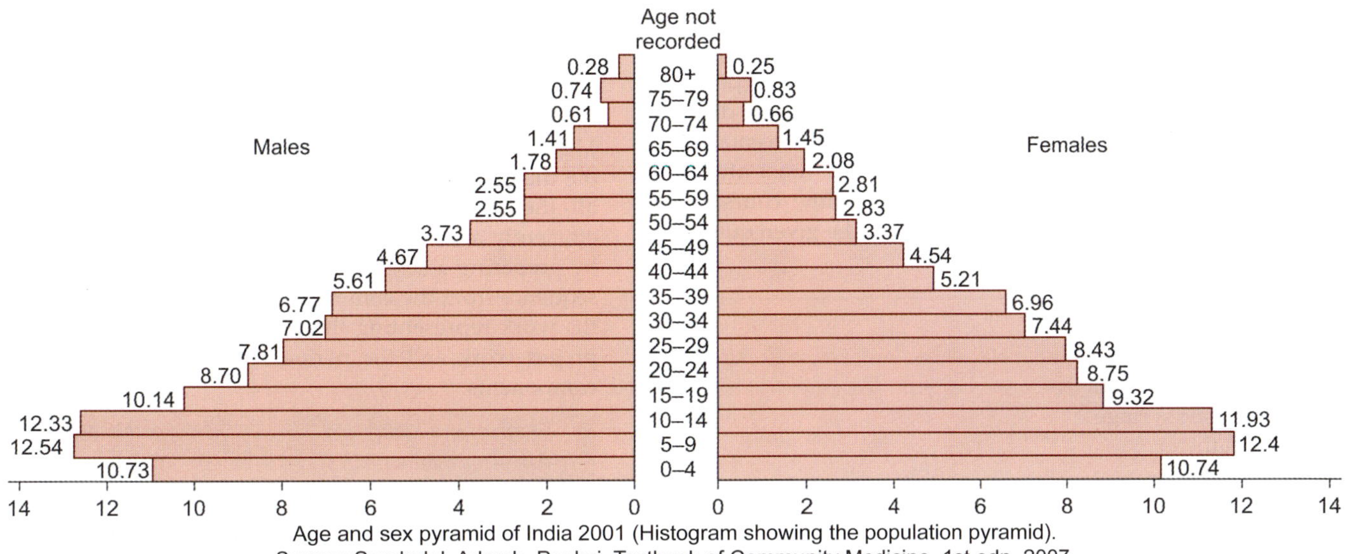

Age and sex pyramid of India 2001 (Histogram showing the population pyramid).
Source: Sunderlal, Adarsh, Pankaj. Textbook of Community Medicine, 1st edn, 2007.

272. There were 50 patients in a ward (20 females and 30 males). 10 females and 20 males require surgery. Probability of each patient selected for surgery is:

a. 1/6 b. 2/6
c. 3/5 d. 6/25

Total patients: 50

Patients requiring surgery: 30 (10 females and 20 males)

So probability of selection: 30/50 = 3/5

273. Mean + 1.96 SD include following % of values in a normal distribution curve:

a. 68% b. 99.5%
c. 88.7% d. 95%

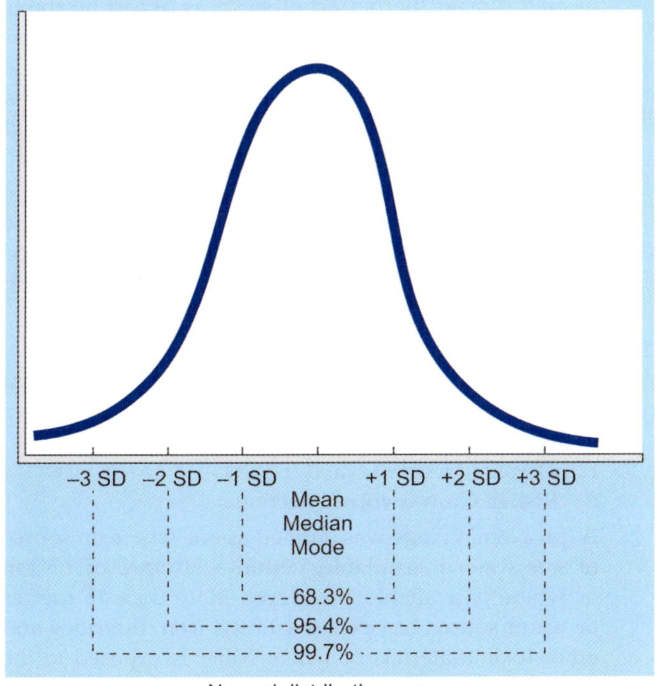

Normal distribution curve.

1.96 is the approximate value of the 97.5 percentile point of the normal distribution used in probability and statistics. 95% of the area under a normal curve lies within roughly 1.96 standard deviations of the mean, and due to the central limit theorem, this number is therefore used in the construction of approximate 95% confidence intervals.

274. The frequently occurring value in a data is:

a. Median b. Mode
c. Standard deviation d. Mean

The **mode** is the value that appears most often in a set of data. The mode of a discrete probability distribution is the value x at which its probability mass function takes its maximum value. In other words, it is the value that is most likely to be sampled. The mode of a continuous probability distribution is the value x at which its probability density function has its maximum value, so the mode is at the peak.

275. When the height and weight is perfectly correlated, coefficient of correlation is:

a. +1 b. –1
c. 0 d. More than 1

The Pearson correlation is +1 in the case of a perfect direct (increasing) linear relationship (correlation), –1 in the case of a perfect decreasing (inverse) linear relationship (**anticorrelation**), and some value between –1 and 1 in all other cases, indicating the degree of linear dependence between the variables. As it approaches zero there is less of a relationship (closer to uncorrelated). The closer the coefficient is to either –1 or 1, the stronger the correlation between the variables.

276. In an outbreak of cholera in a village of 2,000 population, 20 cases have occurred and 5 died. Case fatality rate is:

a. 1% b. 0.25%
c. 5% d. 25%

Ans. 272. **c.** 3/5 273. **d.** 95% 274. **b.** Mode 275. **a.** +1
276. **d.** 25%

A **case fatality rate** (CFR)—or **case fatality risk, case fatality ratio** or just **fatality rate**—is the proportion of deaths within a designated population of "cases" (people with a medical condition), over the course of the disease. A CFR is conventionally expressed as a percentage and represents a measure of risk. CFRs are most often used for diseases with discrete, limited time courses, such as outbreaks of acute infections. In the given question, 5 × 100/20 = 25%.

MISCELLANEOUS

277. All of the following hospital waste must be discarded in blue bag EXCEPT:

a. Plastic syringe
b. Catheter
c. Cannula
d. Placenta

Blue/ white translucent colour

- Type of container: Plastic bag/puncture proof container
- Waste category: 4 (waste sharps) and 7 (waste generated from disposable items other than waste sharp)
- Treatment options: Autoclaving/microwaving/ chemical treatment and destruction/ shedding

278. In xerophthalmia, what does X1A indicates?

a. Conjunctival xerosis
b. Bitots spots
c. Corneal xerosis
d. Corneal ulcer

WHO classification of xerophthalmia

X1A	Conjunctival xerosis
X1B	Conjunctival xerosis with Bitot's spots
X2	Corneal xerosis
X3A	Corneal xerosis with ulceration
X3B	Keratomalacia

279. True statement for lead poisoning:

a. Urinary Coproporphyrin > 100 mcg/ L indicates exposure to lead
b. Greatest source is drinking water from lead pipes
c. Stippling of basophils is a significant finding
d. Can cause blue line on gums

The toxic effects of inorganic lead exposure are abdominal colic, obstinate constipation, loss of appetite, blue line on the gums, stippling of red cells, anaemia, wrist drop and foot drop.

280. All of the following are sterilized by hot air oven EXCEPT:

a. Scalpels b. Glassware
c. Plastic syringes d. Dressings

Hot air is very useful for sterilizing articles such as glasswares, syringes, swabs, dressings, French chalk, oils, Vaseline and sharp instruments.

281. Graphic plan of all events and activities to be completed to reach an end objective is:

a. Job catching b. Work sampling
c. Cost accounting d. Network analysis

Management/network analysis is a process of carrying out the project work of the health care service, involving all the resources to achieve the defined objectives, efficiently and economically by a network analysis, i.e. by preparing a schedule diagrammatically, in a logical sequence from the commencement to the completion of the work representing the different components of the project work and the period required for each of the components.

	Program evaluation and review technique (PERT)	*Critical path method (CPM)*
1.	Design is based on event	Design is based on activity
2.	Time requirement is estimated	Time requirement is taken from previous experience
3.	Main objective is to take shortest time	There is mixture of time and cost
4.	Activity time is not subjective	Activity time is subjective
5.	Slack time* cannot be identified	Slack time can be identified

*Slack time is the difference between the minimum time required and the maximum time taken up for the activity.

282. Extended sickness benefit is given for:

a. 309 days b. 365 days
c. 409 days d. 490 days

Sickness benefit is a benefit given to the insured worker in cash during the period of sickness, when he/she is unable to attend to the work, provided the sickness is duly certified by the Insurance Medical Officer. The benefit consists of 50% of the average daily wage, for a maximum period of 91 days, in any continuous period of 365 days. This is called 'Ordinary Sickness Benefit'. This benefit covers only short term illness.

Employees suffering from long-term illnesses, the benefit of cash is extended beyond 91 days. It is called 'Extended Sickness Benefit'. This benefit is payable up to 309 days.

283. Problem village is all EXCEPT:

a. Where no water source in a distance of 1.6 km from community
b. Water is more than depth of 15 m
c. There is excess of Na, K, F salts
d. Risk of Guineaworm infection

A 'problem' village was defined as one where no source of safe water is available, within a distance of 1.6 km or where is available at a depth more than 15 metres or water source has excess salinity, iron, fluorides and other toxic materials or where water is exposed to the risk of Cholera.

Ans. **277. d.** All of the above **278. a.** Conjunctival xerosis **279. d.** Can cause blue line... **280. c.** Plastic syringes
281. d. Network... **282. a.** 309 days **283. d.** Risk of Guineaworm infection

284. Absolute CONTRAINDICATION for IUCD insertion are all of the following EXCEPT:

a. PID
b. Abnormal uterine bleeding
c. Ca cervix
d. DM

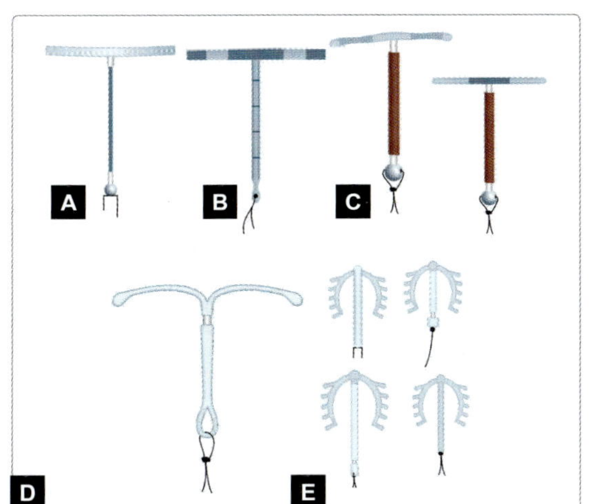

(A) T Cu 200 B, (B) T Cu 220 C, (C) T Cu 380 A and T Cu 380 S, (D) Cu Nova T 200, (E) ML Cu 250 and 375.

Absolute contraindications for IUD use

- Pregnancy
- Significantly distorted uterine anatomy
- Unexplained vaginal bleeding concerning for pregnancy or pelvic malignancy
- Gestational trophoblastic disease with persistently elevated beta-human chorionic gonadotropin levels
- Ongoing pelvic infection

285. OCP protects the woman against all EXCEPT:

a. Menorrhagia
b. Benign breast disease
c. PID
d. Venous thromboembolism

Absolute contraindications to use of OCPs

- < 6 weeks postpartum
- Smoker over the age of 35 (>15 cigarettes per day)
- Hypertension (systolic > 160 mm Hg or diastolic > 100 mm Hg)
- Current of past history of venous thromboembolism (VTE)

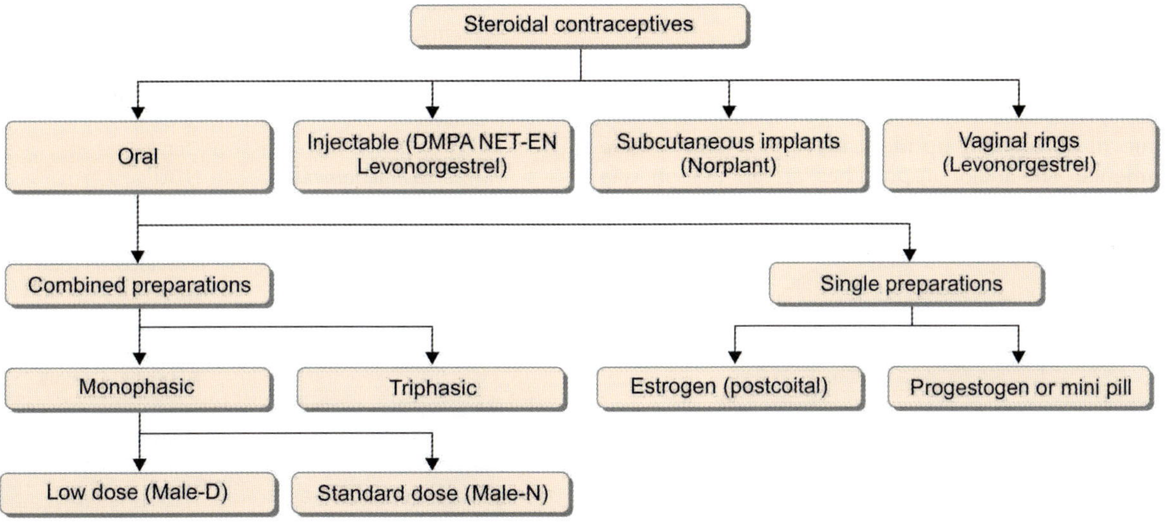

Different steroidal contraceptives.

286. Spermicide used in contraceptive 'TODAY':

a. NET-EN
b. DMPA
c. Nonoxynol
d. Nor-ethinosterol

Nonoxynol-9 is the FDA approved spermicide contained in **Today** Sponge/foam. This paralyzes the sperm. The effect lasts for about 1 hour.

287. Management technique, which is more promising tool for application in health field?

a. Input-output analysis
b. Cost accounting
c. Cost-benefit analysis
d. Cost-effectiveness analysis

Cost-effectiveness analysis (CEA) is a form of economic analysis that compares the relative costs and outcomes (effects) of two or more courses of action. **Cost-effectiveness analysis** is distinct from **cost-benefit analysis,** which assigns a monetary value to the measure of effect. Examples are:

- Health treatment of TB patients vs DOTS (DOTS is cost effective)
- Provision of safe water supply vs treatment of water borne diseases (purification of water is cost-effective).

288. PERT is for:

a. System analysis
b. Input-output analysis
c. Cost-effective analysis
d. Network analysis

Ans. **284. d.** DM **285. d.** Venous... **286. c.** Nonoxynol **287. d.** Cost-effectiveness... **288. d.** Network analysis

The **program** (or **project**) **evaluation and review technique**, commonly abbreviated **PERT**, is a statistical tool, used in project management, which was designed to analyze and represent the tasks involved in completing a given project.

Sl. No.	Activity of the project work	Duration (in weeks)
1.	Preparation of the plan	1
2.	Approval of the plan	2
3.	Preparation of the list of beneficiaries	4
4.	Arrangement of human resources	6
5.	Training of the manpower	3
6.	Education of the community	2
7.	Indent for the equipment	1
8.	Transport arrangement	2
9.	Starting the service	1

289. An example of 2-way discussion:
a. Group discussion
b. Symposium
c. Role playing
d. Seminar

A **discussion group** is a group of individuals (6-12 persons) with similar interest who gather either formally or informally to bring up ideas, solve problems or give comments. The major approaches are in person, via conference call or website.

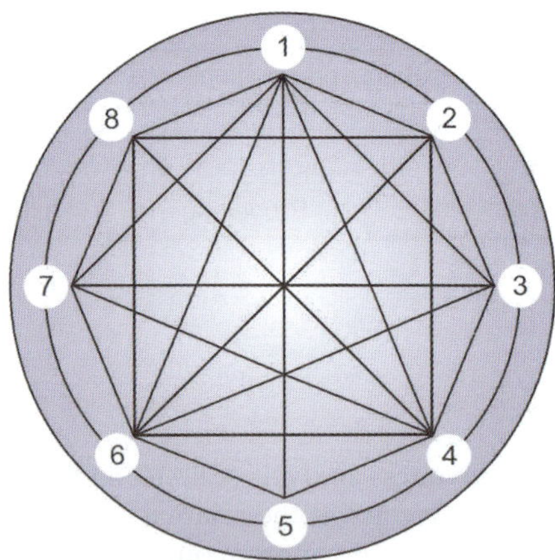

A group discussion.

290. Acculturation is:
a. Cultural history of health and disease
b. Study of various cultures
c. Culture contact
d. All of the above

Acculturation is cultural modification of an individual, group, or people by adapting to or borrowing traits from another culture (a merging of cultures as a result of prolonged contact).

291. Cluster testing is helpful in detecting cases of:
a. Measles
b. Diabetes
c. Cancer
d. STD

In a sense, "cluster testing" is really an extension of contact tracing for sexually transmitted illnesses. It was long ago noted that certain patients, when approached by the venereal disease investigator or the clinician, would offer the suggestion that: "You ought to have a look at Sam Jones, too. He's got a bad rash just like mine." Sometimes the health worker, on one pretext or another, did "have a look at Sam Jones, too." Sometimes Sam had scabies. But sometimes Sam had secondary syphilis.

Classification of STI agents and diseases caused by them.

Agents	Diseases
Bacteriae (including *spirochetes*) *Treponema pallidum*, *Haemophilus ducreyi*, *Neisseria gonorrhoeae*	Syphilis, Yaws, Pinta. Chancroid (Soft sore) Gonorrhea, Urethritis, Cervicitis, Epididymitis, Salpingitis, PID, Ophthalmia neonatorum.
Calymmatobacterium granulomatis	Donovanosis (Granuloma inguinale)
Chlamydia trachomatis (L_1, L_2, L_3)	Lymphogranuloma venereum (LGV)
Chlamydia trachomatis (D to K)	Nongonococcal Urethritis (NGU) Cervicitis
Mycoplasma hominis	NGU
Ureaplasma urealyticum	NGU
Shigella spp.	Proctocolitis (due to anal sex)
Campylobacter spp.	Proctocolitis (due to anal sex)
Bacterial vaginosis–associated organisms	Bacterial vaginosis
Group B streptococci	Vaginitis, Urethritis, Cervicitis, Balanitis, Cystitis
Viral agents	
Human (alpha) herpes virus 1 and 2	Herpes genitalis
Human (beta) herpes virus 5	Cervicitis, NGU
Hepatitis B virus	Serum hepatitis
Human papilloma virus	Genital warts
Molluscum contagiosum virus	Genital molluscum contagiosum
Human immunodeficiency virus (HIV)	AIDS
Protozoal agents	
Entamoeba histolytica	Amoebiasis
Giardia lamblia	Giardiasis
Trichomonas vaginalis	Trichomoniasis (vaginitis)
Fungal agents	
Candida albicans	Vaginal candidiasis
Ectoparasites	
Pthirus pubis	Pubic pediculosis (It is not a disease but infestation)
Sarcoptes scabiei	Genital scabies

Ans. **289. a.** Group discussion **290. c.** Culture contact **291. d.** STD

292. Bagassosis occurs with:

a. Silical fibres
b. Carbon particles
c. Sugarcane fibres
d. Cotton

Bagassosis, an interstitial lung disease, is a type of hypersensitivity pneumonitis attributed to exposure to moldy molasses (bagasse).

Common pneumoconioses, their causative agents and the industries of the occurrence.

Dusts	Disease	Industries
Inorganic (Mineral) dusts		
Silica	Silicosis	Sand stone industry, stone quarrying and dressing, granite industry, pottery and ceramic industry, gold, silver, mica and steel industry
Asbestos	Asbestosis	Asbestos cement factory, fireproof textiles, brake lining gaskets
Iron	Siderosis	Iron ores and mines, iron and steel industries
Coal dust	Anthracosis	Coal mines
Aluminum	Aluminosis	Aluminum industries
Barium	Baritosis	Photography, printing, barium diagnostic works
Beryllium	Berylliosis	Beryllium mining, manufacture of alloys
Stone	Lithosis	Stone industries
Organic (Vegetable) dusts		
Cotton dust	Byssinosis	Textile industries
Sugar cane dust (Bagasse)	Bagassosis	Cane sugar factories, paper and card board factories
Tobacco dust	Tobaccosis	Tobacco factories (Beedi, Cigar, Cigarette)
Mouldy hay (Grain dust)	Farmer's lung	Agricultural industry

293. Sharp instruments may be sterilized with:

a. Radiation
b. Lysol
c. Hot air
d. All of the above

Conventional hot air ovens are very useful for sterilization of glassware articles, syringes, swabs, dressings, powders, oils, Vaseline (petroleum jelly) and sharp instruments.

294. What is the color coding of bag in hospitals to dispose off human anatomical wastes such as body parts?

a. Yellow
b. Black
c. Red
d. Blue

Human anatomical waste is disposed in yellow color container.

Color coding for waste containers.

Type of waste	Contents	Color code of container	Remarks
1. General waste	**All domestic type:** Non-infectious non-hazardous, e.g. (a) recyclable: all kinds of papers, cardboard packing materials, metal or aluminum tins, magazines, newspapers, ledgers. (b) non-recyclable: Kitchen waste.	WHITE Container with black label "for general wastes only".	May be periodically sold at prevailing rates
2. Infectious waste:			Segregate carefully into correct type of bag
(a) Category No. 1	**Human anatomical waste:** Human tissue, organs and body parts.	**Yellow** With biohazard sign	
(b) Category No. 3	**Waste from laboratory**		
(c) Category No. 6	**Soiled waste:** Items contaminated with blood, and body fluids including cotton, dressings, soiled plaster casts, lines, beddings, other material contaminated with blood.	**Red** International infectious substance symbol	
(d) Category No. 4	**Waste sharps:** Needles, syringes, scalpels, blade, glass, etc.		After treatment and multilation these wastes are recyclable
(e) Category No. 7	**Solid waste:** Wastes generated from disposable items IV tubes, catheters, IV and blood bags, etc.	Blue	May be infectious
(f) Category No. 5	Discarded and outdated medicines	Black	

Ans. 292. c. Sugarcane fibres **293. c.** Hot air **294. a.** Yellow

295. Plastic wrapper of surgical syringe should be discarded in:

a. Black bag
b. Yellow bag
c. Red bag
d. Blue bag

General waste like office waste or dry non-infectious waste is segregated in black colour container.

Norms of the color coding containers

Color coding and waste segregation		Waste disposal
Black	General waste: Office waste, dry non-infectious waste	❑ Dispose with regular garbage in a secure sanitary landfill or have incinerated.
Red	Infectious plastic syringe, cannula, catheter	❑ Should be shredded, cut or mutilated. This ensures that they are not recycled/reused. ❑ Should be placed in a sturdy impervious (plastic) bag, tied securely with a twist tie and the contents identified with a label or tag. ❑ Dispose with regular garbage in a secure sanitary landfill or have incinerated.
Yellow	Infectious waste: Pathological specimens anatomical waste	❑ Should be place in leak proof container and the contents identified with a label or tag. ❑ Should either be incinerated or autoclaved before disposal in a secure sanitary landfill.
Blue/ White	Glass waste: Whole and broken glass	❑ Should be placed in disposable, puncture resistant containers. Bottles with a narrow neck are well suited for the purpose. ❑ Disinfected with chemicals or autoclave or incinerated before disposal.
Gray	Sharps; Needles, blades, scalpels	

296. Cytotoxic drug is disposed in:

a. Yellow bag
b. Red bag
c. Blue bag
d. Black bag

Discarded Medicines and cytotoxic waste are disposed in Plastic bag of Black color (category 5).

Schedule I: Categories of biomedical waste.

Option	Waste category
Category 1	Human anatomical waste (Human tissues, organs, body parts, placenta, aborted fetus, amputated parts, tumors, etc.)
Category 2	Animal waste (Animal tissues, organs, body parts, carcasses, waste generated in veterinary hospitals, colleges, discharge from animal house)
Category 3	Microbiology and biotechnology waste (Laboratory cultures, specimens, vaccines, human and animal cell culture, toxins, etc.)
Category 4	Waste sharps (both used and unused) (needles, syringes, scalpels, blades, glass)
Category 5	Discarded medicines and cytotoxic drugs
Category 6	Soiled waste (Waste contaminated with blood and body fluids such as cotton swabs, bedding, dressings, plaster casts, linen, etc.)
Category 7	Solid waste (Catheters, IV sets, tubings, blood bags, etc.)
Category 8	Liquid waste (Waste generated from laboratories and washing, cleaning, housekeeping)
Category 9	Incineration ash (Ash generated from incineration of biomedical waste)
Category 10	Chemical waste (Wastes of disinfectants, insecticides, etc.)

297. Outdated drugs and cytotoxic drugs are disposed of by:

a. Incineration
b. Store for month and burial
c. Destruction and disposal in landfill
d. Dumping

Categorization of wastes.

Category	Waste types	Segregation	Disposal
Cat No. 1	Human anatomical wastes		Incineration/ deep burial
Cat No. 2	Animal wastes		-Do-
Cat No. 3	Microbiology and biotechnology wastes		-Do/ Autoclave
Cat No. 4	Sharps		Autoclave/ destruction/shred
Cat No. 5	Discarded medicine and cytotoxic drugs		Secured landfill
Cat No. 6	Soiled wastes		Incineration/ autoclave
Cat No. 7	Soiled wastes		Autoclave/ destruction/shred
Cat No. 8	Liquid wastes	Drainage	Effluent treatment
Cat No. 9	Incineration ash		Secured landfill
Cat No. 10	Chemical wastes		-Do-

Source: CME on awareness of biomedical waste disposal, 2006.

Ans. **295. a.** Black bag **296. d.** Black bag **297. c.** Destruction and...

Many cytotoxics can be **disposed** of by chemical destruction or disposition in secured landfill.

298. Needles are disposed of in:

a. Black container b. Blue container
c. Yellow container d. Red container

Waste sharp and solid waste should be segregated in blue container.

299. MC side effect of IUCD insertion:

a. Ectopic pregnancy
b. Pelvic infection
c. Pain
d. Bleeding

With a copper **IUD, spotting**, light bleeding, heavier or prolonged bleeding and pain with bleeding are common in the first three to six months of use

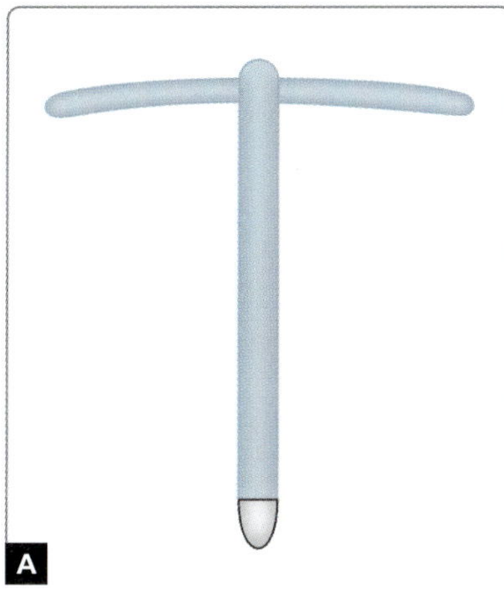

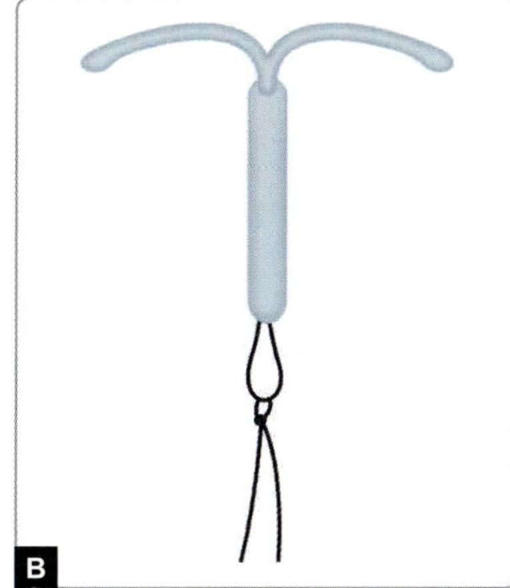

(A) Progestasert; (B) LNG 20.

300. Best index for measuring efficacy of contraceptives:

a. Quetelet index
b. Chandler's index
c. Life-table analysis
d. Pearl index

Life-table methods are often used to study birth control effectiveness. In this role, they are an alternative to the Pearl Index.

As used in birth control studies, a decrement table calculates a separate effectiveness rate for each month of the study, as well as for a standard period of time (usually 12 months). Use of life table methods eliminates time-related biases (i.e. the most fertile couples getting pregnant and dropping out of the study early, and couples becoming more skilled at using the method as time goes on), and in this way is superior to the Pearl Index.

301. Disinfectants used for blood spills:

a. Sodium hypochlorite b. Ethanol
c. Glutaraldehyde d. Phenol

Sodium hypochlorite is a chemical compound with the formula NaClO. It is composed of a sodium cation (Na^{+}) and a hypochlorite anion (ClO^{-}); it may also be viewed as the sodium salt of hypochlorous acid. When dissolved in water it is commonly known as **bleach**, or **liquid bleach**. A 1-in-5 dilution of household bleach with water (1 part bleach to 4 parts water) is effective against many bacteria and some viruses, and is often the disinfectant of choice in cleaning surfaces in hospitals.

302. Method of safe disposal of mercury:

a. Deep burial
b. Chemical treatment
c. Controlled combustion
d. Careful collection and recycle

Spilled mercury and waste mercury-containing equipment and products should be treated as hazardous materials and in many cases as hazardous wastes. This waste must be disposed of in accordance with all relevant requirements and be recycled wherever possible. To help plan for the proper recycling or disposal of mercury-containing products, identify hazardous waste management firms and/or certified carriers and remember to properly package products prior to transport to help prevent breaks or leaks.

303. The maximum number of work hours/week, prescribed under the Factories act is:

a. 42 hours/week b. 48 hours/week
c. 54 hours/week d. 60 hours/week

Section 51 of the **Factories Act**, 1948 prescribes that **no** adult worker shall be required or allowed to work in a factory for more than **forty-eight hours** in any week or not more than 60 hours including over-time.

304. FALSE regarding growth chart:

a. Lowermost line represents children below third percentile
b. Between top 2 lines, it shows road to health
c. The position of dot is more important than direction
d. It is an important tool for educating

By looking at the direction of the child's growth curve, the health worker and the mother can see at a glance whether the child is gaining weight appropriately or not.

Ans. 298. **b.** Blue container 299. **d.** Bleeding 300. **c.** Life-table analysis 301. **a.** Sodium hypochlorite 302. **d.** Careful collect... 303. **b.** 48 hours/week 304. **c.** The position of dot is more important than direction

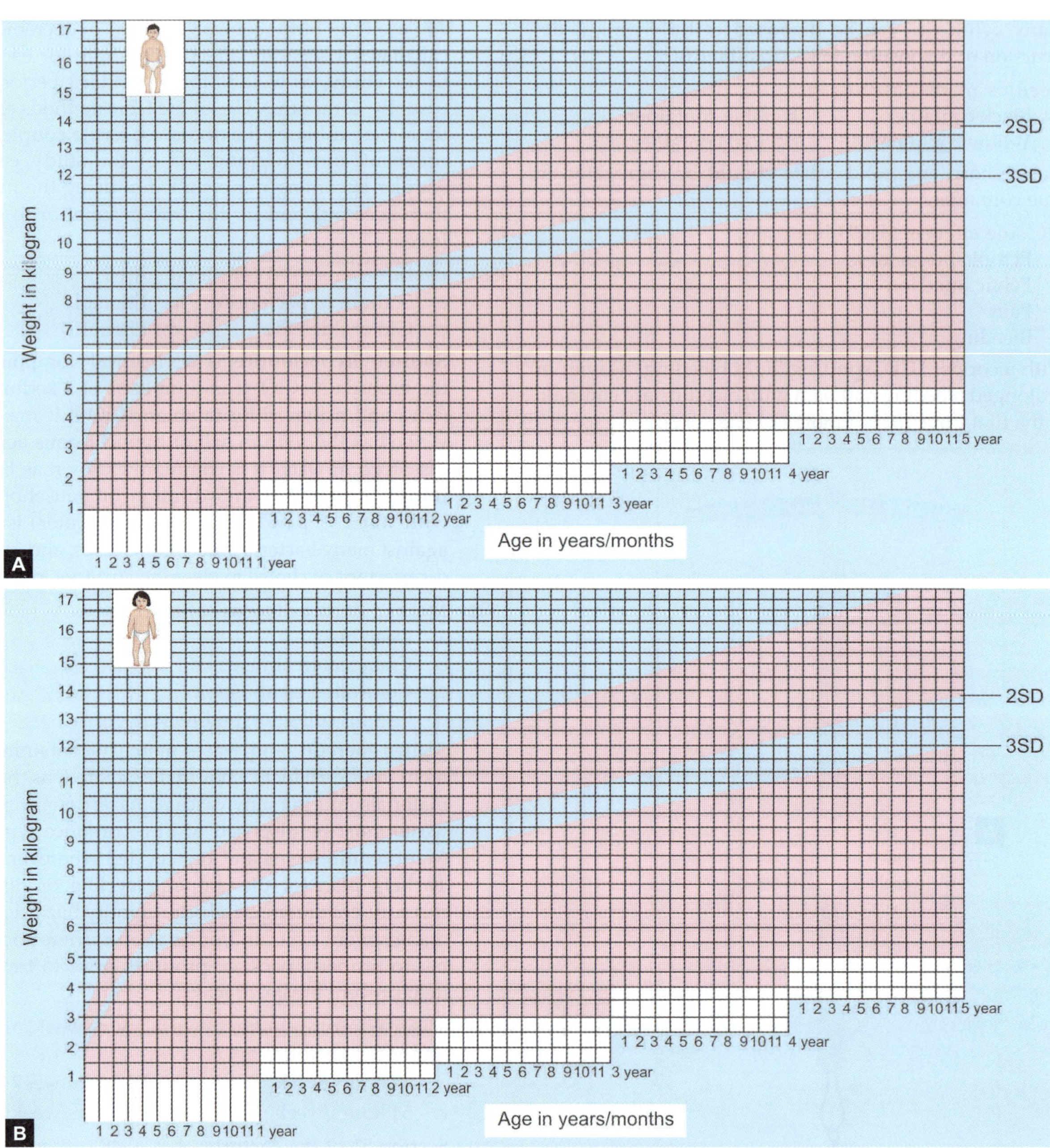

New growth chart used Indian *anganwadis.* (A) For boys; (B) For girls.

305. In triage system for disaster management, which of the following color codes denote 'high priority treatment' and 'transfer'?

a. Red
b. Blue
c. Black
d. Yellow

Triage

- Red tags—(Immediate) are used to label those who cannot survive without immediate treatment but who have a chance of survival.
- Yellow tags—(Observation) for those who require observation (and possible later re-triage). Their condition is stable for the moment and, they are not in immediate danger of death. These victims will still need hospital care and would be treated immediately under normal circumstances.
- Green tags—(Wait) are reserved for the "walking wounded" who will need medical care at some point, after more critical injuries have been treated.
- White tags—(Dismiss) are given to those with minor injuries for whom a doctor's care is not required.
- Black tags—(Expectant) are used for the deceased and for those whose injuries are so extensive that they will not be able to survive given the care that is available.

Ans. 305. a. Red

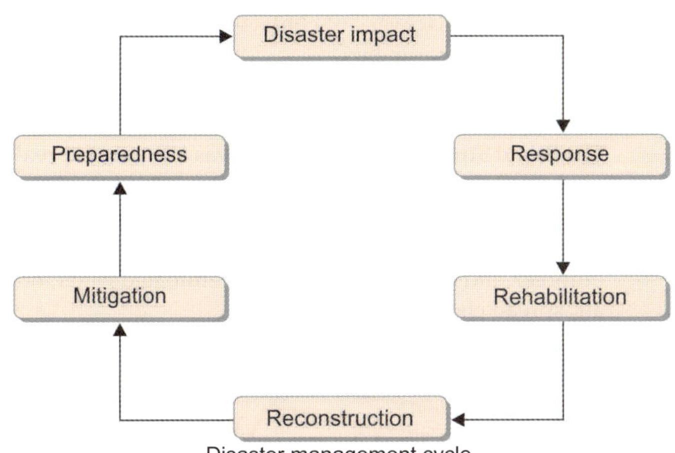

Disaster management cycle.

306. Height independent obesity index:

a. Corpulence index b. Quetelet index
c. Brocca index d. Ponderal index

The **Corpulence Index (CI)** or **Ponderal Index (PI)** is a measure of leanness of a person calculated as a relationship between mass and height. It was first proposed in 1921 as the "Corpulence Index" by Rohrer and hence also known as **Rohrer's Index**. It is similar to the body mass index, but the mass is normalized with the third power of body height rather than the second power.

307. Cut off BMI for obesity:

a. 20 b. 25
c. 30 d. 35

Obese class I has a BMI of 30–34.9 kg/m^2

Classification of obesity according to body mass index.

Classification	*Body mass index (kg/m^2)*
Under weight	< 18.5
Normal range	18.5–24.9
Overweight	> 25
Preobese	25–29.9
Obese class I	30–34.9
Obese class II	35–39.9
Obese class III	> 40

308. Ideal desk recommended for a school child is:

a. 'Plus' desk b. 'Minus' desk
c. 'Zero' desk d. None of the above

Minus desk

- The edge of the chair goes inside the edge of the desk
- **It is the recommended desk for use in schools**
- Advantage—Easy to write on the desk, maintenance of good posture
- Disadvantage—Difficult to get up from the chair as the chair has to be pulled out before the student can stand.

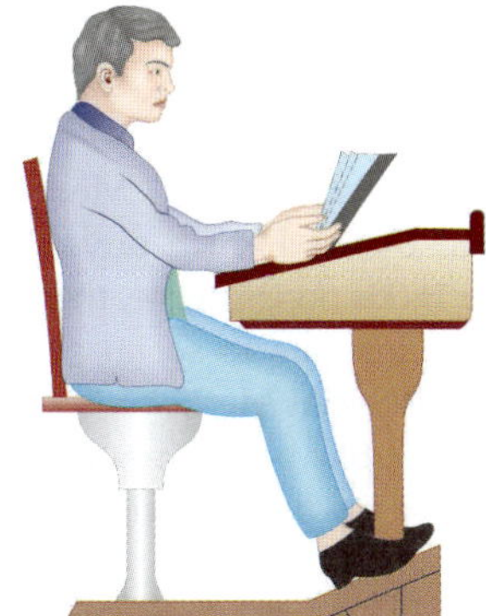
Correct position in a minus desk.

309. Diffuse mesothelioma is seen with:

a. Asbestos b. Arsenic
c. Tobacco use d. TB

Mesothelioma (or, more precisely, **malignant mesothelioma**) is a rare form of cancer that develops from cells of the mesothelium, the protective lining that covers many of the internal organs of the body. Mesothelioma is most commonly caused by exposure to asbestos. The most common anatomical site for mesothelioma is the pleura (the outer lining of the lungs and internal chest wall), but it can also arise in the peritoneum (the lining of the abdominal cavity), the pericardium (the sac that surrounds the heart).

Types of occupational cancers, their carcinogens and related industries.

Type of cancer	*Carcinogen*	*'At risk' group in the industry*
Skin cancer*	Anthracene, coal-tar, soot, pitch, oils and dyes, acids, U-V rays, X-rays.	Farmers, shepherds, fisherman, road-builders oil refiners, dye-stuff makers, radiology department staff, tar distillers, coke-oven workers.
Lung cancer	Arsenic, asbestos, beryllium, chromium, uranium, tobacco, coal tar, nickel.	Asbestos factory, uranium-mines, nickel-refineries, gas industry, tobacco industry.
Bladder cancer #	β-naphthylamine, benzidine, auramine, aromatic amines, para-amino diphenyl, hemo-toxins.	Aniline industry, rubber industry, electric cable industry.
Leukemia	Ionizing radiations (X-rays and gamma rays), radioactive isotopes	Radiology department, atomic energy research station

Note: 'Dhoti-cancer' as described by Khanolkar is not an industrial cancer but caused by mechanical irritation (friction) of dhoti over the skin of waist.

*Occupational skin cancers also include Mule spinner's cancer and Chimney sweeper's cancer (cancer of scrotum).

#Cancer of the bladder resulting from the infestation of Schistosoma hematobium (a biological agent) is not an industrial cancer.

Ans. **306. a.** Corpulence... **307. c.** 30 **308. b.** 'Minus' desk **309. a.** Asbestos

310. The term 'social medicine' was first introduced by:

a. John Snow
b. David Morley
c. Jules Guerin
d. CEA Winslow

Historically, the term "Social Medicine" is known to be first coined by the French physician-journalist Jules Guerin in the 1800s. At this time, the term meant extending Medicine's insights to social problems. Since then, the definition of Social Medicine has evolved to be synonymous with public health, epidemiology, state medicine, community medicine, social pathology.

311. John Snow's discovery of cholera is an example of:

a. Natural experiments
b. Spot map study
c. Randomized trial
d. Short study

The **Broad Street cholera outbreak** was a severe outbreak of cholera that occurred near Broad Street in the Soho district of London, England in 1854. This outbreak is best known for the physician John Snow's study of the outbreak and his discovery that contaminated water, not air, spread cholera.

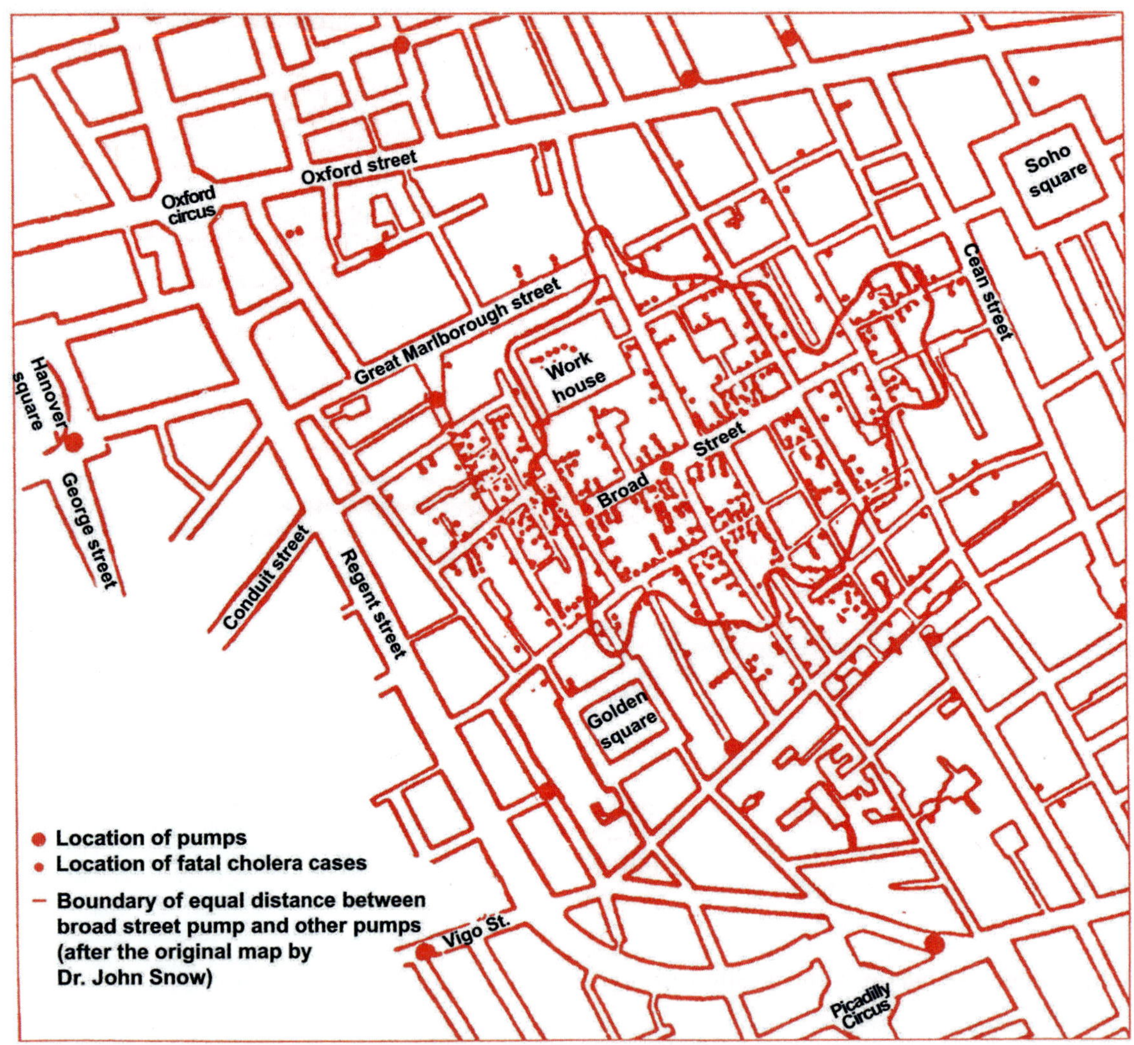

Spot map Asiatic cholera in London.
Source: Park K Park's Textbook of Preventive and Social Medicals 18th edn. 2005.

312. 'Cafeteria approach' is related with:

a. Diet programme
b. Child and maternal health
c. National vector borne disease control programme
d. Contraception

A "Cafeteria Approach" meaning choose whatever method of contraception you like was introduced by the Health and Family welfare minister Prof. Chandrasekhar.

Ans. **310. c.** Jules Guerin **311. b.** Spot map study **312. d.** Contraception

ANSWERS WITH REFERENCES

GENERAL CONCEPTS

1. **Ans. (a)** 26-29
Ref: Park's PSM, 21/e p639t

2. **Ans. (d)** Pathogenesis
Ref: Park's PSM, 21/e p32

3. **Ans. (d)** Associated with antecedent causation
Ref: Park's PSM, 21/e p75

4. **Ans. (c)** Long term changes
Ref: Park's PSM, 21/e p62

5. **Ans. (a)** Hypertension
Ref: Park's PSM, 21/e p37

6. **Ans. (a)** TP/ TP + FP
Ref: Park's PSM, 21/e p128

7. **Ans. (a)** IMR, life expectancy at 1 year of age and literacy rate
Ref: Suryakantha's Community Medicine 3/e p7

8. **Ans. (c)** Prevalence is increased
Ref: Suryakantha's Community Medicine 3/e p245

9. **Ans. (d)** Specificity
Ref: Suryakantha's Community Medicine 3/e p297

10. **Ans. (d)** Exotic
Ref: Suryakantha's Community Medicine 3/e p268

11. **Ans. (b)** Continuous monitoring of occurrence and distribution of a disease
Ref: Suryakantha's Community Medicine 3/e p269

12. **Ans. (d)** Rehabilitation
Ref: Suryakantha's Community Medicine 3/e p20

13. **Ans. (b)** Cohort study
Ref: Suryakantha's Community Medicine 3/e p259 (Table 18.6)

14. **Ans. (c)** Case fatality rate
Ref: Suryakantha's Community Medicine 3/e p247

15. **Ans. (b)** Secondary prevention
Ref: Suryakantha's Community Medicine 3/e p18

16. **Ans. (c)** Proportion
Ref: Suryakantha's Community Medicine 3/e p244

17. **Ans. (b)** To eliminate selection bias
Ref: Suryakantha's Community Medicine 3/e p261

18. **Ans. (d)** Cervical pap smear checking
Ref: Suryakantha's Community Medicine 3/e p18

19. **Ans. (d)** True positive
Ref: Suryakantha's Community Medicine 3/e p296

20. **Ans. (a)** Isolation
Ref: Suryakantha's Community Medicine 3/e p276

21. **Ans. (b)** Randomization
Ref: Suryakantha's Community Medicine 3/e p271

22. **Ans. (b)** Attributable risk
Ref: Suryakantha's Community Medicine 3/e p259

23. **Ans. (b)** Multifactorial cause of Ca lung
Ref: Suryakantha's Community Medicine 3/e p258

24. **Ans. (b)** Cohort study
Ref: Suryakantha's Community Medicine 3/e p260

25. **Ans. (a)** Incidence will not change
Ref: Suryakantha's Community Medicine 3/e p243

26. **Ans. (d)** Verification of diagnosis
Ref: Suryakantha's Community Medicine 3/e p277

27. **Ans. (c)** Odd's ratio can be calculated
Ref: Suryakantha's Community Medicine 3/e p255

28. **Ans. (c)** Primordial prevention
Ref: Suryakantha's Community Medicine 3/e p18

29. **Ans. (d)** Index case
Ref: Internet resources

30. **Ans. (c)** Cohort study
Ref: Suryakantha's Community Medicine 3/e p256

31. **Ans. (a)** Disease is very fatal and/or easily curable
Ref: Suryakantha's Community Medicine 3/e p244

32. **Ans. (a)** Point source epidemic
Ref: Suryakantha's Community Medicine 3/e p250

33. **Ans. (d)** Primordial prevention
Ref: Suryakantha's Community Medicine 3/e p18

34. **Ans. (c)** Ecological
Ref: Internet resources

35. **Ans. (c)** Period of communicability
Ref: Suryakantha's Community Medicine 3/e p276

36. **Ans. (a) Incidence of disease amongst exposed/incidence of disease amongst non-exposed**
Ref: Suryakantha's Community Medicine 3/e p258

37. **Ans. (b) Missed cases**
Ref: Internet resources

38. **Ans. (c) Relative risk**
Ref: Suryakantha's Community Medicine 3/e p258

39. **Ans. (c) Low prevalence and low incidence**
Ref: Suryakantha's Community Medicine 3/e p244

40. **Ans. (a) Field trials**
Ref: Suryakantha's Community Medicine 3/e p263

41. **Ans. (d) Attributable risk can be known**
Ref: Suryakantha's Community Medicine 3/e p256

42. **Ans. (d) Helps in identifying risk factors of a disease**
Ref: Suryakantha's Community Medicine 3/e p253

43. **Ans. (c) It is a risk factor for the disease**
Ref: Internet resources

44. **Ans. (d) Screening for hypertension**
Ref: Suryakantha's Community Medicine 3/e p19

45. **Ans. (b) Case control study**
Ref: Suryakantha's Community Medicine 3/e p225

46. **Ans. (c) Analytical study**
Ref: Suryakantha's Community Medicine 3/e p242

47. **Ans. (b) Measures life expectancy adjusted without disability**
Ref: Internet resources

48. **Ans. (b) Supplements routine notification system**
Ref: Suryakantha's Community Medicine 3/e p271

49. **Ans. (c) Preserving traditional lifestyle**
Ref: Suryakantha's Community Medicine 3/e p18

50. **Ans. (b) Denominator is mid-year population**
Ref: Suryakantha's Community Medicine 3/e p246

51. **Ans. (a) Every person has an equal chance of selection**
Ref: Suryakantha's Community Medicine 3/e p261

52. **Ans. (c) Less time consuming**
Ref: Suryakantha's Community Medicine 3/e p253

53. **Ans. (b) 10 years**
Ref: Internet resources

54. **Ans. (d) Housing**
Ref: Suryakantha's Community Medicine 3/e p707

55. **Ans. (a) Under-5 mortality**
Ref: Suryakantha's Community Medicine 3/e p8

56. **Ans. (b) Useful for rare diseases**
Ref: Suryakantha's Community Medicine 3/e p258

57. **Ans. (c) Secular trend**
Ref: Suryakantha's Community Medicine 3/e p251

58. **Ans. (a) Primordial prevention**
Ref: Suryakantha's Community Medicine 3/e p8

59. **Ans. (a) Incubation period of the disease**
Ref: Suryakantha's Community Medicine 3/e p276

60. **Ans. (a) Point source epidemic**
Ref: Suryakantha's Community Medicine 3/e p250

61. **Ans. (c) Selection bias**
Ref: Internet resources

62. **Ans. (d) Reduce selection bias in allocation of treatment**
Ref: Suryakantha's Community Medicine 3/e p260

63. **Ans. (a) Health**
Ref: Suryakantha's Community Medicine 3/e p7

64. **Ans. (a) Health promotion**
Ref: Suryakantha's Community Medicine 3/e p17

65. **Ans. (b) Agent, host, environment**
Ref: Suryakantha's Community Medicine 3/e p13

66. **Ans. (b) Secondary level**
Ref: Suryakantha's Community Medicine 3/e p19

67. **Ans. (a) To know the total number of cases**
Ref: Suryakantha's Community Medicine 3/e p271

68. **Ans. (d) Per capita income**
Ref: Suryakantha's Community Medicine 3/e p7

69. **Ans. (c) Resting affected limbs in neutral position**
Ref: Suryakantha's Community Medicine 3/e p20

70. **Ans. (d) Clinical trials**
Ref: Suryakantha's Community Medicine 3/e p260

VACCINES

71. **Ans. (b) HIV patients**
Ref: Park's PSM, 21/e p98

72. **Ans. (b) 10 days of vaccination**
Ref: Suryakantha's Community Medicine 3/e p444

73. **Ans. (a) 9 months**
Ref: Suryakantha's Community Medicine 3/e p320

74. **Ans. (b) Active immunity**
Ref: Suryakantha's Community Medicine 3/e p280

75. **Ans. (a) Exotoxin**
Ref: Suryakantha's Community Medicine 3/e p281

76. **Ans. (b) At birth**
Ref: Suryakantha's Community Medicine 3/e p285

77. **Ans. (d) BCG**
Ref: Suryakantha's Community Medicine 3/e p281

78. **Ans. (c) Meningococcal vaccine**
Ref: Suryakantha's Community Medicine 3/e p350

79. **Ans. (a) Influenza**
Ref: Suryakantha's Community Medicine 3/e p281

80. **Ans. (b) Given around 100 yards of a case detected**
Ref: Internet resources

81. **Ans. (c) Typhoid**
Ref: Suryakantha's Community Medicine 3/e p282

82. **Ans. (a) IgG**
Ref: Internet resources

83. **Ans. (b) IgM**
Ref: Internet resources

84. **Ans. (d) Hepatitis B**
Ref: Suryakantha's Community Medicine 3/e p281

85. **Ans. (a) Yellow fever**
Ref: Suryakantha's Community Medicine 3/e p281

86. **Ans. (a) DPT**
Ref: Suryakantha's Community Medicine 3/e p291

87. **Ans. (d) 3 years**
Ref: Suryakantha's Community Medicine 3/e p391

88. **Ans. (a) It is a killed vaccine**
Ref: Suryakantha's Community Medicine 3/e p405

89. **Ans. (c) Aluminium**
Ref: Suryakantha's Community Medicine 3/e p345

90. **Ans. (c) 0, 1, 6 months**
Ref: Suryakantha's Community Medicine 3/e p397

91. **Ans. (a) Immediately after birth**
Ref: Suryakantha's Community Medicine 3/e p285

92. **Ans. (b) Deltoid muscle**
Ref: Suryakantha's Community Medicine 3/e p498

93. **Ans. (a) Normal saline**
Ref: Suryakantha's Community Medicine 3/e p358

94. **Ans. (b) 20 IU/kg**
Ref: Suryakantha's Community Medicine 3/e p500

95. **Ans. (c) Bivalent and quadrivalent**
Ref: Suryakantha's Community Medicine 3/e p543

96. **Ans. (b) 2**
Ref: Suryakantha's Community Medicine 3/e p286

97. **Ans. (c) Live attenuated vaccine**
Ref: Suryakantha's Community Medicine 3/e p320

98. **Ans. (c) 3 days of exposure**
Ref: Suryakantha's Community Medicine 3/e p321

99. **Ans. (c) Immunity against paralytic and wild strains**
Ref: Suryakantha's Community Medicine 3/e p403

100. **Ans. (a) 10 years**
Ref: Suryakantha's Community Medicine 3/e p444

101. **Ans. (a) 1 year**
Ref: Suryakantha's Community Medicine 3/e p398

102. **Ans. (d) A and C**
Ref: Suryakantha's Community Medicine 3/e p350

103. **Ans. (a) MMR**
Ref: Suryakantha's Community Medicine 3/e p281

104. **Ans. (a) 0, 3 and 7**
Ref: Suryakantha's Community Medicine 3/e p500

COMMUNICABLE AND NON-COMMUNICABLE DISEASES

105. **Ans. (c) Oxygen saturation**
Ref: Park's PSM, 21/e p159

106. **Ans. (a) Rocky mountain spotted fever**
Ref: Park's PSM, 21/e p274t

107. **Ans. (a) Bitot spot >0.5%**
Ref: Park's PSM, 21/e p569t

108. **Ans. (b) 200**
Ref: Park's PSM, 21/e p221

109. **Ans. (d) 95**
Ref: Suryakantha's Community Medicine 3/e p321

110. **Ans. (b) Sputum positive**
Ref: Park's Preventive and Social Medicine 21st/e p169

111. **Ans. (d) Rabies**
Ref: Suryakantha's Community Medicine 3/e p490

112. **Ans. (a) Rocky mountain spotted fever**
Ref: Suryakantha's Community Medicine 3/e p272

113. **Ans. (c) Dengue**
Ref: Suryakantha's Community Medicine 3/e p119

114. **Ans. (c) Leishmania tropica**
Ref: Suryakantha's Community Medicine 3/e p440

115. **Ans. (a) Anopheles**
Ref: Suryakantha's Community Medicine 3/e p122

116. **Ans. (c) Individual approach**
Ref: Internet resources

117. **Ans. (b) 0.00002 mg of PPD**
Ref: Suryakantha's Community Medicine 3/e p355

118. **Ans. (b) P. ovale**
Ref: Suryakantha's Community Medicine 3/e p423

119. **Ans. (a) Flea**
Ref: Suryakantha's Community Medicine 3/e p135

120. **Ans. (d) Rate less than 0.1/1000 live births**
Ref: Suryakantha's Community Medicine 3/e p422

121. **Ans. (b) Hook worm**
Ref: Suryakantha's Community Medicine 3/e p415

122. **Ans. (d) None of the above**
Ref: Suryakantha's Community Medicine 3/e p452

123. **Ans. (a) Malaria**
Ref: Suryakantha's Community Medicine 3/e p424

124. **Ans. (d) Step well workers**
Ref: Suryakantha's Community Medicine 3/e p407

125. **Ans. (d) Australia**
Ref: Suryakantha's Community Medicine 3/e p490

126. **Ans. (c) 10-14 days**
Ref: Suryakantha's Community Medicine 3/e p425

127. **Ans. (c) 21st day**
Ref: Suryakantha's Community Medicine 3/e p508

128. **Ans. (b) No. of eggs/gm of stool**
Ref: Suryakantha's Community Medicine 3/e p413

129. **Ans. (c) Secondary attack rate is 30%**
Ref: Suryakantha's Community Medicine 3/e p318

130. **Ans. (d) Infection after 16 weeks of gestation results in major congenital defects**
Ref: Suryakantha's Community Medicine 3/e p323

131. **Ans. (c) Treatment failure**
Ref: Suryakantha's Community Medicine 3/e p363

132. **Ans. (c) Anopheles stephensi**
Ref: Internet resources

133. **Ans. (c) Larvicide**
Ref: Suryakantha's Community Medicine 3/e p126

134. **Ans. (b) Man is the intermediate host**
Ref: Suryakantha's Community Medicine 3/e p432

135. **Ans. (c) Immediately stitch wound under antibiotic coverage**
Ref: Suryakantha's Community Medicine 3/e p496

136. **Ans. (c) Pigs manifest disease**
Ref: Suryakantha's Community Medicine 3/e p449

137. **Ans. (a) Influenza**
Ref: Suryakantha's Community Medicine 3/e p329

138. **Ans. (a) Industrial workers**
Ref: Suryakantha's Community Medicine 3/e p485

139. **Ans. (a) Supplementation of vitamins**
Ref: Internet resources

140. **Ans. (a) Giving TT vaccine between age group 10-15 years girls**
Ref: Suryakantha's Community Medicine 3/e p420

141. **Ans. (b) It is a diagnostic test**
Ref: Suryakantha's Community Medicine 3/e p507

142. **Ans. (a) Spread by sexual transmission**
Ref: Suryakantha's Community Medicine 3/e p521

143. **Ans. (c) Ticks**
Ref: Suryakantha's Community Medicine 3/e p141

144. **Ans. (b) Street virus**
Ref: Suryakantha's Community Medicine 3/e p490

145. **Ans. (c) 6 days**
Ref: Suryakantha's Community Medicine 3/e p445

146. **Ans. (a) Filarial parasite**
Ref: Suryakantha's Community Medicine 3/e p113

147. **Ans. (a) Leishmania donovani**
Ref: Suryakantha's Community Medicine 3/e p440

148. **Ans. (b) Pig**
Ref: Suryakantha's Community Medicine 3/e p448

149. **Ans. (d) Influenza**
Ref: Suryakantha's Community Medicine 3/e p330

150. **Ans. (a) Rabies, tetanus**
Ref: Suryakantha's Community Medicine 3/e p418, 491

151. **Ans. (c) Droplet**
Ref: Suryakantha's Community Medicine 3/e p504

152. **Ans. (d) Ampicillin**
Ref: Internet resources

153. **Ans. (c) Mite**
Ref: Suryakantha's Community Medicine 3/e p456

154. **Ans. (b)** 5 days
Ref: Suryakantha's Community Medicine 3/e p318

155. **Ans. (c)** Polio
Ref: Internet resources

156. **Ans. (c)** Yellow fever
Ref: Suryakantha's Community Medicine 3/e p120

157. **Ans. (b)** Kyasanur forest disease
Ref: Suryakantha's Community Medicine 3/e p455

158. **Ans. (b)** Tuberculin test
Ref: Internet resources

159. **Ans. (c)** Tetanus
Ref: Internet resources

160. **Ans. (c)** 3.5
Ref: Internet resources

161. **Ans. (b)** 10 days
Ref: Suryakantha's Community Medicine 3rd/e

162. **Ans. (a)** Aedes
Ref: Suryakantha's Community Medicine 3/e p120

163. **Ans. (b)** Tick
Ref: Suryakantha's Community Medicine 3/e p142

164. **Ans. (d)** Dog
Ref: Internet resources

165. **Ans. (a)** Pancreatitis
Ref: Suryakantha's Community Medicine 3/e p313

166. **Ans. (a)** Chlamydia
Ref: Suryakantha's Community Medicine 3/e p469

167. **Ans. (d)** Lymphoma
Ref: Suryakantha's Community Medicine 3/e p920

168. **Ans. (b)** 10%
Ref: Internet resources

169. **Ans. (b)** 0.3%
Ref: Internet resources

170. **Ans. (a)** Less than 1/1000 live births
Ref: Suryakantha's Community Medicine 3/e p422

171. **Ans. (b)** Malarial parasite in anopheline mosquito
Ref: Suryakantha's Community Medicine 3/e p113

172. **Ans. (b)** 15 days
Ref: Suryakantha's Community Medicine 3/e p129

173. **Ans. (a)** Epidemic typhus
Ref: Suryakantha's Community Medicine 3/e p137

174. **Ans. (c)** 12–24 days
Ref: Suryakantha's Community Medicine 3/e p324

175. **Ans. (a)** Cyclodevelopmental
Ref: Suryakantha's Community Medicine 3/e p113

176. **Ans. (b)** Tularemia
Ref: Suryakantha's Community Medicine 3/e p142

177. **Ans. (a)** Flea
Ref: Suryakantha's Community Medicine 3/e p134

178. **Ans. (a)** Short term treatment under supervision
Ref: Suryakantha's Community Medicine 3/e p370

179. **Ans. (d)** Man to man transmission is seen
Ref: Suryakantha's Community Medicine 3/e p454

180. **Ans. (a)** Treatment under supervision
Ref: Suryakantha's Community Medicine 3/e p362

DEMOGRAPHY AND PREVENTIVE HEALTH

181. **Ans. (b)** Population <15 years & >65 years
Ref: Park's PSM, 21/e p447

182. **Ans. (b)** Adolescent males
Ref: Park's PSM, 21/e p544

183. **Ans. (b)** Primary school children
Ref: Suryakantha's Community Medicine 3/e p609

184. **Ans. (c)** 50th percentile
Ref: Suryakantha's Community Medicine 3/e p593

185. **Ans. (a)** 11 gm%
Ref: Suryakantha's Community Medicine 3/e p190

186. **Ans. (a)** Annual general marriage rate
Ref: Internet resources

187. **Ans. (d)** Feeding started with 4 hours of birth
Ref: Suryakantha's Community Medicine 3/e p589

188. **Ans. (d)** Perinatal mortality rate
Ref: Suryakantha's Community Medicine 3/e p602

189. **Ans. (c)** Both
Ref: Suryakantha's Community Medicine 3/e p603

190. **Ans. (c)** Mid-year population of women of 15–44 years age
Ref: Suryakantha's Community Medicine 3/e p623

191. **Ans. (b)** Perinatal mortality
Ref: Suryakantha's Community Medicine 3/e p605

192. **Ans. (b)** NRR
Ref: Suryakantha's Community Medicine 3/e p624

193. **Ans. (b)** 1,000 live births [weighing over 1 kg at birth]
Ref: Suryakantha's Community Medicine 3/e p603

194. **Ans. (c)** Total fertility rate
Ref: Suryakantha's Community Medicine 3/e p624

195. **Ans. (b) Crude birth rate – crude death rate**
Ref: Suryakantha's Community Medicine 3/e p621

196. **Ans. (a) 5.0%**
Ref: Internet resources

197. **Ans. (a) Low birth weight**
Ref: Suryakantha's Community Medicine 3/e p577

198. **Ans. (a) 1,00,000 live births**
Ref: Suryakantha's Community Medicine 3/e p601

199. **Ans. (d) Transport facility for referral of pregnant women during pregnancy**
Ref: Suryakantha's Community Medicine 3/e p869

200. **Ans. (a) 6 months**
Ref: Internet resources

201. **Ans. (d) 4 rounds**
Ref: Internet resources

202. **Ans. (d) General fertility rate**
Ref: Suryakantha's Community Medicine 3/e p622

NUTRITION

203. **Ans. (d) Glutamic acid**
Ref: Park's PSM, 21/e p564

204. **Ans. (c) Microcytes**
Ref: Suryakantha's Community Medicine 3/e p191

205. **Ans. (d) Methylene blue reduction test**
Ref: Suryakantha's Community Medicine 3/e p184

206. **Ans. (c) Soybean**
Ref: Suryakantha's Community Medicine 3/e p172

207. **Ans. (a) Wheat**
Ref: Suryakantha's Community Medicine 3/e p170

208. **Ans. (b) Methionine**
Ref: Suryakantha's Community Medicine 3/e p170

209. **Ans. (d) Iron**
Ref: Suryakantha's Community Medicine 3/e p173

210. **Ans. (d) Egg**
Ref: Suryakantha's Community Medicine 3/e p174

211. **Ans. (c) Safflower oil**
Ref: Suryakantha's Community Medicine 3/e p157

212. **Ans. (c) Nyctalopia**
Ref: Suryakantha's Community Medicine 3/e p160

213. **Ans. (c) BOAA**
Ref: Suryakantha's Community Medicine 3/e p181

214. **Ans. (a) Height for age**
Ref: Suryakantha's Community Medicine 3/e p188

215. **Ans. (c) Net protein utilization**
Ref: Suryakantha's Community Medicine 3/e p155

216. **Ans. (d) Egg**
Ref: Suryakantha's Community Medicine 3/e p174

217. **Ans. (b) 150**
Ref: Suryakantha's Community Medicine 3/e p177

218. **Ans. (d) 70 microgram/100 mL of blood**
Ref: Suryakantha's Community Medicine 3/e p222

219. **Ans. (b) 60 kg**
Ref: Suryakantha's Community Medicine 3/e p

220. **Ans. (d) Oxalic acid**
Ref: Internet resources

221. **Ans. (a) Sanguinarine**
Ref: Suryakantha's Community Medicine 3/e p196

222. **Ans. (c) Pyrrolizidine alkaloids**
Ref: Suryakantha's Community Medicine 3/e p197

223. **Ans. (b) 75 grams**
Ref: Suryakantha's Community Medicine 3/e p600

224. **Ans. (b) Vitamin C**
Ref: Suryakantha's Community Medicine 3/e p173

225. **Ans. (b) Calcium**
Ref: Suryakantha's Community Medicine 3/e p173

226. **Ans. (d) Human milk has comparatively less of lactose**
Ref: Suryakantha's Community Medicine 3/e p173

ENVIRONMENT AND SANITATION

227. **Ans. (b) Bagassosis**
Ref: Park's PSM, 21/e p747

228. **Ans. (b) Contact period: 30 minutes**
Ref: Suryakantha's Community Medicine 3/e p32

229. **Ans. (b) 3**
Ref: Suryakantha's Community Medicine 3/e p50

230. **Ans. (a) Activated sludge process**
Ref: Suryakantha's Community Medicine 3/e p88

231. **Ans. (d) SO_2**
Ref: Suryakantha's Community Medicine 3/e p49

232. **Ans. (a) Biological oxygen demand**
Ref: Suryakantha's Community Medicine 3/e p87

233. **Ans. (d) 200 mg/L**
Ref: Suryakantha's Community Medicine 3/e p42

234. **Ans. (d) 160 dB**
Ref: Suryakantha's Community Medicine 3/e p52

235. **Ans. (c) Travellers**
Ref: Suryakantha's Community Medicine 3/e p306

236. **Ans. (d) 70–80%**
Ref: Suryakantha's Community Medicine 3/e p124

237. **Ans. (d) CO_2 is the major greenhouse gas**
Ref: Suryakantha's Community Medicine 3/e p892

238. **Ans. (a) CO_2**
Ref: Suryakantha's Community Medicine 3/e p892

239. **Ans. (a) Plague (Yersinia pestis)**
Ref: Suryakantha's Community Medicine 3/e p890

240. **Ans. (d) 0.5 mg/L**
Ref: Suryakantha's Community Medicine 3/e p32

241. **Ans. (b) 33%**
Ref: Suryakantha's Community Medicine 3/e p30

242. **Ans. (a) Carbon mono-oxide**
Ref: Suryakantha's Community Medicine 3/e p892

243. **Ans. (b) Escherichia coli**
Ref: Suryakantha's Community Medicine 3/e p43

244. **Ans. (b) On the sand bed**
Ref: Suryakantha's Community Medicine 3/e p30

245. **Ans. (b) Per capita space per student should be 6 sq. feet**
Ref: Suryakantha's Community Medicine 3/e p599

246. **Ans. (b) 15 metres**
Ref: Suryakantha's Community Medicine 3/e p78

247. **Ans. (a) Ortho-tolidine test**
Ref: Suryakantha's Community Medicine 3/e p33

248. **Ans. (d) E. coli**
Ref: Suryakantha's Community Medicine 3/e p45

249. **Ans. (b) Air pollution**
Ref: Suryakantha's Community Medicine 3/e p49

250. **Ans. (c) 600 mg litre**
Ref: Suryakantha's Community Medicine 3/e p42

NATIONAL POLICIES AND HEALTH CARE

251. **Ans. (d) Equity of distribution**
Ref: Park's PSM, 21/e p828

252. **Ans. (c) Green**
Ref: Park's PSM, 21/e p397

253. **Ans. (d) Skilled birth attendant**
Ref: Suryakantha's Community Medicine 3/e p778

254. **Ans. (b) Epidemic conjunctivitis**
Ref: Suryakantha's Community Medicine 3/e p852

255. **Ans. (c) Nyay panchayat**
Ref: Suryakantha's Community Medicine 3/e p796

256. **Ans. (c) 5,000**
Ref: Suryakantha's Community Medicine 3/e p760

257. **Ans. (b) Neonatal hypothyroidism**
Ref: Internet resources

258. **Ans. (d) If a patient develops paralysis within 30 days diagnosis of AFP**
Ref: Suryakantha's Community Medicine 3/e p839

259. **Ans. (b) Increasing number of children affected**
Ref: Internet resources

260. **Ans. (b) Formulation of state and district health programme**
Ref: Suryakantha's Community Medicine 3/e p777

261. **Ans. (c) 1 for 1000 children**
Ref: Suryakantha's Community Medicine 3/e p765

262. **Ans. (b) Malaria surveillance**
Ref: Suryakantha's Community Medicine 3/e p771

263. **Ans. (d) 12 feet**
Ref: Internet resources

264. **Ans. (a) 7th April**
Ref: Suryakantha's Community Medicine 3/e p927

265. **Ans. (b) 1 per 10,000 population**
Ref: Suryakantha's Community Medicine 3/e p519

266. **Ans. (b) 100 Villages and population of one lakh**
Ref: Suryakantha's Community Medicine 3/e p797

267. **Ans. (c) Diagnose renal diseases**
Ref: Suryakantha's Community Medicine 3/e p770

268. **Ans. (b) Advice of food, nutrition and rest**
Ref: Suryakantha's Community Medicine 3/e p860

269. **Ans. (c) 3**
Ref: Suryakantha's Community Medicine 3/e p771

BIOSTATISTICS

270. **Ans. (c) 95%**
Ref: Park's PSM, 21/e p

271. **Ans. (c) Both**
Ref: Suryakantha's Community Medicine 3/e p658

272. **Ans. (c) 3/5**
Ref: Suryakantha's Community Medicine 3/e p673

273. **Ans. (d)** 95%
Ref: Suryakantha's Community Medicine 3/e p670

274. **Ans. (b)** Mode
Ref: Suryakantha's Community Medicine 3/e p665

275. **Ans. (a)** +1
Ref: Suryakantha's Community Medicine 3/e p690

276. **Ans. (d)** 25%
Ref: Suryakantha's Community Medicine 3/e p246

MISCELLANEOUS

277. **Ans. (d)** All of the above
Ref: Park's PSM, 21/e p735t

278. **Ans. (a)** Conjunctival xerosis
Ref: Park's PSM, 21/e p568, 592, 836

279. **Ans. (d)** Can cause blue line on gums
Ref: Park's PSM, 21/e p749

280. **Ans. (c)** Plastic syringes
Ref: Park's PSM, 21/e p117

281. **Ans. (d)** Network analysis
Ref: Suryakantha's Community Medicine 3/e p788

282. **Ans. (a)** 309 days
Ref: Suryakantha's Community Medicine 3/e p235

283. **Ans. (d)** Risk of Guineaworm infection
Ref: Suryakantha's Community Medicine 3/e p870

284. **Ans. (d)** DM
Ref: Suryakantha's Community Medicine 3/e p635

285. **Ans. (d)** Venous thromboembolism
Ref: Suryakantha's Community Medicine 3/e p638 (Flow chart 24.1)

286. **Ans. (c)** Nonoxynol
Ref: Suryakantha's Community Medicine 3/e p633

287. **Ans. (d)** Cost-effectiveness analysis
Ref: Suryakantha's Community Medicine 3/e p789

288. **Ans. (d)** Network analysis
Ref: Suryakantha's Community Medicine 3/e p788

289. **Ans. (a)** Group discussion
Ref: Suryakantha's Community Medicine 3/e p726

290. **Ans. (c)** Culture contact
Ref: Internet resources

291. **Ans. (d)** STD
Ref: Suryakantha's Community Medicine 3/e p459

292. **Ans. (c)** Sugarcane fibres
Ref: Suryakantha's Community Medicine 3/e p216

293. **Ans. (c)** Hot air
Ref: Suryakantha's Community Medicine 3/e p299

294. **Ans. (a)** Yellow
Ref: Suryakantha's Community Medicine 3/e p94

295. **Ans. (a)** Black bag
Ref: Suryakantha's Community Medicine 3/e p95

296. **Ans. (d)** Black bag
Ref: Suryakantha's Community Medicine 3/e p94

297. **Ans. (c)** Destruction and disposal in landfill
Ref: Suryakantha's Community Medicine 3/e p95

298. **Ans. (b)** Blue container
Ref: Suryakantha's Community Medicine 3/e p94

299. **Ans. (d)** Bleeding
Ref: Suryakantha's Community Medicine 3/e p636

300. **Ans. (c)** Life-table analysis
Ref: Suryakantha's Community Medicine 3/e p651

301. **Ans. (a)** Sodium hypochlorite
Ref: Suryakantha's Community Medicine 3/e p300

302. **Ans. (d)** Careful collection and recycle
Ref: Internet resources

303. **Ans. (b)** 48 hours/week
Ref: Suryakantha's Community Medicine 3/e p233

304. **Ans. (c)** The position of dot is more important than direction
Ref: Suryakantha's Community Medicine 3/e p592

305. **Ans. (a)** Red
Ref: Suryakantha's Community Medicine 3/e p883

306. **Ans. (a)** Corpulence index
Ref: Suryakantha's Community Medicine 3/e p537

307. **Ans. (c)** 30
Ref: Suryakantha's Community Medicine 3/e p537

308. **Ans. (b)** 'Minus' desk
Ref: Suryakantha's Community Medicine 3/e p599

309. **Ans. (a)** Asbestos
Ref: Suryakantha's Community Medicine 3/e p223

310. **Ans. (c)** Jules Guerin
Ref: Suryakantha's Community Medicine 3/e p4

311. **Ans. (b)** Spot map study
Ref: Suryakantha's Community Medicine 3/e p663

312. **Ans. (d)** Contraception
Ref: Internet resources

PRACTICE QUESTIONS

GENERAL CONCEPTS

1. **Killing power of a disease is known as:**
   a. Serial interval b. Case morbidity rate
   c. Survival rate d. Case fatality rate
2. **All of the following are true for Case control study EXCEPT:**
   a. Bias
   b. Odds ratio can be calculated
   c. Relative risk can be calculated
   d. Less time consuming
3. **Impairment is defined as:**
   a. Inability to carry out certain routine activities
   b. Not able to play the role, expected
   c. Loss or abnormality in structure or function
   d. Inability to walk
4. **First case that comes to the notice of investigator:**
   a. Primary case b. Secondary case
   c. New case d. Index case
5. **Which of the following is the best study:**
   a. Case control studies b. Cohort studies
   c. Both d. None
6. **Sullivan index is:**
   a. Related to hookworm infestation
   b. Depends on per capita income
   c. Disability free life period
   d. Includes infant mortality rate
7. **Which of the following is true for Cohort study:**
   a. Bias
   b. Rare diseases can be studied
   c. Cause to effect
   d. Economical
8. **Generation time is defined as:**
   a. Period between onset of the first/index case and the secondary case
   b. Period between the successful entry of a pathogen and the appearance of the first clinical sign/symptom of the disease
   c. Infection receipt to maximum infectivity
   d. Period during which the reservoir is infectious to others
9. **True positive is:**
   a. Negative predictive value
   b. Positive predictive value
   c. Specificity
   d. Sensitivity
10. **Health promotion is which level of prevention:**
    a. Primary b. Secondary
    c. Tertiary d. Primordial
11. **In 1935 students were admitted to a college where height and weight was taken. Based on previous data, a study was conducted in 1977 in same population to determine how many will develop CAD in 1986. Such study is known as:**
    a. Experimental study b. Cohort study
    c. Retrospective study d. Cross sectional study
12. **Prospective study is done for which of the following:**
    a. 30-year-old female to check for cystic fibrosis
    b. Female >40 years with breast lump
    c. Heel prick test for neonatal tetanus at birth
    d. Illegal migrant screening
13. **All of the following can be calculated from Cohort study EXCEPT:**
    a. Odd's ratio b. Incidence
    c. Relative risk d. Exposure
14. **Which of the following does NOT come under primary prevention?**
    a. Immunization
    b. Specific protection
    c. Early diagnosis and treatment
    d. Contraceptives
15. **Submerged portion in iceberg phenomenon represents:**
    a. Undiagnosed cases in a community
    b. Diagnosed cases of a community
    c. Clinical cases that physician can see
    d. Clinical cases that comes to the knowledge of investigator
16. **Which of the following is NOT included in Physical Quality of Life Index?**
    a. Income
    b. Literacy
    c. Life expectancy at age 1
    d. Infant mortality rate

Ans. 1. **d.** Case fatality rate 2. **c.** Relative risk can... 3. **c.** Loss or abnormali... 4. **d.** Index case
5. **b.** Cohort studies 6. **c.** Disability free life... 7. **c.** Cause to effect 8. **c.** Infection receipt to...
9. **d.** Sensitivity 10. **a.** Primary 11. **b.** Cohort study 12. **b.** Female >40 years...
13. **a.** Odd's ratio 14. **c.** Early diagnosis... 15. **a.** Undiagnosed... 16. **a.** Income

17. Disease recurring after many years shows which type of trend:
a. Secular trend
b. Cyclic trend
c. Seasonal trend
d. Variable trend

18. Which of the following formula is for calculating specificity?
a. True positive × 100/True positive + false positive
b. True negative × 100/True negative + false negative
c. True positive × 100/True positive + false negative
d. True negative × 100/True negative + false positive

19. Calculate specificity of a screening test in which negative result is seen in 50% of non-diseased population and positive results in 10% of healthy population?
a. 0.5
b. 0.6
c. 0.83
d. 0.9

20. NOT a component of epidemiological triad:
a. Agent
b. Environment
c. Host
d. Time

21. Biological environmental changes are recurrent. What should be done to reduce error?
a. Standardization
b. Excessive training of examiner
c. Using 2 examiners
d. Repeated measurement

22. Which of the following condition is NOT notifiable to WHO:
a. Cholera
b. Chickenpox
c. Plague
d. Yellow fever

23. Diagnostic power of a disease is reflected by:
a. Sensitivity
b. Specificity
c. Predictive value
d. Population attributable risk

24. Due to an effective prevention program, the prevalence of an infectious disease in a community has been reduced by 90%. A physician continues to use the same diagnostic test for the disease that she has always used. How have the tests characteristics changed?
a. Its sensitivity has increased
b. Its positive predictive value has increased
c. Its negative predictive value has increased
d. The tests characteristics have not changed

25. Screening test as compared to diagnostic test:
a. Expensive
b. Individual approach
c. Done by physician
d. Done on apparently healthy subjects

VACCINES

26. Rotavirus vaccine can lead to:
a. Seizures
b. Abscess
c. Intussusception
d. Lymph node enlargement

27. First vaccine was developed for:
a. Chickenpox
b. Cholera
c. Smallpox
d. Measles

28. Which of the following vaccine is NOT included in immunization schedule?
a. Kala azar
b. Polio
c. Hepatitis
d. Measles

29. Human specific immunoglobulin/Ig is usually NOT given for:
a. Rabies
b. Tetanus
c. Varicella zoster
d. TB

30. Which of the following set does NOT include all live vaccines?
a. BCG + Oral polio + Oral typhoid
b. Mumps + Rubella + Dakar Yellow fever
c. BCG + Hepatitis A + Influenza live
d. Measles + Mumps + Rubella

COMMUNICABLE AND NON-COMMUNICABLE DISEASES

31. Incubation period for chicken pox:
a. 1–6 days
b. 10–21 days
c. 21–32 days
d. 40–50 days

32. Follow-up programme for AFP, patient is assessed after:
a. 15 days
b. 30 days
c. 60 days
d. 90 days

33. Secondary attack rate/SAR of measles:
a. 70%
b. 80%
c. 90%
d. 100%

34. Which is associated with an increased risk of coronary artery disease?
a. LDL:HDL ratio >5
b. HDL:LDL ratio >5
c. Serum cholesterol <220 md/dL
d. Raised serum HDL levels

Ans. 17. **a.** Secular trend; 18. d. True negative...; 19. **c.** 0.83; 20. **d.** Time; 21. **d.** Repeated measu...; 22. **b.** Chickenpox; 23. **c.** Predictive value; 24. **c.** Its negative predictive...; 25. **d.** Done on appare...; 26. **c.** Intussusception; 27. **c.** Smallpox; 28. **a.** Kala azar; 29. **d.** TB; 30. **b.** Mumps + Rubella...; 31. **b.** 10–21 days; 32. **c.** 60 days; 33. **b.** 80%; 34. **a.** LDL:HDL ratio >5

35. Incubation period of viral hepatitis B:
a. 15–30 day b. 30–45 days
c. 50–150 days d. 150–250 days

36. SAFE, all EXCEPT:
a. Surgery b. Antibiotics
c. Education d. Facial cleanliness

37. A 12-year-old child presented with fever with chills, headache, bodyache and pea soup diarrhoea. He is suffering from:
a. Cholera b. Typhoid fever
c. Amoebiasis d. Shigellosis

38. During epidemic of hepatitis E, fatality is maximum in:
a. Children b. Adults
c. Elderly d. Pregnant women

39. An infant 6 months presented with a respiratory rate of 50/minutes. He is NOT taking food and water for last 7 days. Diagnosis is:
a. Mild ARI b. Very severe ARI
c. Severe ARI d. Moderate ARI

40. Reservoir of typhoid fever:
a. Dog b. Cat
c. Human d. Monkey

41. Risk factor for development of lung carcinoma:
a. Amount of smoking
b. Use of cigarettes with filter
c. Duration of smoking
d. All of the above

42. Which of the following disease has NOT been eradicated?
a. Leprosy
b. Guinea worm
c. Small pox
d. Polio

43. Which of the following is NOT an indicator of prevalence rate of malaria?
a. Child spleen rate
b. Annual parasite index
c. Infant parasite rate
d. Parasite density index

44. Number of hookworm eggs/gram of stool is:
a. Pearl index
b. Sullivan's index
c. Chandler's index
d. PQLI

45. Which is a reservoir in typhoid carriers:
a. Stomach
b. Esophagus
c. Bile duct of human
d. Spleen

46. Scabies is caused by:
a. Reduviid bug
b. Dermatophagoides
c. Sarcoptes scabiei
d. Leptotrombidium

47. Endemic typhus is caused by:
a. R. prowazekii b. R. tsutsugamushi
c. R. typhi d. R. quintana

48. MDR-TB resistance is:
a. Resistance to INH
b. Resistance to IH + rifampicin
c. Resistance to INH + rifampin + Quinolones
d. Resistance to INH + riafmpin + Quinolones + any one second line injectable drug

49. Duration of treatment of multibacillary leprosy:
a. 6 months b. 12 months
c. 18 months d. 24 months

DEMOGRAPHY AND PREVENTIVE HEALTH

50. In rural setup, which of the following encourages eligible couples to adopt family planning services:
a. Doctor
b. Village health guide
c. Female health worker
d. ASHA

51. Demographic cycle stage IV:
a. Late expanding b. Early expanding
c. Low stationary d. High stationary

52. MC cause of neonatal mortality rate:
a. Congenital heart disease
b. Birth trauma
c. Preterm
d. Neonatal jaundice

53. Toddler is:
a. Less than 1 year b. 1–3 years
c. 3–6 years d. 6–9 years

54. MC cause of maternal mortality:
a. Anemia b. Infections
c. Malnutrition d. Bleeding

Ans. **35. c.** 50–150 days **36. c.** Education **37. b.** Typhoid fever **38. d.** Pregnant women
39. b. Very severe ARI **40. c.** Human **41. d.** All of the above **42. a.** Leprosy
43. b. Annual parasite... **44. c.** Chandler's... **45. c.** Bile duct of human **46. c.** Sarcoptes scabiei
47. c. R. typhi **48. d.** Resistance to... **49. b.** 12 months **50. c.** Female health...
51. c. Low stationary **52. c.** Preterm **53. b.** 1–3 years **54. d.** Bleeding

55. What needs to be done if a lady forgets to take 2 pills in last 5 days of starting the pills?
a. Continue taking rest of the pills throwing away the missed pills
b. Take 2 pills on next day and continue taking rest of the pills
c. Used extra measures of contraception along with taking all the missed pills
d. Avoid coitus

56. Number of live births per 1,000 women of reproductive age group is:
a. NFR b. GFR
c. TFR d. GRR

57. In epilepsy, which is CONTRAINDICATED?
a. OCP b. IUCD
c. Barrier methods d. Spermicidal jelly

NUTRITION

58. Water soluble vitamin:
a. Vitamin A b. Vitamin C
c. Vitamin E d. Vitamin K

59. Deficiency of vitamin D results in:
a. Scurvy b. Osteomalacia
c. Osteoporosis d. Osteopetrosis

60. Human milk is essential for neurological development due to:
a. Casein b. Carotene
c. Taurine d. Lactose

61. Adulterant in endemic ascites:
a. BOAA b. Crotolaria seeds
c. Sanguinarine d. Mustard oil

62. Which protein is NOT present in milk?
a. Lactoalbumin b. Casein
c. Lactoglobulin d. Transferrin

63. Richest source of vitamin C:
a. Papaya b. Jaggery
c. Red meat d. Indian gooseberry

64. Prevalence of Bitot's spot as criteria of vitamin A deficiency:
a. >0.01% b. >0.05%
c. >0.5% d. >1%

65. Pulses are deficient in:
a. Methionine + cysteine b. Lysine
c. Tryptophan d. Proteins

66. A paediatric patient who was exclusively fed on breast milk, now presented with joint pains and gum bleeding. He was NOT interested in eating fruits also. He prefers to have animal foods only. Most likely diagnosis:
a. Vitamin A deficiency b. Vitamin D deficiency
c. Vitamin C deficiency d. Vitamin K deficiency

67. Milk is a poor source of which vitamin:
a. Vitamin A
b. Vitamin B
c. Vitamin C
d. Vitamin D

68. Haemorrhagic disease of newborn is because of deficiency of:
a. Vitamin A b. Vitamin E
c. Vitamin K d. Vitamin D

69. Vitamin A deficiency leads to:
a. Scurvy
b. Bleeding at birth
c. Corneal xerosis and keratomalacia
d. Bone pains

70. First clinical sign of vitamin A deficiency:
a. Night blindness
b. Conjunctival xerosis
c. Bitot's spots
d. Corneal xerosis

71. Glycemic index of 90 is for:
a. Ice cream
b. White rice
c. Legumes
d. Potato chips

72. Glycemic index is MINIMUM for:
a. Milk
b. Wheat
c. Fruits
d. Brown rice

73. Serotonin is a precursor of:
a. Lysine
b. Tryptophan
c. Methionine
d. Homocysteine

74. First clinical symptom of vitamin A deficiency:
a. Night blindness
b. Conjunctival xerosis
c. Bitot's spots
d. Corneal xerosis

Ans.				
	55. a. Continue taking...	56. b. GFR	57. a. OCP	58. b. Vitamin C
	59. b. Osteomalacia	60. c. Taurine	61. b. Crotolaria seeds	62. d. Transferrin
	63. d. Indian gooseberry	64. c. >0.5%	65. a. Methionine +...	66. c. Vitamin C...
	67. c. Vitamin C	68. c. Vitamin K	69. c. Corneal xerosis...	70. b. Conjunctival...
	71. d. Potato chips	72. a. Milk	73. b. Tryptophan	74. a. Night blindness

ENVIRONMENT AND SANITATION

75. Asbestosis is associated with:
a. Miners nystagmus
b. Pleural mesothelioma
c. Mottling in chest X-ray
d. Fine nodular density on chest X-ray

NATIONAL POLICIES AND HEALTH CARE

76. How many post-natal visits are made by multipurpose worker female:
a. 1–3
b. 3–5
c. 5–7
d. 7–9

77. In NVBDCP, the disease NOT included is:
a. Malaria b. Yellow fever
c. Filaria d. Leishmaniasis

78. Minimum remuneration is provided to ASHA under JSY scheme:
a. 100 INR b. 200 INR
c. 300 INR d. 400 INR

79. Free medical care by government is called:
a. State medicine b. Socialized medicine
c. Social science d. Social service

80. First referral centre:
a. Subcentre
b. PHC
c. CHC
d. Medical college

81. Who is in charge of PHC?
a. Multipurpose health worker male
b. Multipurpose health worker female
c. Doctor
d. Nurse

82. JSY is to promote:
a. Implement immunization programme effectively
b. Safe childhood
c. Safe deliveries
d. All of the above

83. ASHA, FALSE statement is:
a. Provides nutritional, immunization, family planning and educational services
b. Accountable to Gram panchayat
c. Receive monthly pay
d. Educated till 8th class

84. Which of the following is FALSE about ASHA?
a. Selected by village panchayat/Gram sabha
b. Trained by ANM
c. Minimum 4th class pass
d. A functionary under NRHM 2005–2012

85. Which programme involves services to mothers and their unhealthy newborns?
a. JSY
b. JSSK
c. RCH
d. ICDS

BIOSTATISTICS

86. Which of the following is used to represent the magnitude of a data?
a. Pie diagram
b. Scatter diagram
c. Bar diagram
d. Dot diagram

87. Calculate the mean and mode from 2, 2, 3, 4, 4, 4, 4, 5, 5, 7, 8, 8, 9:
a. 4 and 5
b. 5 and 4
c. 5 and 9
d. 9 and 5

MISCELLANEOUS

88. GOBIFFF is promoted by:
a. WHO
b. UNICEF
c. UNESCO
d. UNAID

89. Blindness is defined as visual acuity less than:
a. 6/30 b. 3/60
c. 6/60 d. 3/30

90. FALSE for critical path method:
a. There is mixture of time and cost
b. Schedule prepared in the form of flowchart
c. Longest time required to complete the task is calculated
d. Design is based on event

91. The scientific study of old age, the process of ageing, and the particular problems of old people is known as:
a. Anthropology
b. Psychology
c. Pathology
d. Gerontology

Ans. **75. b.** Pleural... **76. b.** 3–5 **77. b.** Yellow fever **78. b.** 200 INR
79. a. State medicine **80. c.** CHC **81. c.** Doctor **82. c.** Safe deliveries
83. c. Receive monthly... **84. c.** Minimum 4th... **85. b.** JSSK **86. c.** Bar diagram
87. b. 5 and 4 **88. b.** UNICEF **89. b.** 3/60 **90. d.** Design is based on...
91. d. Gerontology

IMAGE-BASED QUESTIONS

1. Study the following image:

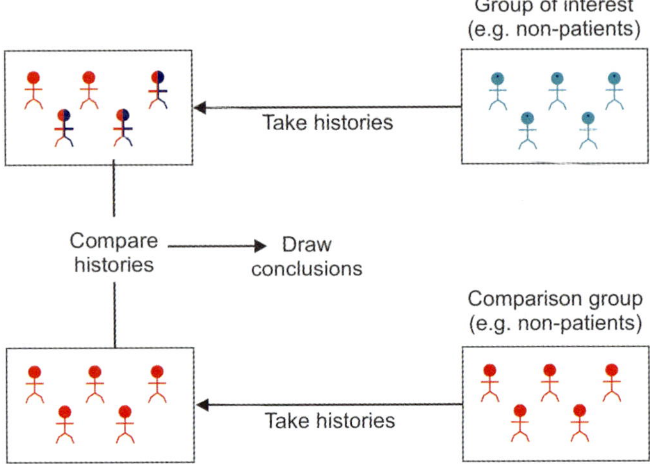

a. Cohort study
b. Prospective study
c. Case control study
d. Randomization

Case control study proceeds backward from effect to cause. Thus, exposure and disease have already occurred at the time of initiation of study. It involves the study between the cases and controls.

2. What is being calculated:

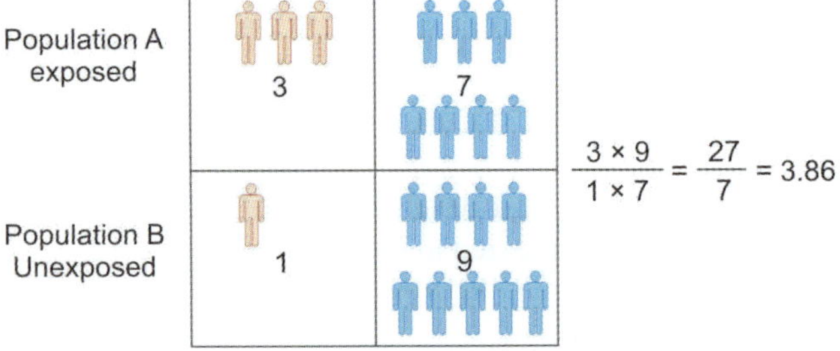

a. Attributable risk
b. Relative risk
c. Incidence
d. Odd's ratio

To know the strength of association between the disease and the suspected factor, an indicator called 'Odd's ratio' (i.e. cross-product ratio) has to be calculated.

3. What can be calculated from this image:

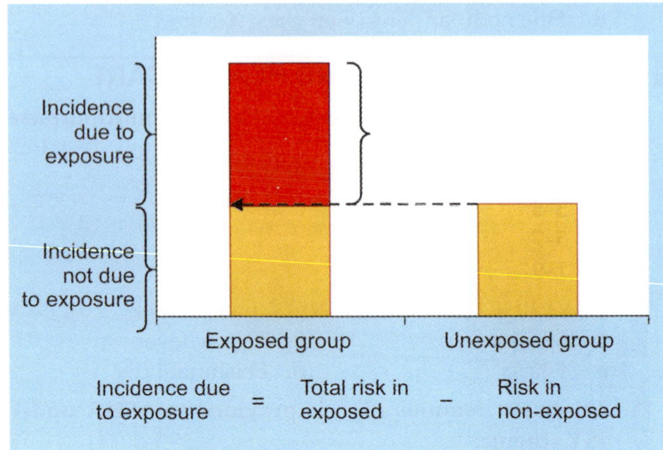

a. Attributable risk
b. Relative risk
c. Incidence
d. Odd's ratio

Attributable risk (AR) is the ratio of risk difference and the incidence of the disease among exposed, often expressed as percentage.

AR = Incidence exposed – Incidence unexposed/ Incidence exposed

4. Temperature employed in this mode of e-waste disposal:

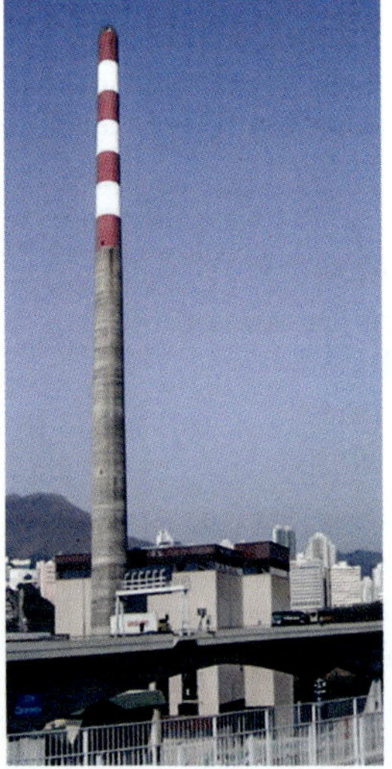

a. 10 degree C
b. 100 degree C
c. 1000 degree C
d. 10000 degree C

In Incineration, the e-waste is burnt in a specially designed in incinerators at a high temperature of about 1000 degree C. It is a complete combustion process.

5. Principle of this mode of sterilization:

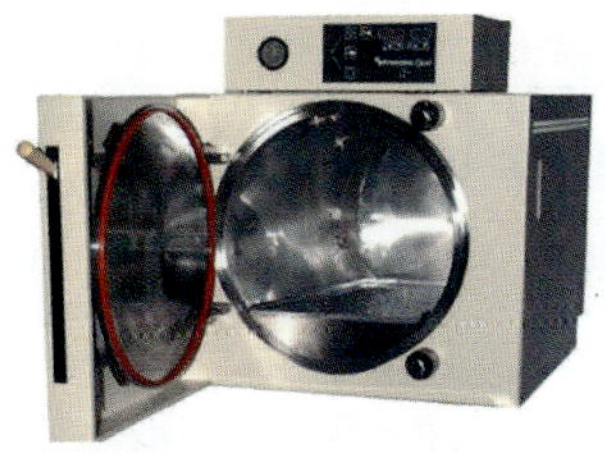

a. Dry heat
b. Moist heat
c. Hot air
d. Radiation

Autoclaves work on the method of sterilization by steam. It is used to sterilize the surgical instruments, OT garments, linen, gloves, masks, gowns, etc. However it is not suitable for plastics.

6. Which mode of biological transmission:

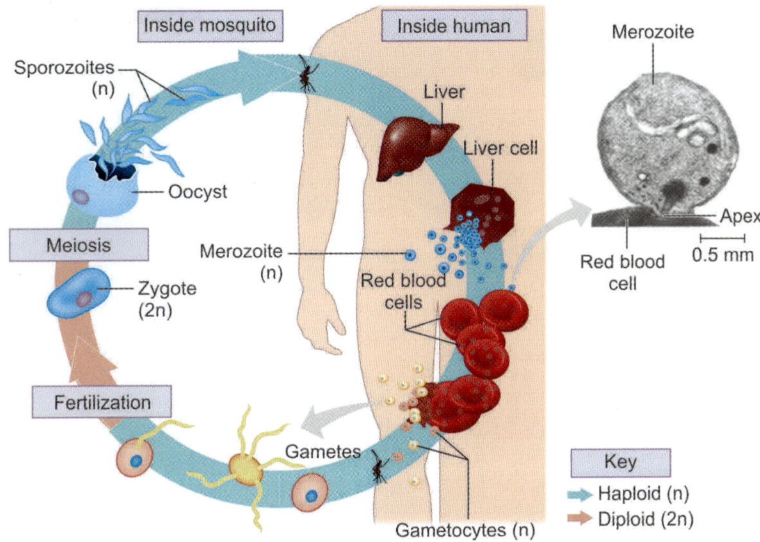

a. Propagative
b. Cyclopropagative
c. Cyclodevelopmental
d. Developmental

Malarial parasite in female anopheles show cyclopropagative type of transmission, where the pathogens undergo not only multiplication, but also cyclic development inside the body of the vector.

7. Which type of biological transmission:

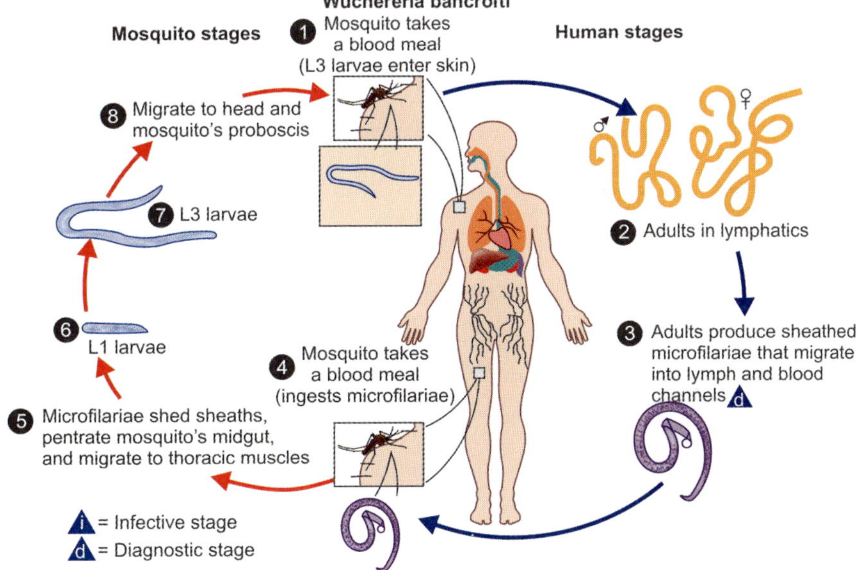

a. Propagative
b. Cyclopropagative
c. Cyclodevelopmental
d. Cyclic

Wucheria bancrofti microfilariae inside female culex mosquito shows cyclodevelopmental type of transmission where pathogens undergo only developmental changes and no multiplication inside the body of the vector.

8. Which vaccine can be given by this route:

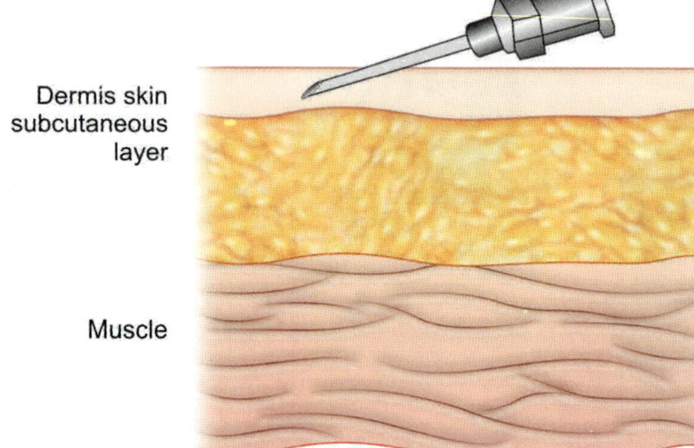

a. IPV
b. DPT
c. MMR
d. BCG

BCG is given intradermally using 'tuberculin syringe' on the upper aspect of left arm above the insertion of deltoid. 0.05 mL for the newborn because skin is thin & 0.1 mL for an infant above 1 month of age

9. Which vaccine is given through this route:

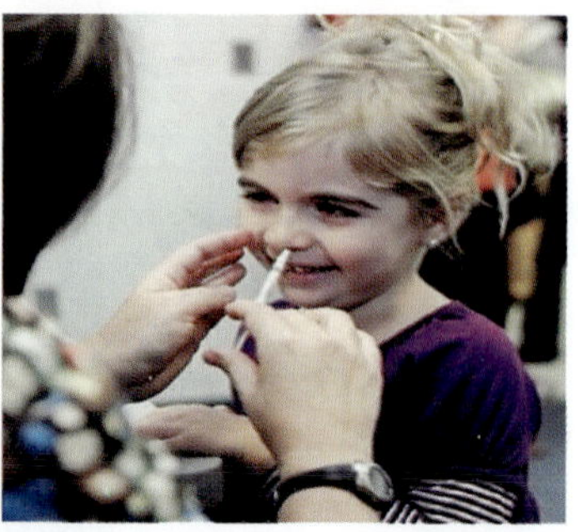

a. BCG
b. OPV
c. Influenza vaccine
d. Rabies

Live attenuated influenza vaccine is administered intranasally as 'nose spray/nose drops'.

10. Such finding is highly suggestive of:

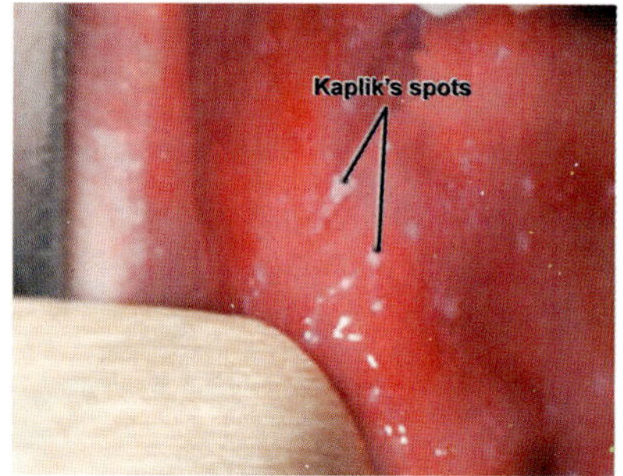

a. Chicken pox
b. Small pox
c. Measles
d. Rubella

One or two days before the appearance of rashes, Koplik's spot appear on the buccal mucous membrane, by the side of the second molar tooth, around the orifice of the Stenson's duct. Koplik's spots are pathognomic of measles.

MCQ POINTS

S. No.	Question statements	Answers
1.	Black colour code in triage system stands for	***Dead/moribund patients***
2.	Cold chain is used for	***Transporting vaccines from hospital to periphery***
3.	Sling psychrometer is used for	***Measuring humidity***
4.	Education, occupation and income are part of which index	***Kuppuswamy index***
5.	Population covered by PHC under plain area	***30,000***
6.	NMEP scheme was recommended by	***Chadha committee***
7.	Expectation of life, free of disability is …index	***Sullivan***
8.	Community health centre covers a population of	***80 thousand to 1.2 lac***
9.	Disinfecting action of chlorine (chlorination) is due to	***Hypochlorous acid***
10.	Most reliable bacteriological indicator of water pollution	***E. coli***
11.	Active form of vitamin D is	***1,25-dihydroxy-cholecalciferol***
12.	Amount of Cereals (in mg) provided in mid-day meal is	***75 mg***
13.	Korsakoff's psychosis results due to deficiency of	***Thiamine/B1***
14.	Richest source of linoleic acid	***Safflower oil***
15.	Rose spots are seen in	***Typhoid***
16.	Casal's necklace is due to deficiency of	***Niacin***
17.	Breast feeding should be initiated within ... hours of delivery by caesarean sections	***4 hours***
18.	Most common indirect cause of maternal mortality in India	***Anemia***
19.	Incubation period of whooping cough	***1-2 weeks***
20.	Causative agent for cutaneous leishmaniasis	***Leishmania tropica***
21.	Dengue is caused by	***Flavivirus***
22.	Vaccine C/I in HIV patient	***All live vaccines***
23.	Serial interval indicates... of disease	***Incubation period***
24.	Sentinel surveillance is done to detect ... cases	***Missed***
25.	Specificity of a test indicates	***True negatives***
26.	A patient takes strict vegetarian diet without consuming any animal product. Likely vitamin deficiency	***B12***
27.	Reverse Cold chain is used for	***Transporting stools samples from periphery to laboratory***
28.	Energy requirement of a heavy worker female (in kcal/ Day)	***2850***
29.	MC antioxidant vitamin	***Vitamin E***
30.	Population covered by subcentre under plain area	***5,000***
31.	MPHW scheme was recommended by	***Kartar Singh***
32.	Maximum permissible noise level in wards (in dB)	***20–35 dB***
33.	Incidence among exposed/incidence among non-exposed is known as	***Relative risk***
34.	During cholera epidemic, wells should be disinfected ...	***Daily***
35.	Most reliable clostridial (bacteriological) indicator of water pollution	***Cl. perfringenes***
36.	Stage of falciparum not seen in peripheral blood smear	***Schizont***
37.	Bagassosis is due to inhalation of	***Sugarcane dust***
38.	High level of parasitemia is seen in which plasmodia	***Falciparum***

S. No.	Question statements	Answers
39.	ASHA is a functionary under which national programme	***National Rural Health MIssion/NRHM***
40.	Yellow fever is transmitted by	***Aedes***
41.	Human anatomical waste is disposed in which color bags	***Yellow color***
42.	Breast feeding should be initiated within ... hours of normal vaginal delivery	***Half***
43.	Most common direct cause of maternal mortality in India	***Haemorrhage***
44.	Population under one PHC in hilly area	***20,000***
45.	Chikungunya fever is transmitted by which mosquito	***Mansonides and Aedes both***
46.	Number of deaths due to a disease/Number of cases of the same disease is known as	***Case fatality rate***
47.	Perinatal period is calculated from ... to of ... days of birth	***28 weeks of gestation to first 7 days of life***
48.	Relative risk can be calculated from ... study	***Cohort***
49.	Most important essential fatty acid	***Linoleic acid***
50.	Validity of certificate of yellow fever lasts... from days to ... years	***10 days to 10 years***
51.	Avoidance of fatty acid in diet comes under which level of prevention	***Primordial***
52.	Repeatedly occurring value (biostatistics) is known as	***Mode***
53.	Psychotherapy for mental disorder prevention comes under ... prevention	***Primary (specific protection)***
54.	Bleaching powder contains ... % of available chlorine	***33%***
55.	Tiger mosquito is another term for which mosquito	***Aedes***
56.	Teaching students about the side effects of medications is what level of prevention	***Primordial***
57.	Chagas disease is caused by	***Trypanosoma cruzi***
58.	Epidemic typhus is transmitted by	***Louse***
59.	Number of flea of each species per rodent is known as	***Specific flea index***
60.	Ragi is rich source of	***Calcium***
61.	Permutit process is done to remove from ... water	***Hardness***
62.	Epidemic dropsy is due to adulteration of mustard oil with ... oil	***Argemone***
63.	... fish is used for biological control of mosquitoes	***Gambusia***
64.	Cafeteria approach is related with	***Contraception under RCH programme***
65.	Food poisoning due to bacillus cereus is seen after consumption of	***Fried rice***
66.	Acrodermatitis enteropathica responds well to	***Zinc***
67.	Minor changes in antigenicity of influenza virus is known as	***Antigenic drift***
68.	Vitamin deficiency in a patient on INH therapy	***Pyridoxine***
69.	Energy yield of egg (in kcal)	***70 kcal***
70.	Causative agent for plague	***Yersinia pestis***
71.	Size of particles considered dangerous for pneumoconiosis	***0.3 to 5 microns***
72.	Hypogonadism, reduced immunity and alopecia may be manifestation of deficiency of which trace metal	***Zinc***
73.	Soiling index is an indicator of pollution of	***Air pollution***
74.	Headquarter of FAO	***Rome, Italy***
75.	BOAA causes	***Lathyrism***
76.	MC cause of infant mortality rate in India	***Prematurity/Low birth weight***
77.	Fertility indicator which gives approximate magnitude of completed family size	***Total fertility rate***
78.	Inhalation of moldy hay leads to which condition	***Farmer's lung***

S. No.	Question statements	Answers
79.	Caplan's syndrome is pneumoconiosis plus which musculoskeletal condition	***Rheumatoid arthritis***
80.	Demyelinating neurological lesion in spinal cord is associated with deficiency of which vitamin	***B12***
81.	WHO day	***7th April***
82.	Chandler index of 200–250 indicates that	***Potential danger***
83.	Duration of surveillance in paucibacillary leprosy is	***2 years***
84.	Case finding in RNTCP is by	***Sputum microscopy***
85.	Requirement of calcium in pregnancy	***1200 mg***
86.	Hooch tragedy was because of consumption of	***Methyl alcohol***
87.	DOC for chemoprophylaxis in cholera	***Tetracycline***
88.	In typhoid, gut perforation usually occurs in which week	***3rd week***
89.	Post-exposure prophylaxis of rabies in a patient is who is previously vaccinated	***0, 3, 7 days***
90.	In living rooms, number of air changes/per hour should be	***2–3***
91.	Number of postnatal visits by a female health worker should be at least	***2***
92.	Most heat sensitive vaccine	***Oral polio vaccine***
93.	MDG are to be achieved by which year	***2015***
94.	Calculate median from 2, 4, 6, 5	***4.5 (arrange like 2, 4, 5, 6 and take average of 4 and 5)***
95.	Exotic disease are	***Diseases which comes to a country from other country***
96.	In triage, which colour indicates high priority treatment and transfer	***Red***
97.	Biological transmission of plasmodium in anopheles	***Cyclopropagative***
98.	Virulence of a disease is indicated by	***Case fatality rate***
99.	Effect of duration of disease on prevalence	***Direct relationship (more the duration, more the prevalence will be)***
100.	Incidence can be calculated from which study	***Cohort***